BIOLOGY OF NEW WORLD *MICROTUS*

SPECIAL PUBLICATIONS

This series, published by the American Society of Mammalogists, has been established for papers of monographic scope concerned with some aspect of the biology of mammals.

Correspondence concerning manuscripts to be submitted for publication in the series should be addressed to the Editor for Special Publications, Hugh H. Genoways (address below).

Copies of Special Publications of the Society may be ordered from the Secretary-Treasurer, Gordon L. Kirkland, Jr., Vertebrate Museum, Shippensburg University, Shippensburg, Pennsylvania 17257.

Price of this issue $55.00

COMMITTEE ON SPECIAL PUBLICATIONS

BIOLOGY OF NEW WORLD *MICROTUS*

EDITED BY

ROBERT H. TAMARIN

Department of Biology
Boston University
Boston, Masschusetts 02215

SPECIAL PUBLICATION NO. 8
THE AMERICAN SOCIETY OF MAMMALOGISTS
PUBLISHED 12 SEPTEMBER 1985

Library of Congress Catalog Card No. 82-73762

ISBN No. 0-943612-07-1

CONTRIBUTORS

SYDNEY ANDERSON
Curator, Department of Mammalogy
American Museum of Natural History
Central Park West and 79th Street
New York, New York 10024

GEORGE O. BATZLI
Department of Zoology
University of Illinois
Urbana, Illinois 61801

ELMER C. BIRNEY
Bell Museum of Natural History
University of Minnesota
Minneapolis, Minnesota 55455

ROSS E. BYERS
Winchester Fruit Research Laboratory
Virginia Polytechnic Institute and State University
Winchester, Virginia 22601

MICHAEL D. CARLETON
Division of Mammals
National Museum of Natural History
Smithsonian Institution
Washington, D.C. 20560

ROBERT A. DIETERICH
Institute of Arctic Biology
University of Alaska
Fairbanks, Alaska 99701

MICHAEL S. GAINES
Department of Systematics and Ecology
University of Kansas
Lawrence, Kansas 66045

LOWELL L. GETZ
Department of Ecology, Ethology, and Evolution
University of Illinois
Urbana, Illinois 61801

ROBERT S. HOFFMANN
Museum of Natural History
University of Kansas
Lawrence, Kansas 66045

BARRY L. KELLER
Department of Biological Sciences
Idaho State University
Pocatello, Idaho 83201

JAMES W. KOEPPL
Museum of Natural History
University of Kansas
Lawrence, Kansas 66045

CHARLES J. KREBS
Institute of Animal Resource Ecology
University of British Columbia
Vancouver, British Columbia,
V6T 1W5 Canada

WILLIAM Z. LIDICKER, JR.
Museum of Vertebrate Zoology
University of California
Berkeley, California 94720

DALE M. MADISON
Biology Department
State University of New York
Binghamton, New York 13901

FRANK F. MALLORY
Biology Department
Laurentian University
Sudbury, Ontario,
P3E 2C6 Canada

JOSEPH H. NADEAU
The Jackson Laboratory
Bar Harbor, Maine 04609

OLIVER P. PEARSON
Museum of Vertebrate Zoology
University of California
Berkeley, California 94720

Carleton J. Phillips
Department of Biology
Hofstra University
Hempstead, New York 11550

Robert K. Rose
Department of Biological Sciences
Old Dominion University
Norfolk, Virginia 23508

Robert W. Seabloom
Department of Biology
University of North Dakota
Grand Forks, North Dakota 58201

Mary J. Taitt
Institute of Animal Resource Ecology
University of British Columbia
Vancouver, British Columbia,
V6T 1W5 Canada

Robert M. Timm
Field Museum of Natural History
Roosevelt Road at Lake Shore Drive
Chicago, Illinois 60605

Jerry O. Wolff
Department of Biology
University of Virginia
Charlottesville, Virginia 22901

Bruce A. Wunder
Department of Zoology and
Entomology
Colorado State University
Fort Collins, Colorado 80523

Richard J. Zakrzewski
Sternberg Memorial Museum
Fort Hays Kansas State College
Hays, Kansas 67601

PREFACE AND ACKNOWLEDGMENTS

In 1979, Hugh H. Genoways, Chairman of the Editorial Committee of the American Society of Mammalogists, asked me if I would be interested in editing a special publication of the society to be titled, "Biology of New World *Microtus*." Knowing that there was an interest in such a volume, and that such a volume could be a valuable resource, I was happy to do it. The successful "Biology of *Peromyscus*," published in 1968 by the society, gave us a model from which to work. The expected date of publication was set at late 1984.

There then followed a meeting with the Editorial Committee of the Society to establish content and authorship. It was decided that the book should be restricted to New World *Microtus* to keep the size of the volume to a manageable length. Because we have many chapters, there is some repetition and fragmentation, but each subject is self-contained and readily available to anyone using the book as a reference source. As did John King, editor of the *Peromyscus* volume, I limited my editorial responsibilities to overseeing the writing and revising the chapters. I hope that each chapter is an up-to-date synthesis of the material in that field, a guideline for future research, and a useful reference. Some chapters, such as Phillips' chapter on microanatomy, contain much new information.

The authors of this book did not take a firm stand on the question of *Microtus* systematics. Anderson, in his chapter on taxonomy and systematics, chose to outline the problems and issues in vole taxonomy rather than making premature "definitive" statements. Hence, a few authors, such as Zakrzewski, consider *Pitymys* as a valid generic name while most consider it to be a synonym of *Microtus*. I think that there is still much to be done in the area of vole systematics, but Anderson points us in the right direction.

Chapters were subjected to anonymous peer review. Although I would like to thank individually the many reviewers who put so much effort into improving the quality of this volume, I obviously cannot and still maintain their anonymity. I thus hope that a general acknowledgment will convey my gratitude. I greatly appreciate their efforts. I would also like to thank Hugh H. Genoways and Timothy E. Lawlor for the many hours of editorial work that they put in after the manuscript for this book left my desk. Lastly, thanks to my family, Ginger, David, and Bonnie, for putting up with an inordinately long 1983.

R. H. T.
16 February, 1984

CONTENTS

THE FOSSIL RECORD *Richard J. Zakrzewski* 1
Abstract 1
Introduction 1
Systematics and the Fossil Record 5
Concluding Remarks 29
Acknowledgments 29
Selected Bibliography 30
Appendix A. Fossil Faunas Containing *Pitymys* and *Microtus* 37
Appendix B. Localities Containing *Pitymys pinetorum, P. ochrogaster,* and *Microtus pennsylvanicus* 48

TAXONOMY AND SYSTEMATICS *Sydney Anderson* 52
Abstract 52
Introduction 53
History of Systematics at the Generic Level 55
History of Systematics at the Species Level 68
Discussion of Systematic Viewpoints 74
Literature Cited 81

ZOOGEOGRAPHY *Robert S. Hoffmann* and *James W. Koeppl* 84
Abstract 84
Introduction 84
Ecological Zoogeography 85
Historical Zoogeography 105
Acknowledgments 113
Literature Cited 113

MACROANATOMY *Michael D. Carleton* 116
Abstract 116
Introduction 117
Integument 118
Skeleton and External Form 121
Musculature 136
Circulatory System 138
Digestive System 140
Reproductive System 155
Discussion 159
Literature Cited 169

MICROANATOMY *Carleton J. Phillips* 176
Abstract 176
Introduction 177
Methods 177
Brain 179
Anterior Pituitary Gland 179
Eyes 180
Tarsal (Meibomian) Glands 193
Integumentary Glands 194
Dentition 196

Salivary Glands 202
Digestive Tract 217
Adrenal Glands 241
Reproductive Tracts 243
Acknowledgments 247
Literature Cited 247

ONTOGENY *Joseph H. Nadeau* 254
Abstract 254
Introduction 254
The Prenatal Period 255
Parturition 262
The Postnatal Period 270
Synthesis 277
Summary 280
Acknowledgment 280
Literature Cited 280

HABITATS *Lowell L. Getz* 286
Abstract 286
Introduction 287
Habitat Factors 288
Responses to Habitat Features 291
Competitive Exclusion and Habitat Utilization 299
Habitat Utilization on Islands 300
Habitat Configuration and Stability 301
Effects of Human Activities on *Microtus* Habitats 302
Agricultural Habitats 304
Literature Cited 305

COMMUNITY ECOLOGY *Robert K. Rose* and *Elmer C. Birney* 310
Abstract 310
Introduction 310
Communities of Small Mammals with *Microtus* 312
The Influence of *Microtus* on Communities 325
The Role of *Microtus* in Small Mammal Communities 329
Conclusions and Perspectives 333
Acknowledgments 334
Literature Cited 335

BEHAVIOR *Jerry O. Wolff* 340
Abstract 340
Introduction 341
Non-social Behavior 341
Social Behavior 344
Literature Cited 366

ACTIVITY RHYTHMS AND SPACING *Dale M. Madison* 373
Abstract 373
Introduction 374
Activity Rhythms 374
Spacing 389
Generalities and Predictions for Future Testing 411
Acknowledgments 413
Literature Cited 413

DISPERSAL *William Z. Lidicker, Jr.* 420
Abstract 420
Introduction 421
Review of Techniques 422
A Classification of Dispersal 425
Characterization of Dispersers 427
Demographic Causes and Consequences 436
Evolutionary Issues 442
Summary and Conclusions 445
Literature Cited 448

PARASITES *Robert M. Timm* 455
Abstract 455
Introduction 456
Mites 457
Ticks 472
Lice 478
Beetles 481
Flies 482
Fleas 484
Directions for Future Research 503
Acknowledgments 504
Literature Cited 504
Appendix A. Endoparasites 528

PREDATION *Oliver P. Pearson* 535
Abstract 535
Introduction 536
Predation by Birds 537
Predation by Mammals 550
Predation by Fish, Amphibians, and Reptiles 558
Discussion 559
Conclusions 562
Literature Cited 563

POPULATION DYNAMICS AND CYCLES *Mary J. Taitt* and *Charles J. Krebs* 567
Abstract 567
Introduction 568
Methods of Study 569
Observed Population Patterns 572
Hypotheses to Explain Population Patterns 588
Tests of Hypotheses 593
Mathematical Models 609
Discussion 610
Literature Cited 612

MANAGEMENT AND CONTROL *Ross E. Byers* 621
Abstract 621
Introduction 621
History of Vole Control in Orchards 623
Environmental Hazards and Chemical Residues 639
Concluding Remarks 641
Literature Cited 642

LABORATORY MANAGEMENT AND PATHOLOGY *Frank F. Mallory* and *Robert A. Dieterich* 647
Abstract 647
Introduction 647
Laboratory Management 652
Pathology 657
Summary 676
Acknowledgments 676
Literature Cited 677

ENDOCRINOLOGY *Robert W. Seabloom* 685
Abstract 685
Introduction 686
Timing of Reproductive Function 686
Estrus and Ovulation 693
Formation and Duration of Corpus Luteum 697
Gestation 698
Post-partum Events 700
Testicular Activity 702
Thyroid 703
Adrenal Cortex 704
Summary and Conclusions 716
Literature Cited 718

REPRODUCTIVE PATTERNS *Barry L. Keller* 725
Abstract 725
Introduction 726
Length of Breeding Season 728
Breeding Intensity 740
Litter Size 751
Discussion 766
Acknowledgments 768
Literature Cited 768

NUTRITION *George O. Batzli* 779
Abstract 779
Introduction 779
The Diets of Microtines 781
Intake, Forage Quality, and Individual Performance 790
Forage Quality and Population Characteristics 803
Conclusions 806
Literature Cited 806

ENERGETICS AND THERMOREGULATION *Bruce A. Wunder* 812
Abstract 812
Introduction 813
Methods 815
Energy Acquisition 817
Energy Allocation 821
Energy-Flow Models: Individuals and Populations 837
Future Studies 838
Literature Cited 839

GENETICS *Michael S. Gaines* 845
Abstract 845
Introduction 845
Pelage Coloration 846
Cytogenetics 849
Allozymic Variation 853
Quantitative Genetics 864
Relationship between Genetics and Population Regulation 870
Conclusions 875
Acknowledgments 878
Literature Cited 878

INDEX 884

THE FOSSIL RECORD

RICHARD J. ZAKRZEWSKI

Abstract

REMAINS of fossils assignable to *Microtus* are known from 241 sites in 39 states and provinces in North America. These sites range in age from early Pleistocene (Irvingtonian-Aftonian?) to Holocene.

Two groups, based in part on the morphology of the m1, can be distinguished: 1) a *Pitymys* group, wherein the m1 consists of three closed triangles; and 2) a *Microtus* group, wherein the m1 consists of four or more closed triangles.

Pitymys is considered a valid genus. It is represented in the fossil record by at least eight extinct species, and two extant species have a fossil record. *Microtus* is represented by two extinct species, and 10 extant species have a fossil record.

Both genera probably originated in Asia and migrated across the Bering Land Bridge into North America. The first migration appears to have taken place about 1.8 m.y.b.p. and is represented by primitive species of both genera. Advanced species represent additional migrations and/or autochthonous development.

Both genera had a wider distribution in the past. Ranges of various species have retracted, in some cases substantially, since mid-Holocene time, probably as a result of climatic change.

Introduction

This chapter deals with the fossil record of *Microtus* in North America, fossil record being defined as all Pleistocene and any Holocene sites wherein any of the recorded taxa are locally extinct. Using this definition, I list 241 sites from 39 states and provinces in North America (Fig. 1 and Appendix A). Additional Holocene records that do not meet this definition can be found in Semken

Dedicated to the late John E. Guilday.

(in press). The distribution of these sites suggests a sampling bias, reflecting both potential deposits and individual interests.

Although the primary function of this chapter is to update the fossil record, I also make some comments regarding systematics. The sole basis for the comments is the morphology of the teeth. The terminology of the teeth follows, or is modified from, van der Meulen (1973) and is shown in Fig. 2.

I have used a standard format in discussing each taxon. This format includes the sites where the taxon is found, the age of the sites, characters used to distinguish the taxon, problems in applying these criteria, general comments regarding interrelationships, distribution, etc. For fossil taxa I have included the type locality and the location, number, and nature of the type specimen.

A number in parentheses follows each site when it is listed under a taxon in the text. This number can be used to find the site on the distribution maps (Figs. 1, 5, 6, 8), in the appendices, and to refer to the pertinent references in the selected bibliography or to personal communications listed in the acknowledgments.

Although Boellstorff (1978) showed that it is no longer reasonable to refer to events in the early Pleistocene by the classical glacial-interglacial terminology, I continue to do so herein (Fig. 3). My major rationale is to avoid confusion. Most non-geologists are familiar with the terminology and most published records use these terms for a time reference.

In compiling these records I relied on published information (most of the citations are primary sources; a few, however, are secondary) and the cooperative spirit of a number of colleagues. I examined small samples of all the extant taxa and some of the extinct ones. I view the results as a "state-of-the-art" statement and as a starting point for subsequent work.

Abbreviations used in text are as follows:

Institutions

- AMNH—American Museum of Natural History, New York
- CM —Carnegie Museum of Natural History, Pittsburgh
- FGS —Florida Geological Survey, Gainesville
- KU —University of Kansas, Museum of Natural History, Lawrence
- UA —University of Alaska, Fairbanks
- UF —University of Florida, Gainesville

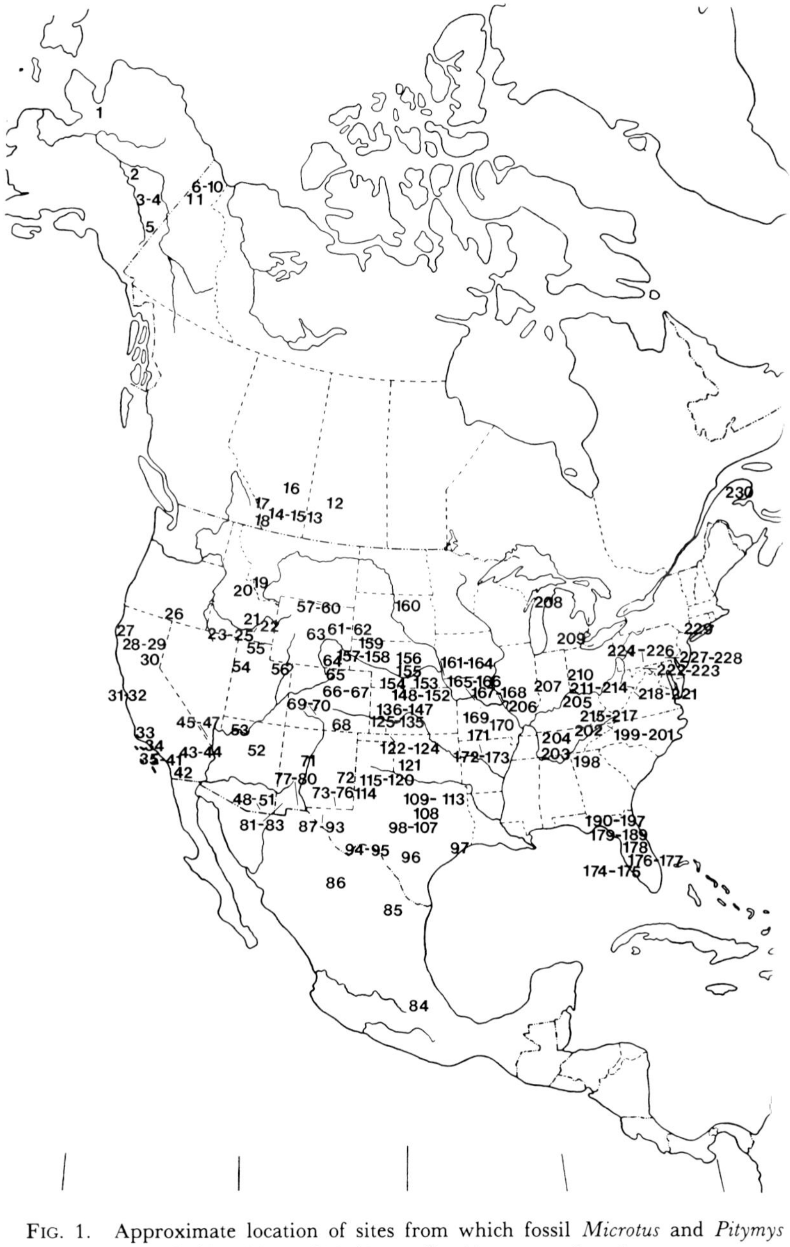

FIG. 1. Approximate location of sites from which fossil *Microtus* and *Pitymys* have been reported. Sites 231 to 241 (Appendix A) are not plotted.

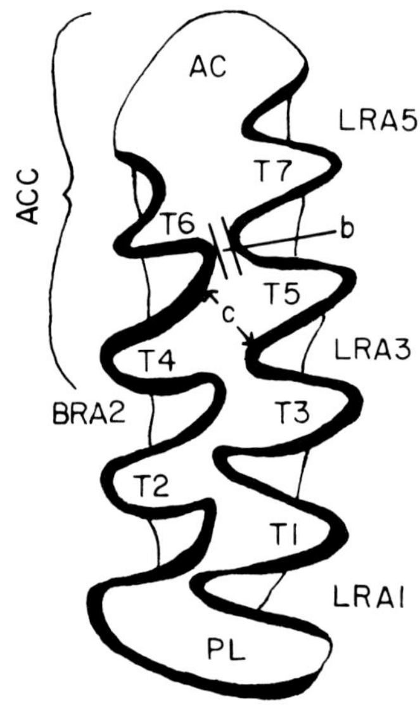

FIG. 2. Terminology employed for teeth. Abbreviations are: AC, anterior cap; ACC, anteroconid complex; BRA, buccal reentrant angle; b, shortest distance between BRA3 and LRA4; c, shortest distance between BRA3 and LRA3; LRA, lingual reentrant angle; PL, posterior loop; T, triangle.

Teeth (see Fig. 2)

ACC	—anteroconid complex
AC	—anterior cap
b	—shortest distance between BRA3 and LRA4
c	—shortest distance between BRA3 and LRA3
BRA	—buccal reentrant angle
LRA	—lingual reentrant angle
PL	—posterior loop
T	—triangle

Ages

B.P.—before present, m.y.b.p.—million years before present, H—Holocene; W—Wisconsin; S—Sangamon; I—Illinoian; Y—Yarmouth; K—Kansan; A—Aftonian; L—Late

Superscripts with Taxa

$^+$—taxon extinct locally

°—taxon extinct

nd—*nomen dubium*

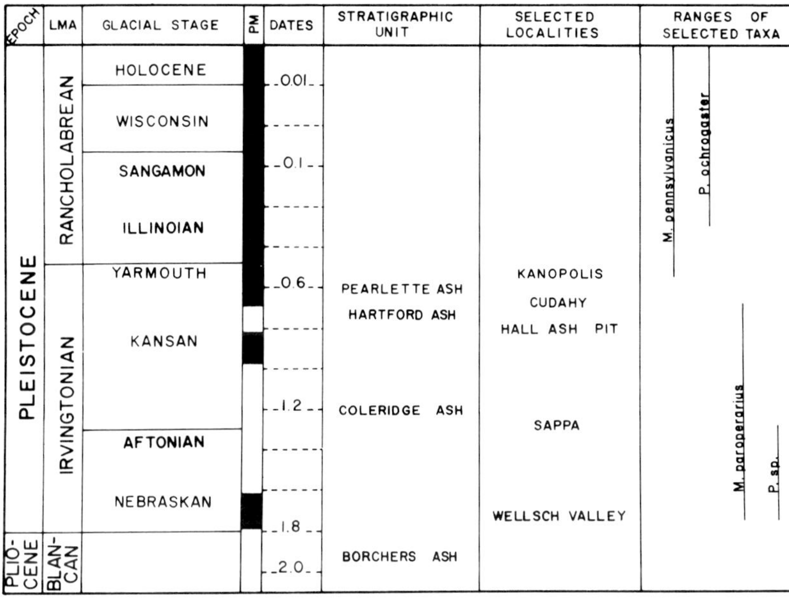

EPOCH
LMA
GLACIAL STAGE
PM
DATES
STRATIGRAPHIC UNIT
SELECTED LOCALITIES
RANGES OF SELECTED TAXA
PLEISTOCENE
PLIO-CENE
RANCHOLABREAN
IRVINGTONIAN
BLAN-CAN
HOLOCENE
WISCONSIN
SANGAMON
ILLINOIAN
YARMOUTH
KANSAN
AFTONIAN
NEBRASKAN
0.01
0.1
0.6
1.2
1.8
2.0
PEARLETTE ASH
HARTFORD ASH
COLERIDGE ASH
BORCHERS ASH
KANOPOLIS
CUDAHY
HALL ASH PIT
SAPPA
WELLSCH VALLEY
M. pennsylvanicus
P. ochrogaster
M. paroperarius
P. sp.

FIG. 3. Time chart showing relationships of different units and selected sites discussed in text. LMA, land mammal age; PM, paleomagnetic stage.

Systematics and the Fossil Record

Microtus is the most advanced of the genera of voles in North America. The molars are evergrowing, contain cement in the reentrant angles, the enamel of the occlusal surface is often differentiated into thick and thin segments, and well-developed dentine tracts are present on the sides of a number of loops or triangles.

Two groups can be distinguished. One consists of taxa that have three closed alternating triangles on the m1, herein considered the *Pitymys* group; the other, taxa that have four or more closed alternating triangles on the m1, herein considered the *Microtus* group. Presently, most workers consider *Pitymys* a subgenus of *Microtus*; however, there is some merit for considering *Pitymys* a distinct genus, a view that I favor and follow herein.

Pitymys *Group*

The *Pitymys* group can be distinguished from the *Microtus* group by its m1, which consists of a PL, three closed alternating triangles, and an ACC that varies in its complexity (Fig. 4). Triangles anterior to the first three are generally confluent and appear to be added in sets of two, rather than individually. The upper molars tend to be less complex, retaining the primitive pattern. The enamel on the occlusal surface is inconsistent in its differentiation into thin and thick segments. Some specimens exhibit differentiation; others do not.

I would include in this group and place in synonymy under *Pitymys* McMurtrie, 1831, the following taxa: *Neodon* Hodgson, 1849; *Pedomys* Baird, 1857; *Phaiomys* Blyth, 1863; and *Allophaiomys* Kormos, 1933. This approach is not novel. One of the more recent variations is that of Martin (1974).

It is nearly impossible to distinguish *Pitymys pinetorum* (Le Conte) from "*Pedomys*" *ochrogaster* (Wagner) on the basis of dental morphology (" " around generic names signify incorrect usage). Although an opinion can be reached if large samples are available (see *Pitymys ochrogaster* section below), the criteria cannot be used to distinguish taxa above the species level.

"*Allophaiomys*" is not distinguishable at the generic level from "*Phaiomys*" (Martin, 1975). Differences that have been found are of the sort that distinguish species, not genera.

"*Allophaiomys*" was probably ancestral to *Pitymys* (van der Meulen, 1973). Although the early members of this lineage are generally distinguishable from the later, it is sometimes difficult to assign individuals from intermediate populations (Hibbard et al., 1978). This lineage is shown by the pattern of the m1, which consists of two major "end" morphotypes with intermediates (Fig. 4A–C, F). These facts suggest that the taxa should be placed in one genus.

Some specimens of "*Neodon*" have two sets of confluent triangles (Fig. 4D). However, others have the typical *Pitymys* pattern (Fig. 4E) and, therefore, should be retained in that genus. This approach is consistent with the approach used in the consideration of other genera, including *Microtus,* that vary in the number of triangles.

Based on the fossil record, *Pitymys* had a wider distribution than it does now. Hinton (1926) suggested that *Pitymys*' present distribution and habits are a result of competition with *Microtus*. An alternative model was suggested by Hibbard (1944), who felt that *Pitymys* may have been forced southward by advancing ice and resorted to burrowing for thermoregulation. Where *Microtus* and *Pitymys* occur together they are not in competition.

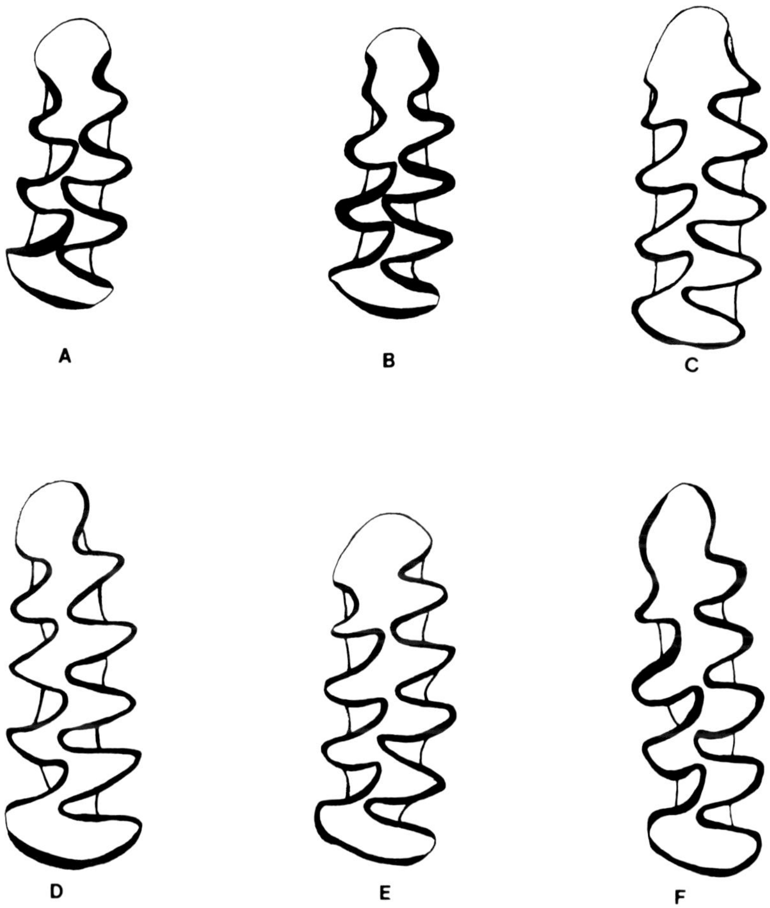

FIG. 4. Selected morphotypes of m1 in *Pitymys*. A, *P.* sp.; B, *P. llanensis*; C, *P. ochrogaster*; D, *P. meadensis*; E, *P. quasiater*; F, *P. pinetorum*. See text for additional explanation.

Pitymys is thought to have descended from *Mimomys* (van der Meulen, 1974), probably in Asia. The first appearance in the New World is near the beginning of the Pleistocene at Wellsch Valley (13) in Saskatchewan (Figs. 1, 3). Later taxa may have resulted from speciation in North America or subsequent migration over the Bering Land Bridge.

Pitymys *sp.*—Remains of this taxon are known from Kansas, Aries (133), Nash (134), Kentuck (147), Wathena (148), Courtland Canal (151); Nebraska, Sappa (154); Saskatchewan, Wellsch Valley (13); South Dakota, Java (160); and Texas, Fyllan Cave (104) (Fig. 5). These sites are considered to be Irvingtonian (Aftonian-Kansan) in age.

The specimens from these sites are at the most primitive grade of evolution. The majority of m1s can be assigned to morphotype 1a (Fig. 4A). I have listed all the records here primarily for convenience. Future work may show that any or all are distinct. Specimens from few of the sites have been critically studied and sample sizes are generally small.

Einsohn (1971) assigned specimens from Kentuck, Wathena, and Sappa to *Microtus llanensis* Hibbard on the basis of size and occlusal pattern. (Hibbard [1952, Fig. 10] figured a m1 with morphotype 1a and assigned it to *M. llanensis.*) Martin (1975) referred the specimens from Kentuck and Java to "*Allophaiomys*" *pliocaenicus* Kormos. Van der Meulen (1978) suggested that the specimens from these three local faunas represent a species different from "*A.*" *pliocaenicus* because the degree of confluency between triangles 4 and 5 and the AC is intermediate in development between "*A.*" *pliocaenicus* and "*A.*" *deucalion* Kretzoi. Van der Meulen (1978) also pointed out that, although all m1s assignable to morphotype 1 exhibit enamel differentiation, the American specimens exhibit greater differentiation of enamel than does "*A.*" *deucalion.* It is perhaps for this reason that Churcher and Stalker (in press) are placing the finds from the Wellsch Valley, Java, and Kentuck in a new species.

I am not convinced that enamel differentiation is a valid character for defining taxa in this group. I have looked at specimens from Fyllan Cave, which I (Zakrzewski, 1975) originally assigned to *Microtus llanensis,* and Wathena, but have examined in detail only some from Kentuck. I was unable to distinguish any enamel differentiation in the Kentuck specimens. Enamel differentiation is a variable character in this group. To learn whether the variability is ontogenetic, individual, or species specific will require more study. However, the Wellsch Valley specimens may represent a valid species because the type series appears to be larger than other specimens; the possibility of a size cline should also be considered.

In addition, while I was examining the Kentuck sample, I observed a number of m1s of morphotype 1b (Fig. 4B). This morphotype is common within samples of more advanced, but extinct, species of *Pitymys*. It can also be found within samples of extant taxa, in which the common morphotype is 1c (Fig. 4C, F). Van der Meulen (1978) admitted that dividing the taxa at the generic level was arbitrary. Because of the chrono-morphocline exhibited, it seems more reasonable to place all morphotype 1 specimens in one genus.

The Wellsch Valley site may have yielded the earliest known specimens of *Pitymys* in North America. Deposits at this site have been dated at 1.75 m.y.b.p. on the basis of paleomagnetic studies. Only the Nash site could be as old or older. The Nash occurs in the upper part of the Crooked Creek formation (fm.) in sediments that were channeled into the part of the Crooked Creek that contains the Borchers Ash dated at 1.96 m.y.b.p. (Fig. 3) (Zakrzewski, 1981). These deposits are overlain by the Kingsdown fm., which contains an ash that has been dated at 1.2 m.y.b.p. (Boellstorff, 1976). Underlying this ash is the Aries site (Honey, pers. comm.). The Coleridge Ash, which is underlain by the Sappa, also has been dated at 1.2 m.y.b.p. The other sites are considered to be approximately equivalent to the Sappa.

If the age of the Wellsch is correct, then *Pitymys* was in North America earlier than previously suspected. This occurrence also supports the hypothesis that *Pitymys* and *Microtus* have a long independent history because *M. paroperarius*, a more advanced taxon, is also recorded from this site.

Pitymys guildayi *(van der Meulen, 1978)*.—This species is known only from Maryland, Cumberland Cave (222) (Fig. 5) of Irvingtonian (Kansan) age [see Pennsylvania (235) in Appendix A for additional record]. The type (CM 20333) is a right dentary with m1–m2.

Pitymys guildayi is approximately intermediate between *Pitymys* sp. from Kentuck and Wathena and *P. llanensis* with respect to the length of the ACC, the width of the AC, and the width of c (van der Meulen, 1978).

Although he conceded that "*Allophaiomys*," "*Phaiomys*," and "*Pedomys*" could not be distinguished on the basis of tooth morphology, van der Meulen (1978) placed *P. guildayi* in "*Pedomys*" because the enamel on the teeth is differentiated and because "*Pedomys*" and "*Phaiomys*" have undergone independent development on their respective continents and, therefore, should be considered separate genera.

I have examined the type of *P. guildayi*, and although I agree

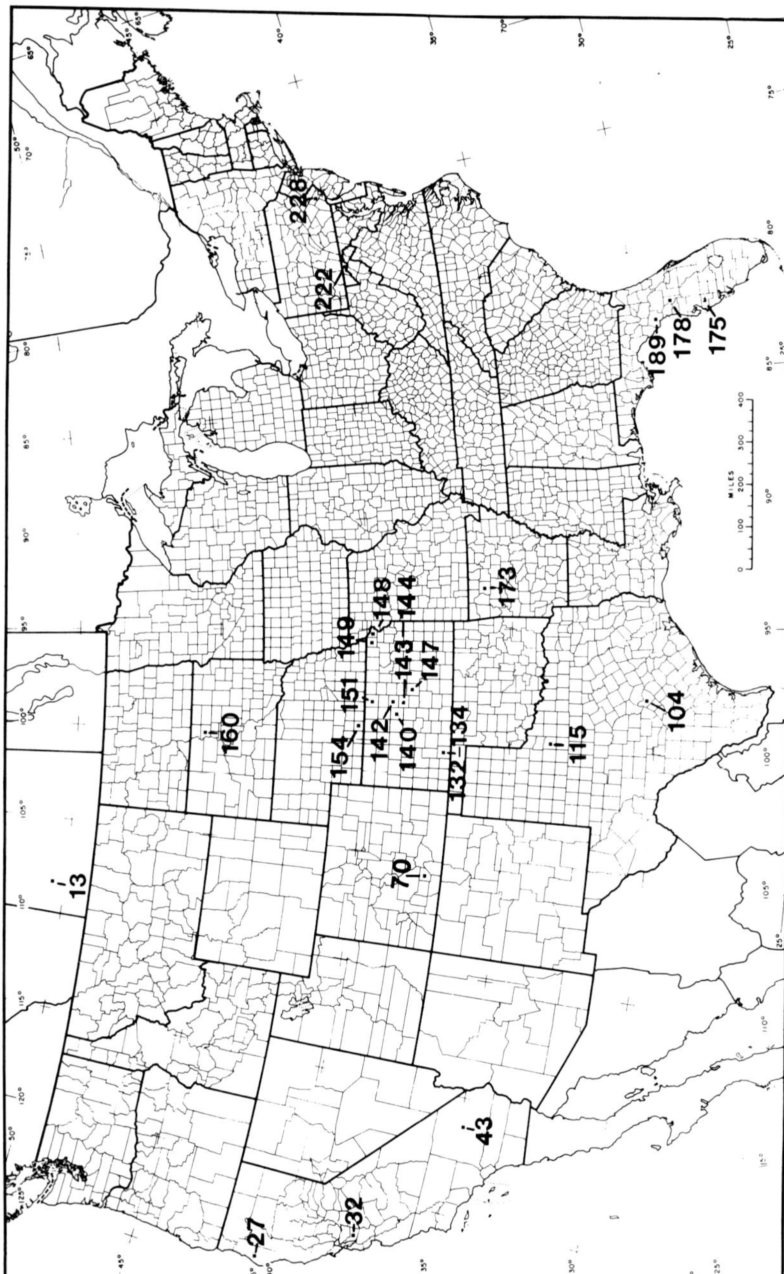

FIG. 5. Approximate location of sites in Canada and contiguous United States from which extinct species of *Pitymys* have been reported. See Appendix A and species accounts for details. Site 235 (Appendix A) is not plotted.

with van der Meulen that the teeth exhibit enamel differentiation, I do not feel that this character can be used to distinguish "*Pedomys*" from any other taxon. Likewise, although the two lineages may have undergone some independent development, their morphology suggests descendancy from a morphotype 1a ancestor; to consistently follow independent development as the sole basis for generic rank would quickly result in a number of morphologically indistinguishable genera.

Pitymys cumberlandensis *van der Meulen, 1978.*—Remains of this species have been reported from Arkansas, Conard Fissure (173); and Maryland, Cumberland Cave (222) (Fig. 5). Both of these sites are considered to be Irvingtonian (Kansan) in age.

The type (CM 20338, right dentary with m1–m3) is from Cumberland Cave. Van der Meulen (1978) characterized *P. cumberlandensis* as showing little enamel differentiation on the teeth, having a m1 with BRA4 and LRA5 that are shallow and rarely contain cement, and unreduced third molars.

Van der Meulen (1978) considered *P. cumberlandensis* to be ancestral to *P. pinetorum, P. parvulus,* and *P. nemoralis,* and judged that these four taxa constitute the genus *Pitymys,* based in part on undifferentiated enamel. He felt that *P. cumberlandensis* was too primitive to have been derived from "*Allophaiomys*." Although these relationships may be correct, I don't think that undifferentiated enamel can be used as one of the diagnostic characters.

Pitymys involutus *(Cope, 1871)*.—Specimens of this taxon have been reported from Pennsylvania, Port Kennedy Cave (228); and Maryland, Cumberland Cave (222) (Fig. 5). Both of these sites are considered to be Irvingtonian (Kansan-Yarmouth) in age.

Cope (1871) described *P. involutus* from Port Kennedy. Subsequently, Gazin (Gidley and Gazin, 1938) referred material from Cumberland Cave to the taxon. The species was considered distinct on the basis of the development of the reentrants on the ACC and its small size.

Since 1938 the teeth from the type specimen (AMNH 8699a, dentary with m1–m3) have been lost (Hibbard, 1955*a*). The specimen that Hibbard (1955*a,* Fig. 2d) suggested might be *P. involutus* appears to be *Microtus paroperarius.* Van der Meulen (1978) stated that he was able to find all three taxa that he recognized from the Cumberland Cave among the small sample available to Gazin. Because van der Meulen was unable to determine which of the three would be synonymous with *P. involutus,* he suggested that the taxon be considered a *nomen dubium.*

Pitymys dideltus *(Cope, 1871)*.—Remains of this taxon are only known from Pennsylvania, Port Kennedy Cave (228) (Fig. 5). The specimens that served as types for *P. dideltus* (AMNH 8694) and its junior synonym *P. "sigmodus"* (AMNH 8696) have disintegrated or are missing (Hibbard, 1955*a*). If the specimens that Hibbard (1955*a*) considered to pertain to *P. dideltus* were assigned correctly the taxon would be valid. The diagnostic criteria would be that the total length of the toothrow falls within the range of *P. pinetorum,* but the length of the m1 exceeds that in either *P. pinetorum* or *P. ochrogaster.* Hibbard (1955*a*) listed an m1 (AMNH 8695) as having an occlusal length of 3.8 mm. Only *P. aratai* has the m1 as large, but the total length of the toothrow exceeds that of *P. pinetorum* (Martin, 1974).

Van der Meulen (1978) considered *P. dideltus* a *nomen dubium,* because the type has been destroyed and the site from which it was collected is no longer accessible.

Pitymys aratai *Martin, 1974.*—This taxon is known only from Florida, Coleman IIA (178) of Rancholabrean (Illinoian?) age (Fig. 5). The species (type UF 11685, right dentary with m1–m3) can be distinguished easily because of the *Pitymys* pattern on the m1 and its large size. The m1 is 3.8 mm long, which is at the upper end of the range of *Microtus xanthognathus* (Leach) and *M. richardsoni* (DeKay) (Martin, 1974: Table 3.8). *Pitymys dideltus* also has a m1 that measures 3.8 mm (Hibbard, 1955*a*), but as mentioned *P. dideltus* is best considered as a *nomen dubium.* Repenning (1983) synonymized *P. aratai* with *P. mcnowni* Hibbard.

Pitymys hibbardi *Holman, 1959.*—Remains of this taxon are known from Florida, Bradenton (175) and Williston (189) (Fig. 5). Both sites are considered to be Rancholabrean (Sangamon) in age. The type (FGS V-5929, left dentary with m1–m3) of *P. hibbardi* was described by Holman (1959) from Williston. It was differentiated primarily on the basis of its large size, which is at the upper limit of the range of extant taxa. *Pitymys hibbardi* has a reduced capsular process on the dentary and is smaller than *P. aratai.* Martin (1974) thought that *P. hibbardi* might have evolved from *P. aratai.*

Pitymys llanensis *(Hibbard, 1944)*.—Remains of this species have been found in Arkansas, Conard Fissure (173); Kansas, Cudahy (132), Kanopolis (143), Unnamed (144), Kentuck? (147); and Texas, Vera (115) (Fig. 5). These sites are all considered to be Irvingtonian (Kansan-Yarmouth) in age.

Hibbard (1944) described *P. llanensis* (type KU 6626, left dentary with m1–m2) from the Cudahy and placed it in "*Pedomys.*" Semken (1966) and van der Meulen (1978) followed this assignment.

Pitymys llanensis can be distinguished from other taxa on the basis of its m1. The ACC is longer and wider than in *P. guildayi.* The tooth is generally shorter than those of *P. pinetorum* and *P. ochrogaster,* and narrower than that of the latter. The b in *P. llanensis* is wider than that of *P. pinetorum.*

The majority of m1s belonging to *P. llanensis* are assignable to morphotype 1b (Fig. 4B). Morphotype 1b is intermediate between 1a (typical of *P.* sp.; Fig. 4A) and 1c (typical of *P. ochrogaster* [Fig. 4C] and *P. pinetorum* [Fig. 4F]). Van der Meulen (1978) stated that these morphotypes occur in different percentages within different fossil populations and used them biostratigraphically. In examining the sample from Kentuck, I was unable to determine whether two taxa or a highly variable population of one taxon were present. This overlapping of morphotypes is one reason that I place all taxa with three closed triangles into *Pitymys.*

The specimens from the Unnamed site may pertain to *Microtus.*

Pitymys mcnowni *Hibbard, 1937.*—This species is known from California, Centerville Beach? (27); and Kansas, Unnamed (149). Paleomagnetic dating places the California site in the Irvingtonian, whereas the Kansas site is probably Rancholabrean.

The type (KU 3851, right dentary with m1–m2) is from Kansas. Hibbard (1937) considered the taxon distinct on the basis of the large size of its m1 (3.3 × 1.3 mm) and the character of the salient angles, which he described as being broader and with rounder apices than in other taxa.

The measurements, especially the length, are at the upper end of the range for *P. ochrogaster* and *P. pinetorum.* Only one *Pitymys* specimen that I have measured (Hibbard et al., 1978, text-fig. 6) was greater than 3.3 mm. Seven specimens were 1.3 mm or wider. I have not examined the type, but suggest that it may represent a large *P. ochrogaster* or *P. pinetorum.*

On the basis of size and dental pattern, Repenning (1983) suggested that *P. mcnowni* is synonymous with *P. aratai* and ancestral to, if not conspecific with, *P. nemoralis* (V. Bailey).

Pitymys ochrogaster *(Wagner, 1842)*.—Specimens of the prairie vole have been reported from 30 to 63 sites in 14 states (Appendix B). These sites range in age from Rancholabrean (Illinoian) to Holocene.

It is very difficult to distinguish *P. ochrogaster* from *P. pinetorum* on the basis of teeth unless large sample sizes are available. I suspect that some of the taxonomic assignments of the fossils are based on the geographic location of the site within the range of the particular taxon rather than on an analysis of the sample. Some workers have accepted the possibility that either one or both taxa might be in their fauna. This latter approach accounts for the range in the number of sites mentioned above and in the *P. pinetorum* section that follows.

Criteria that have been used by paleontologists to separate the taxa include relative thickness of enamel (van der Meulen, 1978), shape of m3 (Hager, 1974), and width of b (Hibbard et al., 1978). The latter character seems to be the most reliable, but even in it there is some overlap between the taxa. Smartt (1977) was able to identify *P. ochrogaster* in New Mexican sites by means of discriminant analysis.

Van der Meulen (1978) stated that "*Pedomys*" can be distinguished from *Pitymys* by the fact that the former has differentiated enamel on the occlusal surface, whereas the latter has enamel of equal thickness. This difference was one of the reasons he named the species *P. guildayi* and *P. cumberlandensis*, respectively, and placed the former in "*Pedomys*" as a subgenus of *Microtus*. *Microtus* is characterized in part by differentiated enamel. Although I agree with this characterization of *Microtus* and have verified the differences in enamel between *P. guildayi* and *P. cumberlandensis*, specimens of *P. ochrogaster* and *P. pinetorum* that I have examined exhibit both conditions. As mentioned above, whether the variation in enamel thickness is a function of the individual's age, geographic location, or some other factor(s) is unknown.

Pitymys pinetorum *(Le Conte, 1830)*.—Fossil remains of the pine vole are known from 38 to 76 sites in 16 states (Appendix B). All of the sites are Wisconsin to Holocene in age and the majority are within the present range of the species.

Pitymys pinetorum has an m1 that is generally longer than that of *P. llanensis*, generally narrower than that of *P. ochrogaster*, and a b that is narrower than in either (Hibbard et al., 1978).

Pitymys pinetorum appears later in the fossil record than *P. och-*

rogaster. I suspect this is a function of sampling; most sites at which it occurs are east of the Mississippi and few of these are older than Wisconsin.

Both van der Meulen (1978) and Repenning (1983) considered *P. pinetorum nemoralis* to be a full species on the basis of size and morphological characteristics. If they are correct, the fossil records of *P. pinetorum* will need to be reexamined in terms of this change.

Pitymys meadensis *Hibbard, 1944.*—Specimens of this taxon have been reported from California, North Livermore Ave. (32), Olive Dell Ranch (43); Colorado, Hansen Bluff (70); Kansas, Cudahy (132), Tobin (140), Wilson Valley (142) (Fig. 5); and Mexico, El Tajo de Tequixquiac (84). With the exception of the site in Mexico, considered to be Rancholabrean (Wisconsin), the localities are of Irvingtonian (Kansan) age.

Pitymys meadensis (type KU 6563, left dentary with m1–m2) was described by Hibbard (1944) from the Cudahy. The species is characterized by the fact that triangles 4 and 5 on the m1 are generally confluent and closed off from the AC. In addition, LRA5 and BRA4 are often deeper than in other species so that a sixth and seventh triangle develop, which are confluent and open into AC (Fig. 4D). This development of the ACC is found in some European taxa and in some specimens of the Mexican species *P. quasiater* (Coues) (Repenning, 1983).

Van der Meulen (1978) placed both *P. meadensis* and *P. quasiater* in *Microtus* because they exhibit differentiated enamel on their occlusal surface. The morphology of the m1 in *P. meadensis* (Fig. 4D) and *P. quasiater* (Fig. 4E) and its closeness to some specimens of *P. pinetorum* (Fig. 4F) suggests the taxa should be retained in *Pitymys.*

Pitymys quasiater is a relict population confined to the southeastern highlands of Mexico, whereas *P. meadensis* was apparently widespread in the past (Fig. 5). Perhaps *P. meadensis* was ancestral to *P. quasiater,* or the two are conspecific. Additional work will be necessary to determine the exact relationship between these two taxa.

Microtus *Group*

This group can be distinguished from the *Pitymys* group by its m1, which consists of a posterior loop, four or more closed alternating triangles, and an AC that varies in its complexity. Triangles on the m1 appear to be added in alternate fashion. The upper molars tend to be more complex as well, with a number of species developing additional triangles. The enamel on the occlusal surface tends to be consistently differentiated into thin and thick segments.

Within the group it is more difficult to assign isolated specimens to individual taxa because of similarities in dentition and the wide range of variation expressed in some species. Two subgroups can be established on the morphology of the m1: a basically four-triangled group (*M. deceitensis, M. paroperarius, M. "speothen"* and *M. oeconomus*) (Fig. 7A); and a five or more triangled group (the remaining taxa) (Fig. 7B).

Other criteria that can be used are size (*M. richardsoni* and *M. xanthognathus* are significantly larger), occlusal pattern of M2 (*M. pennsylvanicus* has an extra triangle), M3 (*M. chrotorrhinus* has additional triangles), and shape of the incisive foramina. The latter character exhibits a great deal of variation owing to age of the individual. Other characters show a great range of variation as well and the best approach for correctly assigning specimens may be to use some appropriate multivariate analysis as was demonstrated by Smartt (1977).

Microtus and *Pitymys* are thought to have separately entered North America from Asia. The first appearance of *Microtus* in the New World is near the beginning of the Pleistocene and is represented by *M. deceitensis* and/or *M. paroperarius*. Advanced species appear to represent subsequent immigrations (van der Meulen, 1978). The genus had a much wider range in the past than it does now. A number of species exhibit a significant retraction of range.

Microtus deceitensis *Guthrie and Matthews, 1971*.—This taxon is known only from its type locality at Cape Deceit (1) Alaska of Irvingtonian (pre or early Kansan) age. Remains of this taxon (type, UA 866, right dentary with m1–m3) are considered to represent the most primitive species in North America assigned to the genus. The absolute age of the deposit is not known and the fauna does not correlate well with any other fauna from North America; therefore, it cannot be determined with certainty whether *M. deceitensis* also represents the earliest record of *Microtus* in the New World. *M. deceitensis* is similar to the extinct *M. paroperarius* Hibbard and the extant *M. oeconomus* Pallas in the possession of a principally four-triangled m1. It differs from the latter two taxa in possessing a more complex m3, in that the second lingual loop tends to be bisected by the LRA2, and a simpler M3, consisting of only two alternating triangles as found in *Pitymys* (Guthrie and Matthews, 1971).

Van der Meulen (1978) felt that *M. deceitensis* represents an extinct side branch of *Microtus* evolution, but also offered the alternative that it may have given rise to *M. xanthognathus*. Repenning (pers. comm.) thinks that *M. deceitensis* represents an Asian relict unrelated to any North American taxon. He places *M. deceitensis* into *Lasiopodomys,* which he raises to generic status on the basis of its *Pitymys*-like M3.

Microtus paroperarius *Hibbard, 1944*.—Remains of *M. paroperarius* are known from Arkansas, Conard Fissure (173); Colorado, Hansen Bluff (70); Iowa, Little Sioux (161); Kansas, Cudahy (132), Holzinger (137), Tobin (140), Wilson Valley (142), Unnamed? (144), Hall Ash Pit (150); Maryland, Cumberland Cave (222); Nebraska, Unnamed (156) and Mullen (157 or 158); Saskatchewan, Wellsch Valley (13); and Texas, Vera (115) [see Pennsylvania (235) in Appendix A for additional record]. The ages of these sites (Fig. 6) range from Irvingtonian (Aftonian?) to Rancholabrean (early Illinoian?).

The type of *M. paroperarius* (KU 6587, partial right dentary with m1–m2) was described by Hibbard (1944) from the Cudahy. It is characterized by its m1, which generally consists of four closed alternating triangles and a fifth triangle that opens broadly into AC (Fig. 7A). A small percentage of specimens may have m1s with five closed triangles. Similar m1s are found in *M. speothen* (Cope) and *M. oeconomus*.

Hibbard (1955*a*) stated that m1s of *M. paroperarius* are smaller than those of *M. speothen* from the Port Kennedy Cave (228). However, the few measurements available for *M. speothen* are just over, or within the range of those obtained for *M. paroperarius*.

Paulson (1961) pointed out that 50% of the m1s of *M. paroperarius* contain cement in LRA4, whereas the LRA4 of *M. oeconomus* lacks cement. Van der Meulen (1978) stated that the two taxa cannot be distinguished on the basis of tooth morphology. Perhaps additional study would show that the taxa are conspecific. If so, a range retraction even greater than that seen in *M. xanthognathus* is indicated.

The Wellsch Valley occurrence is the earliest record of the taxon

(Figs. 3, 6). These specimens were reported as *M. deceitensis* by Kurtén and Anderson (1980). The Mullen occurrence may be the latest. Kurtén and Anderson (1980) reported the specimens from Mullen I, which is Kansan in age, but Martin (1972) reported that they came from Mullen II, which is Illinoian in age, and assigned them to *M. pennsylvanicus* (see Martin, 1972, Fig. 2C) because there were no other indicators of Kansan age. Martin (1972) stated that *M. paroperarius* is ancestral to *M. pennsylvanicus* although he presented no evidence, unless it is the fact that some *M. paroperarius* exhibit five closed triangles. The remaining sites are generally considered to be Kansan in age.

Van der Meulen (1978) suggested that *M. paroperarius* migrated to the New World, along with other taxa, just prior to 0.7 m.y.b.p. However, if the date of 1.75 m.y.b.p for the Wellsch Valley is correct, the migration was much earlier.

Microtus speothen *(Cope, 1871)*.—The remains of this extinct species were known only from the Port Kennedy Cave (228) of Yarmouth age from Pennsylvania. Originally described by Cope as *Arvicola speothen,* he (Cope, 1899) subsequently synonymized the species *A. tetradelta* under *A. speothen* and placed the latter in *Microtus.*

Hibbard (1955*a*) felt that *M. speothen* belonged in the *M. oeconomus* group. He also stated that *M. speothen* was larger than *M. paroperarius.* However, Cope (1899) listed the length of m1 as 3.0 mm, which would fall in the range of *M. paroperarius* m1s (2.6–3.4) reported by Paulson (1961).

Unfortunately, the type of *M. speothen* (AMNH 8689, left dentary with m1–m3) has been destroyed and the site is no longer accessible; therefore, van der Meulen's (1978) suggestion that all of Cope's taxa from Port Kennedy should be considered *nomen dubia* is a reasonable one.

Microtus oeconomus *Pallas, 1778.*—Fossil remains of the tundra vole are known only from the Yukon Territories, Old Crow River Loc. 11 (10) and 12 (8), as well as Bluefish Cave I (11). These sites are Sangamon?, Illinoian, and late Wisconsin, respectively. Similar to the extinct *M. paroperarius* in dental morphology, the two taxa may be conspecific (van der Meulen, 1978). The fossil records of *M. oeconomus* are being studied by Brenda F. Beebe (Jopling et al., 1981) and are the first reports of this taxon as a fossil.

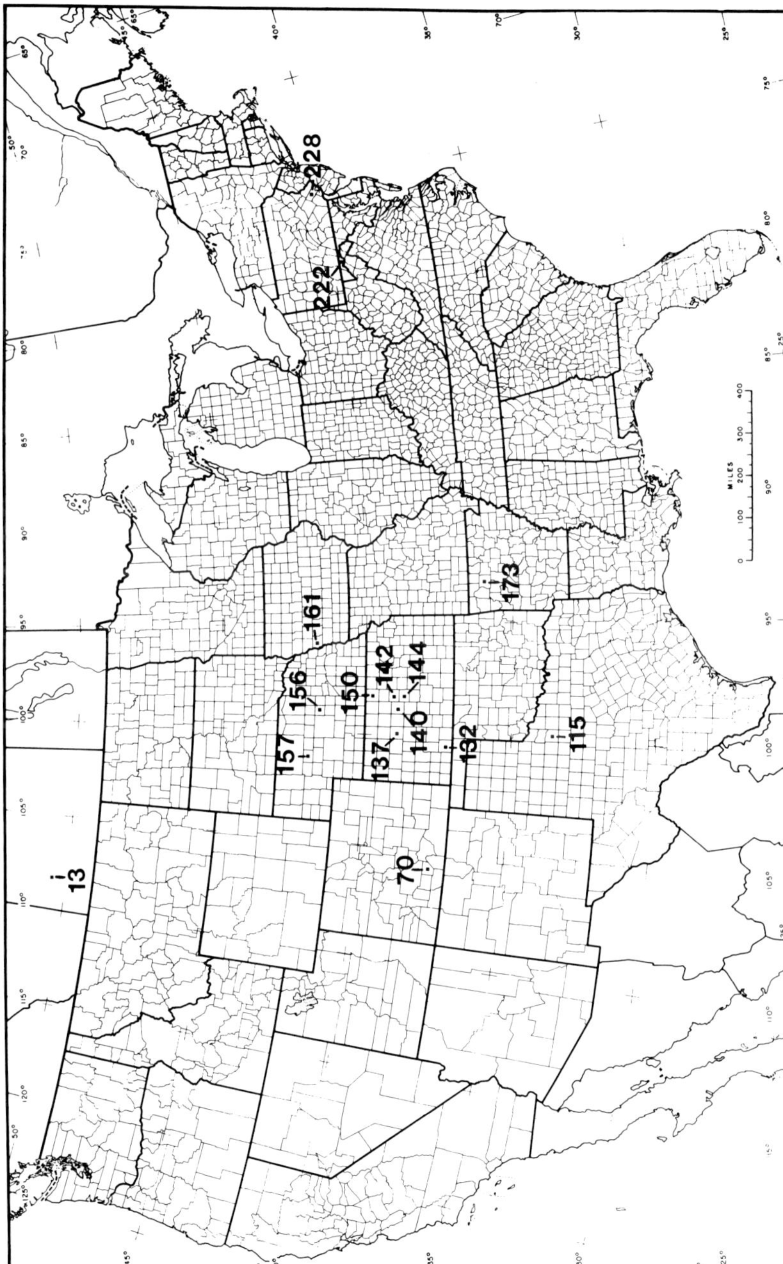

FIG. 6. Approximate location of sites in Canada and contiguous United States from which extinct species of *Microtus* have been reported. See Appendix A and species accounts for details. Site 235 (Appendix A) is not plotted.

Microtus miurus *Osgood, 1901*.—Specimens of the Alaska vole have been reported from Alaska, Sullivan Pit (2), Fairbanks II (3), Fairbanks I (4); and Yukon Territories, Old Crow River Loc. 11 (10), 12 (8 and 9), 14N (7), Bluefish Cave I (11) [see Iowa (238) in Appendix A for additional record]. The sites range in age from Illinoian to Holocene, and with the exception of the Sullivan Pit (Repenning, pers. comm.), the species is not found near any of them today.

Microtus miurus is distinguished by its narrow cranium with a sharp median crest. The former character is used to place *M. miurus* in its own subgenus *Stenocranius*. Kurtén and Anderson (1980) stated that *M. miurus* has a M1 with five triangles and a m1 with a simple trefoil or AC. These two characters could be used to distinguish it from *M. pennsylvanicus*. I found no *M. miurus* with five-triangled M1s and could not distinguish its m1 from that of *M. pennsylvanicus*.

The earliest record of *M. miurus* is from Fairbanks I. Brenda F. Beebe is studying the remains from Bluefish Cave I.

Microtus richardsoni *(DeKay, 1842)*.—Fossil remains of Richardson's vole are known from Alberta, Eagle Cave (18); and Montana, Warm Springs (19). All of these sites are late Wisconsin in age and within the present range of the species. Remains of *M. richardsoni* are relatively easy to recognize. The species is among the largest in the genus, being about the same size as *M. xanthognathus*. It can be distinguished from that and other taxa by the fact that the incisive foramina decrease in size with age, so that in some individuals they are nearly closed. In addition, the M1 and on occasion the M2 possess an additional small triangle (Fig. 7E), although it generally is not closed off from the previous alternating triangle as is the triangle on the M2 of *M. pennsylvanicus* (Fig. 7F).

Microtus californicus *(Peale, 1848)*.—Remains of the California vole are known from California, Samwel Cave (28), Potter Creek Cave (29), cf. Irvington (31), Carpinteria (33), McKittrick (34), Rancho La Brea (35), San Pedro (36), La Mirada (37), Emery Borrow Pit (38), Zuma Creek (39), Costeau Pit (40), Newport Bay Mesa 1067 (41), cf. Vallecito Creek (42), Kokoweef (44); and Nevada, Tule Springs E_1 (45), Glendale? (47). These sites range in age from Irvingtonian (Kansan) to Rancholabrean (Wisconsin).

In assigning specimens to *M. californicus*, some workers (Miller, 1971) have relied on the shape of the incisive foramina, which are wide and unconstricted, and the fact that the teeth of the species seem to be slightly larger than those of other taxa that occur near California. Many M2s of the California vole have the LRA2 directed posteriorly so that it appears a fourth triangle would become isolated if the LRA2 lengthened (Fig. 7D–E).

The oldest remains (if correctly identified) are from the Vallecito Creek and Irvington. In fact one of the specimens from Vallecito could be the oldest record for a *Microtus.* I (Zakrzewski, 1972) questionably assigned an edentulous dentary to *M. californicus* on the basis of the presence of a deep masseteric fossa and alveoli that showed that the teeth were evergrowing. The specimen is from Loc. 6683, which is not in the type section, and is associated with remains of *Synaptomys* (*Metaxomys*) *anzaenis. Metaxomys* is associated with faunas of Blancan age, whereas the extant subgenera with one exception (Dixon l.f., Kansas) are associated with faunas of Irvingtonian and younger age. At that time I suggested two alternative explanations. The specimen represents a genus other than *Microtus* or the *Synaptomys* represent a relict population. Although the former alternative cannot be dismissed, data acquired while preparing this manuscript suggest that the latter interpretation may be closer to the truth.

The other sites are Wisconsin in age. The two sites in Nevada are outside the present range of the taxon and the Glendale record may be *M. montanus* (Kurtén and Anderson, 1980).

Microtus mexicanus *(Saussure, 1861)*.—Fossil remains of the Mexican vole have been reported from Mexico, San Josecito (85); New Mexico, Brown Sand Wedge (72), Dry Cave (73), Burnet Cave (74), Muskox Cave (75), Anthony Cave (77), Conkling Cavern (78), Howells Ridge Cave (82); and Texas, Upper (91) and Lower (92) Sloth Cave, Pratt Cave (93). All of the records ascribed to this taxon are late Wisconsin to Holocene in age. Likewise, all the finds are either in or not substantially distant from the present range.

Smartt (1977) identified the majority of New Mexican records using discriminant analysis. Kurtén and Anderson (1980) stated that the incisive foramina are short, broad, and truncated posteriorly. This character was highly variable in specimens that I examined. In some M1s and M2s the LRA2 is deep and directed posteriorly, so that it appears an additional triangle might form (Fig. 7D). In addition, I observed an M2 of *M. mexicanus* that had a *M. pennsylvanicus* pattern.

Microtus longicaudus *(Merriam, 1888)*.—Specimens of the long-tailed vole have been reported from Alberta, January Cave? (17), Eagle Cave? (18); Colorado, Chimney Rock Animal Trap? (65), Unnamed (69); Idaho, Moonshiner Cave (21), American Falls? (24); New Mexico, Dry Cave (73), Burnet Cave (74); and Wyoming, Agate Basin (62), Little Box Elder Cave (63). They range in age from Sangamon? to Holocene. The oldest and only pre-Wisconsin record of *M. longicaudus* could be from American Falls (the specimen may actually represent *M. pennsylvanicus*). The Alberta and Colorado records may represent *M. montanus.*

There is nothing diagnostic about the teeth of *M. longicaudus.* Some workers feel that this species can be distinguished by its incisive foramina, the borders of which are parallel or taper gradually. However, this feature is not unique to this taxon. Smartt (1977) has used discriminant analysis to identify the long-tailed vole in New Mexican sites.

I have observed an M2 of *M. longicaudus* with a fourth triangle similar to that of *M. pennsylvanicus* and an m1 with a prism fold or "mimomyskante," a feature typical of primitive voles of Blancan age.

Microtus montanus *(Peale, 1848)*.—Remains of the mountain vole are known from Alberta, Eagle Cave? (18), January Cave? (17); Arizona, Salina (52); Colorado, Chimney Rock Animal Trap? (65); Idaho, Jaguar Cave (20), Moonshiner Cave (21), Downey Dump (23), American Falls (24), Rainbow Beach (25); Kansas, cf. Jones (126), Trapshoot (138); Nevada, Glendale? (47); New Mexico, Anthony Cave (77), Shelter Cave (79), Howells Ridge Cave (82); Oregon, Fossil Lake (26); Texas, Navar Ranch #13 (89); Utah, Snowville (55), Silver Creek (56); and Wyoming, Little Canyon Creek Cave (58), Prospects Shelter (59), Natural Trap Cave (60), Little Box Elder Cave (63), Bell Cave (64). These sites range in age from Irvingtonian (Kansan) to Holocene.

The earliest records of *M. montanus* are from Downey Dump and Snowville (Repenning, pers. comm.). The remaining sites range in age from Sangamon to Holocene. The reports from Kansas, Texas, New Mexico, Nevada (if not *M. californicus*), and Alberta (if not *M. longicaudus*) are outside the present range of the taxon.

Smartt (1977) identified specimens of *M. montanus* from New Mexico by using discriminant analysis to differentiate between species that might be present. Davis (1975) recognized the presence of an additional *Microtus* from the Jones site because a number of M2s could not be assigned to *M. pennsylvanicus* even though all of the m1s from the site appeared to be *pennsylvanicus*-like. Davis called his unidentifiable taxon, *Microtus* species *Alpha.* Stewart (1978) suggested that Davis' species *Alpha* might be *M. montanus* on the basis of faunal similarities between the Jones and Trapshoot sites.

Kurtén and Anderson (1980) implied that the posterior constriction of the incisive foramina and an M2 with four closed triangles are diagnostic for this taxon. The posterior constriction is in part a function of the age of the individual, older individuals showing more constriction than younger ones.

I know of no New World *Microtus* for which four closed triangles on the M2 is as typical as it is for *M. pennsylvanicus.* Other species may have a small percentage of individuals that exhibit four closed triangles on M2; however, most non-*pennsylvanicus Microtus* M2s are similar to that shown in Fig. 7C.

Microtus chrotorrhinus *(Miller, 1894).*—Specimens of the yellow-nosed vole have been reported from Pennsylvania, New Paris #4 (224), Hollidaysburg Fissure (225), Bootlegger Sink (227); Québec, Caverne de St. Elzéar (230); Tennessee, Carrier Quarry Cave (199), Baker Bluff (200); Virginia, Back Creek #2 (218), Clark's Cave (219), Natural Chimneys (221); and West Virginia, Eagle Rock Cave (211), Hoffman School Cave (212), Mandy Walters Cave (213), Upper Trout Cave (214). These sites are late Wisconsin to Holocene in age.

Microtus chrotorrhinus is commonly found with *M. xanthognathus* and *M. pennsylvanicus* in cave faunas of the Appalachians. *Microtus chrotorrhinus* is smaller than *M. xanthognathus* and differs from *M. pennsylvanicus* in having a distinctive M3, with two additional triangles. The first and second alternating triangles are generally confluent; however, Guilday (1982) has shown that this pattern is also fairly common in some populations of *M. pennsylvanicus.*

Microtus chrotorrhinus occurs today in the eastern subarctic and as a relict form at high elevations in the central Appalachians. The fossil records with one exception are in or very near to its present range. Graham (1976) listed *M. chrotorrhinus* as a member of the Welsh Cave fauna (205) but this is incorrect.

Guilday et al. (1964) have demonstrated a cline within extant populations. Individuals become larger toward the south. The fossil

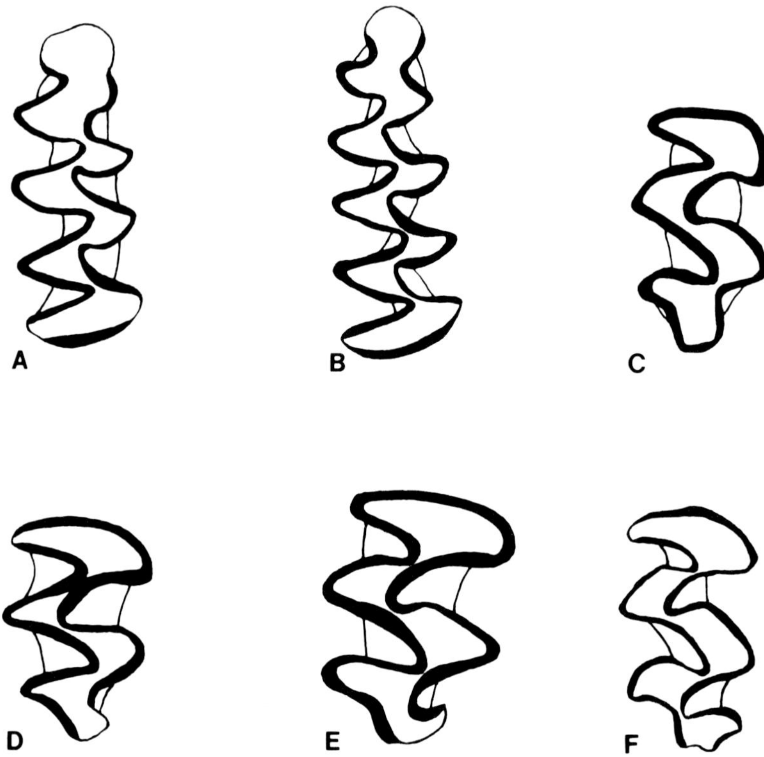

FIG. 7. Selected morphotypes of m1 and M2 in *Microtus*. A, m1 typical of *M. paroperarius* group; B, m1 typical of non-*paroperarius* group of *Microtus*; C, M2 typical of most non-*pennsylvanicus* species of *Microtus*; D, M2 seen in some *M. mexicanus* and *M. californicus* showing incipient development of additional triangle; E, M2 of *M. richardsoni* showing further development of additional triangle; F, M2 typical of *M. pennsylvanicus* showing additional triangle.

specimens from New Paris #4 are equivalent in size to those from extant populations of Labrador and Québec.

Guilday et al. (1977) suggested that *M. chrotorrhinus* was able to survive in the east (in contrast to *M. xanthognathus*) by moving to higher elevations when the climate changed in post-glacial time. It was able to extend its range into northeastern Canada after the ice melted.

Microtus xanthognathus *(Leach, 1815)*.—Fossil remains of the yellow-cheeked vole have been reported from Alaska, Fairbanks II (3), Chicken (5); Arkansas, Peccary Cave (172); Illinois, Meyer Cave (206); Iowa, Waubonsie (164); Kentucky, Welsh Cave (205); Missouri, Bat Cave (170); Pennsylvania, New Paris #4 (224), Bootlegger Sink (227); Québec, Caverne de St. Elzéar (230); Tennessee, Baker Bluff (200), Cheek Bend Cave (203); Virginia, Loop Creek Quarry Cave (215), Gillespie Cliff Cave (216), Back Creek #2 (218), Clark's Cave (219), Natural Chimneys (221); West Virginia, Eagle Rock Cave (211); Wyoming, Prospects Shelter (58); and Yukon Territories, Old Crow River Loc. 44 (6), 12 (8–9), 11 (10), Bluefish Cave I (11) [see Iowa (238, 239) and Wisconsin (241) in Appendix A for additional records]. These sites are all within the Rancholabrean stage ranging in age from late Illinoian [Old Crow River Loc. 12 (8)] to Holocene (Caverne de St. Elzéar).

Microtus xanthognathus can be distinguished from other species of *Microtus,* except for *M. richardsoni,* by its large size. In addition, Hallberg et al. (1974) stated that the BRA3 on the M3 of *M. xanthognathus* lacks cementum, whereas the same reentrant in *M. pennsylvanicus* contains cementum. I have observed cementum in the BRA3 of M3s in adult *M. richardsoni* as well as a narrowing of the incisive foramina with age. These two characters may be useful in separating *M. richardsoni* from *M. xanthognathus.* However, the lack of cementum in the BRA3 should be used with care as Guilday (1982) stated that 10.3% ($n = 113$) of the *M. xanthognathus* from Appalachian caves have cementum, whereas 5.2% ($n = 1,235$) of the *M. pennsylvanicus* lack cementum.

Although still extant across much of northwestern Canada and east-central Alaska, the records of the yellow-cheeked vole from conterminous United States and the Gaspe Peninsula (Fig. 8) are well outside the present range of the species. Guilday et al. (1977) suggested that *M. xanthognathus* dwelled on the taiga. As the climate changed toward the end of the Pleistocene, populations moved northwest following the shifting environment. Populations could not be maintained in the east because of changes in the vegetation. Movement into northeastern Canada was blocked by ice. Biotic evidence from the Ozark region suggested to Hallberg et al. (1974) that *M. xanthognathus* lived in more of a parkland than taiga situation.

Microtus pennsylvanicus *(Ord, 1815)*.—Specimens of the mead-

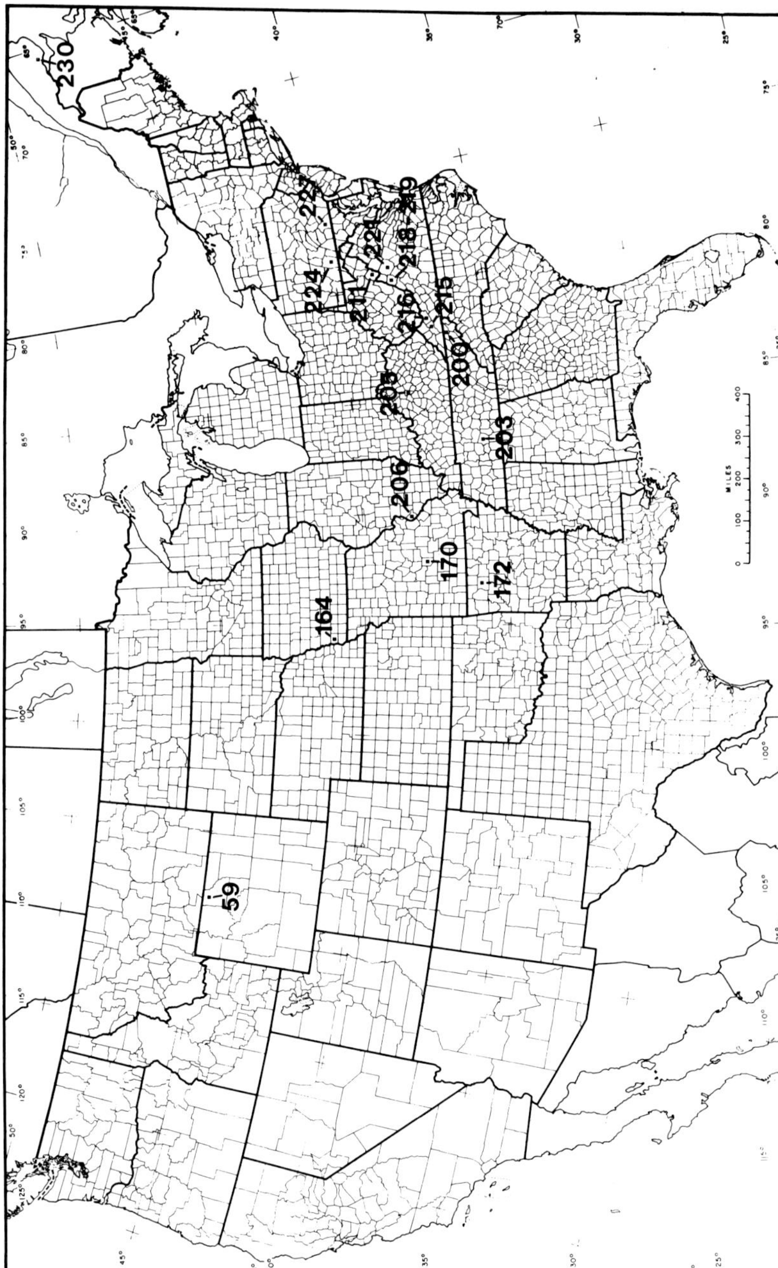

FIG. 8. Approximate location of sites from which *M. xanthognathus* has been reported that are outside of its present range. Sites 238, 239, and 241 (Appendix A) are not plotted.

ow vole have been reported from 91 sites in 24 states and four provinces (Appendix B) that range in age from Irvingtonian (Yarmouth) to Holocene. *M. pennsylvanicus* is the most widely distributed species of *Microtus*. Its distribution was even more extensive in the past as *M. pennsylvanicus* has been reported from more than two dozen sites in seven states south of its present range. The earliest record for the meadow vole is from Kansas, Kanopolis (143).

Microtus pennsylvanicus is closely related to the European field vole, *M. agrestis*. Both taxa have an M2 that exhibits four alternating triangles. This character is considered to be diagnostic for the species and suggested to some workers an additional invasion of microtine stock subsequent to early Kansan time.

The diagnostic fourth alternating triangle of M2 in *M. pennsylvanicus* is much smaller than the other three, in most cases being a small nubbin (Fig. 7F). Although I have never observed an M2 of a meadow vole that lacked the fourth triangle, I have observed a fourth triangle in one specimen each of *M. mexicanus* and *M. longicaudus*. The only difference between the specimens is that in *M. pennsylvanicus* the fourth triangle appears to be closed off from the third, whereas in *M. mexicanus* and *M. longicaudus* a very thin strip of dentine connects the two triangles. *M. mexicanus* and especially *M. californicus* have M2s in which LRA2 is directed posteriorly so that the third triangle appears to be developing a bud and one can visualize how a fourth triangle might develop (Fig. 7D–E).

Guilday (1982) has shown that enough variation exists within the M3s of *Microtus* species common to Appalachian cave faunas that assignment to specific taxa on the basis of a few isolated teeth is unwarranted.

The number of alternating triangles on the m1 in *M. pennsylvanicus* varies from five to seven. Semken (1966) demonstrated an increase in the number of alternating triangles through time for fossil sites in Kansas. Subsequent work by Davis (1975) and McMullen (1978) confirmed this chronocline. Davis (1975) showed that in extant populations, meadow voles with the largest teeth and greatest number of triangles occur on the grasslands of the High Plains where the grass is coarser.

Davis (1975) attempted to relate the present distribution of *M. pennsylvanicus* to the distribution and relative abundance of C-3 and C-4 grasses. Although his results were ambiguous, additional study seems warranted.

Microtus *sp.*—Specimens of *Microtus* not assigned to species are known from Alberta, Medicine Hat M (14) and K (15); Arizona, Choate Ranch (48), Murray Springs (49), Murray Springs Arroyo (50), Papago Springs (51), Vulture Cave^{+} (53); California, Hawver Cave (30); Colorado, Dutton (66), Selby (67); Idaho, Wasden (22); Iowa, Little Sioux$^{+/\circ}$ (161); Kansas, Tobin$^{+/\circ}$ (140); Nebraska, Unnamed^{+} (155); Nevada, Tule Springs $B_2$$^{+}$ (46); New Mexico, Dark Canyon Cave^{+} (76), Palomas Creek Cave^{+} (81), Baldy Peak Cave^{+} (83); Saskatchewan, Ridell^{+} (12); Texas, Tank Trap Wash #1^{+} (87), Huecos Tanks #1^{+} (88), Dust Cave^{+} (90); and Utah, Crystal Ball Cave (54). These sites range in age from Irvingtonian (Kansan) to Holocene. Most of these specimens probably belong to some extant taxon living in or near the area of the site as all but the Little Sioux and Tobin records are Wisconsin and Holocene in age. Some of these specimens are unassignable because of the fragmentary nature of the material. A few of these records were taken from faunal lists where no description or size of sample was noted.

The oldest records are from the Little Sioux and Tobin. The former was reported by Gerald R. Paulson in an unpublished faunal list for the site. Unfortunately, I could not find the specimens in the collections at the University of Michigan. The latter record is represented by an isolated m1 with five closed alternating triangles and a simple anterior cap (Zakrzewski and Kolb, 1982). It could represent the earliest record of an extant taxon as it is very similar to the teeth assigned to *M. pennsylvanicus* from the Kanopolis (143) site (Hibbard et al. 1978). But as discussed above, isolated teeth of *Microtus,* especially m1s, are generally unassignable to a species.

Unless they prove to be of *M. mexicanus,* the records from Texas and New Mexico would substantiate a more extensive range for one or more other species. Other significant extensions at the species level are represented by the non-*pennsylvanicus Microtus* reported by SkwaraWoolf (1980) from the Ridell and the one from the Unnamed site in Nebraska.

Another record of interest is that from Tule Springs B_2 (46). Mawby (1967) stated that the m1 from this site differed in detail with those m1s he examined from site E_1 and those in the mammal collection at the University of California, Berkeley. To learn whether the specimen represents a new taxon or an aberrant individual of some extant taxon requires additional study.

Concluding Remarks

To gain a better understanding of the interrelationships and early history of *Microtus* the following suggestions are offered.

1) Additional sites in all areas need to be found, but especially in those areas for which there are no records.
2) Because of the amount of variation within the taxa, studies on large samples of extant and extinct (when possible) taxa by appropriate multivariate techniques are necessary.
3) When undertaking a systematic study of an extant species, mammalogists should include data that might prove useful regarding isolated teeth as well as other aspects of the anatomy.
4) When dealing with fossils, specimens should not be assigned to an extant taxon solely on the basis of present distribution.

Acknowledgments

I thank the following individuals for allowing me to examine specimens under their care: Jerry R. Choate, Museum of the High Plains, Fort Hays State University; Philip D. Gingerich, Museum of Paleontology, University of Michigan; Robert S. Hoffmann, Museum of Natural History, University of Kansas; Philip Meyers, Museum of Zoology, University of Michigan; and Holmes A. Semken, Department of Geology, University of Iowa (145).

I thank the following individuals for sharing their knowledge of unpublished records (sites in parentheses; see 145 above) or checking the accuracy of the records after compilation: Elaine Anderson (14–15, 38–39, 44, 69, 112, 169), Denver, Colorado; Brenda F. Beebe (11); James A. Burns (17–18), and Rufus S. Churcher, all of the University of Toronto; Walter W. Dalquest, Midwestern University; Ralph E. Eshelman (134, 150–151), Calvert Cliffs Museum, Solomons, Maryland; Shirley Fonda (225), State College, Pennsylvania; Russell W. Graham, Illinois State Museum; the late John E. Guilday (201, 203, 214–216, 235), Carnegie Museum of Natural History; Arthur H. Harris (71, 75–76, 81, 83, 86, 90, 92), University of Texas at El Paso; James Honey (133), Lakewood, Colorado; Ernest L. Lundelius (94, 98, 105–106, 108, 114), University of Texas; Wade Miller (54), Brigham Young University;

Gerald R. Paulson (161), Ann Arbor, Michigan; Charles A. Repenning (23, 52, 55), U.S. Geological Survey, Menlo Park, California; H. A. Semken (164); J. D. Stewart (138, 236), University of Kansas; Danny D. Walker, University of Wyoming; and S. David Webb (174–197), University of Florida. In addition I have listed four unpublished records (135, 136, 144, 155) based on specimens in the Sternberg Memorial Museum. I thank Sydney Anderson, American Museum of Natural History, the late J. E. Guilday, and C. A. Repenning for their constructive comments on an earlier draft of the manuscript. Gwenne Cash drafted the figures and typed the manuscript.

*Selected Bibliography**

ANDERSON, E. 1974. A survey of the late Pleistocene and Holocene mammal fauna of Wyoming. Pp. 78–87, *in* Applied geology and archaeology: the Holocene history of Wyoming (M. Wilson, ed.). Wyoming Geol. Surv. Rept. Invest., 10:79–87. (21, 63)

BOELLSTORFF, J. 1976. The succession of late Cenozoic volcanic ashes in the Great Plains: a progress report. Kansas Geol. Surv. Guidebook, 1:37–71.

———. 1978. North American Pleistocene stages reconsidered in light of probable Pliocene-Pleistocene continental glaciation. Science, 202:305–307.

BURNS, J. A. 1982. Water vole, *Microtus richardsoni* (Mammalia, Rodentia), from the late Pleistocene of Alberta. Canadian J. Earth Sci., 19:628–631. (18)

CHURCHER, C. S., AND A. MAC S. STALKER. In press. Geology and paleontology of the Wellsch Valley site, Saskatchewan. Geol. Surv. Canada. (13)

COPE, E. D. 1871. Preliminary report on the vertebrata discovered in the Port Kennedy bone cave. Proc. Amer. Phil. Soc., 12:73–102. (228)

———. 1899. Vertebrate remains from the Port Kennedy bone deposit. Acad. Nat. Sci. Philadelphia, 11:193–267. (228)

DALQUEST, W. W. 1961. A record of the giant bison (*Bison latifrons*) from Cooke County, Texas. Texas J. Sci., 13:41–44. (231)

———. 1962. The Good Creek formation, Pleistocene of Texas and its fauna. J. Paleontol., 36:568–582. (116–118)

———. 1964. A new Pleistocene local fauna from Motley County, Texas. Trans. Kansas Acad. Sci., 67:499–505. (120)

———. 1965. New Pleistocene formation and local fauna from Hardeman County, Texas. J. Paleontol., 39:63–79. (119)

DALQUEST, W. W., E. ROTH, AND F. JUDD. 1969. The mammal fauna of Schulze Cave, Edwards County, Texas. Bull. Florida State Mus., 13:205–276. (100)

DAVIS, L. C. 1975. Late Pleistocene geology and paleoecology of the Spring Valley Basin, Meade County, Kansas. Unpubl. Ph.D. dissert., Univ. Iowa, Iowa City, 170 pp. (126)

* Numbers in parentheses following citations refer to fossil faunas identified in text and appendices.

DAVIS, L. C., R. E. ESHELMAN, AND J. C. PRIOR. 1973. A primary mammoth site with associated fauna in Pottawattamie County, Iowa. Proc. Iowa Acad. Sci., 79:62–65. (163)

DICE, L. R. 1925. Rodents and lagomorphs of the Rancho La Brea deposits. Carnegie Inst. Washington Publ., 349:119–130. (35)

EINSOHN, S. 1971. The stratigraphy and fauna of a Pleistocene outcrop in Doniphan County, northeastern Kansas. Unpubl. M.S. thesis, Univ. Kansas, Lawrence, 83 pp. (147–148, 154)

ELFTMAN, H. O. 1931. Pleistocene mammals of Fossil Lake, Oregon. Amer. Mus. Novitates, 481:1–21. (26)

FOLEY, R. L. 1984. Late Pleistocene Woodfordian vertebrates from the Driftless Area southwestern Wisconsin, the Moscow local fauna. Illinois State Mus. Rept. Invest., 39:1–50. (241)

FURLONG, E. L. 1906. The exploration of Samwel Cave. Amer. J. Sci., Ser. 4, 22: 235–247. (28)

GIDLEY, J. G., AND C. E. GAZIN. 1938. The Pleistocene vertebrate fauna from Cumberland Cave, Maryland. Bull. U.S. Natl. Mus., 171:1–99.

GRAHAM, R. W. 1976. Late Wisconsin mammalian faunas and environmental gradients of the eastern United States. Paleobiology, 2:343–350. (172, 205)

———. 1981. Preliminary reports on late Pleistocene vertebrates from the Selby and Dutton archeological/paleontological sites, Yuma County, Colorado. Univ. Wyoming Contrib. Geol., 20:33–56. (66–67)

GUILDAY, J. E. 1962*a*. Notes on Pleistocene vertebrates from Wythe County, Virginia. Ann. Carnegie Mus., 36:77–86. (217)

———. 1962*b*. The Pleistocene local fauna of Natural Chimneys, Augusta County, Virginia. Ann. Carnegie Mus., 36:87–122. (221)

———. 1969*a*. A possible caribou-Paleo-Indian association from Dutchess Quarry Cave, Orange County, New York. New York State Archeol. Assoc. Bull., 45:24–29. (229)

———. 1969*b*. Small mammal remains from the Wasden Site (Owl Cave), Bonneville County, Idaho. Tebiwa, 12:47–57. (22)

———. 1977. Sabertooth cat, *Smilodon floridanus* (Leidy), and associated fauna from a Tennessee cave (40 Dv 40), the First American Bank site. J. Tenn. Acad. Sci., 52:84–94. (204)

———. 1982. Dental variation in *Microtus xanthognathus, M. chrotorrhinus,* and *M. pennsylvanicus* (Rodentia: Mammalia). Ann. Carnegie Mus., 51:211–230. (220)

GUILDAY, J. E., AND E. K. ADAM. 1967. Small mammal remains from Jaguar Cave, Lemhi County, Idaho. Tebiwa, 10:26–36. (20)

GUILDAY, J. E., AND H. W. HAMILTON. 1973. The late Pleistocene small mammals of Eagle Cave, Pendleton County, West Virginia. Ann. Carnegie Mus., 44:45–58. (211)

———. 1978. Ecological significance of displaced boreal mammals in West Virginia caves. J. Mamm., 59:176–181. (212–213)

GUILDAY, J. E., H. W. HAMILTON, AND A. D. MCCRADY. 1966. The bone breccia of Bootlegger Sink, York County, Pa. Ann. Carnegie Mus., 38:145–163. (227)

———. 1969. The Pleistocene vertebrate fauna of Robinson Cave, Overton County, Tennessee. Paleovertebrata, 2:25–75. (202)

———. 1971. The Welsh Cave peccaries (*Platygonus*) and associated fauna, Kentucky Pleistocene. Ann. Carnegie Mus., 43:249–320. (205)

GUILDAY, J. E., H. W. HAMILTON, AND P. W. PARMALEE. 1975. Caribou (*Rangifer tarandus* L.) from the Pleistocene of Tennessee. J. Tenn. Acad. Sci., 59: 109–112. (237)

GUILDAY, J. E., P. S. MARTIN, AND A. D. MCCRADY. 1964. New Paris No. 4: a Pleistocene cave deposit in Bedford County, Pennsylvania. Natl. Speleol. Soc. Bull., 26:121–194. (224)
GUILDAY, J. E., P. W. PARMALEE, AND H. W. HAMILTON. 1977. The Clark's Cave bone deposit and the late Pleistocene paleoecology of the central Appalachian Mountains of Virginia. Bull. Carnegie Mus. Nat. Hist., 2:1–87. (162, 218, 219)
GUILDAY, J. E., H. W. HAMILTON, E. ANDERSON, AND P. W. PARMALEE. 1978. The Baker Bluff Cave deposit, Tennessee, and the late Pleistocene faunal gradient. Bull. Carnegie Mus. Nat. Hist., 11:1–67. (199–200)
GUTHRIE, R. D., AND J. V. MATTHEWS. 1971. The Cape Deceit fauna—early Pleistocene mammalian assemblage from the Alaskan Arctic. Quaternary Res., 1:474–519. (1)
HAGER, M. W. 1972. A late Wisconsin-Recent vertebrate fauna from the Chimney Rock Animal Trap, Larimer County, Colorado. Univ. Wyoming Contrib. Geol., 11:63–71. (65)
———. 1974. Late Pliocene and Pleistocene history of the Donnelly Ranch vertebrate site, southeastern Colorado. Univ. Wyoming Contrib. Geol. Spec. Paper, 2:1–62. (68)
HALL, S. A. 1982. Late Holocene paleoecology of the southern plains. Quaternary Res., 17:391–407. (232–234)
HALLBERG, G. R., H. A. SEMKEN, AND L. C. DAVIS. 1974. Quaternary records of *Microtus xanthognathus* (Leach), the yellow-cheeked vole, from northwestern Arkansas and southwestern Iowa. J. Mamm., 55:640–645. (5, 164)
HARINGTON, C. R. 1978. Quaternary vertebrate faunas of Canada and Alaska and their suggested chronological sequence. Syllogeus, 15:1–105. (6)
HARRIS, A. H. 1970. The Dry Cave mammalian fauna and late Pluvial conditions in southeastern New Mexico. Texas J. Sci., 22:3–28. (73)
HAWKSLEY, O., J. F. REYNOLDS, AND R. L. FOLEY. 1973. Pleistocene vertebrate fauna of Bat Cave, Pulaski County, Missouri. Bull. Natl. Speleol. Soc., 35:61–67. (170)
HAY, O. P. 1920. Descriptions of some Pleistocene vertebrates found in the United States. Proc. U.S. Natl. Mus., 58:83–146. (223)
HIBBARD, C. W. 1937. A new *Pitymys* from the Pleistocene of Kansas. J. Mamm., 18:235. (149)
———. 1943. The Rezabek fauna, a new Pleistocene fauna from Lincoln County, Kansas. Univ. Kansas Sci. Bull., 29:235–245. (141)
———. 1944. Stratigraphy and vertebrate paleontology of Pleistocene deposits of southwestern Kansas. Bull. Geol. Soc. Amer., 55:707–754. (132)
———. 1952. Vertebrate fossils from late Cenozoic deposits of central Kansas. Univ. Kansas Paleontol. Contrib., Vertebrata, 2:1–14.
———. 1955*a*. Notes on the microtine rodents from the Port Kennedy Cave deposit. Proc. Acad. Nat. Sci. Philadelphia, 107:87–97.
———. 1955*b*. The Jinglebob interglacial (Sangamon?) fauna from Kansas and its climatic significance. Univ. Michigan Mus. Paleontol. Contrib., 12: 179–228. (127)
———. 1956. *Microtus pennsylvanicus* (Ord) from the Hay Springs local fauna of Nebraska. J. Paleontol., 30:1263–1266. (159)
———. 1963. A late Illinoian fauna from Kansas and its climatic significance. Papers Michigan Acad. Sci., Arts Letters, 48:187–221. (129)
HIBBARD, C. W., AND W. W. DALQUEST. 1966. Fossils from the Seymour formation of Knox and Baylor counties, Texas, and their bearing on the late Kansan climate of that region. Univ. Michigan Mus. Paleontol. Contrib., 21:1–66. (115)

HIBBARD, C. W., AND D. W. TAYLOR. 1960. Two late Pleistocene faunas from southwestern Kansas. Univ. Michigan Mus. Paleontol. Contrib., 16:1–223. (122, 128, 130)

HIBBARD, C. W., J. C. FRYE, AND A. B. LEONARD. 1944. Reconnaissance of Pleistocene deposits in north-central Kansas. Kansas Geol. Surv. Bull., 52: 1–28. (152)

HIBBARD, C. W., ET AL. 1978. Mammals from the Kanopolis local fauna, Pleistocene (Yarmouth) of Ellsworth County, Kansas. Univ. Michigan Mus. Paleontol. Contrib., 25:11–44. (104, 143, 147, 148, 154)

HINTON, C. A. 1926. Monograph of voles and lemmings (Microtinae) living and extinct. British Mus. Nat. Hist., London, 488 pp.

HOLMAN, J. A. 1959. Birds and mammals from the Pleistocene of Williston, Florida. Bull. Florida State Mus., 5:1–25. (189)

———. 1979. New fossil vertebrate remains from Michigan. Michigan Academ., 11:391–397. (209)

HOOD, C. H., AND O. HAWKSLEY. 1975. A Pleistocene fauna from Zoo Cave Taney County, Missouri. J. Missouri Speleol. Surv., 15:1–42. (171)

HOPKINS, M. L., R. BONNICHSEN, AND D. FORTSCH. 1969. The stratigraphic position and faunal associates of *Bison* (*Gigantobison*) *latifrons* in southeastern Idaho, a progress report. Tebiwa, 12:1–8. (24)

IRVING, W. N., AND C. R. HARINGTON. 1973. Upper Pleistocene radiocarbon-dated artefacts from the northern Yukon. Science, 179:335–340. (7)

JAKWAY, G. E. 1958. Pleistocene Lagomorpha and Rodentia from the San Josecito Cave, Nuevo Leon, Mexico. Trans. Kansas Acad. Sci., 61:313–327. (85)

JOPLING, A. V., W. N. IRVING, AND B. F. BEEBE. 1981. Stratigraphic, sedimentological and faunal evidence for the occurrence of pre-Sangamonian artefacts in northern Yukon. Arctic, 34:3–33. (8–10)

KURTÉN, B., AND E. ANDERSON. 1980. Pleistocene mammals of North America. Columbia Univ. Press, New York, 440 pp. (3–4, 47, 210, 214)

LASALLE, P., AND J. E. GUILDAY. 1980. Caverne de Saint-Elzéar-de-Bonaventure. Rapport preliminaire sur les fouilles de 1977 et 1978. Ministere Ener. Res., Québec, 31 pp. (230)

LINDSAY, E. H., AND N. T. TESSMAN. 1974. Cenozoic vertebrate localities and faunas in Arizona. J. Arizona Acad. Sci., 9(1):3–24. (48–51)

LOGAN, L. E., AND C. C. BLACK. 1979. The Quaternary vertebrate fauna of Upper Sloth Cave, Guadalupe Mountains National Park, Texas. Natl. Park Ser. Proc. Trans., 4:141–158. (91)

LUNDELIUS, E. L. 1967. Late-Pleistocene and Holocene faunal history of central Texas. Pp. 287–319, *in* Pleistocene extinctions, the search for a cause (P. S. Martin and H. E. Wright, eds.). Yale Univ. Press, New Haven, Connecticut, 453 pp. (95–96, 98, 101–103, 107–108)

———. 1979. Post-Pleistocene mammals from Pratt Cave and their environmental significance. Natl. Park Serv. Proc. Trans., 4:239–258. (93)

MARTIN, L. D. 1972. The microtine rodents of the Mullen assemblage from the Pleistocene of north central Nebraska. Bull. Univ. Nebraska State Mus., 9:173–182. (157–158)

MARTIN, R. A. 1974. Fossil mammals from the Coleman IIA fauna, Sumter County. Pp. 35–99, *in* Pleistocene mammals of Florida (S. D. Webb, ed.). Univ. Florida Press, Gainesville, 270 pp. (178)

———. 1975. *Allophaiomys* Kormos from the Pleistocene of North America. C. W. Hibbard Mem. Vol. 3. Univ. Michigan Papers Paleontol., 12:97–100. (160)

MARTIN, R. A., AND S. D. WEBB. 1974. Late Pleistocene mammals from the Devil's Den fauna, Levy County. Pp. 114–145, *in* Pleistocene mammals of Florida (S. D. Webb, ed.). Univ. Florida Press, Gainesville, 270 pp. (186)

MAWBY, J. E. 1967. Fossil vertebrates of the Tule Springs Site, Nevada. Nevada State Mus. Anthropol. Papers, 13:107–128. (45–46)

MCDONALD, H. G., AND E. ANDERSON. 1975. A late Pleistocene vertebrate fauna from southeastern Idaho. Tebiwa, 18:19–37. (25)

MCMULLEN, T. L. 1978. Mammals of the Duck Creek local fauna, late Pleistocene of Kansas. J. Mamm., 59:374–386. (139)

MEADE, J. I., AND A. M. PHILLIPS, III. 1981. The late Pleistocene and Holocene fauna and flora of Vulture Cave, Grand Canyon, Arizona. Southwestern Nat., 26:257–288. (53)

MILLER, W. E. 1971. Pleistocene vertebrates of the Los Angeles Basin and vicinity (exclusive of Rancho La Brea). Bull. Los Angeles Co. Mus. Nat. Hist. Sci., 10:1–124. (36–37, 40–41)

———. 1976. Late Pleistocene vertebrates of the Silver Creek local fauna from north central Utah. Great Basin Nat., 36:387–424. (56)

OLSON, E. C. 1940. A late Pleistocene fauna from Herculaneum, Missouri. J. Geol., 48:32–57. (168)

PARMALEE, P. W. 1967. A Recent cave bone deposit in southwestern Illinois. Natl. Speleol. Soc. Bull., 29:119–147. (206)

PARMALEE, P. W., AND W. E. KLIPPEL. 1981. A late Pleistocene population of the pocket gopher, *Geomys* cf. *bursarius,* in the Nashville Basin, Tennessee. J. Mamm., 62:831–835. (203)

PARMALEE, P. W., AND R. D. OESCH. 1972. Pleistocene and Recent faunas from the Brynjulfson Caves, Missouri. Illinois State Mus. Rept. Invest., 25:1–52. (165–166)

PARMALEE, P. W., P. J. MUNSON, AND J. E. GUILDAY. 1978. The Pleistocene mammalian fauna of Harrodsburg Crevice, Monroe County, Indiana. Natl. Speleol. Soc. Bull., 40:64–75. (207)

PARMALEE, P. W., R. D. OESCH, AND J. E. GUILDAY. 1969. Pleistocene and Recent vertebrate faunas from Crankshaft Cave, Missouri. Illinois State Mus. Rept. Invest., 14:1–37. (167)

PATTON, T. H. 1963. Fossil vertebrates from Miller's Cave Llano County, Texas. Texas Mem. Mus. Bull., 7:1–41. (106)

PAULSON, G. R. 1961. The mammals of the Cudahy fauna. Papers Michigan Acad. Sci., Arts Letters, 46:127–153. (132, 156)

PETERSON, O. A. 1926. The fossils of Frankstown Cave, Blair County, Pennsylvania. Ann. Carnegie Mus., 16:249–314. (226)

RASMUSSEN, D. L. 1974. New Quaternary mammal localities in the upper Clark Fork River Valley, western Montana. Northwest Geol., 3:62–70. (19)

RAY, C. E. 1967. Pleistocene mammals from Ladds, Bartow County, Georgia. Bull. Georgia Acad. Sci., 25:120–150. (198)

REPENNING, C. A. 1983. *Pitymys meadensis* Hibbard from the Valley of Mexico and the classification of North American species of *Pitymys* (Rodentia: Cricetidae). J. Vert. Paleontol., 2:471–482. (27, 32, 43, 70, 84)

REPENNING, C. A., D. M. HOPKINS, AND M. RUBIN. 1964. Tundra rodents in a late Pleistocene fauna from the Tofty Placer District, central Alaska. Arctic, 17:177–197. (2)

RHODES, R. S., II. 1984. Paleoecology and regional paleoclimatic implications of the Farmdalian Craigmile and Woodfordian Waubonsie mammalian local faunas southwestern Iowa. Illinois State Mus. Rept. Invest., 49:1–51. (164, 240)

ROSENBERG, R. S. 1983. The paleoecology of the late Wisconsinan Eagle Point local fauna, Clinton County, Iowa. Unpubl. M.S. thesis, Univ. Iowa, Iowa City, 70 pp. (239)

ROTH, E. L. 1972. Late Pleistocene mammals from Klein Cave, Kerr County, Texas. Texas J. Sci., 74:75–84. (99)

SAUNDERS, J. J. 1977. Late Pleistocene vertebrates of the western Ozark Highland, Missouri. Illinois State Mus. Rept. Invest., 33:1–118. (169)

SAVAGE, D. E. 1951. Late Cenozoic vertebrates of the San Francisco Bay region. Univ. California Publ. Bull. Dept. Geol. Sci., 28:215–314. (31)

SCHULTZ, C. B., AND E. B. HOWARD. 1935. The fauna of Burnet Cave, Guadalupe Mountains, New Mexico. Proc. Acad. Nat. Sci. Philadelphia, 87:273–298. (74)

SCHULTZ, C. B., AND L. D. MARTIN. 1970. Quaternary mammalian sequence in the central Great Plains. Pp. 341–353, *in* Pleistocene and Recent environments of the central Great Plains (W. Dort and J. K. Jones, Jr., eds.). Univ. Kansas Dept. Geol. Spec. Publ., Univ. Kansas Press, Lawrence, 3:1–433. (153)

SCHULTZ, G. E. 1969. Geology and paleontology of a late Pleistocene basin in southwest Kansas. U.S. Geol. Surv. Spec. Paper, 105:1–85. (125, 128, 130, 131)

SCHULTZ, J. R. 1938. A late Quaternary mammal fauna from the tar seeps of McKittrick, California. Carnegie Inst. Washington Publ. 487:111–215. (34)

SEMKEN, H. A. 1961. Fossil vertebrates from Longhorn Cavern Burnet County, Texas. Texas J. Sci., 13:290–310. (105)

———. 1966. Stratigraphy and paleontology of the McPherson *Equus* beds (Sandahl local fauna), McPherson County, Kansas. Univ. Michigan Mus. Paleontol. Contrib., 20:121–178. (146–147)

———. 1967. Mammalian remains from Rattlesnake Cave, Kinney County, Texas. Texas Mem. Mus., Pearce-Sellards Ser., 7:1–11. (94)

———. In press. Late Pleistocene/Holocene environmental changes on the northern plains of the United States: mammalian record. *In* Late Pleistocene/Holocene environmental changes in the High Plains: the vertebrate record (R. W. Graham and H. A. Semken, eds.). Illinois State Mus. Rept. Invest.

SINCLAIR, W. J. 1904. The exploration of Potter Creek Cave. Univ. California Publ. Dept. Amer. Archeol. Ethnol., 2:1–27. (29)

SKINNER, M. F. 1942. The fauna of Papago Springs Cave, Arizona, and a study of *Stockoceros*; with three new antilocaprines from Nebraska and Arizona. Bull. Amer. Mus. Nat. Hist., 80:143–220. (51)

SKWARAWOOLF, T. 1980. Mammals of the Riddell local fauna (Floral formation, Pleistocene, late Rancholabrean) Saskatoon, Canada. Saskatchewan Mus. Nat. Hist. Contrib., 2:1–129. (12)

SLAUGHTER, B. H. 1964. Geological survey and appraisal of the paleontological resources of the Cooper Reservoir Basin, Delta and Hopkins counties, Texas. Fondren Sci. Ser., 6:1–11. (109)

———. 1966*a*. The Moore Pit local fauna, Pleistocene of Texas. J. Paleontol., 40:78–91. (111)

———. 1966*b*. The vertebrates of the Domebo local fauna Pleistocene of Oklahoma. Contrib. Mus. Great Plains, 1:31–55. (121)

———. 1975. Ecological interpretation of the Brown Sand Wedge local fauna. Pp. 179–192, *in* Late Pleistocene environments of the southern High Plains (F. Wendorf and J. J. Hester, eds.). Fort Burgwin Res. Center Publ., 9:1–290. (72)

SLAUGHTER, B. H., AND B. R. HOOVER. 1963. Sulphur River formation and the

Pleistocene mammals of the Ben Franklin local fauna. Southern Methodist Univ. J. Grad. Res. Center, 31:132–148. (110)

SLAUGHTER, B. H., AND W. L. MCCLURE. 1965. The Sims Bayou local fauna: Pleistocene of Houston, Texas. Texas J. Sci., 17:404–417. (97)

SLAUGHTER, B. H., AND R. RITCHIE. 1963. Pleistocene mammals of the Clear Creek local fauna, Denton County, Texas. Southern Methodist Univ. J. Grad. Res. Center, 31:117–131. (113)

SMARTT, R. A. 1977. The ecology of late Pleistocene and Recent *Microtus* from south-central and southwestern New Mexico. Southwestern Nat., 22:1–19. (77–80, 82)

STARRETT, A. 1956. Pleistocene mammals of the Berends fauna of Oklahoma. J. Paleontol., 30:1187–1192. (124)

STEPHANS, J. J. 1960. Stratigraphy and paleontology of a late Pleistocene Basin, Harper County, Oklahoma. Bull. Geol. Soc. Amer., 71:1675–1702. (123)

STEWART, J. D. 1978. Mammals of the Trapshoot local fauna, late Pleistocene of Rooks County, Kansas. (Abs.) Proc. Nebraska Acad. Sci., 88th Ann. Meet., pp. 45–46. (126, 138)

STOCK, C. 1918. The Pleistocene fauna of Haver Cave. Univ. California Publ., Bull. Dept. Geol. Sci., 10:461–515. (30)

STORER, J. E. 1976. Mammals of the Hand Hills formation, southern Alberta. Pp. 186–209, *in* Athlon: essays on paleontology in honour of Loris Shano Russell (C. S. Churcher, ed.). Royal Ontario Mus., Life Sci., Misc. Publ., 286 pp. (16)

VAN DEVENDER, T. R., AND D. H. RISKIND. 1979. Late Pleistocene and early Holocene plant remains from Huecos Tanks State Historical Park: the development of a refugium. Southwestern Nat., 24:127–140. (87–89)

VAN DER MEULEN, A. J. 1973. Middle Pleistocene smaller mammals from the Monte Peglia, (Orvieto, Italy) with special reference to the phylogeny of *Microtus* (Arvicolidae, Rodentia). Quaternaria, 17:1–144.

———. 1974. On *Microtus* (*Allophaiomys*) *deucalion* (Kretzoi, 1969), (Arvicolidae, Rodentia), from the upper Villanyian (lower Pleistocene) of Villany-5, S. Hungary. Proc. Koninkl. Nederl. Akad. Wetensch., Series B, 77:259–266.

———. 1978. *Microtus* and *Pitymys* (Arvicolidae) from Cumberland Cave, Maryland, with a comparison of some New and Old World species. Ann. Carnegie Mus., 47:101–145. (147, 148, 173, 222, 228)

WALKER, D.N. 1982. Early Holocene vertebrate fauna. Pp. 274–394, *in* The Agate Basin site: a record of the Paleoindian occupation of the northwestern High Plains (G. C. Frison and D. J. Stanford, eds.). Academic Press, New York, 403 pp.

———. In press. Late Pleistocene/Holocene environmental changes in the northwestern plains of the United States: the vertebrate record. *In* Late Pleistocene/Holocene environmental changes in the High Plains: the vertebrate record (R. W. Graham and H. A. Semken, eds.). Illinois State Mus. (57–60)

WEBB, S. D. 1974. Chronology of Florida Pleistocene mammals. Pp. 5–31, *in* Pleistocene mammals of Florida (S. D. Webb, ed.). Univ. Florida Press, Gainesville, 270 pp. (174–180, 184, 186–189, 191–193, 196–197)

WILSON, R. L. 1967. The Pleistocene vertebrates of Michigan. Papers Michigan Acad. Sci., Arts Letters, 52:197–234. (208)

WILSON, R. W. 1933. Pleistocene mammalian fauna from the Carpinteria asphalt. Carnegie Inst. Washington Publ., 440:59–76. (33)

WOODMAN, N. 1982. A subarctic fauna from the late Wisconsinan Elkader site, Clayton County, Iowa. Unpubl. M.S. thesis, Univ. Iowa, Iowa City, 56 pp. (238)

ZAKRZEWSKI, R. J. 1972. Fossil microtines from late Cenozoic deposits in the Anza-Borrego Desert, California, with the description of a new subgenus of *Synaptomys*. Los Angeles Co. Mus. Nat. Hist. Contrib. Sci., 221:1-12. (42)

———. 1975. The late Pleistocene arvicoline rodent *Atopomys*. Ann. Carnegie Mus., 45:255-261. (104)

———. 1981. Kangaroo rats from the Borchers local fauna, Blancan, Meade County, Kansas. Trans. Kansas Acad. Sci., 84:78-88.

ZAKRZEWSKI, R. J., AND K. K. KOLB. 1982. Late Kansan faunas from central Kansas. Trans. Kansas Acad. Sci., 85:200-215. (137, 140, 142)

ZEIMANS, G., AND D. N. WALKER. 1974. Bell Cave, Wyoming: preliminary archeological and paleontological investigations. Pp. 88-90, *in* Applied geology and archeology: the Holocene history of Wyoming (M. Wilson, ed.). Wyoming Geol. Surv. Rept. Invest., 10:1-127. (64)

Appendix A. Fossil Faunas Containing Pitymys *and* Microtus*

Alaska

Sullivan Pit (2), Tofty Placer District, H/W
M. miurus, M. xanthognathus?+

Fairbanks II (3), Yukon-Tanana Upland, W, 11,735 ± 130 to 40,000 B.P.
M. miurus+, *M. xanthognathus*

Chicken (5), Yukon-Tanana Upland, W
M. xanthognathus

Fairbanks I (4), Yukon-Tanana Upland, I
M. miurus

Cape Deceit (1), Derring Region, K/A
M. deceitensis°

Alberta

Eagle Cave (18), High Rock Range, W, 22,700 ± 1,000 B.P.
M. richardsoni, M. longicaudus or *montanus*+

January Cave (17), Front Range, W, 23,100 ± 860 B.P.
M. longicaudus or *montanus*+

Medicine Hat M (14), Medicine Hat District, W, 25,000 ± 800 to 38,000+ B.P.
M. sp.

Medicine Hat K (15), Medicine Hat District, S
M. sp.

Hand Hills (16), Hand Hills, W/I
M. pennsylvanicus

* Dates ending in B.P. are radio-carbon dates; dates ending in m.y.b.p. are fission-track dates; dates with no postscript are based on paleomagnetic inferences. Abbreviations and symbols: nd, *nomen dubium*; °, taxon extinct; +, taxon extinct locally; #, records from Webb (pers. comm.) and supercede those in Webb (1974).

Arizona

Vulture Cave (53), Coconino Co., W, ≤13,170± B.P.
M. sp.⁺
Papago Springs (51), Santa Cruz Co., W
M. sp.
Choate Ranch (48), Cochise Co., W
M. sp.
Murray Springs (49), Cochise Co., W
M. sp.
Murray Springs Arroyo (50), Cochise Co., W
M. sp.
Salina (52), Navajo Co., W
M. montanus

Arkansas

Peccary Cave (172), Newton Co., W, 16,700 ± 250 B.P.
P. pinetorum, P. ochrogaster⁺, *M. pennsylvanicus*⁺, *M. xanthognathus*⁺
Conard Fissure (173), Newton Co., K
P. llanensis°, *P. cumberlandensis*°, *M. paroperarius*°

California

La Mirada (37), Los Angeles Co., W, 10,690 ± 360 B.P.
M. californicus
Rancho La Brea (35), Los Angeles Co., W, 12,650 ± 160 to 40,000+ B.P.
M. californicus
McKittrick (34), Kern Co., W, 38,000 ± 2,500 B.P.
M. californicus
Samwel Cave (28), Shasta Co., W
M. californicus
Potter Creek Cave (29), Shasta Co., W
M. californicus
Hawver Cave (30), Eldorado Co., W
M. sp.
Carpinteria (33), Santa Barbara Co., W
M. californicus
San Pedro (36), Los Angeles Co., W
M. californicus
Emery Borrow Pit (38), Los Angeles Co., W
M. californicus
Zuma Creek (39), Los Angeles Co., W
M. californicus
Costeau Pit (40), Orange Co., W
M. californicus
Newport Bay Mesa 1067 (41), Orange Co., W
M. californicus
Kokoweef (44), San Bernadino Co., W
M. californicus
North Livermore Ave. (32), Alameda Co., Y, 500,000
P. meadensis°

Irvington (31), Alameda Co., Y/K
M. cf. *M. californicus*
Vallecito Creek (42), San Diego Co., Y/K
M. cf. *M. californicus*
Centerville Beach (27), Humboldt Co., K/A, >730,000 to <900,000
P. mcnowni?°
Olive Dell Ranch (43), San Bernardino Co.
P. meadensis°

Colorado

Chimney Rock Animal Trap (65), Larimer Co., W, 11,908 ± 180 B.P.
M. longicaudus or *M. montanus*
Dutton (66), Yuma Co., W
P. ochrogaster, M. pennsylvanicus, M. sp.
Selby (67), Yuma Co., W
M. sp.
Unnamed (69), Alamosa Co., W
M. longicaudus
Mesa De Maya (68), Las Animas Co., S
P. ochrogaster
Hansen Bluff (70), Alamosa Co., K, ≥0.7 m.y.b.p.
P. meadensis°, *M. paroperarius*°

Florida#

Warm Mineral Springs (174), Sarasota Co., W
P. pinetorum
Devil's Den III (186), Levy Co., W
P. pinetorum, M. pennsylvanicus
Waccasassa IIB (187), Levy Co., W
P. pinetorum, M. pennsylvanicus
Ichetucknee River (197), Columbia Co., W
P. pinetorum
Vero 2 (176) and 3 (177), Indian River Co., W
P. pinetorum
Kendrick IA (179), Marion Co., W
P. pinetorum
Arrendondo I (190), Alachua Co., W
P. pinetorum, M. pennsylvanicus
Arrendondo IB (191), Alachua Co., W
M. pennsylvanicus
Arrendondo II (192), IIA (193), B (194), and C (195), Alachua Co., W
P. pinetorum
Haile XIB (196), Alachua Co., S
P. pinetorum
Reddick IA (180), B (181), C (182), D (183), and IIC (184), Marion Co., S
P. pinetorum
Mefford I (185), Marion Co., S
P. pinetorum
Withlacooche VIIA (188), Levy Co., S
M. pennsylvanicus

Bradenton (175), Manatee Co., S
P. hibbardi°
Williston (189), Levy Co., S
P. hibbardi°
Coleman IIA (178), Sumter Co., I
P. aratai°

Georgia

Ladds (198), Bartow Co., W
P. pinetorum

Idaho

Jaguar Cave (20), Lemhi Co., H/W, 10,370 ± 350 to 11,580 ± 250 B.P.
M. montanus
Rainbow Beach (25), Power Co., W, 21,500 ± 700 to 31,300 ± 2,300 B.P.
M. montanus
Wasden (22), Bonneville Co., W
M. sp.
Moonshiner Cave (21), Bingham Co., W
M. longicaudus, M. montanus
American Falls (24), Power Co., S
M. montanus, M. longicaudus or *M. pennsylvanicus*
Downey Dump (23), Bannock Co., K
M. montanus

Illinois

Meyer Cave (206), Monroe Co., H
P. pinetorum, M. pennsylvanicus^{+}, *M. xanthognathus*$^{+}$

Indiana

Harrodsburg Crevice (207), Monroe Co., S
P. ochrogaster

Iowa

Brayton (162), Audubon Co., W, 12,420 ± 180 B.P.
P. pinetorum, M. pennsylvanicus
Oakland (163), Pottawattamie Co., W
M. pennsylvanicus
Waubonsie (164), Mills Co., W, 14,430 ± 1,030 to 14,830 ± 1,120 B.P.
P. pinetorum, P. ochrogaster, M. pennsylvanicus, M. xanthognathus^{+}
Elkader (238), Clayton Co., W, 20,530 ± 130 B.P.
M. pennsylvanicus, M. xanthognathus^{+}, *M.* cf. *M. miurus*$^{+}$
Eagle Point (239), Clinton Co., W
M. pennsylvanicus, M. xanthognathus^{+}
Craigmile (240), Mills Co., W, 23,200 ± 535 B.P.
P. pinetorum, P. ochrogaster, M. pennsylvanicus

Little Sioux (161), Harrison Co., K, 0.74 m.y.b.p.
M. paroperarius$^{\circ}$, *M.* sp.$^{+/\circ}$

Kansas

Robert (125), Meade Co., W, 11,100 ± 390 B.P.
P. ochrogaster, M. pennsylvanicus^{+}
Jones (126), Meade Co., W, 26,700 ± 1,500 to 29,000 ± 1,300 B.P.
P. ochrogaster, M. pennsylvanicus^{+}, *M.* cf. *M. montanus*$^{+}$
Hill City (236), Graham Co., W
M. sp.
Keiger Creek (135), Clark Co., W
M. pennsylvanicus^{+}
Trapshoot (138), Rooks Co., W
P. ochrogaster, M. pennsylvanicus^{+}, *M. montanus*$^{+}$
Jinglebob (127), Meade Co., W
P. ochrogaster, M. pennsylvanicus^{+}
Unnamed (152), Smith Co., W/S
M. pennsylvanicus
Cragin Quarry (128), Meade Co., S
P. ochrogaster, M. pennsylvanicus^{+}
Mt. Scott (129), Meade Co., I
P. ochrogaster, M. pennsylvanicus^{+}
Butler Spring (130), Meade Co., I
P. ochrogaster, M. pennsylvanicus^{+}
Adams (131), Meade Co., I
M. pennsylvanicus^{+}
Unnamed (136), Trego Co., I
M. pennsylvanicus^{+}
Duck Creek (139), Ellis Co., I
P. ochrogaster, M. pennsylvanicus^{+}
Williams (145), Rice Co., I
P. ochrogaster, M. pennsylvanicus^{+}
Sandahl (146), McPherson Co., I
P. ochrogaster, M. pennsylvanicus^{+}
Unnamed (149), Brown Co., ?
P. mcnowni$^{\circ}$
Rezabek (141), Lincoln Co., I
P. ochrogaster, M. pennsylvanicus^{+}
Kanopolis (143), Ellsworth Co., Y
P. llanensis$^{\circ}$, *M. pennsylvanicus*$^{+}$
Cudahy (132), Meade Co., K, ≥0.6 m.y.b.p.
P. llanensis$^{\circ}$, *P. meadensis*$^{\circ}$, *M. paroperarius*$^{\circ}$
Hall Ash Pit (150), Jewell Co., K, ≥0.74 m.y.b.p.
M. paroperarius$^{\circ}$
Holzinger (137), Trego Co., K
M. paroperarius$^{\circ}$
Tobin (140), Russell Co., K
P. meadensis$^{\circ}$, *M. paroperarius*$^{\circ}$, *M.* sp.$^{+/\circ}$
Wilson Valley (142), Lincoln Co., K
P. meadensis$^{\circ}$, *M. paroperarius*$^{\circ}$
Unnamed (144), Ellsworth Co., K
P. llanensis?$^{\circ}$ or *M. paroperarius*?$^{\circ}$

Aries (133), Meade Co., K, ≥1.2 m.y.b.p.
P. sp.°
Kentuck (147), McPherson Co., K
P. sp.°, *P. llanensis*°
Wathena (148), Doniphan Co., K
P. sp.°
Courtland Canal (151), Jewell Co., K
P. sp.°
Nash (134), Meade Co., A, >1.2, <1.9 m.y.b.p.
P. sp.°

Kentucky

Welsh Cave (205), Woodford Co., W
P. pinetorum and/or *P. ochrogaster, M. pennsylvanicus, M. xanthognathus*[+]

Maryland

Cavetown (223), Washington Co., W
M. pennsylvanicus
Cumberland Cave (222), Allegany Co., L.K.
P. guilday°, *P. cumberlandensis*°, *P. involutus*[nd], *M. paroperarius*°

Mexico

Unnamed (86), Chihuahua, W
M. pennsylvanicus[+]
San Josecito (85), Nuevo Leon, W
M. mexicanus
El Tajo de Tequixquiac (84), Mexico, W
P. meadensis°

Michigan

Sleeping Bear Dune (208), Leelanau Co., H, 730 ± 250 B.P.
P. pinetorum, P. ochrogaster[+], *M. pennsylvanicus*
Adams (209), Livingston Co., W
M. pennsylvanicus

Missouri

Brynjulfson Cave #2 (165), Boone Co., H, 1,400 ± 200 to 2,260 ± 230 B.P.
P. pinetorum and/or *P. ochrogaster, M. pennsylvanicus*[+]
Brynjulfson Cave #1 (166), Boone Co., H/W, 9,440 ± 760 to 34,000 ± 2,100 B.P.
P. pinetorum and/or *P. ochrogaster, M. pennsylvanicus*[+]
Crankshaft Cave (167), Jefferson Co., H/W
P. pinetorum and/or *P. ochrogaster, M. pennsylvanicus*[+]
Boney Spring (169), Benton Co., W, 13,700 ± 600 to 16,580 ± 220 B.P.
P. pinetorum and/or *P. ochrogaster, M. pennsylvanicus*[+]
Herculaneum (168), Jefferson Co., W
P. ochrogaster
Zoo Cave (171), Taney Co., W
P. pinetorum and/or *P. ochrogaster, M. pennsylvanicus*[+]

Bat Cave (170), Pulaski Co., W
P. pinetorum? and/or *P. ochrogaster, M. pennsylvanicus*+, *M. xanthognathus*+

Montana

Warm Springs #1 (19), Silver Bow Co., H/W
M. pennsylvanicus, M. richardsoni

Nebraska

Unnamed (155), Buffalo Co., W/S
M. sp.+
Angus (153), Nuckolls Co., I
P. ochrogaster, M. pennsylvanicus
Hay Springs (159), Sheridan Co., I
M. pennsylvanicus+
Mullen II (158), Cherry Co., I
P. pinetorum+ and/or *P. ochrogaster, M. pennsylvanicus*
Mullen I (157), Cherry Co., K
M. paroperarius°
Unnamed (156), Valley Co., K
M. paroperarius°
Sappa (154), Harlan Co., K, ≥1.2 m.y.b.p.
P. sp.°

Nevada

Tule Springs E_1 (45), Clark Co., W
M. californicus+
Tule Springs B_2 (46), Clark Co., W
M. sp.
Glendale (47), Clark Co., W
M. californicus+ or *M. montanus*+

New Mexico

The Khulo (80), Doña Ana Co., H
M. pennsylvanicus+
Howells Ridge Cave (82), Grant Co., H/W
P. ochrogaster+, *M. pennsylvanicus*+, *M. mexicanus*+, *M. montanus*+
Anthony Cave (77), Doña Ana Co., H/W
M. pennsylvanicus+, *M. mexicanus*+, *M. montanus*+
Conkling Cavern (78), Doña Ana Co., H/W
M. mexicanus+
Shelter Cave (79), Doña Ana Co., H/W
M. montanus+
Burnet Cave (74), Eddy Co., H/W
M. mexicanus+, *M. longicaudus*+
Brown Sand Wedge (72), Roosevelt Co., W, 11,170 ± 360 B.P.
P. ochrogaster+, *M. pennsylvanicus*+, *M. mexicanus*+
Dry Cave (73), Eddy Co., W, 10,730 ± 150 to 33,590 ± 1,150 B.P.
P. ochrogaster, M. mexicanus, M. longicaudus+
Muskox Cave (75), Eddy Co., W
P. ochrogaster+, *M. pennsylvanicus*+, *M. mexicanus*+

Dark Canyon Cave (76), Eddy Co., W
M. sp.$^{+}$
Isleta Cave #1 (71), Bernalillo Co., W
M. pennsylvanicus^{+}
Palomas Creek Cave (81), Sierra Co., W
M. sp.$^{+}$
Baldy Peak Cave (83), Luna Co., W
M. sp.$^{+}$

New York

Dutchess Quarry Cave (229), Orange Co., W, 12,530 ± 370 B.P.
P. pinetorum, M. pennsylvanicus

Ohio

Carter (210), Darke Co., W, 10,230 ± 150 B.P.
M. pennsylvanicus

Oklahoma

Domebo (121), Caddo Co., W, 11,200 ± 500 B.P.
P. pinetorum, P. ochrogaster
Bar M #1 (122), Harper Co., W, 21,360 ± 1,250 B.P.
M. pennsylvanicus^{+}
Doby Springs (123), Harper Co., I
M. pennsylvanicus^{+}
Berends (124), Beaver Co., I
P. ochrogaster, M. pennsylvanicus^{+}

Oregon

Fossil Lake (26), Lake Co., W
M. montanus

Pennsylvania

New Paris #4 (224), Bedford Co., H/W, 9,540 to 11,300 ± B.P.
P. pinetorum, M. pennsylvanicus, M. chrotorrhinus^{+}, *M. xanthognathus*$^{+}$
Hollidaysburg Fissure (225), Blair Co., H/W, 10,000 to 12,000 B.P.
P. pinetorum, M. pennsylvanicus, M. chrotorrhinus^{+}
Bootlegger Sink (227), York Co., W, 11,550 ± 100 B.P.
P. pinetorum, M. pennsylvanicus, M. chrotorrhinus^{+}, *M. xanthognathus*$^{+}$
Frankstown Cave (226), Blair Co., W
M. pennsylvanicus
Port Kennedy Cave (228), Montgomery Co., Y
P. involutus$^{\circ/nd}$, *P. dideltus*$^{\circ/nd}$, *M. speothen*$^{\circ/nd}$
Hanover Quarry Fissure (235), Adams Co., A
P. guildayi$^{\circ}$, *P. cumberlandensis*$^{\circ}$, *M. paroperarius*$^{\circ}$

Québec

Caverne de St. Elzéar (230), Bonaventure Co., H, 5,110 ± 150 B.P.
M. pennsylvanicus, M. chrotorrhinus, M. xanthognathus^{+}

Saskatchewan

Riddell (12), Saskatoon District, W
M. pennsylvanicus, M. sp.
Wellsch Valley (13), Swift Current-S. Saskatchewan Upland, A, $1.75 \cdot 10^6$
P. sp.°, *M. paroperarius*°

South Dakota

Java (160), Walworth Co., K
P. sp.°

Tennessee

First American Bank Site (204), Davidson Co., H/W, 9,410 to 10,034± B.P.
P. pinetorum and/or *P. ochrogaster*
Baker Bluff (200), Sullivan Co., W, 10,560 ± 220 to 19,100 ± 850 B.P.
P. pinetorum and/or *P. ochrogaster*⁺, *M. pennsylvanicus, M. chrotorrhinus*⁺, *M. xanthognathus*⁺
Guy Wilson (201), Sullivan Co., W, 19,700 ± 600 B.P.
M. pennsylvanicus
Carrier Quarry Cave (199), Sullivan Co., W
P. pinetorum and/or *P. ochrogaster, M. pennsylvanicus, M. chrotorrhinus*⁺
Robinson Cave (202), Overton Co., W
P. pinetorum, M. pennsylvanicus
Cheek Bend Cave (203), Maury Co., W
P. ochrogaster, M. pennsylvanicus, M. xanthognathus⁺
Beartown Cave (237), Sullivan Co., W
M. cf. *M. pennsylvanicus*

Texas

Kyle Site (108), Hill Co., H, 389 ± 130 to 1,389 ± 150 B.P.
P. pinetorum⁺ and/or *P. ochrogaster*⁺
Blue Spring Shelter (232), Randall Co., H, 840 to 1,135 B.P.
P. pinetorum⁺ and/or *P. ochrogaster*⁺
Barton Springs Road (103), Travis Co., H, 1,015 ± 105 to 3,450 ± 150 B.P.
P. pinetorum⁺ and/or *P. ochrogaster*⁺
Deadman Shelter (233), Swisher Co., H, 1,240 to 1,485 B.P.
P. pinetorum⁺ and/or *P. ochrogaster*⁺
Canyon Country Club Cave (234), Randall Co., H, 1,270–1,650 B.P.
P. pinetorum⁺ and/or *P. ochrogaster*⁺
Miller's Cave (106), Llano Co., H/LW, 3,008 ± 310 to 7,290± B.P.
P. pinetorum⁺ and/or *P. ochrogaster*⁺
Klein Cave (99), Kerr Co., H, 7,683 ± 643 B.P.
P. pinetorum, M. pennsylvanicus⁺
Felton Cave (101), Sutton Co., H, 7,700 ± 130 B.P.
P. pinetorum⁺ and/or *P. ochrogaster*⁺
Schulze Cave (100), Edwards Co., H/LW, 9,310 ± 310 to 9,680 ± 700 B.P.
P. pinetorum⁺ and/or *P. ochrogaster*⁺
Ben Franklin (110), Delta Co., H/LW, 9,550 ± 375 to 11,135 ± 450 B.P.
P. pinetorum⁺ and/or *P. ochrogaster*⁺, *M. pennsylvanicus*⁺
Lubbock Lake (114), Lubbock Co., H/LW, 9,883 ± 350 to 12,650 ± 350 B.P.
P. pinetorum⁺ and/or *P. ochrogaster*⁺

Levi Shelter (102), Travis Co., H/LW, ≥10,000 B.P.
P. pinetorum^{+} and/or *P. ochrogaster*$^{+}$

Cooper Reservoir (109), Delta and Hopkins cos., H/W
P. pinetorum^{+} and/or *P. ochrogaster*$^{+}$

Huecos Tanks #1 (88), El Paso Co., H/W
M. sp.$^{+}$

Navar Ranch #13 (89), El Paso Co., H/W
M. montanus^{+}

Longhorn (105), Burnet Co., H/W
P. pinetorum^{+} and/or *P. ochrogaster*$^{+}$

Cave Without A Name (98), Kendall Co., W, 10,900 ± 190 B.P.
P. pinetorum?$^{+}$ and/or *P. ochrogaster*$^{+}$, *M. pennsylvanicus*$^{+}$

Howard Ranch (119) = Grosebeck Creek, Hardeman Co., W, 16,775 ± 565 B.P.
P. pinetorum and/or *P. ochrogaster*$^{+}$, *M. pennsylvanicus*$^{+}$

Clear Creek (113), Denton Co., W, 28,840 ± 4,740 B.P.
P. pinetorum and/or *P. ochrogaster*$^{+}$

Tank Trap Wash #1 (87), El Paso Co., W, >33,000 B.P.
M. sp.$^{+}$

Dust Cave (90), Culberson Co., W
M. sp.$^{+}$

Rattlesnake Cave (94), Kinney Co., W
P. pinetorum^{+} and/or *P. ochrogaster*$^{+}$

Montell Cave (95), Uvalde Co., W
P. pinetorum^{+} and/or *P. ochrogaster*$^{+}$

Zesch Cave (107), Mason Co., W
P. pinetorum^{+} and/or *P. ochrogaster*$^{+}$

Upper Sloth Cave (91), Culberson Co., W
M. mexicanus

Lower Sloth Cave (92), Culberson Co., W
M. mexicanus

Pratt Cave (93), Culberson Co., W
M. mexicanus^{+}

Quitaque (120), Motley Co., W
P. pinetorum^{+} and/or *P. ochrogaster*$^{+}$, *M. pennsylvanicus*$^{+}$

Friesenhahn (96), Bexar Co., W
P. pinetorum^{+} and/or *P. ochrogaster*$^{+}$

Moore Pit (111), Dallas and Denton cos., W
P. pinetorum^{+} and/or *P. ochrogaster*$^{+}$

Coppell (112), Dallas and Denton cos., W
P. pinetorum^{+} and/or *P. ochrogaster*$^{+}$

Sims Bayou (97), Harris Co., W
P. ochrogaster

Easely Ranch (116), Foard Co., S
P. pinetorum^{+} and/or *P. ochrogaster*$^{+}$, *M. pennsylvanicus*$^{+}$

Monument (117), Foard Co., S
P. pinetorum^{+} and/or *P. ochrogaster*$^{+}$, *M. pennsylvanicus*$^{+}$

Smith Ranch (118), Foard Co., S
P. pinetorum^{+} and/or *P. ochrogaster*$^{+}$

South Fish Creek (231), Cooke Co., S
P. pinetorum^{+} and/or *P. ochrogaster*$^{+}$

Vera (115), Knox Co., K
P. llanensis$^{\circ}$, *M. paroperarius*$^{\circ}$

Fyllan Cave (104), Travis Co., K
P. sp.$^{\circ}$

Utah

Crystal Ball Cave (54), Millard Co., W
M. sp.
Silver Creek (56), Summit Co., W/S, >40,000 B.P.
M. montanus
Snowville (55), Box Elder Co., K
M. montanus

Virginia

Strait Canyon (220), Highland Co., W, 29,870 + 1,800–1,400 B.P.
M. pennsylvanicus
Loop Creek Quarry Cave (215), Russell Co., W
M. xanthognathus[+]
Gillespie Cliff Cave (216), Tazwell Co., W
M. xanthognathus[+]
Early's Pits (217), Wythe Co., W
M. pennsylvanicus
Back Creek #2 (218), Bath Co., W
M. pennsylvanicus, M. chrotorrhinus[+], *M. xanthognathus*[+]
Clark's Cave (219), Bath Co., W
P. pinetorum, M. pennsylvanicus, M. chrotorrhinus[+], *M. xanthognathus*[+]
Natural Chimneys (221), Augusta Co., W
P. pinetorum, M. pennsylvanicus, M. chrotorrhinus[+], *M. xanthognathus*[+]

West Virginia

Eagle Rock Cave (211), Pendleton Co., W
P. pinetorum, M. pennsylvanicus, M. chrotorrhinus, M. xanthognathus[+]
Hoffman School Cave (212), Pendleton Co., W
P. pinetorum, M. pennsylvanicus, M. chrotorrhinus
Mandy Walters Cave (213), Pendleton Co., W
P. pinetorum, M. pennsylvanicus, M. chrotorrhinus
Upper Trout Cave (214), Pendleton Co., W
P. pinetorum, M. pennsylvanicus, M. chrotorrhinus

Wisconsin

Moscow Fissure (241), Iowa Co., 17,050 ± 1,500 B.P.
P. cf. *P. ochrogaster, M. pennsylvanicus, M. xanthognathus*[+]

Wyoming

Bush Shelter (57), Washakie Co., H, 9,000 B.P.
M. pennsylvanicus[+]
Little Canyon Creek Cave (58), Washakie Co., H/W, 10,170 B.P.
M. pennsylvanicus[+], *M. montanus*
Agate Basin (62), Niobrara Co., H/W, 10,430 to 11,450 B.P.
M. pennsylvanicus[+], *M. longicaudus*[+]
Bell Cave (64), Albany Co., H/W, 12,240 B.P.
P. ochrogaster, M. pennsylvanicus[+], *M. montanus*
Prospects Shelter (59), Bighorn Co., H/W, 10,000 to 27,000 B.P.
P. ochrogaster, M. pennsylvanicus[+], *M. montanus, M. xanthognathus*[+]

Natural Trap Cave (60), Bighorn Co., H/W, 12,000 to 20,000 B.P.
P. ochrogaster, M. pennsylvanicus+, *M. montanus*
Sheaman Site (61), Niobrara Co., W
M. pennsylvanicus+
Little Box Elder Cave (63), Converse Co., W
P. ochrogaster, M. pennsylvanicus+, *M. montanus, M. longicaudus*

Yukon Territories

Bluefish Cave I (11), Bluefish-Porcupine Upland, H/W, 12,900 ± 100 B.P.
M. miurus+, *M. oeconomus, M. xanthognathus*
Old Crow River Loc. 12 (9), Old Crow Basin, W
M. miurus+, *M. pennsylvanicus, M. xanthognathus*
Old Crow River Loc. 44 (6), Old Crow Basin, S?, >54,000 B.P.
M. xanthognathus
Old Crow River Loc. 11 (10), Old Crow Basin, S?
M. miurus+, *M. oeconomus*, cf. *M. xanthognathus*
Old Crow River Loc. 12 (8), Old Crow Basin, I
M. miurus+, *M. oeconomus, M. xanthognathus*
Old Crow River Loc. 14N (7), Old Crow Basin, ?age
M. miurus+

Appendix B. Localities Containing Pitymys pinetorum, P. ochrogaster, *and* Microtus pennsylvanicus

P. pinetorum

Arkansas
Peccary Cave (172)
Florida
Warm Mineral Springs (174)
Vero 2 (176)
Vero 3 (177)
Kendrick IA (179)
Reddick IA (180)
Reddick IB (181)
Reddick IC (182)
Reddick ID (183)
Reddick IIC (184)
Mefford I (185)
Devil's Den (186)
Waccasassa IIB (187)
Arrendondo I (190)
Arrendondo II (192)
Arrendondo IIA (193)
Arrendondo IIB (194)
Arrendondo IIC (195)
Haile XIB (196)
Ichetucknee River (197)
Georgia
Ladds (198)
Illinois
Meyer Cave (206)
Iowa
Brayton (162)
Waubonsie?+ (164)
Kentucky
Welsh Cave? (205)
Michigan
Sleeping Bear Dune (208)
Missouri
Brynjulfson Cave #2? (165)
Brynjulfson Cave #1? (166)
Crankshaft Cave? (167)
Boney Spring? (169)
Bat Cave? (170)
Zoo Cave? (171)

Nebraska
- Mullen II?$^{+}$ (158)

New York
- Dutchess Quarry Cave (229)

Oklahoma
- Domebo (121)

Pennsylvania
- New Paris #4 (224)
- Hollidaysburg Fissure (225)
- Bootlegger Sink (227)

Tennessee
- Carrier Quarry Cave? (199)
- Baker Bluff? (200)
- Robinson Cave (202)
- First American Bank Site? (204)

Texas
- Rattlesnake Cave?$^{+}$ (94)
- Montell Cave?$^{+}$ (95)
- Friesenhahn? (96)
- Cave Without A Name?$^{+}$ (98)
- Klein Cave (99)
- Schulze Cave?$^{+}$ (100)
- Felton Cave?$^{+}$ (101)
- Levi Shelter?$^{+}$ (102)
- Barton Springs Road?$^{+}$ (103)
- Longhorn?$^{+}$ (105)
- Miller's Cave?$^{+}$ (106)
- Zesch Cave?$^{+}$ (107)
- Kyle Site?$^{+}$ (108)
- Cooper Reservoir?$^{+}$ (109)
- Ben Franklin? (110)
- Moore Pit? (111)
- Coppell?$^{+}$ (112)
- Clear Creek? (113)
- Lubbock Lake?$^{+}$ (114)
- Easely Ranch?$^{+}$ (116)
- Monument?$^{+}$ (117)
- Smith Ranch?$^{+}$ (118)
- Howard Ranch? (119)
- Quitaque?$^{+}$ (120)
- South Fish Creek?$^{+}$ (231)
- Blue Spring Shelter?$^{+}$ (232)
- Deadman Shelter?$^{+}$ (233)
- Canyon Country Club Cave?$^{+}$ (234)

Virginia
- Clark's Cave (219)
- Natural Chimneys (221)

West Virginia
- Eagle Rock Cave (211)
- Hoffman School Cave (212)
- Mandy Walters Cave (213)
- Upper Trout Cave (214)

P. ochrogaster

Arkansas
- Peccary Cave^{+} (172)

Colorado
- Dutton (66)
- Mesa de Maya (68)

Indiana
- Harrodsburg Crevice (207)

Iowa
- Waubonsie? (164)

Kansas
- Robert (125)
- Jones (126)
- Jinglebob (127)
- Cragin Quarry (128)
- Mt. Scott (129)
- Butler Spring (130)
- Trapshoot (138)
- Duck Creek (139)
- Rezabek (141)
- Williams (145)
- Sandahl (146)

Kentucky
- Welsh Cave? (205)

Michigan
- Sleeping Bear Dune (208)

Missouri
- Brynjulfson Cave #2? (165)
- Brynjulfson Cave #1? (166)
- Crankshaft Cave? (167)
- Herculaneum (168)
- Boney Spring? (169)
- Bat Cave? (170)
- Zoo Cave? (171)

Nebraska
- Angus (153)
- Mullen II? (158)

New Mexico
- Brown Sand Wedge^{+} (72)
- Dry Cave (73)
- Muskox Cave^{+} (76)
- Howells Ridge Cave^{+} (82)

Oklahoma
- Domebo (121)
- Berends (124)

Tennessee
- Carrier Quarry Cave? (199)

Baker Bluff? (200)
Cheek Bend Cave (203)
First American Bank Site? (204)

Texas
Rattlesnake Cave?$^{+}$ (94)
Montell Cave?$^{+}$ (95)
Sims Bayou (97)
Cave Without A Name?$^{+}$ (98)
Schulze Cave?$^{+}$ (100)
Felton Cave?$^{+}$ (101)
Levi Shelter?$^{+}$ (102)
Barton Springs Road?$^{+}$ (103)
Longhorn?$^{+}$ (105)
Miller's Cave?$^{+}$ (106)
Zesch Cave?$^{+}$ (107)
Kyle Site?$^{+}$ (108)
Cooper Reservoir?$^{+}$ (109)
Ben Franklin?$^{+}$ (110)
Moore Pit?$^{+}$ (111)
Coppell?$^{+}$ (112)
Clear Creek?$^{+}$ (113)
Lubbock Lake?$^{+}$ (114)
Easely Ranch?$^{+}$ (116)
Monument?$^{+}$ (117)
Smith Ranch?$^{+}$ (118)
Howard Ranch?$^{+}$ (119)
Quitaque?$^{+}$ (120)
South Fish Creek?$^{+}$ (231)
Blue Spring Shelter?$^{+}$ (232)
Deadman Shelter?$^{+}$ (233)
Canyon Country Club Cave?$^{+}$ (234)

Wisconsin
Moscow Fissure (241)

Wyoming
Prospects Shelter (59)
Natural Trap Cave (60)
Little Box Elder (63)
Bell Cave (64)

M. pennsylvanicus

Alberta
Hand Hills (16)

Arkansas
Peccary Cave^{+} (172)

Colorado
Dutton (65)

Florida
Devil's Den (186)
Waccasassa IIB (187)
Withlacoochee VIIA (188)
Arrendondo I (190)
Arrendondo IIB (194)

Idaho
American Falls? (24)

Illinois
Meyer Cave^{+} (206)

Iowa
Brayton (162)
Oakland (163)
Waubonsie (164)
Elkader (238)
Eagle Point (239)

Kansas
Robert^{+} (125)
Jones^{+} (126)
Jinglebob^{+} (127)
Cragin Quarry^{+} (128)
Mt. Scott^{+} (129)
Butler Spring^{+} (130)
Adams^{+} (131)
Keiger Creek^{+} (135)
Unnamed^{+} (136)
Trapshoot^{+} (138)
Duck Creek^{+} (139)
Rezabek^{+} (141)
Kanopolis^{+} (143)
Williams^{+} (145)
Sandahl^{+} (146)
Unnamed (152)

Kentucky
Welsh Cave (205)

Maryland
Cavetown (223)

Mexico
Unnamed^{+} (86)

Michigan
Sleeping Bear Dune (208)
Adams (209)

Missouri
Brynjulfson Cave #2^{+} (165)
Brynjulfson Cave #1^{+} (166)
Crankshaft Cave^{+} (167)
Boney Spring^{+} (169)
Bat Cave^{+} (170)
Zoo Cave^{+} (171)

Montana
Warm Springs #1 (19)

Nebraska
Angus (153)
Mullen II (158)
Hay Springs^{+} (159)

New Mexico
Isleta Cave^{+} (71)
Brown Sand Wedge^{+} (72)

Muskox Cave+ (75)
Anthony Cave+ (77)
The Khulo+ (80)
Howells Ridge Cave+ (82)
New York
Dutchess Quarry Cave (229)
Ohio
Carter (210)
Oklahoma
Bar M #1+ (122)
Doby Springs+ (123)
Berends+ (124)
Pennsylvania
New Paris #4 (224)
Hollidaysburg Fissure (225)
Frankstown Cave (226)
Bootlegger Sink (227)
Québec
Caverne de St. Elzéar (230)
Saskatchewan
Riddell (12)
Tennessee
Carrier Quarry Cave (199)
Baker Bluff (200)
Guy Wilson (201)
Robinson Cave (202)
Cheek Bend Cave (203)
First American Bank Site (204)
Beartown (237)
Texas
Cave Without A Name+ (98)
Klein Cave+ (99)
Ben Franklin+ (110)
Easely Ranch+ (116)
Monument+ (117)
Howard Ranch+ (119)
Quitaque+ (120)
Virginia
Early's Pits (217)
Back Creek #2 (218)
Clark's Cave (219)
Strait Canyon (220)
Natural Chimneys (221)
West Virginia
Eagle Rock Cave (211)
Hoffman School Cave (212)
Mandy Walters Cave (213)
Upper Trout Cave (214)
Wisconsin
Moscow Fissure (241)
Wyoming
Bush Shelter+ (57)
Little Canyon Creek+ (58)
Prospects Shelter+ (59)
Natural Trap Cave+ (60)
Sheaman Site+ (61)
Agate Basin+ (62)
Little Box Elder Cave+ (63)
Bell Cave+ (64)
Yukon Territories
Old Crow River Loc. 12 (9)

Symbol: +, taxon extinct locally.

TAXONOMY AND SYSTEMATICS

SYDNEY ANDERSON

Abstract

THE Holarctic arvicoline or microtine rodents have long been recognized as a distinct group at the level of family or subfamily, and are here regarded as a subfamily of the Muridae. The genus with the most species is *Microtus*.

The methods and results of major taxonomic works (Miller in 1896, Bailey in 1900, and Hinton in 1926) are compared. The taxonomy of North American *Microtus* has passed through several historic phases relating to the availability of specimens, increases in knowledge, and changing taxonomic viewpoints. Prior to 1860 scattered explorations resulted in relatively small series of specimens and 34 supposed species were named. From 1860 to 1890 not much happened. The decade ending in 1900 was more productive than any other decade before or since. Most full species now recognized were known by the end of that decade, large series were collected, a polytypic concept of species developed, and the number of monotypic species began to decline. From 1900 to 1920 the new trends continued but at a slower pace. From 1920 to 1950 was a period of further consolidation, the number of recognized species decreased rapidly as monotypic species became subspecies, and the number of subspecies increased rapidly as geographic variation became better known. The period of alpha taxonomy, which focused on the question of what are the species, matured from 1950 to 1980, so that the number of recognized species has approached an equilibrium.

However, if the task of taxonomy is considered to be the elucidation of relationships at all levels, the taxonomic work needed for an adequate understanding of the Arvicolinae lies mostly in the future.

Many natural groups are clustered in ways that give "hollow curve" frequency distributions. For example, within the genus *Microtus,* the subgenus *Microtus* includes about half of the 25 or so North American species and the other half are scattered among six other subgenera. The results of the "artichoke method" are evident in *Microtus* taxonomy as in that of most other groups. No attempt has ever been made to apply numerical taxonomy or contemporary cladistic methods to the study of *Microtus*. What we have is an eclectic mixture of methods and results. I argue that this is not necessarily bad, but that since there is little agreement on systematic methods, it is important that authors explain their assumptions and procedures as well as presenting data and taxonomic results.

Introduction

In this chapter the taxonomic context of arvicoline or microtine rodents is presented and the close connection of Old World and New World arvicoline faunas is noted, then the history of the classification of these rodents at the generic level is summarized, and the classification of New World *Microtus* at the species level is reviewed. Finally, some systematic methods are discussed with the objective of clarifying what has been done and suggesting needs for future work.

The genus *Microtus* consists of several dozen species of "microtine" or "arvicoline" rodents belonging to the family Arvicolidae or subfamily Arvicolinae (within Muridae or Cricetidae). The context of the group within the Class Mammalia (as outlined by Simpson, 1945) is:

Class Mammalia Linnaeus, 1758
Subclass Theria Parker and Haswell, 1897
Infraclass Eutheria Gill, 1872
Order Rodentia Bowdich, 1821

The rodents are the most successful order of living mammals as measured by numbers of species and individuals. Rodents are generally recognized as a monophyletic group based on peculiarities of teeth and skulls related to gnawing. Convergent similarities occur in other orders, such as the Primates and Marsupialia. Because of other characters, however, there is little doubt that the aye-aye is a primate or that a wombat is a marsupial. The Rodentia originated very early in mammalian evolution and there is no clear evidence for the precise relationship of Rodentia among other orders of Mammalia. This is one of the major unresolved problems in mammalian taxonomy.

Suborder Myomorpha Brandt, 1855
Superfamily Muroidea Miller and Gidley, 1918

Carleton (1980) reviewed the history of major classifications of muroid rodents at the familial level. The arvicolines or microtines have been treated at various times as both a family and a subfamily. Chaline et al. (1977) recognized the family Arvicolidae. Carleton and Musser (1984) recognized the subfamily Arvicolinae within the family Muridae. The level as such (subfamily vs. family) is not so important as are the hypotheses of relationships. More explicit diagrams of relationship and more explicit statements of characters and rationale for each branching point and lineage are needed.

Family Muridae Gray, 1821
Subfamily Arvicolinae Gray, 1821

The lemmings and voles, the major groups in Arvicolinae, were thought by Hinton (1926) to have been derived separately from the Murinae. Repenning (1968) analyzed the earliest arvicolines (Pliocene forms not known to Hinton) and likewise noted a possibility of polyphyly, as derivatives of Cricetidae. Martin (1979) analyzed fossil North American arvicolines and implied polyphyly by stressing independent developments of various arvicoline dental specializations in different lines and by a drawing showing 16 unconnected lineages, thus avoiding the question of relationships. Martin argued that, because of the rapidity of changes and similar changes in different lines, arvicolines are useful in biostratigraphy in spite of uncertainty about details of phylogenetic connections.

The systematic relationships of both living and fossil North American arvicolines in general and the genus *Microtus* in particular involve Old World groups as well as North American groups. The following living groups in North America presumably have their nearest relatives in Eurasia rather than in North America, and perhaps other groups within North American *Microtus* also do:

Dicrostonyx torquatus, Lemmus sibiricus, and *Clethrionomys rutilis* inhabit both continents.

Lagurus curtatus is related to *Lagurus lagurus* and *L. luteus* of the Old World.

Microtus miurus and the insular form *M. abbreviatus* are related to *M. gregalis* of the Old World. All are placed in the subgenus *Stenocranius.*

If the subgenus *Pitymys* is monophyletic, then the New World species are related to the Old World species of *Pitymys* more closely than to other New World *Microtus*.

Microtus richardsoni has been placed in the subgenus *Arvicola* which allies it with Old World species of that subgenus.

Microtus pennsylvanicus and its close insular relatives in North America have been allied with *Microtus agrestis* of the Old World on the basis of a posterior loop on m2.

Microtus chrotorrhinus has a giant chromosome that suggests a possible relationship with *Microtus agrestis* (Kirkland and Jannett, 1982).

Microtus longicaudus and its insular near relative *Microtus coronarius* have some similarities with the Old World subgenus *Chionomys*.

Some of these affinities are generally agreed upon, some are very tentative hypotheses, and some are controversial. For example, the teeth of *Microtus richardsoni* are more complex than those of the Old World species of *Arvicola* and this leads some paleontologists, whose attention is focused on dental traits, to reject the hypothesis of monophyly and consider resemblences in other features as convergences. There is considerable uncertainty about the affinities of species of *Pitymys, Neodon,* and *Pedomys,* with each other and with other species of *Microtus*. This is good, because it indicates that people are reexamining and refining the classification. Much remains to be done.

History of Systematics at the Generic Level

The pivotal study in the systematics of arvicoline rodents at the generic level is Miller's (1896) revision. It is pivotal in the sense that no comparably comprehensive study had been done earlier or has been done since. In general, prior studies were more limited in scope, geographically, taxonomically, or in characters considered. Miller considered all arvicolines, both Old World and New World, and reviewed and attempted to synthesize all relevant characters.

The content of the genus *Microtus* as recognized by Miller (1896) was greater than that of most later authors. There has been a tendency to elevate Miller's subgenera to genera. The "essential characters" of the genus *Microtus* (Miller, 1896:44) were considered to be as follows.

1) "Upper incisors without grooves." Such grooves normally oc-

cur in *Synaptomys* and *Promethiomys* and may appear as infrequent variants in individuals of other genera including *Microtus.*

2) "Lower incisors with roots [partly] on outer side of molar roots." Posteriorly, the incisor root passed from the lingual side to the labial side of the molar roots between the second and third molars. This is the general condition among voles. In the lemmings *Synaptomys, Myopus, Lemmus,* and *Dicrostonyx,* the root of the incisor lies medial to the roots of all three lower molars.

3) "Molars rootless." Among the lemmings, this condition of persistent growth occurs in all four genera. Among the living New World voles, it occurs only in *Microtus* (as treated by Miller, including *Lagurus* and *Neofiber*), not in *Phenacomys* (including *Arborimus*), *Clethrionomys* (then called *Evotomys*), or *Ondatra* (then called *Fiber*). Persistent growth is the final stage in the development of hypsodonty, which is found in varying degrees in all Arvicolinae.

4) "Enamel pattern characterized by approximate equality of reentrant angles." This differs from the condition of the lower molars in *Phenacomys* which have much deeper inner reentrant angles than outer reentrant angles. Inequality of depth of angles occurs also in the upper molars of *Synaptomys, Myopus,* and *Lemmus,* which have deeper outer reentrant angles than inner ones, and to a lesser degree also in their lower molars, which have deeper inner angles.

5) "First lower molar usually with five closed or nearly closed triangles." Within *Microtus* the fourth and fifth triangles of m1 are confluent rather than closed in subgenera *Pitymys, Pedomys,* and *Neodon.* This differs from the conditions in lemmings, among which *Synaptomys, Myopus,* and *Lemmus* have three closed triangles and two transverse loops, or four transverse loops and no closed triangles, and *Dicrostonyx* has seven closed triangles and two transverse loops.

6) "Upper third molar with one, two, or three closed triangles." *Phenacomys* has two or three, *Clethrionomys* has three, *Dicrostonyx* has three or four and two transverse loops, and *Synaptomys, Myopus,* and *Lemmus* have four transverse loops and no closed triangles.

7) "Tail nearly always longer than hind foot, terete." The tail is shorter than the hindfoot in *Lemmus, Myopus,* and *Dicrostonyx* (and in Asiatic *Lagurus* among Miller's *Microtus*). The tail is somewhat flattened laterally in *Ondatra.*

8) "Feet, fur, eyes, and ears very variable." All of the other

genera (about 18) of arvicolines combined contain fewer species (about 60) than *Microtus* (about 68; Honacki et al., 1982) and exhibit less variation within any one genus in these features. The hindfeet of *Ondatra* are modified for aquatic locomotion and the feet of the arctic lemmings, *Lemmus* and *Dicrostonyx,* have peculiarities not seen in *Microtus.*

9) "Thumb never with a well-developed ligulate nail." A nail of this sort is present in *Lemmus.*

Names of genera and subgenera that have been used for living North American species of *Microtus* at one time or another, and that are synonyms by virtue of the fact that their type species belong to *Microtus,* in Miller's (1896) broadest sense, are as follows.

Microtus Schrank, 1798, type species *Microtus terrestris* of Schrank, a synonym of *Mus arvalis* Pallas, now *Microtus arvalis,* of the Old World, and not *Mus terrestris* of Linnaeus. Miller (1896) initiated the wide use of the name *Microtus.* Prior to 1896 *Arvicola* was used. *Microtus* is the central genus and subgenus in the complex, and the group with the most species.

Arvicola Lacépède, 1799, type species *Mus amphibius* Linnaeus, a synonym of *Microtus terrestris* (Linnaeus). The American species *Microtus richardsoni* has been referred to *Arvicola* in the narrower subgeneric sense by some authors, although this referral is not universally accepted. *Arvicola* includes two Old World species.

Mynomes Rafinesque, 1817, type species *Mynomes pratensis* Rafinesque, a synonym of *Mus pennsylvanicus* Ord, now *Microtus pennsylvanicus.*

Psammomys LeConte, 1830, type species *Psammomys pinetorum* LeConte, now *Microtus pinetorum,* not *Psammomys* Cretzschmar, 1828, which is a gerbil.

Pitymys McMurtrie, 1831, type species *Psammomys pinetorum* LeConte.

Ammomys Bonaparte, 1831, type species *Psammomys pinetorum* LeConte, hence an objective synonym of *Pitymys* McMurtrie.

Lagurus Gloger, 1841, type species *Mus lagurus* Pallas, now treated as *Lagurus lagurus*; the genus includes the American species *Lagurus curtatus.*

Pedomys Baird, 1857, type species *Arvicola austerus* LeConte, now a subspecies of *Microtus ochrogaster.*

Chilotus Baird, 1857, type species *Arvicola oregoni* Bachman, now *Microtus oregoni.*

Neofiber True, 1884, type species *Neofiber alleni* True, now separated from *Microtus.*

Aulacomys Rhoads, 1894, type species *Aulacomys arvicoloides* Rhoads, now a subspecies of *Microtus richardsoni.*

Tetramerodon Rhoads, 1894, type species *Arvicola tetramerus* Rhoads, now a subspecies of *Microtus townsendii.*

Orthriomys Merriam, 1898, type species *Microtus umbrosus* Merriam, proposed as subgenus, later used as genus.

Herpetomys Merriam, 1898, type species *Microtus guatemalensis* Merriam, proposed as subgenus, later used as genus.

Stenocranius Kastschenko, 1901, type species *Arvicola slowzowi* Poliakoff, a synonym of *Mus gregalis* Pallas, now *Microtus gregalis*; valid as a subgenus including *Microtus miurus* and *M. abbreviatus* of the New World.

Chionomys Miller, 1908, type species *Arvicola nivalis* Marins, now *Mictotus nivalis,* Old World; *Microtus longicaudus* was referred to this subgenus by Anderson (1960) but this has been generally ignored.

Lemmiscus Thomas, 1912, type species *Arvicola curtata* Cope, now *Lagurus curtatus.*

Sumeriomys Argyropulo, 1933, type species *Mus socialis* Pallas, now *Microtus socialis*; cited here because of its involvement with *Suranomys*; the name *Sumeriomys* has not been specifically applied to any New World *Microtus.*

Suranomys Chaline, 1972, p. 142, type species *Microtus malei* Hinton, a Pleistocene species. *Microtus ratticeps, M. nivalis, M. gud,* and *M. roberti* were also assigned to the subgenus. Later, *M. operarius, M. oeconomus, M. socialis,* and *M. oregoni* were also assigned (Chaline, 1974). The type species of *Chilotus, Chionomys,* and *Sumeriomys* were all assigned to *Suranomys* and all are older names than *Suranomys.* The oldest is *Chilotus.*

Arvalomys Chaline, 1974, type species by original designation (Chaline, 1974:450) *Microtus arvalis. Arvalomys* included Old and New World species generally referred to the subgenus *Microtus* and has the same type species as *Microtus. Arva-*

lomys is therefore an objective junior synonym of *Microtus* as a subgenus.

References above that are not included in the Literature Cited section may be found in Hall (1981) or Miller (1896).

In 1912, Miller treated *Pitymys* and *Arvicola* as genera separate from *Microtus* in his book on the mammals of western Europe. He characterized *Microtus* as "restricted to the species with normal skull, palate, and enamel folding, 8 mammae, 6 plantar tubercles, and no special modifications of external form" (p. 659). In the "essential characters" of the subgenus *Microtus* in 1896, Miller also had given the following: third lower molar (m3) without closed triangles; first lower molar (m1) with five closed triangles and nine salient angles; third upper molars (M3) with three closed triangles and seven or eight salient angles; sole moderately hairy (contrasting with naked in *Neofiber,* nearly naked in *Arvicola,* thickly haired between heel and tubercles in *Pedomys,* hairy in *Eothenomys, Alticola,* and *Hyperacrius,* and very hairy in *Lagurus* and *Phaiomys*); and claws of hindfeet longest (those of forefeet longest in *Pitymys,* very long and about equal on all four feet in *Phaiomys*).

In 1926, Hinton published the first volume of a planned two volume monograph on the Microtinae (=Arvicolinae as used here). The second volume, which would have included *Microtus,* was never published, but the first volume is of interest here for several reasons. Repenning (1968) evaluated it as "the most significant single contribution to the development of an understanding of the evolution of these rodents." In it the Old World species of *Arvicola* were treated as a distinct genus. *Microtus richardsoni* of the New World was excluded from *Arvicola.* All of the subgenera recognized by Miller in 1896 were raised to genera. The Old World genus *Ellobius* was assigned to the Microtinae. The resemblence of the Malagasy genus *Brachytarsomys* to microtines was described. Hinton recognized 31 genera and subgenera (including fossil forms) in the subfamily.

The concept of arvicoline rodents as a distinct subfamily originated much earlier (Coues, *in* Coues and Allen, 1877; Gray, 1821). Hinton (1926:2) related the distinctive features of the microtines to diet and burrowing habit. Included as "general characters" (p. 5) were the following: 1) robust or thickset build; 2) head broad and flattened; 3) muzzle bluntly rounded; 4) eyes small; 5) ears small;

6) skin of trunk largely enclosing moderately long and powerful limbs (this contributes to character 1); 7) pentadactyl, but thumb reduced in size; 8) tail never very long, reaching two-thirds of the length of head and body; 9) fur tending to be soft and dense; 10) skull of firm construction (in some cases massive); 11) sagittal sutures between paired frontal, premaxillary, maxillary, and palatine bones generally fusing early (before or just after birth); 12) rostrum short; 13) eyes forward of vertical plane touching the front edges of the anterior molars; 14) zygomatic arches strongly built and more or less widely bowed laterally, zygomatic plate stout and obliquely oriented to long axis of skull; 15) palatine processes of maxillary and palatine bones enormously thickened, in correlation with hypsodonty of molars and powerful development of the jaw musculature; 16) auditory bullae well developed; 17) mandible stout, in correlation with the hypsodonty and muscular development noted under 15; 18) cheekteeth hypsodont; and 19) worn surfaces of cheekteeth displaying a pattern of triangles and transverse loops, produced by the truncation by wear of the ends of tall prismatic columns.

The above list is abstracted from detailed discussions of these and many related features. Diagnostic characters are here mingled with characters that are not peculiar to the subfamily (in the current terminology, synapomorphies are mingled with plesiomorphies). Hinton was quite aware of the difference between the concepts of apomorphy and plesiomorphy (but not the newer words, of course) and his discussion of evolution provides many interesting ideas about evolutionary changes in the group. On page 26 he summarized the most prominent characters that "sharply define" the subfamily as: the firm construction of the skull, shortened rostrum, forwardly placed orbits, peculiarly formed zygomatic plates, presence of postorbital squamosal crests or processes, the thickened palatal process of the maxillaries and palatines, and the hypsodont prismatic cheekteeth.

Although Hinton (1926) did not draw an explicit diagram of phylogenetic relationships of microtine rodents he did discuss them in sufficient detail that such a diagram can be drawn, and I have done so (Fig. 1). The broader scope of the entire subfamily represented by the diagram is helpful in considering the content of the genus *Microtus* alone, because the content is not generally agreed upon and because the same principles and characters apply at various taxonomic levels.

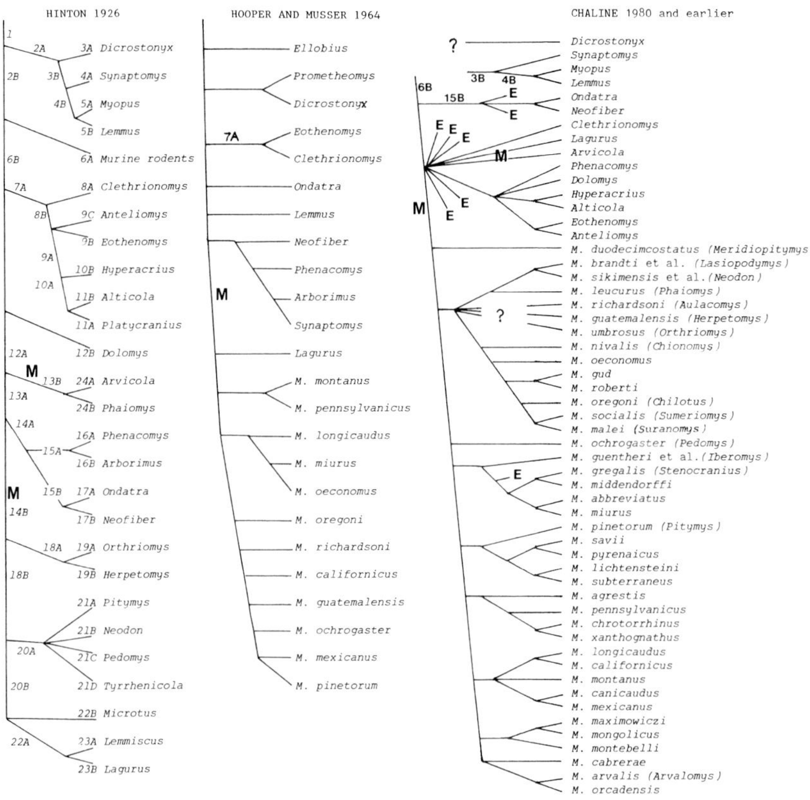

FIG. 1. Cladograms indicating hypothesized branching sequences (the reader should not infer any other meaning from the diagrams) in the evolution of Arvicolinae according to Hinton (1926; based on all characters), Hooper and Musser (1964; based on anatomy of the glans penis), and Chaline (1980; based on teeth). The lines that are labelled are for reference to selected specific characters given in text. Clades that coincide in content between the three diagrams are few and are labelled. Current authors would generally switch the positions of clades 2A and 6A and thus consider the arvicolines to be monophyletic rather than polyphyletic. Extinct lines shown are indicated by E; not all extinct lines are shown. The clade(s) labelled M belong to *Microtus* in the broad sense.

Hinton agreed with his mentor, Forsyth Major, in favoring the "multituberculate theory" of eutherian origins. The theory is that all orders of eutherian mammals descended from the multituberculates of the extinct order Allotheria and that the major trend in evolutionary change in molariform teeth was from longitudinally complex teeth to simpler teeth. This view was controversial in 1926 and no one advocates it in exactly this form today. Simplification may have occurred in some phylogenetic lineages, of course. Hinton (1926:34) reported in a footnote that "As long ago as 1914 Winge and I were comparing our views on this subject, and he told me that I had got everything upside down. No doubt others will be of the same opinion today!" Much of Hinton's discussion of evolutionary trends is quite acceptable, but in regard to the trend of molar evolution Winge (1941) may have been correct.

The evolutionary changes that Hinton postulated in each lineage of Fig. 1 (or the synapomorphies that are the basis for the hypothesis of monophyly for the lineage, in current cladistic terminology) are outlined here (in the form of a key for convenience, although it is not a key and cannot be used to identify specimens). The phylogeny is mostly dichotomous but there are multichotomies in lines 9A and 20A. Each alternative coincides with the initial lineage of a clade in the diagram. A clade is defined as any one line and all of its descendent lines. The numbers of living species noted in different groups are from Corbet and Hill (1980), Hall (1981), or Honacki et al. (1982), rather than from Hinton.

1. Skull lightly built; rostrum moderately long; temporal ridges widely separated; palate thin and flat; medial sutures of skull persistent; eyes and ears large; tail moderately long; lower incisor inferior or lingual to molars, short, not extending back of m3; cheekteeth low-crowned, rooted, multitubercular, and longitudinally complex; jaw motion transverse or oblique; incisors narrow and orthodont or opisthodont; enamel of incisors pigmented; enamel of cheekteeth even in thickness (there is no dichotomy here, these are postulated characters of primitive ancestral murine rodent) 2

2(1). A. Skull more heavily built; rostrum shortened; palate thickened and concave; medial sutures tending to fuse in skull; eyes and ears reduced; tail shortened; molar teeth becoming prismatic and occlusal surface flat, reentrant folds lacking cement, becoming hypsodont and then persistent in growth (never rooted in old age); roots of molar capsules extend on labial side of incisor root of lower jaw .... Lemmings, 3

B. Molar teeth remaining as in 1 above (no synapomorphic characters; this is what remains after the lemmings are removed) 6

3(2). A. Fur thickened and seasonally variable; limbs and tail shortened; ears reduced to mere fold; feet broadened, soles furred, pads reduced; claws enlarged, claws of manal digits 3 and 4 undergoing seasonal change in form; ulna powerfully built; incisors becoming proodont; skull becoming even heavier .... Genus *Dicrostonyx,* ten species

B. Molars simplified longitudinally, cement added in reentrant folds, strengthening teeth; incisors and other teeth broadened; salient angles of lower molars reduced on outer side and those of upper molars reduced on inner side 4

4(3). A. Incisors becoming grooved (regarded as a "memorial" of primitive cuspidate incisor); palate like that of *Microtus* .... Genus *Synaptomys,* two New World species

B. Build becoming heavier (as in 3A); palate like that of *Clethrionomys* 5

5(4). A. Bullae globular .... Genus *Myopus* (or subgenus of *Lemmus*), one Old World species; recently placed in the genus *Lemmus*

B. Size larger; skull much heavier; squamosals tending to converge anteriorly; eyes smaller; feet larger and broader; thumb nail large and flat; palmar and plantar surfaces hairy; bulla not greatly inflated, spongy within .... Genus *Lemmus,* three species

6(2). A. Molars simplified longitudinally .... Murine rodents

B. Molars becoming prismatic and flat on occlusal surface, molars becoming hypsodont, eight mammae present (presumably the characteristics of the subfamily appear here as well as in 2A, such as heavy skull, short rostrum, smaller eyes and ears, shorter tail, thicker palates, and fusion of medial cranial sutures) .... Voles, 7

7(6). A. Posterior palate shelf-like 8

B. Posterior palate with sloping median septum and lateral pits, at first septum broad and ill-defined, pits small and shallow, lateral bridges incompletely developed 12

8(7). A. Molars becoming persistent in growth 9
B. Molars rooted in adults (symplesiomorphy only) .... Genus *Clethrionomys,* seven species
9(8). A. Reentrant angles wide, teeth appear "drawn out," with little cement .... Genus *Alticola,* seven Old World species, 10
B. Mammae reduced to four .... Genus *Eothenomys,* 12 Old World species
C. Temporal ridges tending to fuse in interorbital area, complex "primitive" M3 with five or six salient angles on each side, median spine on posterior of palate .... Genus *Anteliomys*; now put in *Eothenomys*
10(9). A. (No synapomorphy postulated) 11
B. Fossorial specialization; m3 reduced in size and simplified in structure .... Subgenus *Hyperacrius*; recently treated as separate genus
11(10). A. Skull much flattened .... Subgenus *Platycranius,* one species
B. (No synapomorphy postulated) .... Subgenus *Alticola,* three species
12(7). A. Progressive hypsodonty in time; temporal ridges not meeting palate as in *Arvicola* .... Extinct genus *Mimomys,* 13
B. Tail long, fur soft .... Genus *Dolomys,* one Old World species; now called *Dinaromys*
13(12). A. (This dichotomy was only vaguely defined by Hinton, as separate discussions of a *Mimomys* to *Arvicola* line and another line from *Phenacomys*-like to *Microtus* and other genera). Eyes and ears moderately large; feet normal; tail moderately long; rostrum moderately long; interorbital region broad; temporal ridges separate (these are all primitive traits listed under initial lineage 1) 14
B. Molars growing persistently; palate further developed to *Microtus*-form; temporal ridges meeting; bullae developing some internal bony trabeculae; stapedial artery enclosed in bone (all of these traits are present also in one or more of the branches of 13A) 24

14(13). A. Bullae small and globular, without internal trabeculae; stapedial artery naked as it nears stapes; m3 not displaced by shaft of lower incisor which passes below it 15
B. Molars becoming persistent in growth .... Genus *Microtus* in a broad sense, 18
15(14). A. Lower molars with long inner salient angles; groove between alveoli of cheekteeth and ascending ramus not "pocketed" .... New World Genus *Phenacomys* in its broadest sense, 16
B. Palate simple; stapedial artery in bony tube; interorbital area narrow; aquatic modifications of feet and fur; size large 17
16(15). A. (No synapomorphies) .... Genus *Phenacomys,* one New World species
B. Arboreal; tail long .... Genus *Arborimus,* two New World species
17(15). A. Size larger .... Genus *Ondatra,* one New World species
B. Molars becoming persistent in growth .... Genus *Neofiber,* one New World species
18(14). A. Median interorbital crest; m3 has closed triangles; m1 with variable number of triangles, three to five; inguinal mammae lost .... "Mexican line," 19
B. m3 without closed triangles 20
19(18). A. Bullae smaller .... Subgenus *Orthriomys, Microtus umbrosus* only
B. Bullae larger (derived feature) .... Subgenus *Herpetomys, Microtus guatemalensis* only
20(18). A. m1 with only three closed triangles, triangles 4 and 5 are confluent .... *Pitymys* generic group, 21
B. m1 with five closed triangles .... *Microtus-Lagurus* line, 22
21(20). A. Fossorial specialization; eyes small; ears small; tail short; large hands; moderately hairy soles; pelage short and dense; four or six mammae; skull rather smooth; braincase more or less depressed .... Genus *Pitymys*
B. Temporal ridges fused in interorbital region in adults; eight mammae; fur full and soft; ears evident above fur; bullae moderately large; mastoid not inflated .... Genus *Neodon,* one Old World species

C. Temporal ridges fused; six mammae; fur long and coarse; ears concealed in fur; bullae small; mastoid inflated .... Genus *Pedomys,* one New World species
D. Face long; bullae small .... Extinct genus *Tyrrhenicola*

22(20). A. Bullae enlarged, cancellous; reentrant angles lack cement; soles hairy .... Genus *Lagurus,* 23
B. (No synapomorphies; this is what is left after the distinctive *Lagurus* is removed) .... Genus *Microtus* (in a restricted sense)

23(22). A. Lemming-like externally, with short tail; m3 with four closed triangles and two outer salient angles (synapomorphies) .... Subgenus *Lagurus,* two Old World species; three species have been recognized recently and two of these have been placed in a separate genus, *Eolagurus*
B. Less lemming-like, tail not so short; m3 with 3 closed triangles and two outer salient angles .... Subgenus *Lemmiscus,* one New World species

24(13). A. Size medium to large; skull massive, strongly ridged when adult; squamosals approach each other anteriorly; bullae small, few trabeculae within; aquatic modifications; palms and soles naked .... Subgenus *Arvicola,* two Old World species
B. Size small to medium; skull less massive; squamosals well separated; bullae large, dense spongy bone within; fossorial modifications; fur long and soft; palms and soles densely haired, pads concealed .... Genus *Phaiomys,* one species; placed with *Pitymys* by Corbet and Hill (1980)

Hinton's phylogeny has some questionable features, beyond the need to add newer knowledge and to reevaluate many of the characters used. It postulates a polyphyletic derivation of the Arvicolinae from murine rodents, "much later divergence from the primitive Murine stock by Microti than by Lemmi" (Hinton, 1926:40). This conclusion results from the weight accorded the multituberculate theory and results in the necessity of postulating multiple origins of various characters, including most of the diverse features that characterize the Arvicolinae. This raises the question as to which, if any, taxa should be polyphyletic. The development of persistently growing molar teeth is postulated to have occurred at least five different times (in lineages 2A, 8A, 13B, and 14B). This raises the usual questions about relative importance ("weighting") of different characters and about the role of parsimony in classification. Some of the taxa recognized are not defined by synapomorphies, but are what is left after small monophyletic groups are removed from larger monophyletic groups. For example, the genus *Microtus* (as represented by 22B) is merely what is left after *Lagurus* (22A) is removed from 20B; the genus *Clethrionomys* (8B) is what is left after 8A is removed from 7A; and the subgenus *Alticola* (11B) is what is left after 10B and 11A are removed from 9A. These are examples of results achieved by what I will describe as the "artichoke method."

In 1941, Ellerman published volume 2 in his monumental compilation on the families and genera of living rodents. In regard to names that have been used for North American *Microtus,* he largely followed Hinton in treating the following as separate genera: *Neofiber, Lagurus, Orthriomys, Herpetomys, Pitymys, Arvicola* (excluding *Microtus richardsoni*), *Pedomys,* and *Microtus.* Ellerman used the following as subgenera within the genus *Microtus*: *Microtus, Aulacomys* (for *M. richardsoni*), *Stenocranius,* and *Chilotus. Chionomys* was disregarded in his classification as being poorly defined.

In 1953, Hall and Cockrum published a synopsis of North American microtine rodents. They recognized *Neofiber, Lagurus,* and *Microtus* as separate genera and recognized within *Microtus* the subgenera *Microtus, Herpetomys, Orthriomys, Aulacomys, Chilotus, Stenocranius, Pitymys,* and *Pedomys.* Subsequent American authors have tended to follow this grouping.

Because of uncertainty as to the limits of the genus, the planners of this volume arbitrarily agreed to use the content of the genus *Microtus* in North America as treated by Hall and Cockrum (1953) and after them Hall and Kelson (1959) in order that the coverage of the different chapters would be comparable.

Hall subsequently (1981) dropped the use of the subgeneric names *Herpetomys, Orthriomys,* and *Chilotus,* and changed *Aulacomys* back to synonymy in *Arvicola.*

Hooper and Musser (1964) published a phylogenetic diagram for arvicolines based on the anatomy of the glans penis alone (mostly following Hooper and Hart, 1962). The diagram was drawn rather subjectively in order to summarize general clusters and different degrees of phenetic distinctness as well as branching sequences. The characters that were the bases for each detail of the diagram were not explicitly listed. For purposes of comparison and discussion I extracted the very tentative cladistic relationships implied by the branching sequence alone (ignoring lengths of side branches and distances between branching points) and compared this cladogram with that drawn from Hinton's work. Other than the terminal twigs (mostly genera and subgenera), only one postulated clade coincided (7A from Hinton was represented by a common clade for *Eothenomys* and *Clethrionomys,* the only twigs examined among the six twigs of 7A).

Kretzoi (1969) outlined a phylogeny for arvicolines but did not include any diagram of branching relationships.

In an essay outlining the evolutionary branching of arvicolines based on dental morphology (mostly not described in the essay), Chaline (1980) presented a pattern combining anagenesis (in which a fossil taxon changes into another taxon without branching) and cladogenesis (in which one line branches into two or more, in one case about 10 and in another about 15). I drew a branching diagram to represent Chaline's phylogeny based on this and earlier papers (Chaline, 1974, 1975*a,* 1975*b*) and compared it with the diagrams drawn from Hinton (1926) and Hooper and Musser (1964). Other than the terminal twigs themselves, only four clades coincided (see Fig. 1).

Since there presumably was only one actual phylogeny and since we have more than one hypothetical phylogeny and little agreement among them, it is clear that more work is needed here.

History of Systematics at the Species Level

The pivotal study at the level of species in the systematics of North American *Microtus* was Bailey's (1900) revision. Bailey used the same generic content and subgenera that Miller (1896) used and set the stage for a reduction in the number of recognized species by defining ten species groups within the subgenus *Microtus* and by recognizing a number of subspecies. Bailey's own words (1900: 9) clearly summarized the nature of his contribution to the advancement of systematic knowledge of the genus: "It is not many years since certain prominent writers treated as mere varieties, or subspecies, animals that belong to widely different subgenera, while

TABLE 1

THE DEVELOPMENT OF TAXONOMY FOR NORTH AMERICAN *Microtus* AS DEMONSTRATED BY A SERIES OF COMPREHENSIVE SUMMARIES OF NUMBERS OF TAXA*

Taxon	Number			
	Bailey (1900)	Miller (1923)	Hall and Cockrum (1953)	Hall (1981)
Species	48	52	25	22
Monotypic species	37	37	10	8
Subspecies	29	57	122	131

* *Lagurus* and *Neofiber* are excluded.

others described and named with full specific rank every different condition of pelage in a single species. In some cases the original type was not preserved, or no type was designated by the describer, or still worse, the type locality was not given, so that subsequent writers renamed these same species or confounded them with others. The resulting confusion can now be cleared up by means of series of specimens collected within the past ten years at most of the known type localities, and in the general region of those not definitely known. The series of specimens available, and the number of localities represented, make it possible to define almost every North American species from typical specimens, and in most cases to give the various changes of pelage due to season and age."

For the benefit of the readers who may not be familiar with examples of the earlier taxonomic treatments to which Bailey was referring, "certain prominent writers" who "treated as mere varieties, or subspecies, animals that belong to widely different subgenera" probably referred to Coues and Allen (1877). Other writers who "described and named with full specific rank every condition of pelage in a single species" can be found listed in the synonymy (Hall, 1981) of *Microtus pennsylvanicus pennsylvanicus* where the names themselves, such as *hirsutus, alborufescens,* and *fulva,* suggest that trivial features of the pelage were involved.

The developing taxonomy for North American *Microtus* may be examined by comparing a series of comprehensive summaries: Bailey in 1900, Miller in 1923, Hall and Cockrum in 1953, and Hall in 1981 (Table 1).

The number of names that had been proposed as species names

prior to 1900 was 74, of which 26 were reduced to subspecific status or synonymized by Bailey (1900). Prior to Bailey's (1900) revision, and mostly in the three years before 1900, 11 names had been proposed as subspecies of previously recognized species (not counting the nominate subspecies created thereby) and one species had been reduced to subspecies. Other names had lapsed into complete synonymy, not being recognized as subspecies.

Between 1900 and 1953 the following changes occurred. In Bailey's (1900) *pennsylvanicus*-group of seven species, revisionary changes reduced the number of recognized species to three. In 1908, Bangs named a new species in this group, *M. provectus*. New subspecies were named in 1901, 1920, 1940, 1948, and in 1951. (The taxonomic names, authors, and bibliographic references are readily available in Hall, 1981, and other sources and need not be given here. The dates are given to provide a general view of the chronology.) Bailey's *montanus*-group of five species was reduced to a single species, and new subspecies were named in 1914, 1935, 1938, 1941, and 1952. Bailey's *californicus*-group of three species was reduced to one species in 1918 and new subspecies were named in 1922, 1926, 1928, 1931, 1935, and 1937. In Bailey's (1900) *operarius*-group of seven species, reductions in recognized species were made in 1942 by Zimmermann who regarded it as conspecific with *Microtus oeconomus* of the Old World. New subspecies were described in 1909, 1932, and 1952. The two species in Bailey's *townsendii*-group were treated as subspecies in 1936. New subspecies were recognized in 1936, 1940, and 1943. In Bailey's *longicaudus*-group of five species, a reduction in recognized species was made in 1938. Several new subspecies were named between 1922 and 1938. In 1911 a new insular species in this group, *M. coronarius,* was named. In Bailey's *mexicanus*-group of three species, a reduction in recognized species was made in 1932 and new subspecies were named in 1902, 1934, 1938, and 1948. Bailey's *xanthognathus*-group has never included anything except *Microtus xanthognathus*. His *chrotorrhinus*-group was essentially redundant with his species *Microtus chrotorrhinus,* which included two subspecies. A third subspecies was named in 1932. In regard to Bailey's subgenus *Pitymys,* we note that in 1898 he named *Microtus pinetorum nemoralis,* but in his revision of 1900, perhaps as a lapsus, he used the name *Microtus nemoralis*. In 1916, Howell named *Pitymys parvulus*. New subspecies of *Pitymys* were named in 1941 and 1952. In 1912, Thomas removed *Lagurus* from the genus *Microtus,* and this treatment has been followed by other authors since. The three species of Bailey's subgenus *Chilotus* were treated as subspecies of *Microtus oregoni* in 1920. New subspecies were named in 1908 and 1920. Three of the four species in Bailey's subgenus *Pedomys* were treated as subspecies of *Microtus ochrogaster* in 1907. New subspecies of *M. ochrogaster* were named in 1942 and 1943.

In 1920, Howell and Harper both used *Neofiber* as a genus separate from *Microtus* as Chapman had done in 1889. Merriam (1891) had reduced *Neofiber* to a subgenus of *Microtus.* Miller (1896) and Bailey (1900) treated *Neofiber* as a subgenus of *Microtus* and provided diagnostic characters and comparisons. Subsequent authors who used *Neofiber* as a genus (including Harper, 1920; Howell, 1920; and Schwartz, 1953) did not state why it should be treated as a genus instead of a subgenus. As noted above, Ellerman (1941) and Hinton (1926) raised most of Miller's subgenera of *Microtus* to separate genera, including *Neofiber.* Martin (1979) did not connect the base of the phylogenetic line leading to *Neofiber* with either *Microtus* or *Ondatra.*

In 1901, Osgood named *Microtus miurus* and in 1907 he named a subspecies thereof. New species of similar *Microtus* from the same region (Alaska and vicinity) were named in 1931, 1945, and 1947. In 1952, Hall and Cockrum reduced these all to subspecies of *M. miurus.*

In the years from 1953 to 1981 the following taxonomic changes were made. The species *Microtus provectus* was reduced to a subspecies of *M. pennsylvanicus* in 1954. New subspecies of *M. pennsylvanicus* were named in 1956, 1967, and 1968. Youngman (1967) considered *breweri* and *nesophilus* to be subspecies of *M. pennsylvanicus.* The species *Microtus canicaudus* was separated from *M. montanus* in 1970. New subspecies of *M. montanus* were named in 1954. In *Microtus californicus* a new subspecies was named in 1961. In 1966, Goodwin named a new species, *Microtus oaxacensis.*

In *Microtus townsendii,* a new subspecies was named in 1955. The species *Microtus oeconomus* was revised in 1961 by Paradiso and Manville. Hall (1981) pointed out that *oeconomus* may not be the correct name for the North American populations now referred to *Microtus oeconomus.* The correct name may be *ratticeps* or *kamtschaticus,* but until the question can be resolved it may be desireable to continue with *oeconomus.* In 1960 a new subspecies of *Microtus longicaudus* was named. *Microtus ludovicianus* was reduced to subspecific status in *M. ochrogaster* in 1972 and in 1977 a new subspecies of *M. ochrogaster* was named. *Microtus fulviventer* was reduced to subspecific status in *M. mexicanus* in 1964 and in 1955 a new subspecies of *M. mexicanus* was named. *Microtus parvulus* was made a subspecies of *M. pinetorum* in 1952. A new subspecies of *Microtus richardsoni* was named in 1959. *Microtus miurus* was regarded as conspecific with *Microtus gregalis* of the Old World by some authors but was again treated as a separate species in 1970 by Fedyk. *Microtus nemoralis* was regarded by Repenning (1983) as a species separate from *M. pinetorum* and more closely related to *M. quasiater, M. meadensis* (fossil), and Old World *Pitymys,* which was regarded as a genus separate from *Microtus.*

The taxonomic history described above and represented in Fig. 2 exhibits several rather different phases, as follows.

1) 1815 to 1860. Initial scattered exploration in which about half of the full species now recognized were discovered—34 supposed species were named; a rather typological view was common; and adequate series of specimens to enable workers to escape the typological (small sample) perspective were not available.

2) 1860 to 1890. Not much happened—few new names were proposed; and few specimens were obtained.

3) 1890 to 1900. The most productive decade in the taxonomic history of North American *Microtus*—most of the remaining full species now recognized were discovered; the mass produced break-back mouse trap was available; the U.S. Government was persuaded by C. Hart Merriam to launch the great explorations of the Biological Survey; large series of specimens were obtained; variation within and between populations became obvious; a polytypic concept of the species supplanted the typological concept; subspecies names were used more often; the winnowing process began, the number of monotypic species began to decline, and the number of recognized species increased noticeably more slowly than the number of names being proposed for species.

4) 1900 to 1920. The new forces initiated just before 1900 continued their development but at a slower rate—revisionary work continued on a species by species basis; the numbers of proposed species increased more slowly than before, and the numbers of recognized species increased slowly and then ceased to increase; the number of monotypic species did not change; and the number of

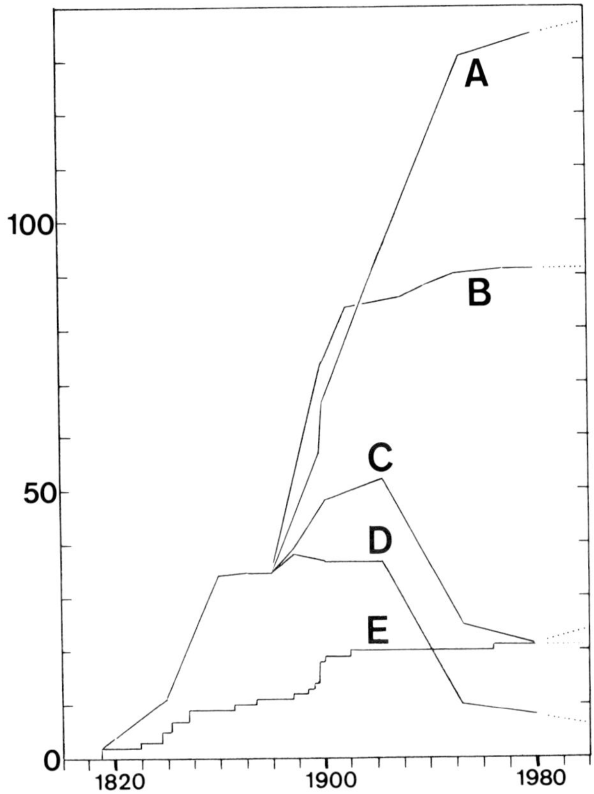

FIG. 2. Taxonomic history of North American *Microtus* (excluding *Lagurus* and *Neofiber*, as most authors have done in recent decades). A, cumulative number of recognized subspecies and monotypic species; B, cumulative number of names of species proposed; C, number of species recognized as valid at different times; D, number of monotypic species recognized at different times; E, cumulative number of species proposed among those recognized as valid in 1980.

recognized subspecies continued to increase rapidly as continued field work filled in details of geographic variation within species.

5) 1920 to 1950. Further consolidation—the number of recognized species decreased rapidly as monotypic species became subspecies of polytypic ones following the discovery of intergradation; few new species were proposed and these were quickly synonymized; and the numbers of recognized subspecies continued to increase rapidly.

6) 1950 to 1980. Maturation of the period of alpha taxonomy—fewer distinctive subspecies were discovered and a reaction against continued subspecific splitting occurred; only one new species was proposed; and the decline in numbers of recognized species continued gradually and now approaches an equilibrium.

Discussion of Systematic Viewpoints

In this section I examine the systematic approaches that Miller, Hinton, and others have used in classifying Arvicolinae, outline some needs for future taxonomic research, and discuss the effect upon taxonomy of a major pattern of macroevolution.

Miller (1896:24) rationalized his synthesis of genera in the following terms: "In the present paper the classification used is based on an assemblage of characters. The more important of these, or the ones least adapted to the special needs of the different animals, and hence least likely to vary, are: Form of skull, structure of bony palate, pattern of enamel folding, number of mammae, number of plantar tubercles, and presence or absence of musk glands on the sides. Characters of less importance, because more readily modified to fit a species to the special requirements of its environment, and hence more unstable, are: Quality of fur, hairiness of soles, length of tail, form of front feet, size of eyes, and form of external ear. It is only through careful consideration of all these that a satisfactory arrangement of the species can be obtained."

This is certainly better than no explanation, which is what many authors have provided when creating and changing rodent taxonomy. Nevertheless, Miller's statement does not provide any explicit guidelines on how "careful consideration" will lead to "a satisfactory arrangement." The systematic theory was still murky.

In contrast, Hinton's (1926) point of view seems almost contemporary in theory. He wrote (1926:5) that "if the more or less substantial mask of specialization be stripped off from each species one finds the primitive core of each animal underneath; if the primitive characters so found be used as the bases of comparison there is no difficulty either in arranging species, genera, and families in natural order, or in conceiving what the essential characters of the ancestor common to any given group must have been. That is what I have attempted to do in this chapter. The stripping process is, however, by no means easy, and it reveals many a disconcerting gap in our knowledge." I take it that "the essential characters of the ancestor common to any given group" means about the same as "synapomorphies" in much of the current cladistic literature (see Nelson and Platnick, 1981, for a comprehensive summary).

Hinton, however, did not complete his work on the genus *Microtus* and he did not apply the theory in order to postulate relationships other than the contents of groups recognized by names in his formal classification.

Bailey (1900) dealt with problems of alpha taxonomy. What are the species? How do they vary geographically? What are their polytypic morphological limits? Exactly where do they occur geographically and ecologically? The theory here relates to the nature of biological species, whether they exist and, if so, how they may be recognized? These questions have attracted most of the taxonomic attention in the genus *Microtus* since 1900.

Less attention has been given to examining relationships above the species level in *Microtus* or among arvicoline rodents generally, either in theory or practice.

One method commonly used in arvicoline taxonomy (and in most other groups for that matter) I call the "artichoke method." The analogy is to the fact that the outer leaves of an artichoke are more conspicuous than the inner ones and when one takes an artichoke apart one usually begins with the most conspicuous part, then takes the next most conspicuous leaf, etc. Some taxonomists follow the same pattern. For example, if the keys to Murinae or Microtinae in Ellerman (1941) are examined, it seems that the most peculiar and thus conspicuous form is pulled off first, then the next most conspicuous, etc. Since the species that are unusually conspicuous morphologically tend to be rare in nature and since the most common specimens tend to be of some less conspicuous species, the keys are inefficient and frustrating to use for most identifications. There is no agreement as to how many successively less conspicuous species one should remove from the core of the genus and call subgenera. As the degree of distinctness becomes less and less, the decision as to which of the remaining species is most distinct becomes more and more difficult to make. Eventually, even the most ardent splitter usually gives up before the final split is made and complete redundancy of species and subgenus is reached.

The artichoke method is generally phenetic in that the most conspicuously different item or small subset of items in the cluster is singled out for separation. The taxonomist is usually not hypothesizing a cladistic relationship, although in some cases this is done.

The existing classification of most groups of mammals, and of the genus *Microtus* in particular, has resulted from an eclectic interaction of several different procedures: 1) an initial recognition and naming of distinctive (and presumably often monophyletic) groups at various levels (for example, the subclass Eutheria, the order Rodentia, the subfamily Arvicolinae, the genus *Microtus*); 2) the singling out and naming of species (or small groups of species that are unusually distinctive in a phenetic sense, without any necessary hypothesis of cladistic relationship (the artichoke method; for example, the subgenera *Chilotus, Pedomys, Aulacomys, Orthriomys*); 3) the naming of "left-over groups" for consistency rather than because of any clearcut hypothesis of monophyly (for example, after the presumably distinctive and mostly monotypic subgenera in the genus *Microtus* are named, what is left, which is most of the species in the genus, is called the subgenus *Microtus*). The tradition of "consistency" is practiced at all of the non-obligatory levels of the classification. One is not obligated to use subgenera, but if any subgenus is recognized in a genus all of the species must be put in some subgenus. The "left-over" subgenus may have no distinctive features in common except the shared derived features of the genus. In this case, the subgeneric arrangement does not necessarily imply anything about geneological or cladistic relationships among the species within the genus. It indicates only that a few are phenetically more peculiar than the others. The left over groups may be paraphyletic and in one sense are permitted by our ignorance rather than sustained by our knowledge. They are not exactly comparable to what have been called "wastebasket" groups, which may be admittedly polyphyletic or paraphyletic, but like the "wastebasket" groups they are not conceived to be strictly monophyletic (holophyletic).

There is still much interesting work to be done in refining the analyses of geographic variation within species whether or not one chooses to use subspecies names. Slightly differentiated but nonetheless distinct sibling species probably remain to be detected by a combination of old and new methods of study. Relationships between populations in the Old World and the New World need careful examination at the species level.

The major unfinished taxonomic tasks, however, are above the species level in the hierarchy of classification. In my opinion, the role of taxonomy should be to describe and interpret relationships at all levels from local populations or demes on up. The traditional levels such as genus, subgenus, species, and subspecies are somewhat arbitrary and their existence may lead to unwarranted emphases, such as the idea that something with a name is more important than something without a name. This leads either to the disregard of important things or to a stultifying and unstable proliferation of names. If there are 20–25 species of *Microtus* in North America and if that number is not likely to change much, our task has not ended. What needs to be done now is to study the relationships at all levels among these species, a task that has barely begun.

Many published reports of newly studied biological features are sufficiently comparative to have taxonomic implications. The authors have generally avoided the sort of uncritical enthusiasm for single characters that led to some of the classifications proposed for arvicolines prior to Miller's (1896) major revision. There has been no major taxonomic synthesis of these fascinating newer developments. The needed syntheses may be conducted either among all arvicolines or within smaller groups such as *Microtus*, and should integrate a number of different features. It is not possible to do it all at once. Any reasonably comprehensive and careful synthesis can serve as the hypothesis of relationships for further testing with other characters. It will be better if authors do not feel compelled to express all of the hypothesized relationships in a formal classification. I suspect that knowledge of the fate of earlier single-character classification combined with the deplorable idea that only formal named taxa are important in taxonomy (which is equivalent to the current view of some cladists that all hypothesized relationships *should* be expressed in formal classification) may actually inhibit progress in arvicoline taxonomy.

The following is merely a sample of papers on diverse features recently studied in rodents that might eventually be used in these taxonomic syntheses: myology (Repenning, 1968); male reproductive anatomy, including bacula, soft parts, and accessory glands (Anderson, 1960; Arata, 1964; Hooper and Hart, 1962); meibomian glands in eyelids (Hrabě, 1978; Quay, 1954*a*); skin glands (Jannett, 1975; Quay, 1968); diastemal palate (Quay, 1954*b*); behavior (Gray and Dewsbury, 1975; Jannett and Jannett, 1974); chromosomes, including gross karyology and finer structure seen in

G- and C-banding studies (Matthey, 1957); cranial foramina (Wahlert, 1978); basicranial circulation (Bugge, 1974); stomach anatomy (Carleton, 1981); blood chemistry, including enzymes and hemoglobin (Nadler et al., 1978); and DNA sequencing.

Characters used in older classifications need reexamination also. Potentially useful systematic information may come from any comparative biological study.

Since 1950, considerable thought and verbiage have been devoted to taxonomic methods and objectives. The ideas of numerical taxonomy burst upon the scene in the 1950s, emanating chiefly from the University of Kansas, where I was at the time. The ideas of cladistic taxonomy burst upon the scene in the 1970s, emanating chiefly from the American Museum of Natural History, where I was at the time. My presence was a coincidence, and I was, and still am, somewhat skeptical about some of the assumptions, methods, and goals of each school. Both schools have contributed importantly to systematics. In any event, no one has yet published applications of the precepts and methods of either numerical phenetics or present day cladistics to the classification of *Microtus*.

My taxonomic viewpoint is basically phylogenetic or cladistic, but it differs in some ways from other cladistic viewpoints, such as those summarized by Cracraft (1981) in a recent discussion of bird classification. His references or the book by Nelson and Platnick (1981) will lead the interested reader to the chief summaries of the cladistic school, so I will not document these sources. A recent study by Marshall (1980) of caenolestid marsupials illustrates a useful application of the method, in my opinion.

Assuming that a convincing case for the monophyletic status of the genus *Microtus* can be made, it will be quite valuable to attempt to develop a complete phylogenetic hypothesis of the relationships of the species. Eventually this will need to include all species, both New and Old World. This is a challenging task, but cannot be done here. I attempted earlier in this chapter to abstract from Hinton's extended discussions the phylogenetic gist and I found that some lines were defined by shared primitive (symplesiomorphic) characters only.

A group now defined by shared primitive features may have unnoted synapomorphies. If these are discovered, the group may then be regarded as monophyletic. The point here is that primitive and derived states have different meanings in taxonomy. Other things being equal (which they rarely are in reality), it might be better to have monophyletic taxa than paraphyletic or polyphyletic taxa, and it might be better to postulate a more parsimonious phylogeny than one with parallelisms and character reversals. Nevertheless, uncertainties do exist about character states and directions of evolutionary change, and paraphyletic taxa will continue to be recognized. I see no way to avoid these problems. What is important is to have a reasonably clear understanding of our concepts. If our present concept of the genus *Microtus* seems to be paraphyletic, we should acknowledge this. We can continue to use the concept, at least until we have something better.

In regard to parsimony, I am neither a numerical cladist nor numerical pheneticist. I do not think that since it is difficult to decide which, if any, characters are more important it is better to regard all characters as equally important. The most parsimonious phylogeny for a given set of characters may not be the most acceptable one. One very peculiar feature may outweigh three simple features.

A nested hierarchy of taxa in biological classification preceded any explicit notion of evolution and was not, therefore, conceptually dependent upon evolution. The evolutionary idea of a branching tree is, however, not only consistent with a nested hierarchy, but seems to provide the best general explanation for the occurrence of the hierarchy of characters and taxa. The degree to which it is possible to hypothesize or to know what the actual phylogenetic tree may have been and the degree to which this understanding should be or can be expressed in classification are moot points. In the classification of mammals (and of arvicoline rodents in particular), it is my impression that authors with fairly definite ideas about the existence of monophyletic groups have tended to name these groups in their classifications, but not all named groups are accompanied by explicit hypotheses of monophyly.

Let us now briefly consider the nearly universal "hollow curve" frequency distribution found in nature, including the nested sets of our biological classifications, and how this relates to the artichoke method in taxonomy.

The prevalence of hollow-curve frequency distributions in taxonomic data sets was documented in some detail by me earlier (Anderson, 1974). In general, if within some larger group the numbers of subgroups (at any given level of the hierarchy) containing different numbers of items are plotted as a frequency diagram, a deeply concave or "hollow" curve will result. For example, if the numbers of genera of living mammals containing different numbers of species are plotted, half of the genera contain one species, and most of the species are included in a small percentage of the genera. The pattern exists in nature; it is not an artifact of the method of clustering for the same pattern is seen in the results of phenetic study, cladistic study, or eclectic study. The pattern is apparent in North American *Microtus* where about half the species belong to the subgenus *Microtus* and the other six subgenera share the other half. Given the pattern it is possible to predict how many successive branching points are likely to be present in a maximally resolved cladogram for a group of any size (Anderson, 1975). Given 61 species of *Microtus* (New and Old World, and including *Pitymys*; Corbet and Hill, 1980), about 11 categories would be needed between species and genus if all branchings in the phylogeny were to be expressed in a formal classification.

To summarize where I think the taxonomy of *Microtus* should go from here, I note the following. To ask whether *Pitymys* should be considered a distinct genus or a subgenus of *Microtus* is not an especially interesting question, to me. Some interesting questions are: 1) Do the species of *Pitymys* share distinctive peculiarities? 2) If so, is this because they have descended from a common ancestor that had those peculiarities? 3) Or (as an alternative) are the species of *Pitymys* the ends of a number of separate lineages of *Microtus* that have become more fossorial than most *Microtus*? These may or may not be easy questions to answer, but they should be examined and answered to whatever degree possible. The focus of the investigation should be on the characters and on relationships rather than on names or arbitrary categories. After a reasonably well-established hypothesis of relationships exists, nomenclature and classification should be addressed. Sometimes, I think, we taxonomists get the cart before the horse.

There will be differences of opinion about what is interesting or important, about phenetic versus cladistic criteria for "relationships," about the value of stability, and about other matters in this entire procedure. I don't think a general consensus now exists in systematic mammalogy in regard to these details. I would not insist that everyone agree with me. What I would try to encourage, however, as an author, reviewer, and editor, is that assumptions, viewpoints, objectives, and methods be indicated clearly. When this is done, a person with a different point of view can at least evaluate the author's accomplishment in terms of the author's goals and also relate the study to different viewpoints.

Literature Cited

ANDERSON, S. 1960. The baculum in microtine rodents. Univ. Kansas Publ. Mus. Nat. Hist., 12:181-216.

———. 1974. Patterns of faunal evolution. Quart. Rev. Biol., 49:311-332.

———. 1975. On the number of categories in biological classifications. Amer. Mus. Novitates, 2584:1-9.

ARATA, A. 1964. The anatomy and taxonomic significance of the male accessory reproductive glands of muroid rodents. Bull. Florida State Mus., Biol. Sci., 9:1-42.

BAILEY, V. 1900. Revision of American voles of the genus *Microtus*. N. Amer. Fauna, 17:1-88.

BUGGE, J. 1974. The cephalic arterial system in insectivores, primates, rodents and lagomorphs, with special reference to the systematic classification. Acta Anat., Suppl., 62:1-160.

CARLETON, M. D. 1980. Phylogenetic relationships in neotomine-peromyscine rodents (Muroidea) and a reappraisal of the dichotomy within New World Cricetinae. Misc. Publ. Mus. Zool., Univ. Michigan, 157:1-146.

———. 1981. A survey of gross stomach morphology in Microtinae (Rodentia: Muroidea). Z. Saugetierk., 46:93-108.

CARLETON, M. D., AND G. G. MUSSER. 1984. Muroid rodents. *In* Orders and families of recent mammals of the world (S. Anderson and J. K. Jones, Jr. eds.). Wiley, New York, 686 pp.

CHALINE, J. 1972. Les rongeurs du Pléistocène moyen at supérieur de France. Cah. Paléontol., Cent. Natl. Rech. Sci., 410 pp. + 17 plates.

———. 1974. Esquisse de l'evolution morphologique, biométrique, et chromosomique du genre *Microtus* (Arvicolidae, Rodentia) dans le Pléistocene de l'hemisphere Nord. Bull. Soc. Geol. France, 16:440-450.

———. 1975*a*. Evolution et rapports phylétiques des Campagnols (Arvicolidae, Rodentia) apparentés à *Dolomys* et *Pliomys* dans l'hémisphère Nord. Compt. Rend. hebd. Seanc. Acad. Sci., Paris, Ser. D, 281:33-36.

———. 1975*b*. Taxonomie des Campagnols (Arvicolidae, Rodentia) de la sous-famille des Dolomyinae no. dans l'hémisphère Nord. Compt. Rend. hedb. Seanc. Acad. Sci., Paris, Ser. D, 281:115-118.

———. 1980. Essai de filiation des campagnols et des lemmings (Arvicolidae, Rodentia) en zone Holarctique d'apres la morphologie dentaire. Palaeovertebrata, Montpellier, Mem Jubil. R. Lavocat, pp. 375-382.

CHALINE, J., P. MEIN, AND F. PETTER. 1977. Les grandes lignes d'une classification évolutive des Muroidea. Mammalia, 41:245-252.

CORBET, C. B., AND J. E. HILL. 1980. A world list of mammalian species. Cornell Univ. Press, Ithaca, New York, 226 pp.

COUES, E., AND J. A. ALLEN. 1877. Monographs of North American Rodentia. *In* Report of the United States geological survey of the territories (F. V. Hayden, ed.), 11:1-1091.

CRACRAFT, J. 1981. Toward a phylogenetic classification of the Recent birds of the world (Class Aves). Auk, 98:681–714.

ELLERMAN, J. R. 1941. The families and genera of living rodents. Volume II. Family Muridae. British Museum, London, 690 pp.

GRAY, G. D., AND D. A. DEWSBURY. 1975. A quantitative description of the copulatory behavior of meadow voles (*Microtus pennsylvanicus*). Anim. Behav., 23:261–267.

GRAY, J. E. 1821. On the natural arrangement of vertebrose animals. London Med. Reposit., 15(1):296–310.

HALL, E. R. 1981. The mammals of North America. John Wiley, New York, 2:601–1181 + *90*.

HALL, E. R., AND E. L. COCKRUM. 1953. A synopsis of the North American microtine rodents. Univ. Kansas Publ. Mus. Nat. Hist., 5:373–498.

HALL, E. R., AND K. R. KELSON. 1959. The mammals of North America. Ronald Press, New York, 2:547–1083 + *79*.

HARPER, F. 1920. The Florida water-rat (*Neofiber alleni*) in Okefinokee Swamp, Georgia. J. Mamm., 1:65–66, plate 3.

HINTON, M. A. C. 1926. Monograph of the voles and lemmings (Microtinae) living and extinct. British Museum, London 488 pp. + 15 plates.

HONACKI, J. H., K. E. KINMAN, AND J. W. KEOPPL (EDS.). 1982. Mammal species of the world. Allen Press and Association of Systematics Collections, Lawrence, Kansas, 694 pp.

HOOPER, E. T., AND B. S. HART. 1962. A synopsis of Recent North American microtine rodents. Misc. Publ. Mus. Zool., Univ. Michigan, 151:1–68.

HOOPER, E. T., AND G. G. MUSSER. 1964. The glans penis in Neotropical cricetines (Family Muridae) with comments on the classification of muroid rodents. Misc. Publ. Mus. Zool., Univ. Michigan, 123:1–57.

HOWELL, A. H. 1920. Description of a new race of the Florida water-rat (*Neofiber alleni*). J. Mamm., 1:79–80.

HRABĚ, V. 1978. Tarsal glands of voles of the genus Pitymys (Microtidae, Mammalia) from southern Austria. Folia Zool., 27:123–128.

JANNETT, F. J., JR. 1975. 'Hip glands' of *Microtus pennsylvanicus* and *M. longicaudus* (Rodentia: Muridae), voles without hip glands. Syst. Zool., 24:171–175.

JANNETT, F. J., JR., AND J. Z. JANNETT. 1974. Drum-marking by *Arvicola richardsoni* and its taxonomic significance. Amer. Midland Nat., 92:230–234.

KIRKLAND, G. L., AND F. J. JANNETT, JR. 1982. *Microtus chrotorrhinus*. Mamm. Species, 180:1–5.

KRETZOI, M. 1969. Skize einer Arvicoliden-Phylogenie Stand 1969. Vertebrata hungarica, 11/1-2:155–193.

MARSHALL, L. G. 1980. Systematics of the South American marsupial family Caenolestidae. Fieldiana (Geol.), 5:1–145.

MARTIN, L. D. 1979. The biostratigraphy of arvicoline rodents in North America. Trans. Nebraska Acad. Sci., 7:91–100.

MATTHEY, R. 1957. Cytologie comparée, systématique at phylogénie des Microtinae (*Rodentia-Muridae*). Rev. Suisse, Zool., 64:39–71.

MERRIAM, C. H. 1891. Results of a biological reconnaissance of south-central Idaho. 2. Annotated list of mammals, with descriptions on new species. N. Amer. Fauna, 5:31–87.

MILLER, G. S., JR. 1896. Genera and subgenera of voles and lemmings. N. Amer. Fauna, 12:1–78.

———. 1912. Catalogue of the mammals of western Europe. British Mus., London, 1019 pp.

———. 1923. List of North American Recent mammals. Bull. U.S. Natl. Mus., 128:1–673.

NADLER, C. F., ET AL. 1978. Biochemical relationships of the Holarctic vole genera (*Clethrionomys, Microtus,* and *Arvicola* (Rodentia: Arvicolinae)). Canadian J. Zool., 56:1564–1575.

NELSON, G., AND N. PLATNICK. 1981. Systematics and biogeography, cladistics and vicariance. Columbia Univ. Press, New York, 567 pp.

QUAY, W. B. 1954*a*. The meibomian glands of voles and lemmings (Microtinae). Misc. Publ. Mus. Zool., Univ. Michigan, 82:1–23.

———. 1954*b*. The anatomy of the diastemal palate in microtine rodents. Misc. Publ. Mus. Zool., Univ. Michigan, 86:1–49.

———. 1968. The specialized posterolateral sebaceous glandular regions in microtine rodents. J. Mamm., 49:427–445.

REPENNING, C. A. 1968. Mandibular musculature and the origin of the subfamily Arvicolinae (Rodentia). Acta Zool. Cracoviensis, 13(3):1–72.

———. 1983. *Pitymys meadensis* Hibbard from the Valley of Mexico and the classification of North American species of *Pitymys* (Rodentia: Cricetidae). J. Vert. Paleontol., 2:1–482.

SCHWARTZ, A. 1953. A systematic study of the water rat (*Neofiber alleni*). Occas. Papers Mus. Zool., Univ. Michigan, 547:1–27.

SIMPSON, G. G. 1945. The principles of classification and a classification of mammals. Bull. Amer. Mus. Nat. Hist., 85:1–350.

WAHLERT, J. H. 1978. Cranial foramina and relationships of the Eomyoidea (Rodentia, Geomorpha). Skull and upper teeth of Kansasimys. Amer. Mus. Novitates, 2645:1–16.

WINGE, H. 1941. The interrelationships of the mammalian genera. Vol. II. Rodentia, Carnivora, Primates. C. A. Reitzels Forlag, Copenhagen, 376 pp.

YOUNGMAN, P. M. 1967. Insular populations of the meadow vole, *Microtus pennsylvanicus,* from northeastern North America, with descriptions of two new subspecies. J. Mamm., 48:579–588.

ZOOGEOGRAPHY

ROBERT S. HOFFMANN AND

JAMES W. KOEPPL

Abstract

THE genus *Microtus* is less species-rich in the New World than the Old, perhaps reflecting the origin and longer residence of the genus in the Palearctic. While *Microtus* are usually thought of as grassland species, most species are mainly associated with successional meadow facies of forest and woodland biomes. The 19 species and four insular allospecies occupying the New World may be classified ecologically; three are primarily tundra inhabitants; nine are primarily taiga species, equally divided among boreal, montane, and Pacific coastal sections; two are southwestern chaparral or woodland species; one is primarily Great Plains grassland; one eastern deciduous forest; and four are relict species with small ranges scattered through cloud forest communities in the Mexican mountains. Patterns of Pleistocene occurrence of New World *Microtus* are correlated with these ecological patterns. The oldest lineages are apparently represented by the Mexican cloud-forest relicts; chaparral, grassland, and eastern deciduous forest lineages are somewhat more recent; and taiga- and tundra-inhabiting voles represent the most recent, late-Pleistocene lineages to appear in the New World. Certain allospecies pairs probably diverged only in the Wisconsinan–Holocene period, a few thousand years ago.

Introduction

Twenty-three species of *Microtus* currently are recognized from the New World (Anderson, this volume). The extratropical portion of the New World is termed the Nearctic, a biogeographic region first defined by Sclater (1858) and Wallace (1876). The genus *Microtus* is found throughout much of the Nearctic, and in the New World virtually is restricted therein; various species of these voles are important components of most Nearctic mammal faunas. The Nearctic often is combined with its Old World counterpart, the Palearctic, to form the Holarctic, a circumboreal biogeographic region.

The number of species of *Microtus* in the Palearctic is greater than in the Nearctic. If one includes the species of *Pitymys* and *Proedromys,* as in the broad generic concept employed in this volume, there are 48 species of Old World voles (Honacki et al., 1982). The difference is increased if the four species confined to small islands in the New World are eliminated; most or all are sometimes considered subspecies of closely related mainland species. The three insular species of the Palearctic (*M. kikuchii, M. montebelli,* and *M. sachalinensis*) occupy extensive ranges on large islands—Taiwan, Japan (Kyushu, Honshu, Sado; perhaps Shikotan), and Sakhalin, respectively—and thus differ from New World insular taxa.

The difference in species richness—48 versus 19—may be accounted for in part by the larger area of the Palearctic, approximately 14 million square miles as compared to six and a half million for the Nearctic. Nevertheless, whereas the Palearctic is about double the area of the Nearctic, it possesses about two and a half times as many species of *Microtus.* Of this total of 67 species, only one, *M. oeconomus,* occurs on both sides of the Bering Strait and thus displays a Holarctic, or amphiberingian, distribution. Relationships between other Palearctic and Nearctic species at higher taxonomic levels are, in many cases, not well understood.

Biogeography and its subfield, zoogeography, can be divided into two areas of inquiry. Ecological biogeography is concerned with present interrelationships of species or higher taxa as members of associations of organisms. Historical biogeography examines the question of past origins and relationships of species or higher taxa as members of biotas (Wiley, 1981). These two approaches are not mutually exclusive, but it is convenient to review them separately.

Ecological Zoogeography

Biomes and Biogeographic Provinces

Attempts to classify associations of organisms (communities, life zones, biomes, and smaller associations) have a long history (Allee et al., 1951; Shelford, 1963; Udvardy, 1969). Voles of the genus

TABLE 1
BIOMES AND BIOGEOGRAPHIC PROVINCES OF THE NEARCTIC IN WHICH *Microtus* OCCUR

Biome	Biogeographic province[1]	Mammal province[2]
Tundra		
Low Arctic	Alaskan Tundra	Alaskan
		Western Eskimoan
	Aleutian	Aleutian
	Canadian Tundra	Eastern Eskimoan
		Ungavan
Alpine	—	—
Taiga		
Boreal	Yukon Taiga	Yukonian
	Canadian Taiga	Western Hudsonian-Canadian
		Eastern Hudsonian-Canadian
Coastal	Sitkan	Vancouverian
	Oregonian	Oregonian (part)
		Humboldtian (part)
Montane[3]	Rocky Mountains	Montanian
		Coloradan
		Uintian
	Sierra-Cascade	Oregonian (part)
		Humboldtian (part)
		Sierran
Montane Pine-Oak	Madrean-Cordilleran (part)	Navahonian
		Yaquinian
		San Matean
Temperate Grassland	Grasslands	Saskatchewanian
		Kansan
		Texan
Temperate Deciduous Forest		
Northern-Upland		Alleghenian
		Illinoian
		Carolinian (part)
Southern-Lowland	Austroriparian	Carolinian (part)
		Louisianan (part)
Broad Sclerophyll	Californian	Diablan
		Californian
		San Bernardian
Cold Desert	Great Basin	Columbian
		Artemesian

TABLE 1
CONTINUED

Biome	Biogeographic province[1]	Mammal province[2]
Tropical Forest		
Cloudforest	Madrean-Cordilleran (part)	—

[1] From Udvardy (1975).
[2] From Hagmeier (1966).
[3] Montane taiga in the Appalachian Mountains is included with Udvardy's Eastern Forest Province and Hagmeier's Alleghanian Province.

Microtus occupy particular habitats (Getz, this volume), but these habitats occur within biomes (a concept based on climax vegetation) or biotic provinces (a concept based on both systematic resemblance of the biota and ecogeographic similarity). *Microtus* can thus be considered to occupy not only habitats, but also biomes or biotic provinces.

Biomes have been classified differently by different authors, but there is general agreement on the major biomes of North America. These include (generally from north to south and from west to east) the following: 1) arctic tundra, including polar desert, high arctic tundra, and low arctic tundra; 2) alpine; 3) coniferous forest, or taiga, including boreal taiga, Pacific coastal taiga, and montane taiga; 4) temperate grassland, or steppe, including the northern and southern Great Plains; 5) temperate deciduous forest, including a northern-upland region and southern-lowland region; 6) broad sclerophyll, or chaparral-oak woodland; 7) cold desert; 8) hot desert; 9) pinyon-juniper-oak woodland; 10) montane pine-oak forest; 11) subtropical-tropical deciduous forest; 12) tropical rainforest, including cloud forest (modified from Shelford, 1963). Different permutations of these elements have been suggested by other authors (see Kendeigh, 1961; and Odum, 1971). Biomes are related to biotic provinces in a general way: although biomes may be geographically discontinuous, biotic provinces are continuous, and usually are contained within, a given biome. Table 1 lists those biomes (see above), biogeographic provinces (Udvardy, 1975), and "mammal provinces" (Hagmeier, 1966) in which *Microtus* occurs in the New World, as a guide to terminology employed in this section. All maps are polyconic oblique conic conformal projections.

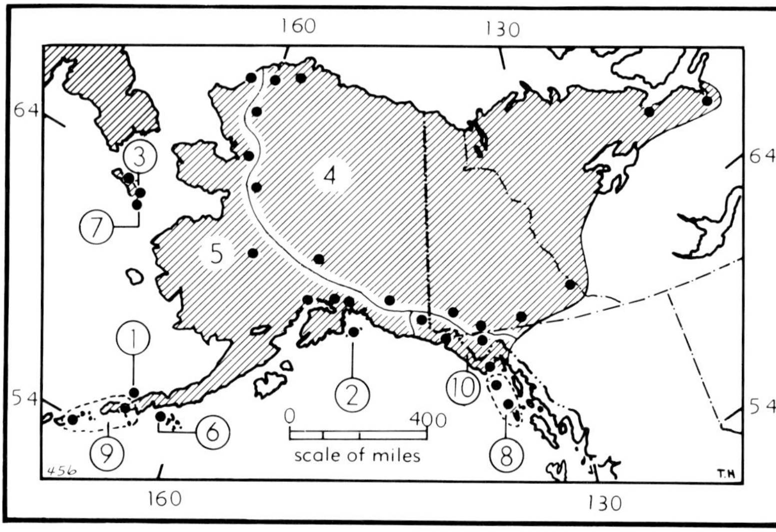

FIG. 1. Distribution of *Microtus oeconomus* in North America (modified from Hall, 1981). Subspecies are: 1, *M. o. amakensis*; 2, *M. o. elymocetes*; 3, *M. o. innuitus*; 4, *M. o. macfarlani*; 5, *M. o. operarius*; 6, *M. o. popofensis*; 7, *M. o. punukensis*; 8, *M. o. sitkensis*; 9, *M. o. unalascensis*; 10, *M. o. yakutatensis*.

Voles of the genus *Microtus* range northward into the tundra biome or Western Eskimoan province in Alaska and Canada, and southward into montane pine-oak, subtropical deciduous, and cloud-forest formations (Madrean-Cordilleran province) in the montane highlands of central Guatemala, and inhabit all but the most xeric of the biomes enumerated above. In the following section we discuss their distribution by major biomes.

Tundra.—The northernmost records are of the tundra vole, *M. oeconomus*, which is known to occur (Bee and Hall, 1956) on the northern slope of the Brooks Range in Alaska to 71°N latitude about 50 mi S of Pt. Barrow (Fig. 1). As its North American common name implies, this species regularly inhabits the tundra biome in mesic meadow habitats (Getz, this volume) of the low arctic (in the Palearctic, however, *M. oeconomus* has a much broader distribution both geographically and ecologically). No *Microtus* inhabits the more severe high arctic or polar desert associations that are occupied by the lemmings (*Lemmus* and *Dicrostonyx*). The only other species of *Microtus* to occur regularly in arctic tundra habitats

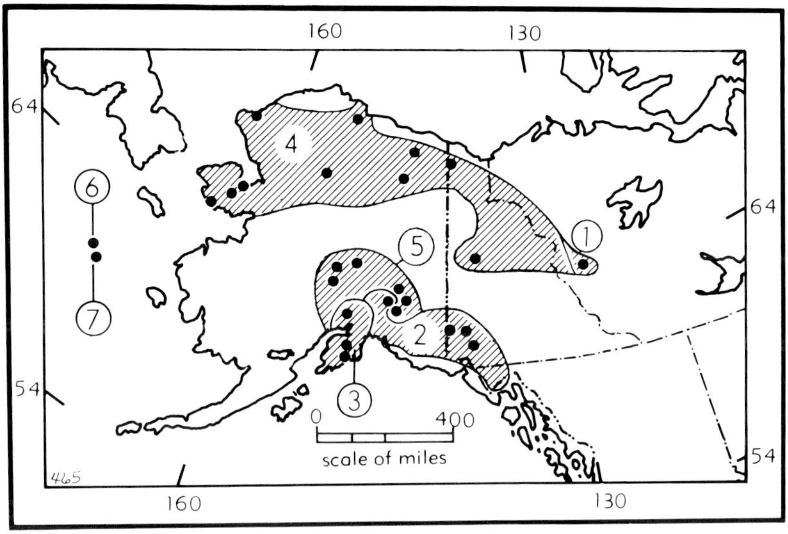

FIG. 2. Distribution of *Microtus miurus* (mainland) and its insular allospecies *M. abbreviatus* (modified from Hall, 1981). Subspecies are: 1, *M. m. andersoni*; 2, *M. m. cantator*; 3, *M. m. miurus*; 4, *M. m. muriei*; 5, *M. m. oreas*; 6, *M. a. abbreviatus*; 7, *M. a. fisheri*.

(Fig. 2) are the singing vole, *M. miurus* (and its insular allospecies, the St. Matthew Island vole, *M. abbreviatus*), and the meadow vole, *M. pennsylvanicus* (Fig. 3). *Microtus miurus* and *M. abbreviatus* are classified in the subgenus *Stenocranius* together with the Palearctic narrow-skulled vole (*M. gregalis*). *Stenocranius* has an amphiberingian distribution, like *M. oeconomus,* and both taxa are thought to have occupied the Bering land bridge during the latest (Wisconsinan) glacial period until the land bridge was flooded by rising sea level about 7,500 years ago (Hoffmann, 1976). The populations of voles found on islands in the Bering Strait (*M. abbreviatus* on St. Matthew and Hall islands; *M. oeconomus* on St. Lawrence, Unalaska, Kodiak, and adjacent small islands) thus represent refugial survivors of the late Pleistocene land-bridge populations (Hoffmann, 1981). The singing vole is found in more xeric tundra habitats than the tundra vole (Getz, this volume), and often is associated with dwarf and riparian willow stands (Bee and Hall, 1956). *Microtus pennsylvanicus* is found only sporadically in arctic tundra. Available distributional records suggest that it may range north-

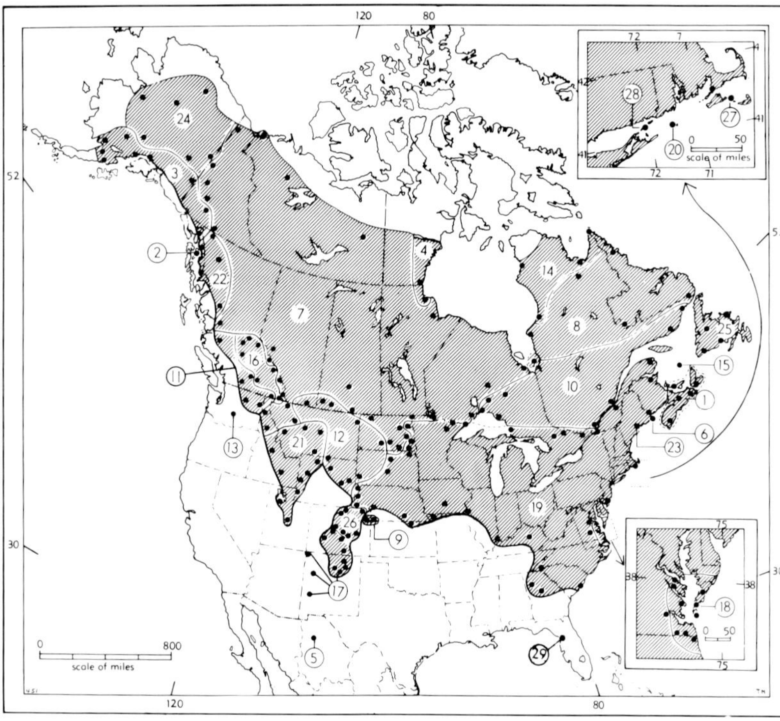

FIG. 3. Distribution of *Microtus pennsylvanicus* and its insular allospecies *M. breweri* (27) and *M. nesophilus* (28; extinct) (modified from Hall, 1981). Subspecies of *M. pennsylvanicus* are: 1, *M. p. acadicus*; 2, *M. p. admiraltiae*; 3, *M. p. alcorni*; 4, *M. p. aphorodemus*; 5, *M. p. chihuahensis*; 6, *M. p. copelandi*; 7, *M. p. drummondii*; 8, *M. p. enixus*; 9, *M. p. finitus*; 10, *M. p. fontigenus*; 11, *M. p. funebris*; 12, *M. p. insperatus*; 13, *M. p. kincaidi*; 14, *M. p. labradorius*; 15, *M. p. magdalenensis*; 16, *M. p. microcephalus*; 17, *M. p. modestus*; 18, *M. p. nigrans*; 19, *M. p. pennsylvanicus*; 20, *M. p. provectus*; 21, *M. p. pullatus*; 22, *M. p. rubidus*; 23, *M. p. shattucki*; 24, *M. p. tananaensis*; 25, *M. p. terraenovae*; 26, *M. p. uligocola*; 27, *M.* [*p.*] *breweri*; 28, *M.* [*p.*] *nesophilus*; 29, *M. p. dukecampbelli*.

ward into the tundra more regularly in the Canadian Arctic east of the range of *M. oeconomus* (Fig. 3), suggesting the possibility of competitive interaction between the species. Youngman (1975) reported both species "utilizing the same runways" in the Yukon.

Taiga.—South of the arctic tundra in North America extends a broad transcontinental belt of northern coniferous forest, or boreal taiga. The western and southwestern margin of the boreal taiga merges into the structurally rather similar Pacific coastal taiga and Cascade-Sierra-Rocky Mountain montane taiga, whereas in the east there is a transition through the mixed coniferous-deciduous forest of the Great Lakes-New England region to the montane taiga and mixed forests of the Appalachians. The vole with the widest distribution in the taiga biome of North America is *M. pennsylvanicus* (Fig. 3). Its vernacular name—meadow vole—suggests a contradiction; meadow voles, though widely distributed in taiga, occur mainly in grassy meadow habitats within the coniferous forest (Getz, this volume). Along the northwestern margin of their range, they are syntopic in taiga meadows with *M. oeconomus* (see above). Meadow voles extend southward in the Appalachian (Alleghenian province) and Rocky Mountains (Montanian, Coloradan provinces), and also into the eastern deciduous forest and in the grasslands of the northern Great Plains. In the Pacific coastal taiga association, however, there occurs the similar and probably related *M. townsendii* (Fig. 4). Townsend's vole, like the meadow vole, inhabits meadows within the coastal taiga (Getz, this volume) from Vancouver Island to northern California (Oregonian, Humboldtian provinces), and is completely allopatric with *M. pennsylvanicus* (Cowan and Guiguet, 1956; Dalquest, 1948).

Two other voles are restricted to the Pacific coastal taiga biome. The creeping vole, *M. oregoni* (Fig. 5), is a species of strongly fossorial habits that inhabits forest as well as meadow habitats (Getz, this volume). It is sufficiently distinctive to be placed in its own monotypic subgenus (*Chilotus*), and probably represents a relict distribution of a relatively old lineage (see below). In contrast, the gray-tailed vole, *M. canicaudus,* probably is a recently derived, peripheral isolate of the widely distributed montane vole, *M. montanus* (Fig. 6); it is restricted to grassy meadows and prairies (Getz, this volume) in and around the Willamette Valley in northwestern Oregon and perhaps adjacent Washington. This Pacific coastal area thus is one center of species richness for the genus; other vole genera—*Arborimus* and *Clethrionomys*—also have species restricted to this region.

The putative parental lineage to the gray-tailed vole is the montane vole (*M. montanus*), which is found in montane taiga throughout the Cascade-Sierra and Rocky Mountain ranges and the distribution of which also includes the intervening riparian meadows, arid grasslands and shrub steppe and semi-deserts (Getz, this vol-

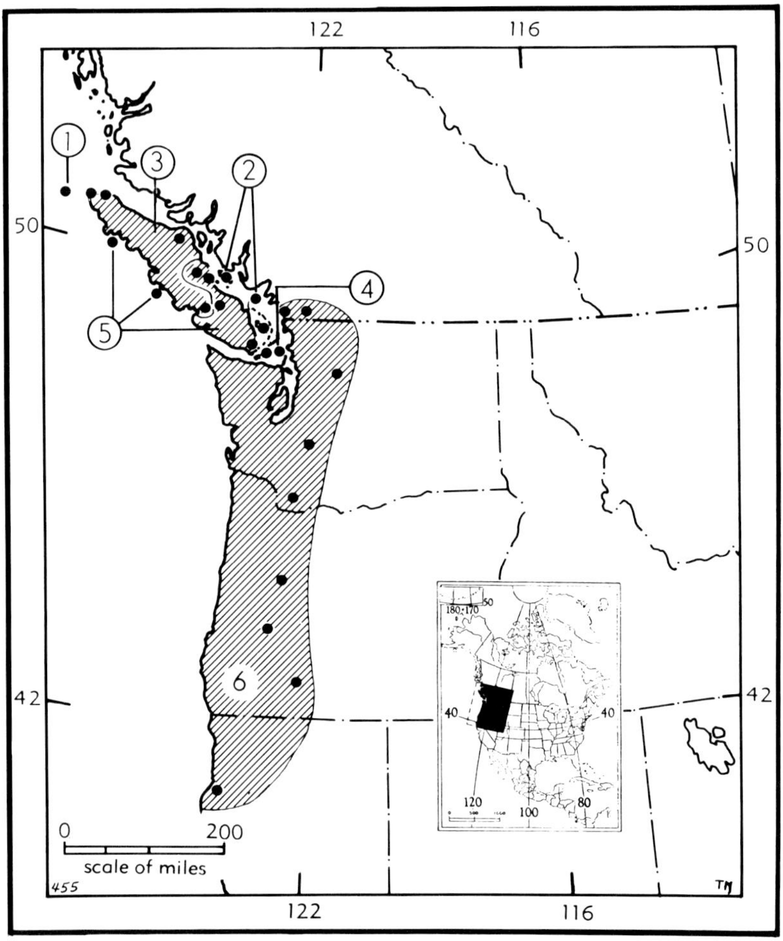

FIG. 4. Distribution of *Microtus townsendii* (from Hall, 1981). Subspecies are: 1, *M. t. cowani*; 2, *M. t. cummingi*; 3, *M. t. laingi*; 4, *M. t. pugeti*; 5, *M. t. tetramerus*; 6, *M. t. townsendii*.

ume) of the Columbia Plateau, Snake River Plains, and northern Great Basin (Fig. 6). Another species whose range primarily is within the montane taiga biome and cold desert biomes is the long-tailed vole, *M. longicaudus* (Fig. 7). This vole occupies not only the area in which the montane vole is found, but also extends westward to the Pacific coastal taiga in Oregon and northern California and

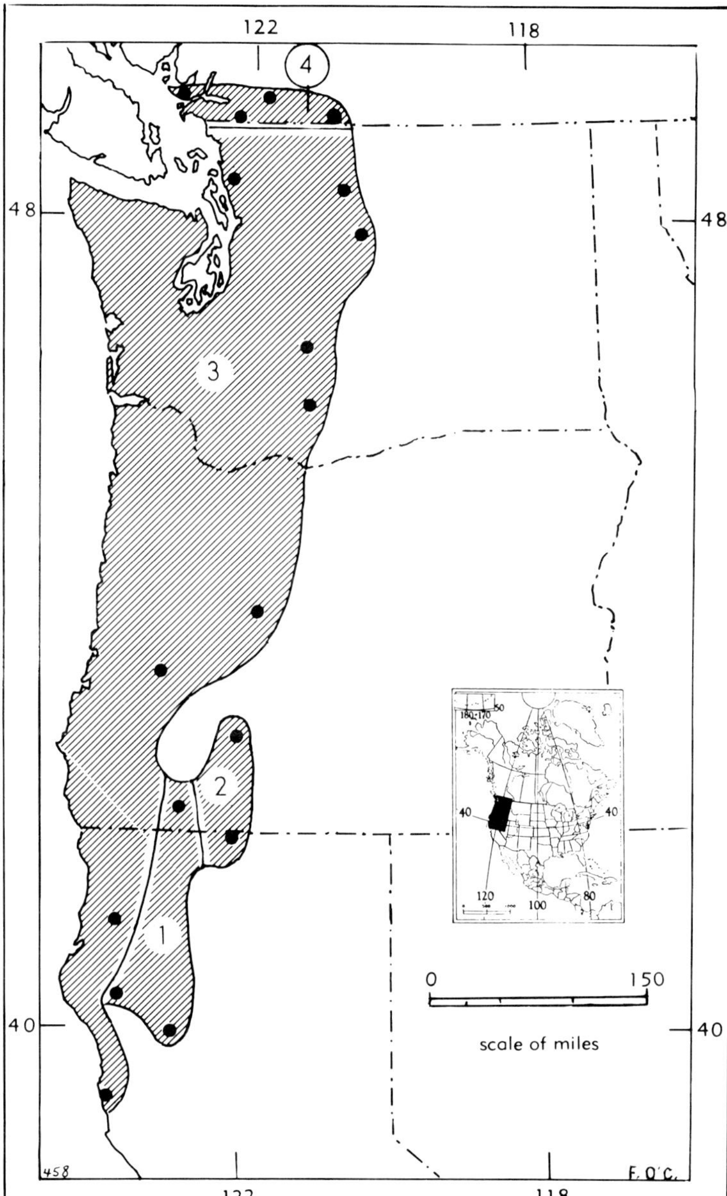

FIG. 5. Distribution of *Microtus oregoni* (from Hall, 1981). Subspecies are: 1, *M. o. adocetus*; 2, *M. o. bairdi*; 3, *M. o. oregoni*; 4, *M. o. serpens*.

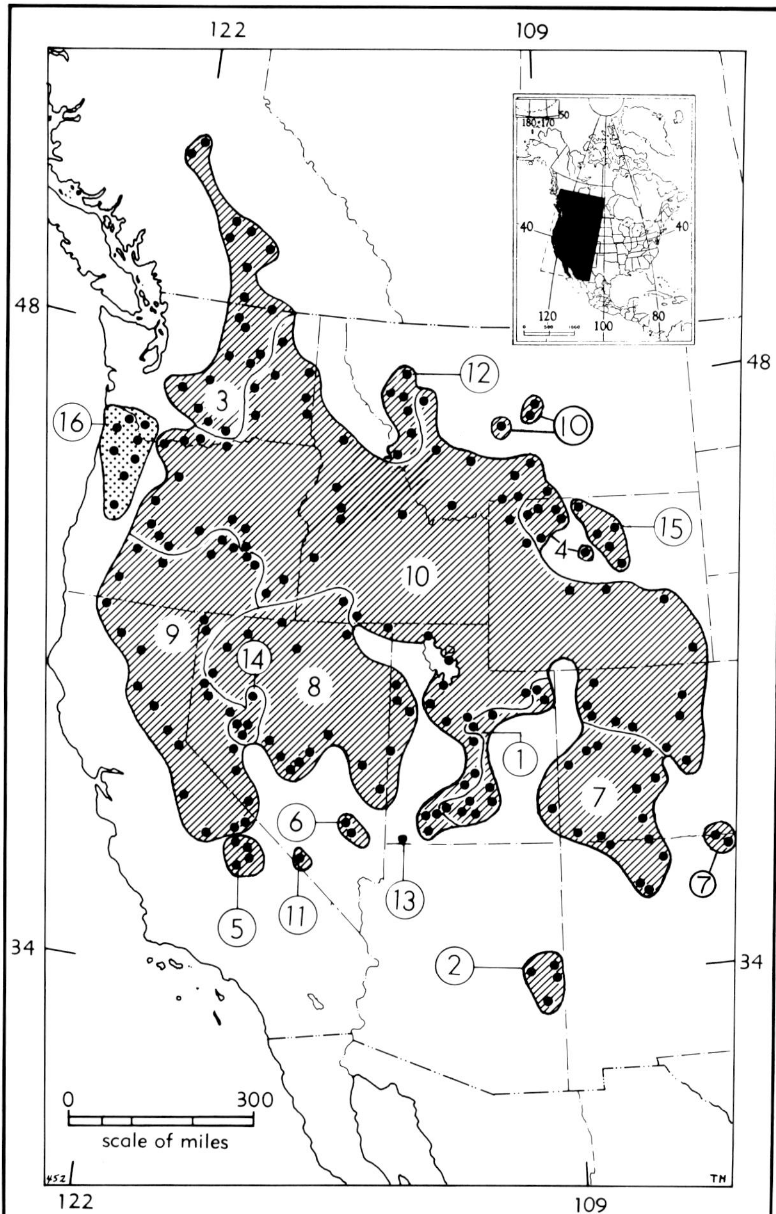
122
109
48
48
34
34
122
109
1
2
3
4
5
6
7
7
8
9
10
10
11
12
13
14
15
16
0
300
scale of miles
40
40
120
100
80
180-170
50
TN
452

northward into the coastal and boreal taiga as far as northeastern Alaska.

Microtus montanus and *M. longicaudus* thus occupy habitats in taiga biomes south and west of the range of *M. pennsylvanicus,* but all three species are geographically sympatric in a considerable portion of the central and southern Rocky Mountains. Here, then, is another center of species richness for the genus.

The species discussed so far are medium-sized voles that have rather general habitat requirements. Another group contains three species that apparently are more specialized in their habitat requirements, and two of the three are large in body size. The taiga vole, *M. xanthognathus,* is known from scattered localities in the boreal taiga zone from the west coast of Hudson Bay northwestward to central Alaska, and south to central Alberta (Fig. 8) (Western Hudsonian and Canadian, Yukonian provinces). From central Alberta southward in the Rocky Mountains to central Utah (Montanian, Coloradan provinces), and in the Cascade Mountains (Oregonian province), the almost equally large water vole, *M. richardsoni,* occurs in the alpine and in subalpine taiga stands (Fig. 9). Finally, in the eastern boreal taiga from northeastern Minnesota to Labrador and southward in the Appalachian Mountains to North Carolina (Alleghenian province), the smaller rock vole, *M. chrotorrhinus,* has been found sparingly (Fig. 10). All three of these species seem to be specialists, found only where a particular combination of habitat conditions are met (Getz, this volume), but their combined ranges encompass most of the taiga biome. In all, then, nine species of *Microtus* have ranges that are primarily associated with the taiga biome in North America.

South of the taiga biome and its montane extensions, a smaller number of species of *Microtus* is to be found, each occupying sharply defined habitats. Moreover, the systematic relationships of these

---

←

FIG. 6. Distribution of *Microtus montanus* and *M. canicaudus* (16) (modified from Hall, 1981). Subspecies of *M. montanus* are: 1, *M. m. amosus*; 2, *M. m. arizonensis*; 3, *M. m. canescens*; 4, *M. m. codiensis*; 5, *M. m. dutcheri*; 6, *M. m. fucosus*; 7, *M. m. fusus*; 8, *M. m. micropus*; 9, *M. m. montanus*; 10, *M. m. nanus*; 11, *M. m. nevadensis*; 12, *M. m. pratincola*; 13, *M. m. rivularis*; 14, *M. m. undosus*; 15, *M. m. zygomaticus.*

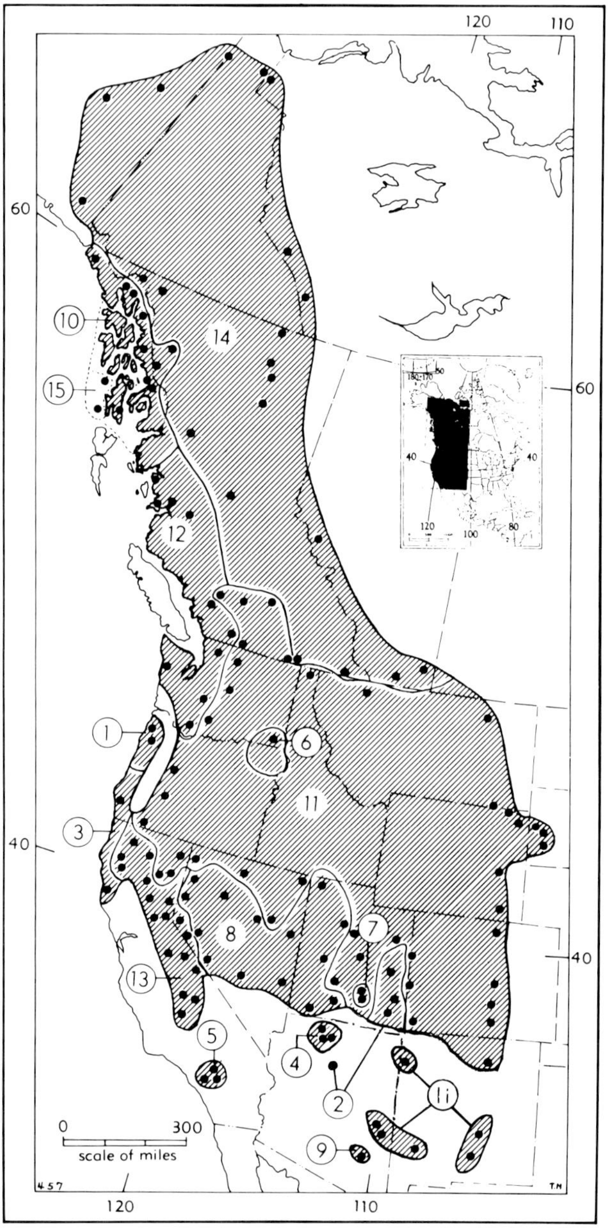
120
110
60
60
40
40
14
10
15
12
1
6
11
3
8
7
13
5
4
2
11
9
0
300
scale of miles
120
110
457
T.H

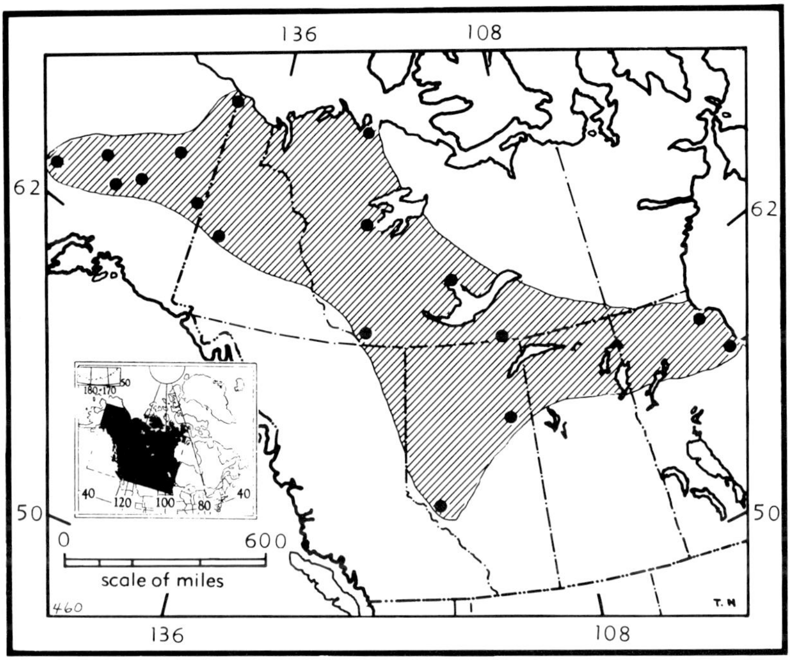

FIG. 8. Distribution of *Microtus xanthognathus* (from Hall, 1981).

species are controversial, and many of them have at one time or another been affiliated with the genus *Pitymys*.

Shrubland and woodland.—Southwestern North America is occupied by two allopatric species. The California vole, *M. californicus*, occurs in the broad sclerophyll (chaparral) oak woodlands and grassland of the Pacific coast from central Oregon (where it is geographically sympatric with several other species of *Microtus*) southward to northern Baja California (Fig. 11) (Humboldtian,

---

←

FIG. 7. Distribution of *Microtus longicaudus* and its insular allospecies *M. coronarius* (15) (modified from Hall, 1981). Subspecies of *M. longicaudus* are: 1, *M. l. abditus*; 2, *M. l. alticola*; 3, *M. l. angusticeps*; 4, *M. l. baileyi*; 5, *M. l. bernardinus*; 6, *M. l. halli*; 7, *M. l. incanus*; 8, *M. l. latus*; 9, *M. l. leucophaeus*; 10, *M. l. littoralis*; 11, *M. l. longicaudus*; 12, *M. l. macrurus*; 13, *M. l. sierrae*; 14, *M. l. vellerosus*.

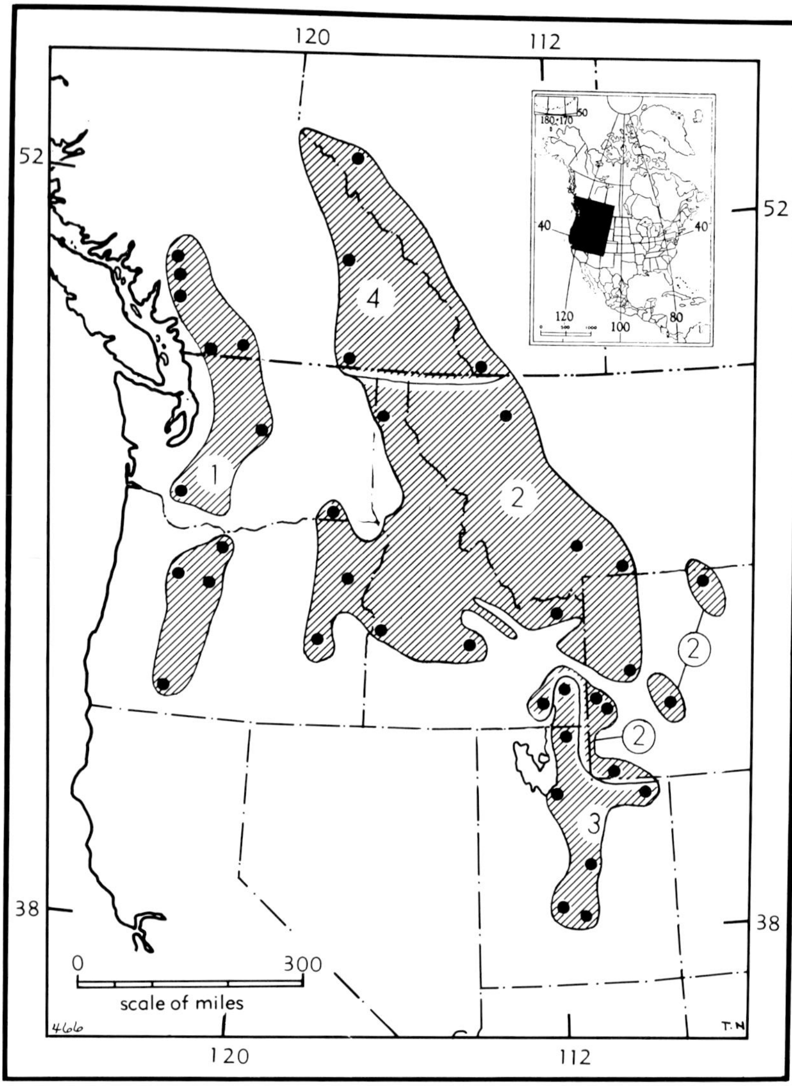

FIG. 9. Distribution of *Microtus richardsoni* (modified from Hall, 1981). Subspecies are: 1, *M. r. arvicoloides*; 2, *M. r. macropus*; 3, *M. r. myllodontus*; 4, *M. r. richardsoni*.

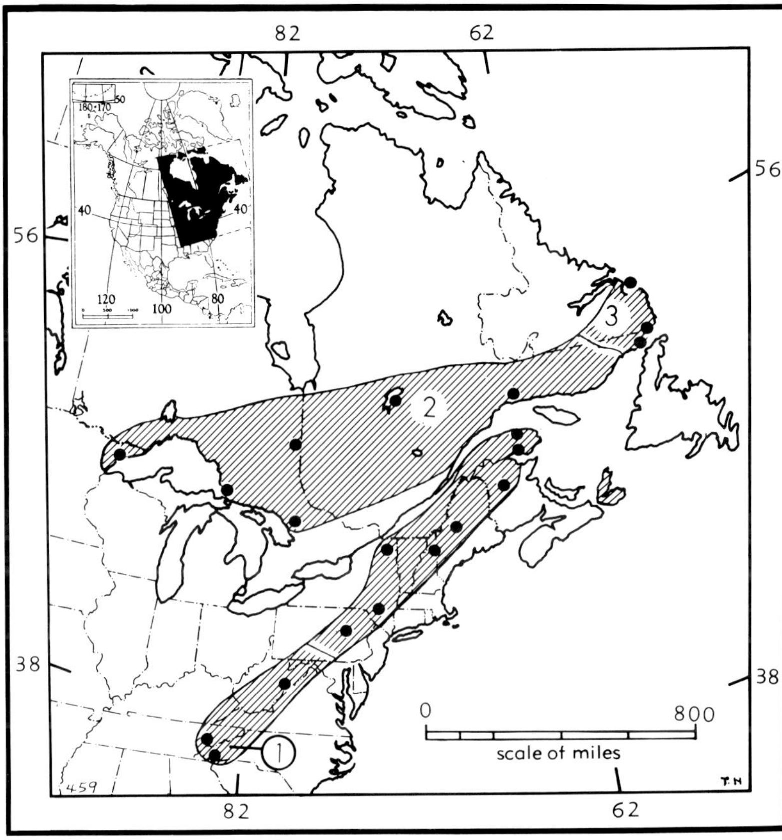

FIG. 10. Distribution of *Microtus chrotorrhinus* (modified from Hall, 1981). Subspecies are: 1, *M. c. carolinensis*; 2, *M. c. chrotorrhinus*; 3, *M. c. ravus*.

Diablian, Californian, San Bernardinian provinces). The Mexican vole, *M. mexicanus,* occurs from the southern Rocky Mountains southward in the Sierra Madre of Mexico to central Oaxaca (Madrean-Cordilleran province) (Fig. 12). Both species usually inhabit grassy habitats within or adjacent to, oak and pine woodlands, respectively (Getz, this volume). The Mexican vole occupies one of the most xeric habitats among Nearctic *Microtus,* although it also may live in cool, moist sites (Getz, this volume).

Grassland.—Farther east, the prairie vole, *M. ochrogaster,* is con-

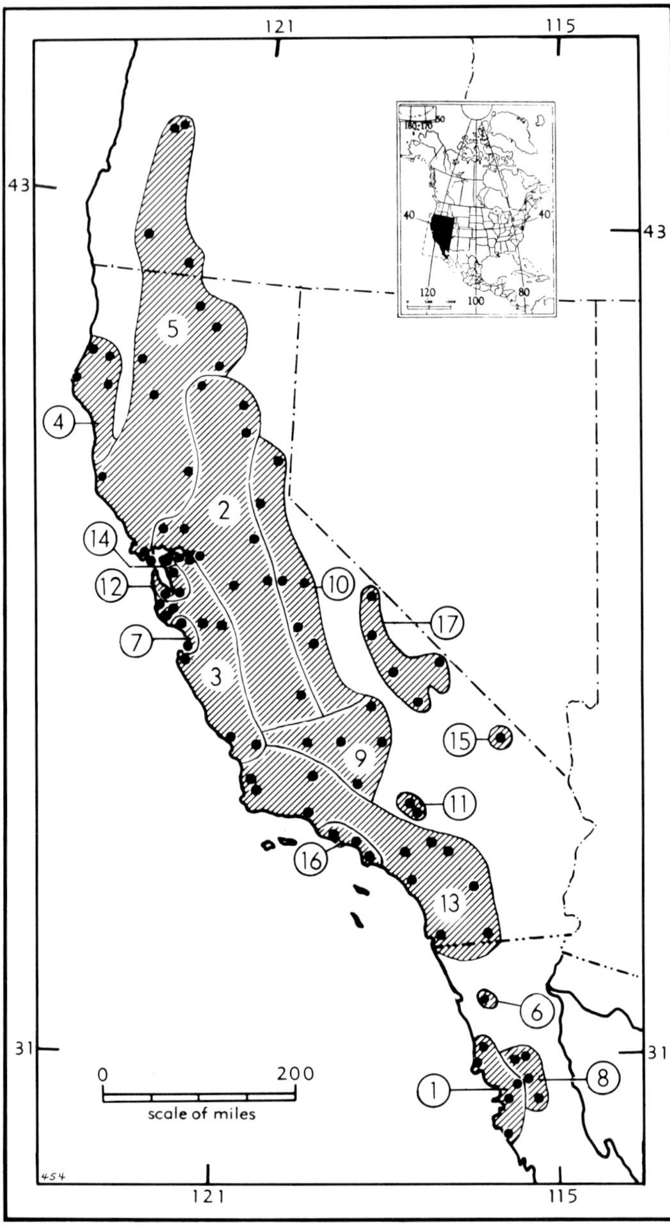
121
115
43
43
31
31
121
115
5
4
2
14
12
10
17
7
3
15
9
11
16
13
6
1
8
0
200
scale of miles
454

tinuously distributed in both mesic and xeric grasslands of the eastern half of the northern and central Great Plains, from the southern Prairie Provinces of Canada south to Oklahoma, and eastward through the "Prairie Peninsula" to western West Virginia (Fig. 13) (Saskatchewanian, Kansan, Illinoian provinces). An isolated relict population (*M. o. ludovicianus*) once inhabitated the Gulf Coast prairies of eastern Texas and western Louisiana, but it may now be extinct.

Temperate deciduous forest.—The temperate deciduous forest biome provides habitat for the woodland vole, *M. pinetorum* (Fig. 14). This is a highly fossorial species that inhabits both meadow and forest habitats; *M. pinetorum* and *M. ochrogaster* are broadly sympatric in the broad ecotone between deciduous forest and grassland biomes. The two species tend to segregate by habitat (Getz, this volume), but may use the same runways. A widely disjunct relict, the Jalapan woodland vole, *M. quasiater,* is known only from a small area in the Sierra Madre Occidental of central Mexico (Fig. 15). It may represent a peripheral isolate of *M. pinetorum,* or a relict of an earlier arvicolid invasion of the New World. Its principal habitat is meadow and grassland within the "oak forest association of tropical vegetation" (Hall and Dalquest, 1963). Thus, it may more properly belong to the next biome.

Cloud forest.—The remaining three species also are poorly known. The Oaxacan vole, *M. oaxacensis,* is known only from evergreen "cloud forest" habitat in the vicinity of Vista Hermosa, in the Sierra Madre Occidental of Oaxaca (Fig. 16). The Zempoaltepec vole, *M. umbrosus,* is known only from the vicinity of Zempoaltepec and Totontepec, also in the mountains of central Oaxaca (Fig. 16). Finally, the Guatemalan vole, *M. guatemalensis,* has been found on several isolated mountain ranges from central Chiapas to central Guatemala (Fig. 16); both *M. umbrosus* and *M. guatemalensis* are

---

←

FIG. 11. Distribution of *Microtus californicus* (modified from Hall, 1981). Subspecies are: 1, *M. c. aequivocatus*; 2, *M. c. aestuarinus*; 3, *M. c. californicus*; 4, *M. c. constrictus*; 5, *M. c. eximius*; 6, *M. c. grinnelli*; 7, *M. c. halophilus*; 8, *M. c. huperuthrus*; 9, *M. c. kernensis*; 10, *M. c. mariposae*; 11, *M. c. mohavensis*; 12, *M. c. paludicola*; 13, *M. c. sanctidiegi*; 14, *M. c. sanpabloensis*; 15, *M. c. scirpensis*; 16, *M. c. stephensi*; 17, *M. c. vallicola*.

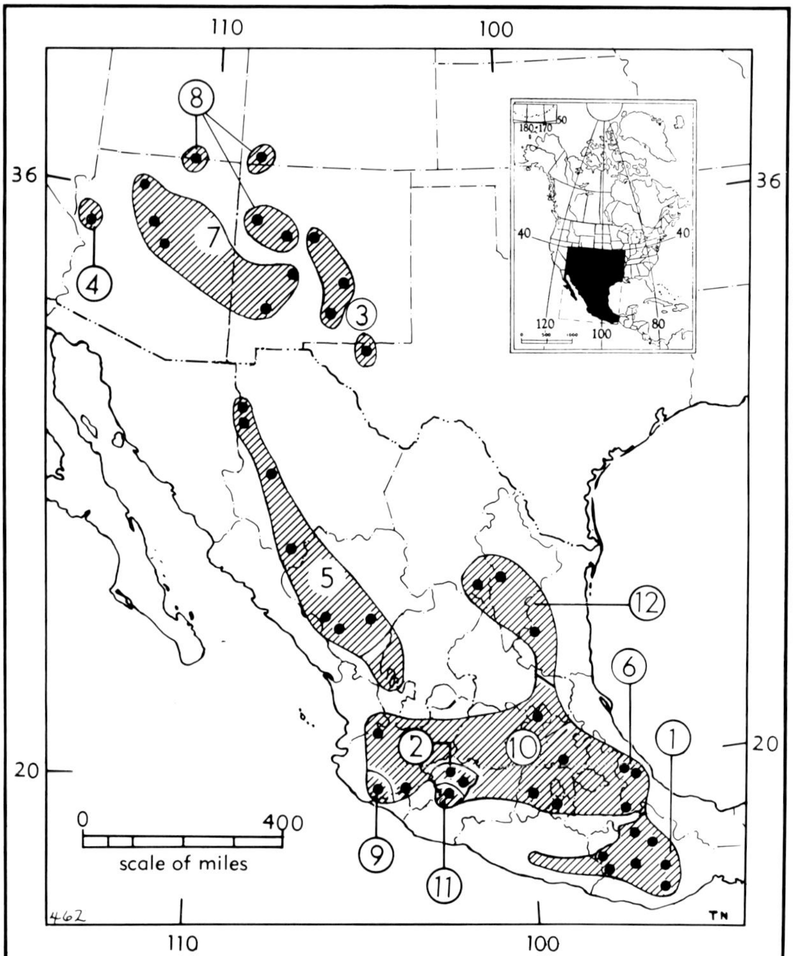

FIG. 12. Distribution of *Microtus mexicanus* (modified from Hall, 1981). Subspecies are: 1, *M. m. fulviventer*; 2, *M. m. fundatus*; 3, *M. m. guadalupensis*; 4, *M. m. hualpaiensis*; 5, *M. m. madrensis*; 6, *M. m. mexicanus*; 7, *M. m. mogollonensis*; 8, *M. m. navaho*; 9, *M. m. neveriae*; 10, *M. m. phaeus*; 11, *M. m. salvus*; 12, *M. m. subsimus*.

found in montane pine-oak and evergreen cloud-forest biomes. None of the three shows any obvious close relationship to more northerly species of *Microtus*, and all probably are best regarded as relicts of early arvicolid invasions of the New World (see below).

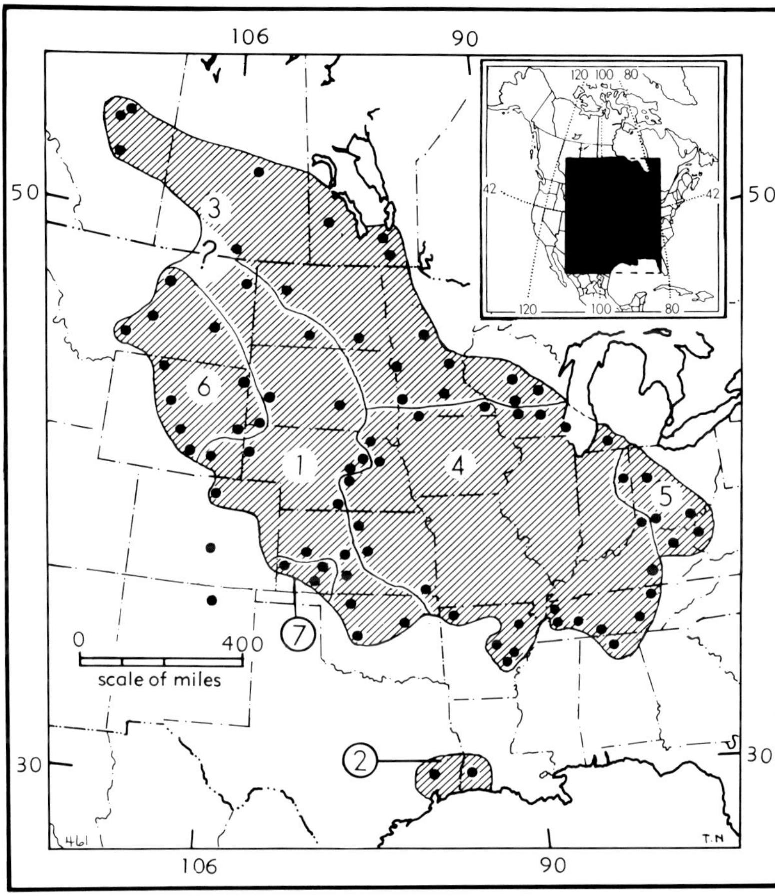

FIG. 13. Distribution of *Microtus ochrogaster* (modified from Hall, 1981). Subspecies are: 1, *M. o. haydenii*; 2, *M. o. ludovicianus*; 3, *M. o. minor*; 4, *M. o. ochrogaster*; 5, *M. o. ohionensis*; 6, *M. o. similis*; 7, *M. o. taylori*.

Summary of Ecological Zoogeography

It is clear from the foregoing that the largest number of species of *Microtus* in the New World (nine) are found in ecological formations associated with coniferous forest (taiga) biomes. Of these, three species occur primarily within boreal taiga (*M. chrotorrhinus, M. pennsylvanicus, M. xanthognathus*), three species within Pacific coastal taiga (*M. canicaudus, M. oregoni,* and *M. townsendii*), and

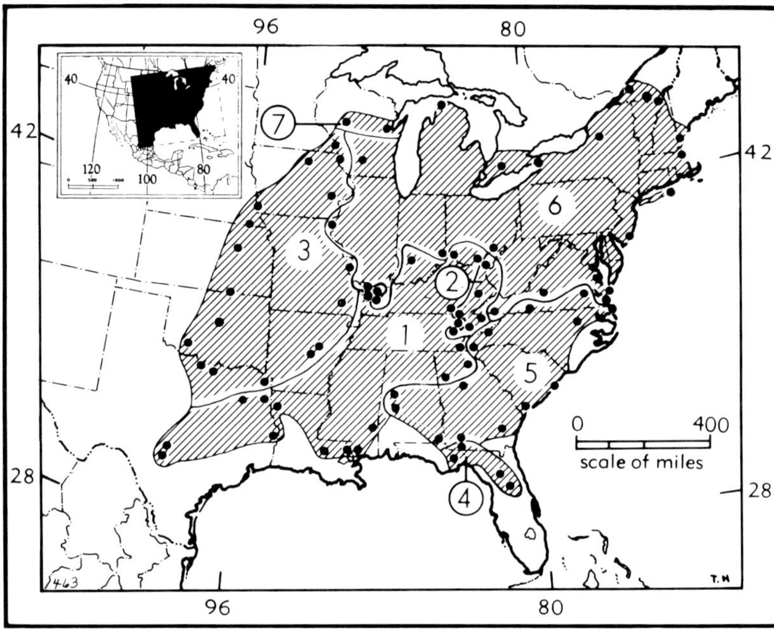

FIG. 14. Distribution of *Microtus pinetorum* (from Hall, 1981). Subspecies are: 1, *M. p. auricularis*; 2, *M. p. carbonarius*; 3, *M. p. nemoralis*; 4, *M. p. parvulus*; 5, *M. p. pinetorum*; 6, *M. p. scalopsoides*; 7, *M. p. schmidti*.

three species within Rocky Mountain montane taiga (*M. longicaudus, M. montanus,* and *M. richardsoni*). The southwestern pine-oak forest inhabitant, *M. mexicanus,* also might be included either here or with the three relict species (*M. guatemalensis, M. oaxacensis,* and *M. umbrosus*) that inhabit montane cloud forest, which includes a pine-oak forest aspect; these constitute the next largest ecological group. Tundra-dwelling voles comprise two species (*M. miurus* and *M. oeconomus*), both Beringian in distribution (see below), and recent entrants into the New World. In contrast, the two deciduous forest species (*M. pinetorum* and *M. quasiater*) probably are much more ancient. Finally, the broad-leaf sclerophyll woodland-shrubland of the Pacific Coast ("chaparral") and its associated grassland harbors one species (*M. californicus*), as does the temperate grassland of the Great Plains (*M. ochrogaster*).

Thus, whereas most species of *Microtus* inhabit meadows and

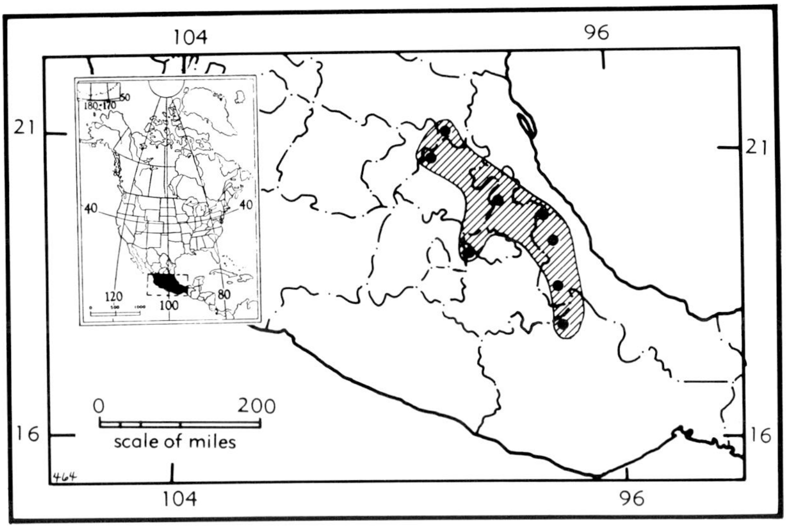

FIG. 15. Distribution of *Microtus quasiater* (from Hall, 1981).

similar grassy habitats (Getz, this volume), in a broader sense most are forest and woodland species in terms of the biomes they inhabit. From their predominance in taiga biomes it also is possible to infer that *Microtus* long has been associated with northern forest and woodland environments. It is this historical dimension that we shall examine next.

Historical Zoogeography

Early Pleistocene

"Modern" voles, including *Microtus* in the broad sense of this volume, first appeared in the New World in the early Pleistocene (Irvingtonian—Martin, 1979; Repenning, 1980; Zakrzewski, this volume), about 1.8–2.0 m.y.b.p. These first modern voles with rootless molars are placed in *Allophaiomys* (=*Pitymys*; see Zakrzewski, this volume), an extinct Holarctic genus thought by some to be ancestral either to modern *Pitymys* (van der Meulen, 1978; Zakrzewski, this volume) or to all later rootless cheektoothed voles (Chaline, 1974). According to Repenning (1980), these modern voles dispersed into the Nearctic from the Palearctic across the Bering

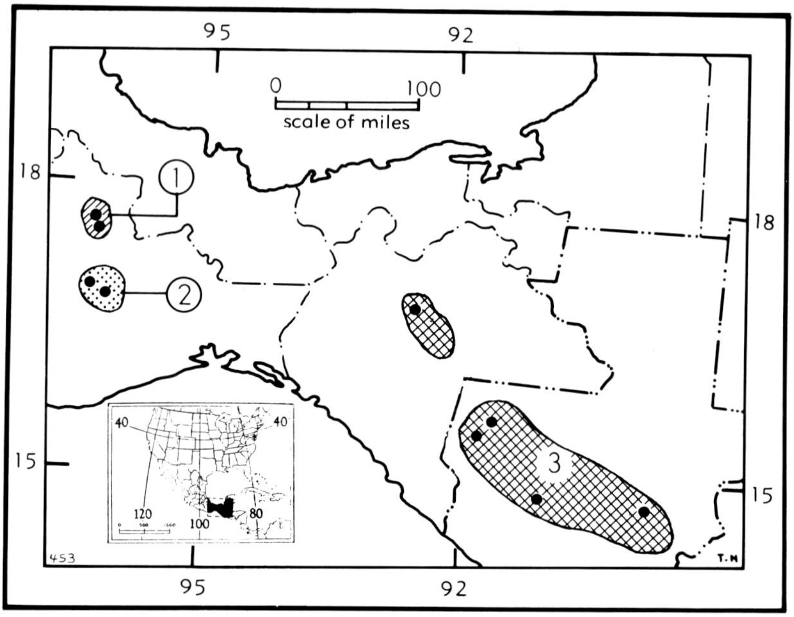

FIG. 16. Distributions of *M. oaxacensis* (1), *M. umbrosus* (2), and *Microtus guatemalensis* (3) (modified from Hall, 1981).

land bridge. However, Martin (1979) was more cautious, and suggested that the earliest records in North America might predate those in Eurasia. In any event, the lineages of this early radiation probably include the subgenera *Phaiomys* (now restricted to the Old World) and early *Neodon* (Martin, 1974; Repenning, 1980). Survivors of this early radiation in the New World may include *M. umbrosus* (Martin, 1974) and perhaps *M. guatemalensis* (Repenning, 1980), both of which exhibit relict distributions in the montane cloud forests of Mexico and Guatemala (Fig. 16).

Middle Pleistocene

A later dispersal event, about 1.2 m.y.b.p., brought "even-more-modern-looking forms" (Repenning, 1980), including later *Neodon*, and the subgenus *Pitymys* (L. W. Martin [1979] and R. Martin [1974] placed the first appearance of *Pitymys* later, around 0.6

m.y.b.p.). Survivors of these lineages may include *M. quasiater* (Repenning, 1980) and *M. oaxacensis* (Martin, 1974, who also included *M. guatemalensis* here). Again, these are species with relict montane distributions at the southern extreme of the range of the genus (Fig. 16). The *Pitymys* lineage in North America subsequently differentiated into at least two others, leading to *M.* (*Pitymys*) *pinetorum,* the temperate deciduous forest species (Fig. 14), and *M.* (*Pedomys*) *ochrogaster,* the temperate grassland species (Fig. 13) (see Martin, 1974; van der Meulen, 1978; and Kurtén and Anderson, 1980).

The earliest appearance of *Microtus* (sensu stricto) in the New World is controversial. Until recently, this was thought to be in the Middle Irvingtonian (*M. paroperarius*; Martin, 1979; van der Meulen, 1978), but Repenning (1980) claimed that not only *M. paroperarius* but also *M. californicus* first appeared around 1.8 m.y.b.p., at the beginning of the Pleistocene (see Zakrzewski, this volume). Another controversial, possibly early, date is for *Microtus deceitensis,* first described from Alaska (Guthrie and Matthews, 1972) and later from Saskatchewan (Harington, 1978), but referred to *M. paroperarius* by Zakrzewski (this volume). These faunas also are considered early Pleistocene by some (Kurtén and Anderson, 1980) or even late Pliocene (Repenning, 1980). That it is a *Microtus* with a primitive dental pattern is agreed, but whether it is a "side branch" (Kurtén and Anderson, 1980), or an early evolutionary stage "possibly leading to *M. xanthognathus*" (van der Meulen, 1978), is not (see Zakrzewski, this volume).

In either event, species of *Microtus* (sensu stricto) are common, either as immigrants or autochthons, in the late Pleistocene. Repenning (1980) spoke of a "dispersal wave about 0.47 m.y.b.p., [when] *Microtus pennsylvanicus* floods North America east of the Rocky Mountains . . . ." Subsequently, all other living species are found as fossils, except *M. canicaudus, M. oregoni, M. townsendii,* and insular forms (Zakrzewski, this volume).

If *M. californicus* did indeed appear in North America at the beginning of the Pleistocene, its restricted, possibly relict, distribution (Fig. 11) and its unusual habitat (broad-leafed sclerophyll vegetation) are understandable. However, its phylogenetic relationships to other *Microtus,* New or Old World, remain obscure. The same is true of another Pacific coast endemic, *M. oregoni* (Fig. 5). It has been placed in the subgenus *Chilotus,* which usually is regarded as monotypic, though Ognev (1950) proposed a close relationship between *M. oregoni* and the Old World *M. socialis.* Given its restricted range, ecological specialization, and isolated position among New World *Microtus,* it probably represents an early immigration or evolutionary divergence.

Another species possibly related to an otherwise Old World subgenus is *M. longicaudus* which, with its insular allospecies, *M.* [*l.*] *coronarius* (Fig. 7), has been allocated to *Chionomys* (Anderson, 1960). The subgenus *Chionomys* also includes *M. nivalis, M. gud,* and *M. roberti* of the western Palearctic, eastward to the Kopet Dag Mountains, and Lawrence (1982) implied that the eastern Palearctic *M. millicens* and *M. musseri* also might be related to this group. These latter two probably are relict species now restricted to the mountains of western China (Lawrence, 1982), but their ranges might be evidence of a biogeographic track (Wiley, 1981) if they and *M. longicaudus* do belong to *Chionomys.* Such a relationship would imply a fairly early dispersal of the ancestor of *M. longicaudus* across Beringia into the New World, but an alternative hypothesis is that *M. longicaudus* is convergent with *Chionomys* and evolved more recently from a New World lineage.

The history of the New World water vole, *M. richardsoni,* is plagued by similar uncertainty. Hooper and Hart (1962), Jannett and Jannett (1974), and others allocated this species to the genus (or subgenus; see Hall, 1981) *Arvicola.* However, it is difficult to account for *M. richardsoni* as a late Pleistocene immigrant from the Old World *Arvicola* lineage, and it may be an evolutionary lineage paralleling *Arvicola* but from an early Blancan *Mimomys*-like New World lineage (Hoffmann, 1980). A third alternative is that *richardsoni* represents a "long independent history [and] separate derivation from *Allophaiomys* . . ." (Martin, *in* Honacki et al., 1982). Finally, it has been suggested (Repenning, in litt.) that *M. richardsoni* is a late Pleistocene peripheral isolate of the *M. xanthognathus* lineage. Of these different possibilities, the last one now seems to us to be most likely. If so, and if *M. xanthognathus* is derived from *M. deceitensis,* then the three species of taiga-inhabiting voles (*M. chrotorrhinus, M. richardsoni,* and *M. xanthognathus*) that are now allopatric (Figs. 8–10) may represent a lineage that has been evolving in North America since at least mid-Pleistocene, and perhaps earlier.

Late Pleistocene

The most widespread species of New World *Microtus* is *M. pennsylvanicus* (Fig. 3); its history goes back to late mid-Pleistocene, about 500,000 years ago. It may be a descendant of *M. paroperarius* (Guthrie, 1965; Martin, 1972), an earlier immigrant and one of the first *Microtus* (sensu stricto) in North America (see above). This lineage in turn may have given rise to other lineages adapted to taiga meadows, such as *M. montanus-M. canicaudus* in the Rocky Mountains-Sierra-Cascade (Fig. 6), *M. mexicanus* in the southern Rocky Mountains-Sierra Madre (Fig. 12), and *M. townsendii* in the Pacific coastal taiga (Fig. 4). The superspecies *Microtus [pennsylvanicus]* has a distribution characterized by several insular allospecies, *M. [p.] breweri* on Muskeget, and *M. [p.] nesophilus* on Gull Island (extinct); *M. [p.] provectus* on Block Island sometimes has been given species rank, and several insular subspecies have been named. In addition, a series of geographically isolated populations occur along the margin of the species' range, south to Florida (Fig. 3) (Woods et al., 1982) and Chihuahua (Bradley and Cockrum, 1968). According to Repenning (1980), *M. pennsylvanicus,* although apparently abundant and widely distributed in the late Pleistocene, was found only east of the Rocky Mountains (see also Martin, 1968). Presently, an isolated relict population (*M. p. kincaidi*) is found at Moses Lake in central Washington (Fig. 3).

Farther west and south, taiga meadows are inhabited by the allopatric *M. townsendii* (Fig. 4). Rand (1954) was the first to suggest that Pleistocene isolation in taiga refugia south of the continental ice might have led to divergence of an ancestral *M. pennsylvanicus,* thus giving rise to *M. townsendii* by peripheral isolation. The karyotype of living *M. pennsylvanicus* is 2n = 46 (FN = 50), whereas that of *M. townsendii* is entirely uniarmed with 2n = 50 (FN = 48). The two karyotypes are derivable from one another by a combination of fusion/fission and inversion mechanisms (Gaines, this volume).

Microtus mexicanus, which inhabits montane coniferous forest meadows to the south of the range of *M. pennsylvanicus,* has a distribution that suggests it also might have diverged from the ancestral lineage through Pleistocene isolation (Fig. 12). The Mexican vole has a karyotype of 2n = 44 (FN = 54), and thus has six biarmed autosomal pairs as compared with three in *M. pennsylvanicus* (Gaines, this volume). It has diverged considerably from *M. pennsylvanicus* and *M. townsendii* in its habitat relationships, being adapted to more xeric conditions than the other two (Getz, this volume), and this suggests an earlier divergence.

Of the small taiga meadow-dwelling voles, the one exhibiting the greatest amount of range overlap with *M. pennsylvanicus* is *M. montanus* (Fig. 6). The two species are geographically sympatric in the central and southern Rocky Mountains, but are segregated ecologically. The meadow vole, where it co-occurs with the montane vole, usually is restricted to mesic grassland, whereas the latter is found in more xeric situations (Getz, this volume). Where *M. montanus* lives in the absence of *M. pennsylvanicus,* it regularly inhabits mesic habitats as well (intermountain basins, Cascade-Sierra ranges). This habitat segregation probably is due to a combination of habitat selection and competitive interaction (Koplin and Hoffmann, 1968; Murie, 1969, 1971). Its present distribution is completely allopatric to that of *M. townsendii*; only where it takes the mesic habitat does it slightly and marginally overlap with *M. mexicanus* (Findley, 1969).

The montane vole also possesses one of the most derived karyotypes found among New World *Microtus,* with 2n = 24 (FN = 44), and a completely biarmed complement (Gaines, this volume). This, plus the extent of sympatry, suggests that *M. montanus* has had a long and independent history. Whether it represents an early offshoot of the *M. paroperarius-M. pennsylvanicus* lineage, or perhaps instead is derived from another New World lineage, is not presently resolvable.

Microtus canicaudus has been regarded as a subspecies of *M. montanus,* but differs karyotically, electrophoretically, and morphologically (Hsu and Johnson, 1970). Its allopatric distribution (Fig. 6) and the fact that it shares a highly derived (though slightly different) karyotype with *M. montanus* indicates that it is a recently diverged allospecies that probably evolved as a result of peripheral isolation in the late Pleistocene.

The two lineages of New World *Microtus* (Figs. 1, 2) yet to be discussed are tundra specialists, *M. oeconomus* and *M. miurus* (together with its insular allospecies, *M. abbreviatus*). Both are restricted to the northwestern corner of North America, and are not known to occur in suitable lowland tundra or alpine habitats to the east or south of their present ranges, even though no obvious physiographic barriers restrict their distribution. In the Old World, *M. oeconomus* has a much wider range, both geographically and ecologically. It occurs throughout Siberia, southward into Mongolia and China, and westward through eastern Europe to the Baltic, Scandinavia, and Hungary, with an isolated relict population in the Netherlands (Honacki et al., 1982; Saint Girons, 1973). Within this range it occupies not only tundra, but also wet meadow and marsh habitats throughout the taiga, mixed forest, and forest-steppe zones.

The Palearctic sister species of continental *M. miurus* is the narrow-skulled vole, *M. gregalis,* and until recently the two often were considered conspecific (Rausch, 1964; Rausch and Rausch, 1968). Fedyk (1970) demonstrated chromosomal and morphological differences, and discussed the evolutionary history of the group. In the Old World, *M. gregalis* has a large range, being found throughout Siberia, south to Mongolia, China, and Tadzhikistan, and west to the Ural Mountains and the White Sea. Within this area it is found in upland tundra and rocky, montane habitats, but also occupies forest meadows, forest steppe, various grassland-steppe habitats, and even semi-arid steppe (Ognev, 1950).

Thus, the New World representatives of these Holarctic taxa are much more limited in habitat than Old World representatives, and restricted geographically to within or near the limits of the ice-free refugium of East Beringia. New World populations of *M. oeconomus* have differentiated little from eastern Siberian populations (Nadler et al., 1976, 1978), and their occurrence on St. Lawrence Island (a surviving part of the Bering land-bridge) suggests that the species is a recent immigrant to the New World, probably within Wisconsin time (about 70,000 years ago; but see Zakrzewski, this volume). The New World narrow-skulled voles exhibit greater differentiation, and this might indicate a somewhat earlier divergence, perhaps during late Illinoian time (about 170,000 years ago). Narrow-skulled voles are reported from pre-Wisconsinan glacial deposits in Beringian Alaska (Kurtén and Anderson, 1980; Zakrzewski, this volume).

Summary of Historical Zoogeography

A clear relationship between evolutionary history, ecological association, and systematic position is indicated by the foregoing analyses. The earliest appearance of *Microtus* in the New World was in the early Pleistocene; these were primitive voles represented by surviving lineages of species with relict distributions in montane cloud forests at the southern edge of the Nearctic. They either are referred to monotypic subgenera (*Orthriomys, Herpetomys*) within *Microtus,* or are members of the subgenera (or genera) *Pitymys* or *Neodon* (Martin, 1974).

The appearance in the middle Pleistocene of more modern lineages also may be related to other montane relict species surviving in central and southern Mexico (*M. oaxacensis* and *M. quasiater*) that also have been placed in *Pitymys* or *Neodon.* However, these pitymyine lineages also gave rise to the temperate deciduous forest vole, *M.* (*Pitymys*) *pinetorum,* and to the grassland vole, *M.* (*Pedomys*) *ochrogaster. Microtus californicus,* a broad sclerophyll relict, also may have appeared at this time.

The late Pleistocene saw repeated appearance (immigrations) of *Microtus* lineages. The first of these, about half a million years ago, was associated with Kansan glaciation. Paleogeographic evidence suggests that, at that time, taiga covered at least part of the Bering landbridge (Hoffmann, 1976), whereas more temperate vegetation may have been present earlier. The lineage leading to the taiga-dwelling specialists—*M. xanthognathus, M. chrotorrhinus,* and *M. richardsoni*—probably appeared then, as did the lineage leading to the less specialized *M. pennsylvanicus.* Other vole species found in taiga biomes also might have appeared about this time, such as *M.* (*Chilotus*) *oregoni* and *M.* (*Chionomys*) *longicaudus.*

Later in the late Pleistocene, climatic conditions on the Bering landbridge became more severe (Hoffmann, 1976), and only cold tundra and steppe-tundra species probably were able to survive Beringian conditions. There is evidence that, in the Illinoian glacial period, the lineage leading to *M.* (*Stenocranius*) *miurus* reached East Beringia but no farther. Finally, in the Wisconsinan glacial period *M. oeconomus* also crossed Beringia.

These last two or three major glacial periods were also characterized by displacement and fragmentation of taiga biomes south of the glacial ice (Hoffmann, 1976, 1981). This resulted in isolation and subsequent speciation in one or more of the *Microtus* lineages already present in North America, and to the evolution of *M. montanus* and *M. mexicanus* in the Rocky Mountains-Sierra-Cascade-Great Basin and the Madrean-Cordilleran provinces, respectively, probably in the Illinoian. It also resulted in isolation and speciation of *M. townsendii* and *M. canicaudus* in the Oregonian Province, probably in the Wisconsinan. Also during (or at the end of) the Wisconsinan, the several insular allospecies probably evolved: *M. abbreviatus* from *M. miurus, M. coronarius* from *M. longicaudus,* and *M. breweri* and *M. nesophilus* from *M. pennsylvanicus.*

The above scenario is a testable evolutionary hypothesis in that it predicts the time and place of occurrence of the various lineages as fossils; it also makes certain predictions concerning phylogenetic relationships.

Acknowledgments

Research upon which this review was based in part was supported by National Science Foundation grants DEB 80-04148 and 80-07246 as part of a joint research project co-sponsored by the Academies of Sciences of the U.S. and U.S.S.R., and the bilateral Environmental Protection Agreement (Project 0.2.05-7104). Assistance in field and laboratory was provided by R. R. Patterson, R. L. Rausch, T. Pearson, J.-P. Airoldi, P. B. Robertson, C. F., N. W., C., R., and C. F. Nadler, Jr.; S. A., J. F., D. R., and B. E. Hoffmann, H. Levenson, L. R. Heaney, A. E. Kozlovskii, V. N. Orlov, V. E. Sokolov, M. N. Meier, A. Gill, M. Johnson, M. Gaines, and L. Deutsch. We also acknowledge the cooperation of the several state and provincial game departments in granting us permission to collect.

Literature Cited

Allee, W. C., A. E. Emerson, O. Park, T. Park, and K. P. Schmidt. 1951. Principles of animal ecology. W. B. Saunders, Philadelphia, 337 pp.

Anderson, S. 1960. The baculum in microtine rodents. Univ. Kansas Publ. Mus. Nat. Hist., 12:181–216.

Bee, J. W., and E. R. Hall. 1956. Mammals of northern Alaska. Misc. Publ. Mus. Nat. Hist., Univ. Kansas, 8:1–309.

Bradley, W. G., and E. L. Cockrum. 1968. A new subspecies of the meadow vole (*Microtus pennsylvanicus*) from northwestern Chihuahua, Mexico. Amer. Mus. Novitates, 2325:1–7.

Chaline, J. 1974. Esquisse de l'évolution morphologique biométrique et chromosomique du genre *Microtus* (*Arvicolidae, Rodentia*) dans le Pléistocène de l'hémisphère nord. Bull. Soc. Geol. France, 16:440–450.

Cowan, I. McT., and C. J. Guiguet. 1956. The mammals of British Columbia. Handb. British Columbia Prov. Mus., 11:1–413.

DALQUEST, W. W. 1948. The mammals of Washington. Univ. Kansas Publ., Mus. Nat. Hist., 2:1–444.

FEDYK, S. 1970. Chromosomes of *Microtus* (*Stenocranius*) *gregalis major* (Ognev, 1923) and phylogenetic connections between sub-arctic representatives of the genus *Microtus* Schrank, 1798. Acta Theriol., 15:143–152.

FINDLEY, J. S. 1969. Biogeography of southwestern boreal and desert mammals. Pp. 113–128, *in* Contributions in mammalogy (J. K. Jones, Jr., ed.). Misc. Publ. Mus. Nat. Hist., Univ. Kansas, 51:1–428.

GUTHRIE, R. D. 1965. Variability in characters undergoing rapid evolution, an analysis of *Microtus* molars. Evolution, 19:214–233.

GUTHRIE, R. D., AND J. V. MATTHEWS, JR. 1972. The Cape Deceit fauna—early Pleistocene mammalian assemblage from the Alaskan arctic. Quaternary Res., 1(for 1971):474–510.

HAGMEIER, E. M. 1966. A numerical analysis of the distribution patterns of North American mammals. II. Re-evaluation of the provinces. Syst. Zool., 15: 279–299.

HALL, E. R. 1981. The mammals of North America. Second ed. John Wiley, New York, 2:601–1181 + *90* pp.

HALL, E. R., AND W. W. DALQUEST. 1963. The mammals of Veracruz. Univ. Kansas Publ., Mus. Nat. Hist., 14:165–362.

HARINGTON, C. R. 1978. Quaternary vertebrate faunas of Canada and Alaska and their suggested chronological sequence. Natl. Mus. Canada, Syllogeus, 15: 1–105.

HOFFMANN, R. S. 1976. [An ecological and zoogeographical analysis of animal migration across the Bering land-bridge during the Quaternary period.] Pp. 354–367, *in* Beringia in Cenozoic (V. L. Kontrimavichus, ed.). Acad. Sci., Vladivostok, 594 pp. (In Russian, with English summary).

———. 1980. Of mice and men: Beringian dispersal and the ice-free corridor. Canadian J. Anthrol., 1:51–52.

———. 1981. Different voles for different holes: environmental restrictions on refugial survival of mammals. Pp. 25–45, *in* Evolution today (G. G. E. Scudder and J. L. Reveal, eds.), Proc. Second Internatl. Congr. Evol. Biol., Vancouver, B.C., 486 pp.

HONACKI, J. H., K. E. KINMAN, AND J. W. KOEPPL. 1982. Mammal species of the world. Allen Press and Assoc. Syst. Coll., Lawrence, Kansas, 694 pp.

HOOPER, E. T., AND B. S. HART. 1962. A synopsis of Recent North American microtine rodents. Occas. Pap. Mus. Zool., Univ. Michigan, 120:1–68.

HSU, T. C., AND M. L. JOHNSON. 1970. Cytological distinction between *Microtus montanus* and *Microtus canicaudus*. J. Mamm., 51:824–826.

JANNETT, F. J., JR., AND J. Z. JANNETT. 1974. Drum-marking by *Arvicola richardsoni* and its taxonomic significance. Amer. Midland Nat., 92:230–234.

KENDEIGH, S. C. 1961. Animal ecology. Prentice-Hall, Englewood Cliffs, New Jersey, 468 pp.

KOPLIN, J. R., AND R. S. HOFFMANN. 1968. Habitat overlap and competitive exclusion in voles (*Microtus*). Amer. Midland Nat., 80:494–507.

KURTÉN, B., AND E. ANDERSON. 1980. Pleistocene mammals of North America. Columbia Univ. Press, New York, 442 pp.

LAWRENCE, M. A. 1982. Western Chinese arvicolines (Rodentia) collected by the Sage Expedition. Amer. Mus. Novitates, 2745:1–19.

MARTIN, L. D. 1972. The microtine rodents of the Mullen assemblage from the Pleistocene of north central Nebraska. Bull. Univ. Nebraska State Mus., 9:173–182.

MARTIN, L. W. 1979. The biostratigraphy of arvicoline rodents in North America. Trans. Nebraska Acad. Sci., 7:91–100.

MARTIN, R. A. 1968. Late Pleistocene distribution of *Microtus pennsylvanicus*. J. Mamm., 49:265–271.

———. 1974. Fossil mammals from the Coleman IIA fauna, Sumter County. Pp. 35–99, *in* Pleistocene mammals of Florida (S. D. Webb, ed.). Univ. Presses Florida, Gainesville, 270 pp.

MURIE, J. O. 1969. An experimental study of substrate selection by two species of voles (*Microtus*). Amer. Midland Nat., 82:622–625.

———. 1971. Behavioral relationships between two sympatric voles (*Microtus*): relevance to habitat segregation. J. Mamm., 52:181–186.

NADLER, C. F., V. R. RAUSCH, E. A. LYAPUNOVA, R. S. HOFFMANN, AND N. N. VORONTSOV. 1976. Chromosomal banding patterns of the Holarctic rodents, *Clethrionomys rutilus* and *Microtus oeconomus*. Z. Saugetierk., 41: 137–146.

NADLER, C. F., ET AL. 1978. Biochemical relationships of the Holarctic vole genera (*Clethrionomys, Microtus,* and *Arvicola* (Rodentia: Arvicolinae)). Canadian J. Zool., 56:1564–1575.

ODUM, E. P. 1971. Fundamentals of ecology. Third ed. W. B. Saunders Co., Philadelphia, 574 pp.

OGNEV, S. I. 1950. Zveri SSSR i prilezhashchikh stran. vol. 7, Glires. Acad. Sci. Moscow-Leningrad. 706 pp. + 15 maps (Engl. Transl. Off. Tech. Serv., 1963).

RAND, A. L. 1954. The ice age and mammal speciation in North America. Arctic, 7:31–35.

RAUSCH, R. L. 1964. The specific status of the narrow-skulled vole (subgenus *Stenocranius* Kashchenko) in North America. Z. Saugetierk., 29:343–358.

RAUSCH, R. L., AND V. R. RAUSCH. 1968. On the biology and systematic position of *Microtus abbreviatus* Miller, a vole endemic to the St. Matthew Islands, Bering Sea. Z. Saugetierk., 33:65–99.

REPENNING, C. A. 1980. Faunal exchanges between Siberia and North America. Canadian J. Anthropol., 1:37–44.

SAINT GIRONS, M.-C. 1973. Les mammifères de France et du Benelux. Doin, Paris, 481 pp.

SCLATER, P. L. 1858. On the general geographical distribution of the members of the class Aves. J. Proc. Linn. Soc. (Zool.), 2(for 1857):130–145.

SHELFORD, V. E. 1963. The ecology of North America. Univ. Illinois Press, Urbana, 610 pp.

UDVARDY, M. D. F. 1969. Dynamic zoogeography with special reference to land animals. Van Nostrand Reinhold Co., New York, 445 pp.

———. 1975. World biogeographic provinces. Map, *in* A classification of the biogeographic provinces of the world. Internatl. Union Conserv. Nature and Nat. Resour. (IUCN), Occas. Paper, 18.

VAN DER MEULEN, A. J. 1978. *Microtus* and *Pitymys* (Arvicolidae) from Cumberland Cave, Maryland, with a comparison of some New and Old World species. Ann. Carnegie Mus., 47:101–145.

WALLACE, A. R. 1876. The geographical distribution of animals. Harper and Bros., New York, 1:1–503; 2:1–607.

WILEY, E. O. 1981. Phylogenetics. J. Wiley and Sons, New York, 439 pp.

WOODS, C. A., W. POST, AND C. W. KILPATRICK. 1982. *Microtus pennsylvanicus* (Rodentia: Muridae) in Florida: a Pleistocene relict in a coastal salt marsh. Bull. Florida State Mus., 28:25–52.

YOUNGMAN, P. M. 1975. Mammals of the Yukon Territory. Natl. Mus. Nat. Sci. (Canada), Publ. Zool., 10:1–192.

MACROANATOMY

MICHAEL D. CARLETON

Abstract

OUR basic knowledge of the morphology of *Microtus* has accumulated incidentally in the pursuit of greater taxonomic understanding of the genus, its morphological limits, and its position within the web of kinship to other Arvicolidae. Although systematists have focussed by far their greatest attention on variation in the dentition and cranial skeleton of *Microtus,* a rich amount of information is available for less traditional character complexes, such as the musculature, alimentary canal, and reproductive tract. In this chapter, that morphological information is reviewed under the headings of six organ systems—Integument, Skeleton and External Form, Musculature, Circulatory System, Digestive System, and Reproductive System—and presented within both a functional context and a phylogenetic framework. Many aspects of *Microtus* anatomy, particularly the cranial skeleton, associated masticatory musculature, and dentition, have been linked directly or indirectly to selection for exploitation of a herbivorous trophic niche, and species of *Microtus* are generally viewed as among the more derived of Arvicolidae with respect to character state development of such features. Curiously though, the genus *Microtus* as currently recognized seemingly lacks any uniquely derived traits that serve to unambiguously distinguish it from other Arvicolidae. Of the approximately 71 characters that have been distilled from various morphological and taxonomic investigations of Arvicolidae, the character states exhibited by specimens of *Microtus* are either primitive for Muroidea (22) or Arvicolidae (27), or variously shared with other arvicolid genera (22). Instead, the identification of *Microtus* historically has been defined polythetically. These observations lend support to the viewpoint that *Microtus* is at best a paraphyletic taxon.

Introduction

Perhaps no other group of rodents within Muroidea, an assemblage numbering some 250 genera and over 1,000 species, possesses so distinctive a form as the Arvicolidae. Whether one considers species so disparate as the muskrat and bog lemming, the quality of "microtineness" is nonetheless penetrative: robust animals with short legs and tails, blunt muzzles, diminutive pinnae, and small eyes. The prismatic, hypsodont cheekteeth are definitive. Despite the priority of the family-group name Arvicolidae, voles of the genus *Microtus,* by their speciosity and ecological abundance, qualify as the morphotypical representatives of the family. This chapter explores the macroanatomy of that genus.

Mere description of form, the repetition of morphological terms and facts, is an unenlightening, not to mention boring, exercise. Morphology finds its heuristic expression in the taxonomic and functional insights that it provides to systematic biology, and it is this dualistic quality that keeps the study of morphology fresh and dynamic. As this chapter demonstrates, much of our knowledge of the gross anatomy of *Microtus* was incidentally generated in the pursuit of greater taxonomic comprehension of the group. Function, as a separate consideration, more often seemed to emerge as an afterthought from such taxonomically motivated discovery of morphological variety. Accordingly, in reviewing the morphological literature on *Microtus,* I seek to present information within both a phylogenetic framework and a functional context. Several hierarchical levels of relationship are pertinent to our morphological conception of the taxon *Microtus.* Of particular interest here are the anatomical variation exhibited by species constituting the genus, the diagnostic properties of *Microtus* with respect to other genera of Arvicolidae, and the distinctive attributes shared by *Microtus* and other Arvicolidae as members within the broader sphere of the vast and diverse Superfamily Muroidea.

The cranial and dental illustrations that grace these pages were rendered by Janine Higgins, whose careful work and attention to detail I much appreciate. The figures are based on specimens housed in the National Museum of Natural History. Jean Smith patiently typed the various drafts of the manuscript. I dedicate this chapter to David J. Klingener, former major professor, who first introduced me to the delights of rodent anatomy through a manuscript for a chapter he had written on *Peromyscus* anatomy. The invitation to author this chapter on *Microtus* was consequently received and accepted with pleasure and a sense of somehow coming full circle.

Integument

Species of *Microtus* are a rather sombre-colored lot. The pelage of most matches some shade of brown, varying from light, sometimes grayish, to very dark, almost blackish. Bright splashes of color are primarily limited to the yellow or rust-colored noses observed in *M. chrotorrhinus* and *M. xanthognathus*. The fur texture is likewise unremarkable, being moderately thick, long, and lax in the majority of species. The longer guard hairs and dense, wooly underfur of the water vole (*M. richardsoni*) and the short, finely-dense, "molelike" pelt of species of the subgenus *Pitymys,* constitute the prinicipal textural variants within the genus. Unlike pelage texture and color, more systematic attention has been focussed upon other cutaneous features, namely skin glands, the Meibomian glands of the eyelids, and the plantar footpads.

Skin Glands

Differences in pelage texture, color, density, and length usually indicate the location of hypertrophied sebaceous glands, which exude an odiferous, lipidic substance. The glands undergo rapid differentiation coincident with puberty, are typically better developed in males but may be equally pronounced in both sexes, are highly sensitive to androgen levels, and function in dispersing scents that mediate many crucial aspects of arvicolid behavior (for example, individual recognition, territory, social dominance, reproductive condition, and breeding status).

Early students of arvicolid systematics, such as Bailey (1900) and Miller (1896), accorded taxonomic significance to the presence–absence and location of the skin glands and incorporated this variation into their identification keys, a variation still used in taxonomic keys (Hall, 1981). Howell (1924) detailed the size, age, and sexual variation of the hip glands in a population of *Microtus montanus.*

Quay (1968) provided the first exhaustive collation of sebaceous patches in Arvicolidae. He identified four zones on the posterolateral region of a vole's trunk where the glands occur: caudal, rump, hip, and flank. Caudal glands exist only in *Dicrostonyx* and rump glands in *Lemmus* and *Myopus* (Claussen, 1975; Quay, 1968). Other arvicolid genera have either flank (most) or hip glands or lack posterolateral glandular development altogether (*Ondatra, Ellobius,* and *Prometheomys*). *Microtus* encompasses species in each of the last three categories, but the glandular occurrence does not accord with current subgeneric alignments. Quay documented hip glands in *Pitymys* and some *Microtus*; flank glands in *Aulacomys, Stenocranius,* some *Microtus,* and possibly *Herpetomys* and *Pedomys*; but discovered no posterolateral glands in *Chilotus, Orthriomys,* and certain *Microtus.* Quay reported that, at high latitudes, all adult male and female *M. oeconomus* possessed well developed hip glands; yet, at more southern localities, the percentage of voles with highly developed glands decreased, especially among females. Quay suggested that this cline may generally apply to North American *Microtus* at the specific and populational levels. Jannett (1975), however, cautioned that, in view of the responsiveness of cutaneous glands to hormonal titres, variation in their development within species could relate to populational differences in the timing and extent of reproductive activity.

The question of the polarity of evolution of glandular zones in Arvicolidae is an interesting one. Quay (1968) reasoned that the breadth of representation of skin glands among arvicolids argues for their early acquisition, probably as flank patches, during their evolution. While the presence of some sebaceous zone in the ancestral arvicolid seems probable, the decreasing histological complexity of the posterior glands and the occurrence of caudal and rump glands only in lemmings, forms otherwise thought to be primitive, suggest that a transformation series from caudal to rump to hip to flank is a plausible alternative. The diverse anatomical locations of the glandular zones presuppose different postures and motions assumed when animals dispense their scents (see, for instance, Jannett and Jannett, 1974; Quay, 1968; Wolff and Johnson, 1979) and may reflect the radiation of arvicolids into dissimilar structural habitats (for example, open tundra, boreal forest floor, grass runways, subterranean tunnels, and river banks). The absence of skin glands in some *Microtus* is considered a derived trait (Jannett, 1975; Quay, 1968). Jannett (1975) stimulated an atypical differentiation of hip glands in *M. longicaudus* and *M. pennsylvanicus,* species which normally lack such glands, by administering large dosages of exogenous testosterone. He interpreted these results as additional proof that the progenitors of these two voles possessed skin glands and that the cutaneous target zones had lost their sensitivity to physiologically normal androgen levels. His study also underscores the possible evolutionary plasticity of these glandular features and the potential for reversals and convergences. Recently, Boonstra and Youson (1982) and Tamarin (1981) have found hip glands in field populations of *M. pennsylvanicus.*

Meibomian Glands

The eyelids of arvicolids, like those of other mammals, contain modified sebaceous glands, called Meibomian or tarsal glands. Several authors have revealed differences among arvicolids involving the number, size, and position of these glands, differences which do not correlate with season of capture, sex, or age of the animals (Dearden, 1959; Hrabě, 1977, 1978; Quay, 1954*a*). Quay's (1954*a*) study is the broadest taxonomically and encompasses most subgenera of North American *Microtus.* In the primitive condition, the glands are smaller, more evenly spaced, and numerous; species of *Dicrostonyx, Lemmus, Synaptomys, Clethrionomys, Lagurus,* and *Phenacomys* fall into this category (Dearden, 1959; Quay, 1954*a*). Fewer Meibomian glands with large, uneven gaps between them characterize the progressive condition, as observed in *Arvicola, Ondatra,* and species of *Microtus.* The reduction in glandular number seems to be compensated by an increased size of those that remain, especially the posterior ones which extend beyond the eyelid margin (=extrapalpebral glands). *Microtus* species are surprisingly uniform and generally average between three and six tarsal glands; *M.* (*Stenocranius*) *miurus* is the most divergent, having a mean of nine glands. The functional or ecological correlates of this reductional trend remain obscure.

Plantar Footpads

The number, size, and position of plantar pads or tubercles have been used in taxonomic keys of Arvicolidae (Bailey, 1900; Dukelski, 1927; Hinton, 1926; Miller, 1896). Most genera have either five or six metatarsal pads, but the densely furry soles of *Dicrostonyx* apparently lack pad definition. The maximum number of six pads, probably the plesiomorphic state, consists of four interdigitals, situated near the phalangeal bases, and the thenar and hypothenar, set closer to the heel. Although most genera exhibit a constant number of plantar pads, *Microtus* contains species with either five or six. Miller (1896) and Bailey (1900) employed this variable at the subgeneric level in *Microtus,* identifying *Aulacomys, Chilotus, Herpetomys, Orthriomys, Pedomys,* and *Pitymys* as having five pads, and *Microtus* and *Stenocranius* as having six. The stability of this character within *Microtus* should be more thoroughly documented. Howell (1924), for instance, reported substantial variation in a single population of *M. montanus,* whereas Dukelski (1927) concluded that plantar pad morphology was appropriately conservative for application at lower taxonomic levels. In addition to their obvious functional connotation with respect to locomotion and type of substrate, the plantar pads are sites where sweat glands are localized (Griffiths and Kendall, 1980).

Skeleton and External Form

Cranial and External Morphometrics

Mensural data on the skull and external form of *Microtus* is diffusely spread through the literature. The compilation in Table 1 is intended only to introduce the more comprehensive studies that contain tabulations of cranial and external variables; many more sources of measurements exist, particularly in faunistic accounts. Earlier studies often provided measurements of individual specimens but lacked sample statistics. Although many dimensions have been used historically, only some dozen have been consistently recorded (Table 1). Perhaps the preeminence of these variables followed the precedent set by their employment in early studies (for example, Howell, 1924; Kellogg, 1918). More likely, their popularity stems from their repeatability and the ease of positioning the caliper's jaws about the anatomical landmarks which characterize the arvicolid skull (Figs. 1, 2).

Morphological heterogeneity between and within population samples generally has been partitioned into geographic and nongeographic sources of variation, the latter subdivided into variation associated with age, secondary sexual dimorphism, seasonal influ-

TABLE 1
CRANIAL DIMENSIONS AND SOURCES OF MENSURAL DATA FOR NEW WORLD *Microtus*

Dimension	Literature source and species*
Lengths	
Alveolobasilar	2, 6
Angular process	2
Basilar	1, 5, 12
Bony palate	1, 5, 12
Condyloalveolar	3
Condylobasal	1, 4, 8, 9, 10, 11, 12
Condylobasilar	1, 2, 3, 6
Condyloincisive	3, 7, 13
Condylopalatal	2
Condylozygomatic	2, 3, 14
Dentary	1, 12
Diastema	3, 7, 8, 14
Incisive foramen	2, 3, 5, 7, 10, 14
Maxillary toothrow (alveolar)	1, 2, 3, 4, 5, 6, 8, 9, 10, 11, 12
Nasal	1, 2, 4, 5, 7, 8, 9, 10, 12, 14
Occipitonasal	1, 4, 8, 12
Palatilar	4, 6, 8, 14
Rostral	7, 13, 14
Total toothrow (I1–M3)	13
Widths	
Alveolar (across toothrows)	2, 3
Braincase	7, 8
Interorbital	1, 2, 3, 4, 5, 6, 7, 8, 9, 10, 11, 12, 13, 14
Interparietal	1
Lambdoidal	2, 3, 6, 8, 9, 10, 11, 14
Mastoid	1, 4, 5, 8, 12, 13
Postpalatal	5
Prelambdoidal	6, 8, 11, 13, 14
Rostral	4, 8, 14
Zygomatic	1, 2, 3, 4, 5, 6, 7, 8, 9, 10, 11, 12, 13, 14
Miscellaneous	
Cranial capacity	2, 3
Depth of braincase	6, 14
Height of skull	1, 2, 3, 7, 9, 12, 14
Palatofrontal height	8

* 1. Kellogg (1918): *M. californicus*.
2. Howell (1924): *M. montanus*.

ences, and a vague category usually labelled "individual." There are other ways to categorize and view biological variation (see, for example, Mayr, 1969; Yablokov, 1974), but the above divisions illustrate the approach commonly adopted by systematists who have interpreted continuous variation of the skull and external form of *Microtus*. For an appreciation of the evolving treatment of population variation in taxonomic studies of *Microtus*, the reader should consult Anderson (1959), Howell (1924), Snyder (1954), and Choate and Williams (1978). Howell's (1924) exhaustive exposition of variation in a population of *M. montanus yosemite* warrants special mention and, although antiquated in some regards, could serve in any mammalogy course as a didactic introduction to sources of variation in a mammalian species population.

Cranial changes during growth are frequently striking in muroid rodents and especially so in arvicolids. The authors above have qualitatively described the suite of ontogenetic changes in *Microtus*: the skull loses its rounded, fragile conformation and becomes heavier and "squared"; bony processes and ridges, especially the postorbital process and lambdoidal ridge, become strongly expressed and cranial sutures disappear; as the skull enlarges, the proportional relationship of the facial and cranial regions shifts from relatively short rostrum and wide braincase to an elongate, narrower configuration; the weak, narrow zygoma expand and bow laterally; the dorsal curvature of the skull progressively flattens. To reduce age-related biases, investigators have grouped skulls into growth-age cohorts. Because the molars of *Microtus* continuously erupt, stages of tooth wear, used as age indices in other muroid studies,

---

←

3. Goin (1943): *M. pennsylvanicus.*
4. Hall (1946): *M. longicaudus, M. montanus.*
5. Durrant (1952): *M. longicaudus, M. mexicanus, M. montanus, M. richardsoni.*
6. Anderson (1954, 1956, 1959): *M. montanus, M. pennsylvanicus.*
7. Snyder (1954): *M. pennsylvanicus.*
8. Bee and Hall (1956): *M. miurus, M. oeconomus.*
9. Jones (1964): *M. ochrogaster, M. pinetorum, M. pennsylvanicus.*
10. Rausch (1964); Rausch and Rausch (1968): *M. abbreviatus, M. miurus.*
11. Armstrong (1972): *M. longicaudus, M. mexicanus, M. montanus, M. ochrogaster, M. pennsylvanicus.*
12. Kirkland (1977): *M. chrotorrhinus.*
13. Choate and Williams (1978): *M. ochrogaster.*
14. Wilhelm (1982): *M. mexicanus.*

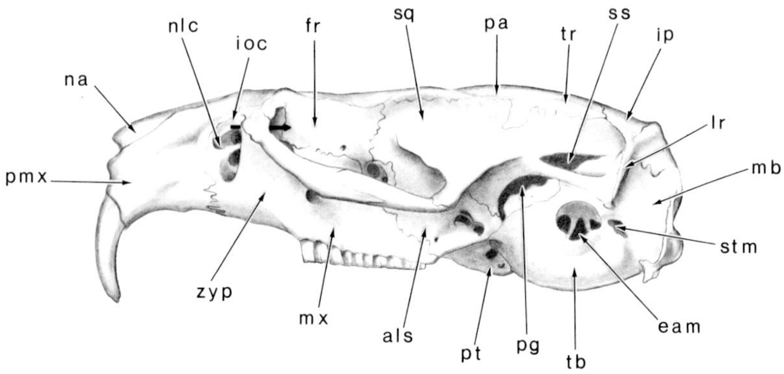

FIG. 1. Lateral view of cranium of male *Microtus* (*Stenocranius*) *miurus,* Alaska. The key that follows defines abbreviations that appear in this figure and in Figs. 2–4.

Foramina and Fossae

alc—alisphenoid canal
eam—external auditory meatus
fm—foramen magnum
fo—foramen ovale
foa—foramen ovale accessorius
hg—hypoglossal
icf—internal carotid fissure
inc—incisive
ioc—infraorbital canal
ipm—interpremaxillary
jg—jugular
ml—middle lacerate
mpf—mesopterygoid fossa
ms—masticatory
nlc—nasolacrimal canal
op—optic
pg—postglenoid
plpp—posterolateral palatal pits
ppf—parapterygoid fossa
ppl—posterior palatine
smx—sphenomaxillary
sph—sphenoidal fissure
spv—sphenopalatine vacuities
ss—subsquamosal
st—stapedial
stm—stylomastoid

Bones and Processes

als—alisphenoid
alst—strut of alisphenoid
bo—basioccipital
bs—basisphenoid
fr—frontal
ip—interparietal
ju—jugal
lbr—lateral bridge
lr—lambdoidal ridge
mb—mastoid bulla
mr—median ridge
mx—maxilla
na—nasal
os—orbitosphenoid
pa—parietal
pl—palatine
pmx—premaxilla
pop—postorbital process
ps—presphenoid
pt—pterygoid
sq—squamosal
tp—tympanic bulla
tr—temporal ridge
ts—transverse shelf
zya—zygomatic arch
zyp—zygomatic plate

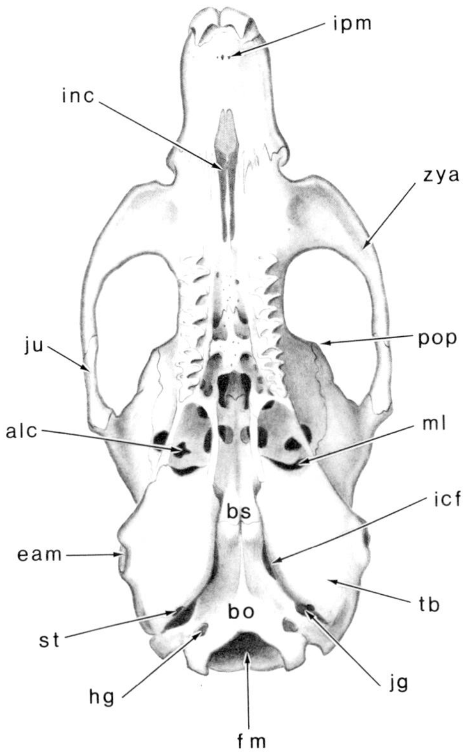

FIG. 2. Ventral view of cranium of male *Microtus* (*Stenocranius*) *miurus,* Alaska. For abbreviations, see Fig. 1.

cannot be assigned. As a result, systematists have relied upon cranial dimensions (Howell, 1924), ratios compounded therefrom (Anderson, 1959), or suture closure and ridge development (Choate and Williams, 1978; Klimkiewicz, 1970; Snyder, 1954) in their recognition of age classes. Snyder (1954) and Anderson (1959) constructed ratio diagrams of several cranial variables to portray the amount of age-related change and to identify which variables most quickly attain "adult" dimensions. Cranial breadth, prelambdoidal breadth, height of skull, and interorbital width undergo relatively little modification with age, while rostral, condylobasilar, and alveolobasilar length and zygomatic breadth change dramatically. Gebczynska

(1964) monitored growth in cranial dimensions using laboratory-raised *M. agrestis* and verified the same pattern of allometric changes.

Engels (1979) nicely elucidated these allometric properties in the skull of *M. arvalis* by tracing the growth of individual bones. Using discriminant function and canonical variate analyses, he demonstrated that the growth rates of the toothrows and bones of the braincase, orbits, and bullae abate by the postnatal day 22; consequently, their dimensions are comparatively age-invariant following weaning. In contrast, facial bones (nasals, premaxillae, and maxillae) and those of the basicranial axis continue growth over a longer period, contributing a significant age factor to their variability in populations. An axis of decreasing duration of growth exists from anterior to posterior for the dermal roofing bones. The interaction of these developmental tendencies imparts the proportional readjustments that contrast the skulls of juvenile and adult voles as described above.

Secondary sexual differences in size are not conspicuous in *Microtus,* but where such disparity exists, males are the larger sex. Slight size dimorphism has been recorded in *M. chrotorrhinus* (Kirkland, 1977), *M. longicaudus* (Findley and Jones, 1962), *M. mexicanus* (Findley and Jones, 1962), *M. miurus* (Bee and Hall, 1956), *M. montanus* (Anderson, 1959; Howell, 1924), *M. oeconomus* (Bee and Hall, 1956), and *M. pennsylvanicus* (Goin, 1943; Snyder, 1954). Although males consistently average larger than females, the hiatus is usually insignificant statistically, leading investigators to combine measurements of the sexes for analytic purposes (Anderson, 1959; Choate and Williams, 1978; Findley and Jones, 1962; but see Snyder, 1954, for an exception). In addition to averaging larger, authors have commented that males exhibit greater extremes of development, an observation supported by the higher coefficients of variation derived for most cranial variables of the male gender in *M. montanus* and *M. pennsylvanicus* (Anderson, 1959; Goin, 1943; Howell, 1924). In view of the size differences observed in other species, it is interesting that Choate and Williams (1978) discovered no significant sexual dimorphism in *M. ochrogaster,* nor did either sex average consistently larger among their samples. The degree or presence of sexual dimorphism in size should be verified for other species of *Microtus,* and the association of species' mating systems with the extent of dimorphism should be explored.

The contribution of seasonal effects to non-geographic heterogeneity of population samples has been addressed infrequently but may account for appreciable inter- and intralocality variation, especially among species having northern distributions. Bee and Hall (1956) substantiated remarkable seasonal differences in cranial size and shape for populations of *M. oeconomus* and *M. miurus* inhabiting the arctic slope of Alaska. *Microtus miurus* born in spring and summer possess the narrow braincase and elongate skull characteristic of the subgenus *Stenocranius*, whereas individuals born in late fall and winter resemble the nominate subgenus in cranial conformation. Bee and Hall (1956) attributed these dissimilarities to the rapid growth of spring- and summer-reared animals, fostered by the richer diet and less stressful climate, and cautioned that understanding variation in these northern *Microtus* requires equal assessment of seasonal and geographic effects. Conceivably, the importance of seasonal influences diminishes in more southern and presumably more equable environments, a relationship that could be evaluated by comparing locality samples of a species such as *M. pennsylvanicus*, which has a broad latitudinal distribution.

The residual population variation not explained by age, sexual dimorphism, or season of capture is characterized as "individual," and the sample statistic Coefficient of Variation is often used to convey the amount of this variation. Coefficients of variation for cranial dimensions are usually less than 10.0 and frequently fall between 2.5 and 6.0, but those for external measurements are typically greater (Choate and Williams, 1978; Goin, 1943; Howell, 1924; Snyder, 1954; Wilhelm, 1982). These values fit the broad pattern of variability of linear skeletal measurements distilled from studies of numerous kinds of mammals (Yablokov, 1974). The investigations of Goin (1943) and Snyder (1954) employed the same locality sample of *M. pennsylvanicus* but disclosed quite different magnitudes of individual variation. Snyder noted that this discrepancy probably arose from his use of more restricted age classes and the consequent elimination of some age-related size increases. Rather than an explanatory source of population heterogeneity, variation termed "individual" is more often an all-other category tailored to the convenience and purpose of a specific study and cannot be assumed to reflect the underlying genetic variability intrinsic to the population. Still other factors, either procedural or biological, may be contributive.

The number of subspecies recognized for most species of *Microtus* bears testimony to the occurrence of geographic variation (see Hoffmann and Koeppl, this volume). In his study of Californian *M. montanus,* Kellogg (1922*a*) observed that his samples are recognizable colonies whose center of differentiation corresponds to separate marshy areas. Fortunately, he concluded that formal identification of each variant would only create a nomenclatural morass. Snyder (1954) performed analyses of variance on samples of *M. pennsylvanicus pennsylvanicus* and demonstrated significant locality effects for most external and cranial measurements within a restricted geographic area of northwestern Pennsylvania. Furthermore, samples of several subspecies of *M. pennsylvanicus* from northeastern North America collectively exhibited the range of variation documented for just the localized samples of *M. p. pennsylvanicus,* a result which led Snyder to question the purpose of so many subspecies. Findley and Jones (1962) examined patterns of variation among disjunct populations of *M. longicaudus, M. mexicanus,* and *M. montanus* from montane regions of the southwestern U.S. and observed a positive correlation between the amount of geographic variation within a species and the degree of geographical or ecological restriction of its constitutive populations. Snell and Cunnison (1983) assessed patterns of interpopulational cranial variation of *M. pennsylvanicus* from throughout its range and found that phenetic distances among populations did not correspond to geographic distances. They concluded that geographic proximity is not a good estimate of isolation of populations, but that other factors (for example, topographical complexity, intervening unfavorable habitats, and sensitivity to local selection pressures) probably account for the disruption of genetic continuity and maintenance of morphological differences among geographically close populations of *M. pennsylvanicus.*

These four cases, drawn from different times and exemplifying different methods and perspectives, are cited not to revive debate on the subspecies concept but to emphasize the demic nature of geographic variation that characterizes populations of *Microtus* and that is expressed in the subtle but demonstrable differences in size and shape between those populations.

As is true for the subspecific category as applied to other mammals, the recognition of geographic races of *Microtus* species rests primarily on differences in size, proportion, and pelage color. Few taxonomic studies, however, have attempted to quantify broad geographic trends and objectively delimit subspecific boundaries. Anderson (1959) qualitatively scored coat color in *M. pennsylvanicus* using an exemplar method, mapped the distribution of mean color values, and discerned geographical groupings that aided his delineation of subspecies. Reflectance analyses of pelage color in *M. ochrogaster* from the central Great Plains, however, disclosed no meaningful trends or patterns of racial differentiation (Choate and Williams, 1978). In *M. montanus,* Anderson (1959) detected a geographic trend toward larger-bodied voles from the southern part of its range, a reversal of Bergmann's generalization on ecophysiological affects on body size. Choate and Williams (1978) noted a similar body-cline in *M. ochrogaster.* Snell and Cunnison (1983) more thoroughly explored the relationship of climate and cranial variation in *M. pennsylvanicus,* using several multivariate techniques to assess the effects of 15 climatic variables. They too noted an inverse correlation of size and temperature, extreme low temperature and mean annual number of days with frost being two of the most significant climatic factors explaining cranial variation.

The studies of Choate and Williams (1978), Snell and Cunnison (1983), and Wilhelm (1982) constitute the first extensive use of multivariate methods in collating geographic variation of morphometric variables used to describe *Microtus* populations.

Qualitative Cranial Features

Besides size and shape, other aspects of cranial morphology have commanded attention in systematic studies of *Microtus,* among them the condition of the posterior palatal area, the occurrence of cranial foramina, and the septal development of the bullar chambers. Although the variation observed in these traits is described as discontinuous, especially as dogmatically used in binary keys, extensive examination has revealed intermediate stages at some hierarchical level of comparison. Some of this heterogeneity fits Berry and Searle's (1963) picture of epigenetic polymorphism, in which variation is realized during ontogeny, perhaps as a result of developmental thresholds for character expression that result in discrete adult phenotypes. Such epigenetic traits may be constant in some species, or even in certain populations of a species, but they exhibit polymorphic variation in others. Hilborn (1974) surveyed the occurrence of some cranial foramina in *M. californicus* and concluded that the

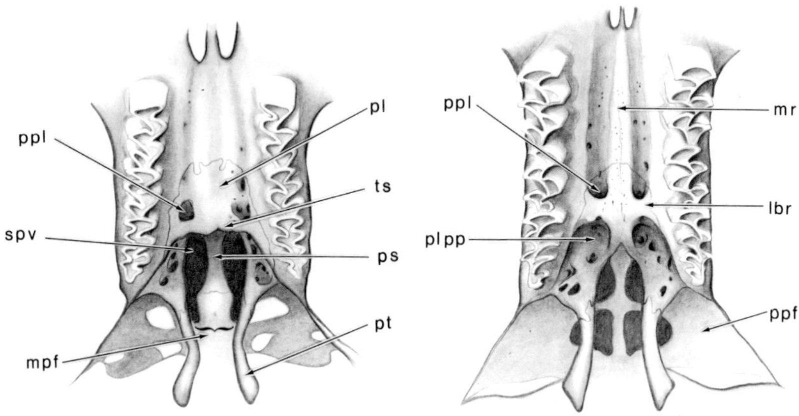

FIG. 3. Ventral view of two common palatal arrangements observed in Arvicolidae: left, simple condition as exemplified by *Clethrionomys gapperi,* Virginia; right, complicated configuration as exhibited by *Microtus pennsylvanicus,* Wisconsin. For abbreviations, see Fig. 1.

prevalence of such traits could be used to measure genetical differences between local populations.

In their pioneering studies of arvicolids, Hinton (1926) and Miller (1896) attached particular taxonomic import to the bony architecture of the posterior palatal region. Bailey (1900:10) gave palatal development as a trenchant generic character in his diagnosis of *Microtus*: "Palate with median ridge, distinct lateral pits, complete lateral bridges (not terminating in posterior shelf in any American species)." His description characterizes the more prevalent of the two basic anatomical plans recognized in Arvicolidae (Fig. 3). In the other, the palate terminates as a transverse shelf, with or without a median spine, and the palatal pits extend anteriorly and above the palatal shelf. This arrangement is seen in *Clethrionomys, Eothenomys,* and, to a lesser degree, in *Lemmus.* Although the palatal types seem clearly defined, assignment of genera, species, and sometimes individuals to one condition or the other is sometimes equivocal. Thus, Hooper and Hart (1962) stated that all degrees of intermediacy are found within Arvicolidae, and Rausch (1964) illustrated gradations between the extreme palatal configurations once thought to distinguish Old World *M. gregalis* from New World *M. miurus.* Hinton (1926:16) drew attention to the thick processes of the maxillary and palatine bones and emphasized this feature as an integral characteristic of arvicolids. The degree of thickness varies within Arvicolidae, however, and this variation seemingly relates to posterior palatal development. As recognized by Hinton, the thickness of the palatal extensions of the maxillaries and palatines correlates with the hypertrophied alveolar cavities of the high-crowned molars. And like the incremental development of hypsodonty observed between genera of arvicolids, it is not surprising that a corresponding gradation in palatal structure exists also.

The incisive foramina in *Microtus* are either broad and oval-shaped at both ends or constricted posteriorly. Anderson (1959) recognized seven states of foraminal shape bridging these extremes and tabulated their frequency of occurrence in 11 species representing five subgenera of *Microtus*. Most species' histograms spanned several character states but always displayed a clear-cut modality. Quay (1954*b*) demonstrated that the posterior constriction is confined to the maxillary portion of the incisive foramina and may become expressed strongly in older animals. In *M.* (*Aulacomys*) *richardsoni*, the posterior closure is so complete that the absolute length of the incisive foramina decreases with age; a slight increase in length represents the normal growth pattern in other *Microtus*. Quay did not speculate on the functional significance of this phenomenon.

The patency of foramina that pierce the base of the alisphenoid bone varies among arvicolids (terminology follows Wahlert, 1974). In the hypothesized primitive state, a strut of the alisphenoid demarcates a medial masticatory foramen, which transmits the masticatory and buccinator branches of the trigeminal nerve (V3), and a posterolateral foramen ovale accessorius, which conducts other branches of V3. This condition obtains in *Ellobius*, *Eothenomys*, and the lemmings *Lemmus*, *Myopus*, and *Synaptomys*. In the remaining genera, including most species of *Microtus*, the base of the alisphenoid has a single, spacious opening (Fig. 4), presumably derived by loss of the alisphenoid strut. Berry and Searle (1963) scored the double-foramina condition in 83% of the *Lemmus lemmus* examined, but in only 1% of one population of *Microtus agrestis* and none of another. In conformance with Berry and Searle's results, I discovered that a single opening prevails in most *Microtus* (32 of 35 species examined). Nevertheless, two Old World species, *M. majori* and *M. montebelli*, generally possess discrete masticatory and

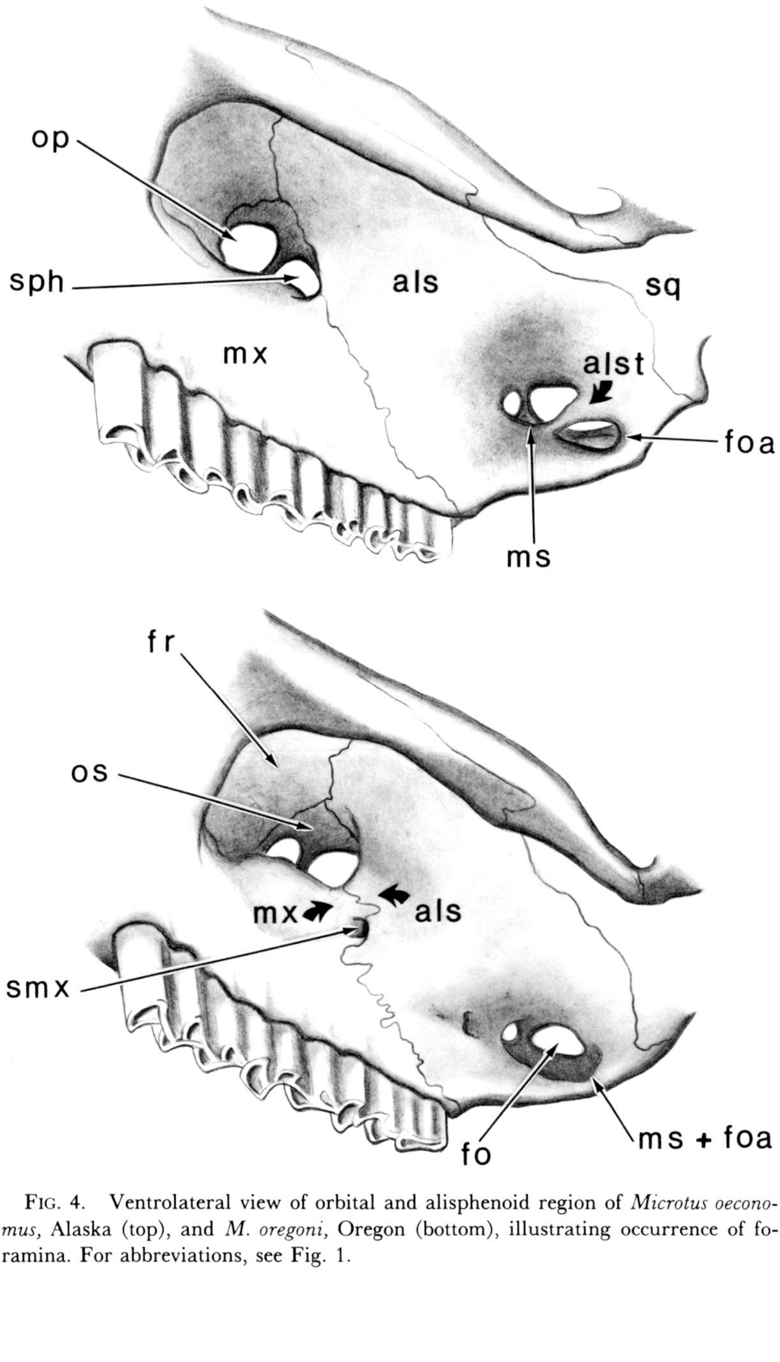

FIG. 4. Ventrolateral view of orbital and alisphenoid region of *Microtus oeconomus*, Alaska (top), and *M. oregoni*, Oregon (bottom), illustrating occurrence of foramina. For abbreviations, see Fig. 1.

ovale foramina, and one trans-Beringean species, *M. oeconomus* (Fig. 4), commonly exhibits both, but I did not assay frequencies in detail.

Some uncertainty has attended the identity of another cranial foramen, a small one situated between the maxillary and alisphenoid bones and ventral to the sphenoidal fissure. This foramen transmits a branch of the internal maxillary artery, its continuation in the lower orbit evidenced by a faint groove across the maxillary bone. Within Arvicolidae, the foramen occurs in *Myopus, Synaptomys, Lagurus* (*Lemmiscus*), *Arvicola,* and most species of *Microtus.* Among North American *Microtus,* it is uniformly lacking in *M. oeconomus* (Fig. 4) and variable in *M. pinetorum* and *M. quasiater.* The variable extent of contiguity between the alisphenoid and maxillary bones that encircle this foramen suggests a plausible transformation series associated with the degree of hypsodonty and complementary height of the molar alveolar capsules (Fig. 4). Both Guthrie (1963) and Hinton (1926) observed that the space enclosed by the maxillary-alisphenoid junction is homologous with the ventrolateral portion of the sphenoidal fissure in those arvicolids which lack this accessory foramen. The dorsal extension of the alveolar capsules that accompanied the evolution of extreme hypsodonty resulted in contact of the maxillary palisades with the alisphenoid, thereby sequestering the ventrolateral part of the sphenoidal fissure as a new foramen. Howell (1924) termed the opening the foramen rotundum, but Hill (1935) noted the incorrectness of Howell's designation and instead called it the alisphenoid foramen. Because the latter name invites confusion with the alisphenoid canal, because the opening is not strictly homologous with the anterior end of the alisphenoid canal of other rodents, and because the foramen apparently evolved as a neomorphic trait only in certain arvicolids, I suggest the positional term sphenomaxillary foramen.

The auditory bullae of arvicolids are globose structures (Fig. 2), appearing moderately inflated compared to most cricetines but not matching the outsized proportions seen in many gerbillines. Hooper (1968) examined serial cranial sections of *Lemmus, Synaptomys, Clethrionomys, Neofiber,* and three species of *Microtus,* and discerned three types of middle ear systems, termed the open, intermediate, and closed. In examples of the first (for example, *Clethrionomys*), a large accessory tympanum is present, and the walls of the mastoid and tympanic bullae lack osseous internal septa and spicules, thus presenting an open bullar chamber. In forms exhibiting the closed system (for example, *Lemmus*), an accessory tympanum is absent, and the interior walls of the mastoid and tympanic capsules bear thick masses of spongy bone that greatly restrict the free space of the chambers. *Microtus* possesses the intermediate type, in which the accessory tympanum consists of a minute arc between the dorsal lamina of the tympanic bone, and the bullar walls have moderate amounts of cancellous partitions and struts. Even within the "intermediate" category, species of *Microtus* vary appreciably in the density and completeness of these bony projections: sparse in the subgenus *Orthriomys*; moderate in *Aulacomys, Herpetomys, Pedomys,* and some *Microtus*; and high in *Chilotus, Pitymys, Stenocranius,* and many *Microtus.*

The bony meshwork of the bullae reduces the unobstructed space behind the tympanic membrane. Simkin (1965) postulated that the cancellous bone functions as an acoustic filter, dampening out biologically unimportant frequencies from the animal's environment. His suggestion seems compatible partially with Fleischer's (1978) idea that the cancellous network acts to suppress undesirable resonances in a middle ear with a reduced cavity volume. Simkin (1965) associated the spongy bullae with mammals living in close habitats, such as the bogs, grassy tunnels, and subnivean galleries occupied by arvicolids; however, Hooper (1968) concluded that the ecological correlates of arvicolids with dissimilar middle ear anatomies were ambiguous. The presence of an accessory tympanum augments the receptor surface of the tympanic membrane and probably enhances the middle ear transformer ratio. Comparative studies of auditory sensitivity using *Clethrionomys, Microtus,* and *Lemmus,* may offer some insight to these variations.

Two configurations of the malleus, denoted as the parallel and perpendicular types, have been documented in Muroidea (Cockerell et al., 1914; Fleischer, 1978). The two anatomical plans derive their names from the parallel or perpendicular orientation of the blade of the manubrium to the rotational axis of the malleus-incus complex. The parallel type characterizes New World cricetines and murines, whereas the perpendicular morphology occurs in gerbillines and arvicolids. Cockerell et al. (1914) considered the parallel malleus as primitive, but Fleischer (1978) derived both kinds from a state called the "ancestral type," which resembles the parallel morphology except for the lack of an orbicular apophysis. The conformational rearrangements that define the perpendicular malleus, such as found in *Microtus,* lessen the tortional stiffness of the malleus-incus complex, suggesting a middle ear complex better attuned to low frequency sounds (Fleischer, 1978).

Postcranial Skeleton

Compared to the cranium the postcranial skeleton of arvicolid rodents has attracted less attention in systematic and functional studies. Carleton (1980) found that *M. pennsylvanicus* possess 13 thoracic and 6 lumbar vertebrae, a count typical of other arvicolids and Old and New World cricetines, and suggested that this ratio represents the primitive condition in Muroidea. The numbers of thoracics (and associated ribs) and lumbars in other muroids range from 12 to 15 and 6 to 7, respectively. The reason for this diversity in vertebral and rib number has not been explored. Another feature of the axial skeleton shared by all arvicolids is the lack of a pronounced vertebral spine on the neural arch of the second thoracic vertebra (Carleton, 1980). An hypertrophied spine arises from the second thoracic vertebra in other muroids and serves as the origin of the nuchal ligament and part of the splenius muscle, which inserts along the lambdoidal ridge of the skull. The loss of this spine in *Microtus* and other arvicolids intimates changes in posture and mobility of the head.

Investigators have demonstrated the utility of the pelvis for identifying, sexing, and aging *Microtus* recovered from owl pellets (Brown and Twigg, 1969; Dunmire, 1955; Guilday, 1951; Hecht, 1971). Brown and Twigg (1969) and Dunmire (1955) were able to discriminate adult male and female *Microtus* using dimensions and ratios of the innominate bones, which undergo slight modifications at sexual maturity in males but change dramatically in females as a result of resorption and remodelling at the pubic symphysis. Mensural overlap and consequent uncertainty of gender were restricted to prepubertal individuals. The pelvic changes that signal pregnancy and parturition allowed Brown and Twigg (1969) to define non-parous, uniparous, and multiparous female cohorts. Brown and Twigg also identified several pelvic features that distinguish British Muridae from Arvicolidae.

Carleton (1980) noted that *Microtus pennsylvanicus* lack an entepicondylar foramen on the humerus. All arvicolids examined (14 genera, including 22 species of *Microtus*) support this observation, suggesting that foramen loss is characteristic of the family. Its occurrence in other Muroidea is sporadic: present in gerbillines, most Old World cricetines, most North American cricetines, and many murines; absent in arvicolids, South American cricetines, and many murines. Anatomists have debated whether the foramen protects the filiform structures (median nerve and sometimes the brachial artery) that traverse it, or whether its occurrence reflects muscular-skeletal changes affecting the distal humerus. Landry (1958) rejected both notions and argued that the foramen acts as a retinaculum, which restrains the median nerve from sagging across the elbow joint, especially in mammals with a deep, loose axilla. Although his explanation may account for the foramen's variation in some mammals, it inadequately accommodates the Muroidea, species of which generally have a loose investiture of skin about the axilla but nonetheless vary in foramen occurrence.

Stains (1959) examined the calcanea of *M. pennsylvanicus, M. ochrogaster,* and *M. pinetorum,* and remarked on the distal placement of the trochlear process, a shelf-like buttress for the peroneus longus tendon, in arvicolids as compared to other muroids. The distal shift of the trochlear shelf intimates adjustments in the lever action of the peroneus longus, an important flexor of the foot.

Musculature

Studies of arvicolid musculature have emphasized the branchiomeric complex because of interest in masticatory accommodations associated with a herbivorous trophic niche. Howell (1924) provided brief descriptions of the jaw muscles in *Microtus montanus* and concluded that adult cranial morphology mirrors the mechanical forces exerted during ontogenetic development of muscular attachments, which in turn are related to the animal's food and feeding mode. Repenning (1968) presented a more detailed picture of the masticatory musculature of *M. longicaudus.* In particular, he noted that the insertion of the masseter medialis, pars anterior, onto the ascending mandibular ramus imparted a conspicuous depression, which he designated the "arvicoline groove." Repenning stressed the importance of this character as a marker to discriminate early microtines from dentally progressive cricetines in the fossil record. The bulk of our knowledge of myological variation in the Arvicolidae issues from the work of Kesner (1977, 1980).

In his functional analysis of jaw muscles, Kesner (1980) identified correlates of the propalinal mastication (motion of the mandible primarily in an anterior-posterior direction) so highly evolved in arvicolids. In contrast to a generalized cricetine pattern, he concluded that the anterior vector component of the superficial masseter, masseter lateralis profundus, and internal pterygoid and the vertical component of the medial temporalis are strongly pronounced. These differences in muscle action, achieved through changes in fiber orientation and muscle bulk, shifts in origins and insertions, and remodeling of the cranium and dentary, synergistically operate to enhance the longitudinal grinding of the dental batteries in arvicolids. Kesner highlighted the role played by the central tendon of the medial temporalis in propounding his "propalinal swing" hypothesis of arvicolid feeding mechanics. The central tendon attaches to the postorbital process, a bony crest on the squamosal of arvicolids; muscle fibers originating from this tendon insert into the temporal fossa of the dentary. He postulated that the postorbital-crest tendon of the temporalis functions as a suspensory sling for the mandible, uniformly transmitting vertical compressive forces throughout the arc of mandibular excursion, while other muscles (superficial masseter, masseter lateralis profundus, and internal pterygoid) supply the major protrusive action of the lower jaw. Species of *Microtus,* as well as *Ondatra* and *Neofiber,* have a long, well-developed postorbital-crest tendon compared to the shorter condition observed in *Phenacomys* and *Lagurus.*

The attachment of the hyoid apparatus to the cranium occurs by two basic kinds of suspensory arrangements among Muroidea, although some intermediate conditions have been described (Kesner, 1977; Klingener, 1968; Rinker, 1954; Sprague, 1941). In the plesiomorphic state, a stylohyal cartilage forms a ligamentous connection to the wall of the stylomastoid foramen, a discrete jugulohyoideus muscle inserts upon the end of the stylohyal, and the stylohyoideus originates broadly from the same cartilage. This configuration typifies *Clethrionomys, Phenacomys, Lemmus, Synaptomys,* and *Dicrostonyx* within Arvicolidae (Kesner, 1977). In the derived state, the stylohyal is absent or greatly reduced, as is the jugulohyoideus, and the stylohyoideus muscle originates from the paroccipital process and a fascial sheet that now supports the hyoid complex. This morphology is exemplified by *Ondatra, Lagurus,* and *Microtus.* The functional consequences of these evolutionary transformations are unknown; one can only surmise that they relate to powers of vocalization or perhaps to mastication and deglutition.

In his study of generic affinities, Kesner (1977) sampled myological diversity of the jaw, hyoid, and pectoral limb regions. He determined character state polarities for 47 muscles in *Microtus* (three North American species) and nine other arvicolid genera and performed several multivariate analyses. Compared to representative cricetines, arvicolids possess synapomorphies in the presence of a medial insertion of the masseter lateralis profundus, development of the postorbital-crest tendon of the temporalis, a robust internal pterygoid, reduction of the tendinous arcade of the digastric, and the insertion of the pectoralis minor onto the coracoid process. Of the species of *Microtus* examined (*pennsylvanicus, pinetorum,* and *richardsoni*), *M. richardsoni* is the most differentiated and Kesner supported its transfer to *Arvicola.* He further recommended that the complexity of relationships suggested by muscular variation is best conveyed by a multitribal classification of Arvicolidae.

Circulatory System

Our comparative anatomical knowledge of the circulatory system in Muroidea is mostly limited to the cephalic arterial blood supply, probably a reflection of the desire to establish homologies and functions of the cranial foramina often employed as taxonomic characters in studies of Rodentia. Variations in carotid circulatory patterns, particularly the branching of the stapedial artery, critically bear on the occurrence of some cranial foramina as detailed in the studies of Bugge (1970) and Guthrie (1963).

A complete carotid circulation is thought to represent the ancestral muroid condition. The stapedial artery separates from the internal carotid near the tympanic bulla, which it enters via the stapedial foramen. Inside the bulla, the stapedial bifurcates: the opthalmic branch crosses the inner surface of the squamosal bone, its pathway marked by a faint groove, and enters the orbit through the sphenofrontal foramen; the internal maxillary branch emerges from the bulla at the petrotympanic fissure, reenters the skull through the alisphenoid canal, and passes into the orbit through the sphenoidal fissure. This circulatory arrangement characterizes Old World cricetines, many New World cricetines, and some nesomyines. For a thorough depiction of the intricate carotid circulation, the reader should consult Bugge (1970), Guthrie (1963), and Klingener (1968).

Reductions of the stapedial artery occur in the Arvicolidae, Gerbillinae, Murinae, and some New World Cricetinae. Guthrie (1963) portrayed the carotid circulation of *Microtus pennsylvanicus,* and Bugge (1970) dissected *M. agrestis* plus examples of *Lemmus, Clethrionomys,* and *Arvicola.* In all, the proximal portion of the opthalmic artery is absent and so too are the sphenofrontal foramen and squamosal groove. Instead, the distal part of the opthalmic originates from the internal maxillary and exits the cranium through the lower part of the sphenoidal fissure. The stapedial artery and foramen remain large since the internal maxillary constitutes the continuation of the stapedial outside of the tympanic bulla. Examination of skulls of other arvicolids suggests that this pattern is found in all except *Synaptomys, Myopus,* and *Lemmus.* These lack a stapedial foramen and may therefore have an arterial configuration resembling that reported in *Sigmodon* (Bugge, 1970), in which both the opthalmic and internal maxillary anastomose with the internal carotid but still emerge via the sphenoidal fissure. In this condition, the importance of the stapedial artery to the orbital circulation is greatly diminished.

No other mammalian order exhibits variation in carotid circulation like that encountered in the Rodentia (Bugge, 1970), but the reason for this diversity is poorly understood. Guthrie (1963) implicated the freer movement of the mandible in the glenoid fossa and the consequent stress this masticatory innovation applied to the primitive carotid arrangement. His explanation focussed on variation in the origin of the internal maxillary artery across all Rodentia and seems inapplicable to the patterns observed in Muroidea. However, his account of the probable mechanism whereby this diversity was realized phylogenetically is pertinent. In rodents, the embryonic carotid vessels consist of remnants of the primitive aortic arch circulation. Interspecific variation in the adult circulatory pattern partly results from the persistence of certain embryonic connections and the atrophy of others (Bugge, 1970; Guthrie, 1969). Thus, the existence of alternative pathways permits some developmental plasticity in the configuration of the blood circuit. In this light, it is instructive to remember that selection for propalinal mastication and bullar hypertrophy, as exemplified by *Microtus,* has produced major restructuring of the cranium, particularly involving those skull regions where bifurcation of the carotid arteries occurs. The enlarged pulp cavities of the hypsodont teeth, the excavation of the parapterygoid fossae for the internal pterygoid muscles, and the expansion of the tympanic bullae have profoundly affected the morphology of the alisphenoid and otic regions, which contain the critical foramina for several primary carotid branches. Perhaps the search for a functional explanation for the variability in carotid circulation among Muroidea will lie in the specific skeletal and muscular adaptations peculiar to each group and the circulatory accommodations such evolutionary changes have imposed.

A large venous plexus continuous with veins of the nasal chamber occupies the maxillary (posterior) portion of the incisive foramina. Quay (1954*b*) termed this network the nasopalatine venous plexus and noted that its branches penetrate the incisive papillae, which elevate the openings of the nasopalatine ducts. The nasopalatine complex is drained by the posterior palatine veins, which course along furrows on the bony palate and conjoin the internal maxillary via the posterior palatine foramina. Modification of the nasopalatine venous plexus is suggested for those *Microtus* (for example, *richardsoni* and *montanus*) with posteriorly constricted incisive foramina.

Digestive System

Dentition

Whether viewed from a paleontological or neontological perspective, the meristic quality of cheektooth variations has continually appealed to students of arvicolid evolution and early established this character suite as the *sine qua non* of their systematics. Hinton (1926:22) succinctly catalogued the dental features that investigators have relied upon, to one degree or another, over the past century:

> The difference in the number, form, and relative size of the triangles and salient angles, the degree to which the dentinal spaces are open to or closed off from each other, the greater or less complexity of the anterior loop in M_1 and of the posterior loop in M^3, the distribution and nature of the enamel sheet in different parts of the periphery, the presence or absence of cement, and above all the circumstance whether the cheek-teeth are

> of persistent or of limited growth *i.e.,* rooted or rootless;—all these, when used with discretion, afford excellent characters for the distinction of genera and species.

With regard to each of these characters, *Microtus* is among the more progressive genera in the family.

The molar teeth of Arvicolidae stand as the foremost example of hypsodont development within the Muroidea. Their hypsodonty involves a vertical elongation of the entire crown (denoted coronal hypsodonty) in contrast to a pronounced extension of the individual cusps, or tubercular hypsodonty. The transformation from a rooted, high-crowned tooth to an "evergrowing" one, in which the pulp cavity of the root retains its generative function throughout an individual's lifetime marked a major threshold in the evolution of the arvicolid molar. The few arvicolids that now possess rooted molars, generally viewed as an indicator of primitiveness, include *Clethrionomys, Dinaromys, Ellobius, Ondatra, Phenacomys,* and *Prometheomys*; some of these develop closed roots only as old adults. The remaining taxa, including all species of *Microtus,* have continuously growing, "rootless" cheekteeth. Early fossil arvicolids lacked cement in the reentrant folds, a condition which persists in several extant genera (for example, in *Dicrostonyx* and *Lagurus*); however, prominent cement buttresses line the reentrant angles of *Microtus* molars. For discussion of the complex histological rearrangements that necessarily accompanied selection for persistently-growing, hypsodont molars, see Phillips (this volume).

The occlusal surfaces of the molars consist of dentine basins enclosed by enamel triangles, the number, shape, and completeness of which have been stressed in studies of arvicolid relationships. Generally a tooth has an anterior loop (also called the "trefoil"), a series of alternating salient angles and reentrant folds, and a posterior loop (Fig. 5). If the enamel border of a salient angle extends across the tooth to contact its opposite member, the wholly enclosed enamel prism is termed a closed triangle; if the dentine of contiguous salient angles remains confluent, those prisms are designated open triangles. The metameric nature of arvicolid cheekteeth has discouraged attempts to homologize cusps following the Cope-Osbornian tritubercular system. Instead, an alphanumeric system has been employed to designate the molar components and to facilitate comparisons (Hinton, 1926; Klimkiewicz, 1970; Koenigswald, 1980; Martin, 1973; Oppenheimer, 1965). Most meristic conventions have

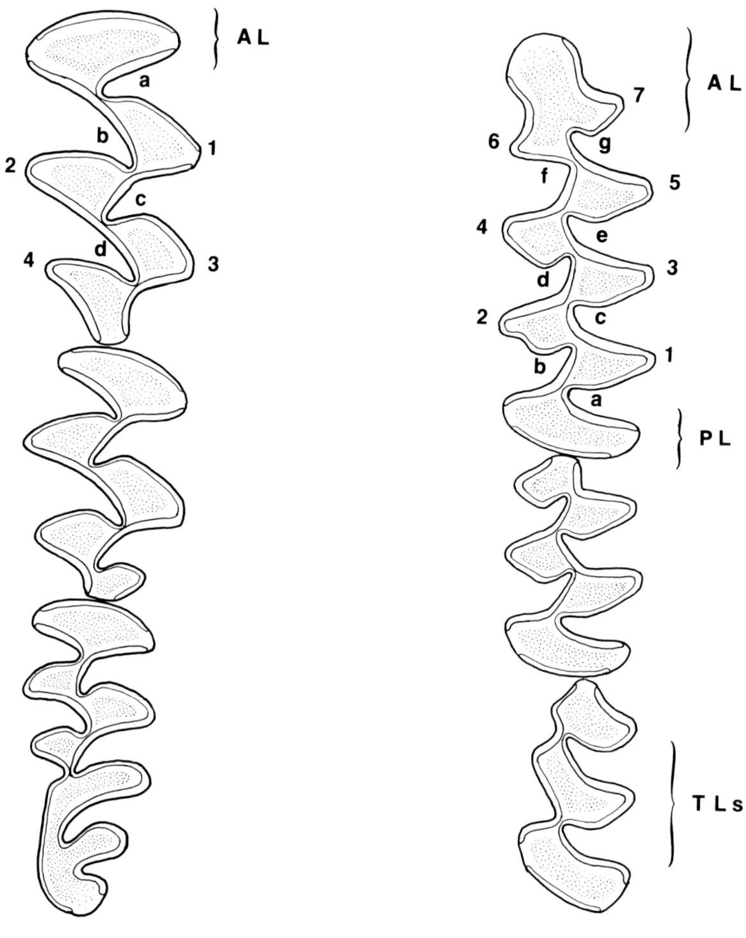

FIG. 5. Occlusal view of the upper right (left) and lower left (right) molar toothrows of *Microtus pennsylvanicus* (from Virginia) illustrating one possible alphanumeric labelling scheme. Abbreviations are: AL, anterior loop; PL, posterior loop; TLs, transverse loops; a–g, reentrant folds; 1–5, salient angles of closed triangles; 6–7, salient angles of open triangles.

followed Hinton's (1926) scheme for labelling the triangles, salient angles, and reentrant angles from anterior to posterior in the upper molars and from posterior to anterior in the lowers, after first indicating the anterior and posterior loops (Fig. 5).

Variation in the upper third and lower first and second molars broadly defines two occlusal patterns among North American *Microtus*. One pattern, as exemplified by the subgenera *Herpetomys, Orthriomys, Pedomys,* and *Pitymys* consists of two closed and one open triangle in M3, only three closed triangles in m1, and two closed and two open triangles in m2 (Table 2). The subgenera *Aulacomys, Microtus,* and *Stenocranius,* on the other hand, are characterized by at least three closed triangles in M3, usually five entire triangles in m1, and four closed triangles in m2 (Table 2). In each pairwise comparison, the presumably homologous elements are identifiable for each tooth (Fig. 6). These two patterns represent the primary foci of dental variation in the genus and were used traditionally to delineate the subgenera (Bailey, 1900; Miller, 1896). Still other molar configurations have been recognized as taxonomically important, especially the presence of two closed triangles in the m3 of *Orthriomys* and *Herpetomys,* the development of a posteromedial loop in the M2 of some *Microtus,* and the greater complexity of the M3 of *M. chrotorrhinus* (Table 2, Fig. 6). The presence of poorly developed triangles has been cited frequently for the separate generic status of *Pitymys,* a taxonomic opinion more often espoused by paleontologists and European workers (for example, Corbet 1978; Zakrzewski, this volume) than by North American mammalogists (for example, Anderson, this volume; Hall, 1981). However, the gradational character of dental variation in the group complicates such a diagnostic yardstick for generic limits, for it at once brings to issue the status and relationship of other subgenera (for example, *Chilotus, Herpetomys,* and *Pedomys*) and even species of typical *Microtus* (for example, *M. oeconomus*), whose dentition exhibits comparable degrees of divergence.

In view of the taxonomic weight traditionally accorded arvicolid dental morphology, it appears somewhat incongruous that every author who has scrutinized their dentition has remarked upon the tremendous individual variation, sometimes seen bilaterally on an individual, and the fine structural gradations within and between populations. Nonetheless, species and populations display a sharp modality in occlusal configuration, and the conspicuous variation typically involves only particular areas of two molars. Hinton's (1926) claim that the dental pattern of an individual's cheekteeth became altered with age and wear was disproved by Oppenheimer (1965), who found no appreciable difference in the pattern of a

TABLE 2
PRINCIPAL DENTAL VARIATION IN NEW WORLD *Microtus*

Subgenus and species	M2			M3				m1				m2		m3		
	3cT	3cT + 1oT	4cT	2cT	2c + 1oT	3cT	3c + 2oT	3cT	4cT	5cT	6cT	2c + 2oT	4cT	3TL	2TL + 2oT	2TL + 2cT
Aulacomys																
richardsoni	X				X	(X)				X	(X)		X	X		
Chilotus																
oregoni	X				X					X		X		X		
Herpetomys																
guatemalensis	X					X		X					X			X
Microtus																
breweri			X			X				X			X	X		
californicus		X	(X)			X				X			X	X	(X)	
canicaudus	X					X				X			X	X		
chrotorrhinus	X						X			X		X	(X)	X		
longicaudus	X					X				X	(X)		X	X		
mexicanus	X					X				X			X	X		
montanus		X	(X)			X				X	(X)		X	X		
nesophilus		X			X					X			X	X		
oaxacensis	X						X			X			X	X		
oeconomus	X					X			X	(X)			X	X		
pennsylvanicus		(X)	X			X				X	(X)		X	X		
townsendii	X					X				X			X	X		
xanthognathus	X					X				X			X	X		

TABLE 2
CONTINUED

Subgenus and species	M2			M3				m1				m2		m3		
	3cT	3cT + 1oT	4cT	2cT	2c + 1oT	3cT	3c + 2oT	3cT	4cT	5cT	6cT	2c + 2oT	4cT	3TL	2TL + 2oT	2TL + 2cT
Orthriomys																
umbrosus	X				X			X				X	(X)			X
Pedomys																
ochrogaster	X			X				X				X			X	(X)
Pitymys																
pinetorum	X			X				X				X		X		
quasiater	X			(X)	X			X				X		X		
Stenocranius																
abbreviatus	X				X					X		X		X		
miurus	X				X					(X)	X	(X)	X	X		

Abbreviations: c, closed; o, open; T, triangles; PL, posterior loop; TL, transverse loop; X, prevalent character state of species; (X), common variant of species.

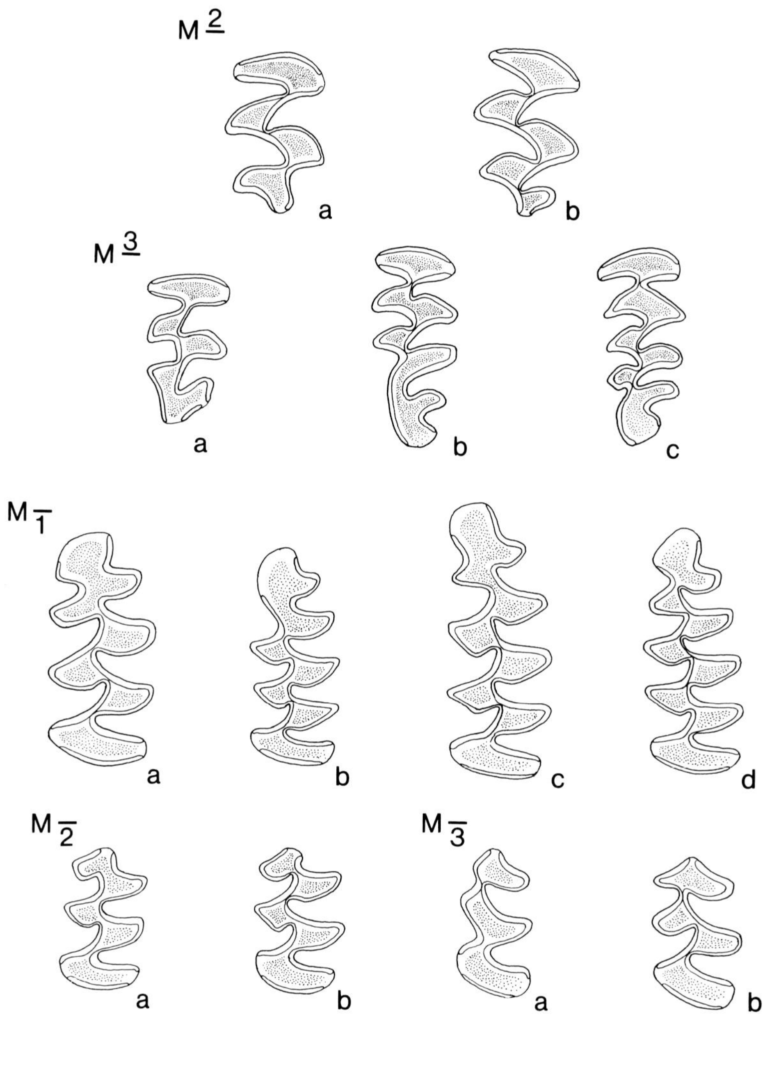

FIG. 6. Occlusal view of principal molar variants in species of *Microtus* (see also Table 2). M^2 (=M2): a, *M.* (*Pedomys*) *ochrogaster*; b, *M.* (*Microtus*) *pennsylvanicus*. M^3 (=M3): a, *M.* (*Pedomys*) *ochrogaster*; b, *M.* (*Microtus*) *pennsylvanicus*; c, *M.* (*Microtus*) *chrotorrhinus*. M_1 (=m1): a, *M.* (*Orthriomys*) *umbrosus*; b, *M.* (*Microtus*) *oeconomus*; c, *M.* (*Microtus*) *pennsylvanicus*; d, *M.* (*Stenocranius*) *miurus*. M_2 (=m2): a, *M.* (*Pedomys*) *ochrogaster*; b, *M.* (*Microtus*) *pennsylvanicus*. M_3 (=m3): a, *M.* (*Microtus*) *pennsylvanicus*; b, *M.* (*Orthriomys*) *umbrosus*.

single tooth abraded to simulate various stages of wear. In his seminal classification of voles and lemmings, Miller (1896) estimated that 75 percent of the individuals of a given species conform to a "normal" pattern. Figures and frequency tabulations of molar variation are available for *M. chrotorrhinus* (Guilday, 1982; Martin, 1973), *M. longicaudus* (Kellogg, 1922*b*), *M. montanus* (Howell, 1924; Kellogg, 1922*a*), *M. pennsylvanicus* (Goin, 1943; Guilday, 1982; Guthrie, 1965; Klimkiewicz, 1970; Miller, 1896; Oppenheimer, 1965), and *M. xanthognathus* (Guilday, 1982) among New World *Microtus*.

The notion of a polarity of variation has emerged from these studies, as witnessed by the greater variability repeatedly affirmed for the lower first and upper third molars. Thus, an axis of increasing variation exists from front to back in the upper toothrow and from back to front in the lower one; in addition, the same direction of variation obtains for the anterior and posterior moieties of the individual molars composing the toothrows. The magnitude of these polarities was exhaustively verified by Guthrie (1965), who measured 42 dimensions of the molars in *M. pennsylvanicus*. He recorded higher variation coefficients for the posterior halves of the upper molars and anterior halves of the lowers, and found those of the posterior part of M3 and front part of m1 to be extraordinarily high. Guthrie concluded that the extreme variation is confined to those molar segments experiencing the most phylogenetic change and hypothesized that such variation is exposed as a result of directional selection breaking up previously balanced, polygenic linkage systems. Hinton (1926) opined that the greater variability of m1 and M3 correlated with their terminal position in the toothrows, but his explanation failed to account for the stability of M1 and m3 at the opposite ends. Guthrie (1965) modified Hinton's surmise by observing that it is the inherently labile primordia of m1 and M3 which remain unobstructed, whereas the homologous sections of the other molars abut the stable loop of the contiguous teeth. Niethammer (1980) shifted the causal explanation to a functional basis, noting that the surfaces of m1 and M3 do not continuously occlude during a chewing orbit; as a result of less masticatory involvement in use of these teeth, their terminal portions are, in some sense, functionally unencumbered and more sensitive to selection for increased complexity and length.

Several studies have documented clinal variation in molar pattern. In the Eurasian vole *M. arvalis,* Stein (1958) showed that northern populations have a greater frequency of simpler upper third molars (fewer salient angles) compared to southern populations, where a relatively complex pattern dominates. He related the geographic trend to habitat quality, the northern populations occupying more forested areas and the southern ones mostly inhabiting grassland biomes. Jorga (1974) observed greater molar variation in populations of *M. oeconomus* from the southern periphery of its range, where one might presume the habitat to be suboptimal. Semken (1966) discovered that the incidence of *M. pennsylvanicus* with six closed triangles is less in samples from the northeastern United States than in those from the Great Plains. The apparent association of dental complexity, and perhaps variability, with ecological setting needs to be rigorously evaluated, a seemingly tractable study given the abundance of *M. pennsylvanicus* deposited in North American collections.

In light of the undisputed origin of arvicolids from some brachyodont cricetid stock, there exists an unexpected amount of disagreement over the direction of evolution of arvicolid molars. Hinton's (1926) commitment to a multituberculate origin of the Rodentia persuaded him to view simplification (that is, the loss of enamel loops and triangles) as the major trend of dental modification in Arvicolidae. His conclusions apparently influenced others in their interpretations of patterns of variation at lower taxonomic levels. For example, Goin (1943) considered the M3 of *M. pennsylvanicus* as undergoing reduction and that of *M. chrotorrhinus* as resembling the primitive state. Klimkiewicz (1970), Oppenheimer (1965), and Zimmermann (1956) similarly affirmed that the variation in their species' samples validated the reductional trend in size and complexity of arvicolid cheekteeth. The alternative hypothesis of molar evolution, that is, augmentation of enamel loops and triangles, rests on more substantial evidence (Guthrie, 1965, 1971; Koenigswald, 1980; Phillips and Oxberry, 1972). For example, Pleistocene forms of *Microtus* exhibit weaker triangulation, suggesting phyletic increase in enamel complexity leading to Recent species (Guthrie, 1965; Semken, 1966). Moreover, straightforward outgroup comparisons and examination of early Pliocene fossils confute the idea of dental simplification as the derivative morphology. That arvicolid molar diversification historically followed a trend of multiplication of enamel folds and angles does not eliminate the possibility of reversal to a simpler state in some lineages. However, identification of such evolutionary reversals will require more definitive corroboration than has been marshalled to date.

The syndrome of dental innovations that appeared in arvicolids is believed to enhance propalinal grinding and thereby to allow greater utilization of the harsh, siliceous grasses that compose the bulk of their diet (Guthrie, 1965, 1971; Hinton, 1926; Koenigswald, 1980; Phillips and Oxberry, 1972; Vorontsov, 1979). The longitudinal orientation of wear scratches on the enamel (Guthrie, 1971) and the erosional profile etched into the dentine basins (Greaves, 1973) substantiate the dominant propalinal motion of the mandible. Although authors have referred to the grinding surface of arvicolid toothrows as a plane, close inspection reveals that their longitudinal occlusal outlines trace gentle curves that are convex in the uppers and concave in the lowers. Kesner (1980) demonstrated that the degree of toothrow curvature varies—pronounced in *Microtus,* for example, and flatter in *Phenacomys*—and correlates with the length of the postorbital-crest tendon of the temporalis muscle. The latter relationship supports his propalinal hypothesis, indicating that the excursion of the mandible during propalinal chewing describes an arc whose limits and curvature are constrained by the postorbital-crest tendon.

Guthrie (1971) viewed the origin and elaboration of the arvicolid cheektooth as meeting two general requirements for comminution of abrasive foods: prolonged resistance to crown wear and increased complexity of the grinding surface. The maintenance of an effective grinding surface was advanced by the attainment of continually growing molars, as demonstrated by Koenigswald and Golenishev (1979), who measured eruption rates using fluorescent tetracycline as a growth marker. In *M. fortis* and *M. mandarinus,* the M1 and M2 erupt 0.5–0.7 mm per week, and the whole vertically elongate crown can regenerate in eight to twelve weeks. As remarked by Guthrie (1971), resistance to dental abrasion is incidentally achieved through increased complexity of the occlusal plane. Nevertheless, the enhanced coronal complexity also relates to masticatory efficiency because it augments the number of enamel cutting blades. Guthrie enumerated the derived features that constitute the "greater complexity" of dentally advanced arvicolids such as *Microtus*: increase in degree of penetration and decrease in width of reentrant angles; increase in acuteness of the salient angles; addition of angles;

more pronounced alternation of salient angles; and redistribution of enamel thickness. These modifications, in concert with a propalinal mode of chewing, create a system of opposing, interdigitating shearing blades, neatly designed for slicing and cutting coarse food items. Koenigswald (1980) considered the conformation of arvicolid molars from the aspect of biomechanical stresses imparted during propalinal mastication and observed the predictable orientation of enamel structures perpendicular to the direction of jaw motion. In species with apomorphic dentitions, the leading edge of an enamel triangle is thicker and convex, whereas the trailing edge is thinner and concave. He further noted that the deepening of reentrant angles until they abut the opposite enamel border appreciably lengthens the shearing edges without broadening the molar rows. In *M. chrotorrhinus,* Martin (1973) found that third molars with more convoluted posterior loops are absolutely longer than those with simpler configurations and may indicate that the phylogenetic formation of more triangles materially increased the length of the dental batteries as well as their complexity. Guthrie (1971) discussed the influence of competition, habitat, and other selective pressures controlling the extent of dental complexity and variation.

The enamel face of the incisors of *Microtus* lacks longitudinal grooves as found in some other arvicolid genera (for example, in *Synaptomys*). The absence of incisive sulci has been considered so diagnostic of the genus that individual exceptions have been deemed noteworthy (Fish and Whitaker, 1971; Jones, 1978). In most species, the upper incisors are orthodont or opisthodont; only *M.* (*Aulacomys*) *richardsoni* has noticeably proodont incisors (Bailey, 1900). The earlier recognition of the lemming and vole divisions within Arvicolidae was based partly on the length and course of the lower incisors (Hinton, 1926; Miller, 1896). In the Lemmi, the lower incisors terminate before or at the level of the m3 and lie to the lingual side of the molar row; in the Microti, the incisors extend dorsally into the condylar process and pass between the bases of the m2 and m3 to cross from the lingual to the labial side of the mandible.

Oral Cavity

Quay (1954*b*) studied the diastemal palate in Arvicolidae (including 12 species of New World *Microtus*) and documented variation in the development of furred infoldings of the upper lip (inflexi pelliti labii superioris) in relation to the occurrence of the anterior longitudinal ridge and other palatal rugae and to the position of the nasopalatine openings. The inflexed lobes of the upper and lower lips presumably function to obstruct extraneous material from the masticatory area of the mouth when the animal is gnawing. The inflexi of *Microtus* are moderately extensive, abutting at the diastemal midline but not fusing as in *Ellobius,* the most fossorially adapted arvicolid. Arvicolids with small medial folds of the upper lip (for example, *Dicrostonyx, Clethrionomys*) have a keel-like ridge of palatal epithelium, the anterior longitudinal ridge, which protrudes between the widely separated inflexi. In conjunction with their extensive labial inflexi, *Microtus* lack an anterior longitudinal ridge. Quay (1954*b*) discerned a posterior displacement of the nasopalatine ducts relative to the length of the diastemal palate. Most species of *Microtus* are intermediate in the position of the nasopalatine apertures, but *M.* (*Aulacomys*) *richardsoni* is extreme in its posterior location of these openings. The nasopalatine canals pass dorsally through the premaxillary portion of the incisive foramina and into the floor of the nasal chambers, where they are anatomically closely associated with the vomeronasal, or Jacobson's, organ (Meredith, 1980; Wohrmann-Repenning, 1980). The probable function of Jacobson's organ as an extra-oral gustatory site and the dominating importance of chemical communication in mediating much of rodent behavior (Eisenberg and Kleiman, 1972) make the variable position of the nasopalatine ducts an attractive morphological and behavioral system for investigation.

Vorontsov (1962, 1979) surveyed the kinds and distribution of sensory papillae on the tongue, and in particular, circumvallate papillae. Gerbillines, sigmodontines, cricetines, murines, and all arvicolids possess a single circumvallate papilla, centrally located behind the elliptical prominence of the tongue. Nesomyines and cricetomyines are the only muroids known to have three circumvallate papillae, a condition thought to be primitive because it is shared with Sciuromorpha and some Hystricomorpha. Golley (1960) stated that the tongue of *M. pennsylvanicus* lacks foliate papillae.

Spacious internal cheek pouches, like those found in Old World hamsters (Cricetinae) and African pouched rats (Cricetomyinae), are lacking in *Microtus* and other arvicolids.

Midgut

The ancestral gastric morphology in muroids has been interpreted as a simple, single-chambered sac having approximately equal distributions of glandular and cornified mucosal linings (Carleton, 1973; Vorontsov, 1962, 1979). Such a hemiglandular gastric plan occurs in numerous species and all major groups of Muroidea, even characterizing entire subfamilies (for example, Gerbillinae), but is known only in the lemmings (*Lemmus, Myopus,* and *Synaptomys*) within Arvicolidae.

Compared to the unilocular-hemiglandular condition, the stomach of *Microtus* displays many derived features. As Toepfer (1891) and Tullberg (1899) noted for Old World *M. arvalis* and *M. agrestis,* the glandular area in *Microtus* consists of a small circular patch restricted to the greater curvature opposite the esophageal orifice (discoglandular type following Carleton, 1973). Carleton (1981) substantiated the uniformity of *Microtus* (including 18 North American species representing all subgenera except *Orthriomys*) with respect to the discoglandular pattern of their gastric mucosae and the persistence of a thin strip of glandular tissue at the pylorus. A bordering fold of cornified epithelium (=Grenzfalten of Toepfer, 1891; pediculated squamous flap of Dearden, 1969) surrounds the discoglandular zone. The left rim of this bordering fold is fimbriated, a condition peculiar to *Microtus* and some other arvicolid genera (Carleton, 1981; Vorontsov, 1979). Externally, the stomach of specimens of *Microtus* is bilocular. This appearance results both from the elaboration of the incisura angularis, a muscular fold on the lesser curvature, and the expansion craniad of the left half of the stomach. The latter forms a thin-walled, highly distensible fornix (=esophageal sac; forestomach; fornix ventricularis of Vorontsov, 1979), capable of accommodating large amounts of food. The anatomical modifications associated with the bilocular-discoglandular stomach seen in *Microtus* reflect changes in the composition of the digestive glands and the architecture of the smooth musculature, which in turn imply profound differences in gastric digestion and motility (see, for example, Dearden, 1966, 1969; Golley, 1960; Luthje, 1976).

Two functional themes have been reiterated to explain the trend of keratinization and glandular reduction observed in muroid stomachs. Bensley (1902) and Tullberg (1899) emphasized the mechanical effect wrought by abrasive foodstuffs, such as the chitinous exoskeleton of insects or the siliceous fibers of grasses. Toepfer (1891) and Vorontsov (1962, 1979), on the other hand, interpreted the modifications as adaptations for symbiotic digestion of cellulose-rich foods. The latter hypothesis, with its obvious analogy to ruminant digestive processes, seems more intuitively logical, especially in light of the herbivory demonstrated for many arvicolids, particularly *Microtus*. Nevertheless, much basic data on gastric histology, motility, physiology, and microbial symbionts must be gathered before one of these hypotheses, or yet other plausible interpretations (see Carleton 1973, 1981), can be accepted.

All arvicolids examined have a discrete saccular gall bladder, but it is sporadically absent in other muroid assemblages (Carleton, 1980; Vorontsov, 1979). Why some rodents lack a gall bladder is unclear. Vorontsov (1979) speculated that a gall bladder should be expected in forms that feed opportunistically and infrequently on foods high in protein and fat to ensure that a large supply of bile is in reserve and can be mobilized quickly, whereas in species that feed more frequently and regularly, bile secretion occurs more or less continuously, obviating the need for large volumes of concentrated bile and an organ for storage. The largely herbivorous regimen and polyphasic activity patterns of *Microtus* seem to refute this hypothesis. The liver in species of *Microtus* is divided into seven lobes, which Vorontsov (1979) interpreted as derived from the eight-lobed state characteristic of some other arvicolids and muroids.

Hindgut

Species of *Microtus*, and arvicolids in general, possess a short small intestine in relation to the length of the large intestine and caecum. Mean relative lengths of the small intestine, large intestine, and caecum (expressed as a percentage of total intestinal length) are 45, 37, and 18, respectively, for eight Old World species of *Microtus* (Vorontsov, 1962, 1979). In contrast, muroid species whose diet predominantly consists of insects or seeds exhibit a comparatively long small intestine and short large intestine and caecum, generally in the range of 62, 28, and 10 percent of total length (Vorontsov, 1962).

As cautioned by Barry (1977), these simple proportions do not reflect accurately the available surface area for nutrient absorption in the hindgut. In terms of mucosal surface area, the small intestine, with its villous projections and submucosal folds, is still the primary section for nutrient assimilation among the small mammals examined, including *Microtus ochrogaster* and *M. pennsylvanicus*. Thus, in *M. ochrogaster,* the small intestine, large intestine, and caecum constitute 44, 35, and 21 percent, respectively, of total intestinal length, but the three compose 73, 14, and 13 percent of the total absorptive surface of the hindgut. Although the ratios do not accurately convey their potential importance for absorption within a species, differences between species, whether in relative lengths or surface areas, are in the direction predicted by their food habits. The mucosal surface area of the caecum in *Microtus,* for instance, substantially exceeds that observed in *Peromyscus*; in fact, the difference in caecal capacity suggested by relative surface areas (about 3.9 times) is more impressive than that (about 2.5 times) calculated from relative lengths (Barry, 1977: Table 1). The greater length and capacity of the caecum in *Microtus* and other arvicolids assume functional significance in view of the large amount of herbaceous matter they consume and the documented role of the caecum as the hindgut site for cellulose fermentation (Moir, 1968).

Aside from relative intestinal lengths, other structural modifications undoubtedly affect absorptive surface area. Barry (1976) observed that the small intestinal villi of *M. pennsylvanicus* and *M. ochrogaster* are characteristically short, broad, and less dense than those of *Peromyscus* and *Mus*. He also derived a positive correlation between mucosal surface area of the small intestine and the percent animal material in the diet, a finding consistent with the activity of the duodenum in absorbing amino acids and the low-protein fare of *Microtus*. The proximal section of the large intestine is coiled upon itself to form a tapered series of loops, which number 10 to 12 coils in *Lemmus* and *Ondatra* but only three to five in species of *Microtus*; most muroid species either lack colic loops or have only one or two (Vorontsov, 1979). Compared to other Arvicolidae, the caeca found in *Microtus* are moderately sacculated, but they easily surpass in complexity the shorter, smooth-walled caeca observed in most cricetines, murines, and gerbillines. Long villi occur in the caecum of *Phenacomys* and *Dicrostonyx* but have not been discovered in the one species of *Microtus* examined (*californicus*) nor in *Clethrionomys, Lagurus, Ondatra, Lemmus,* and *Synaptomys* (Voge and Bern, 1949, 1955). Coprophagy has been documented for *M. penn-*

sylvanicus (Ouellette and Heisinger, 1980). The prevalence of this nutritional strategy within the genus and the possible correspondence to morphological specializations of the hindgut, such as colic loops or caecal sacculae, should be explored.

Reproductive System

Male

The architecture of the baculum and glans penis has received considerable attention from systematists in their assessments of relationships within Arvicolidae. Hamilton (1946) examined four North American species of *Microtus,* but subsequent investigators have increased that number to seventeen, representing all North American subgenera except *Orthriomys* (Anderson, 1960; Burt, 1960; Dearden, 1958; Hooper and Hart, 1962; Martin, 1979). This representation, together with those Old World genera and species examined (Askenova and Tarasov, 1974; Didier, 1954; Ognev, 1950), establishes the Arvicolidae as the most thoroughly surveyed group of muroids in regard to phallic morphology.

The baculum in *Microtus* generally consists of four parts, a proximal bony shaft tipped distally with three cartilaginous digits or processes. Arata et al. (1965) characterized the junction between the shaft and distal processes as a synovial joint. Species of *Microtus* differ in the occurrence and development of the lateral bacular processes: they are conspicuous in the subgenera *Chilotus* and *Herpetomys* and most species of the nominate subgenus; diminutive in the subgenera *Aulacomys, Pedomys, Pitymys,* and *Stenocranius*; and absent in *M.* (*Microtus*) *californicus* and *M. mexicanus* (Anderson, 1960; Hamilton, 1946). Anderson (1960) constructed a key to North American arvicolids based on bacular traits, but cautioned that species of *Microtus* were especially difficult to accommodate because of the variable pronouncement of the lateral bacular digits.

Arata et al. (1965) traced the ontogenetic development of the baculum of *Microtus montanus* from week-old neonates to adults. They found that the proximal shaft is true bone, a perichondral ossification formed from dense aggregations of mesenchyme cells in the manner described for the rat (Ruth, 1934). However, the reputed "ossifications" of the distal bacular digits mentioned by previous authors are in fact calcifications of hyaline or fibrocartilage, a process appearing first in the medial bacular digit and later in the lateral ones. Marked expansion of the proximal shaft and calcification of the distal elements proceeded rapidly after day 35, approximately coincident with the threshold of reproductive maturity in *M. montanus*. The ontogeny of bacular morphology in *M. montanus* basically conforms to that observed in other arvicolids with trident bacula (Artimo, 1969; Tarasov, 1974). These studies reveal the large variation in bacular conformation associated with age and physiological state of the animal and emphasize the need for cautious taxonomic interpretation of differences between samples consisting of few specimens and incomparable age profiles.

As demonstrated by Hooper and Hart (1962), the interspecific variability of the soft parts of the glans penis surpasses that seen in the bacular infrastructure. Species of *Microtus* have a short, broad glans with a moderately deep terminal crater, the ventral rim of which is usually papillose. The ornate appearance of the glans is enhanced further by other soft tissue structures that project from the floor of the crater into its interior: the dorsal papilla; the urethral process; and the medial and lateral bacular mounds. Hooper and Hart (1962) sorted the species of *Microtus* into two groups based upon the structure of the dorsal papilla, the length of the lateral bacular mounds, and lobulation of the urethral process, and recommended that *M.* (*Aulacomys*) *richardsoni* be allocated to *Arvicola*. At a higher taxonomic level, they arranged *Microtus* with *Lagurus* and *Arvicola* in a tribal assemblage. The data from both bacular and penile morphology favors a multitribal classification of the arvicolids, a major departure from the traditional dual tribal system (Lemmi and Microti) adopted by Hinton (1926) and Miller (1896).

The trident baculum, glans penis with a crater and assorted crater embellishments, and intricate phallic vascular supply found in *Microtus* and other arvicolids characterize a fundamental morphological plan termed the "complex" type by Hooper (1960). Attributes of the contradistinctive "simple" phallic scheme, which occurs in relatively few muroid genera, include a baculum consisting of a single element, the absence of a terminal crater and crater processes, and an uncomplicated vascular system (Hooper and Musser, 1964). Possession of a complex phallus broadly allies arvicolids with such muroid groups as Old World cricetines, South American cricetines, gerbillines, and murines (Hooper and Hart, 1962; Hooper and Musser, 1964). Anderson (1960) and Hooper and Hart (1962) considered the well-developed bacula and relatively ornate glandes penes of *Clethrionomys* and *Phenacomys*, voles with rooted molars, to represent the primitive condition of the phallus in Arvicolidae, and viewed absence of lateral bacular digits and a comparatively simple glans penis as derived morphologies. Their hypotheses agree with the conventional interpretation of the complex to simple transformation of the phallus, as advocated for the Muroidea as a whole (Hershkovitz, 1966; Hooper and Musser, 1964).

The male accessory reproductive glands of muroid rodents constitute a richly variable organ-system, typically consisting of five sets of glands: preputial, bulbourethral, ampullary, vesicular, and prostate. Three pairs of prostates are conventionally recognized and designated by their position with respect to the urethra: anterior, dorsal, and ventral; the last pair usually is subdivided into lateral ventral and medial ventral lobes. A complete array of accessory reproductive glands is believed to represent the plesiomorphic arrangement in Muroidea (Arata, 1964; Carleton, 1980; Voss and Linzey, 1981).

Such an array typifies the accessory reproductive glands in species of *Microtus* examined to date. Hamilton (1941) described and figured the tract of *M. pennsylvanicus*, and Arata (1964) included *M. ochrogaster* and *M. pinetorum*. In addition, the 12 Old World *Microtus* reported conform to the hypothesized primitive complement (Askenova, 1973; Indyk, 1968), although Askenova (1973) did detect slight but consistent differences in size and form of the preputials and lateral ventral prostates among nine species studied. Except for the larger size of their preputial glands, the accessory reproductive glands found in arvicolids are indistinguishable from those characteristic of many New World cricetines, murines, and some gerbillines (Arata, 1964; Voss and Linzey, 1981). The homogeneity in accessory gland morphology exists primarily among forms with a complex penis and presents a stark contrast to the elaborate modification or loss of particular accessory glands documented for forms with a simple phallus (Arata, 1964; Linzey and Layne, 1969).

Female

The number and distribution of mammary glands have been applied taxonomically at the subgeneric level in *Microtus* and considered suitably diagnostic to employ in keys (Bailey, 1900; Miller, 1896). Indeed, species of *Microtus* collectively exhibit the gamut of variation recorded in the entire family. The common number of mammae, eight (two pectoral pairs and two inguinal pairs), occurs in the subgenera *Aulacomys, Chilotus, Stenocranius,* and most *Microtus,* as well as the majority of other arvicolid genera. Niethammer (1972) interpreted this as the primitive number and pattern in Arvicolidae and viewed reductions in mammary count as derivations. Two distributional patterns have been described for *Microtus* with six nipples: one pectoral pair and two inguinal pairs in *Pedomys,* and two pectoral pairs but just one inguinal pair in *Herpetomys.* Three arrangements are known for *Microtus* having only four mammae: two inguinal pairs in *Pitymys,* one pectoral pair and one inguinal pair in *M.* (*Microtus*) *mexicanus,* and two pectoral pairs in *Orthriomys.* Voles that have fewer than eight nipples but that retain the pectoral pairs constitute an interesting exception among muroid rodents to the conventional trend, which involves loss of the anterior pairs and retention of the inguinal ones (Arvy, 1974). This condition raises questions about the position of the female when nursing and the tenacity of nipple-clinging by the young. Niethammer (1972) demonstrated a positive correlation between number of mammae and average litter size for species of Arvicolidae and commented that species with fewer nipples occupy the southern periphery of the global arvicolid distribution, a generalization which holds for North American *Microtus.*

Aside from variation in the mammary gland formula, the female reproductive system has received scant attention in systematic investigations. Ziegler (1961) documented the presence of a baubellum (os clitoridis) in some individuals of *M. longicaudus* and *M. californicus* and suggested that it was not as uniform in appearance and occurrence as the baculum. Arata et al. (1965) failed to discover a baubellum in 21 *M. montanus* but demonstrated the presence of three cartilaginous lobes of the clitoris, presumably homologous to the distal processes of the complex penis. Hamilton (1941) illustrated the female urogenital tract of adult *M. pennsylvanicus,* noting the duplex uterine structure characteristic of most Rodentia. The need for detailed comparative studies of the female reproductive tract complementary to those performed on the male tract is readily apparent.

The need to augment our understanding of function associated with variations in both male and female reproductive morphologies is similarly indicated. The role of preputial gland secretions in advertising reproductive status and modulating agonistic and territorial behavior is well established (Brown and Williams, 1972), but the purposes of the other male accessory reproductive glands are less easily interpretable. The probable interaction of accessory glands in the formation of copulatory plugs, which have been reported for species of *Microtus,* and the hypothesis of copulatory plugs as a mechanism of chastity enforcement offer exciting research opportunities linking morphology and breeding systems in muroid rodents (see Hartung and Dewsbury, 1978; Voss, 1979). In discussing the adaptive significance of the baculum of the hamster, Callery (1951:206) allowed that ". . . detailed studies of copulation may show that this structure is of significance in reproduction." While this prediction may seem vacuous, it nonetheless conveys our very elementary appreciation of function in regard to phallic morphology, especially those variations which define the simple versus complex penes of muroid rodents. Hershkovitz (1966) advanced a lock and key hypothesis to explain muroid phallic diversity, and Long and Frank (1968) related the structure of the baculum to facilitation of vaginal penetration and stimulation. Dewsbury and colleagues (see review by Dewsbury, 1975) have revealed a correspondence of penile shape and certain aspects of copulatory patterns, but their correlation pertains only to muroids with a simple phallus. Except in a most general sense, these hypotheses offer little insight toward understanding the functional importance of details of muroid penile morphology (for example, the dorsal papilla, urethral flaps, bacular mounds) to copulatory behavior and female reproductive anatomy. Blandau (1945), on the other hand, meticulously verified that the bacular mounds of the glans penis of the lab rat are reciprocally oriented to engage similar lappets guarding the vaginal cervix and described how their contact during copulation stimulated cervical relaxation and exposure of the uterine orifices just prior to ejaculation. Investigations of this kind, together with further elucidation of female neuroendocrine mechanisms associated with ovulation and pregnancy initiation, will provide greater illumination of muroid reproductive adaptations.

Discussion

The morphological attributes surveyed in the preceding sections compose the known phenotypic landscape of the genus *Microtus* and may be viewed from the standpoint of their antiquity. Hennig (1966) spoke of the "Age of Origin" of a group of organisms, and, in an analogous sense, I am looking at the relative age of origin of the various anatomical features exhibited by living species of *Microtus.* To review the morphology of *Microtus* from this perspective involves both an assessment of the characters' evolutionary polarity and some estimate of their initial appearance in phylogeny. My rationale for determining the ancestral or derived nature of the various traits (see Table 3) may be found in the previous discussions or the literature sources cited. Only certain characters are of interest here. The observation that all *Microtus* possess hair, are viviparous, and have evergrowing incisors attests to past evolutionary events (cast in our taxonomic hierarchy as the Class Mammalia, Subclass Theria, and Order Rodentia, respectively) so distantly removed as to be inappropriate to a discussion of this volume's subject. Within Rodentia, four hierarchical levels, presumably corresponding to major adaptive radiations, seem pertinent to an understanding of the heritage of characters seen in extant *Microtus.* These levels are the Muroidea, the Arvicolidae, a tribal-level clade including *Microtus,* and the cladogenesis of species assigned to the genus *Microtus* itself.

The Superfamily Muroidea embraces some 250 genera and 1,100 Recent species, or about one-quarter of all living mammals. Their speciosity, virtually world-wide distribution, and immense ecological diversity qualify them as the most successful radiation of contemporary rodents. Although many of the Recent muroid groups may not have differentiated until the late Oligocene or Miocene, muroids certainly appeared by early Oligocene times, over 40 m.y.b.p. The late Eocene form *Simimys* may be the earliest known muroid; however, this enigmatic genus has been variously shuffled between Muroidea and Dipodoidea (see Emry, 1981, for an overview). The voles and lemmings, Family Arvicolidae, constitute one of the more recently evolved assemblages of the 13–15 that are conventionally recognized within Muroidea (see Carleton, 1980, for a review of muroid classifications). The earliest indisputable arvicolids, *Microtoscoptes* and *Paramicrotoscoptes,* date from the latest Miocene (early Hemphillian) of North America, about 6–8 m.y.b.p. (Martin, 1975; Repenning, 1980). Despite the comparative recency of their appearance, arvicolids have radiated explosively into some 17 genera representing approximately 125 species, much of this diversification occurring from the late Pliocene or early Pleistocene onwards. Sometime during this period, the ancestor of *Microtus* and related genera emerged. Formal tribes have been erected for the genera of Arvicolidae, but I have refrained from specifying one that embraces *Microtus* because disagreement exists over the content of such a tribe. Nevertheless, the differentiation of a tribal-level group including *Microtus* and some unspecified number of other genera probably transpired in the upper Pliocene, about 2.5–4.0 m.y.b.p. The genus *Microtus,* which contains over half of the 125 living species of arvicolids, arose comparatively recently. The transition from its putative antecedent *Allophaiomys* is recognized as very early Pleistocene, 1.6 to 1.8 m.y.b.p. (Chaline, 1966, 1977; Repenning, 1980).

Consideration of the antiquity of the characters of *Microtus* from these four taxonomic ages of origin imposes the stratification presented in Table 3. Several points of clarification are warranted regarding interpretation of the table. I was obviously constrained in assigning a character to one of the four taxonomic levels which I initially deemed pertinent to include. Consequently, the placement of a trait under a particular column connotes its appearance at least at that given taxonomic level; the trait's origin may have been earlier. For instance, the smooth-faced upper incisors observed in *Microtus* may antedate Muroidea and probably characterized the ancestral myomorph or even the primordial rodent. In instances where several character states are found among species of *Microtus,* I listed only the plesiomorphic condition and indicated the existence of more apomorphic states by an arrow. The extent of these derived morphologies is addressed in the preceding anatomical review. I do not mean to imply that a character is necessarily uniquely derived for the taxonomic level at which it is listed, only that it must have originated at that level at least once in the genealogical pathway leading to extant *Microtus.* Numerous examples of suspected parallelism may be cited among the characters surveyed.

The literature covering various aspects of arvicolid anatomy encompasses six major organ systems and some 71 characters. Of these 71, most states (49) exhibited by *Microtus* are interpreted as ancestral either at the level of the Muroidea or Arvicolidae (Table 3), and therefore are inappropriate for assessing the near generic relatives of *Microtus* or the basis of its generic recognition. A superficial appraisal of the 22 traits listed under the tribal-level clade (Table 3) suggests that many of them cladistically affiliate *Microtus*

TABLE 3

HIERARCHICAL LEVELS OF HERITAGE OF CHARACTERS EXHIBITED BY *Microtus*

	Character state origin at the taxonomic level of:			
Organ systems and characters	Muroidea	Arvicolidae	Tribal-level clade	*Microtus*
Integument				
Skin glands		Flank →	[Hip →]	
Meibomian glands			<10 glands	
Plantar footpads	Six →			
Pollex	Lacks broad nail			
Skeleton				
Tail		<head + body		
Nasals and rostrum		Short		
Zygomatic notch	Absent			
Zygomatic plate		Oriented obliquely		
Postorbital process		Present		
Interorbit	Lacks shelf			
Mesopterygoid fossae		Extends between M^3s		
Parapterygoid fossa		Compressed, cavernous		
Bony palate			Ridge + bridge	
Palatal pits		Present		
Incisive foramen		Oval ends →		
Masticatory foramen	Present →			
Foramen ovale accessorius	Present →			
Sphenofrontal foramen		Absent		
Sphenomaxillary foramen	Absent →			
Stapedial foramen	Present			

TABLE 3
CONTINUED

Organ systems and characters	Character state origin at the taxonomic level of: Muroidea	Arvicolidae	Tribal-level clade	*Microtus*
Auditory bullae			Osseus septa	
Bullar inflation		Moderate		
Accessory tympanum			Minute	
Malleus		Perpendicular		
Angular process		Pointed laterad		
Mandibular temporal fossa			Excavated	
Arvicoline groove		Present		
Thoracolumbar ratio	13:6	[13:6]		
Neural spine of 2nd thoracic		Absent		
Entepicondylar foramen		Absent		
Trochlear process of calcaneum		Placed distally		
Musculature				
Postorbital crest tendon			Long, robust	
Masseter lateralis profundus		Medial insertion		
Internal pterygoid		Large		
Digastric tendinous arcade		Reduced		
Pectoralis minor insertion		Corocoid process		
Jugulohyoideus			Absent	
Stylohyoideus origin			Paroccipital	
Circulatory system				
Opthalmic artery origin		Internal maxillary		

TABLE 3
CONTINUED

Organ systems and characters	Character state origin at the taxonomic level of: Muroidea	Arvicolidae	Tribal-level clade	*Microtus*
Digestive system				
Molar crown		Hypsodont, prismatic		
Molar roots			Absent, evergrowing	
Cement			Present	
Depth of reentrant angles	Equal			
Second upper molar			3 closed Δs →	
Third upper molar			2 closed Δs →	
First lower molar			3 closed, 2 open Δs →	
Second lower molar			2 closed, 2 open Δs →	
Third lower molar			3 transverse loops →	
Upper incisor grooves	Absent			
Lower incisor path			Long labiad	
Inflexii labii superioris			Abut, not fused	
Anterior longitudinal ridge			Absent	
Circumvallate papillae		One present		
Cheek pouches	Undeveloped			
Stomach form			Bilocular	
Glandular region			Discoglandular	
Bordering fold			Fimbriated	
Liver			Seven-lobed	
Gall bladder	Present			
Caecum		Long, sacculate		

TABLE 3
CONTINUED

Organ systems and characters	Character state origin at the taxonomic level of: Muroidea	Arvicolidae	Tribal-level clade	*Micro-tus*
Colic loops		3–5 coils		
Caecal villi	Absent			
Reproductive system				
Baculum	Trident	[Medial digit →]		
Crater rim		Papillose	[Papillose]	
Glans penis	Complex type	[Complex type]		
Preputial glands	Present			
Bulbourethral glands	Present			
Ampullary glands	Present			
Vesicular glands	Present			
Prostate glands	3 pairs			
Mammary glands	4 pairs →			
	22	27	22	0

[= alternative interpretation of character state polarity; → = even more derived conditions found in some species of *Microtus*.

with *Arvicola* and *Lagurus* (*Lemmiscus*), a notion which received support in some studies (for example, Hinton, 1926; Hooper and Hart, 1962) but not others (Dearden, 1959; Koenigswald, 1980). At this stage of our understanding, however, the morphological similarity of *Microtus* to other genera cannot be reliably segregated into that due to parallelism and that consequent to descent from a common ancestor. A surprising paradox emerges from this exercise: given the currently accepted contents of *Microtus,* the genus itself seemingly lacks any uniquely derived character states that unambiguously diagnose it from other genera of Arvicolidae (Table 3). This finding indirectly acknowledges that the derived features observed in *Microtus* may have been independently acquired in multiple lineages of arvicolids or may indeed represent synapomorphies uniting *Microtus* in a tribal group. Whatever the case, the existence of synapomorphic features that circumscribe *Microtus* to the exclusion of other arvicolids is not eminently apparent.

What attributes, then, lend identity to *Microtus*? Miller's (1896) synopsis of the arvicolids (then viewed as the subfamily Microtinae) stressed (p. 24) a ". . . classification . . . based on an assemblage of characters." In this attitude, his systematic approach was decidedly more enlightened than that of his predecessors, such as Blasius and Lataste, who erected their systems of classification largely around single morphological features (Miller [1896] reviewed the early history of *Microtus* taxonomy). Miller (1896:44) enumerated nine "essential characters" for *Microtus* (see also Anderson, this volume):

1) upper incisors without grooves;
2) lower incisors with roots on the outer side of molar series;
3) molars rootless;
4) enamel pattern characterized by approximate equality of reentrant angles;
5) m1 usually with five closed or nearly closed triangles;
6) M3 with one, two, or three closed triangles;
7) tail nearly always longer than hindfoot, terete;
8) feet, fur, eyes, and ears very variable;
9) thumb never with a well-developed ligulate nail.

Characters 1, 4, 7, and 9 are symplesiomorphies and attest to nothing more than the common heritage of species of *Microtus* as muroids. In effect, these attributes separated species of *Microtus* from some anatomically distinctive forms which Miller retained as genera, namely *Dicrostonyx, Lemmus, Synaptomys,* and *Ondatra.* Characters 2, 3, 5, and 6 stand as apomorphies relative to their condition in the ancestral arvicolid, yet they are shared by several genera. Moreover, the variable definition of numbers 5 and 6 renders them difficult to apply in specific cases. And condition 8 cannot really be considered a diagnostic character, but rather Miller's (1896) acknowledgement of the immense variation of these features within the genus as he perceived it. In his revision of North American *Microtus,* Bailey (1900) repeated most of Miller's generic characters, namely 1–4, 7, and 9. Bailey, however, deleted characters 5, 6, and 8 from his generic definition and added one other: palate with median ridge, lateral pits, and complete lateral bridges. The topography of the palatal region in *Microtus* is considered derived, but like the apomorphic states which compose parts of Miller's diagnosis, it characterizes several genera of arvicolids.

The recognition of *Microtus,* therefore, has traditionally rested upon a mixture of ancestral and derived features, the latter derived only relative to the ancestor or early representatives of Arvicolidae but not strictly synapomorphic for *Microtus.* The taxon's cohesiveness issues not from the joint possession of uniquely derived features but from the unique combination of traits exhibited by most of its members, a property which qualifies it as a polythetic entity (sensu Sneath and Sokal, 1973). This observation provides some credence to the viewpoint that *Microtus* is at best a paraphyletic taxon (sensu Ashlock, 1972); that is, not all descendants of the most recent common ancestor of the genus *Microtus* are contained within it. Whether the genus is polyphyletic also remains a possibility. One may argue that evaluation of the status of *Microtus* based upon the antiquated (presumably) studies of Bailey (1900) and Miller (1896) presents a specious perspective; after all, the generic limits of *Microtus* have changed substantially since the year 1900. This is true. Of the 14 subgenera allocated to *Microtus* by Miller (1896) and Bailey (1900), six are currently established as genera (*Alticola, Arvicola, Eothenomys, Hyperacrius, Lagurus,* and *Neofiber*) and one is considered synonymous with another genus (*Anteliomys* of *Eothenomys*). Yet despite the restriction in generic scope, the characters used today (see, for example, Hall, 1981; Ognev, 1950) are remarkably the same basic ones set forth by Miller and Bailey, a realization which further strengthens the interpretation of *Microtus* as (at best) a paraphyletic group.

What this observation portends for future phylogenetic studies of *Microtus* is unclear. Further analyses may result in division of the taxon, identifying smaller and, ideally, monophyletically delineated groups. In fact, investigators subsequent to Miller and Bailey followed this course and raised most of their subgenera to genera. Thus, Hinton (1926) and Ellerman (1941) treated *Chilotus, Herpetomys, Orthriomys, Pedomys,* and *Pitymys* as genera distinct from *Microtus,* together with the six now recognized as valid, and even Miller later accorded generic status to several forms which he originally had arranged as subgenera in 1896 (Miller, 1912, 1924; Miller and Kellogg, 1955). Alternatively, pursuance of the criterion of monophyly may recommend the subordination of certain genera to their former rank as subgenera of *Microtus,* a course which holds a certain attraction. The distant phyletic affinity perceived today for some former subgenera of Miller's (1896) *Microtus* (that is, *Alticola, Eothenomys, Hyperacrius,* and *Neofiber*) seems to ratify maintenance of their generic separateness, but the isolation of *Arvicola* and *Lagurus* deserves reappraisal in this light. Possibly, the unequivocal establishment of a monophyletic concept for *Microtus* will prove to be an elusive goal. The genus may remain a polythetically defined assemblage whose cladistic stature relative to other genera of Arvicolidae is always suspected of being paraphyletic. Such a pragmatic taxonomic stance may be inescapable in view of the rife parallelism that has apparently attended the radiation of arvicolids and the difficulty of distilling synapomorphic traits in a complex of persistent sister species. These evolutionary circumstances apply particularly to *Microtus,* a genus in which parallelism seemingly represents an historical fact of the group's cladogenesis (Chaline, 1966, 1974), and one whose period of differentiation occurred as recently as the early Pleistocene (Chaline, 1977; Repenning, 1980).

Any of the systematic courses outlined above will hinge on careful and rigorous analysis of the characters which form the essence of our phylogenetic inference and classificatory reference system. Such analysis must include the continued exploration of other anatomical systems and discovery of new characters, potentially valuable for testing current estimates of relationship. And there exists a need to extend character surveys of non-traditional anatomical systems that have received cursory attention to date. For example, the muscular and reproductive systems of too few species of *Microtus* have been examined, disallowing definitive assessments of a character's ubiquity within the genus and its value as a synapomorphy. Throughout the chapter, I have referred somewhat casually and dogmatically to "characters" as if their basis and recognition are intrinsically self-evident. The documentation of correlation among and unsuspected variation of several hallowed "characters" used in arvicolid systematics reveals the weakness of any such assertion. Perhaps the number of triangles is less important than some term that simultaneously conveys the shape of those triangles and the orientation of their cutting surfaces. The former difference is countable and easily expressed; the latter lacks familiarity and a formulated language of comparison. Therefore, in addition to searching out other taxonomically useful features and augmenting previous anatomical studies, the primacy of character analysis to the construction of phylogenies and classifications obligates us to continually refine our character definitions.

Literature Cited

ANDERSON, S. 1954. Subspeciation in the meadow mouse, *Microtus montanus,* in Wyoming and Colorado. Univ. Kansas Publ., Mus. Nat. Hist., 7:489–506.

———. 1956. Subspeciation in the meadow mouse, *Microtus pennsylvanicus,* in Wyoming, Colorado, and adjacent areas. Univ. Kansas Publ., Mus. Nat. Hist., 9:85–104.

———. 1959. Distribution, variation, and relationships of the montane vole, *Microtus montanus.* Univ. Kansas Publ., Mus. Nat. Hist., 9:415–511.

———. 1960. The baculum in microtine rodents. Univ. Kansas Publ., Mus. Nat. Hist., 12:181–216.

ARATA, A. 1964. The anatomy and taxonomic significance of the male accessory reproductive glands of muroid rodents. Bull. Florida State Mus., Biol. Sci., 9:1–42.

ARATA, A., N. C. NEGUS, AND M. S. DOWNS. 1965. Histology, development, and individual variation of complex muroid bacula. Tulane Studies Zool., 12:51–64.

ARMSTRONG, D. M. 1972. Distribution of mammals in Colorado. Monogr. Mus. Nat. Hist., Univ. Kansas, 3:1–415.

ARTIMO, A. 1969. The baculum of the wood lemming, *Myopus schisticolor* (Lilljeb.), in relation to sexual status, size and age. Ann. Zool. Fennici, 6:335–344.

ARVY, L. 1974. Contribution a la connaissance de l'appareil mammaire chez les rongeurs. Mammalia, 38:108–138.

ASHLOCK, P. D. 1972. Monophyly again. Syst. Zool., 21:430–438.

ASKENOVA, T. G. 1973. The structure of accessory male glands in some species of the genus *Microtus* (Rodentia, Cricetidae). Zool. Zhur., 52:1843–1848.

Askenova, T. G., and S. A. Tarasov. 1974. Structural patterns of os penis in some species of the genus *Microtus* (Rodentia, Cricetidae). Zool. Zhur., 53:609–615.

Bailey, V. 1900. Revision of American voles of the genus *Microtus*. N. Amer. Fauna, 17:1–88.

Barry, R. E. 1976. Mucosal surface areas and villous morphology of the small intestine of small mammals: functional interpretations. J. Mamm., 57: 273–290.

———. 1977. Length and absorptive surface area apportionment of segments of the hindgut for eight species of mammals. J. Mamm., 58:419–420.

Bee, J. W., and E. R. Hall. 1956. Mammals of northern Alaska on the arctic slope. Misc. Publ. Mus. Nat. Hist., Univ. Kansas, 8:1–309.

Bensley, R. R. 1902. The cardiac glands of mammals. Amer. J. Anat., 2:105–156.

Berry, R. J., and A. G. Searle. 1963. Epigenetic polymorphism of the rodent skeleton. Proc. Zool. Soc. London, 140:577–615.

Blandau, R. J. 1945. On the factors involved in sperm transport through the cervix uteri of the albino rat. Amer. J. Anat., 77:253–272.

Boonstra, R., and J. Youson. 1982. Hip glands in field populations of *Microtus pennsylvanicus*. Canadian J. Zool., 60:2955–2958.

Brown, J. C., and G. I. Twigg. 1969. Studies on the pelvis in British Muridae and Cricetidae (Rodentia). J. Zool., 158:81–132.

Brown, J. C., and J. D. Williams. 1972. The rodent preputial gland. Mamm. Rev., 2:105–147.

Bugge, J. 1970. The contribution of the stapedial artery to the cephalic arterial supply in muroid rodents. Acta Anat., 76:313–336.

Burt, W. H. 1960. Bacula of North American mammals. Misc. Publ. Mus. Zool., Univ. Michigan, 113:1–76.

Callery, R. 1951. Development of the os genitale in the golden hamster, *Mesocricetus* (*Cricetus*) *auratus*. J. Mamm., 32:204–207.

Carleton, M. D. 1973. A survey of gross stomach morphology in New World Cricetinae (Rodentia, Muroidea), with comments on functional interpretations. Misc. Publ. Mus. Zool., Univ. Michigan, 146:1–43.

———. 1980. Phylogenetic relationships in neotomine-peromyscine rodents (Muroidea) and a reappraisal of the dichotomy within New World Cricetinae. Misc. Publ. Mus. Zool., Univ. Michigan, 157:1–146.

———. 1981. A survey of gross stomach morphology in Microtinae (Rodentia, Muroidea). Z. Saugetierk., 46:93–108.

Chaline, J. 1966. Un example d'evolution chez les Arvicolides (Rodentia): les lignees *Allophaiomys-Pitymys* et *Microtus*. Comptes Rendus, Ser. D, 263: 1202–1204.

———. 1974. Palingenese et phylogenese chez les campagnols (Arvicolidae, Rodentia). Comptes Rendus, Ser. D, 278:437–440.

———. 1977. Rodents, evolution, and prehistory. Endeavour, 1:44–51.

Choate, J. R., and S. L. Williams. 1978. Biogeographic interpretation of variation within and among populations of the prairie vole, *Microtus ochrogaster*. Occas. Papers Mus., Texas Tech Univ., 49:1–25.

Claussen, C. P. 1975. Der caudale Ruckenfleck des Waldlemmings, *Myopus schisticolor* L. Z. Saugetierk., 40:368–371.

Cockerell, T. D., L. I. Miller, and M. Printz. 1914. The auditory ossicles of American rodents. Bull. Amer. Mus. Nat. Hist., 33:347–380.

Corbet, G. B. 1978. The mammals of the Palaearctic Region: a taxonomic review. British Mus. (Nat. Hist.) and Cornell Univ. Press, London and Ithaca, New York, 314 pp.

DEARDEN, L. C. 1958. The baculum in *Lagurus* and related microtines. J. Mamm., 39:541–553.

———. 1959. Meibomian glands in *Lagurus*. J. Mamm., 40:20–25.

———. 1966. Histology of the gastroesophageal junction in certain microtine rodents. J. Mamm., 47:223–229.

———. 1969. Stomach and pyloric sphincter histology in certain microtine rodents. J. Mamm., 50:60–68.

DEWSBURY, D. A. 1975. Diversity and adaptation in rodent copulatory behavior. Science, 190:947–954.

DIDIER, R. 1954. Etude systematique de l'os penien des Mammiferes (suite), Rongeurs: Murides. Mammalia, 18:237–256.

DUKELSKI, N. M. 1927. External characters in the structure of the feet and their value for classification of voles. J. Mamm., 8:133–140.

DUNMIRE, W. W. 1955. Sex dimorphism in the pelvis of rodents. J. Mamm., 36: 356–361.

DURRANT, S. D. 1952. Mammals of Utah. Taxonomy and distribution. Univ. Kansas Publ., Mus. Nat. Hist., 6:1–549.

EISENBERG, J. F., AND D. G. KLEIMAN. 1972. Olfactory communication in mammals. Ann. Rev. Ecol. Syst., 3:1–32.

ELLERMAN, J. R. 1941. The families and genera of living rodents. Vol. II. British Mus. (Nat. Hist.), London, 689 pp.

EMRY, R. J. 1981. New material of the Oligocene muroid rodent *Nonomys*, and its bearing on muroid origins. Amer. Mus. Novitates, 2712:1–14.

ENGELS, H. 1979. Das postnatale Schadelwachstum bei der Hausmaus *Mus musculus* Linne, 1758, und bei zwei verscheiden groben Unterarten der Feldmaus *Microtus arvalis* Pallas, 1779. Gegenbaurs Morph. Jahrb., Leipzig, 125:550–571.

FINDLEY, J. S., AND C. J. JONES. 1962. Distribution and variation of voles of the genus *Microtus* in New Mexico and adjacent areas. J. Mamm., 43:154–166.

FISH, P. G., AND J. O. WHITAKER. 1971. *Microtus pinetorum* with grooved incisors. J. Mamm., 52:827.

FLEISCHER, G. 1978. Evolutionary principles of the mammalian middle ear. Adv. Anat. Embryol. Cell Biol., 55:1–70.

GEBCZYNSKA, Z. 1964. Morphological changes occurring in laboratory *Microtus agrestis* with age. Acta Theriol., 9:67–76.

GOIN, O. B. 1943. A study of individual variation in *Microtus pennsylvanicus pennsylvanicus*. J. Mamm., 24:212–223.

GOLLEY, F. B. 1960. Anatomy of the digestive tract of *Microtus*. J. Mamm., 41: 89–99.

GREAVES, W. S. 1973. The inference of jaw motion from toothwear facets. J. Paleontol., 47:1000–1001.

GRIFFITHS, J., AND M. D. KENDALL. 1980. Structure of the plantar sweat glands of the bank vole *Clethrionomys glareolus*. J. Zool., 191:1–10.

GUILDAY, J. E. 1951. Sexual dimorphism in the pelvic girdle of *Microtus pennsylvanicus*. J. Mamm., 32:216–217.

———. 1982. Dental variation in *Microtus xanthognathus, M. chrotorrhinus,* and *M. pennsylvanicus* (Rodentia: Mammalia). Ann. Carnegie Mus., 51:211–230.

GUTHRIE, D. A. 1963. The carotid circulation in the Rodentia. Bull. Mus. Comp. Zool., 128:455–481.

———. 1969. The carotid circulation in *Aplodontia*. J. Mamm., 50:1–7.

GUTHRIE, R. D. 1965. Variability in characters undergoing rapid evolution, an analysis of *Microtus* molars. Evolution, 19:214–233.

———. 1971. Factors regulating the evolution of microtine tooth complexity. Z. Saugetierk., 36:37–54.

Hall, E. R. 1946. Mammals of Nevada. Univ. California Press, Berkeley, 710 pp.

———. 1981. The mammals of North America. John Wiley and Sons, New York, 2:601–1181 + *90.*

Hamilton, W. J. 1941. Reproduction of the field mouse *Microtus pennsylvanicus* (Ord.). Mem. Cornell Univ. Agric. Exp. Sta., 237:1–23.

———. 1946. A study of the baculum in some North American Microtinae. J. Mamm., 27:378–387.

Hartung, T. G., and D. A. Dewsbury. 1978. A comparative analysis of copulatory plugs in muroid rodents and their relationship to copulatory behavior. J. Mamm., 59:717–723.

Hecht, P. 1971. Vergleichende anatomische und biometrische Untersuchungen an Os coxae, Scapula, Femur und Humerus bei Waldmaus (*Apodemus sylvaticus*), Gelbhalsmaus (*Apodemus flavicollis*), Feldmaus (*Microtus arvalis*) und Rotelmaus (*Clethrionomys glareolus*). Saugetierk. Mitt., 19:132–157.

Hennig, W. 1966. Phylogenetic systematics. Univ. Illinois Press, Urbana, 263 pp.

Hershkovitz, P. 1966. South American swamp and fossorial rats of the Scapteromyine Group (Cricetinae, Muridae) with comments on the glans penis in murid taxonomy. Z. Saugetierk., 31:81–149.

Hilborn, R. 1974. Inheritance of skeletal polymorphism in *Microtus californicus.* Heredity, 33:87–121.

Hill, J. E. 1935. The cranial foramina in rodents. J. Mamm., 16:121–129.

Hinton, M. A. C. 1926. Monograph of the voles and lemmings (Microtinae) living and extinct. Vol. I. British Mus. Nat. Hist., London, 488 pp.

Hooper, E. T. 1960. The glans penis in *Neotoma* (Rodentia) and allied genera. Occas. Papers Mus. Zool., Univ. Michigan, 618:1–21.

———. 1968. Anatomy of middle ear walls and cavities of microtine rodents. Occas. Papers Mus. Zool., Univ. Michigan, 657:1–28.

Hooper, E. T., and B. S. Hart. 1962. A synopsis of Recent North American microtine rodents. Misc. Publ. Mus. Zool., Univ. Michigan, 120:1–68.

Hooper, E. T., and G. G. Musser. 1964. The glans penis in Neotropical cricetines (Family Muridae) with comments on classification of muroid rodents. Misc. Publ. Mus. Zool., Univ. Michigan, 123:1–57.

Howell, A. B. 1924. Individual and age variation in *Microtus montanus yosemite.* J. Agric. Res., 28:977–1015.

Hrabě, V. 1977. Tarsal glands in *Microtus agrestis* (Microtidae, Mammalia) from the territory of Austria. Folia Zool., 26:229–235.

———. 1978. Tarsal glands of voles of the genus *Pitymys* (Microtidae, Mammalia) from southern Austria. Folia Zool., 27:123–128.

Indyk, F. 1968. The structure of the prostatic part of the urethra and of its glands in some Microtinae. Acta Theriol., 13:261–276.

Jannett, F. J. 1975. "Hip glands" of *Microtus pennsylvanicus* and *M. longicaudus* (Rodentia: Muridae), voles "without" hip glands. Syst. Zool., 24:171–175.

Jannett, F. J., and J. Z. Jannett. 1974. Drum marking by *Arvicola richardsoni* and its taxonomic significance. Amer. Midland Nat., 92:230–234.

Jones, G. S. 1978. *Microtus longicaudus* with grooved incisors. Murrelet, 59:104–105.

Jones, J. K. 1964. Distribution and taxonomy of mammals of Nebraska. Univ. Kansas Publ., Mus. Nat. Hist., 16:1–356.

Jorga, W. 1974. On the variability of the molar enamel pattern of the northern vole, *Microtus oeconomus* (Pallas, 1776). Z. Saugetierk., 39:220–229.

KELLOGG, R. 1918. A revision of the *Microtus californicus* group of meadow mice. Univ. California Publ. Zool., 21:1–42.

———. 1922*a*. A study of the Californian forms of the *Microtus montanus* group of meadow mice. Univ. California Publ. Zool., 21:245–274.

———. 1922*b*. A synopsis of the *Microtus mordax* group of meadow mice in California. Univ. California Publ. Zool., 21:275–302.

KESNER, M. H. 1977. Myology of the cranial and pectoral appendicular regions of rodents of the subfamily Microtinae. Unpubl. Ph.D. dissert., Univ. Massachusetts, Amherst, 197 pp.

———. 1980. Functional morphology of the masticatory musculature of the rodent subfamily Microtinae. J. Morphol., 165:205–222.

KIRKLAND, G. L. 1977. The rock vole, *Microtus chrotorrhinus* (Miller) (Mammalia: Rodentia), in West Virginia. Ann. Carnegie Mus., 46:45–53.

KLIMKIEWICZ, M. K. 1970. The taxonomic status of the nominal species *Microtus pennsylvanicus* and *Microtus agrestis* (Rodentia: Cricetidae). Mammalia, 34:640–665.

KLINGENER, D. J. 1968. Anatomy. Pp. 127–147, *in* Biology of *Peromyscus* (Rodentia) (J. A. King, ed.). Spec. Publ., Amer. Soc. Mamm., 2:1–593.

KOENIGSWALD, W. VON. 1980. Schmelzstruktur und Morphologie in den Molaren der Arvicolidae (Rodentia). Abh. Senckenb. Naturforsch. Ges., 539:1–129.

KOENIGSWALD, W. VON, AND F. N. GOLENISHEV. 1979. A method for determining growth rates in continuously growing molars. J. Mamm., 60:397–400.

LANDRY, S. O. 1958. The function of the entepicondylar foramen in mammals. Amer. Midland Nat., 60:100–112.

LINZEY, A. V., AND J. N. LAYNE. 1969. Comparative morphology of the male reproductive tract in the rodent genus *Peromyscus* (Muridae). Amer. Mus. Novitates, 2355:1–47.

LONG, C. A., AND T. FRANK. 1968. Morphometric variation and function in the baculum, with comments on the correlation of parts. J. Mamm., 49: 32–43.

LUTHJE, B. 1976. Comparative investigations on the stomach of central European Murinae (Murray 1866) and Microtinae (Miller 1896) (Rodentia) in respect to functional anatomy and histochemistry. Zool. Jb. Anat., 96:451–512.

MARTIN, L. D. 1975. Microtine rodents from the Ogallala Pliocene of Nebraska and the early evolution of the Microtinae in North America. Papers Paleontol., Univ. Michigan Mus. Paleontol., 12:101–110.

MARTIN, R. L. 1973. The dentition of *Microtus chrotorrhinus* (Miller) and related forms. Univ. Connecticut Occas. Papers, Biol. Sci., 2:183–201.

———. 1979. Morphology, development and adaptive values of the baculum of *Microtus chrotorrhinus* (Miller, 1894) and related forms. Saugetierk. Mitt., 27:307–311.

MEREDITH, M. 1980. The vomeronasal organ and accessory olfactory system in the hamster. Pp. 303–326, *in* Chemical signals, vertebrates and aquatic invertebrates (D. Müller-Schwarze and R. M. Silverstein, eds.). Plenum Press, New York, 445 pp.

MILLER, G. S. 1896. The genera and subgenera of voles and lemmings. N. Amer. Fauna, 12:1–84.

———. 1912. Catalogue of the mammals of western Europe in the collection of the British Museum. British Mus., London, 1,019 pp.

———. 1924. List of North American Recent mammals. Bull. U.S. Natl. Mus., 128:1–673.

MILLER, G. S., AND R. KELLOGG. 1955. List of North American Recent mammals. Bull. U.S. Natl. Mus., 205:1-954 pp.
MOIR, R. J. 1968. Ruminant digestion and evolution. Handbook of physiology, alimentary canal, 5 (chap. 126):2673-2694.
NIETHAMMER, J. 1972. Die Zahl der Mammae bei *Pitymys* und bei den Microtinen. Bonner Zool. Bietr., 23:49-60.
———. 1980. Eine Hypothese zur Evolution microtoider Molaren bei Nagetieren. Z. Saugetierk., 45:234-238.
OGNEV, S. I. 1950. Mammals of the U.S.S.R. and adjacent countries. Rodentia. Israel Program for Scientific Translations, Jerusalem (1964), 3:1-626.
OPPENHEIMER, J. R. 1965. Molar cusp pattern variations and their interrelationships in the meadow vole, *Microtus p. pennsylvanicus* (Ord). Amer. Midland Nat., 74:39-49.
OUELLETTE, D. E., AND J. F. HEISINGER. 1980. Reingestion of feces by *Microtus pennsylvanicus*. J. Mamm., 61:366-368.
PHILLIPS, C. J., AND B. OXBERRY. 1972. Comparative histology of molar dentitions of *Microtus* and *Clethrionomys*, with comments on dental evolution in microtine rodents. J. Mamm., 53:1-20.
QUAY, W. B. 1954*a*. The Meibomian glands of voles and lemmings (Microtinae). Misc. Publ. Mus. Zool., Univ. Michigan, 82:1-17.
———. 1954*b*. The anatomy of the diastemal palate in microtine rodents. Misc. Publ. Mus. Zool., Univ. Michigan, 86:1-41.
———. 1968. The specialized posterolateral sebaceous glandular regions in microtine rodents. J. Mamm., 49:427-445.
RAUSCH, R. L. 1964. The specific status of the narrow-skulled vole (subgenus *Stenocranius* Kashchenko) in North America. Z. Saugetierk., 29:343-358.
RAUSCH, R. L., AND V. R. RAUSCH. 1968. On the biology and systematic position of *Microtus abbreviatus* Miller, a vole endemic to the St. Matthew Islands, Bering Sea. Z. Saugetierk., 33:65-99.
REPENNING, C. A. 1968. Mandibular musculature and the origin of the subfamily Arvicolinae (Rodentia). Acta Zool. Cracoviensa, 13:1-72.
———. 1980. Faunal exchanges between Siberia and North America. Canada J. Anthropol., 1:37-44.
RINKER, G. C. 1954. The comparative myology of the mammalian genera *Sigmodon, Oryzomys, Neotoma,* and *Peromyscus* (Cricetinae), with remarks on their intergeneric relationships. Misc. Publ. Mus. Zool., Univ. Michigan, 83:1-124.
RUTH, E. B. 1934. The os priapi: a study in bone development. Anat. Rec., 60: 231-249.
SEMKEN, H. A. 1966. Stratigraphy and paleontology of the McPherson *Equus* beds (Sandahl local fauna), McPherson County, Kansas. Contrib. Mus. Paleontol., Univ. Michigan, 6:121-178.
SIMKIN, G. N. 1965. Types of ear cavities of mammals in relation to distinctive features of their mode of life. Zool. Zhur., 44:1538-1545.
SNEATH, P. H. A., AND R. R. SOKAL. 1973. Numerical taxonomy. The principles and practice of numerical classification. W. H. Freeman and Co., San Francisco, 573 pp.
SNELL, R. R., AND K. M. CUNNISON. 1983. Relation of geographic variation in the skull of *Microtus pennsylvanicus* to climate. Canadian J. Zool., 61: 1232-1241.
SNYDER, D. P. 1954. Skull variation in the meadow vole (*Microtus p. pennsylvanicus*) in Pennsylvania. Ann. Carnegie Mus., 13:201-234.

SPRAGUE, J. M. 1941. A study of the hyoid apparatus of the Cricetinae. J. Mamm., 22:296–310.

STAINS, H. J. 1959. Use of the calcaneum in studies of taxonomy and food habits. J. Mamm., 40:392–401.

STEIN, G. H. W. 1958. Uber den Selektionswert der simplex-Zahnform beider Feldmaus *Microtus arvalis* (Pallas). Zool. J. Syst., 86:27–34.

TAMARIN, R. H. 1981. Hip glands in wild-caught *Microtus pennsylvanicus*. J. Mamm., 62:421.

TARASOV, S. A. 1974. Postnatal development of os penis in some voles (Rodentia, Cricetidae). Zool. Zhur., 53:1109–1111.

TOEPFER, K. 1891. Die morphologie des magens der Rodentia. Morphol. Jb. Leipzig, 17:380–407.

TULLBERG, T. 1899. Ueber das system der Nagethiere, eine phylogenetische studie. Nova Acta R. Soc. Scient. Upsaliensis, Ser. 3, 18:1–514.

VOGE, M., AND H. A. BERN. 1949. Cecal villi in the red tree mouse *Phenacomys longicaudus*. Anat. Rec., 104:477–482.

———. 1955. Cecal villi in *Dicrostonyx torquatus* (Rodentia: Microtinae). Anat. Rec., 123:124–131.

VORONTSOV, N. N. 1962. The ways of food specialization and evolution of the alimentary system in Muroidea. Pp. 360–377, *in* Symposium Theriologicum (J. Kratochvbil and J. Pelikban, eds.). Publ. House Czechoslovak Acad. Sci., Praha, 383 pp.

———. 1979. Evolution of the alimentary system in myomorph rodents. Amerind Publ. Co., New Delhi, 346 pp.

VOSS, R. S. 1979. Male accessory glands and the evolution of copulatory plugs in rodents. Occas. Papers Mus. Zool., Univ. Michigan, 689:1–27.

VOSS, R. S., AND A. V. LINZEY. 1981. Comparative gross morphology of male accessory glands among Neotropical Muridae (Mammalia: Rodentia) with comments on systematic implications. Misc. Publ. Mus. Zool., Univ. Michigan, 159:1–41.

WAHLERT, J. H. 1974. The cranial foramina of protrogomorphous rodents; an anatomical and phylogenetic study. Bull. Mus. Comp. Zool., 146:363–410.

WILHELM, D. D. 1982. Zoogeographic and evolutionary relationships of selected populations of *Microtus mexicanus*. Occas. Papers Mus., Texas Tech Univ., 75:1–30.

WOHRMANN-REPENNING, A. 1980. The relationship between Jacobson's organ and the oral cavity in a rodent. Zool. Anz. Jena, 204:391–399.

WOLFF, J., AND M. JOHNSON. 1979. Scent marking in Taiga voles, *Microtus xanthognathus*. J. Mamm., 60:400–404.

YABLOKOV, A. V. 1974. Variability of mammals. Amerind Publ. Co., New Delhi, 350 pp.

ZIEGLER, A. C. 1961. Occurrence of os clitoridis in *Microtus*. J. Mamm., 42:101–103.

ZIMMERMANN, K. 1956. Zur evolution der Molar-Strukur der Erdmaus, *Microtus agrestis* (L.). Zool. Jb. Syst., 84:269–274.

MICROANATOMY

CARLETON J. PHILLIPS

Abstract

A small selection of tissues from species of New World *Microtus* have been investigated in detail at the light microscopic level; at the ultrastructural level *Microtus* is virtually unknown. Most previous histological studies have been in conjunction with analyses of the evolutionary process, systematics, populations, and ontogeny. In particular, light microscopic data are available in the literature for such features as the dentition, integumentary glands, tarsal glands, adrenal glands, ovaries and testes, and digestive tracts. Microanatomical studies of the dentition have revealed likely steps or phases and preadaptive characteristics involved in the evolution of evergrowing molars. The histology, histochemistry, and actual presence or absence of both tarsal and integumentary glands have been used successfully in systematic investigations. The adrenal glands of *Microtus* have been shown to undergo histological changes in correlation with population density and reproductive status. Ovarian microanatomy has allowed for estimation of prenatal mortality; histology of both ovaries and testes has been used previously to demonstrate the effects of variables such as light intensity, photoperiod, and crowding on sexual maturation. Previously unavailable ultrastructural descriptions of the retinal pigment epithelium and photoreceptor cells, the parotid and submandibular salivary glands, and the esophagus, stomach, and small intestine are provided in this chapter. The eye in *Microtus* has approximately 10% cone and 90% rod photoreceptors; ultrastructurally the retina resembles that found in fossorial pocket gophers, *Geomys*. The parotid salivary gland is serous and has secretory intercalated ducts, whereas the submandibular has mucous acini, secretory intercalated ducts, and granular intralobular ducts. The ultrastructure of the esophagus, gastric mucosa, and small intestine generally resembles that of laboratory rodents. Although *Microtus* is not known to have a symbiotic microbial relationship, rod-type bacteria nevertheless are found attached to the keratinized, non-glandular surface of the forestomach.

Introduction

With three major exceptions, organ systems in species of New World *Microtus* have not been described in detail at either the light microscopic or transmission electron microscopic levels. The exceptions—dentition, stomachs, and certain skin glands—previously have been described and discussed in considerable histological (light microscopic) detail with reference to systematics, evolution, and ecology. The light microscopic histology of several other organs—especially adrenal glands and ovaries and testes—has been used fairly frequently, particularly in the course of ecological and populational studies. Somewhat surprisingly, however, these tissues never have been described qualitatively or quantitatively to the point where intergeneric or interspecific histological comparisons can be made with precision.

The absence of complete, descriptive, microanatomical data for *Microtus,* and other microtines as well, is not particularly surprising in view of the fact that microanatomical compendia are available only for laboratory mice (*Mus*), rats (*Rattus*), and golden hamsters (*Mesocricetus*). The amount of previously published descriptive microanatomical data for *Microtus* necessitated that this chapter be somewhat limited in scope. Consequently, not all organ systems are represented here and, among those that are, some are described and illustrated at the ultrastructural level for the first time.

The main goals of this chapter are: 1) to help establish a data base that will allow for comparisons between *Microtus* and other genera of rodents; 2) to stimulate further study by illustrating the sparseness of current knowledge; 3) to summarize the existing microanatomical data and sources of information; and 4) to present structural information useful to those engaged in other areas of research in which knowledge of microanatomy, particularly at the ultrastructural level, could be valuable to analysis and interpretation of data.

Methods

Both light and electron microscopic techniques were used to obtain microanatomical data that are presented for the first time in this chapter. New data are based on five specimens of *Microtus pennsylvanicus* (two males, three females) collected in Franklin and

Aroostook Counties, Maine. Voucher specimens from these localities are deposited in the collection at the Carnegie Museum of Natural History.

The standard light micrographs of molar dentition were taken with an Olympus Vanox photomicroscope with Nomarski interference-contrast optics (IOC). The jaws were fixed in 10% non-buffered formalin and decalcified in Decal (Scientific Products); a calcium precipitant test (Lillie, 1965) was used to determine total decalcification. The jaws then were embedded in Paraplast and sectioned and stained according to routine, widely used techniques (see Humason [1972] and Lillie [1965] for detailed descriptive information).

Cellular ultrastructure, as studied with transmission electron microscopy (TEM), is heavily emphasized in this chapter. Although much remains to be learned from light-level histochemistry, ultrastructure probably will prove to be a better basic source of information suitable for comparative investigations. The techniques employed for TEM analysis are less well standardized than are histological techniques, and for that reason I present here a reasonably complete description of methodology. I found trialdehyde fixative to be very well suited to ultrastructural analysis of microtines and, with minor changes in protocol, it can be used easily under field conditions (Phillips, in press).

Specimens were anaesthetized with 0.25 cc of sodium pentobarbital (50 mg/ml) and intubated by means of polyethylene tubing that was passed via the mouth and esophagus into the stomach. The primary fixative (based on Kalt and Tandler, 1971) consisted of 3% glutaraldehyde, 2% formaldehyde (made fresh each day from paraformaldehyde powder), 1% acrolein, 2.5% dimethyl sulfoxide (DMSO), and 1 mM $CaCl_2$ in 0.05 M cacodylate buffer at pH 7.2 with 0.1 M sucrose. For digestive tract tissues, fixative was introduced to the lumina by attaching a 1 cc syringe to the free end of the tubing. Meanwhile, other tissues, such as eyes and salivary glands, were removed and either hemisectioned (eyes) or diced in fixative. After 5 min the digestive tract tissues were removed from the visceral cavity and diced in fixative. All tissues were stored in primary fixative for 20 h and then placed in fresh buffer with 3% glutaraldehyde and stored at 4°C. For processing, tissues were washed for 1 h in 0.05 M cacodylate buffer (pH 7.2) with 0.1 M sucrose (three changes, 10 min each) and post-fixed for 1 h in 1%

OsO_4 with cacodylate buffer and sucrose. Tissues then were dehydrated in an ETOH series (50, 70, 90, and 95%) for 20 min each followed by three changes in 100% ETOH (10 min each) and then three changes (10 min each) in propylene oxide. Lastly, tissues were left overnight in a propylene oxide-Epon 812 mixture (1:1) and vacuum infiltrated for 6 h in fresh Epon 812. The resin was allowed to polymerize for 48 to 60 h at 60°C. Thin sections were studied and micrographed with a Philips TEM 201 operated at 60 KV. "Thick" sections (0.5 μm) of Epon-embedded tissue were stained with toluidine blue and micrographed with an Olympus Vanox and Nomarski IOC.

Brain

Histological study of the brain of any mammal is extremely complex and requires not only careful fixation but also careful orientation. Indeed, stereoscopic histological atlases are available only for common laboratory rodents such as rats and golden hamsters (for example, see Knigge and Joseph, 1968). Insofar as *Microtus* is concerned, the brain has not been described at either the light or electron microscopic level and, therefore, nothing definitive can be said about the microanatomy of the brain. However, Quay (1969) reported that he sectioned and examined histologically the brains of 12 specimens of *Microtus pennsylvanicus.* Quay's investigation was a follow-up of an earlier study of the collared lemming (Quay, 1960) and dealt with the occurrence of colloid deposits in the brains of microtine rodents collected in western Canada. Although Quay (1969) did not find birefringent colloid deposits in the brain of any of the specimens of *Microtus,* 12 of 16 captive specimens of *Dicrostonyx* and one wild-caught specimen of *Phenacomys* did exhibit these unusual, possibly pathological, features in their brain tissue.

Anterior Pituitary Gland

The ultrastructure of the anterior pituitary gland has been studied and described only for an Old World species, *Microtus agrestis* (Charlton and Worth, 1975), but deserves mention here because of Hinkley's (1966) earlier investigation of the effects of plant extracts on cell types in the anterior pituitary of *M. montanus.* In the study by Charlton and Worth (1975), the pituitary cell types were identified by fine structural criteria and comparisons were made to homologous cells in laboratory rats. Prolactotrophs, somatotrophs, gonadotrophs, corticotrophs, thyrotrophs, and follicular cells were all found to be very similar to the presumably homologous cells in *Rattus,* even after a series of experimental manipulations (Charlton and Worth, 1975). One unusual feature, which possibly is unique to the anterior pituitary of *Microtus,* was an "organelle" of unknown function found in the adenohypophysial cells. The authors (Charlton and Worth, 1975) described the structure as a complex array of closely appressed granular endoplasmic reticulum (GER) located adjacent to the Golgi complex. From this discription it seems likely that the structure is related to protein synthesis. Although the gonadotrophic cells from sexually mature individuals most commonly contained this "organelle," it also was found in all of the other types of granular cells. The discovery of an unusual feature in gonadotrophs is especially noteworthy in terms of Hinkley's (1966) report that in male *Microtus montanus,* gonadotrophic (delta) cells increased by 41% following a diet of acetone-ether extract from sprouted wheat.

Eyes

The structure of the eye in *Microtus* previously has been investigated only superficially (for example, Chase, 1972); and because the following account covers only the retinal pigment epithelium (RPE) and neural retina, many relatively basic questions will remain unanswered. Even though microtines have not been studied in detail, enough other species of rodents have been subjects of developmental, functional, histological, and ultrastructural investigations for one to conclude that probably no other mammalian order approaches the Rodentia in structural diversity of the eye. This should not be particularly surprising because the behavioral and ecological diversity among rodents clearly sets them apart from other orders. Indeed, it is for these very reasons that attention is called to the eye in species of *Microtus.*

A basic assumption in constructing an understanding of the evolution of visual-system microanatomy is, of course, that *Microtus* relies on visual cues as well as on olfactory and auditory input.

Although the eyes in *Microtus* are small in comparison to the bulging eyes that are so obviously characteristic of most nocturnal cricetids, it nevertheless is safe to assume that vision is an important component of the total sensory system in microtines. Particularly significant in this regard is the finding that *Microtus pennsylvanicus* uses a sun-compass system in orientation, at least in homing females (Fluharty et al., 1976). They demonstrated that experimental shifts in photoperiod would alter orientation in a predictable, clock-wise fashion. Thus, the eyes in *M. pennsylvanicus* apparently serve as the receptors in a fundamentally important, integrated behavioral-physiological process that includes some type of "biological clock." The level of visual activity in *Microtus* is unknown, but it possibly is significant that most, or perhaps all, of the species are highly susceptible to predation by owls. Consequently, future studies in which different roles of the visual system (for example, integrated sensory receptors in comparison to "sight") can be analyzed and then compared will be of special interest.

Microanatomical examination of the eye of light-adapted individuals reveals that the choroid layer and retinal pigment epithelium are relatively thick in *Microtus*. The stroma of the choroid is compact, densely pigmented, and contains relatively few macrophages (Fig. 1). The prominent chorio-capillary zone is highly innervated (Fig. 1) in *Microtus* and is set in a dense matrix of connective tissue fibers. When viewed in a plane perpendicular to the RPE, Bruch's membrane has a compressed, dense appearance with elastic fibers scattered throughout. A complex network of interlaced individual collagen fibers and reticular fibrils is readily apparent in oblique views (Fig. 2).

The retinal pigment epithelium (RPE) is a monolayer of cells that developmentally are derived from the neuroectoderm. The function, role, and cytochemistry of the RPE have been investigated fairly intensively in vertebrates and presently these cells are known to: 1) serve as a blood-retina barrier; 2) interact with the photoreceptor cells through phagocytosis and degradation of age membrane discs at the tips of the outer segments; 3) produce pigment granules in varying numbers; and 4) serve in ocular defense through their immunophagocytic capacity (Elner et al., 1981; Nguyen-Lagros, 1978; Young, 1971). Among these roles, the best known and most studied is that of phagocytosis and degradation of outer membrane discs.

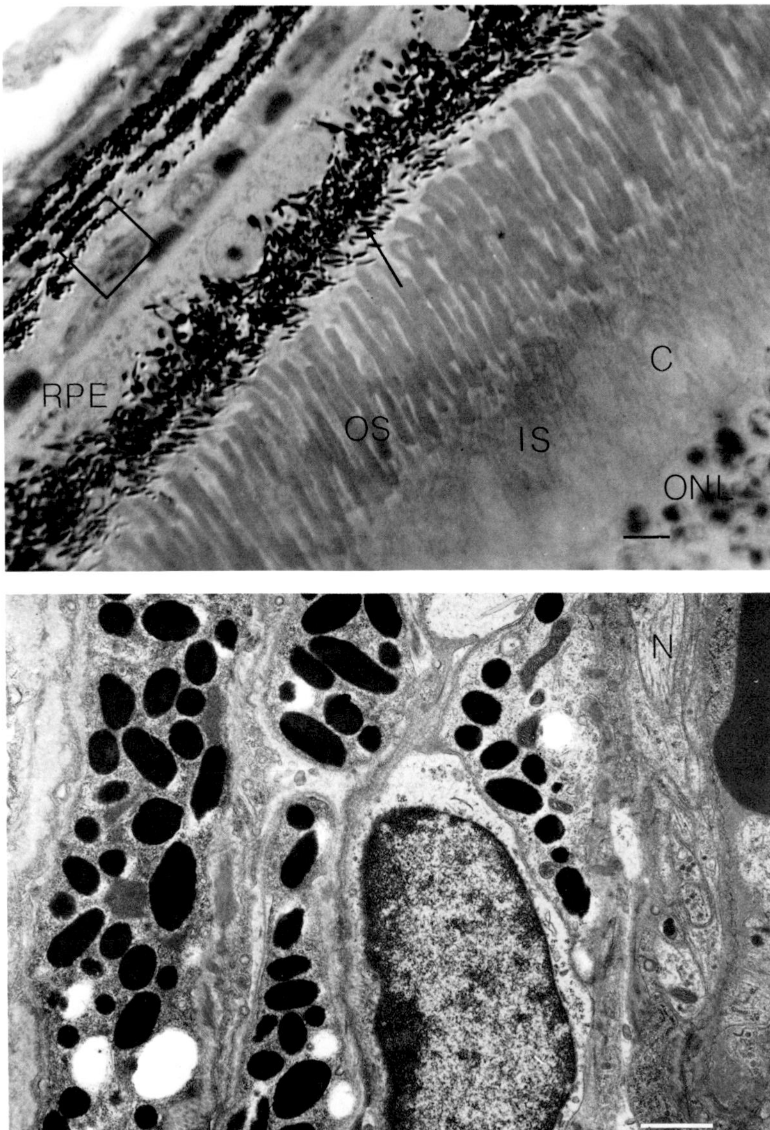

FIG. 1. Top: light micrograph showing several principal retinal components in *Microtus*. Note extreme abundance of melanolysosomes (arrow) in the retinal pigment epithelium (RPE). Area enclosed in box is roughly equivalent to the area shown below. Abbreviations are: OS, outer segments of photoreceptors; IS, inner

The RPE cells in *Microtus* are characterized by their unusual height, extreme abundance of spherical and ovoid melanin granules, and by the presence of osmophilic droplets that are not membrane-bound and apparently lipid in nature (Figs. 1, 2). The RPE basal membrane is complexly infolded; coated vesicles commonly are found within the adjacent cytoplasm but other cytoplasmic constituents, such as free polyribosomes and smooth endoplasmic reticulum (SER), are virtually absent from this area. The remaining cytoplasm, however, is densely filled with tubular SER and polyribosomes (Figs. 2, 3). Lamellar Golgi complexes also are common constituents of the middle zone of RPE cytoplasm (Fig. 2). The RPE mitochondria are found throughout the cell; the mitochondrial profiles either are elongate or nearly round and have both tubular and lamellar cristae.

Given the role of RPE in degradation of outer disc membranes, it is not at all surprising that the cytoplasm of the RPE cells in *Microtus* contains large numbers of phagosomes (Fig. 2), lysosomes, and pigment granules. The pigment granules, which more accurately can be termed "melanolysosomes" because of their acid phosphatase activity (Leuenberger and Novikoff, 1975), are extremely abundant in the RPE cell cytoplasm in *Microtus* (Fig. 1). Analysis of TEM micrographs of *Microtus* RPE provides ultrastructural data that seem to both support and correspond well with the cytochemical studies of Novikoff et al. (1979). Examples of continuity between tubular SER and plasma membranes encasing melanolysosomes, particularly in mature forms of the latter, are fairly common (Fig. 2). Additionally, in instances in which membrane surrounding melanolysosomes is sectioned within about 30° of a perpendicular plane, the surrounding plasma membrane can be demonstrated to be unusually thick and apparently tripartite. In the example illustrated in Fig. 2, the melanolysosomes are in the physical proximity of a Golgi complex and tubular SER, which can be characterized as GERL. The GERL in turn apparently is directly involved in production of RPE lysosomes. Cytochemical

---

←

segments; C, cone photoreceptor; ONL, outer nuclear layer. Scale bar = 3.5 μm. Bottom: transmission electron micrograph (TEM) of choroid showing melanin granules and choroidal innervation (N). Scale bar = 0.5 μm.

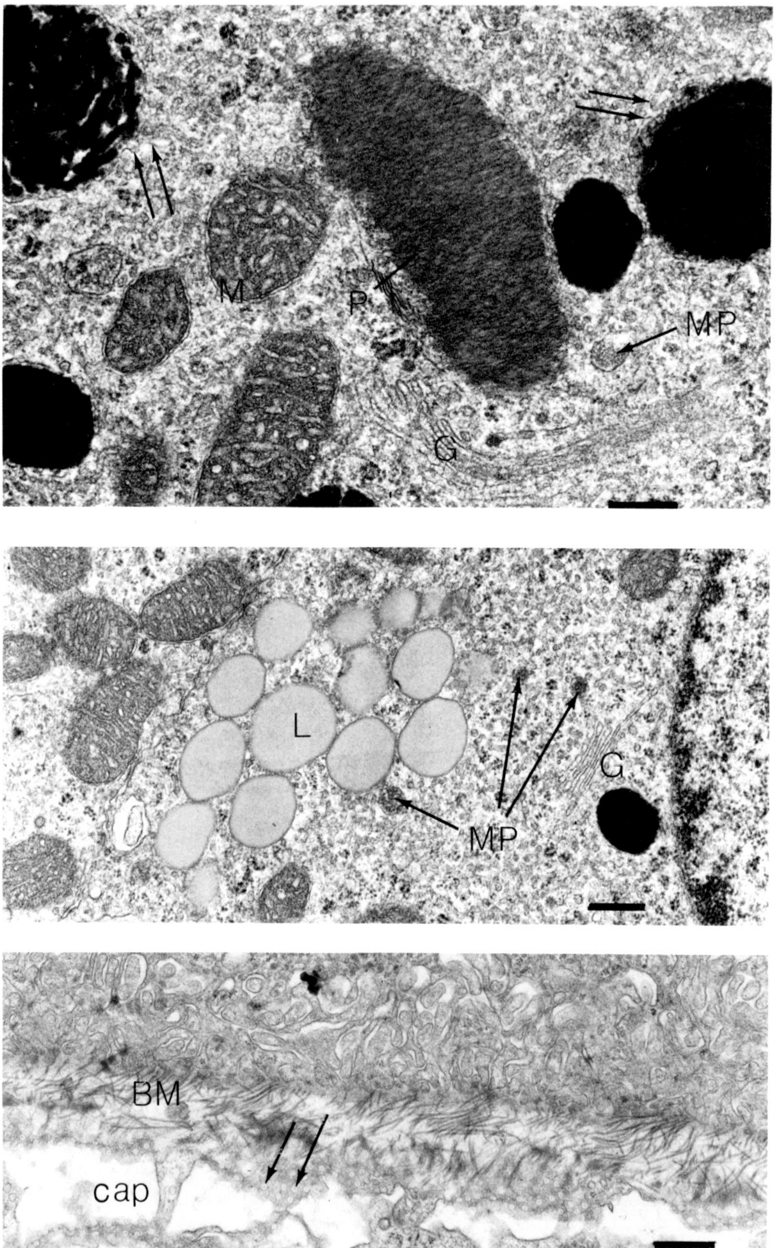
M
P
MP
G
L
MP
G
BM
cap

studies of this organelle have shown it to be both rich in hydrolase and the site of tyrosinase and acid phosphatase activity as well (Eppig and Dumont, 1972; Novikoff, 1976; Novikoff et al., 1979). Microperoxisomes also are abundant in *Microtus* RPE cell cytoplasm. These small spherical bodies are encased in thick, electron dense membrane and internally have a granular appearance (Fig. 2). Previous catalase cytochemical analysis of *Mus* RPE cells has revealed frequent continuity between microperoxisomes and SER (Leuenberger and Novikoff, 1975), and the same sort of TEM images can be found in *Microtus*.

The RPE apical microvilli are highly elaborate and contain abundant ovoid pigment granules (Fig. 1) that are interspersed among the tips of the photoreceptor cell outer segments (Fig. 3). The RPE lateral cell membranes are straight and unspecialized except in the apical zone where adjacent cells have a dense terminal web and desmosomes that form a circumferential ring-like structure within the cytoplasm (Fig. 3).

The neural retina of *Microtus* contains both rod and cone photoreceptor cells (approximately 10% cones, 90% rods). The cells are extremely numerous and densely packed as evidenced by the fact that the outer nuclear layer is 11–14 nuclei deep. According to Chase (1972), in *M. ochrogaster* the RPE, bacillary layer, and outer nuclear layer measure, respectively, 13, 30, and 34 μm.

The cone photoreceptors can be distinguished from the rods by virtue of: 1) their larger inner segments (both in height and width); 2) slightly paler cytoplasm (both in TEM thin sections and in toluidine blue-stained "thick" sections); 3) significantly larger and paler mitochondria; 4) their large, spherical, euchromatic nuclei; and 5) their complex pedicle-type synaptic bases (Figs. 1, 4, 5). Additionally, the cone photoreceptors in *Microtus* are of particular interest because of the extremely large and broad calyx that extends

---

←

FIG. 2. Top: cell cytoplasm in retinal pigment epithelium (RPE) of *Microtus*. Note relationship between smooth endoplasmic reticulum and developing melanolysosomes (see arrows). Abbreviations are: P, phagosome; MP, microperoxisome; G, Golgi complex; M, mitochondrion. Scale bar = 0.25 μm. Middle: lipid droplets (L) in RPE. Scale bar = 0.5 μm. Bottom: Bruch's membrane (BM) and capillary (cap) adjacent to basal surface of an RPE cell. Note pore-like fenestrae in the capillary wall (arrows). Scale bar = 0.25 μm.

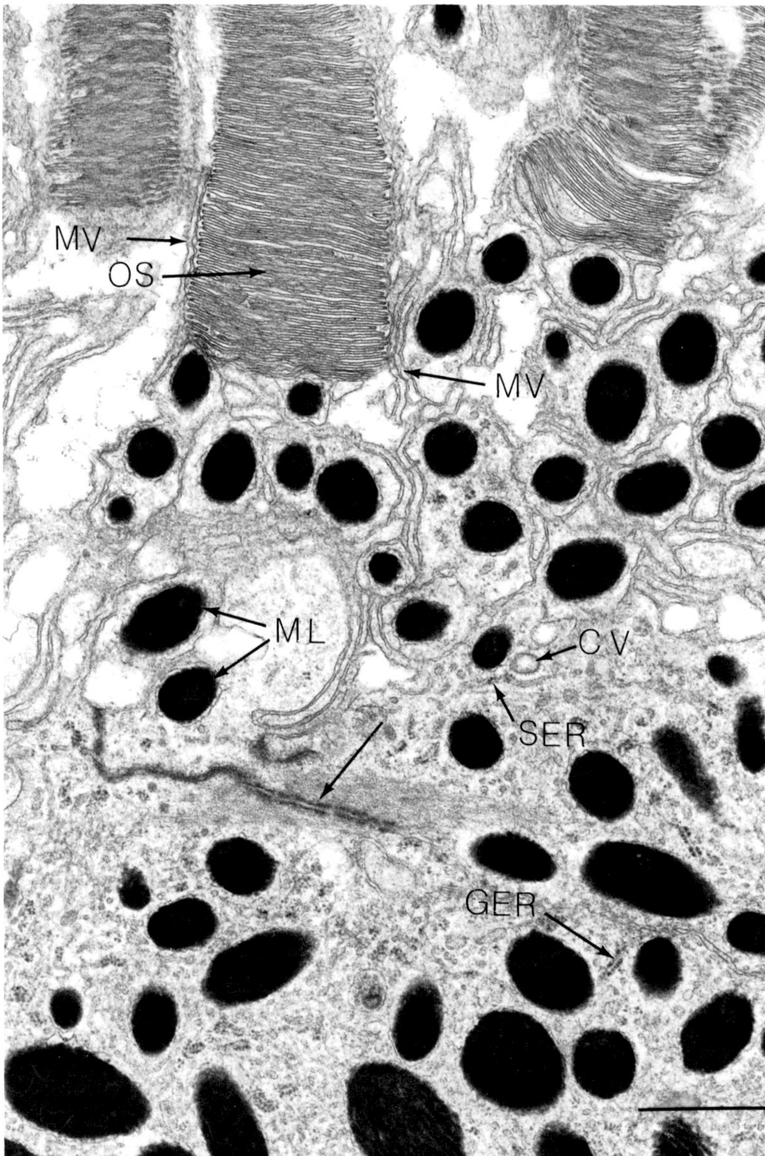

FIG. 3. A slightly oblique cut through the apical surface of a retinal pigment epithelial (RPE) cell showing the relationship between RPE microvilli (MV) and photoreceptor outer segments (OS). Note also the cell junction with dense fibrils

well beyond the ciliary stalk and appears to cradle the entire basal portion of the outer segment (Fig. 5). In at least some examples the calyx clearly forms a type of cytoplasmic bridge so that the inner and the outer segments of a given cell have a continuity that is additional to the non-motile cilium (Fig. 5). Without serial sections it is impossible to determine whether or not such cytoplasmic bridging is characteristic of all the individual cone photoreceptor cells in *Microtus*. In a previous report of cytoplasmic bridging (Richardson, 1969), it was concluded that such bridges were a regular feature of both cones and rods in the thirteen-lined ground squirrel (*Spermophilus tridecemlineatus*).

In contrast to the cones, the abundant rod photoreceptors in *Microtus* are narrow in outline, and the nuclei are somewhat ovoid and characteristically nearly filled with heterochromatin and the synaptic terminals are of the spherule type (Figs. 4, 5). As in the cone photoreceptors, cytoplasmic bridging also is found in the rods but probably because the rods are so narrow, examples are more scarce than they are among the cones. The potential importance of cytoplasmic bridging between the inner and outer segments of rods and cones lies in the question of how new membrane discs are formed by the photoreceptors and how these discs come to contain visual pigment. The most widely accepted model for origin of disc membranes is one in which new discs are thought to originate from invagination of plasma membrane of the outer segment (Sjöstrand and Kreman, 1979). Originally it was assumed that opsin was synthesized in the cytoplasm of the inner segment and then transported directly to the outer segment in membranous vesicles. Such a model viewed membrane as "fixed," and thus proposed that opsin-containing vesicles moved through the cytoplasm and would of necessity use the ciliary stalk as an access route to the outer segment (Fig. 4). Therefore, the presence of cytoplasmic bridging (Fig. 5) would seem to be particularly important because it would result in increased cytoplasmic contact between inner and outer segments (see Richardson, 1969). However, in our more current view of mem-

---

←

(arrow), the large, coated vesicle (CV), tubular smooth endoplasmic reticulum (SER), sparse granular endoplasmic reticulum (GER), and melanolysosomes (ML). Scale bar = 1 μm.

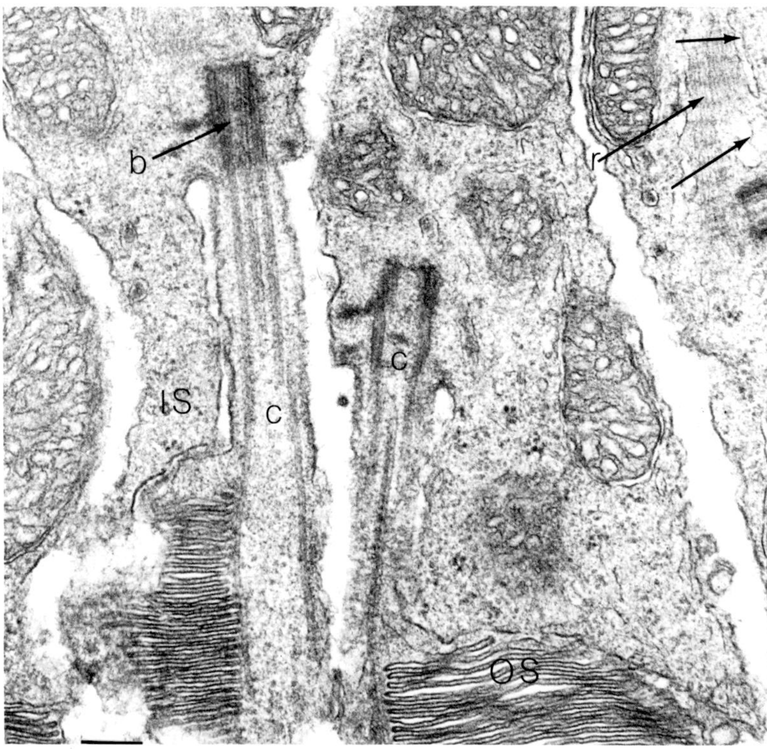
b
r
IS
c
c
c
OS

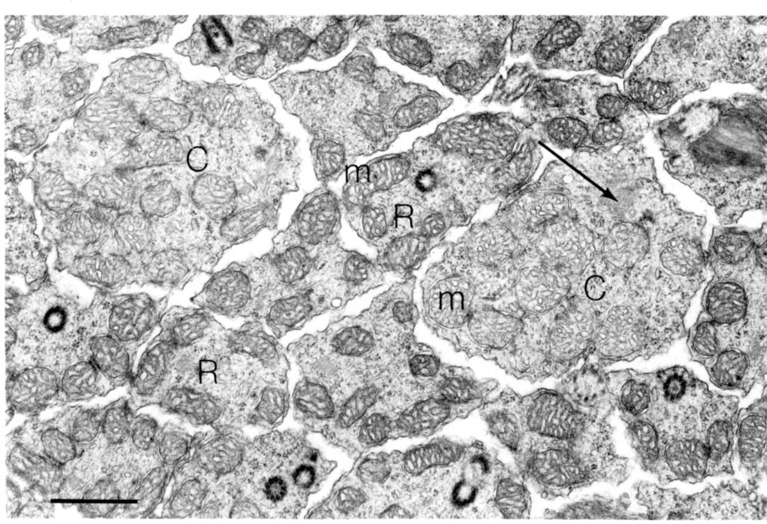
C
m
R
m
C
R

brane structure the possibility of compartmentalized zones within the membrane, as well as constituent flow, allows for non-cytoplasmic transport to the outer segment discs. Such a view is supported by findings from freeze-fracture studies (Besharse and Pfenninger, 1980; Röhlich, 1975; Sjöstrand and Kreman, 1979). Presently it is known that visual pigment apoprotein originates in the GER and Golgi complex of the inner segment, passes through the ellipsoid in association with membrane, is incorporated into the inner segment plasmalemma in the periciliary region, and flows over the cilium into the outer segment where it is incorporated into newly formed discs (Besharse and Pfenninger, 1980; Papermaster et al., 1975; Röhlich, 1975; Young and Droz, 1968). Fundamental structural changes in the plasma membrane take place when the discs actually form from the outer segment membrane (Sjöstrand and Kreman, 1979). It also has been speculated that lipid synthesis takes place in the narrow "growth" zone where discs arise from the outer segment membrane (Sjöstrand and Kreman, 1979). In view of our current understanding of the disc renewal process, the significance of the cytoplasmic bridges found in *Microtus,* and some other rodents as well, could well be the fact that mitochondria are a common feature of the bridges (Fig. 5).

Although membrane flow and the freeze-fracture data per se do not require cytoplasmic continuity between inner and outer segments and do not restrict exchange to the internal portion of the cilium, fundamental alterations in membrane structure and synthesis of lipids would require energy and thus could be facilitated by the immediate presence of mitochondria. Lastly, it is of particular interest that typical mitochondrial profiles located within the cytoplasmic bridges usually are associated physically with tubular SER that sometimes is organized in layers similar to those that characterize a Golgi complex (Fig. 5). The details of the entire renewal process obviously remain to be elucidated and the possibility of species-specific differences also must be considered.

←

FIG. 4. Top: junction of outer segment (OS) and inner segment (IS), showing cilium (c) and associated basal body (b) in the neural retina of *Microtus*. Note also the membrane (arrows) associated with the cross-striated fibril (r). Scale bar = 0.25 μm. Bottom: cross-sections through rods (R) and cone (C) photoreceptors. Compare the mitochondria (m) and note cross-striated fibril (arrow). Scale bar = 1 μm.

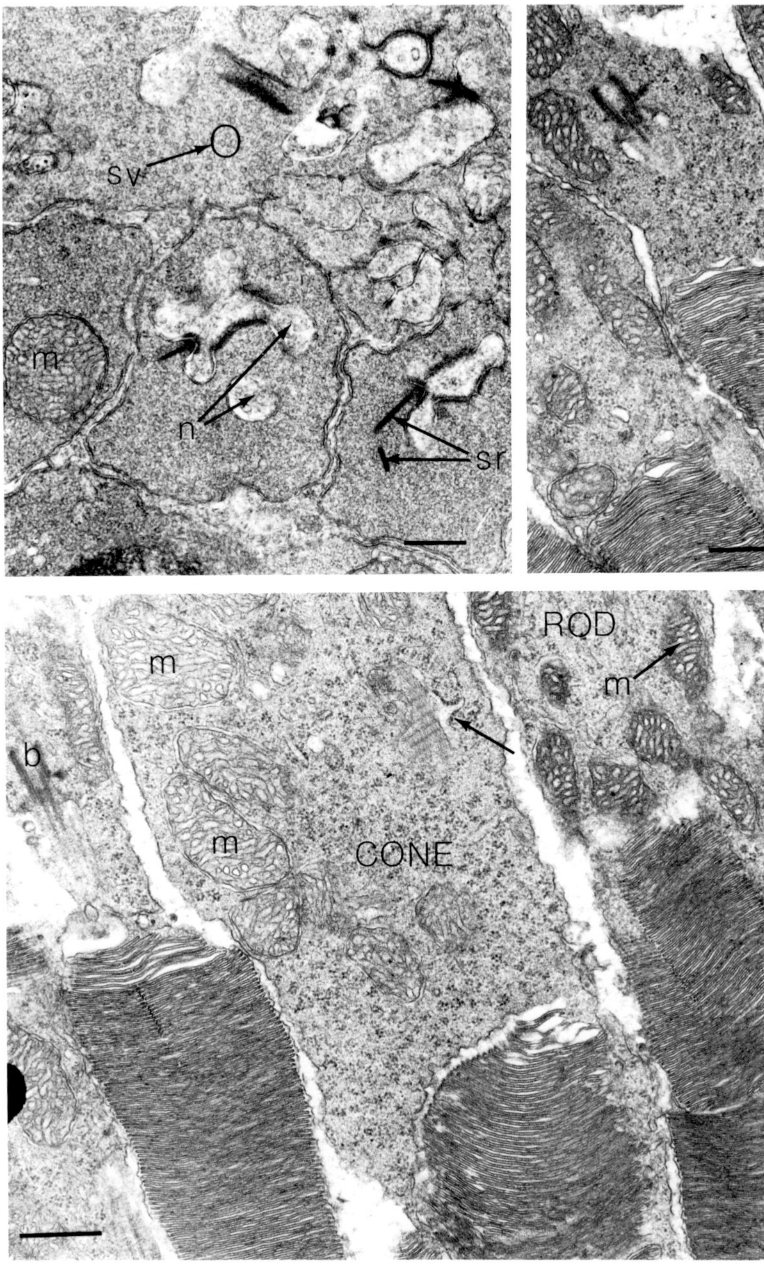
sv
m
n
sr
ROD
m
b
m
m
CONE

The inner segment in both types of photoreceptor cells contains abundant polyribosomes but only a few vesicles and relatively little SER. Both types of photoreceptor cells have cross-striated fibrils that are prominent near the base of the ciliary stalk (Fig. 4). The cross-striated fibrils usually are associated with membrane that either is smooth or, occasionally, studded with ribosomes (Fig. 5). These fibrils are structurally similar to those found in other rodents, such as the guinea pig (*Cavia*), and presumably extend from the cilium to the synaptic terminal as they do in *Cavia* (Spira and Milman, 1979). The exact function of cross-striated fibrils remains unknown, although their morphology and non-random associations with mitochondria and with membrane systems certainly implies that they are more than a ciliary anchoring system. Perhaps cross-striated fibrils aid in propagation of changes in membrane potential or serve as part of a system with contractile capability (Spira and Milman, 1979).

The synaptic layer in *Microtus* retina is vascularized. Broad-based cone pedicles can be distinguished readily from the rod spherules. The cone pedicles are characterized by numerous invading processes from bipolar and horizontal cells; the latter two kinds of cells have a much paler cytoplasm than do the photoreceptors. The similar rod spherules usually contain two to four pale profiles (Fig. 5). Both rod and cone terminals typically contain at least one mitochondrial profile and one or more synaptic ribbon (Fig. 5). Electron dense zones denote synaptic junctions within the terminals as well as between adjacent cones and rods (Fig. 5).

In summary, microanatomical analysis of the retinal pigment epithelium and neural retina in *Microtus* reveals a complex, mixed cone-rod photoreceptor system suggestive of both scotopic and photopic vision. In comparison to other studied rodents, *Microtus* ap-

---

←

FIG. 5. Top left: synaptic layer in the neural retina of *Microtus* showing rod spherules filled with synaptic vesicles (sv). The pale profiles (n) are sections through connecting bipolar and horizontal neurons. Note the single mitochondrial profile (m) and pairs of synaptic ribbons (sr). Scale bar = 0.5 μm. Top right: Bases of outer segments of rod (left) and cone (right) photoreceptors. Scale bar = 1 μm. Bottom: longitudinal sections comparing rod and cone photoreceptors. Compare the mitochondrial profiles (m) and note the ribosomes (arrow) attached to membrane associated with the rootlet fiber; b, basal body. Scale bar = 1 μm.

pears to be unique in a number of ways. Firstly, the RPE not only is thick but also densely filled with melanolysosomes that occupy the apical zone of cytoplasm. Although such comparisons have not been made previously, examination of micrographs published in Kuwabara (1979) and elsewhere clearly indicate that melanolysosome abundance is far greater in *Microtus* than in *Rattus, Mus, Cavia,* and *Mesocricetus.* The greatest morphological similarity is between *Microtus* and the diurnal ground squirrels, *Spermophilus,* and the fossorial plains pocket gopher, *Geomys bursarius* (Feldman and Phillips, 1984; Jacobs et al., 1976; Kuwabara, 1979). However, *Microtus* differs from even these species; in light-adapted *Microtus* the melanolysosomes are confined to the apical RPE cytoplasm and the microvilli are relatively short, whereas in the other two genera the long microvilli contain most of the granules. One possible explanation is that this apparent difference is the result of light or dark adaptation prior to sacrifice, but the data presently are inadequate for such a determination.

The relative percentages of rods and cones (90/10) places *Microtus* toward the nocturnal end of a broad category of rodents possessing mixed retinas. In nocturnal rodents such as Norway rats (*Rattus norvegicus*), pigmented laboratory mice, and the eastern woodrat (*Neotoma floridana*) the retinas essentially are all rod (99%), whereas in diurnal ground squirrels (*Spermophilus* and *Cynomys*), cones comprise about 95% of the photoreceptor cells (Cohen, 1960; Feldman and Phillips, 1984; Jacobs et al., 1976; West and Dowling, 1975). Overall, *Microtus* joins a group of species that includes the gray squirrel (*Sciurus carolinensis*), which has about 60% cones, and the plains pocket gopher (*Geomys bursarius*), which has about 25% cones (Feldman and Phillips, 1984; West and Dowling, 1975). Indeed, from a purely morphological point-of-view, *Microtus* is closest to *Geomys.* If additional study upholds these apparent similarities, the likelihood is that either both of these species share some common features because their eyes are less derived from the early ancestral state, or that the similarities are indicative of convergent evolution toward a fossorial or a semi-fossorial behavior. Indeed, *Microtus pennsylvanicus* spends considerable time in dark burrows and seems to prefer light intensities ranging from twilight to total darkness (Kavanau and Havenhill, 1976). Future study of the microanatomy of rodent eyes undoubtedly will be valuable in elucidation of systematic relationships and evolutionary patterns.

Future study will be required to determine such salient aspects of *Microtus* as visual acuity, spectral sensitivity, and the details of the inner nuclear and inner plexiform layers. The latter aspect in particular is totally unknown as of this writing and represents a topic that cannot easily be inferred from other work and, thus, will require considerable primary research.

Tarsal (Meibomian) Glands

The eyelids of mammals consist of an integumentary covering over a dense connective tissue support (called a "tarsal plate") and skeletal muscle fibers from the orbicularis oculi muscle. Typical sebaceous glands are associated with the hair follicles and, in both the upper and lower lids, hypertrophied sebaceous glands referred to as tarsal, Meibom, or Meibomian glands are positioned within the dermis (see Carleton, this volume). Tarsal glands in the eyelids of a variety of microtine rodents (both New and Old World species) have been described by several authors (Hrabě, 1974; Quay, 1954; Šulc, 1929; Veselý, 1923).

Quay (1954) found interspecific differences among the microtines and suggested that the distribution and abundance of tarsal glands might be of taxonomic value. Hrabě (1974) agreed with this assessment and with the idea that the evolutionary trend was one of reduction (that is, the more "primitive" microtines might be expected to have more glandular units). Both authors (Hrabě, 1974; Quay, 1954) found that although the tarsal glands were reduced in number in some microtines (including *Microtus*), the individual glands nevertheless were significantly larger in size than in those species having more glands. Quay (1954) hypothesized that the apparent evolutionary decrease in numbers of individual glands was related to the trend toward reduction in size of the eye evidenced by many microtines, whereas the increase in size of the individual glands could be correlated with an increased need for protective secretions during burrowing and other activities associated with a semi-fossorial life.

Histologically, the tarsal glands essentially are hypertrophied sebaceous glands that secrete a substance rich in lipids. Apparently the glands found in *Microtus* do not differ notably from homologous glands in other rodents or mammals in general. Quay (1954) did note, however, that within the upper eyelid the lateral-most tarsal gland was not only larger than the others but also had an excretory duct that followed the course of the extraorbital lacrimal gland. He referred to this particular tarsal gland as an extrapalpebral sebaceous gland (Quay, 1954).

Integumentary Glands

Many species of microtine rodents are characterized by localized pads of hypertrophied glandular tissue that underly the epidermis in specific areas of the posterior integument. Although the exact positions of these integumentary glands can vary both generically and specifically, the glands nevertheless always seem to be restricted to four limited areas: 1) the dorsal base of the tail; 2) the rump; 3) bilaterally on the hips and upper thighs; and 4) bilaterally on the flanks (Quay, 1968). Histologically, these glands may be described as "sebaceous" and, thus, at the light microscopic level they resemble or perhaps are identical with much smaller, less concentrated, glandular units normally associated with mammalian hair follicles. Although neither electron microscopic data nor complete biochemical analysis of the secretory product(s) presently are available, lipids clearly are one major product of the microtine skin glands (Quay, 1968). Insofar as function is concerned, there is general agreement that these integumentary glands have a communicative role not only in microtines but also in the other mammals that possess them (see Eisenberg and Kleiman, 1972; Müller-Schwarze, 1983; Ralls, 1971; Wolff and Johnson, 1979).

In *Microtus,* hypertrophied sebaceous glands are particularly interesting for several reasons. Firstly, within the genus these glands apparently do not occur naturally in all of the many recognized species (Quay, 1968). Based on specimens that he examined, Quay (1968) identified a provisional group of seven nominal species in which skin glands had not been found. Among these, the common and widespread *M. pennsylvanicus* is noteworthy because recently Boonstra and Youson (1982) reported the common occurrence of these glands in voles of both sexes. This discovery suggests the possibility of an ontogenetic component to the presence or apparent "absence" of integumentary glands in some species of *Microtus.*

Secondly, it is noteworthy that microtine skin glands can be influenced by androgens (Jannett, 1975). In a series of experiments, Jannett (1975) investigated the responses of both male and female specimens of *M. longicaudus* and male *M. pennsylvanicus* to either injections or subcutaneous implants of testosterone. His experimental animals included both wild-caught and laboratory progeny and were either castrated or ovariectomized. Although neither *M. longicaudus* nor *M. pennsylvanicus* "normally" has skin glands in the wild (excepting Boonstra and Youson's [1982] report discussed above), nearly all of the males and all of the females developed glands following administration of testosterone (Jannett, 1975). Left unanswered by these experiments is the question of why skin glands would develop after stimulation with exogenous testosterone but not as a consequence of endogenous androgens. Quay (1968) earlier had hypothesized a role for androgens and suggested that differential androgen levels or tissue sensitivity might account for species or population differences in the presence or absence of the integumentary glands. Jannett (1975) mentioned the possibility of "different" androgens and the role of other interacting sebotrophic hormones. Regardless of the reasons for specific differences, it seems clear that although some species of *Microtus* seem to lack glands, they nevertheless actually possess the capacity for glandular hypertrophy if given an appropriate stimulation. This finding in itself is significant because it illustrates that the mere absence of a structural feature does not prove that the feature has been "lost" in a genetic or evolutionary sense.

Lastly, the presence or absence and distribution of skin glands in *Microtus* and other microtines clearly has a taxonomic usefulness. Indeed, in his classic revision of voles and lemmings, Miller (1896) not only introduced the subject but set the stage for continuing interest in these unusual integumentary features. Quay (1952, 1968) and Jannett (1975) both have added substantially to the subject.

Histologically, the best description of integumentary glands at the light level may be found in Quay (1968). Using *M. oeconomus* as an example, Quay reported as follows. In comparison with the sebaceous glands of typical hair follicles, the individual sebaceous gland units of the hypertrophied integumentary glands are greatly increased in size and cell count and are branched and multi-lobed. The epidermis that overlies the gland is thickened irregularly, especially in the center of the glandular area. Hair follicles and hair growth itself seem to be reduced or distorted. In association with this finding, the arrector pili muscles within the area of a typical gland either are absent or, at least, difficult to find. The gland ducts within the central area of the gland frequently become cystic and contain keratin that has been sloughed off from the surface as well as cellular debris. Lastly, lipid droplets detected through staining with Sudan Black B (without acetone extraction) tend to increase in both number and size from the periphery of the gland toward the center.

Many questions remain unanswered even though previous studies of integumentary glands have provided a sound foundation. Biochemiocal analysis of secretory product would provide one set of data crucial to additional interpretation of the functional role of the glands. Detailed study of the ontogeny of the glands as well as comparisons between typical hair follicle glands and hypertrophied glands might also be valuable. For example, it would be interesting to know whether or not the sebaceous secretory cells undergo changes when stimulated by testosterone. Either *M. longicaudus* or *M. pennsylvanicus* would be valuable as a model for such research.

Dentition

Microtus is characterized by having both evergrowing incisors and molars. Although the microanatomy of the incisors has not been investigated specifically, the complex molars have been the subjects of histological, histochemical, autoradiographic, and genetic studies (Gill and Bolles, 1982; Koenigswald and Golenishev, 1979; Oxberry, 1975; Phillips and Oxberry, 1972). The evolutionary history of the molars in *Microtus* is fairly well documented in the fossil record (see Carleton, this volume; Zakrzewski, this volume); indeed, microtine dentition in general has been used as an index for both Eurasian and North American Pleistocene deposits (Hibbard, 1959; Kowalski, 1966).

The crowns of *Microtus* molars consist of a series of salient and re-entrant angles that result in an extremely complex, nearly flat, grinding surface (Fig. 6). The occlusal pattern, extreme crown height (hypsodonty), cementoid buttressing, and continuous growth that characterize the molars, all have been associated with an evolutionary shift to an abrasive diet (Guthrie, 1965, 1971; Phillips and Oxberry, 1972; White, 1959). According to Zimmerman (1965), even interspecific differences in degree of occlusal complexity can be correlated with relative percentage of grasses in the diets of *M. pennsylvanicus* and *M. ochrogaster*.

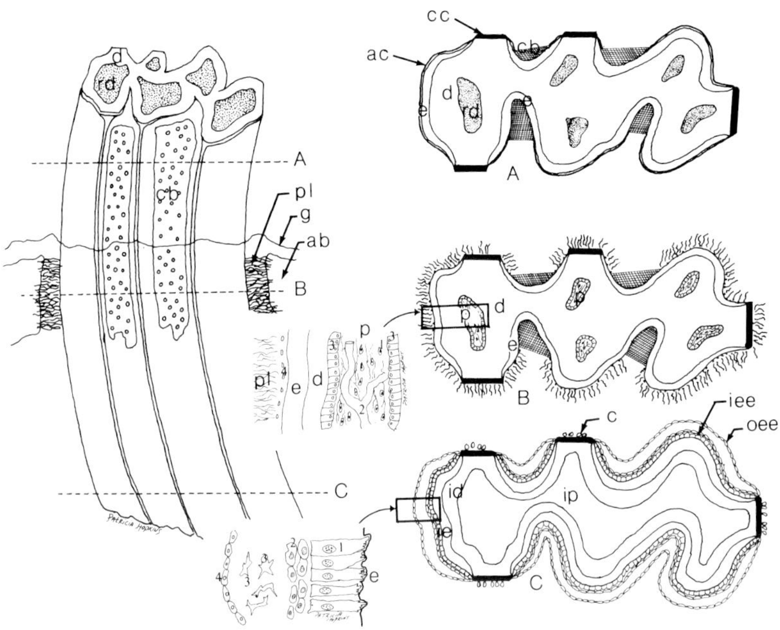

FIG. 6. Diagrammatic representation of an evergrowing molar; transverse sections A, B, and C on right correspond to dotted section lines on the molar shown at left. The overview shows the relationship between molars and periodontal ligaments (pl), gingivum (g), and alveolar bone (ab). Section A: intra-oral "crown." Abbreviations are: ac, thin layer of acellular cement; e, mature enamel; d, mature dentin; cc, cellular cement (major point of attachment); rd, reparative dentin; cb, cementoid buttress. Section B: middle, mature segment of the molar that serves as a "root." Abbreviation: p, pulp. Inset shows histological features of enclosed area, including periodontal ligaments (pl), fibroblasts (1), pulpal blood vessels (2), odontoblasts (3), and cementoblasts (4) on mature enamel (e). Section C: formative apical end of "rooted" portion. Abbreviations are: ie, immature enamel; id, immature dentin; ip, immature pulp; c, cementoblasts; iee, inner enamel epithelium; oee, outer enamel epithelium. Inset shows histological details of enamel epithelium, including ameloblasts (1), stratum intermedium (2), stellate reticulum (3), and outer enamel epithelium.

Microanatomical analyses of evergrowing molars have proven useful in elucidating structural features and in formulating a theoretical concept of evolutionary mechanisms involved with their origin (Phillips and Oxberry, 1972). The major difference between evergrowing molars and typical rooted molars is that crown formation is continuous in the former. Essentially, therefore, the molars in *Microtus* are examples of a morphogenetic system in which the developmental process never ceases (although the rate may change). Histologically, the "rooted" portion of the molar crown concurrently resembles the proliferation, morphodifferentiation, histodifferentiation, and apposition "stages" (Fig. 6) found sequentially in development of typical rooted teeth (Bhaskar, 1976; Phillips and Oxberry, 1972).

Two of the key questions in the evolution of evergrowing molars are: 1) how can a continuously growing crown be held in place; and 2) why is it that attrition from abrasion and thegosis (tooth to tooth contact) does not eventually expose the pulpal chamber?

The first question was investigated in detail by Oxberry (1975), who demonstrated variability in the morphology of the coronal surfaces of the molars. He pointed out that each molar had "major points of attachment" where enamel was lacking and "minor points of attachment" where enamel was present. In the former, the primary dentin is covered by a thick layer of cellular cement that in turn is connected to adjacent alveolar bone by dense periodontal ligaments having an extensive indifferent fiber plexus (Figs. 6, 7). In the latter, the mature enamel is covered by a thin layer of acellular cementum that is deposited shortly before eruption (Phillips and Oxberry, 1972) and which allows for attachment of principal fiber bundles of the periodontal ligaments (Fig. 7).

In addition to special attachment points, the evergrowing molars also are "buttressed" by cellular cement that "grows" within their interstices. This cement has not yet been analyzed histochemically, but its decalcified histological appearance differs from that of typical cellular cement by having dense arrays of collagenous fibers (Figs. 7, 8). One implication of an obvious fibrous appearance under such circumstances is that the ground substance is sparse. The fact that

---

→

FIG. 7. Top: transverse section through rooted portion of an upper molar. Note the cellular cement (CC) serving as a major point of attachment in an area of the tooth lacking enamel (E). Other abbreviations are: D, dentin; P, pulp; PL, periodontium; AC, thin, acellular cement covering enamel; CB, cementoid buttress. Enclosed area is shown at higher magnification below. Nomarski interference-contrast optics; scale bar = 30 μm. Bottom: a major point of attachment showing cellular cement (CC) over dentin (D). Note how periodontal ligaments are invested into the cementum (arrows). Nomarski interference-contrast optics; scale bar = 11 μm.

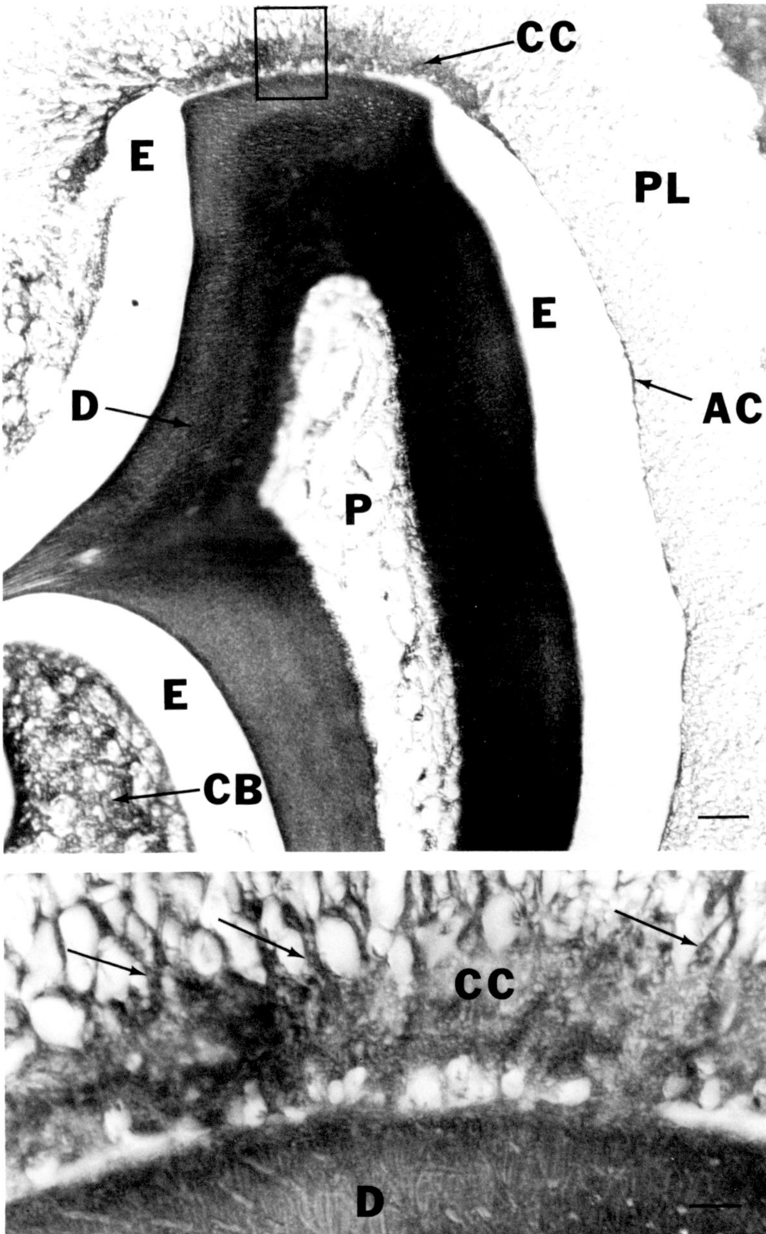
CC
E
PL
E
AC
D
P
E
CB
CC
D

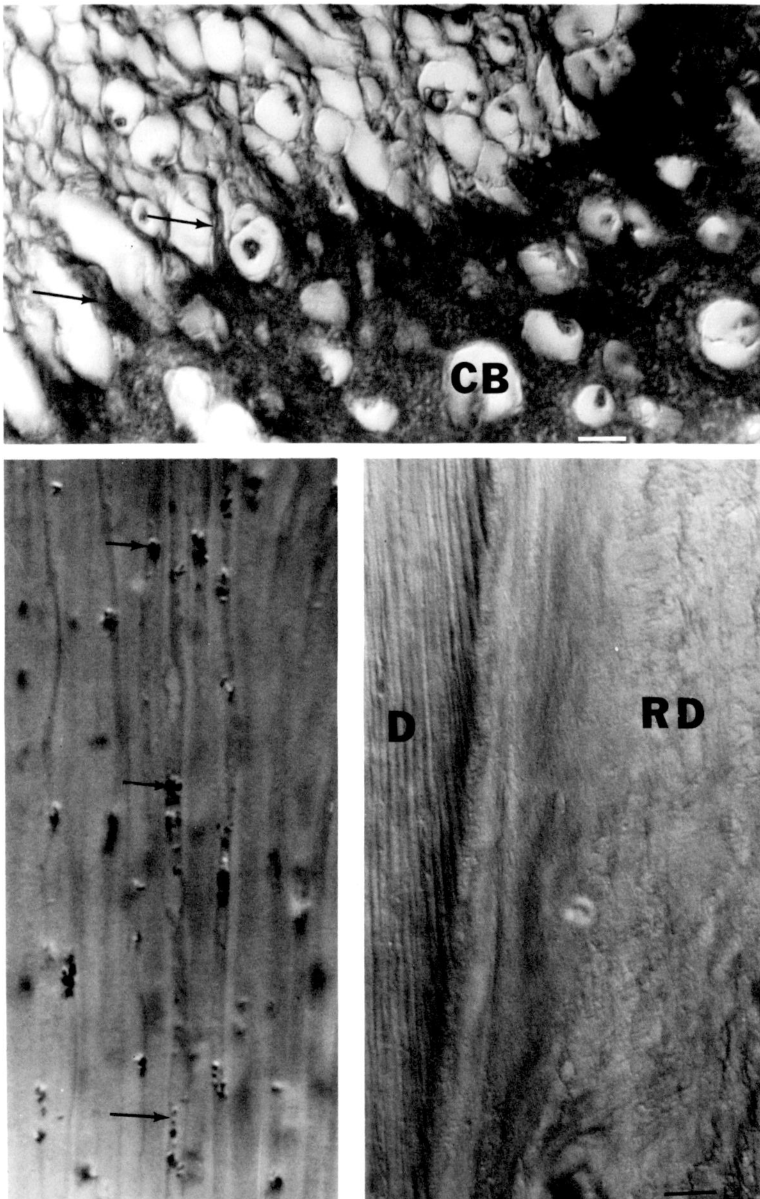

FIG. 8. Top: Nomarski interference-contrast optics view of cellular cementoid buttress (CB) invested by collagen fibers (arrows) of periodontium. Scale bar = 11

the buttresses "grow" from a basal zone where cementoblasts proliferate and become incorporated within the cementum also is unique (Oxberry, 1975; Phillips and Oxberry, 1972). Typically, cementum (both cellular and acellular) is deposited as a layer on freshly mineralized surfaces (either dentin or enamel) rather than as a periodontal deposit having directional growth (see Bhaskar, 1976). Tritiated glycine has been used to monitor incorporation of an amino acid and thus demonstrate the growth zone of the cementoid buttresses (Oxberry, 1975). Within 15 min after injection, Oxberry (1975) found reduced silver grains at the base of the buttresses and after 2 h he found the glycine within newly formed cement. The porous structure of the cementoid buttresses results in the absorption of saliva, oral microflora, and food debris, which give the intraoral coronal surfaces of *Microtus* molars their characteristicially dark-stained appearance.

As the occlusal surfaces of molars are worn away, dentinal tubules become exposed to the oral cavity, fill with debris (Fig. 8), and the associated odontoblasts either die or, at least, have impaired function. Exposure of the cytoplasmic processes of the odontoblasts might be one mechanism that triggers a repair response. Although attrition is difficult to measure, tetracycline-stained molars in two Old World species (*M. fortis* and *M. mandarinus*) have been shown to erupt at between 0.5 and 0.7 mm per week (Koenigswald and Golenishev, 1979). The extreme attrition of evergrowing molars might be expected to also expose the soft dental pulp but does not because of production of reparative (irregular) dentin (Fig. 8) that plugs the coronal pulpal chamber (Oxberry, 1975; Phillips and Oxberry, 1972). Oxberry (1975) demonstrated incorporation of tritiated glycine into newly formed reparative dentin at 1 h after injection, thus suggesting that the process of formation of reparative dentin is fairly rapid. Whether or not the reparative dentin is elaborated solely by odontoblasts is as yet unknown, but possibly other pulpal cells (such as fibroblasts) also are involved.

In summary, microanatomical analysis of the molars in *Microtus*

←

μm. Bottom left: debris-filled dentinal tubules (arrows) exposed to the oral cavity because of attrition of the occlusal surface of a molar. Nomarski interference-contrast optics; scale bar = 29 μm. Bottom right: primary dentin (D) and adjacent irregular, reparative dentin (RD). Nomarski interference-contrast optics; scale bar = 29 μm.

has enabled development of a model for understanding the evolution of evergrowing molars in rodents.

Salivary Glands

Among the variety of major and minor salivary glands in *Microtus,* microanatomical data presently are available for the parotid and submandibular glands, which are only two of the three major glands located outside of the oral cavity. None of the numerous minor salivary glands, located within the lining of the oral cavity and within the tongue, has been studied. No histochemical data presently are available for any microtine salivary glands so knowledge of the chemical composition of the secretory products can be inferred only by comparison of structural features and histological staining reactions to comparable features in salivary glands of laboratory rodents on which more detailed sudies have been undertaken. Presumably, salivary glands have the same roles in *Microtus* as in other mammals and, therefore, they most certainly not only secrete digestive enzymes but probably also secrete IgA, hormones, and lubricating mucoid substances (Dawes, 1978; Hand, 1976; Phillips et al., 1977). It also is likely that salivary glands in rodents have some additional, presently unknown, biological roles. For example, sexual dimorphism in the morphology of secretory portions of the submandibular intralobular duct system has been reported in both *Mus* and *Rattus* (Junqueira et al., 1949; Srinivasan and Chang, 1975). Sexual differences in mucins have been described in the hamster, *Mesocricetus* (Shackleford and Klapper, 1962), and sexual differences in rates of enyzme biosynthesis have been demonstrated in *Mus* (Calissano and Angeletti, 1968).

Limited dynamic interpretations of static ultrastructural images of *Microtus* salivary glands can be developed because the secretory process and general physiology of salivary glands have been investigated in considerable detail in recent years (for a summary, see Tandler, 1978). For example, pulse-chase experiments, often using tritiated leucine, have been employed to develop an understanding of serous secretory cells. It has been demonstrated that protein synthesized in the cisternae of the granular endoplasmic reticulum (GER) is assembled into immature product at the Golgi complex following energy-requiring transfer from the GER (Bogart, 1977; Castle et al., 1972; Palade, 1975). Although details of secretory cell

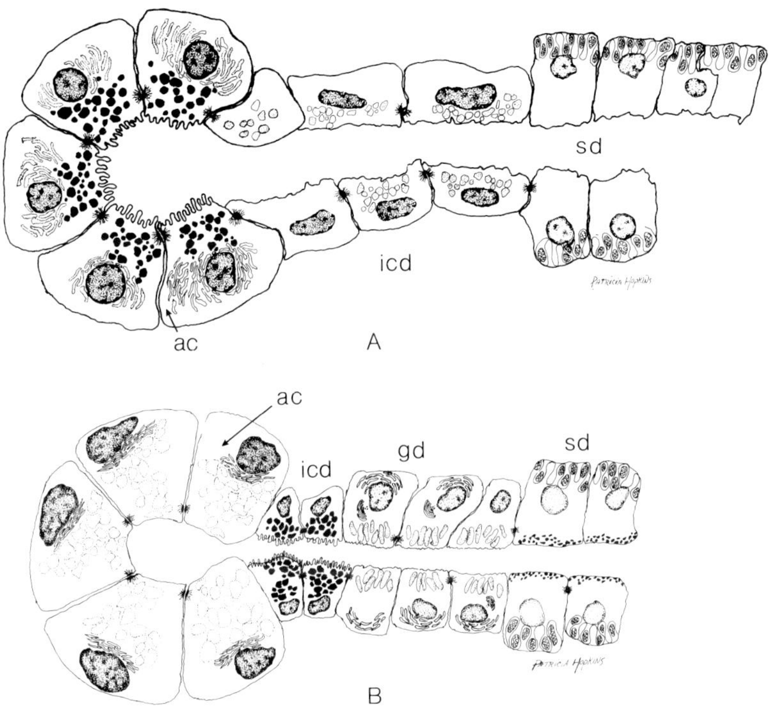

FIG. 9. Diagrammatic representation of parotid (A) and submandibular (B) salivary glands. Abbreviations are: ac, acinar cells; icd, intercalated duct; gd, granular duct; sd, striated duct.

membrane synthesis and membrane recycling processes have remained somewhat elusive, it is known that membrane enclosing secretory granules arises *de novo* concomitantly with the product and differs biochemically from other membrane (Amsterdam et al., 1971). Secretory granules are exported in an orderly, chronological fashion; the granule membrane fuses to the outer cell membrane just prior to release of secretory product into the adjacent lumen (Satir, 1974; Tandler and Poulsen, 1976). Excess membrane subsequently is resorbed in the secretory cell (Amsterdam et al., 1971).

The small parotid salivary gland in *Microtus* is positioned at the base of the ear. It consists of bulbous serous secretory acini, short secretory intercalated ducts, and non-secretory intralobular (striated) ducts (Fig. 9). The pyramidal serous cells are characterized by

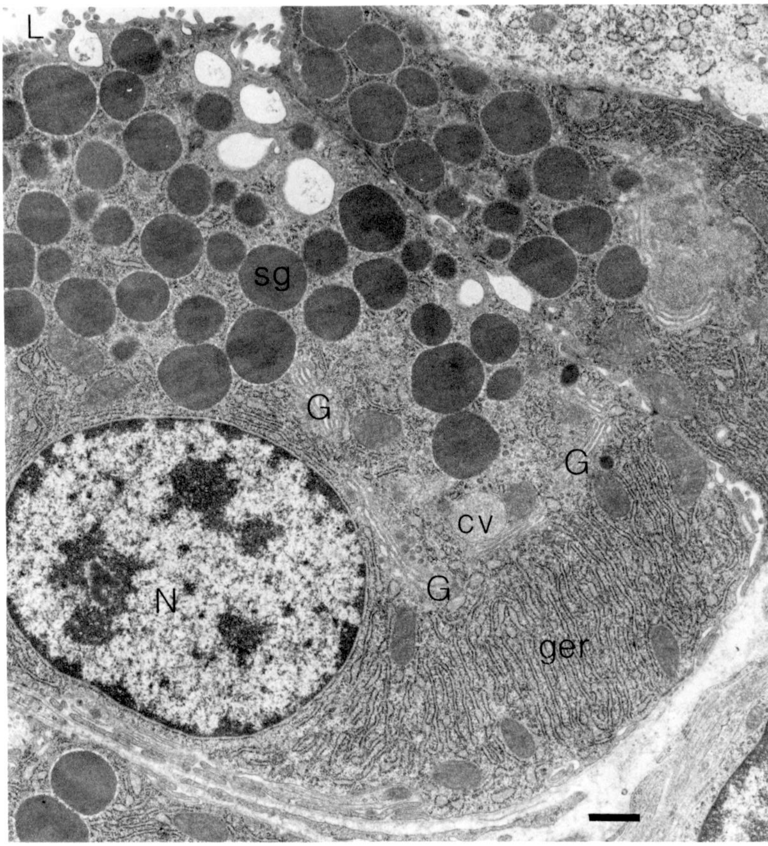
L
sg
G
G
cv
G
N
ger

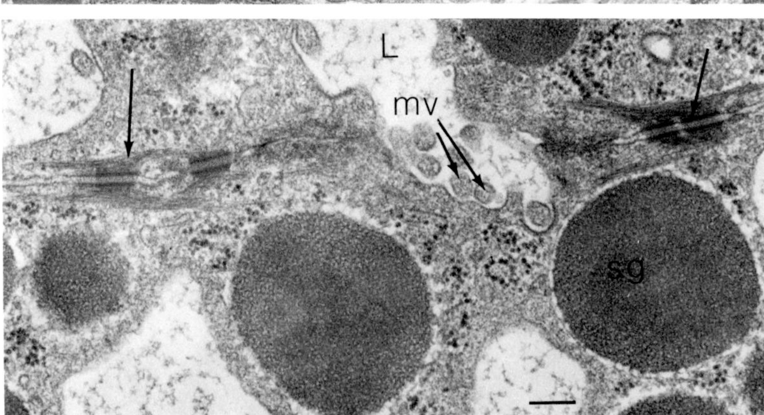
L
mv
sg

large, spherical euchromatic nuclei cradled by abundant lamellar granular endoplasmic reticulum (GER). The basal plasma membrane is relatively smooth, whereas the basal one-half of the lateral membrane typically is slightly interdigitated with that of adjacent secretory cells (Fig. 10). Nerve terminals are associated with these membrane surfaces, being positioned in shallow indentations on the basal surface as well as wedged between adjacent cells (Fig. 11). The apical one-half of the lateral membranes of the serous cells include intercellular canaliculi and, immediately adjacent to the lumen, a zona adherens. The apical membrane, when secretory product is released, is irregular and has short microvilli (Fig. 10).

The serous-cell Golgi complexes are prominent cytoplasmic features; at the inner face of the flat lamellar structures are found coated vesicles and immature secretory granules containing moderately electron dense material (Fig. 10).

The intercalated ducts in parotid salivary glands of *Microtus* apparently are secretory. Although the product has not been chemically categorized, its appearance in the TEM differs significantly from the appearance of the serous granules; intercalated duct cell secretory product is only moderately electron dense and the images suggest that individual granules can coalesce into larger, irregularly shaped granules. Although the coalesced images might be artifactual, they nevertheless are not found in serous cells processed in the same way and therefore can be taken as indicative of some physiochemical difference between secretory granules. Additionally, the intercalated duct cells are characterized by elongate euchromatic nuclei, have very little GER relative to that found in the serous cells, and the Golgi complexes are inconspicuous (Fig. 11). Secretory intercalated ducts also have been reported in the hamster parotid (Shackleford and Schneyer, 1964); however, in this species the product is said to be extremely electron dense.

The intralobular (striated) parotid ducts in *Microtus* are non-

---

←

FIG. 10. Top: secretory acinar cell from the parotid salivary gland. Note the extensive Golgi complex (G), associated condensing vesicles (cv), and mature secretory granules (sg). Other abbreviations are: L, lumen; N, nucleus; ger, granular endoplasmic reticulum. Scale bar = 1 μm. Bottom: higher magnification of lumen (L), secretory granules (sg), and apical and apico-lateral cell surfaces. Note apical microvilli (mv) and adjacent cell junctions (arrows). Scale bar = 0.25 μm.

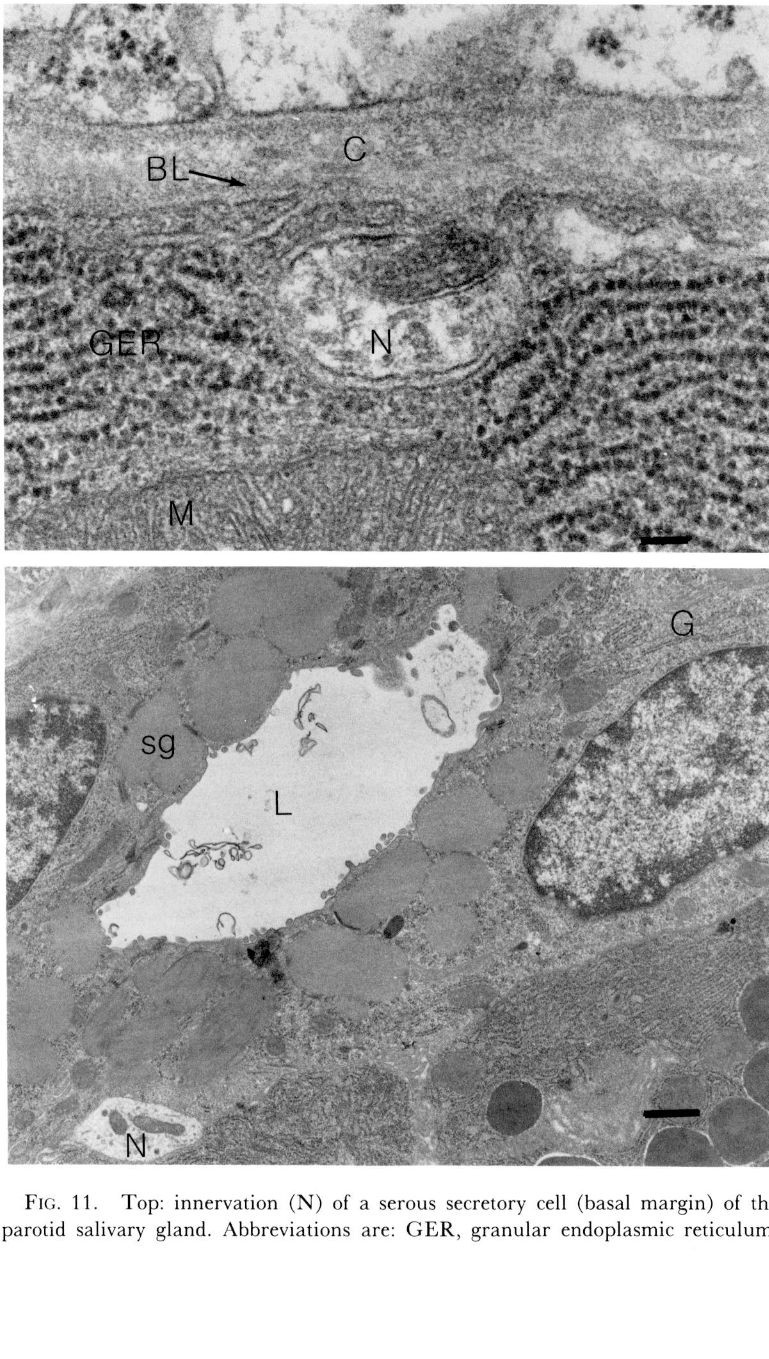

FIG. 11. Top: innervation (N) of a serous secretory cell (basal margin) of the parotid salivary gland. Abbreviations are: GER, granular endoplasmic reticulum;

secretory, at least to judge from their histological and ultrastructural appearance. At least two ultrastructurally distinctive cell types are found in these ducts; each might represent different functional states of the other. The most prominent image is one of a large columnar cell with a spherical, centrally placed euchromatic nucleus. With the trialdehyde fixative and processing techniques used by me, these cells have an extremely pale cytoplasm. Indeed, the cytoplasm is so pale that cytoskeletal features such as microtubules and fibrils that ordinarily are difficult to discern among other cytoplasmic constituents, are seen easily and their relationships to organelles are apparent (Fig. 12). The basal cytoplasm of these pale cells contains large mitochondrial profiles and the basal plasma membrane invaginates deeply into the cell (Fig. 12). The second cellular profile is one in which the cells appear to be a somewhat condensed version of the pale cells, differing from the latter in being smaller, typically wedged between pale cells, and in having a darker cytoplasm and an irregularly shaped nucleus. The luminal membranes of both cell types are characterized by irregular, pleiomorphic microvilli (Fig. 12), and neither contains secretory product, although in both the apical cytoplasm does contain a variety of pale vesicles (Fig. 12).

The submandibular salivary gland in *Microtus* is much larger than the parotid, more complex in structure, and apparently more complex in function as well. The submandibular has large, bulbous acini containing mucous secretory cells (Fig. 9). These mucous cells, which are a large and prominent feature of the gland, are characterized by pale coalescing secretory granules containing flocculent material (Fig. 13). The nuclei tend toward being heterochromatic, are basally positioned, and are irregular or flattened in appearance. The peripheral cytoplasm of the mucous cells is filled with lamellar GER and has a dark, condensed appearance. Coated and smooth vesicles, which are a common feature of serous cells, essentially are lacking in the mucous cells. The Golgi complexes are prominent. The cell outer plasma membrane generally is smooth except at the luminal surface, where a few small microvilli typically are found.

←
M, mitochondrion; C, intercellular collagen; BL, basal lamina. Scale bar = 0.12 μm. Bottom: secretory intercalated duct adjacent to acinus (lower right). Abbreviations are: sg, secretory granules; G, Golgi; L, lumen; N, nerve terminal. Scale bar = 1 μm.

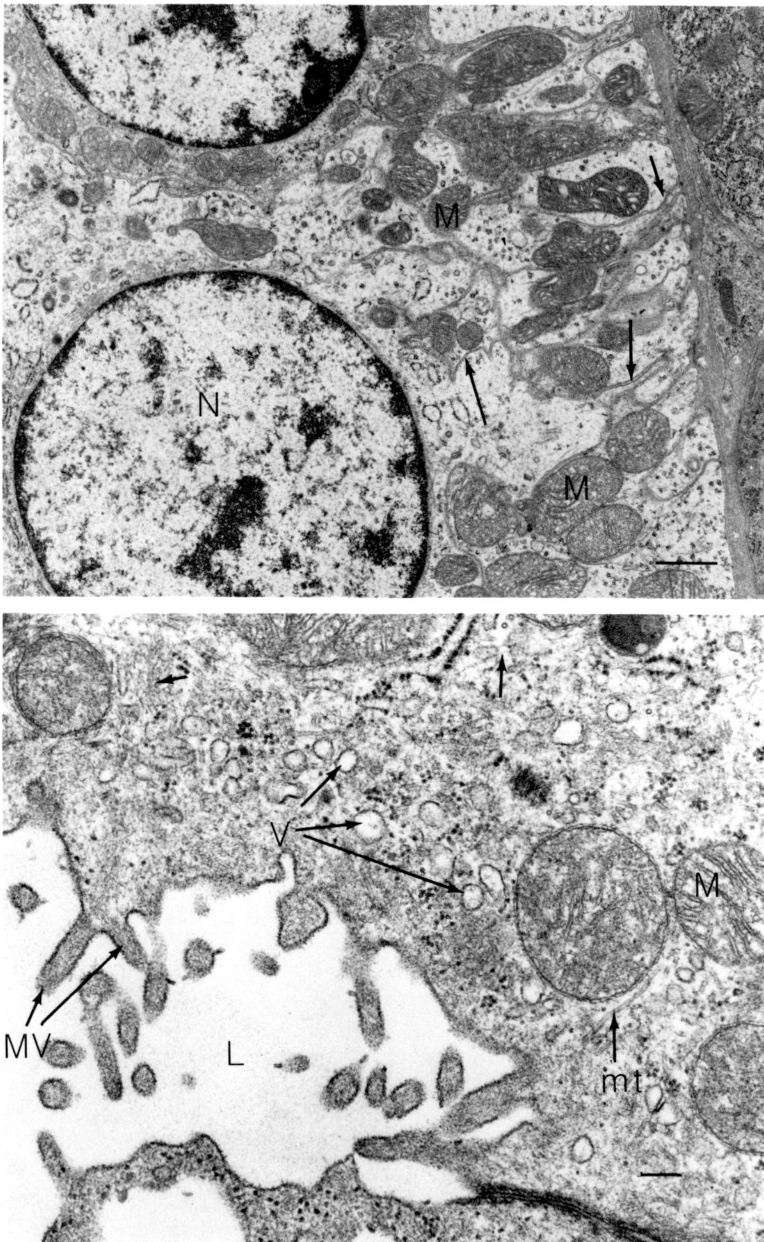
M
N
M
V
M
MV
L
mt

The short intercalated duct is of special interest because it consists of low, cuboidal cells that typically are packed with electron dense secretory granules (Fig. 13). These granules differ from typical serous granules in that they have an irregular rather than spherical shape. The intercalated duct cells have ovoid, basally restricted nuclei containing moderate amounts of heterochromatin. The GER, Golgi complexes, and mitochondria in the intercalated duct cells are sparse but apparently scaled to the overall small size of the cell (Fig. 13). The granular intralobular duct system in the submandibular is secretory in *Microtus* as it is in most other rodents (Fig. 9). The ultrastructure of the granular duct cells somewhat resembles that seen in the intercalated duct cells of the parotid salivary gland of *Microtus*. The cytoplasm is packed densely with round or ovoid secretory granules, many of which are coalesced into larger, more irregularly shaped granules (Figs. 13, 14). One or more large Golgi complexes are in a supranuclear location; the ovoid nucleus itself is not restricted to the basal ergastoplasm, is euchromatic, and is cradled in extensive lamellar GER. The basal and apical cell membranes are unspecialized; the basal membrane is relatively smooth, whereas the apical membrane, which borders on the lumen of the duct, generally is smooth with only a few microvilli (Fig. 14). The lateral membranes are characterized by a prominent gap junction (Fig. 14). The chemical composition of the secretory product produced in the granular duct is unknown. The ultrastructure of the cells, however, might be categorized as sero-mucoid (Shackleford and Wilborn, 1968) because the granules are pale and appear to coalesce, whereas the organellar arrangement and morphology are more nearly similar to that associated with serous secretory cells.

The intralobular striated ducts, to which the granular ducts lead (Fig. 9), are characterized by large, pale cells having spherical, centrally placed euchromatic nuclei (Fig. 15). Unlike the homologous cells of the parotid, the striated duct cells in the submandibular

←

FIG. 12. Top: basal portion of parotid striated duct cell showing infolded basal membrane (arrows), associated mitochondrial profiles (M), and characteristically euchromatic nucleus (N). Scale bar = 1 μm. Bottom: apical surface of striated duct cell. Note microvilli (MV) and collection of vesicles (V) in adjacent cytoplasm. Other abbreviations are: L, lumen; M, mitochondrial profile; mt, microtubule; arrows, cytoskeletal fibrils. Scale bar = 0.25 μm.

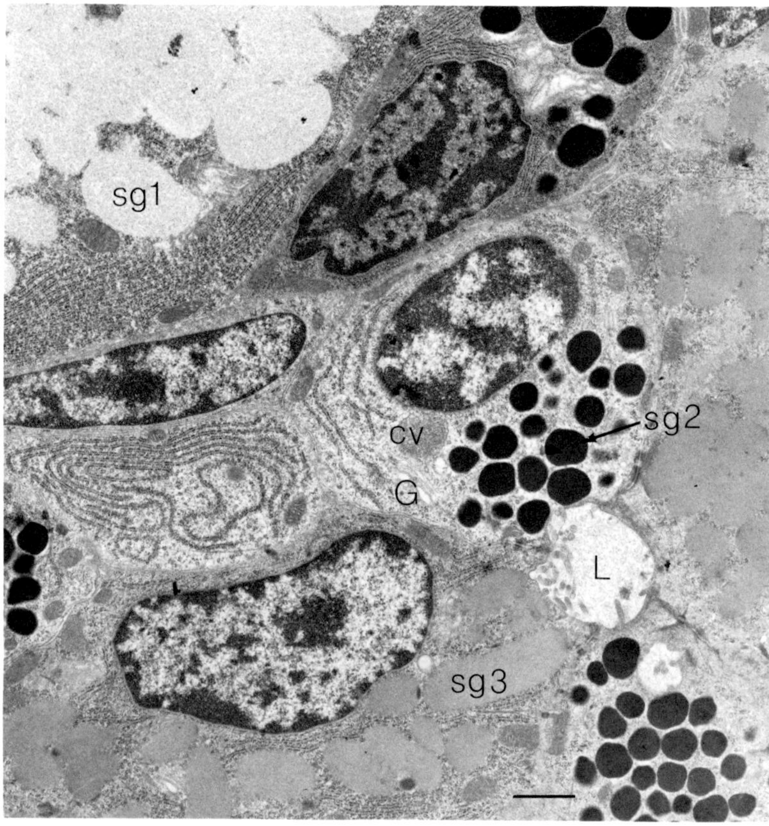
sg1
sg2
cv
G
L
sg3

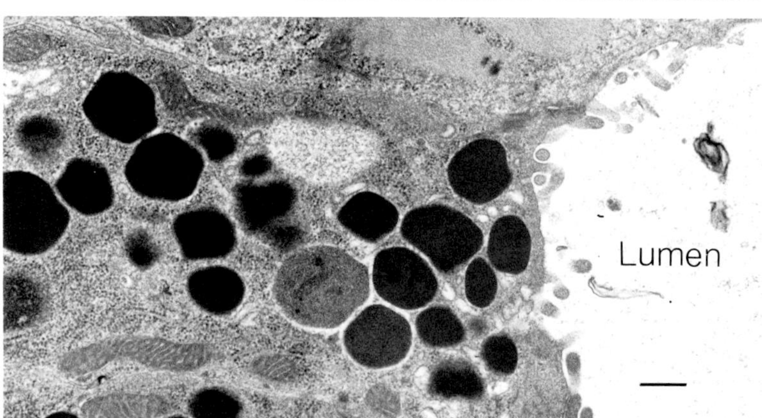
Lumen

salivary gland frequently have accumulations of electron-dense granules in a cytoplasmic zone immediately adjacent to the lumen (Fig. 15). These granules possibly suggest that the striated duct cells in the submandibular are secretory; however, the ultrastructural data in themselves are not unequivocal and, therefore, it also is possible that the granules are associated with an absorptive function of these cells (Rhodin, 1974).

The parotid salivary gland in mammals generally is more conservative in structure than is the submandibular (Phillips et al., 1977). This principle is underscored by *Microtus,* in which the parotid is similar to that found in *Rattus, Mus,* and other species, whereas the submandibular appears to be considerably different from that of other rodents for which data are available. Serous acinar cells such as those found in *Microtus* appear to be typical of rodent parotid glands (Hand, 1976; Shackleford and Schneyer, 1964). Comparisons among rodents are hampered somewhat by differences in fixation technique. In the early (1950–1960) TEM literature on rodent salivary glands, most micrographs were of material fixed with osmium tetroxide and the secretory granules had a pale appearance. The more recent aldehyde fixation techniques preserve cellular proteins and glycoproteins to a different extent and typically the granules appear as illustrated for *Microtus* (Fig. 10). The extreme electron density of the serous secretory granules in aldehyde-fixed tissue samples thus is indicative of the highly proteinaceous nature of the parotid acinar product.

Pulse-chase radioautographic analyses have demonstrated that synthesis and assembly of product of acinar serous cells in rabbits are similar to that found in the zymogen-producing pancreatic cells, with the exception that the process is slower in the parotid cells (Castle et al., 1972). In the absence of data for *Microtus* and other rodents, it only can be inferred that their parotid serous cells are similar functionally to those of rabbits.

The submandibular salivary gland in rodents has attracted far

---

←

FIG. 13. Top: survey view of three types of secretory cells found in submandibular salivary gland. Compare the secretory product of the sero-mucous acinar cells (sg1), the small intercalated duct cells (sg2), and the granular duct (sg3). Other abbrevations are: L, lumen; G, Golgi complex; cv, condensing vesicle. Scale bar = 1 μm. Bottom: higher magnification of intercalated duct cells. Scale bar = 0.5 μm.

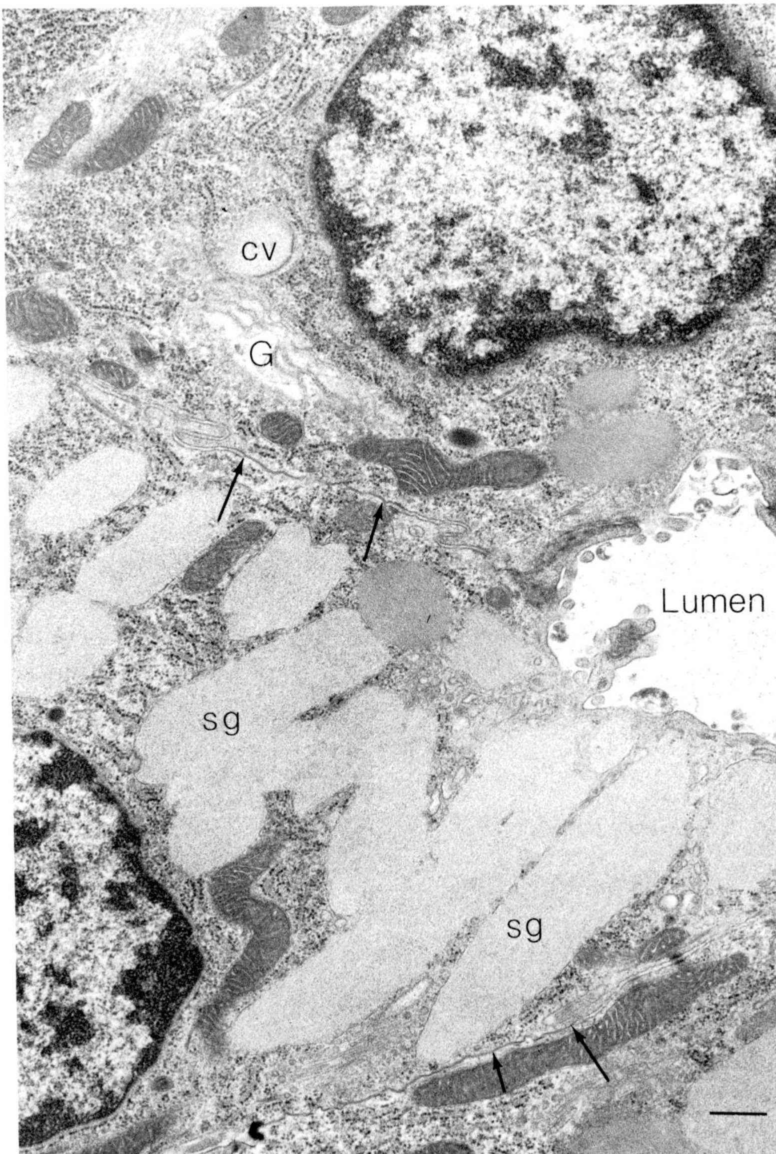

FIG. 14. Cross-section through a granular duct of submandibular salivary gland. Note unusual zones of occluded cell junction (arrows) positioned on lateral cell surfaces. Abbreviations are: sg, secretory granule; G, Golgi complex; cv, condensing vesicle. Scale bar = 0.5 μm.

more attention than has the parotid. In large measure this is due to: 1) its size and location, which make it convenient for developmental studies (for example, see Spooner, 1973); 2) its tendency in rodents to be sexually dimorphic (for example, see Srinivasan and Chang, 1975); and 3) its well-known capacity to produce a variety of compounds, including nerve growth factor (NGF), epidermal growth factor (EGF), renin, and kallikrein, which one would not expect to find in saliva (Hand, 1976; Murphy et al., 1980).

The acinar secretory cells of the submandibular in *Microtus* are similar, ultrastructurally, to those of all other rodents for which comparative data are available. Such secretory cells are described as mucous or, occasionally, seromucous, depending upon selection of ultrastructural criteria and fixative (Hand, 1976; Shackleford and Wilborn, 1968; Simson et al., 1978; Tamarin and Sreebny, 1965). Given the ultrastructural characteristics of these cells, it is not surprising that the acinar cell product differs from that secreted by the parotid in a number of ways, including having a lower level of amylase (Shackleford and Schneyer, 1964). Functional differences between parotid and submandibular acinar cells were demonstrated by Bogart (1977), who used tritiated leucine to investigate intracellular kinetics in *Rattus*. The major kinetic difference was in the greater time spent by the developing product in the vicinity of the Golgi complex (Bogart, 1977), which probably is reflective of the "mucoid" nature of the secretory product. A number of cytochemical studies have provided data that demonstrate that sugar moieties and sulfate can be incorporated into secretory cells and added to a protein secretologue directly at the Golgi complex (Berg and Austin, 1976; Bogart, 1977).

The secretory intercalated duct and granular duct are the most notable features of the submandibular salivary gland in *Microtus*. At sexual maturity in all studied species of rodents, except ground squirrels (*Spermophilus*), a segment of intralobular duct positioned between the intercalated duct and the typical "striated" duct undergoes a specialized differentiation and develops into a "granular" duct that secretes a complex product (Hand, 1976; Shackleford and Schneyer, 1964; Srinivasan and Chang, 1975). Androgenic hormones influence development of the granular duct, which generally is much larger in males than it is in females (Calissano and Angeletti, 1968; Hand, 1976; Junqueira et al., 1949). Recent histochemical investigations have established that nerve growth factor (NGF) and epithelial growth factor (EGF) are two of the secretory

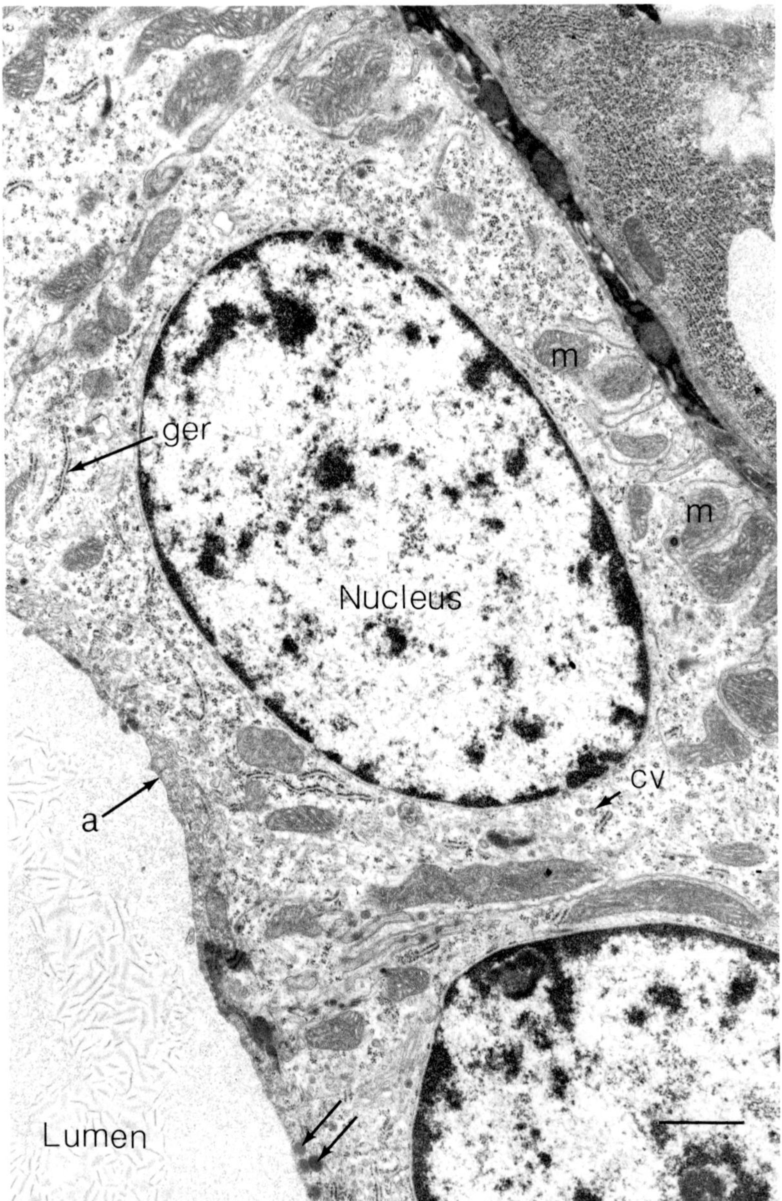
ger
m
m
Nucleus
cv
a
Lumen

products of these granular ducts (Murphy et al., 1980). Unlike the submandibular acinar secretory product, export of growth factors is not triggered by cholinergic secretagogues. Indeed, both alpha and beta adrenergic agents stimulate the release of NGF and EGF into the ductal lumen (Wallace and Partlow, 1976). Because the granular duct serves as an exocrine rather than an endocrine organ (Byyny et al., 1974), one significant question is: how do the growth factors reach the blood? One plausible answer is that the salivary growth factors are swallowed and absorbed in the gastrointestinal tract (Murphy et al., 1980). A second question, which is directly applicable to *Microtus,* is: what are the functions of such growth factors in adult animals? Although essentially all of the research so far has been done with *Mus* as the experimental animal, it is not unreasonable to assume that the granular duct in *Microtus* also secretes NGF or EGF or both. One hypothesis, applicable at least to EGF, is that the capacity to produce considerable quantities of this protein is somehow linked to evergrowing teeth. Previous studies have demonstrated that EGF promotes early eye-opening in young mice (*Mus*) when given orally (Taylor et al., 1972) and, furthermore, stimulates eruption of incisors (Hand, 1976). Although for now we can only speculate, it seems clear that future investigations of the relationships among EGF, salivary glands, and growth could cast light on the basic mechanisms that allowed for evolution of evergrowing teeth.

The apparent microanatomical and ultrastructural differences between the submandibular of *Microtus* and those of other studied rodents is of special interest. *Microtus* is the only rodent genus (among those studied) in which a secretory intercalated duct is interposed between the acinus and granular duct; in other rodents the intercalated duct consists of non-secretory, low cuboidal cells.

←

FIG. 15. Striated duct of submandibular salivary gland. Compare with Fig. 12 and note differences in apical surfaces (a). In submandibular striated duct cells, apical microvilli and cytoplasmic vesicles are lacking; instead, the apical surface is smooth and the apical cytoplasm contains small, electron-dense bodies (arrows). Also notice the fixed formative saliva within the lumen. Abbreviations are: m, mitochondrial profile; cv, coated vesicles; ger, granular endoplasmic reticulum. Scale bar = 1 μm.

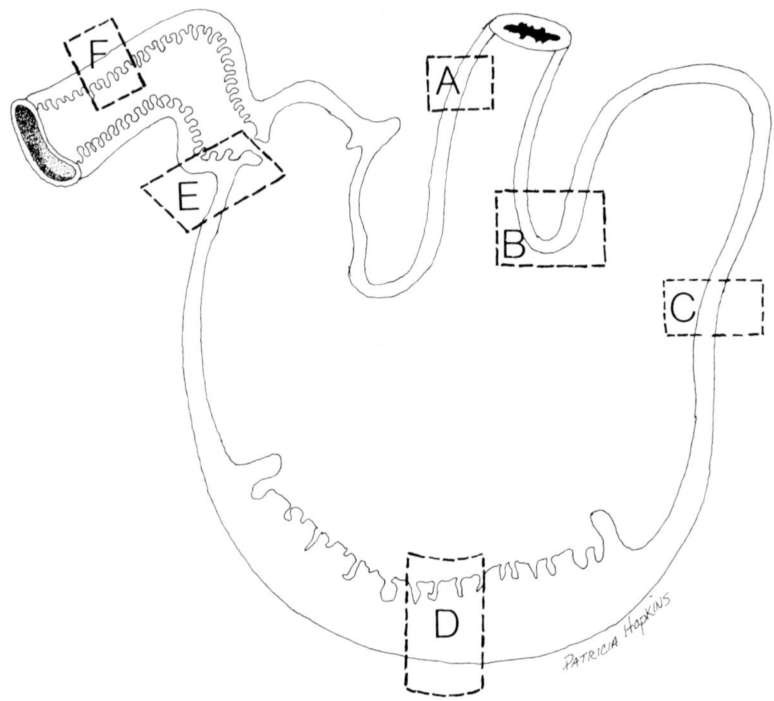

FIG. 16. Diagrammatic view of locations in the digestive tract of *M. pennsylvanicus* from which tissues were taken for EM analysis: A, esophagus; B, cardiac vestibule; C, non-glandular forestomach; D, glandular stomach; E, junction of pylorus and duodenum; F, small intestine.

Additionally, the ultrastructure and secretory product of aldehyde-fixed submandibular intercalated duct cells in *Microtus* (Fig. 13) are similar to granular duct cells in *Mus* (see Murphy et al., 1980). On the other hand, the granular duct cells in the *Microtus* submandibular are similar in appearance to the intercalated duct cells in *Microtus* parotid salivary glands (Figs. 11, 14). Taken together, all of these ultrastructural differences demonstrate the well-known evolutionary plasticity of salivary glands (Phillips et al., 1977). Unfortunately, however, such structural and organizational differences in themselves tell us relatively little about similarities and differences in secretory product.

The possibility that heterochrony has occurred is yet another aspect that deserves consideration when making comparisons between the submandibular of *Microtus* and that of other studied rodents. In the developmental dynamics of the submandibular salivary gland in *Rattus,* the morphology and secretory products of several different cell "types" undergo significant transitions before reaching a final, presumably fully differentiated and stable configuration (Chang, 1974; Srinivasan and Chang, 1975). There is some evidence that in neonate rats the formative intercalated duct cells (whose morphology is generalized) serve as a "stem" cell population from which "striated" and possibly even acinar cells can develop (Chang, 1974). Furthermore, Chang (1974) also found that no fewer than three different cell types (acinar, proacinar, and terminal tubule), each with its own morphology and histochemically distinctive product, participate chronologically in a differentiation pattern that results in the single type of mucous acinar cell characteristic of the submandibular of adult rats. Such developmental data certainly provide the theoretical basis for explaining the striking organizational differences between *Microtus, Rattus, Mus,* and other rodents. If morphological differentiation were to stop prematurely in any of the progenitor cell types, the "mature" gland would appear to have two rather than one secretory cell type in the terminal acinar-intercalated duct zone in the gland. Such is the case in *Microtus,* and the presence of an "extra" type of secretory cell that appears to be a part of the intercalated duct thus may be a result of a heterochronic alteration in developmental sequence.

Digestive Tract

The microanatomy of the digestive tract has been examined histologically in a surprising variety of wild rodents including *Microtus* and several other microtine genera. I review the available information in the following paragraphs and describe and illustrate many ultrastructural features of the digestive tract of *M. pennsylvanicus* for the first time. The locations from which tissues were obtained for TEM analysis are shown diagrammatically in Fig. 16.

An understanding of diet and nutritional requirements is a key component in interpretation of microanatomical features of the digestive tract. Because of the broad interest in ecology, energetics, and population dynamics of *Microtus,* considerable ancillary data are available on feeding habits. Although more detailed information relative to nutritional requirements can be found elsewhere (Batzli, this volume), several aspects bear repeating here.

All species of *Microtus* can be categorized as herbivores; for example, in *M. ochrogaster,* more than 90% of the diet by volume is herbaceous (Zimmerman, 1965). Given the variability in digestibility of grasses and seeds (Batzli and Cole, 1979), the efficiency of the digestive system in *Microtus* is remarkable; in a 46-g *M. pennsylvanicus* with a daily intake of 28.1 g, the total fecal weight was 2.8 g, giving an efficiency of 90% (Golley, 1960). Actual composition of the average diet of individual species varies considerably, however, in accordance with habitat and geography. Additionally, different species of *Microtus* have significantly different nutritional requirements. Batzli and Cole (1979) found that prairie voles (*M. ochrogaster*) could digest grasses as well as could *M. californicus,* but when fed on a strict grass diet, the prairie vole lost weight and eventually died. These rather striking interspecific differences probably are reflected also in the microanatomy of the digestive tract. Hints of such differences certainly are found in the histological studies of Dearden (1966, 1969) and Barry (1976).

Esophagus

The histology of the esophagus at the gastro-esophageal junction has been described and discussed by Dearden (1966). In *Microtus* the abdominal esophagus is characterized by a moderately keratinized, thin lamina mucosae that thickens appreciably at the junction of the cardiac vestibule (Dearden, 1966). The presence of keratin in the stratified squamous epithelium seems to be typical of rodents; generally it is thought that keratinization of the esophagus and cardiac stomach are correlated with a harsh type of diet (Forman, 1972; Horner et al., 1964). Two ultrastructurally distinct types of basal cell are found in the stratum germinativum of the esophagus in *Microtus*; one cell type is characterized by a slightly irregular, largely euchromatic nucleus, whereas the other, which overall has a dark, condensed appearance, is characterized by an extremely irregular, largely heterochromatic nucleus. Hemi-desmosomes are common along the basal plasma membrane in both types of basal cell. Extracellular aggregations of glycogen granules appear to fill pouch-like pockets between adjacent basal cells. These granules apparently are incorporated into the basal cell cytoplasm prior to cellular migration into the stratum spinosum. The stratum spinosum itself is very thin (only 2–3 cells deep) and gives way abruptly to a stratum granulosum.

The esophageal epithelial cells undergo a profound transition between the basal layer and the luminal surface. Dense aggregations of tonofilaments, degrading mitochondria, and clumps of glycogen granules become the most conspicuous features of the cytoplasm (Fig. 17). Membrane-coating granules (multi-lamellar bodies) and keratohyalin granules are present but not particularly abundant in the esophageal epithelium (Fig. 17). The outer cell membrane in the superficial cells take on a thickened, electron-dense appearance that possibly results from deposition of material from the membrane-coating granules (Rhodin, 1974). A somewhat amorphous, osmophilic material fills the intercellular spaces between adjacent squamous cells (Fig. 17). On occasion this material appears to be organized into a fibrillar formation that extends from the outer surface of one cell to the outer surface of another (Fig. 17). Although keratin filaments are found in the esophageal epithelium in *Microtus,* this protein never attains abundance adequate for formation of a true stratum corneum. Consequently, although keratohyalin granules and clumps of glycogen disappear, the outermost layers of cells (7–10 deep) never become electron dense and the cytoplasm clearly contains bundles of tonofilaments (Fig. 17). It is of additional interest that the outermost cells appear to retain enough cell-to-cell adherence so that the layers are not disrupted by fixation-preparation techniques and thus a stratum disjunctium is lacking in the esophagus (Fig. 17).

The esophageal lamina propria in *Microtus* (and other microtines) has been described histologically as a "narrow zone of rather loose connective tissue containing numerous elastic fibers" (Dearden, 1966). One particularly interesting feature of the lamina propria in *Microtus* is the presence of interlacing ligament-like bundles of collagen that underly the basal lamina of the stratum germinativum (Fig. 18). Such esophageal structures apparently have not been described previously in mammals. In 1-μm "thick" sections cut in a plane oblique to the epithelium, the ligament-like bundles are clearly visible because they stain intensely with toluidine blue. Ultrastructural analysis reveals that they consist of highly organized, twisted bundles of collagen and reticulum (Fig. 18). The intense staining reaction cannot be attributed to these visible components alone because in typical loose connective tissue neither one

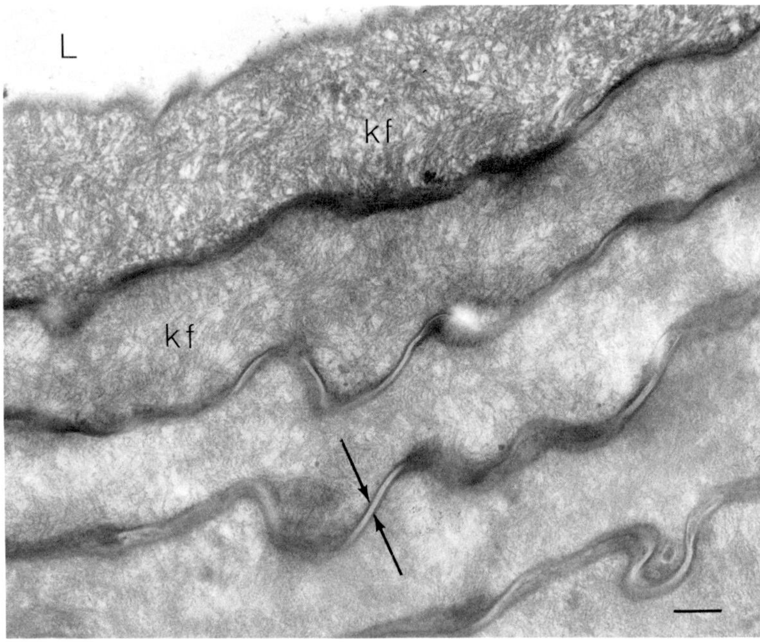
L
kf
kf

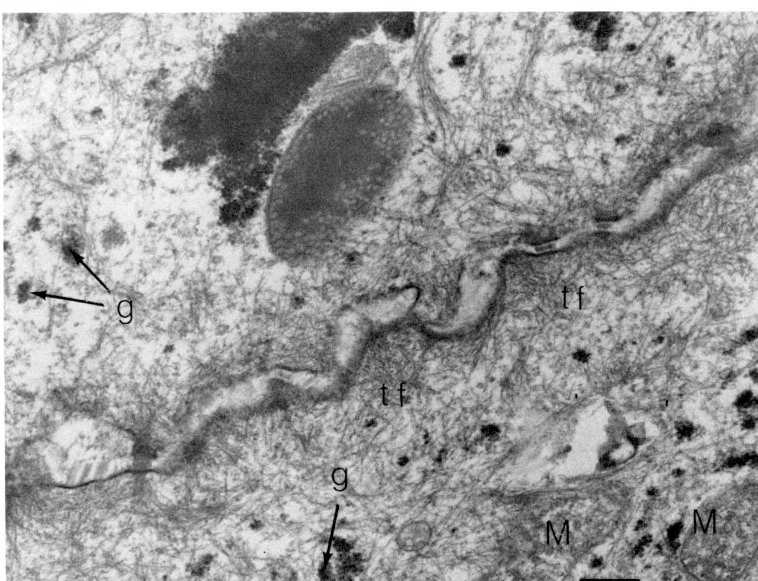
g
tf
tf
g
M
M

normally stains so intensely. In addition to these ligament-like fiber bundles, the connective tissue of the lamina propria also contains fibroblasts, macrophages, and elastic fibers. Mucus-secreting esophageal glands, which have been reported in the lamina propria of a variety of mammalian species (Rhodin, 1974), are lacking in *Microtus* (Dearden, 1966).

The esophageal musculature is of particular interest in *Microtus*. Three layers of muscles—an inner-striated circular, outer-striated longitudinal, and a smooth circular layer—compose the lamina muscularis externa and lamina muscularis mucosae (Fig. 18). In *Microtus* the outer-striated muscle layer extends from the esophagus to the stomach, terminating in the corpopyloric fold (Dearden, 1966). In two other microtines, the collared lemming (*Dicrostonyx groenlandicus*) and the steppe vole (*Lagurus lagurus*), it is the inner-striated layer that has continuity with the corpopyloric fold (Dearden, 1966). The overall anatomical design of the gastro-esophageal junction in *Microtus* and other microtines suggested to Dearden (1966) that a variety of cardiac valves or sphincters are found in mammals. The exact relationship of such valve-like structures in *Microtus* to feeding habits is as yet unclear but should be a focal point for future work.

Stomach

Histologically, the stomach of *Microtus* consists of three distinctive zones (Fig. 16): one, the forestomach, is characterized by non-glandular keratinized squamous epithelium; the second is an area of glandular mucosa; and the third, the pylorus, also is non-glandular and is lined with keratinized squamous epithelium (Dearden, 1969; Golley, 1960). Non-glandular gastric mucosa is typical of rodent stomachs but varies considerably in extent among different species (Ito, 1967). The presence of non-glandular epithelium apparently is correlated with diets that include large quantities of food

---

←

FIG. 17. Top: top five layers of epithelial cells lining the esophagus. Note keratin filaments (kf) and intercellular layers (arrows); L, esophageal lumen. Scale bar = 0.12 μm. Bottom: Cells in an early stage of the keratinization process. Note degenerating mitochondria (M), glycogen (g), and abundant tonofilaments (tf). Scale = 0.25 μm.

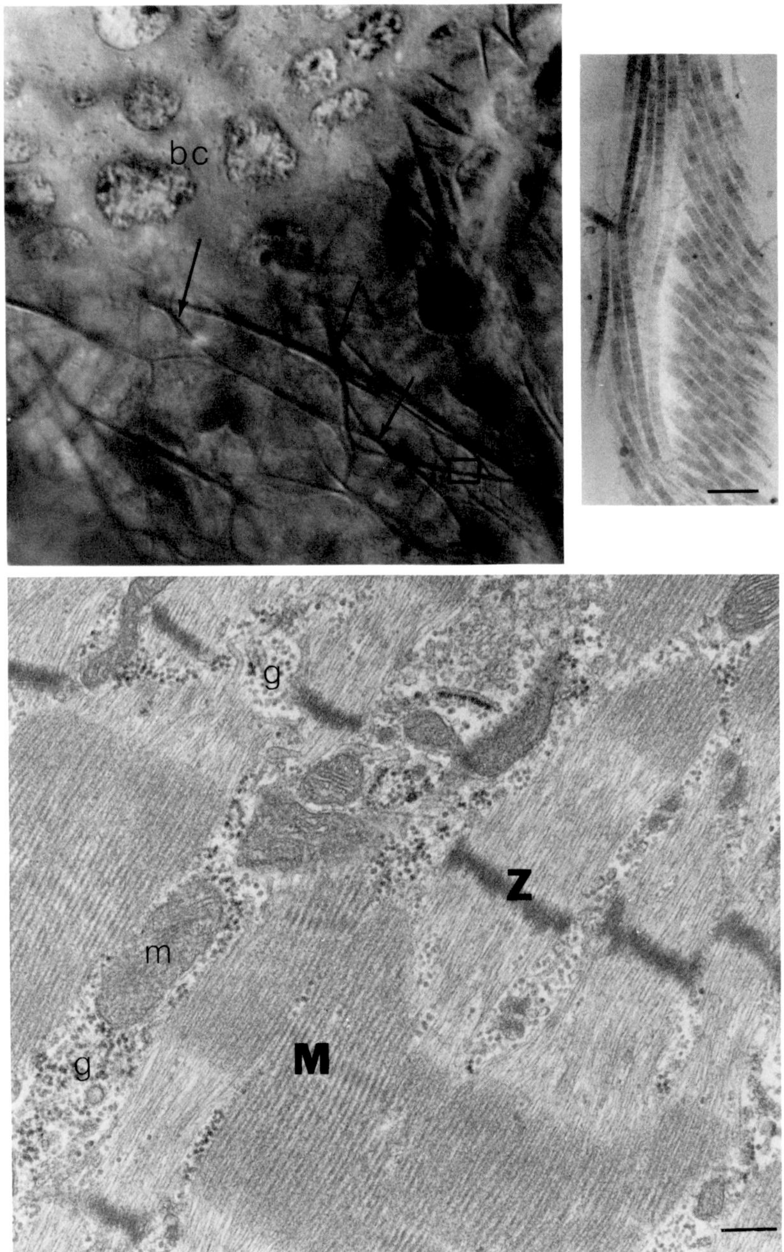
bc
g
Z
m
g
M

having low nutritional value (Ito, 1967). Probably the most extreme example is in the grasshopper mouse, *Onychomys,* in which the bilocular stomach is almost totally lined with stratified squamous epithelium (Horner et al., 1964). Among studied microtines, the glandular-nonglandular ratio varies considerably; *Lemmus* has the most extensive glandular zone, whereas *Dicrostonyx* has the most extensive non-glandular zone (Dearden, 1969). In *Microtus* the glandular gastric mucosa is restricted to a narrow zone of the greater curvature (Fig. 16), which is surrounded by keratinized epithelium and bordered by pediculated squamous flaps (Dearden, 1969).

The ultrastructure of the non-glandular and glandular stomach in *Microtus* has not been described previously. The following description is based on *M. pennsylvanicus.*

Although the non-glandular gastric epithelium is relatively uniform at the histological level and generally is described simply as "cornified" (Dearden, 1969; Golley, 1960), subtle differences are detectable at the ultrastructural level. Both the cardiac vestibule and remaining non-glandular stomach differ from the squamous epithelium of the esophagus at the gastro-esophageal junction. Unlike the esophagus, the stratified squamous epithelium of the stomach is heavily keratinized and thus characterized by both a stratum corneum and a stratum disjunctum (Fig. 19). A typical stratum spinosum is lacking in the non-glandular stomach (Fig. 19). Instead, irregularly-shaped basal cells are overlaid by layers (5–7 cells deep) of flattened cells having elongate nuclei and abundant tonofilaments, keratohyalin granules, and membrane-coating granules. Also in the non-glandular stomach, lipid-like droplets accumulate in the intercellular spaces between the outermost cells of the stratum granulosum and dark inner cells of the stratum corneum. These droplets also are found between cells composing the stratum corneum (Fig. 19). Although these foregoing structural and organizational differences in esophageal and gastric epithelium are not

---

←

FIG. 18. Top left: light microscopic survey showing esophageal basal cell layer (bc) and ligament-like fibers (arrows) attached at base of the epithelium. Boxed area is similar to that shown in TEM view at top right. Scale bar = 13 μm. Top right: braided collagen ligament found in lamina propria of esophagus. Scale bar = 0.25 μm. Bottom: skeletal muscle of esophagus, with prominent Z and M bands. Other abbreviations are: g, glycogen; m, mitochondrial profiles. Scale bar = 0.25 μm.

obvious except with the transmission electron microscope, they nevertheless are not particularly surprising. The stratified squamous epithelium of this portion of a digestive tract appears relatively uniform (except in thickness) at the light microscopic level, and one easily can have the impression that the non-glandular stomach is a continuation of the esophagus. However, developmental and comparative studies have shown that the non-glandular gastric epithelium is derived from the same source as is the glandular mucosa and, therefore, is not a continuation of esophagus (Ito, 1967; Kammeraad, 1942).

The cardiac vestibule differs from the non-glandular forestomach in that the epithelium clearly is closely associated with smooth muscle of the muscularis mucosa (Figs. 20, 21, 22). Epithelial basal cells of both the non-glandular forestomach and esophagus overlie loose connective tissue, whereas in the cardiac region these cells are only narrowly separated from the smooth muscle by densely packed collagen, elastic fibers, and fibroblasts (Fig. 20). These differences in the positional relationships between smooth muscle and stratified squamous epithelium probably are reflective of different functional roles. As pointed out by Dearden (1966), the thick smooth muscle layer associated with the gastro-esophageal junction is consistent with the idea that this zone is capable of serving as a valve.

→

FIG. 19. Top: survey view of cardiac vestibule epithelium of the stomach, showing outer, keratinized, stratum corneum (1), a granular layer (2) containing keratohyalin (kh), the basal layer (3), and stratum disjunctum (outermost thin layers at upper left). Scale bar = 17 μm. Bottom: TEM view of junction between stratum corneum and stratum granulosum. Note the densely packed keratin filaments (area within the rectangle), lipid-like intercellular material (arrow), and the keratohyalin granule (kh). Scale bar = 0.25 μm.

FIG. 20. Top: transition from basal cells (left) to granular cells (right) in the stomach. Note the dense accumulation of glycogen (g), small keratohyalin granules (kh), and tonofilaments (tf). Other abbreviations are: m, mitochondrial profile; d, desmosome; N, nucleus. Scale bar = 1 μm. Middle: subepithelial components of cardiac vestibule. Note unusual presence of a cilium (arrow) on a fibroblast. Scale bar = 1 μm. Bottom: hemi-desmosomes (arrows) on basal cells. Note the basal lamina (BL). Scale bar = 0.25 μm.

FIG. 21. Top: keratinization process in the non-glandular stomach, showing large keratohyalin granules (kh), glycogen (g), and masses of tonofilaments (tf). Scale bar = 0.25 μm. Bottom: high magnification view of a membrane coating granule (such as the one shown in the rectangle at top). Scale bar = 0.10 μm.

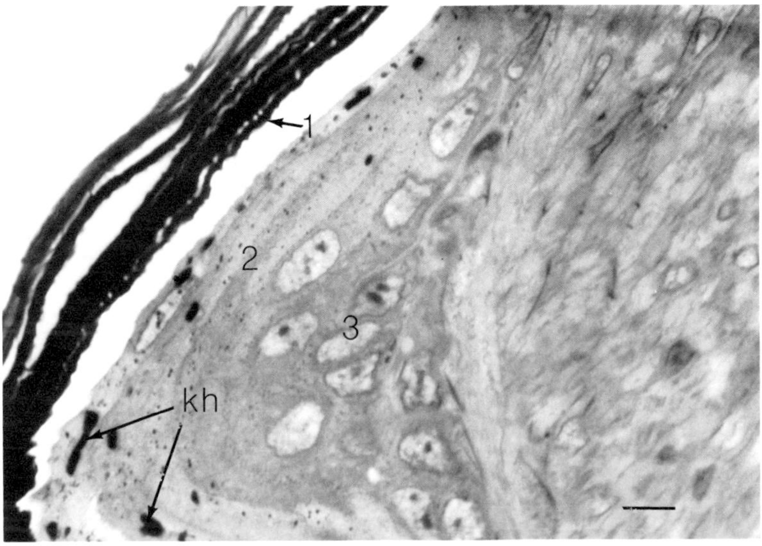
1
2
3
kh

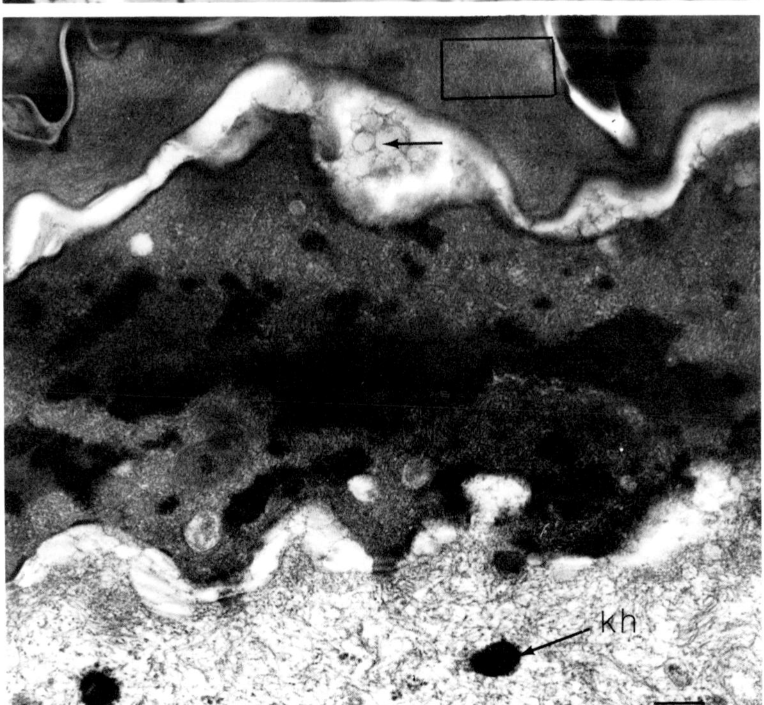
kh

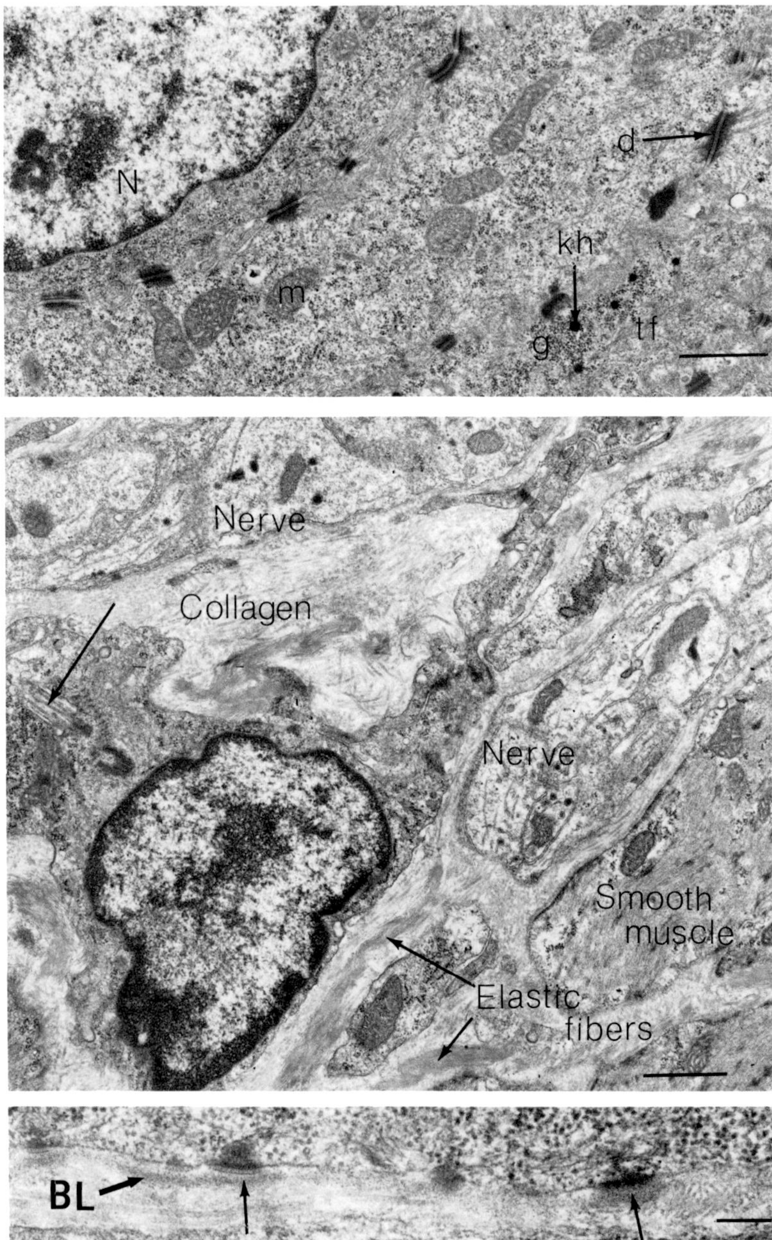
N
d
kh
m
g
tf
Nerve
Collagen
Nerve
Smooth muscle
Elastic fibers
BL

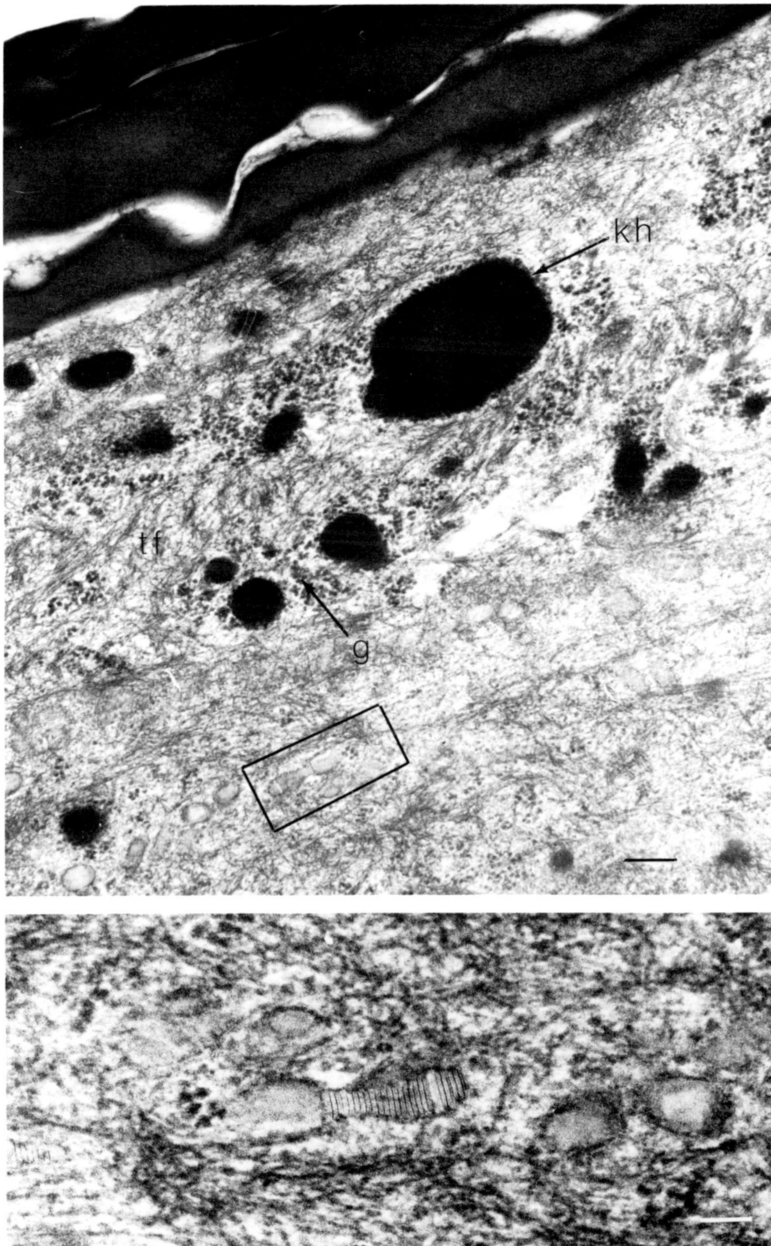
kh
tf
g

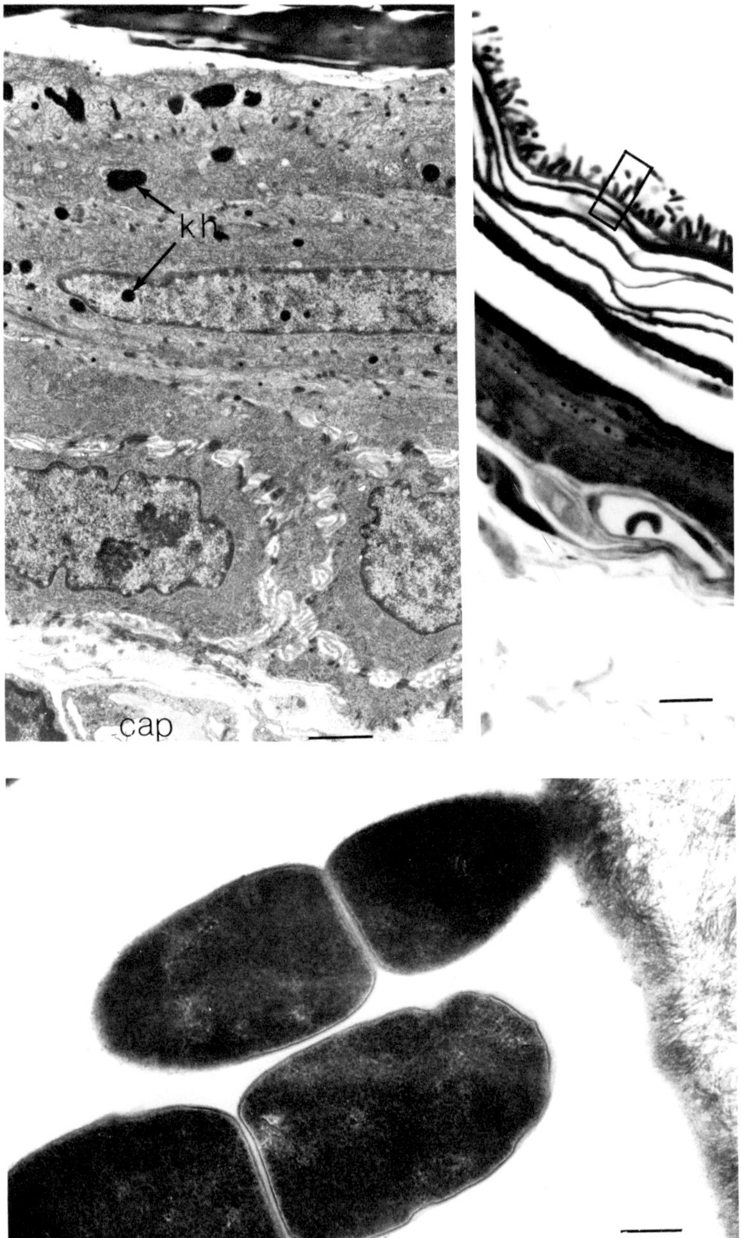
kh
cap

The forestomach in *Microtus* is of special interest because light microscopic analysis of 1-mm "thick" sections as well as TEM views, typically reveals rod-type bacteria within this area (Fig. 22). The fact that these bacteria nearly always (about 90%) are attached and oriented with their long axes perpendicular to the outermost layer of the stratum disjunctium suggests the existence of an association with this portion of the stomach. Symbiotic microbial relationships are relatively common in herbivorous mammals; generally such bacteria are involved in pregastric fermentation of otherwise undigestible plant polymers such as cellulose (for example, see Ito, 1967). Davis and Golley (1963) earlier expressed doubts about microbial fermentation in *Microtus* because "the contents from the esophageal stomach are usually fresh and do not give any evidence that digestion or fermentation has taken place." Although the occurrence of rod-type bacteria in the forestomach of *M. pennsylvanicus* does not in itself prove that microbial fermentation takes place, the microscopic data certainly are consistent with a symbiotic relationship and reflect the importance of future study.

The glandular gastric mucosa in *Microtus* is similar histologically to that found in a variety of other rodents, including laboratory species as well as wild species for which data are available (Dearden, 1969; Horner et al., 1964; Hummel et al., 1966; Ito, 1967). According to Dearden (1969) the gastric pits in *Microtus* are shallow and the gastric glands consist of only parietal (=oxyntic) cells and chief (=peptic) cells. The gastric glands are relatively uniform in depth with chief cells being found in the basal portion and parietal cells occupying the middle region and extending to just below the overlying epithelium (Dearden, 1969). Although parietal and chief cells are indeed a prominent feature of the gastric glands (Figs. 23, 24), two other cell types—mucous neck cells and entero-endocrine cells—also are found within the glands, albeit in smaller num-

---

←

FIG. 22. Top left: survey view of keratinized epithelium of the forestomach. Note the "spiny" nature of the basal cells and presence of keratohyalin granules (kh), including some within a nucleus. Capillaries (cap) are found directly below the basal layer. Scale bar = 1 μm. Top right: light microscopic view of the forestomach showing bacteria attached to the surface. Scale bar = 17 μm. Bottom: TEM view of two bacteria; area shown corresponds to area outlined in micrograph of top right. Scale bar = 0.25 μm.

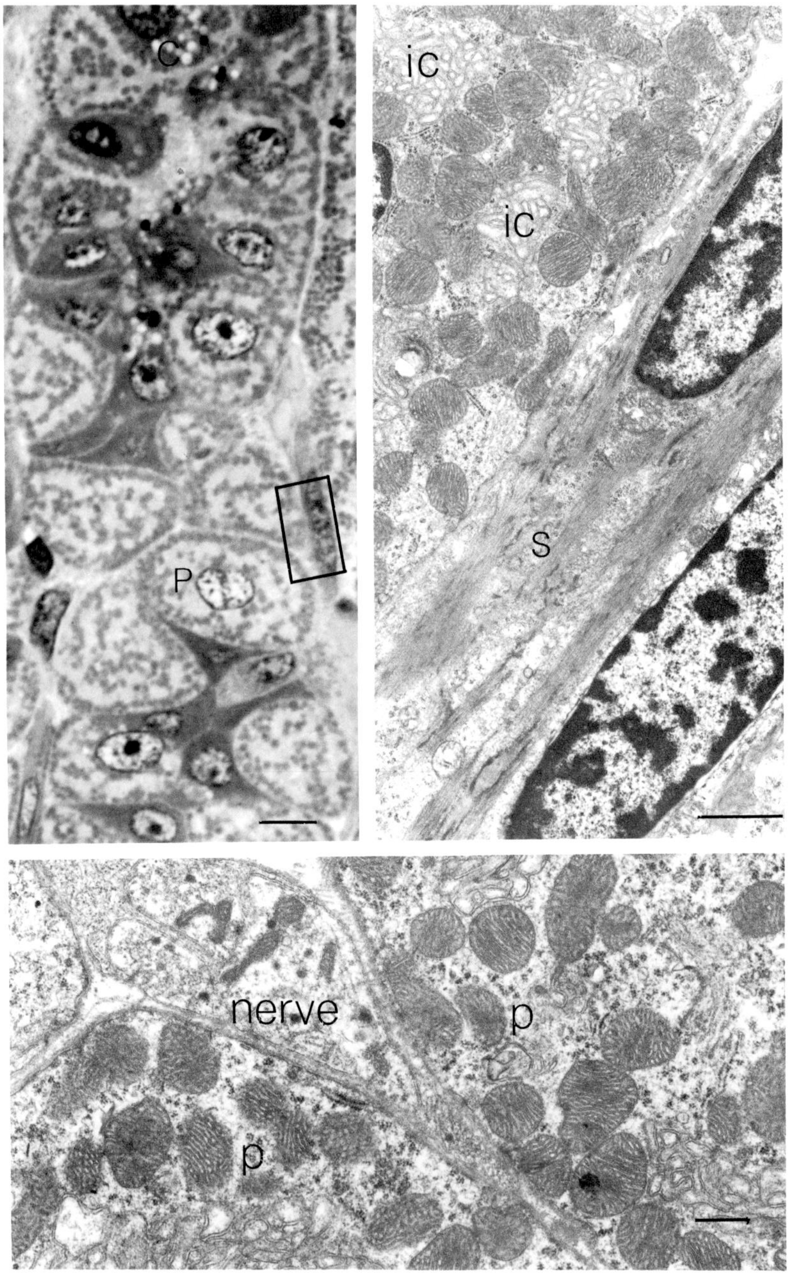
C
P
ic
ic
S
nerve
p
p

bers. Additionally, both light microscopic and ultrastructural views do not necessarily support the idea that chief cells are restricted to the basal portion of the gland (Fig. 23).

Ultrastructurally, the chief cells in *Microtus* are characterized by large, round, basally positioned euchromatic nuclei, abundant GER, prominent Golgi complexes, and immature and mature stored secretory product (Fig. 24). Chief cells synthesize and export pepsinogen which is altered to pepsin in the presence of HCL produced by the parietal cells. The high protein content of the fully developed chief cell product is reflected by its electron dense appearance (Fig. 24). Other granules, presumably immature product, also are a common feature of chief cell cytoplasm. These immature granules are large and pale, contain clumps of electron-dense material, and often are found adjacent to the forming face of the Golgi. The appearance of the immature granules as well as their tendency to coaelesce (Fig. 24) probably partly are due to the primary trialdehyde fixation followed by OsO_4 post-fixation used for the present investigation (Simson et al., 1978).

The secretory function of parietal cells has been studied in considerable detail and, consequently, it is possible to estimate levels of activity as well as functional states of parietal cells from static TEM micrographs of the glandular gastric mucosa in *Microtus* (Black et al., 1980; Forte et al., 1977; Ito and Schofield, 1978; Ito et al., 1977; Schofield et al., 1979). In the animal illustrated (Fig. 23), most of the visible parietal cells were actively secreting HCL as evidenced by the presence of extensive intracellular canaliculi. The canaliculi typically invade deeply into the parietal cell cytoplasm and are easily recognizable by their irregular, loosely organized microvilli and by their thick plasma membrane (Fig. 23). Abundant parietal cell mitochondrial profiles usually are restricted to a zone of cytoplasm immediately around the nucleus and to another zone peripheral to the canaliculi. Parietal cells in *Microtus* typically are situated among chief cells and mucous neck cells (Fig.

←

FIG. 23. Top left: light microscopic survey view of glandular stomach showing parietal cells (P) and chief cells (C). Area within the rectangle is similar to area show in TEM view at right. Scale bar = 17 μm. Top right: smooth muscle cell (s) adjacent to parietal cell. Note the intracellular canaliculi (ic) in the parietal cell. Scale bar = 1 μm. Bottom: Innervation of parietal cells (p). Scale bar = 0.5 μm.

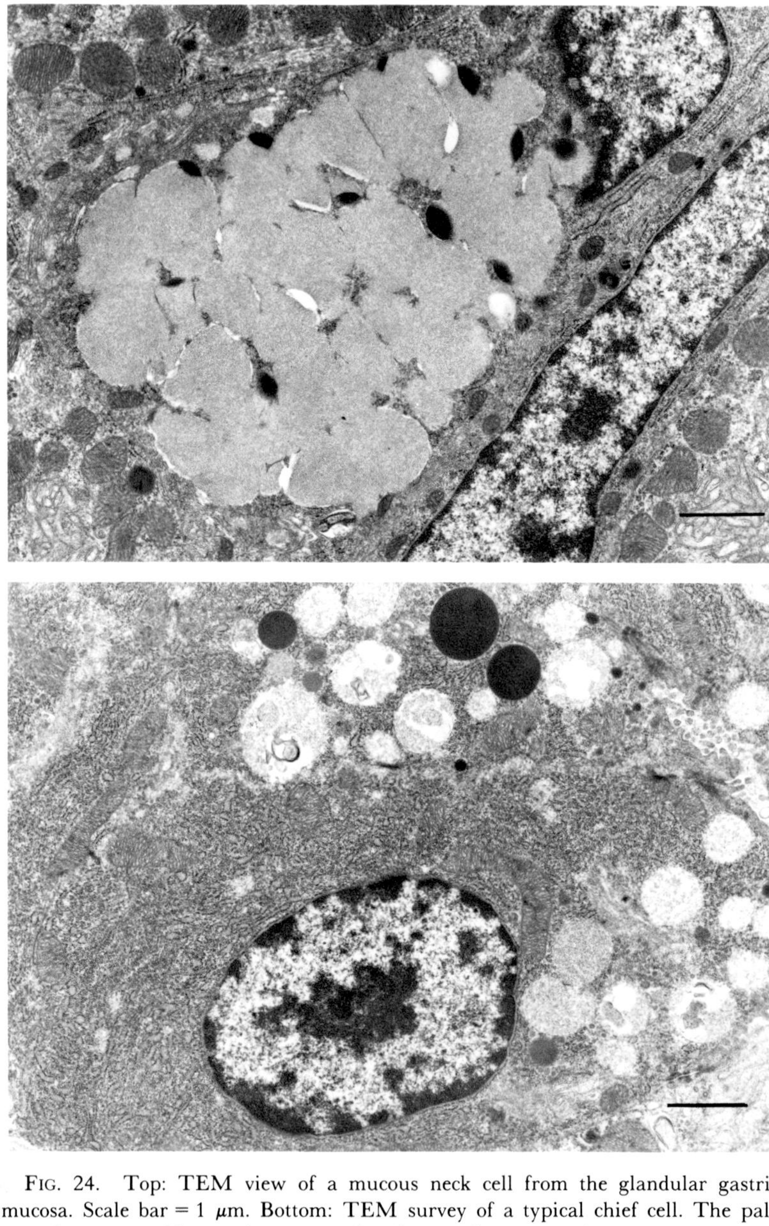

FIG. 24. Top: TEM view of a mucous neck cell from the glandular gastric mucosa. Scale bar = 1 μm. Bottom: TEM survey of a typical chief cell. The pale granules presumably are immature; the electron-dense granules represent mature secretory product. Scale bar = 1 μm.

23). The basal surfaces of parietal cells are in contact with both smooth muscle cells and nerve terminals, although no specialized morphological interrelationship is obvious with the latter (Fig. 23). Inhibition and stimulation of HCL production are noteworthy aspects of parietal cell physiology that have not been explored fully in rodents or in other mammals. However, EGF, which is produced by rodent submandibular salivary glands (see section on Salivary Glands), has been shown to inhibit acid secretion by affecting parietal cell cytoskeleton (Gonzalez et al., 1981). Kusumoto et al. (1979) demonstrated that somatostatin-producing entero-endocrine cells (D cells) are found in juxtaposition with parietal cells in dog stomachs. Somatostatin is an inhibitory molecule that can block gastric acid secretion. In *Microtus,* and apparently other studied rodents as well, such entero-endocrine-cell and parietal-cell relationships have not been found. Instead, only glucagon-producing A cells have been seen thus far in *Microtus* and, although these entero-endocrine cells are not common, the ones examined by me were located among both parietal and chief cells. Because glucagon also has been demonstrated experimentally to inhibit acid secretion while promoting glucose-6-phosphate dehydrogenase activity in the mucous neck cells in humans (Stachura et al., 1981), it seems possible that A cells have a dual role in *Microtus.*

Mucous neck cells in *Microtus* are found interspersed among the parietal cells. Ultrastructurally they are characterized by accumulations of coalescing secretory granules that mostly contain moderately electron-dense material, although many granules also contain small amounts of electron-dense product (Fig. 24). The GER typically is sparse; the nucleus is euchromatic and basally positioned. The large Golgi complexes are unusual in that they are positioned in peripheral cytoplasm and from a lateral perspective appear as layers of membrane-bound electron-dense material (Fig. 24). The surface mucous cells differ from the mucous neck cells in having a more electron-dense secretory product within the apical cytoplasm and in having short microvilli with sparse glycocalyx.

Small Intestine

The pylorus in *Microtus* is non-glandular, consisting instead of a muscular sphincter that Dearden (1969) thought would have an almost symmetrically circular action. The proximal portion of the duodenum is characterized by glands of Brunner, which are con-

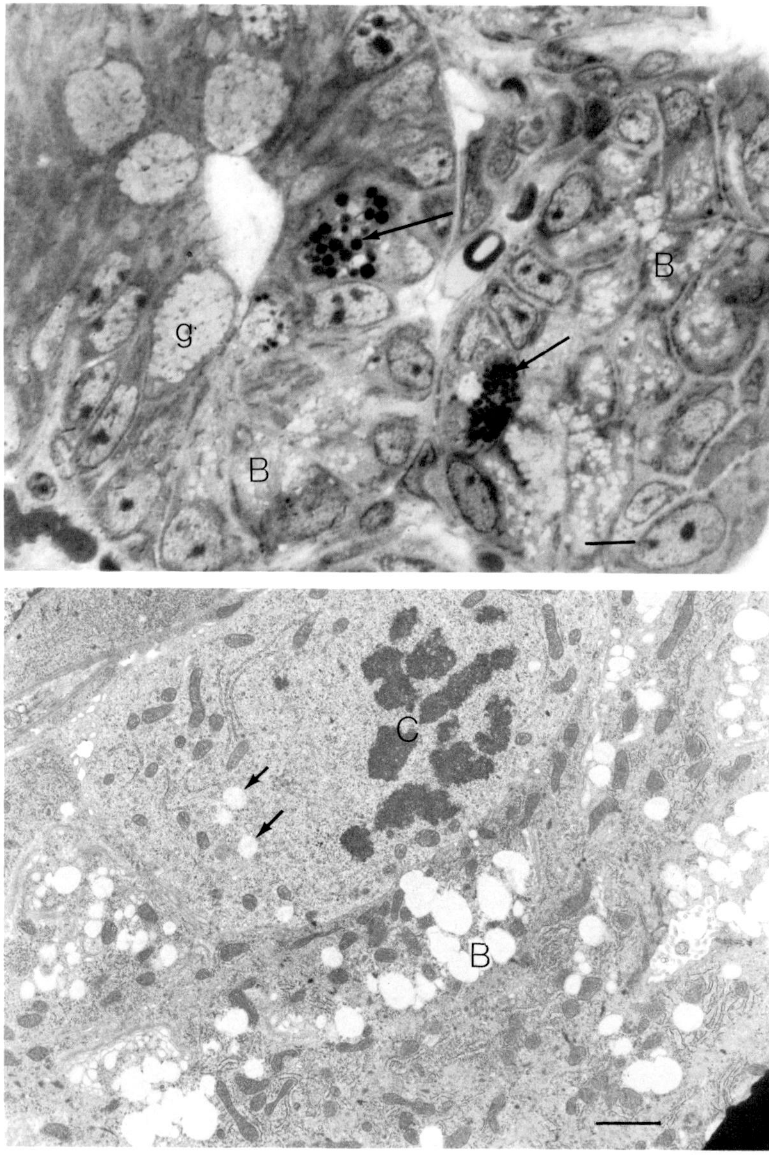

FIG. 25. Top: survey of junction between pylorus and duodenum. Note variety and abundance of secretory cells including goblet cells (g), mucus-producing cells of Brunner's gland (B), and cells containing a dark-staining product (arrows). Scale

sidered as the source of protective alkaline mucins. In *Microtus* the typical secretory cells composing this glandular mass at the junction between "stomach" and "intestine" are mucus-producing but differ ultrastructurally from mucus-producing goblet cells and surface epithelial cells also found in this region (Figs. 25, 26). Cells of the glands of Brunner have large euchromatic nuclei, lamellar GER with swollen cisternae filled with strands of electron-dense material, and large numbers of spherical (sometimes coalescing) pale secretory granules containing a dispersed flocculent secretion product (Figs. 25, 26). The Golgi complexes in these cells are extraordinary; newly formed granules of a variety of sizes are found at the concave face. The outer, convex surface is characterized by flattened saccules containing electron-dense material similar to that found within the GER cisternae (Fig. 26). Numerous mitotic figures within the glands of Brunner in *Microtus* are interesting because they suggest a turnover of secretory cells in these glands. Additionally, in most examples the dividing cells contain at least some secretory product within their cytoplasm (Fig. 25). One type of cell occasionally found within the glands of Brunner is distinctive in that it contains a product that has an electron-dense core with a less dense surrounding halo (Fig. 26). The surface epithelium of the proximal duodenum consists of absorptive cells, goblet cells, and occasional "surface mucous cells" resembling those found in the glandular mucosa of the stomach (Fig. 27). The latter cells probably reflect a slight interdigitation between "gastric" and "intestinal" epithelium.

The small intestine in *Microtus* is characterized by low, broad villi, which is a morphology commonly associated with herbivorous diets (Barry, 1976). The villar pattern, perpendicular to the long axis of the intestine, probably enables the villi to slow the transport of chyme and thus contributes to the high digestive efficiency reported for meadow voles (Barry, 1976; Golley, 1960). A relatively narrow lamina propria is the most striking microanatomical feature of the small intestine in *Microtus* (Fig. 28) and possibly is related

---

←

bar = 17 μm. Bottom: dividing cell (note chromatin, C) with secretory product (arrows). Presumably this is a mucus-producing cell in the Brunner's gland (B). Scale bar = 1 μm.

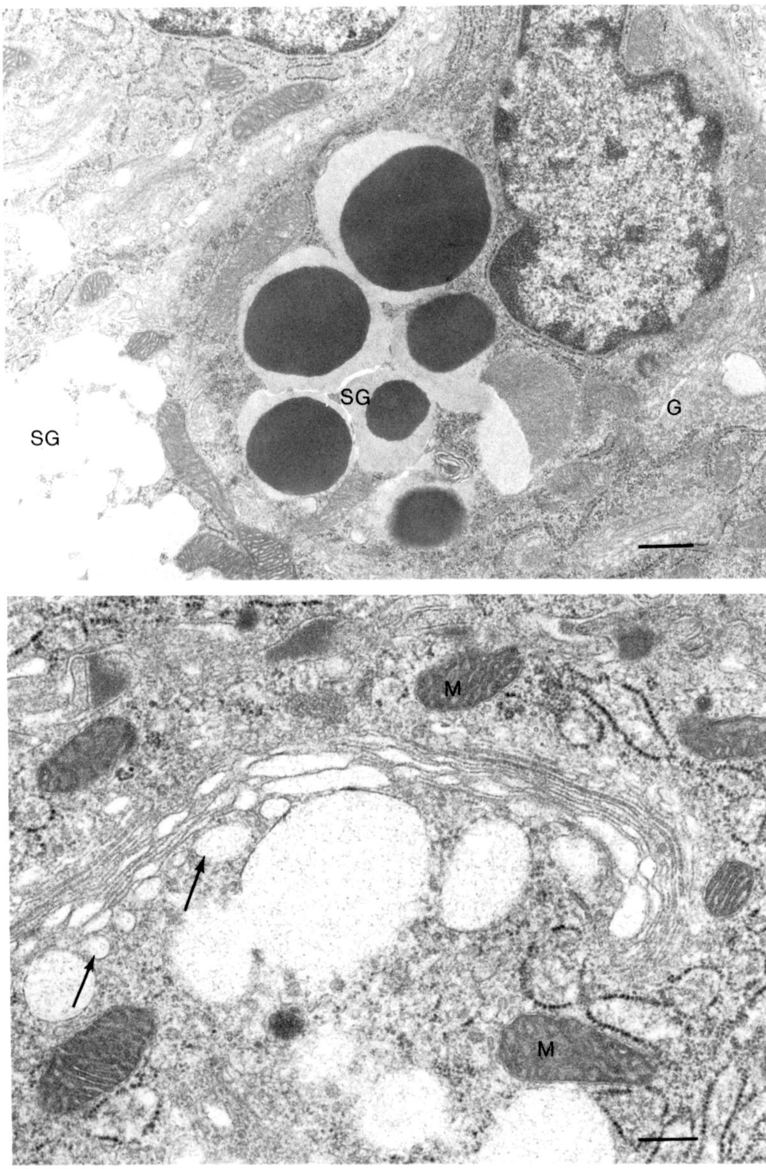

FIG. 26. Top: a comparison of secretory products of Brunner's gland cells (SG on left) and the electron-dense type (SG on right) also found in the duodenum. Note relatively small Golgi (G) and sparse granular endoplasmic reticulum (GER) in the

to villar morphology. Two other considerations are the low intestinal surface area, body-weight ratio and relative uniformity of the absorptive surface as demonstrated in an analysis of mucosal surface area per cm serosal length (Barry, 1976). Barry (1976) thought that in *Microtus* less absorption takes place at the small intestine than in the colon and caecum, which have comparatively great surface areas. Another aspect is the fact that *Microtus* eat large amounts (volume) of food having relatively low nutritional value; possibly passage is slow enough that nutrients can be absorbed gradually over the length of the intestine (Barry, 1976).

Ultrastructurally, the absorptive cells (enterocytes) in the proximal small intestine of *M. pennsylvanicus* are very similar to those of other rodents such as laboratory strains of the Syrian hamster (*Mesocricetus auratus*), house mouse (*Mus musculus*), and Norway rat (*Rattus norvegicus*) (for example, see Buschmann and Manke, 1981*a*, 1981*b*; Rhodin, 1974). The mid-region of a villus is the most appropriate location for interspecies comparison because lower on the villus the absorptive cells presumably are less fully differentiated (at least in ultrastructural morphology), whereas toward the villar apex the cells undergo radical changes as they are about to be extruded from the epithelium (Potten and Allen, 1977). Mid-region absorptive cells in *Microtus* are columnar and have an extensive brush-border of elongate microvilli (Figs. 28, 29, 30). The apices and sides of the apical microvilli have a sparse glycocalyx coating (Fig. 28). Lateral borders of adjacent absorptive cells are characterized by junctional complexes apically and wide intercellular spaces basally (Figs. 28, 29, 30). As illustrated in Fig. 28, from the apical margin the absorptive cell junctional complexes typically are: 1) zonula occludens; 2) zonula adherens; and 3) macula adherens (Fig. 28). The basal intercellular space is interesting in that in non-fasted specimens of *Microtus*, the space nearly always contains accumulations of chylomicrons (Figs. 29, 30) representing the results of lipid absorption in the proximal intestine (Sabesin and Frase, 1977). The mid-lateral region of many active absorptive

---

←

second cell type. Scale bar = 0.5 μm. Bottom: Golgi complex in a Brunner's gland cell. Note immature granules forming along inner face of the Golgi (arrows). Mitochondrial profiles (M) are abundant in this region of the cell. Scale bar = 0.25 μm.

cells also is characterized by complex infoldings of the plasma membrane that result in a zone that can be described as a shallow intracellular canaliculus. The abundance in this zone of coated vesicles both isolated within the cytoplasm and fused on the inner face of the plasma membrane suggests that this is a primary site for exocytosis leading to chylomicron formation. The large amount of chylomicrons (Fig. 30) typically found in non-fasted *Microtus* is significant in view of the general belief that relatively little absorption takes place in the proximal small intestine. It should be noted, however, that the animals illustrated in this chapter had been fed *ad libidum* on a Purina rodent laboratory chow.

The cytoplasm of absorptive cells clearly is organized into compartments. Apically, mitochondrial profiles, vesicles, and flattened strands of GER are the major components. This is followed by a distinctive Golgi zone, another region of mitochondria and GER, the euchromatic nucleus, and, basally, a third region of mitochondria, GER, and free ribosomes (Figs. 28, 29).

With the exception of goblet cells, which are illustrated here (Fig. 28), the other cellular components of the proximal intestine, as well as all of the colon and caecum, are as yet microscopically unstudied in *Microtus.* Future ultrastructural analysis of the caecum in *Microtus,* particularly interspecies comparisons, could prove to be extremely interesting because Lombardi (1978) showed that the caecum has a significant physiological role in osmoregulation. This particularly is true in *M. breweri,* which occurs on Muskeget Island, Massachusetts, where available water cannot be used because of its mineral content. According to Lombardi (1978), the caecum is significantly more elaborate (it has a relatively greater surface area) in *M. breweri* than it is in specimens of *M. pennsylvanicus* from adjacent mainland populations where water is readily available. Whether or not such differences carry through to the fine structure of the epithelial cells remains to be learned.

→

FIG. 27. Top: surface mucous cell found in the proximal duodenum. Note sparse glycocalyx (Gly). Scale bar = 0.5 μm. Bottom: high magnification TEM view of goblet cell mucus (MUC) being released into the duodenal lumen. Note apparent fusion (isolated arrow) of secretory granule membrane (SGM) and the cell membrane (CM) and microvilli (MV) on the adjacent cell. Scale bar = 0.12 μm.

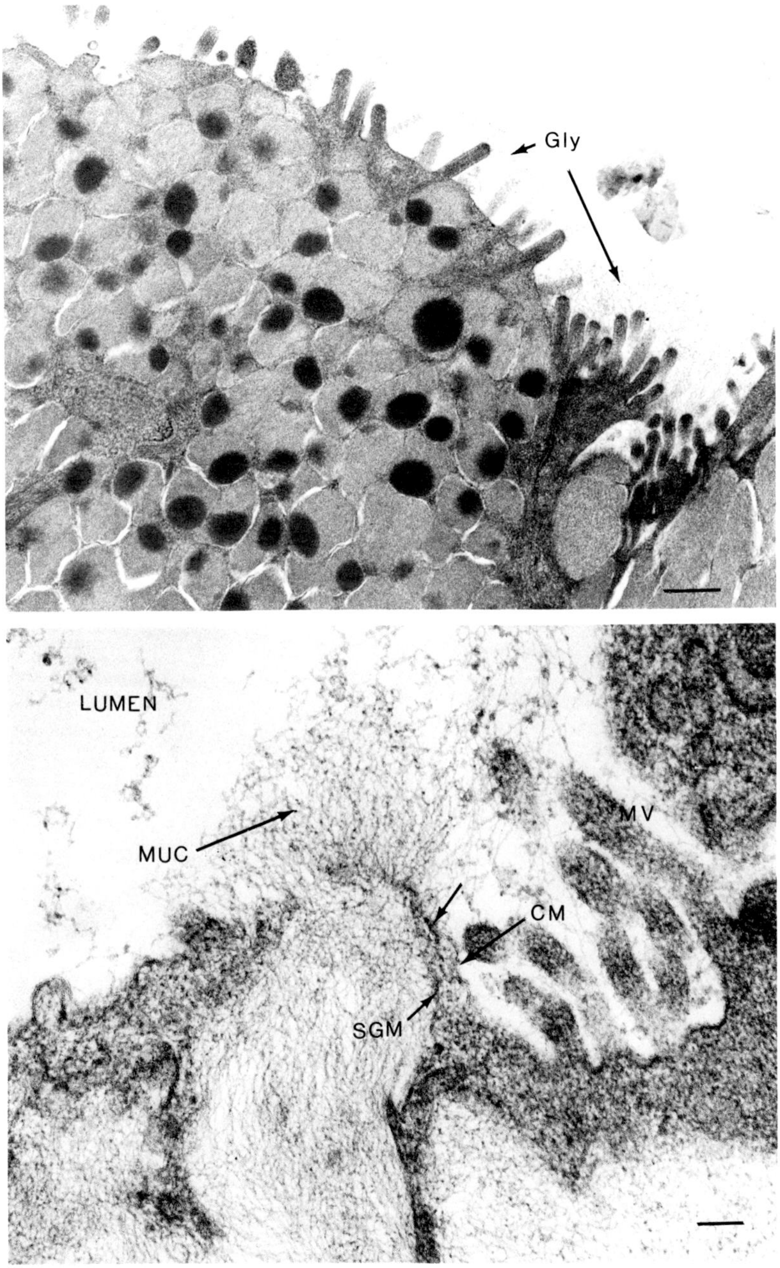
Gly
LUMEN
MUC
MV
CM
SGM

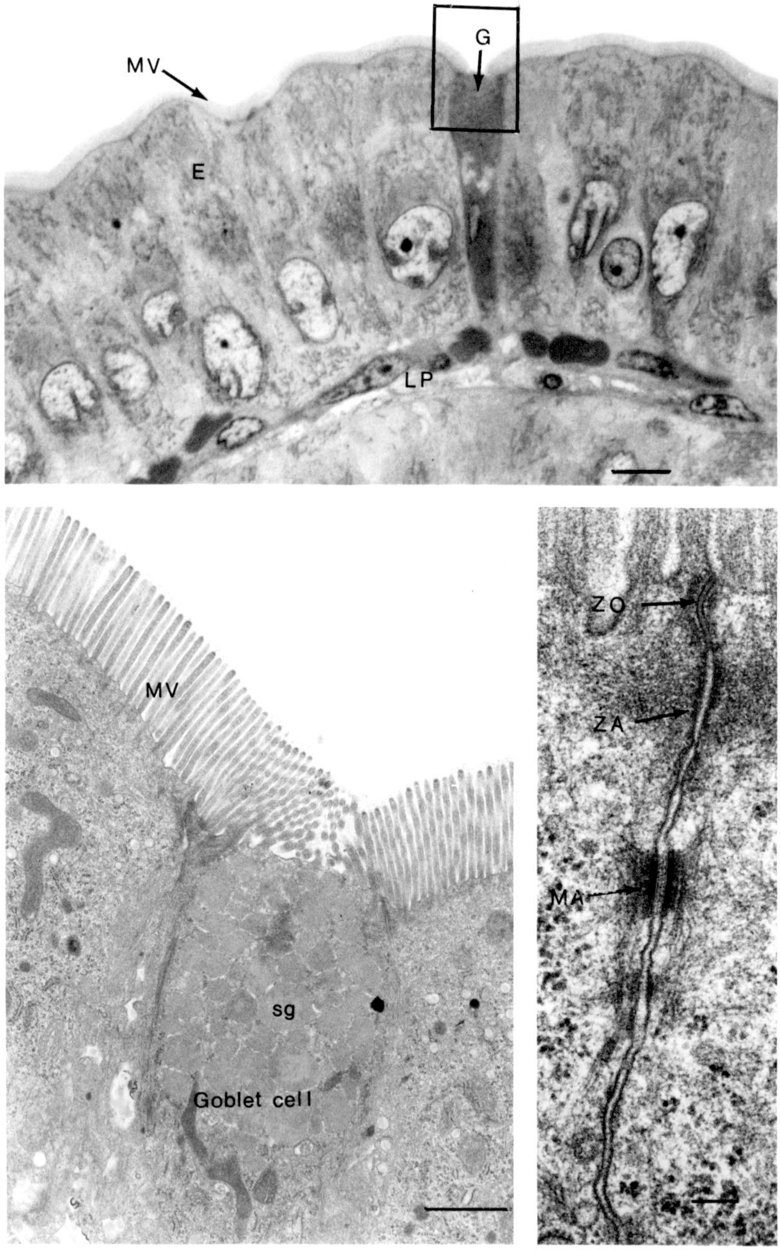
G
MV
E
LP
MV
sg
Goblet cell
ZO
ZA
MA

Adrenal Glands

The adrenal glands are complex components of the mammalian endocrine system. Structurally they consist of two histologically recognizable zones, the outer cortex and the inner medulla. The cortex can be subdivided into three zones that are characterized by cellular and, to some extent, functional differences: 1) the outermost is the zona glomerulosa, consisting of a thin layer of epithelial cells; 2) the middle layer is the zona fasciculata, consisting usually of cells rich in cytoplasmic lipid droplets; and 3) the inner, juxtamedullary, layer is the zona reticularis (Rhodin, 1974). Corticosteroids are synthesized within the cortex, whereas epinephrine and norepinephrine are produced by cells of the medulla.

Insofar as *Microtus* is concerned, most of the interest in the microanatomy of the adrenal gland has resulted from efforts to understand the well-documented population cycles that characterize at least some of the species. A complete review of this particular subject may be found elsewhere (Taitt and Krebs, this volume) and, thus, only relevant histological aspects are described in this brief section.

Christian and Davis (1966) provided fairly detailed data on histological changes in the adrenal glands of female specimens of *M. pennsylvanicus* in response to both population density and reproductive status. These authors were particularly interested in the adrenal cortex and undertook a quantitative analysis of the areas of each of the cortical zones by projecting drawings and using planimetry (Christian and Davis, 1966). Changes in adrenal weight in *Microtus* were found to result from increases or decreases in size of the potentially hyperplastic zona fasciculata and zona reticularis. During an increase in size of these zones caused by adrenal stimulation, cells of both contained abundant lipid (Chitty and Clarke, 1963; Christian and Davis, 1966). One interesting histological

---

←

FIG. 28. Top: light microscopic survey of small intestine showing typical mid-villous enterocytes (E), their microvilli (MV), a goblet cell (G), and the lamina propria (LP). Scale bar = 17 μm. Bottom left: TEM view of area outlined in rectangle at top. Note typical goblet cell secretory granules (sg). Scale bar = 1 μm. Bottom right: typical enterocyte cell junctions. Abbreviations are: ZO, zonula occludens; ZA, zonula adherens; MA, macula adherens. Scale bar = 0.12 μm.

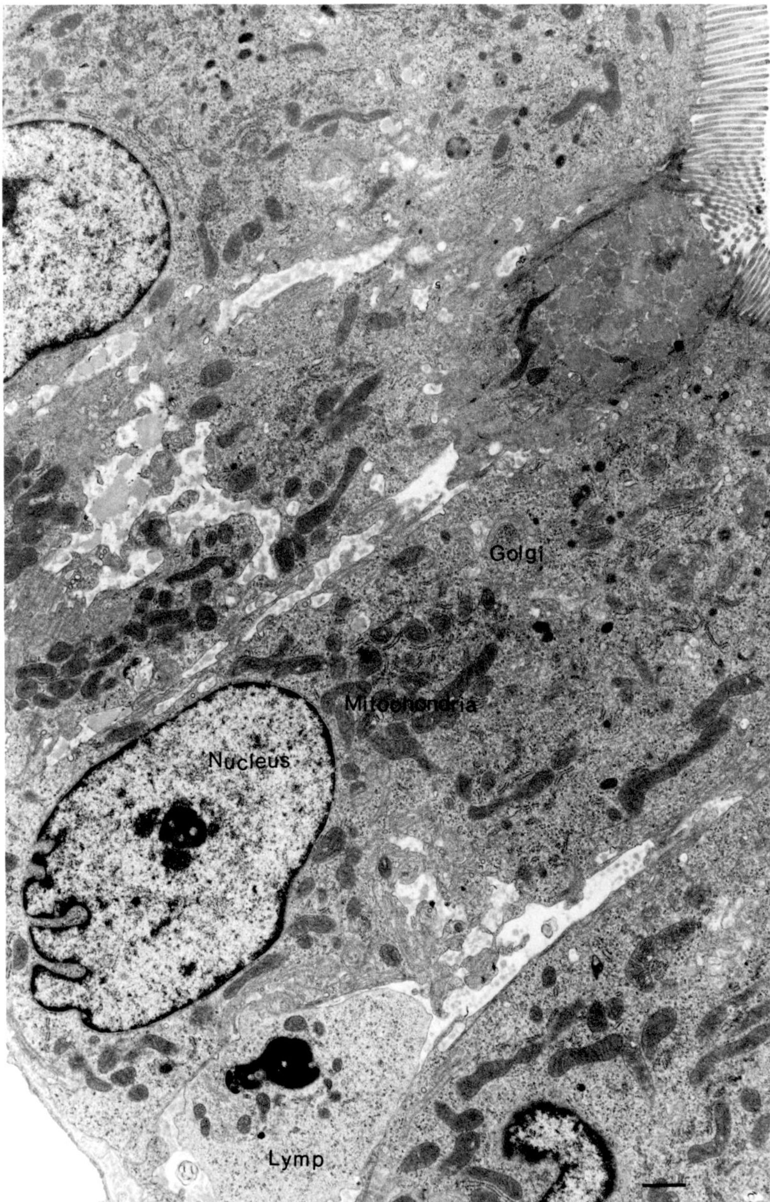

FIG. 29. TEM survey of typical enterocytes in small intestine of *Microtus*. Note also the small infiltrating lymphocyte (Lymp). Scale bar = 1 μm.

question that has arisen from this work is whether or not an X-zone is found in the adrenal glands of *Microtus*. Christian and Davis (1966) concluded that such a zone is lacking, at least in mature female *Microtus*. However, more recently, To and Tamarin (1977) reported finding histological evidence of a transitory X-zone in some nulliparous female *M. breweri* and in subadult, non-breeding males of both *M. breweri* and *M. pennsylvanicus*. Although the functional significance of the X-zone remains unknown, its presence or absence is regarded as important in making comparisons of adrenal weights in animals.

In summary, although the adrenal glands of *Microtus* have not been described in such a way as to make possible microanatomical comparisons with the same glands in other mammals, the histology of the glands nevertheless has been used as an indicator of population stresses and reproductive status. Additionally, *Microtus* possibly could serve as a useful model for future studies of the transitory nature of the X-zone.

Reproductive Tracts

Reproduction and ontogeny in many species of microtine rodents (both Old and New World Species) have been studied from a variety of perspectives. In general, the reproductive biology of microtines is an unusually complex and extremely interesting story that is made even more significant by the tendency of populations to cycle or fluctuate and by the economic importance of some microtines to agriculture. Insofar as the microanatomy of the reproductive tracts is concerned, neither males nor females have been described histologically in such a way as to facilitate comparison with other types of rodents or with other mammals in general. Nevertheless, histology of both testes and ovaries frequently has been employed as an adjunct to investigations of reproductive biology and some published light-level micrographs are available in the literature (see Schadler [1980] for examples of testes and ovaries of *Microtus pinetorum*). Reproduction and ontogeny are discussed in considerable detail elsewhere in this book (Keller, this volume; Seabloom, this volume; Nadeau, this volume), and, therefore, only a few examples of the use of histology are offered here as a brief introduction to the microanatomy of reproductive tracts.

Even though most microtine species spend significant amounts of

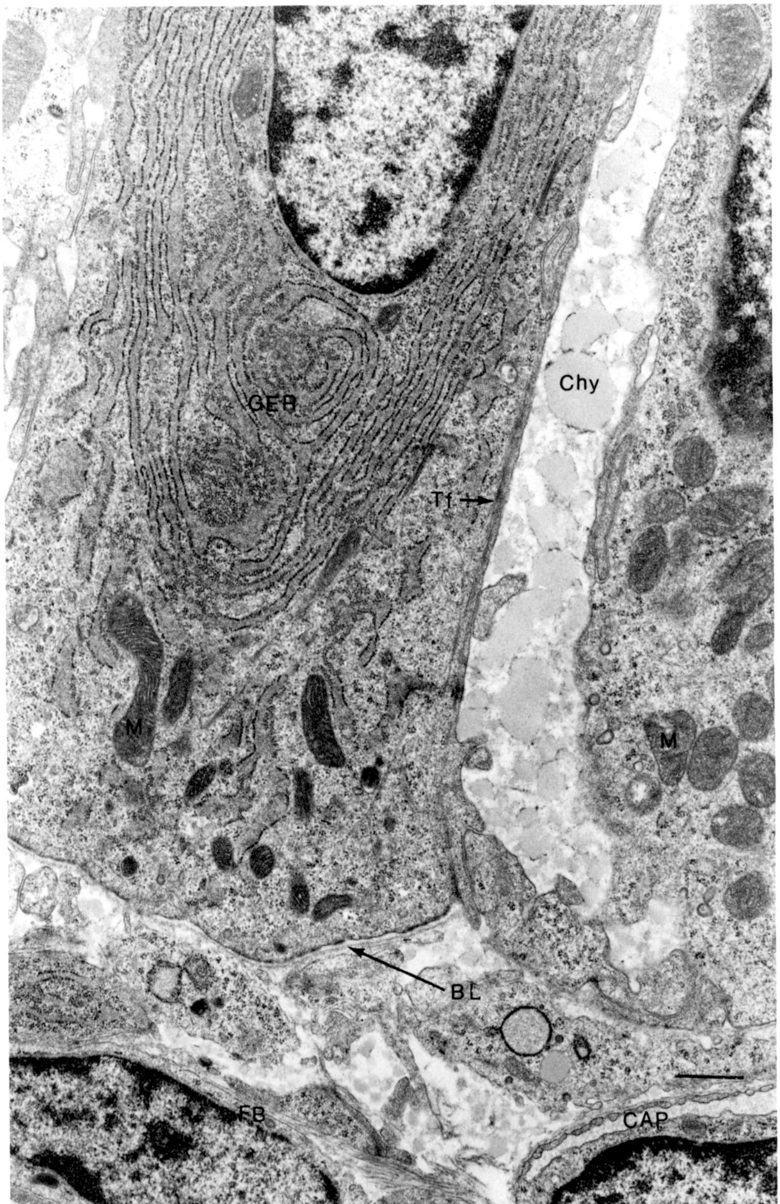
GER
Chy
Tf
M
M
BL
FB
CAP

time in dark burrows and seem to prefer either twilight or complete darkness (Kavanau and Havenhill, 1976), light intensity nevertheless is inversely related to reproductive performance, at least in *Microtus pinetorum* (Geyer and Rogers, 1979). Several investigators have studied the possible effects of light intensity and photoperiod on both development of the gonads and onset of puberty. Basically, a lengthened photoperiod can increase the rate at which puberty is attained, at least in *M. montanus* (Vaughan et al., 1973). Additionally, in two Old World species, *M. agrestis* and *M. arvalis* (Breed and Clarke, 1970*a*; Clarke and Kennedy, 1967), increased photoperiod was shown to both accelerate puberty and enhance glandular development. In regard to onset of puberty, Schadler and Butterstein (1979) presented some useful histological data for *Microtus pinetorum*. According to these authors, in animals maintained at a photoperiod of 12L:12D, testes from 6-week-old animals lacked sperm, whereas those from 8-week-old males had mature spermatozoa in both the testes and the epididymides. Insofar as females are concerned, Schadler and Butterstein (1979) found that in 8-week-old animals the ovaries contained occasional tertiary ovarian follicles but lacked pre-ovulatory follicles and corpora lutea. At 12 weeks, however, 89% of the examined ovaries showed either corpora lutea or ovarian follicles.

Reproductive patterns and comparative fertility have been investigated by histological analysis of ovaries. For example, Hagen and Forslund (1979) used ovarian histology to compare female *Microtus canicaudus* of different age classes. They found that the fetus-corpus luteum ratio was significantly higher in young (18-day) females than in old (70+ days). The apparent value in using ovarian microanatomy in this instance is that it allows one to estimate prenatal (embryonic) mortality. Consequently, comparisons can be made to determine relative success rates among species or age classes. For example, in one study of *Microtus californicus* the corpora lutea were

---

←

FIG. 30. TEM survey of basal portion of *Microtus* enterocytes showing elaborate granular endoplasmic reticulum (GER) and cytoskeletal tonofilaments (Tf). Note accumulation of chylomicrons (Chy) in the intercellular space. Other abbreviations are: M, mitochondria; BL, basal lamina; FB, fibroblast; CAP, fenestrated capillary. Scale bar = 1 μm.

found to greatly exceed the embryo count (Greenwald, 1956), whereas in the Old World *M. agrestis* the corpora lutea did not greatly outnumber embryos during the course of pregnancy (Breed and Clarke, 1970*b*).

As with the case of adrenal gland histology, reproductive-tract microanatomy has been studied in relation to crowding (Schadler, 1980). In this interesting investigation, Schadler (1980) compared a group of crowded and uncrowded individuals of *Microtus pinetorum* and used the histological criteria of Clermont (1972) and Grocock and Clarke (1974) to analyze germinal elements and to determine sperm indices (SI) in the testes. For the ovaries she followed Pederson and Peters (1968) in measuring follicle size. Under crowded conditions, male *M. pinetorum* matured significantly more slowly than did animals kept in less crowded quarters. For example, among crowded males, the following histological features were noted (Schadler, 1980). In 7% the SI was 1 and testes contained mostly sertoli cells with some spermatogonia and occasional spermatocytes. In 12% the SI was 2, the tubules were "small," and secondary spermatocytes and round spermatids were found. Additionally, in this grouping Schadler (1980) also reported finding large eosinophilic cells with pyknotic nuclei. In 39% of the crowded males the SI was 3 and the testes contained elongated spermatids but not spermatozoa. Among the remaining animals, 32% were SI = 1 and, although the testes contained spermatozoa, the tubules were "small"; only 9% were SI = 5. In uncrowded males, 85% were SI = 5 and only 15% were SI = 4. Insofar as the females were concerned, none of those kept in crowded conditions had ovulated and no corpora lutea were found (Schadler, 1980). On the other hand, 21% of uncrowded females had corpora lutea.

The relationship of diet and reproductive performance is yet another example of an area of research in which reproductive organs have been studied histologically. In this intance, the number of maturing ovarian follicles has been shown to increase significantly when green plant food is added to the diet of *Microtus montanus* (Negus and Pinter, 1966; Pinter and Negus, 1965). Gonadal hypertrophy also has been demonstrated in relationship to diet (Negus and Berger, 1971).

In summary, although the histological details of the reproductive tracts in *Microtus* have not been described in a traditional sense, reproductive tract histology nevertheless frequently has been used to measure a variety of environmental variables and physiological parameters.

Acknowledgments

Financial support for the original research reported in this chapter came from the Department of Biology, Hofstra University, and an HCLAS grant (Hofstra University) to the author. Several persons, in particular Dr. Gary W. Grimes, Nadine M. Sposito, and Keith Studholme, offered me their time, ideas, and technical assistance with various aspects of this project. My daughter, Kathrin N. Phillips, collected the specimens of *Microtus* from which the published electron micrographs were made. Lastly, I thank the Hofstra University Special Secretarial Services, headed by Stella Sinicki, for their outstanding assistance with this manuscript.

Literature Cited

AMSTERDAM, A., M. SCHRAMM, I. OHAD, Y. SALOMON, AND Z. SELINGER. 1971. Concomitant synthesis of membrane protein and exportable protein of the secretory granule in rat parotid gland. J. Cell Biol., 50:187–200.

BARRY, R. E., JR. 1976. Mucosal surface areas and villous morphology of the small intestine of small mammals: functional interpretations. J. Mamm., 57:273–290.

BATZLI, G. O., AND F. R. COLE. 1979. Nutritional ecology of microtine rodents: digestibility of forage. J. Mamm., 60:740–750.

BERG, N. B., AND B. P. AUSTIN. 1976. Intracellular transport of sulfated macromolecules in parotid acinar cells. Cell Tissue Res., 165:215–226.

BESHARSE, J. C., AND K. H. PFENNINGER. 1980. Membrane assembly in retinal photoreceptors. I. Freeze-fracture analysis of cytoplasmic vesicles in relationship to disc assembly. J. Cell Biol., 87:451–463.

BHASKAR, S. N. 1976. Orban's oral histology and embryology. C. V. Mosby Co., St. Louis, 470 pp.

BLACK, J. A., T. M. FORTE, AND J. G. FORTE. 1980. Structure of oxyntic cell membranes during conditions of rest and secretion of HCL as revealed by freeze-fracture. Anat. Rec., 196:163–172.

BOGART, B. I., 1977. Electron microscopic autoradiographic analysis of the uptake and intracellular transport of H^3-leucine by the rat submandibular gland acinar cells in tissue slices. Anat. Rec., 187:367–382.

BOONSTRA, R., AND J. H. YOUSON. 1982. Hip glands in a field population of *Microtus pennsylvanicus*. Canadian J. Zool., 60:2955–2958.

BREED, W. G., AND J. R. CLARKE. 1970*a*. Effects of photoperiod on ovarian function in the vole, *Microtus agrestis*. J. Reprod. Fert., 23:189–192.

———. 1970*b*. Ovarian changes during pregnancy and pseudopregnancy in the vole, *Microtus agrestis*. J. Reprod. Fert., 23:447–456.

BUSCHMAN, R. J., AND O. J. MANKE. 1981*a*. Morphometric analysis of the membranes and organelles of small intestinal enterocytes. I. Fasted hamster. J. Ultrastruct. Res., 76:1–14.

———. 1981*b*. Morphometric analysis of the membranes and organelles of small intestinal enterocytes. II. Lipid-fed hamster. J. Ultrastruct. Res., 76:15-26.

BYYNY, R. L., D. N. ORTH, S. COHEN, AND S. DOYNE. 1974. Epidermal growth factor. Effects of androgens and adrenergic agents. Endocrinology, 95:776–782.

CALISSANO, P., AND P. U. ANGELETTI. 1968. Testosterone effect on the synthetic rate of two esteropeptidases in the mouse submaxillary gland. Biochem. Biophys. Acta, 156:51–58.

CASTLE, J. D., J. D. JAMIESON, AND G. E. PALADE. 1972. Radioautographic analysis of the secretory process in the parotid acinar cell of the rabbit. J. Cell Biol., 53:290–311.

CHANG, W. W. L. 1974. Cell population changes during acinus formation in the postnatal rat submandibular gland. Anat. Rec., 178:187–202.

CHARLTON, H. M., AND R. W. WORTH. 1975. The ultrastructure of the anterior pituitary gland of the vole, *Microtus agrestis,* in normal and experimental manipulated animals. J. Anat., 120:69–79.

CHASE, J. 1972. The role of vision in echolocating bats. Unpubl. Ph.D. dissert., Indiana Univ., Bloomington, 191 pp.

CHITTY, H., AND J. R. CLARKE. 1963. The growth of the adrenal gland of laboratory and field voles, and changes in it during pregnancy. Canadian J. Zool., 41:1025–1034.

CHRISTIAN, J. J., AND D. E. DAVIS. 1966. Adrenal glands in female voles (*Microtus pennsylvanicus*) as related to reproduction and population size. J. Mamm., 47:1–18.

CLARKE, J. R., AND J. P. KENNEDY, 1967. Effect of light and temperature upon gonad activity in the vole (*Microtus agrestis*). Genet. Comp. Endocrinol., 8:474–488.

CLERMONT, Y. 1972. Kinetics of spermatogenesis in mammals: seminiferous epithelium cycle and spermatogonial renewal. Physiol. Rev., 52:198–236.

COHEN, A. I. 1960. The ultrastructure of the rods of the mouse retina. Amer. J. Anat., 107:23–48.

DAVIS, D. E., AND F. B. GOLLEY. 1963. Principles in mammalogy. Reinhold Book Corp., New York, 335 pp.

DAWES, C. 1978. The chemistry and physiology of saliva. Pp. 593–629, *in* Textbook of oral biology (J. H. Shaw, E. A. Sweeney, C. C. Cappuccino, and S. M. Meller, eds.). W. B. Saunders, Philadelphia, 1178 pp.

DEARDEN, L. C. 1966. Histology of the gastro-esophageal junction in certain rodents. J. Mamm., 47:223–229.

———. 1969. Stomach and pyloric sphincter histology in certain microtine rodents. J. Mamm., 50:60–68.

EISENBERG, J. F., AND D. G. KLEIMAN. 1972. Olfactory communication in mammals. Ann. Rev. Ecol. Syst., 3:1–32.

ELNER, V. M., T. SCHAFFNER, K. TAYLOR, AND S. GLAGOV. 1981. Immunophagocytic properties of retinal pigment epithelium cells. Science, 211:74–76.

EPPIG, J. J., JR., AND J. N. DUMONT. 1972. Cytochemical localization of tyrosinase activity in pigmented epithelial cells of *Rana pipiens* and *Xenopus laevis* larvae. J. Ultrastruct. Res., 39:397–410.

FELDMAN, J. L., AND C. J. PHILLIPS. 1984. Comparative retinal pigment epithelium and retinal ultrastructure in nocturnal and fossorial rodents: the eastern woodrat, *Neotoma floridana,* and the plains pocket gopher, *Geomys bursarius.* J. Mamm., 65:231–245.

FLUHARTY, S. L., D. H. TAYLOR, AND G. W. BARRETT. 1976. Sun-compass orientation in the meadow vole, *Microtus pennsylvanicus*. J. Mamm., 57:1–9.

FORMAN, G. L. 1972. Comparative morphological and histochemical studies of stomachs of selected American bats. Univ. Kansas Sci. Bull., 49:591–729.

FORTE, T. M., T. E. MACHEN, AND J. G. FORTE. 1977. Ultrastructural changes in oxyntic cells associated with secretory function: a membrane-recycling hypothesis. Gastroenterology, 73:941–955.

GEYER, L. A., AND J. G. ROGERS, JR. 1979. The influence of light intensity on reproduction in pine voles, *Microtus pinetorum*. J. Mamm., 60:839–841.

GILL, A. E, AND K. BOLLES. 1982. A heritable tooth trait varying in two subspecies of *Microtus californicus* (Rodentia: Cricetidae). J. Mamm., 63:96–103.

GOLLEY, F. B. 1960. Energy dynamics of a foodchain of an old-field community. Ecol. Monogr., 30:187–206.

GONZALEZ, A., J. GARRIDO, AND J. D. VIAL. 1981. Epidermal growth factor inhibits cytoskeleton-related changes in the surface of parietal cells. J. Cell Biol., 88:108–114.

GREENWALD, G. S. 1956. The reproductive cycle of the field mouse, *Microtus californicus*. J. Mamm., 37:213–222.

GROCOCK, C. A., AND J. R. CLARKE. 1974. Photoperiodic control of testis activity in the vole, *Microtus agrestis*. J. Reprod. Fert., 39:337–347.

GUTHRIE, R. D. 1965. Variability in characters undergoing rapid evolution, an analysis of *Microtus* molars. Evolution, 19:214–233.

———. 1971. Factors regulating the evolution of microtine tooth complexity. Z. Saugetierk., 36:37–54.

HAGEN, J. B., AND L. G. FORSLUND. 1979. Comparative fertility of four age classes of female gray-tailed voles, *Microtus canicaudus*. J. Mamm., 60:834–837.

HAND, A. R. 1976. Salivary glands. Pp. 328–360, *in* Orban's oral histology and embryology (S. N. Bhaskar, ed.). C. V. Mosby Co., St. Louis, 470 pp.

HIBBARD, C. W. 1959. Late Cenozoic microtine rodents from Wyoming and Idaho. Papers Michigan Acad. Sci. Arts Letters, 44:3–40.

HINKLEY, R. 1966. Effects of plant extracts in the diet of male *Microtus montanus* on cell types of the anterior pituitary. J. Mamm., 47:396–400.

HORNER, B. E., J. M. TAYLOR, AND H. A. PADYKULA. 1964. Food habits and gastric morphology of the grasshopper mouse. J. Mamm., 45:513–535.

HRABĚ, V. 1974. Tarsal glands in Pitymys subterraneus (de Sél.-Long) and Pitymys tatricus Krat. (Microtinae, Mammalia). Zool. Listy, 23:97–105.

HUMASON, G. L. 1972. Animal tissue techniques. W. H. Freeman, New York, 468 pp.

HUMMEL, K. P., RICHARDSON, F. L., AND E. FEKETE. 1966. Anatomy. Pp. 247–307, *in* Biology of the laboratory mouse (E. L. Green, ed.). McGraw-Hill Book Co., NewYork, 706 pp.

ITO, S. 1967. Anatomic structure of the gastric mucosa. Pp. 705–741, *in* Hand book of physiology (C. F. Code, ed.), Amer. Physiol. Soc., Washington, D.C., 2:463–1095.

ITO, S., AND G. C. SCHOFIELD. 1978. Ultrastructural changes in mouse parietal cells after high H+ secretion. Acta Physiol. Scand., Spec. Suppl., pp. 25–34.

ITO, S., D. R. MUNRO, AND G. C. SCHOFIELD. 1977. Morphology of the isolated mouse oxyntic cell and some physiological parameters. Gastroenterology, 73:887–898.

JACOBS, G. H., S. K. FISHER, D. H. ANDERSON, AND M. S. SILVERMAN. 1976. Scotopic and photopic vision in the California ground squirrel: physiological and anatomical evidence. J. Comp. Neurol., 165:209–228.

JANNETT, F. J., JR. 1975. "Hip glands" of *Microtus pennsylvanicus* and *M. lon-*

gicaudus (Rodentia: Muridae), voles "without" hip glands. Syst. Zool., 24: 171–175.

JUNQUEIRA, L. C., A. FAJER, M. RABINOVITCH, AND L. FRANKENTHAL. 1949. Biochemical and histochemical observations on the sexual dimorphism of mice submaxillary glands. J. Cell. Comp. Physiol., 34:129–158.

KALT, M. R., AND B. TANDLER. 1971. A study of fixation of early amphibian embryos for electron microscopy. J. Ultrastruct. Res., 36:633–645.

KAMMERAAD, A. 1942. The development of the gastro-intestinal tract of the rat. I. Histogenesis of the epithelium of the stomach, small intestine and pancreas. J. Morphol., 70:323–351.

KAVANAU, J. L., AND R. M. HAVENHILL. 1976. Compulsory regime and control of environment in animal behavior. III. Light level preferences of small nocturnal mammals. Behaviour, 59:203–225.

KNIGGE, K. M., AND S. A. JOSEPH. 1968. A stereotaxic atlas of the brain of the golden hamster. Pp. 285–319, *in* The golden hamster—its biology and use in medical research (R. A. Hoffman, P. F. Robinson, and H. Magalhaes, eds.). Iowa State Univ. Press, Ames, 545 pp.

KOENIGSWALD, W. V., AND F. N. GOLENISHEV. 1979. A method for determining growth rates in continuously growing molars. J. Mamm., 60:397–400.

KOWALSKI, K. 1966. The stratigraphic importance of rodents in the studies on the European Quaternary. Folia Quaternaria, 22:1–16.

KUSUMOTO, Y., T. IWANAGA, S. ITO, AND T. FUJITA. 1979. Juxtaposition of somatostatin cell and parietal cell in the dog stomach. Arch. Histol., Japan, 42:459–465.

KUWABARA, T. 1979. Species differences in the retinal pigment epithelium. Pp. 58–82, *in* The retinal pigment epithelium (K. M. Zinn and M. F. Marmor, eds.). Harvard Univ. Press, Cambridge, Massachusetts, 521 pp.

LEUENBERGER, P. M., AND A. B. NOVIKOFF. 1975. Studies on microperoxisomes. VII. Pigment epithelial cells and other cell types in the retina of rodents. J. Cell Biol., 65:324–334.

LILLIE, R. D. 1965. Histopathologic technic and practical histochemistry. McGraw-Hill Book Co., New York, 715 pp.

LOMBARDI, R. T. G. 1978. A comparison of the osmoregulatory abilities of the beach vole, *Microtus breweri,* and its mainland counterpart, *Microtus pennsylvanicus.* Unpubl. M.A. thesis, Boston Univ., Boston, 111 pp.

MILLER, G. S. 1896. Genera and subgenera of voles and lemmings. N. Amer. Fauna, 12:1–85.

MÜLLER-SCHWARZE, D. 1983. Scent glands in mammals and their functions. Pp. 150–197, *in* Advances in the study of mammalian behavior (J. F. Eisenberg and D. G. Kleiman, eds.). Spec. Publ. Amer. Soc. Mamm., 7:1–753.

MURPHY, R. A., A. Y. WATSON, J. METZ, AND W. G. FORSSMANN. 1980. The mouse submandibular glands: an exocrine organ for growth factors. J. Histochem. Cytochem., 28:890–902.

NEGUS, N. C., AND P. J. BERGER. 1971. Pineal weight response to a dietary variable in *Microtus montanus.* Experientia, 27:215–216.

NEGUS, N. C., AND A. J. PINTER. 1966. Reproductive responses of *Microtus montanus* to plants and plant extracts in the diet. J. Mamm., 47:596–601.

NGUYEN-LEGROS, J. 1978. Fine structure of the pigment epithelium in the vertebrate retina. Internatl. Rev. Cytol., Suppl. 7, 287–328.

NOVIKOFF, A. B. 1976. The endoplasmic reticulum: a cytochemist's view (a review). Proc. Natl. Acad. Sci., 73:2781–2787.

NOVIKOFF, A. B., P. M. LEUENBERGER, P. M. NOVIKOFF, AND N. QUINTANA. 1979. Retinal pigment epithelium. Interrelations of endoplasmic reticulum and melanolysosomes in the black mouse and its beige mutant. Lab. Invest., 40:155–165.

OXBERRY, B. A. 1975. An anatomical, histochemical, and autoradiographic study of the ever-growing molar dentition of *Microtus* with comments on the role of structure in growth and eruption. J. Morph., 147:337–354.

PALADE, G. 1975. Intracellular aspects of the process of protein synthesis. Science, 189:347–358.

PAPERMASTER, D. S., C. A. CONVERSE, AND J. SIU. 1975. Membrane biosynthesis in the frog retina: opsin transport in the photoreceptor cell. Biochemistry, 14:1343–1352.

PEDERSEN, T., AND H. PETERS. 1968. Proposal for a classification of oocytes and follicles in the mouse ovary. J. Reprod. Fert., 17:555–557.

PHILLIPS, C. J. In press. Field fixation and storage of museum tissue collections suitable for electron microscopy. Acta Zool. Fennica.

PHILLIPS, C. J., AND B. A. OXBERRY. 1972. Comparative histology of molar dentitions of *Microtus* and *Clethrionomys*, with comments on dental evolution in microtine rodents. J. Mamm., 53:1–20.

PHILLIPS, C. J., G. W. GRIMES, AND G. L. FORMAN. 1977. Oral biology. Pp. 121–246, *in* Biology of bats of the New World family Phyllostomatidae, Part II (R. J. Baker, J. K. Jones, Jr., and D. C. Carter, eds.). Spec. Publ. Mus., Texas Tech Univ., Lubbock, 364 pp.

PINTER, A. J., AND N. C. NEGUS. 1965. Effects of nutrition and photoperiod on reproductive physiology of *Microtus montanus*. Amer. J. Physiol., 208:633–638.

POTTEN, C. S., AND T. D. ALLEN. 1977. Ultrastructure of cell loss in intestinal mucosa. J. Ultrastruct. Res., 60:272–277.

QUAY, W. B. 1952. The skin glands of voles and lemmings (Microtinae). Unpubl. Ph.D. dissert., Univ. Michigan, Ann Arbor, 153 pp.

———. 1954. The Meibomian glands of voles and lemmings (Microtinae). Misc. Publ. Mus. Zool., Univ. Michigan, 82:1–7.

———. 1960. Neural and hypophyseal colloid deposition in the collared lemming. Science, 131:42–43.

———. 1968. The specialized posterolateral sebaceous glandular regions in microtine rodents. J. Mamm., 49:427–445.

———. 1969. Comparative occurrence of brain colloid deposits in microtine rodents from Churchill, Manitoba. J. Mamm., 50:21–27.

RALLS, K. 1971. Mammalian scent marking. Science, 171:443–449.

RHODIN, J. A. G. 1974. Histology a text and atlas. Oxford Univ. Press, New York, 803 pp.

RICHARDSON, T. M. 1969. Cytoplasmic and ciliary connections between the inner and outer segments of mammalian visual receptors. Vision Res., 9:727–731.

RÖHLICH, P. 1975. The sensory cilium of retinal rods is analogous to the transitional zone of motile cilia. Cell Tissue Res., 161:421–430.

SABESIN, S. M., AND S. FRASE. 1977. Electron microscopic studies of the assembly, intracellular transport, and secretion of chylomicrons by rat intestine. J. Lipid Res., 18:496–511.

SATIR, B. 1974. Ultrastructural aspects of membrane fusion. J. Supramolecular Struct., 2:529–537.

SCHADLER, M. H. 1980. The effect of crowding on the maturation of gonads in pine voles, *Microtus pinetorum*. J. Mamm., 61:769–774.

SCHADLER, M. H., AND G. M. BUTTERSTEIN. 1979. Reproduction in the pine vole, *Microtus pinetorum*. J. Mamm., 60:841–844.

SCHOFIELD, G. C., S. ITO, AND R. P. BOLENDER. 1979. Changes in membrane surface areas in mouse parietal cells in relation to high levels of acid secretion. J. Anat., 128:669–692.

SHACKLEFORD, J. M., AND C. E. KLAPPER. 1962. A sexual dimorphism of hamster submaxillary mucin. Anat. Rec., 142:495–504.

SHACKLEFORD, J. M., AND C. A. SCHNEYER. 1964. Structural and functional aspects of rodent salivary glands including two desert species. Amer. J. Anat., 115:279–308.

SHACKLEFORD, J. M., AND W. H. WILBORN. 1968. Structural and histochemical diversity in mammalian salivary glands. Alabama J. Med. Sci., 5:180–203.

SIMSON, J. A. U., R. M. DOM, P. L. SANNES, AND S. S. SPICER. 1978. Morphology and cytochemistry of acinar secretory granules in normal and isoproterenol-treated rat submandibular glands. J. Microsc., 113:185–203.

SJÖSTRAND, F. S., AND M. KREMAN. 1979. Freeze-fracture analysis of structure of plasma membrane of photoreceptor cell outer segments. J. Ultrastruct. Res., 66:254–275.

SPIRA, A. W., AND G. E. MILMAN. 1979. The structure and distribution of the cross-striated fibril and associated membranes in guinea pig photoreceptors. J. Anat., 155:319–338.

SPOONER, B. S. 1973. Microfilaments, cell shape changes, and morphogenesis of salivary epithelium. Amer. Zool., 13:1007–1022.

SRINIVASAN, R., AND W. W. L. CHANG. 1975. The development of the granular convoluted duct in the rat submandibular gland. Anat. Rec., 182:29–40.

STACHURA, J., A. TARNAWSKI, J. BOGDAL, W. KRAUSE, AND K. IVEY. 1981. Effect of glucagon on human gastric mucosa: histochemical studies. Gastroenterology, 80:474–481.

ŠULC, K. 1929. O zmenšeném počtu tarsálních žláz u hrabošů (Microtinae). Biol. Spisy Vgs. ŠK zvěr., 8:1–14.

TAMARIN, A., AND L. M. SREEBNY. 1965. The rat submaxillary salivary gland: a correlative study by light and electron microscopy. J. Morph., 117:295–352.

TANDLER, B. 1978. Salivary glands and the secretory process. Pp. 547–592, *in* Textbook of oral biology (J. H. Shaw, E. A. Sweeney, C. C. Cappuccino, and S. M. Meller, eds.). W. B. Saunders Co., Philadelphia, 1178 pp.

TANDLER, B., AND J. H. POULSEN. 1976. Fusion of the envelope of mucous droplets with the luminal plasma membrane in acinar cells of the cat submandibular gland. J. Cell Biol., 68:775–781.

TAYLOR, J. M., W. M. MITCHELL, AND S. COHEN. 1972. Epidermal growth factor: physical and chemical properties. J. Biol. Chem., 247:5928–5934.

TO, L., AND R. H. TAMARIN. 1977. The relation of population density and adrenal gland weight in cycling and noncycling voles (*Microtus*). Ecology, 58:928–934.

VAUGHAN, M. K., G. M. VAUGHAN, AND R. J. REITER. 1973. Effect of ovariectomy and constant dark on the weight of reproductive and certain other organs of the female vole, *Microtus montanus*. J. Reprod. Fert., 32:9–14.

VESELÝ, V. 1923. Die Hilfsteile des Sehorgans von Microtus arvalis. Biol. Spisy Acad. Vet., Brno, 2:277–292.

WALLACE, L. J., AND L. M. PARTLOW. 1976. Adrenergic regulation of secretion of mouse saliva rich in nerve growth factor. Proc. Natl. Acad. Sci., 73: 4210–4214.

WEST, R. W., AND J. E. DOWLING. 1975. Anatomical evidence for cone and rod-like receptors in the gray squirrel, ground squirrel, and prairie dog retinas. J. Comp. Neurol., 159:439–460.

WHITE, T. E. 1959. The endocrine glands and evolution, no. 3: os cementum, hypsodonty, and diet. Contrib. Mus. Paleontol., Univ. Michigan, 13:211–265.

WOLFF, J. O., AND M. F. JOHNSON. 1979. Scent marking in the taiga voles, *Microtus xanthognathus*. J. Mamm., 60:400–404.

YOUNG, R. W. 1971. Shedding of discs from rod outer segments in the rhesus monkey. J. Ultrastruct. Res., 34:190–203.

YOUNG, R. W., AND B. DROZ. 1968. The renewal of protein in retinal rods and cones. J. Cell Biol., 39:169–184.

ZIMMERMAN, E. G. 1965. A comparison of habitat and food of two species of *Microtus*. J. Mamm., 46:605–612.

ONTOGENY

JOSEPH H. NADEAU

Abstract

THE literature on growth and development from conception to sexual maturity of New World *Microtus* is reviewed. The following characters and processes are described: 1) the prenatal period—spermatozoa, ova, ovulation, fertilization, pre- and post-implantation growth and development, implantation, trophoblastic giant cells, and mortality; 2) parturition—gestation period, stage of development, weight and length of neonates, litter size, sex ratio, and parental behavior towards neonates; and 3) postnatal period—growth, development, mortality, molting, and sexual maturation. The contribution of these ontogenetic attributes to a species' "ecological strategy" is evaluated.

Introduction

It could be argued that ontogeny occupies a central position in the description of the biology of any species. The basis for this argument is that growth and development are the processes whereby genetic information is translated into the anatomy, physiology, and behavior of adults. Changes that alter the patterns of ontogeny produce inherited variation in the ways of life of an organism. By studying the ontogeny of particular morphological, metabolic, or neurological attributes, an understanding can be gained not only of the causes and consequences of ontogenetic variation but also of the ways in which phylogenetic diversity is achieved. Indeed, the dependence of phylogenetic diversity on ontogenetic variation was one of the most important rules that Darwin recognized.

The variation in anatomy, physiology, and behavior exhibited by New World *Microtus* makes these species particularly well-suited for ontogenetic studies. The ontogeny of New World *Microtus*, however, has been studied unevenly. For example, a considerable literature exists on litter size (reviewed by Innes, 1978; Krebs and

Myers, 1974; Stenseth and Framstad, 1980). In addition, Hasler (1975) reviewed the literature on gestation period, ovulation, litter size, and sexual maturation, as well as several other aspects of reproduction. Most aspects, however, have hardly been studied. For example, Ozdzenski and Mystkowska's (1976*a*, 1976*b*) studies of *Clethrionomys glareolus* represent the only published descriptions of the stages of prenatal development of any New World or Old World microtine rodent.

The purpose of this chapter is to review the literature on growth and development from conception to sexual maturation of New World *Microtus*. I have tried to include all relevant observations, but I have not tried to include every reference for each observation.

The Prenatal Period

Of the various aspects of the ontogeny of New World *Microtus*, the prenatal period is least studied. As a result, the following descriptions are sketchy. To compensate for these deficiencies, relevant information for Old World *Microtus* is occasionally included.

Spermatozoa

Spermatozoa in New World *Microtus* have not been described in the published literature. In Old World *Microtus* such as *M. agrestis*, spermatozoa are hooked and have a strongly recurved head (Austin, 1957). The mean length of spermatozoa is 103.5 μm, mean head length 6.9 μm, and mean neck and midpiece length 27.4 μm.

Ova

The diameter of the ovum ranges from 65 to 70 μm at ovulation in *M. californicus* (Greenwald, 1956) and is 60 μm in *M. montanus* (Cross, 1971).

Fertilization

In Old World *Microtus* such as *M. agrestis*, there are an average of 4.1 ova in the oviduct at fertilization of nulliparous females (Austin, 1957). The mean number of spermatozoa in the ampulla of the oviduct is 124 (range 28 to 360). An average of 82% of ova are fertilized and only 2% of fertilized ova are polyspermic. The

TABLE 1
PRE-IMPLANTATION DEVELOPMENT IN *Microtus*. TIME IS MEASURED FROM COPULATION

Day of development		Stage of development
Day 0	0 h	Copulation.
	<15 h	Ovulation in *M. californicus* (Greenwald, 1956).
		Meiotic divisions begin after ovulation.
	15–18 h	Two-celled ova (Greenwald, 1956).
Day 2	48–72 h	In *M. californicus,* most ova have 16 cells (Greenwald, 1956).
Day 5		Implantation occurs in *M. pennsylvanicus* (Mallory and Clulow, 1977).

second maturation division in *M. californicus* is completed after fertilization (Greenwald, 1956).

Pre-implantation Growth and Development

The age of embryos is usually measured from the time of copulation (day 0, hour 0), and presence of spermatozoa in vaginal smears is considered evidence for recent copulation. The error involved is usually no more than 12–24 h. A summary of pre-implantation growth and development is provided in Table 1. Cleavage divisions begin about 40 h after copulation. Cells multiply rapidly and in some cases three to four cell divisions have occurred within 48 h. The average rate of cell division is therefore less than one division every 2–3 h.

Post-implantation Growth

Mallory and Clulow (1977, fig. 13) provide a key to the changes in uterine size and shape during gestation in *M. pennsylvanicus.* The average embryonic growth rate in *M. pennsylvanicus* is 0.25 to 0.40 g/day (Barbehenn, 1955).

The patterns of post-implantation growth of representative small rodents from day 10 to parturition are presented in Fig. 1. Before day 10, the embryo is too small and embedded too deeply in extraembryonic and uterine membranes to permit ready measure-

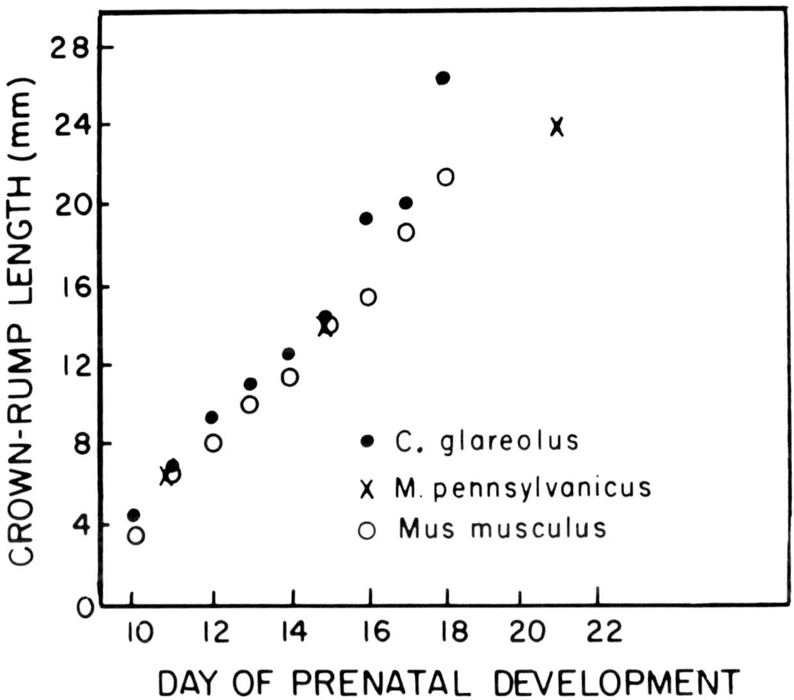

FIG. 1. Relation between crown–rump length and day of prenatal development in *Microtus pennsylvanicus, Mus musculus,* and *Clethrionomys glareolus.* Data are from Mallory and Clulow (1977), Theiler (1972), and Ozdzenski and Mystkowska (1976a), respectively.

ment. Data for *Clethrionomys glareolus* and *Mus musculus* are included for comparative purposes. Crown–rump length was used as a measure of size because more published data were available for crown–rump length than for body weight in *Microtus, Mus,* and *Clethrionomys.* However, crown–rump length and weight are highly correlated (*M. breweri*: r = 0.97, n = 6; *M. pennsylvanicus*: r = 0.98, n = 6; J. H. Nadeau, P. H. Kohn, and R. H. Tamarin, pers. comm.).

The rates of growth in *M. pennsylvanicus, C. glareolus,* and *Mus musculus* are lower and less variable between species during the early portion of prenatal development than during the late portion (Fig. 1). For example, the average growth rates between day 10 and day 16 for *M. pennsylvanicus, C. glareolus* and *Mus musculus* are 1.6, 2.0 and, 1.9 mm per day, respectively, whereas the average rates after day 16 for these three species are 2.0, 4.0 (after day 15), and 3.0 mm per day, respectively. The latter rates are 1.25- to 2-fold higher and relatively more variable than the former. These patterns of growth suggest that rates of embryonic growth for the early portion of prenatal development are highly conserved during rodent evolution and that the neonatal size (weight) characteristic of each species are realized only during the late portion of prenatal development.

The stage in development at which the rate of growth changes does not appear to be related to the appearance of any particular developmental feature. For example, the change in growth rate in *Mus musculus* occurs after most of the major external morphological features have appeared, whereas in *C. glareolus* the change occurs at a slightly earlier stage of morphological development.

The growth rates characteristic of each species show the expected high correlation with both the length of gestation and neonatal weight. Of the three species, *C. glareolus* has the highest growth rate, the lowest neonatal weight and the shortest gestation period, whereas *M. pennsylvanicus* has the lowest growth rate, the highest neonatal weight, and the longest gestation period. It is not known which, if any, of these three parameters is the independent variable. Despite these differences in growth rates, neonatal weights, and gestation periods, however, fetuses of these three species are born at about the same developmental stage; there is no evidence for precocity.

Post-implantation Development

I am not aware of any published description of post-implantation development in New World *Microtus* and therefore have included a summary of Ozdzenski and Mystkowska's (1976*a,* 1976*b*) description of development in *C. glareolus.* Their description focuses on external morphological characters primarily. Neither organogenesis nor the development of sexual characters appear to be described in the literature. Although *C. glareolus* is not a New World *Microtus,* the two are closely related and their ontogenies should be comparable. Moreover, although rates of development sometimes vary between species, the sequence in which developmental features appear is highly conserved, at least among rodents. Thus, post-implantation development in *C. glareolus,* a summary of which is provided in Table 2, may be representative of most microtine rodents.

Trophoblastic Giant Cells

In contrast to the corresponding cells in *Mus musculus,* the trophoblastic giant cells of *Microtus agrestis* (Copp, 1980), *M. arvalis* (Disse, *in* Copp, 1980), *Arvicola amphibius* (Sansom, 1922), and *Clethrionomys glareolus* (Ozdzenski and Mystkowska, 1976*a*) can be found at all levels of the endometrium, including the implantation site. In addition, microtine trophoblastic giant cells are of two types: non-migratory cells that remain at the implantation site and migratory cells of which there are in turn two types, small migratory cells and large migratory cells. One function of non-migratory cells is to anchor Reichert's membrane to the decidua. Reichert's membrane is an extraembryonic membrane covering the outer layer of trophectoderm and is secreted by the parietal endoderm (Snell and Stevens, 1966). Small migratory cells are not highly polypoid as are non-migratory cells and large migratory cells in *Microtus* and trophoblastic giant cells in *Mus.* The function of migratory giant cells is unknown. It is tempting to speculate that these cells might be related to the dispersed alkaline phosphatase activity observed in the endometrium of certain microtine rodents but not in other rodents such as *Mus* (Mohi Aldeen and Finn, 1970).

Prenatal Mortality

Pre-implantation mortality is usually measured as the difference between the number of corpora lutea and the number of implantation sites (including resorbing embryos) and is expressed as this difference divided by the number of corpora lutea ($\times 100$). It is assumed that all ova ovulated are fertilized. Other potential biases in the estimation of mortality rates include corpora lutea that are difficult to identify, accessory corpora lutea, polyovular follicles, twinning, and loss of entire litters. Hoffmann (1958) presents a thorough discussion of the problems associated with measurement of pre-implantation mortality.

A summary of the data on pre-implantation mortality is presented in Table 3. The average percentage of ova lost prior to

TABLE 2

POST-IMPLANTATION DEVELOPMENT OF *Clethrionomys glareolus* (DATA FROM OZDZENSKI AND MYSTKOWSKA, 1976*a*, 1976*b*)

Day of development	Stage of development
Day 4	Blastocyst elongates and implants. Decidual reaction occurs at site of attachment. Inner cell mass orients towards mesometrium. Egg cylinder divides into embryonic and extraembryonic portions. Migrating giant cells appear. Swelling is visible at implantation site. Amnionic cavity forms. Trophoblastic giant cells appear.
Day 5	Ectoplacental cone forms. Endoderm differentiates into embryonic and extraembryonic portions.
Day 6	Primitive streak forms. Mesodermal cells begin to migrate. Amnion and chlorion form. Implantation site is round and embryo is visible through uterine wall.
Day 7	Allantois forms and joins with chorion to form chorio-allantoic placenta.
Day 8	Embryo inverts germ layers to assume shape characteristic of most mammalian embryos. Brachial arches are visible. Eye, auditory vesicles, and heart are visible. Forelimb buds appear as small swellings. There are 13 to 21 somites.
Day 9	In some cases eye lens is visible. Forelimb bud is paddle-shaped. Hindlimb bud swelling is apparent. Trunk and tail are segmented.
Day 10	Maxillae are separated from head. Fore- and hindlimb buds begin to divide into limbs and feet. Retinal pigment is barely apparent. Digits begin to demarcate but are not yet separated.
Day 11	Retinal pigment is obvious. Pinnae are visible. Umbilical hernia appears. Limbs elongate.
Day 12	Eyelids partly cover eyes. Rudiments of vibrissae are visible. Digits are well demarcated.
Day 13	Pinnae cover auditory openings. Limb joint rudiments are apparent.
Day 14	Hair follicles are widely distributed over body. All digits are separated.
Day 15	Eyelids completely cover eyes. Pinnae attaches to skin opposite auditory meatus. Claws are visible. Pigment on head and dorsum is deposited. Umbilical hernia is lost.
Day 16	Skin folds are prominent. Secondary fusion of digits is complete.
Day 17	Fetuses are larger and skin folds are more prominent.
Day 18	Parturition.

TABLE 3
PRENATAL MORTALITY (NOT INCLUDING LOSS OF ENTIRE LITTERS) IN NEW WORLD *Microtus*

Species	Percent of ova lost: Pre-implantation mortality	Post-implantation mortality	References
Microtus breweri	10.9	8.1	Tamarin (1977)
M. californicus	—	7	Greenwald (1957)
	—	4.7	Lidicker (1973)
M. montanus	5.9	2.6–3.9	Hoffmann (1958)
M. ochrogaster	11.0	—	Corthum (1967)
	6.6 (range 3.4–12.9)	7.0	Keller and Krebs (1970)
	9.5	1.6	Rose and Gaines (1978)
M. pennsylvanicus	7.3	8.4	Beer et al. (1957)
	7	—	Corthum (1967)
	9 (range 4.7–45.5)	6.4	Keller and Krebs (1970)
	6.1	2.2	Tamarin (1977)
	—	3.6	Innes (1978)

implantation is 8.14% ($SD = 2.00$). The highest reported rate of mortality is in *Microtus ochrogaster,* the lowest in *M. montanus.*

Post-implantation mortality is usually measured as the difference between the number of resorptions and number of living and resorbing embryos and is expressed as the number of resorptions divided by the number of living and resorbing embryos ($\times 100$). At least three factors represent potential biases in comparison of the numbers of ovulated eggs and litter size. These factors include transmigration of pre-implantation embryos from one uterine horn to the other, ovulation of more than one ovum from a single ovarian follicle, twinning, and loss of entire litters. In *M. pennsylvanicus,* the average number of transmigrated ova per litter is 0.07, the average number of embryos resulting from multiple ovulation per litter is 0.05, and the average number of twins per litter is 0.02 (Beer et al., 1957).

A summary of the data on post-implantation mortality is presented in Table 3. The average percentage of embryos lost after implantation but before parturition is 5.42% (*SD* = 2.53). Among New World *Microtus* the highest reported rate of mortality occurs in *M. pennsylvanicus,* the lowest in *M. ochrogaster.* In *M. townsendii,* 68.2% of unsuccessful litters are lost during gestation or at parturition (Anderson and Boonstra, 1979).

The rate of prenatal mortality depends on parity. In some species (*M. breweri,* for example), the rate is correlated negatively with parity (Tamarin, 1977), whereas in other species (*M. arvalis,* for example) the rate is correlated positively with parity except for the smallest females (Pelikan, 1970).

Parturition

Gestation Period

The average length of gestation in New World *Microtus* and other representative rodents is given in Table 4. The average period is 21.4 days (*SD* = 1.29). The shortest gestation periods are less than 20 days in some populations of *M. ochrogaster* (Fitch, 1957), the longest about 24 days in both *M. oregoni* (Cowan and Arsenault, 1954) and *M. pinetorum* (Kirkpatrick and Valentine, 1970). In some species (*M. agrestis* and *Dicrostonyx groenlandicus,* for example), gestation can be prolonged if the female is lactating (Breed, 1969; Manning, 1954). This effect, however, does not increase the length of gestation considerably. In most cases, it is not clear whether the delay results from delayed post-partum mating, delayed implantation, or decreased post-implantation growth.

Stage of Development

Neonatal *Microtus* are hairless and unpigmented, their eyes and ears are closed, their teeth have not erupted, their anus is not patent, but their vibrissae are apparent. These descriptions apply to neonatal *M. breweri* (Rothstein, 1976), *M. californicus* (Hatfield, 1935; Selle, 1928), *M. montanus* (Bailey, 1924), *M. ochrogaster* (Kruckenberg et al., 1973; Richmond and Conaway, 1969), *M. pennsylvanicus* (Innes and Millar, 1979; Lee and Horvath, 1969), and *M. oregoni* (Cowan and Arsenault, 1954). There is no evidence that fetuses of these species are born at different stages of development.

TABLE 4
LENGTH (DAYS) OF GESTATION IN NEW WORLD *Microtus**

Species	Mean (*SD*)	References
Microtus abbreviatus	21.5	Morrison et al. (1976)
M. californicus	21	Greenwald (1956); Hatfield (1935); Selle (1928)
M. miurus	21	Morrison et al. (1976)
M. montanus	21	Bailey (1924); Hoffmann (1958)
M. ochrogaster	<20	Fitch (1957)
	21	Morrison et al. (1976); Richmond and Conaway (1969)
	22.8	Kenny et al. (1977)
M. oeconomus	20.5	Dieterich and Preston (1977); Morrison et al. (1976)
M. oregoni	24	Cowan and Arsenault (1954)
M. pennsylvanicus	21	Lee and Horvath (1969)
	21	Lee et al. (1970); Mallory and Clulow (1977)
	21.0 (0.2)	Kenny et al. (1977)
	20	Innes and Millar (1981)
M. pinetorum	24	Kirkpatrick and Valentine (1970)
M. townsendii†	22	MacFarlane and Taylor (1982)

* Further data can be found in Hasler (1975).
† Twenty-four days in lactating females.

Weight and Length of Neonates

Weights of neonatal *Microtus* are given in Table 5. Little variation in weight is observed in species such as *M. californicus* (range 2.7 to 2.8 g) and *M. ochrogaster* (range 2.8 to 3.1 g). By contrast, average weight of *M. pennsylvanicus* varies by more than one g among samples (range 1.9 to 3.2). Few data are available for other species.

Neonatal weight often depends on litter size and maternal weight. In some populations of *M. pinetorum,* weight of the entire litter is correlated with maternal weight and therefore, because litter size is independent of maternal weight, weight of each neonate in a litter depends on maternal weight (Paul, 1970). In other populations of *M. pinetorum,* correlations have not been found between

TABLE 5
WEIGHT (G) AT BIRTH IN NEW WORLD *Microtus*

Species	Mean weight (*SD*)	Stage of develop-ment	References
Microtus breweri	3.5	Neonate	J. H. Nadeau, P. H. Kohn, and R. H. Tamarin (pers. comm.)
M. californicus	2.7	Neonate	Selle (1928)
	2.8	Neonate	Hatfield (1935)
M. miurus	2.9	Neonate	Morrison et al. (1977)
M. montanus	2.5	Full term	Hoffmann (1958)
	3.9	Neonate	Bailey (1924)
M. ochrogaster	2.8	Neonate	Richmond and Conaway (1969)
	2.9 (0.1)	—	Fitch (1957)
	2.8 (0.4)	Neonate	Martin (1956)
	3.1	Neonate	Kruckenberg et al. (1973)
M. oeconomus	3.0	Neonate	Morrison et al. (1977)
M. oregoni	1.7 (range 1.6–2.2)	Neonate	Cowan and Arsenault (1954)
M. pennsylvanicus	1.9	Full term	Hamilton (1937)
	2.1 (range 1.6–2.9)	Neonate	Hamilton (1937)
	2.1 (range 1.6–3.0)	Neonate	Hamilton (1941)
	2.3 ± 0.1	Neonate	Innes and Millar (1981)
	2.0–3.0	Neonate	Lee and Horvath (1969)
	2.3	Neonate	Innes and Millar (1979)
	3.2*	Neonate	Morrison et al. (1977)
M. pinetorum	2.0	Neonate	Lochmiller et al. (1982*a*)
	2.2	Neonate	Hamilton (1938)

* Pups were weighed 0–3 days after parturition.

litter size (weight) and maternal weight, or between litter size (weight) and neonatal weight (Lochmiller et al., 1982*a*). In *M. ochrogaster,* total litter weight increases linearly with increasing litter size from litters of one to four, whereas litters of five and six do not weigh significantly more than litters of four (Richmond and Conaway, 1969).

By comparison, individual pup weight is inversely dependent on litter size. Here, the mean weight of pups in litters of size one to

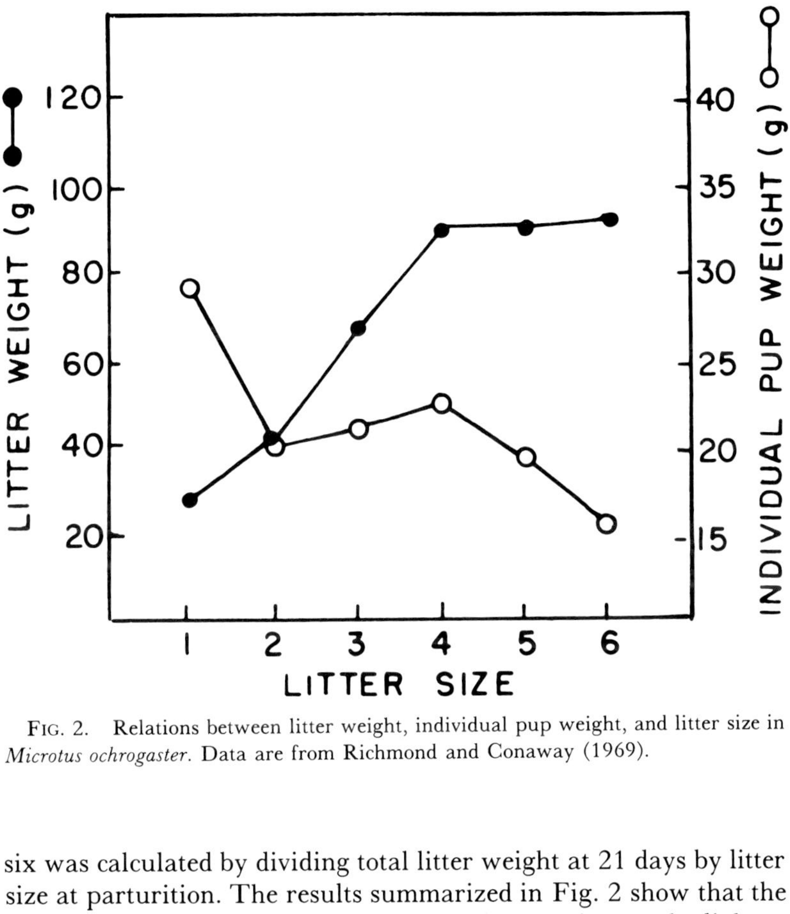

FIG. 2. Relations between litter weight, individual pup weight, and litter size in *Microtus ochrogaster*. Data are from Richmond and Conaway (1969).

six was calculated by dividing total litter weight at 21 days by litter size at parturition. The results summarized in Fig. 2 show that the heaviest pups were found in the smallest litters whereas the lightest pups were found in the largest litters. This relationship is not linear as would be expected if mothers invested similar amounts of energy in each pup regardless of the number of pups in the litter. Instead, the observed relationship between the weight of the entire litter and of individual pups (Fig. 2) suggests that reproductive efficiency is optimized with litters of size 4. In fact, in the population from which these data were collected, the mean litter size was 3.8 (Richmond and Conaway, 1969). Unfortunately, most studies do not present the necessary data to determine whether such variation in neonatal weight is a general pattern.

TABLE 6
LITTER SIZE IN NEW WORLD *Microtus*

Species	Mean (*SD*)	Range	Origin	References
Microtus abbreviatus	3.0	—	Lab	Morrison et al. (1976)
M. breweri	3.4 (1.1)	—	Field	Tamarin (1977)
M. californicus	4.7 (0.1)	1–9	Lab	Colvin and Colvin (1970); Selle (1928)
	4.6 (0.5)	1–9	Field	Greenwald (1956, 1957); Hoffmann (1958); Lidicker (1973)
M. chrotorrhinus	3.6 (0.1)	2–5	Field	Timm et al. (1977); Coventry (1937); see also references in Timm et al. (1977)
M. longicaudus	4.0	1–7	Lab	Colvin and Colvin (1970)
	4.9	4–6	Field	Hoffmeister (1956)
M. miurus	3.9	—	Lab	Morrison et al. (1976)
	8.2	—	Field	References in Hoffmann (1958)
M. montanus	6.0	3–9	Lab	Colvin and Colvin (1970)
	6.0 (0.4)	1–10	Field	Hoffmann (1958); Howell (1924); Negus and Pinter (1965); Negus et al. (1977); Vaughan (1969)
M. ochrogaster	3.9 (0.4)	1–8	Lab	Colvin and Colvin (1970); Kenney et al. (1977); Richmond and Conaway (1969); Thomas and Birney (1979)
	3.5 (0.4)	1–8	Field	Jameson (1947); Martin (1956); Fitch (1957); Layne (1958); Corthum (1967); Keller and Krebs (1970); Cole and Batzli (1978); Rose and Gaines (1978); see also references in Hoffmann (1958)
M. oeconomus	4.0 (0.1)	—	Lab	Morrison et al. (1976)
	6.6 (1.0)	—	Field	Whitney (1977); references in Hoffmann (1958)
M. oregoni	3.3 (0.7)	1–6	Lab	Colvin and Colvin (1970); Cowan and Arsenault (1954)
M. pennsylvanicus	4.4 (0.9)	1–9	Lab	Beer et al. (1957); Colvin and Colvin (1970); Lee and Horvath (1969); Kenney et al. (1977); Morrison et al. (1976); Poiley (1949)

TABLE 6
CONTINUED

Species	Mean (*SD*)	Range	Origin	References
	4.9 (0.6)	1–11	Field	Corthum (1967); Coventry (1937); Hamilton (1941); Innes and Millar (1981); Keller and Krebs (1970); Kott and Robinson (1963); Storm and Sanderson (1968); Tamarin (1977)
	3.1 (0.1)	—	Field	Cowan and Arsenault (1954); references in Hoffmann (1958)
M. pinetorum	1.9 (0.2)	1–3	Lab	Gentry (1968); Kirkpatrick and Valentine (1970)
	2.1 (0.2)	1–5	Field	Gentry (1968); Glass (1949); Goertz (1971); Kirkpatrick and Valentine (1970); Linsdale (1928)
	2.2	—	Lab	Lochmiller et al. (1982*a*); Paul (1970)
	3.1 (0.1)	—	Lab	Schadler and Butterstein (1979)
M. richardsoni	6.0	—	Field	Anderson et al. (1976)
	7.3	7–8	Field	Anderson and Rand (1943)
M. townsendii	4.8	2–6	Lab	MacFarlane and Taylor (1982)
	5.4	2–7	Field	MacFarlane and Taylor (1982)
M. xanthognathus	8.4 (0.6)	6–13	Field	Wolff and Lidicker (1980); Youngman (1975)

Litter Size

Mean litter sizes for fifteen species of New World *Microtus* are given in Table 6. The mean litter size (field samples only) was 4.9 (*SD* = 2.0). Some species have exceptional litter sizes: *M. pinetorum* has an exceptionally small litter size, *M. miurus* (field sample) and *M. xanthognathus* exceptionally large litter sizes (Table 6).

Litter size in microtine rodents depends on a number of factors including parity, age, season, year, and conditions in the mating colony (Innes, 1978; Stenseth and Framstad, 1980). Usually the first litter is the smallest. Few other generalizations are possible, however. Litter size increases with age and parity in some species (*M. montanus* [Negus and Pinter, 1965], *M. californicus* [Greenwald, 1957; Hoffmann, 1958]), but not in others (*M. pennsylvanicus* [Keller and Krebs, 1970; Poiley, 1949; Storm and Sanderson, 1968], *M. ochrogaster* [Keller and Krebs, 1970; Rose and Gaines, 1978], and *M. townsendii* [Anderson and Boonstra, 1979]). Litter size depends on parity in some populations of a species (Negus and Pinter, 1965), but not in others (Hoffmann, 1958). Litter size often increases in the first few litters and then declines, such as in *M. oregoni* (Cowan and Arsenault, 1954) and *M. ochrogaster* (Richmond and Conaway, 1969). Litter size sometimes varies considerably between field and laboratory estimates. For example, *M. oeconomus* in laboratory colonies has a mean litter size of 4.0 pups ($SD = 0.1$), whereas in natural populations mean litter size is 6.6 ($SD = 1.0$). Another striking example is *M. miurus,* which has a mean litter size of 3.9 pups in laboratory colonies and 8.2 pups in natural populations. Clearly, litter size is subject to a variety of influences.

Sex Ratio

With four exceptions the sex ratio among species of New World *Microtus* is approximately 1:1 (Table 7). The first exception involves *M. montanus* in which there is a significant deficiency of males born in laboratory colonies (Vaughan et al., 1973). The origin of the deficiency has not been determined. The second exception occurs in at least one population of *M. pennsylvanicus* (J. H. Nadeau and R. H. Tamarin, pers. comm.). Pregnant females in samples of live-trapped mice from a low-density population near Natick, Massachusetts, were autopsied and the morphological sex of the fetuses determined. There were significantly more males among fetuses than among adults (Table 8). At least two factors affect sex ratio in the Natick population; the first results in an excess of males among fetuses and the second restores an equal sex ratio among adults. Two other populations in southeastern Massachusetts had a 1:1 sex ratio among both fetuses and adults. An important implication of these data is that the usual assumption that an even sex ratio at recruitment reflects an even primary sex ratio may not be supported. Because sex ratio is not usually estimated among fetuses, it is impossible to determine whether skewed prenatal sex ratios are exceptional.

The third and fourth (possible) exceptions are found in *M. agres-*

TABLE 7
ADULT SEX RATIOS (♂♂:♀♀) IN NEW WORLD *Microtus*

Species	Sex ratio	Stage of development	Origin	References
Microtus breweri	1.2:1	Adult	Field	Tamarin (1977)
M. californicus	0.6:1	Neonate	Lab	Selle (1928)
	1:1	Fetus and neonate	—	Greenwald (1957)
	1:1	Adult	Field	Lidicker (1973)
M. montanus	0.40:1*	—	Lab	Vaughan et al. (1973)
M. oregoni	1.1:1	Neonate	Lab	Cowan and Arsenault (1954)
M. pennsylvanicus	1.1:1	Adult	Field	Myers and Krebs (1971); J. H. Nadeau and R. H. Tamarin (pers. comm.); Tamarin (1977)
M. xanthognathus	1:1	Juvenile	Lab and field	Wolff and Lidicker (1980)
M. agrestis	1:1	Fetus and adult	Field	Myllymäki (1977)

* $P < 0.05$.

tis (Myllymäki, 1977) and in *M. richardsoni* (Anderson et al., 1976) in which the sex ratio at recruitment of the first litters of the breeding season are skewed towards females, whereas the ratio was 1:1 later in the year. There are two explanations for these observations: either the primary sex ratio is uneven, or weanling males emigrate or die more often than weanling females early but not late in the season. Because the primary sex ratio in the populations studied by Myllymäki (1977) was even, the explanation for the biased sex ratio must involve differential emigration or mortality. In the study by Anderson et al. (1976), the primary sex ratio was not measured and as a result these explanations were not evaluated.

The sex ratios observed in natural populations of New World *Microtus* do not support Stenseth's (1977) contention that sex ratios are biased slightly towards females in low-density populations and are biased heavily towards females in high-density populations because of inbreeding effects. On the contrary, in the examples given, an even sex ratio or an excess of males are found in both low- and high-density populations (Tables 7, 8).

Some autosomal genotypes are associated with biased sex ratios: certain transferrin genotypes are associated with an excess of males in *M. pennsylvanicus* (Myers and Krebs, 1971). The mechanism by which transferrin, or loci linked to transferrin, and sex ratio are associated is unknown.

Parental Behavior at Parturition and during Postnatal Development

In *M. ochrogaster,* both parents clean up afterbirth and groom young (Fitch, 1957; Thomas and Birney, 1979). In some cases, post-partum breeding, which is common in some microtine rodents (Gustafsson et al., 1980; Kirkpatrick and Valentine, 1970; Lee and Horvath, 1969; Lee et al., 1970; Morrison et al., 1976), occurs before parturition is complete (Richmond and Conaway, 1969).

Wilson (1982) demonstrated that *M. ochrogaster* pups receive more bodily contact than *M. pennsylvanicus* pups. She hypothesized that these differences in social environments during early development could have important effects on adult social systems (for reviews, see Madison, 1980; Thomas and Birney, 1979).

The Postnatal Period

Postnatal Growth

Hoffmeister and Getz (1968) provided a detailed description of growth and age-classes in *M. ochrogaster.* The descriptions included five external, eleven cranial, and two limb measurements, eye-lens weight, and closure of sutures. Most growth and development occurs in the first 2 months. A summary of growth patterns from birth to 1 year of age in laboratory colonies of *M. pennsylvanicus, M. oeconomus, M. miurus,* and *M. abbreviatus* is provided by Morrison et al. (1977).

The average rate of growth between parturition and day 21 of postnatal development is 1.1 g/day in *M. californicus* (Selle, 1928) and 1.0 g/day in *M. montanus* (Bailey, 1924); the mean adult weight for these two species are 50.1 g (Selle, 1928) and 50.0 g (Bailey, 1924), respectively. Lochmiller et al. (1982*b*) found that between days 22 and 46, *M. pinetorum* gained an average of 0.8 g/day; they concluded that the metabolic efficiency of *M. pinetorum* was high

TABLE 8

PRENATAL SEX RATIOS (♂♂:♀♀) IN NATURAL POPULATIONS OF *Microtus breweri* AND *M. pennsylvanicus* IN EASTERN MASSACHUSETTS

Species	Observed ratio	Expected ratio*	χ^2_1
Microtus breweri			
Muskeget Island	41:25 (1.64:1)	36:30	1.53 ($P > 0.05$)
M. pennsylvanicus			
Plymouth	16:12 (1.33:1)	15:13	0.14 ($P > 0.05$)
Natick	22:4 (5.5:1)	14:12	9.90 ($P < 0.005$)

* Expected ratios were based on number of adult males and females. For *M. breweri*, 54.5% of live-trapped voles were males (Tamarin, 1977), and for *M. pennsylvanicus*, 53% were males (Myers and Krebs, 1971).

relative not only to other species of *Microtus* but also to other representative rodents.

The average rate of growth in the first 21 days obscures changes in the growth rate during development (Fig. 3). In some species (*M. pennsylvanicus*, for example), the growth rate remains relatively constant throughout the first 21 days of postnatal development. The mean growth rate is 0.38 g/day ($SD = 0.07$) (Innes and Millar, 1979). In other species, the growth curve appears to be biphasic; the growth rate in early development is higher than in later development. In *M. californicus*, for example, the average growth rate is 1.07 g/day ($SD = 0.17$) from parturition to day 7 and 0.76 g/day ($SD = 0.20$) from day 8 to day 21 (Hatfield, 1935). By contrast, the pattern is reversed in at least two populations of *M. ochrogaster* (Kruckenberg et al., 1973; Lee and Horvath, 1969); that is, the growth rate in early development is lower than in later development. From parturition to day 10, for example, the mean growth rate is 0.58 g/day ($SD = 0.9$), whereas from day 11 to day 14 the mean growth rate is 1.45 g/day ($SD = 0.57$) (Lee and Horvath, 1969). A similar pattern occurs in *M. oregoni* (Cowan and Arsenault, 1954) and in some populations of *M. pennsylvanicus* (Hamilton, 1941). The age at which the change in growth rate occurs also varies. The change occurs between days 12 and 13 in *M. ochrogaster*, between days 7 and 8 in *M. californicus*, and days 10 and 11 in *M. pennsylvanicus*. The change invariably occurs, however, when pup weight is between 8 and 10 g. The significance

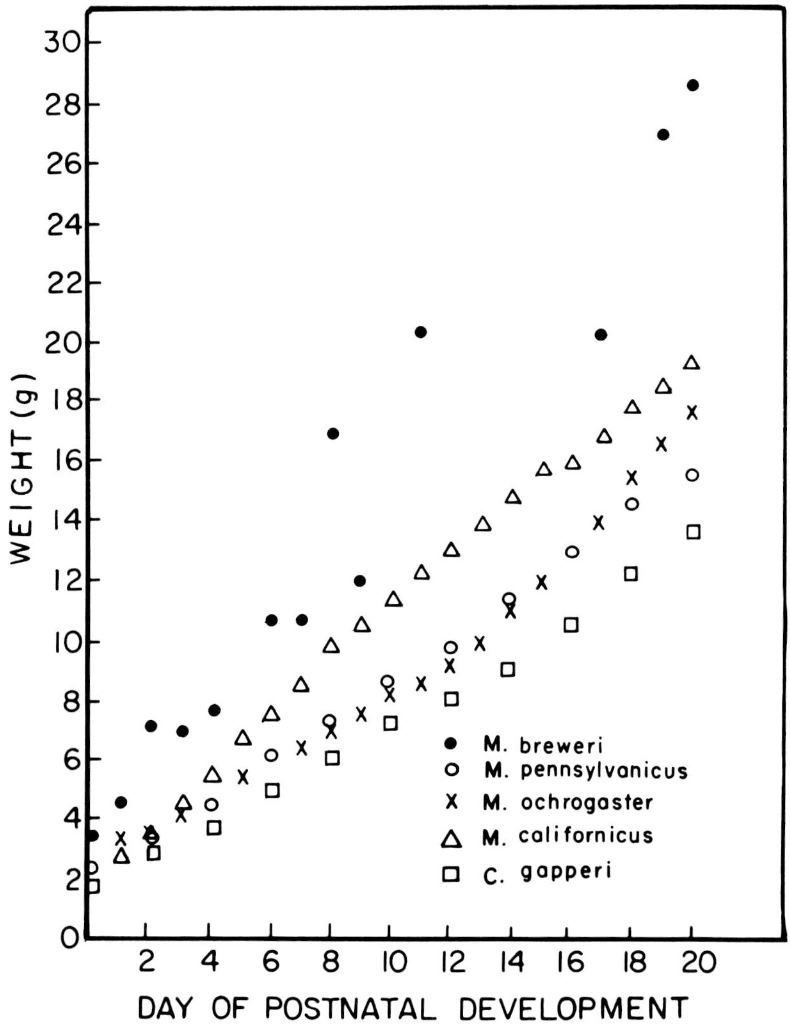

FIG. 3. Patterns of postnatal growth in representative New World *Microtus*. The pattern for *Clethrionomys gapperi* is presented for comparison. Data are from the following sources: *Microtus breweri* (P. H. Kohn, J. H. Nadeau, and R. H. Tamarin, pers. comm.); *M. pennsylvanicus* (Innes and Millar, 1979); *M. californicus* (Hatfield, 1935); *M. ochrogaster* (Kruckenberg et al., 1973).

of these patterns is not known. Because descriptions of the stages of development of these three species were not published, it is impossible to determine whether the change in growth rate is related to the appearance of a particular developmental character or reflects an adaptation to particular demographic or environmental conditions.

Postnatal Development

Data on postnatal development in New World *Microtus* are summarized in Table 9. In addition, Pépin and Baron (1978) described the development of locomotor activity during postnatal development of *M. pennsylvanicus*. Three stages were recognized: 1) the nest stage (days 0 to 7), characterized by random movements; 2) a transitional stage (days 8 to 10), in which crawling was first observed and pups first left the nest; and 3) third stage (days 11 to 21), in which coordination of movement was refined.

Postnatal Mortality

Postnatal mortality is usually calculated by comparing the number of young at week t and the number of lactating females at week $t - 3$. Death, emigration, or immigration of mothers or young, and unrecognized pregnancies can influence these calculations. In *M. townsendii*, approximately 7.5% of young are lost before recruitment (Anderson and Boonstra, 1979). The loss occurs primarily in litters of average size. Of the entire litters that are lost, 13.6% are lost during the first week of lactation and 9.1% are lost during each of the next two weeks. Mortality often depends upon season. In *M. ochrogaster*, for example, the ratio of juveniles to pregnant females ranges from 0.69 in spring to 2.85 in fall (Cole and Batzli, 1978). It should be noted that this ratio is subject to a number of other influences such as emigration (see section on sex ratios above).

Molting

New World *Microtus* have two molts, a juvenile molt and an adult molt. There is considerable variation in the timing of these molts. Ecke and Kinney (1956) studied the molting pattern during the development of *M. californicus* collected in the field. The first or juvenile molt occurred at 23–25 days after parturition when pups

TABLE 9
POSTNATAL DEVELOPMENT IN NEW WORLD *Microtus*

Character	Day of development character appears	Species	References
Gray or black dorsum and pink ventrum	1	*M. breweri*	Rothstein (1976)
		M. californicus	Hatfield (1935)
		M. ochrogaster	Richmond and Conaway (1969)
		M. oregoni	Cowan and Arsenault (1954)
		M. pennsylvanicus	J. H. Nadeau, P. H. Kohn, and R. H. Tamarin, (pers. comm.)
Brown fur	2	*M. breweri*	Rothstein (1976)
		M. ochrogaster	Fitch (1957)
	3	*M. californicus*	Hatfield (1935)
		M. oregoni	Cowan and Arsenault (1954)
		M. pennsylvanicus	Hamilton (1941)
	5	*M. montanus*	Bailey (1924)
Incisors emerge	1–2	*M. ochrogaster*	Fitch (1957); Kruckenberg et al. (1973)
	3–6	*M. breweri*	Rothstein (1976)
	5	*M. montanus*	Bailey (1924)
	5.5	*M. oregoni*	Cowan and Arsenault (1954)
	6–7	*M. pennsylvanicus*	Hamilton (1941)
Molars emerge	7	*M. montanus*	Bailey (1924)
	8	*M. pennsylvanicus*	Hamilton (1941)
	11.5	*M. oregoni*	Cowan and Arsenault (1954)
Crawl	3–4	*M. breweri*	Rothstein (1976)
	4–5	*M. ochrogaster*	Fitch (1957); Richmond and Conaway (1969)
	6.5	*M. oregoni*	Cowan and Arsenault (1954)
	9	*M. pennsylvanicus*	J. H. Nadeau, P. H. Kohn, and R. H. Tamarin (pers. comm.)
Eyes open	5–6	*M. breweri*	Rothstein (1976)
	5–10	*M. ochrogaster*	Fitch (1957); Kruckenberg et al. (1973); Lee and Horvath (1969)
	8–11 (7.1–8.9 g)	*M. montanus*	Bailey (1924); Fitch (1957); Jannett (1978); Kruckenberg et al. (1973); Richmond and Conaway (1969)

TABLE 9
CONTINUED

Character	Day of development character appears	Species	References
	8–9 (10.2 g)	*M. pennsylvanicus*	Hamilton (1937, 1941); Innes and Millar (1979, 1981)
	9–10 (8.3–11.4 g)	*M. californicus*	Greenwald (1956); Hatfield (1935); Selle (1928)
	9 (7.3 g)	*M. oeconomus*	Morrison et al. (1954)
	10–11	*M. oregoni*	Cowan and Arsenault (1954)
	12 (7.0 g)	*M. pinetorum*	Hamilton (1938)
Pinnae unfold	1	*M. breweri*	Rothstein (1976)
	2–3	*M. ochrogaster*	Kruckenberg et al. (1973)
		M. pennsylvanicus	J. H. Nadeau, P. H. Kohn, and R. H. Tamarin (pers. comm.)
	2.5	*M. oregoni*	Cowan and Arsenault (1954)
Eat solid food	8	*M. pennsylvanicus*	Hamilton (1941)
	10–14	*M. ochrogaster*	Richmond and Conaway (1969)
Weaning	8–9	*M. breweri*	Rothstein (1976)
	11–14 (15 g)	*M. pennsylvanicus*	Hamilton (1937, 1941); Innes and Millar (1979, 1981); Lee and Horvath (1969)
	12–17 (10.7–13.1 g)	*M. montanus*	Bailey (1924); Fitch (1957); Jannett (1978); Kruckenberg et al. (1973); Richmond and Conaway (1969)
	13	*M. oregoni*	Cowan and Arsenault (1954)
	14 (14 g)	*M. californicus*	Greenwalt (1956); Hatfield (1935)
	15–17 (11.9–13.1 g)	*M. montanus*	Fitch (1957); Kruckenberg et al. (1973); Jannett (1978)
	17 (11 g)	*M. pinetorum*	Hamilton (1938)
	11.9–18.4 g	*M. ochrogaster*	Cole and Batzli (1979)

were 110 to 120 mm long and was complete by day 45. The second or adult molt began by day 50 and was complete by day 60. The first molt in *M. pinetorum* begins by day 35 and the second at day 50 (Hamilton, 1938). In *M. ochrogaster,* the first molt begins between day 21 and day 28 and the second molt between day 40 and day 84 (Jameson, 1947; Richmond and Conaway, 1969). In *M. californicus,* the first molt begins by day 21 and the second by day 56 (Hatfield, 1935). In *M. breweri,* the first molt occurs when mice are 136–150 mm long and the second when mice are 161–165 mm long (Rowsemitt et al., 1975). Many of these studies also described the pattern of molting.

Sexual Maturation

Spermatogenesis in New World *Microtus* has not been studied, but it was described in at least one species of Old World *Microtus* (Grocock, 1972). On day 1 after parturition, only gonocytes and supporting cells are found in the seminiferous tubules. On day 3 spermatogonia are found, on day 12 primary spermatocytes, and on day 24 round spermatids. The first meiotic divisions begin on day 21 and mature spermatozoa are first found on day 37.

The criterion usually used for determining sexual maturity in males is the presence of mature sperm in the epididymis. The weight, but not necessarily the age, at which male New World *Microtus* become sexually mature appears to be similar among species. Maturity is attained at 35–41 g in *M. californicus* (Greenwald, 1956; Hoffmann, 1958), at 35 g in *M. montanus* (Hoffmann, 1958), at 25–35 g in *M. pennsylvanicus* (Hamilton, 1937; Lee and Horvath, 1969), and at 30 g in *M. townsendii* (MacFarlane and Taylor, 1981). Males first mate at 42 days of age in *M. californicus* (Hatfield, 1935) and at 6–8 weeks in *M. pinetorum* (MacFarlane and Taylor, 1981). *M. pinetorum* first sire at 52 days of age, but the average age is 60 days (Schadler and Butterstein, 1979).

In females, the presence corpora lutea, embryos, or lactation tissue is evidence for sexual maturity. On the average, females become sexually mature at 25–35 g in *M. californicus* (Greenwald, 1956; Hoffmann, 1958), at 33 g in *M. montanus* (Hoffmann, 1958), at 25 g in *M. pennsylvanicus* (Hamilton, 1937), at 70–100 g in *M. richardsoni* (Anderson et al., 1976), and at 25–45 g in *M. townsendii* (MacFarlane and Taylor, 1981). It should be noted that, because adult weight varies considerably between these species, comparisons of weights at sexual maturity may not be particularly informative. In *M. ochrogaster* females, the first mating occurs at 33–34 days of age but the first litter is not produced until females are 60 days old (Richmond and Conaway, 1969). Cole and Batzli (1979) found that female *M. ochrogaster* first reproduce at 81–100 days of age. Fitch (1957) reported *M. ochrogaster* females that were pregnant at 4 weeks of age and Beer et al. (1957) found *M. pennsylvanicus* females that bred at 25 days of age. Schadler and Butterstein (1979) found that, although female *M. pinetorum* first conceive at 77 days of age, the average age at first conception was 105 days. Sterile matings (usually the first mating) have been described in *M. oeconomus* (Hoyte, 1955), *M. californicus* (Greenwald, 1956), *M. pinetorum* (Kirkpatrick and Valentine, 1970), and *M. pennsylvanicus* (Mallory and Clulow, 1977).

In *M. montanus,* the age and weight at sexual maturity in females varies considerably between years (Negus et al., 1977). In some years, most females become sexually mature at 13–14 g, with the lowest weight at pregnancy of 18 g. In other years, females became sexually mature at 24–29 g, with the lowest weight at pregnancy of 30 g. The estimated age at sexual maturity was 2–3 weeks in some years and 7–8 weeks in others.

The age at which females become sexually mature depends on a number of factors including nutrition and social conditions. Greenwald (1956) and Negus and Pinter (1966) showed that sexual maturation in *M. montanus* is significantly influenced by diet. Social factors are also important. In *M. ochrogaster,* the vagina opens earlier and the first litter is born sooner when females are paired with adult males than when paired with male littermates (Hasler and Nalbandov, 1974).

Synthesis

One of the more useful ways to evaluate these diverse ontogenetic attributes as part of a species' "ecological strategy" involves r- and K-selection. According to the theory of r- and K-selection (MacArthur and Wilson, 1967), attributes such as occurrence in uncertain climates and high productivity are typical of r-selected species, whereas occurrence in more certain climates and high efficiency are typical of K-selected species (Pianka, 1970; Southwood et al., 1974). There are several reasons for applying the theory of r- and K-selection to ontogenetic data for New World *Microtus*. First, r- and K-selection is one of the few theories that combines ontogeny and reproduction into a single argument. Second, and perhaps more importantly, it has been argued that the strength of population cycles in microtine rodents depends in part on the location of a species' overall ecological strategy on an r-K continuum (Tamarin, 1978). Although there are difficulties in its application and evaluation, the theory was nevertheless applied to the ontogenetic data for New World *Microtus* to determine whether the ontogenetic attributes are consistent with the theory of r- and K-selection.

Only those species and ontogenetic attributes were included that provided the most complete set of data for analysis. This set consisted of six species and four attributes. For each species, the character of each attribute was identified as being that expected of an r-selected species, or alternatively, that of a K-selected species. r-Selected species were expected to have high rates of prenatal mortality, low neonatal weights, large litter sizes, and high rates of postnatal development; K-selected species were expected to have converse attributes (Pianka, 1970; Southwood et al., 1974). To determine whether a particular attribute in a given species was more r- or more K-selected relative to the same attribute in other species, the following procedure, which is illustrated with the data for neonatal weight, was used. If more than one estimate of neonatal weight was available for a species, an average weight was calculated. An average for all species was then calculated. If less than the mean weight for all species, the weight for a given species was considered to be r-selected, whereas if the weight was greater than the mean weight for all species, the weight for a given species was considered to be K-selected. This procedure was also applied to data for litter size. For prenatal mortality and postnatal development, modifications in this procedure were necessary. For estimating the rate of prenatal mortality, the sum of the rates of pre-implantation and of post-implantation mortality was calculated for each species. These sums were then used to calculate a mean rate for all species and to assign the r or K status for each species as described above. For the rate of postnatal development, each species was given a score corresponding to the time of appearance of a given developmental feature, such as emergence of incisors; a low score corresponded to

TABLE 10
R-K PROFILE OF CERTAIN ONTOGENETIC ATTRIBUTES IN SELECTED SPECIES OF NEW WORLD *Microtus*

Species	Prenatal mortality	Neonatal weight	Litter size	Rate of postnatal development
Microtus breweri	r	K	K	r
M. montanus	K	K	r	r
M. ochrogaster	K	K	K	r
M. oregoni	—	r	K	K
M. pennsylvanicus	r	r	r	K
M. pinetorum	—	r	K	K

early appearance, a high score to later appearance, and a tie score to similar times of appearance. The developmental features included appearance of fur, emergence of incisors, emergence of molars, crawling, opening of eyelids, unfolding of pinnae, and weaning. For each species an average of these scores was calculated and these averages were used as described above to determine the r or K status for each species.

Results of the analysis are presented in Table 10. If each attribute is assumed to contribute equally to a species ecological strategy, then none of the species included in the analysis were uniformly r-selected or uniformly K-selected. Species such as *M. breweri* and *M. pinetorum,* which are thought to be among the more K-selected species of *Microtus,* were r-selected for certain attributes. By contrast, other species such as *M. pennsylvanicus,* which is thought to be relatively r-selected, was K-selected for certain attributes. There are at least two complementary explanations for the absence of uniformity. The first involves the assumption that each of these four attributes contributes equally to a species ecological strategy. It is more likely that some attributes are more important than others. Litter size, for example, is certainly more important than prenatal mortality, because the rate of prenatal mortality is only one of several factors determining litter size; litter size is therefore a composite measure of several attributes. Indeed, litter size shows the expected pattern of r- and K-selection (Table 10). Likewise, neonatal weight is a composite attribute determined by both the rate of growth and length of gestation. Determining the relative importance of each of these ontogenetic attributes to a species' ecological strategy represents an important problem to be studied.

The second explanation for the absence of uniformity involves differences in the response of attributes to selection. Schaffer and Tamarin (1973) have shown that when an organism encounters an ecological challenge, the attribute responding most rapidly to selection will be used to meet the challenge. Among *Microtus* and many other species, litter size is thought to be one of the diagnostic features of a species' location on the r-K continuum. According to Schaffer and Tamarin's argument, litter size is one of the attributes responding most rapidly and perhaps most often to selection.

Summary

Despite the extensive literature on certain aspects of the ontogeny of New World *Microtus,* much remains to be learned. The list of undescribed processes and unanswered questions is very long: there is no published description of the prenatal development of any New World *Microtus*; the factors determining the rates of prenatal and postnatal growth, development, and mortality remain to be identified; the significance of migratory giant cells and interspecific variation of litter size are unknown. In summary, although we recognize the distinguishing characteristics of New World *Microtus,* we have very little knowledge about the ontogenetic processes by which these characteristics are produced. In other words, we can describe *Microtus* but we know little about how growth and development occur. Until some of these problems are solved, the relationship between ontogenetic variation and phylogenetic diversity in New World *Microtus* will remain obscure.

Acknowledgment

This work was supported by general funds of the Jackson Laboratory.

Literature Cited

Anderson, J. L., and R. Boonstra. 1979. Some aspects of reproduction in the vole *Microtus townsendii.* Canadian J. Zool., 57:18–24.

ANDERSON, P. K., P. H. WHITNEY, AND J. P. HUANG. 1976. *Arvicola richardsoni*: ecology and biochemical polymorphism in the front ranges of southern Alberta. Acta Theriol., 21:425–468.

ANDERSON, R. M., AND A. L. RAND. 1943. Status of the Richardson vole (*Microtus richardsoni*) in Canada. Canadian Field-Nat., 57:106–107.

AUSTIN, C. R. 1957. Fertilization, early cleavage and associated phenomena in the field vole (*Microtus agrestis*). J. Anat., 91:1–11.

BAILEY, V. 1924. Breeding, feeding, and other life habits of meadow mice (*Microtus*). J. Agric. Res., 27:523–535.

BARBEHENN, K. R. 1955. A field study of growth in *Microtus pennsylvanicus*. J. Mamm., 36:533–543.

BEER, J. R., C. F. MACLEOD, AND L. D. FRENZEL. 1957. Prenatal survival and loss in some cricetid rodents. J. Mamm., 38:392–402.

BREED, W. G. 1969. Oestrus and ovarian histology in the lactating vole (*Microtus agrestis*). J. Reprod. Fert., 18:33–42.

COLE, F. R., AND G. O. BATZLI. 1978. Influence of supplemental feeding on a vole population. J. Mamm., 59:809–819.

———. 1979. Nutrition and population dynamics of the prairie vole, *Microtus ochrogaster,* in central Illinois. J. Anim. Ecol., 48:455–470.

COLVIN, M. A., AND D. V. COLVIN. 1970. Breeding and fecundity of six species of voles (*Microtus*). J. Mamm., 51:417–419.

COPP, A. J. 1980. The development of field vole (*Microtus agrestis*) and mouse blastocysts in vitro: a study of trophoblast cell migration. Placenta, 1: 47–59.

CORTHUM, K. W., JR. 1967. Reproduction and duration of placental scars in the prairie vole and the eastern vole. J. Mamm., 48:287–292.

COVENTRY, A. F. 1937. Notes on the breeding of some Cricetidae in Ontario. J. Mamm., 18:489–496.

COWAN, I. M., AND M. G. ARSENAULT. 1954. Reproduction and growth in the creeping vole, *Microtus oregoni serpens* Merriam. Canadian J. Zool., 32: 198–208.

CROSS, P. C. 1971. The dictyate oocyte of *Microtus montanus*. J. Reprod. Fert., 25:291–293.

DIETERICH, R. A., AND D. J. PRESTON. 1977. The tundra vole (*Microtus oeconomus*) as a laboratory animal. Lab. Anim. Sci., 27:500–506.

ECKE, D. H., AND A. R. KINNEY. 1956. Aging meadow mice, *Microtus californicus,* by observation of molt progression. J. Mamm., 37:249–254.

FITCH, H. S. 1957. Aspects of reproduction and development in the prairie vole (*Microtus ochrogaster*). Univ. Kansas Publ., Mus. Nat. Hist., 10:129–161.

GENTRY, J. B. 1968. Dynamics of an enclosed population of pine mice, *Microtus pinetorum*. Res. Population Ecol., 10:21–30.

GLASS, B. P. 1949. Reproduction in the pine vole, *Pitymys nemoralis*. J. Mamm., 30:72–73.

GOERTZ, J. W. 1971. An ecological study of *Microtus pinetorum* in Oklahoma. Amer. Midland Nat., 86:1–12.

GREENWALD, G. S. 1956. The reproductive cycle of the field mouse, *Microtus californicus*. J. Mamm., 37:213–222.

———. 1957. Reproduction in a coastal California population of the field mouse, *Microtus californicus*. Univ. California Publ. Zool., 54:421–446.

GROCOCK, C. A. 1972. A study of spermatogenesis in the developing and mature vole (*Microtus agrestis*). J. Reprod. Fert., 29:153–154.

GUSTAFSSON, T., B. ANDERSSON, AND L. WESTLIN. 1980. Reproduction in a laboratory colony of bank vole, *Clethrionomys glareolus*. Canadian J. Zool., 58:1016–1021.

HAMILTON, W. J., JR. 1937. Growth and life span of the field mouse. Amer. Nat., 71:500–507.

———. 1938. Life history notes on the northern pine mouse. J. Mamm., 19:163–170.

———. 1941. Reproduction of the field mouse *Microtus pennsylvanicus.* Cornell Univ. Agric. Exper. Sta. Mem., 237:1–23.

HASLER, J. F. 1975. A review of reproduction and sexual maturation in the microtine rodents. The Biologist, 57:52–86.

HASLER, M. J., AND A. V. NALBANDOV. 1974. The effect of weanling and adult males on sexual maturation in female voles (*Microtus ochrogaster*). Gen. Comp. Endocrinol., 23:237–238.

HATFIELD, D. M. 1935. A natural history study of *Microtus californicus.* J. Mamm., 16:261–267.

HOFFMAN, R. S. 1958. The role of reproduction and mortality in population fluctuations of voles (*Microtus*). Ecol. Monogr., 28:79–108.

HOFFMEISTER, D. F. 1956. Mammals of the Graham (Pinaleno) Mountains, Arizona. Amer. Midland Nat., 55:257–288.

HOFFMEISTER, D. F., AND L. L. GETZ. 1968. Growth and age-class in the prairie vole, *Microtus ochrogaster.* Growth, 32:57–69.

HOWELL, A. B. 1924. Individual variation in *Microtus montanus yosemite.* J. Agric. Res., 28:977–1016.

HOYTE, H. M. D. 1955. Observations on reproduction in some small mammals of arctic Norway. J. Anim. Ecol., 24:412–425.

INNES, D. G. L. 1978. A re-examination of litter size in some North American microtines. Canadian J. Zool., 56:1488–1496.

INNES, D. G. L., AND J. S. MILLAR. 1979. Growth of *Clethrionomys gapperi* and *Microtus pennsylvanicus* in captivity. Growth, 43:268–217.

———. 1981. Body weight, litter size, and energetics of reproduction in *Clethrionomys gapperi* and *Microtus pennsylvanicus.* Canadian J. Zool., 59:785–789.

JAMESON, E. W., JR. 1947. Natural history of the prairie vole (mammalian Genus *Microtus*). Univ. Kansas Publ., Mus. Nat. Hist., 1:125–151.

JANNETT, F. J., JR. 1978. The density-dependent formation of extended maternal families of the montane vole, *Microtus montanus nanus.* Behav. Ecol. Sociobiol., 3:245–263.

KELLER, B. L., AND C. J. KREBS. 1970. *Microtus* population biology. III. Reproductive changes in fluctuating populations of *M. ochrogaster* and *M. pennsylvanicus* in southern Indiana. 1965–1967. Ecol. Monogr., 40:263–294.

KENNEY, A. M., R. L. EVANS, AND D. A. DEWSBURY. 1977. Postimplantation pregnancy disruption in *Microtus ochrogaster, M. pennsylvanicus,* and *Peromyscus maniculatus.* J. Reprod. Fert., 49:365–367.

KIRKPATRICK, R. L., AND G. L. VALENTINE. 1970. Reproduction in captive pine voles, *Microtus pinetorum.* J. Mamm., 51:779–785.

KOTT, E., AND W. L. ROBINSON. 1963. Seasonal variation in litter size of the meadow vole in southern Ontario. J. Mamm., 44:467–470.

KREBS, C. J., AND J. H. MYERS. 1974. Population cycles in small mammals. Adv. Ecol. Res., 8:267–399.

KRUCKENBERG, S. M., H. T. GIER, AND S. M. DENNIS. 1973. Postnatal development of the prairie vole, *Microtus ochrogaster.* Lab. Anim. Sci., 23:53–55.

LAYNE, J. N. 1958. Notes on mammals of southern Illinois. Amer. Midland Nat., 60:219–254.

LEE, C., AND D. J. HORVATH. 1969. Management of the meadow vole (*Microtus pennsylvanicus*). Lab. Anim. Care, 19:88–91.

LEE, C., D. J. HORVATH, R. W. METCALFE, AND E. K. INSKEEP. 1970. Ovulation in *Microtus pennsylvanicus* in a laboratory environment. Lab. Anim. Care, 20:1098–1102.

LIDICKER, W. Z., JR. 1973. Regulation of numbers in an island population of the California vole, a problem in community dynamics. Ecol. Monogr., 43: 271–302.

LINSDALE, J. 1928. Mammals of a small area along the Missouri River. J. Mamm., 9:140–146.

LOCHMILLAR, R. L., J. B. WHELAN, AND R. L. KIRKPATRICK. 1982*a*. Energetic cost of lactation in *Microtus pinetorum*. J. Mamm., 63:475–481.

———. 1982*b*. Postweanling energy requirements of juvenile pine voles, *M. pinetorum*. Amer. Midland Nat., 108:412–415.

MACARTHUR, R. H., AND E. O. WILSON. 1967. The theory of island biogeography. Princeton Univ. Press, Princeton, New Jersey, 203 pp.

MACFARLANE, J. D., AND J. M. TAYLOR. 1981. Sexual maturation in female Townsend's voles. Acta Theriol., 26:113–117.

———. 1982. Pregnancy and reproductive performance in the Townsend's vole, *M. townsendii* (Bachman). J. Mamm. 63:165–168.

MADISON, D. M. 1980. An integrated view of the social biology of *Microtus pennsylvanicus*. The Biologist, 62:20–33.

MALLORY, F. F., AND F. V. CLULOW. 1977. Evidence of pregnancy failure in the wild meadow vole, *Microtus pennsylvanicus*. Canadian J. Zool., 55:1–17.

MANNING, T. H. 1954. Remarks on the reproduction, sex ratio, and life expectancy of the varying lemming, *Dicrostonyx groenlandicus*, in nature and captivity. Arctic, 7:36–48.

MARTIN, E. P. 1956. A population study of the prairie vole (*Microtus ochrogaster*) in northeastern Kansas. Univ. Kansas Publ., Mus. Nat. Hist., 1:125–151.

MOHI ALDEEN, K., AND C. A. FINN. 1970. The implantation of blastocysts in the Russian steppe lemming (*Lagurus lagurus*). J. Exp. Zool., 173:63–78.

MORRISON, P. R., R. DIETERICH, AND D. PRESTON. 1976. Breeding and reproduction of fifteen wild rodents maintained as laboratory colonies. Lab. Anim. Care, 26:237–243.

———. 1977. Body growth in 16 wild rodent species and subspecies maintained in laboratory colonies. Physiol. Zool., 50:294–310.

MORRISON, P. R., F. A. RYSER, AND R. L. STRECKER. 1954. Growth and development of temperature regulation in the tundra redback vole. J. Mamm., 35:376–386.

MYERS, J. H., AND C. J. KREBS. 1971. Sex ratios in open and enclosed vole populations: Demographic implications. Amer. Nat., 105:325–344.

MYLLYMÄKI, A. 1977. Demographic mechanisms in the fluctuating populations of the field vole *Microtus agrestis*. Oikos, 29:468–493.

NEGUS, N. C., AND A. J. PINTER. 1965. Litter sizes of *Microtus montanus* in the laboratory. J. Mamm., 46:434–437.

———. 1966. Reproductive responses of *Microtus montanus* to plants and plant extracts in the diet. J. Mamm., 47:596–601.

NEGUS, N. C., P. J. BERGER, AND L. G. FORSLUND. 1977. Reproductive strategy of *Microtus montanus*. J. Mamm., 58:347–353.

OZDZENSKI, W., AND E. T. MYSTKOWSKA. 1976*a*. Implantation and early postimplantation development of the bank vole *Clethrionomys glareolus* (Schreber). J. Embryol. Exp. Morphol., 35:535–543.

———. 1976*b*. Stages of pregnancy of the bank vole. Acta Theriol., 21:279–286.

PAUL, J. R. 1970. Observations on the ecology, populations and reproductive biology of the pine vole, *Microtus pinetorum,* in North Carolina. Illinois State Mus. Rept. Invest., 20:1–28.

Pelikan, J. 1970. Embryonic resorption in *Microtus arvalis* (Pall.). Zool. Listy, 19:93–102.

Pépin, F.-M., and G. Baron. 1978. Development postnatal de l'activite motrice chez *Microtus pennsylvanicus.* Canadian J. Zool., 56:1092–1102.

Pianka, E. 1970. On r- and K-selection. Amer. Nat., 104:592–597.

Poiley, S. M. 1949. Raising captive meadow voles (*Microtus pennsylvanicus*). J. Mamm., 30:317–318.

Richmond, M. E., and C. H. Conaway. 1969. Management, breeding and reproductive performance of the vole, *Microtus ochrogaster* in a laboratory colony. Lab. Anim. Care, 19:80–87.

Rose, R. K., and M. S. Gaines. 1978. The reproductive cycle of *Microtus ochrogaster* in eastern Kansas. Ecol. Monogr., 48:21–42.

Rothstein, B. 1976. Selected aspects of the behavioral ecology of *Microtus breweri.* Unpubl. Ph.D. dissert., Boston University, 87 pp.

Rowsemitt, C., T. H. Kunz, and R. H. Tamarin. 1975. The timing and patterns of molt in *Microtus breweri.* Occas. Papers Mus. Nat. Hist., Univ. Kansas, 34:1–11.

Sansom, G. S. 1922. Early development and placentation in *Arvicola* (*Microtus*) *amphibius,* with special reference to the origin of placental giant cells. J. Anat., 56:333–365.

Schadler, M. H., and G. M. Butterstein. 1979. Reproduction in the pine vole, *M. pinetorum.* J. Mamm., 60:841–844.

Schaffer, W. M., and R. H. Tamarin. 1973. Changing reproductive rates and population cycles in lemmings and voles. Evolution, 27:111–124.

Selle, R. M. 1928. *Microtus californicus* in captivity. J. Mamm., 9:93–98.

Snell, G. D., and L. C. Stevens. 1966. Early embryology. Pp. 205–245, *in* Biology of the laboratory mouse (E. L. Green, ed.). McGraw-Hill, New York, 706 pp.

Southwood, R., R. May, N. Hassell, and G. Conway. 1974. Ecological strategies and population parameters. Amer. Nat., 108:791–804.

Stenseth, N. C. 1977. Evolutionary aspects of demographic cycles: the relevance of some models of cycles for microtine fluctuations. Oikos, 29:522–538.

Stenseth, N. C., and E. Framstad. 1980. Reproductive effort and optimal reproductive rates in small rodents. Oikos, 34:23–34.

Storm, G. L., and G. C. Sanderson. 1968. Housing and reproductive performance of an outdoor colony of voles. J. Mamm., 49:322–324.

Tamarin, R. H. 1977. Reproduction in the island beach vole, *Microtus breweri,* and the mainland meadow vole, *Microtus pennsylvanicus,* in southeastern Massachusetts. J. Mamm., 58:536–548.

———. 1978. Dispersal, population regulation, and K-selection in field mice. Amer. Nat., 112:545–555.

Theiler, K. 1972. The house mouse. Springer-Verlag, Berlin, 168 pp.

Thomas, J. A., and E. C. Birney. 1979. Parental care and mating system of the prairie vole, *Microtus ochrogaster.* Behav. Ecol. Sociobiol., 5:171–186.

Timm, R. M., L. R. Heaney, and D. D. Baird. 1977. Natural history of rock voles (*Microtus chrotorrhinus*) in Minnesota. Canadian J. Zool., 91:177–181.

Vaughan, M. K., G. M. Vaughan, and R. J. Reiter. 1973. Effect of ovariectomy and constant dark on the weight, reproductive and certain other organs in the female vole, *Microtus montanus.* J. Reprod. Fert., 32:9–14.

VAUGHAN, T. A. 1969. Reproduction and population density in a montane small mammal fauna. Misc. Publ. Mus. Nat. Hist., Univ. Kansas, 51:51–74.

WHITNEY, P. 1977. Seasonal maintenance and net production in two sympatric species of subarctic microtine rodents. Ecology, 58:314–325.

WILSON, S. C. 1982. Parent-young contact in prairie and meadow voles. J. Mamm., 63:300–306.

WOLFF, J. O., AND W. Z. LIDICKER, JR. 1980. Population ecology of the taiga vole, *Microtus xanthognathus,* in interior Alaska. Canadian J. Zool., 58. 1800–1812.

YOUNGMAN, P. M. 1975. Mammals of the Yukon territory. Natl. Mus. Nat. Sci. (Ottawa) Publ. Zool., No. 10, 192 pp.

HABITATS

LOWELL L. GETZ

Abstract

IN North America members of the genus *Microtus* are generally associated with habitats dominated by graminoid vegetation. Species that occur in forested areas are frequently restricted to grassy clearings or to sites in which there is an understory of grasses or sedges. *M. xanthognathus, M. longicaudus,* and *M. richardsoni* are found in coniferous forests, but are most abundant where there is at least some grassy vegetation present on the forest floor. Another forest species, *M. oregoni,* is most often found in forest clearings dominated by forbs; that is, in early successional stages in clearcut forest sites.

Microtus pinetorum, M. oaxacensis, M. umbrosus, and *M. guatemalensis* commonly occur in forested habitats where there is little graminoid vegetation; but *M. pinetorum* is also abundant in orchards where it may be associated with dense grassy cover. *M. chrotorrhinus* is characteristically found in rocky talus within deciduous and coniferous forests, but occurs in grassy balds in the southern Appalachians.

Most species of *Microtus* are associated with mesic or wet habitats; several species occur in marshes or other wet areas where the voles readily enter the water and swim. Only *M. mexicanus* is routinely found in arid habitats. Other species, including *M. montanus, M. longicaudus, M. californicus,* and *M. townsendii* are found in well-drained and sometimes arid habitats as well as in wet places. Individuals that occur in arid habitats, well-drained mesic sites, or in salt marshes obtain their water from the green vegetation upon which they feed.

Graminoid vegetation serves both as the primary cover and as the major food source for most species of *Microtus*. Whether the voles construct underground or surface nests, most *Microtus* traffic occurs on the soil surface; however, *M. pinetorum* and *M. parvulus* are subfossorial, constructing tunnels 2–3 cm below the surface. Where the vegetation growth is sufficiently dense, voles frequently make well-formed surface runways through the green vegetation or dead surface litter.

Most species of *Microtus* feed on green vegetation; seeds, roots, dead vegetation, and insects may be eaten when green vegetation is not available. Although some species (for example, *M. ochrogaster*) may require forbs in their diet, most species feed extensively on grasses and sedges.

Few species of *Microtus* are associated with agricultural situations in North America. The frequent disturbance of vegetative cover during tillage and harvesting activities renders agro-ecosystems unsuitable habitats for most species of *Microtus*. Some species may become abundant in unharvested forage crops (alfalfa, clover and timothy). Major vole (primarily *M. montanus*) "outbreaks" in agricultural systems in North America occurred in Nevada and California in 1906–1908 and throughout the western United States in 1957–1958.

Introduction

Descriptions of the habitats utilized by the various species of *Microtus* are scattered throughout the literature. Most such information is included as anecdotal or descriptive accounts in papers dealing with geographic distributions, regional species lists, or population studies. Relatively few studies concentrate specifically on factors responsible for occurrence of a species in given habitat types. In addition, because of the focus of different studies on specific habitat types, there are often conflicting conclusions as to the responses of a species to a particular habitat feature, such as vegetation type, cover conditions, and moisture regime. Since many species of *Microtus* are capable of utilizing rather wide ranges of habitat conditions, availability of information from a limited array of sites located in different regions complicates generalizations concerning habitat requirements of a species. That most species of *Microtus* display frequent ("periodic") fluctuations in abundance further confuses recognition of their preferred habitats. At times of regionally high population densities, individuals of a species may be crowded out of preferred habitats and be found (albeit temporarily) in relatively high numbers in otherwise marginal habitats. There is seldom information as to phase of the local population cycle at the time of a given study or observation.

The primary approach of this review is, therefore, to emphasize specific habitat features with which given species have been associated rather than to enumerate the various specific habitat types utilized by each species. The latter approach would require lengthy accounts of habitats in which a species has been found throughout its range. Table 1 lists the primary references used to categorize the habitats of each species. Although these references are not all-inclusive, they provide details of specific situations or general summaries of habitat utilization of given species. Other references are cited where appropriate within the text.

I grouped the species of *Microtus* in regard to what appears to be their most generalized responses to specific habitat factors. Species with a wide range of responses appear in more than one category. Wherever possible I included the range of response of a species to given habitat factors. In addition, I rank-ordered responses of sympatric species to habitat factors whenever comparative data were available. A section on competitive exclusion addresses in a more analytical manner comparative responses of sympatric species to given habitat factors.

Habitat Factors

The habitat factors that appear most important in influencing local distribution of *Microtus* are: vegetation type, moisture conditions, and amount of cover.

Herbaceous vegetation has a dual role as a habitat factor: provision of both food and cover. The diet of most species of *Microtus* comprises primarily green vegetation. New growth, inflorescences or seed heads are the preferred parts of plants. Where the vegetation is dense, voles normally must cut the stems into numerous short segments so as to get to the upper parts of the plants. Piles of 4 to 6-cm long clippings of grass and other plant stems indicate the presence of voles.

Species occupying habitats in which green vegetation is seasonally absent or reduced in quantity (for example, in winter or dry season) may feed on dead plant material, seeds, roots, or on insects and other small animals during the period when green vegetation is not available. A few species (for example, *M. pinetorum, M. californicus, M. pennsylvanicus,* and *M. ochrogaster*) feed on the bark of young trees in forestry plantations or on the bark and roots of orchard

TABLE 1

SELECTED REFERENCES PROVIDING INFORMATION ABOUT HABITATS OF SPECIES OF *Microtus*

Species	References
M. abbreviatus	Rausch and Rausch (1968)
M. breweri	Tamarin and Kunz (1974)
M. californicus	Ingles (1965); Krebs (1966)
M. canicaudus	See references for *M. montanus*
M. chrotorrhinus	Goodwin (1929); Hamilton and Whitaker (1979); Kirkland (1977*a*, 1977*b*); Kirkland and Knipe (1979); Martell and Radvanyi (1977); Timm et al. (1977)
M. coronarius	Swarth (1911)
M. guatemalensis	Smith and Jones (1967)
M. longicaudus	Borell and Ellis (1934); Dalquest (1948); Findley (1951); Findley and Jones (1962); Hall (1946); Ingles (1954, 1965); Ivey (1957)
M. ludovicianus†	Lowery (1974)
M. mexicanus	Baker and Phillips (1965); Brown (1968); Davis (1944, 1960); Davis and Robertson (1944); Davis and Russell (1954); Findley and Jones (1962); Hall and Dalquest (1963); Koestner (1944)
M. miurus	Osgood (1901); Peterson (1967); Quay (1951)
M. montanus	Borell and Ellis (1934); Dalquest (1948); Findley (1951); Findley and Jones (1962); Hall (1946); Hoffmann et al. (1969); Ingles (1965)
M. nesophilus†	Miller (1899)
M. oaxacensis	Goodwin (1969); Jones and Genoways (1967)
M. ochrogaster	Hamilton and Whitaker (1979); Jackson (1961)
M. oeconomus	Peterson (1967); Quay (1951)
M. oregoni	Dahlquest (1948); Gashwiler (1972); Ingles (1965); Sullivan (1981)
M. parvulus	Howell (1916); Neill and Boyles (1955)
M. pennsylvanicus	Dalquest (1948); Getz (1961, 1970); Hamilton and Whitaker (1979); Harris (1953); Jackson (1961); Peterson (1966); Woods et al. (1982)
M. pinetorum	Barbour and Baker (1950); Benton (1955); Davis (1960); Fisher and Anthony (1980); Glass and Halloran (1961); Hamilton and Whitaker (1979); Hanson (1944); Jackson (1961); Jameson (1949); Lowery (1974); Miller (1964); Miller and Getz (1969); Peterson (1967)
M. quasiater	Davis (1944)
M. richardsoni	Dalquest (1948); Findley (1951); Hooven (1973); Ingles (1965); Wright (1950)
M. townsendii	Cowan and Guiguet (1965); Dalquest (1940, 1948); Ingles (1965)
M. umbrosus	Goodwin (1969)
M. xanthognathus	Lensink (1954); Wolff and Lidicker (1980)

† Extinct.

trees. In general, however, food in the form of herbaceous vegetation is a necessary habitat requirement for most species of *Microtus*. Food habits may be involved in the preference of some species (for example, *M. ochrogaster*) for habitats with forbs; graminoid vegetation alone may not fulfill the dietary requirements of the species (Cole and Batzli, 1978).

Except for the subfossorial *Microtus pinetorum, M. parvulus* and perhaps *M. chrotorrhinus,* voles are active on the surface. In habitats where the vegetation is dense, voles usually construct distinct surface runways through the base of the vegetation or in the detritus. The greater the vegetation and detritus cover, the more protected are the runways. In habitats with sparse or more open vegetation growth, voles may form "paths" on the surface, or may move more randomly through their home ranges (personal observations in marsh habitats in Michigan, Wisconsin, and Connecticut, and in tall grass prairie and alfalfa habitats in Illinois).

The more dense the vegetation cover, the greater the protection of voles from predators, especially from avian predators (Birney et al., 1976). Vegetation cover also moderates the microclimate (humidity and temperature) of the site (Getz, 1965, 1970, 1971). The more dense the vegetation cover, the greater the moderation of the microclimate, thus reducing potential temperature and moisture stresses upon voles. Protection from predation appears more likely to contribute to higher numbers of voles in dense vegetation. Microclimatic stresses have not been shown to be sufficient to account for differences in local distribution in those species for which data are available (Getz, 1971).

Most species of *Microtus* occur in mesic or wet habitats. Although water balance of few species has been studied, kidney inefficiency appears to be a major reason for restriction to mesic or wet areas (Getz, 1963). Evaporative water losses at humidities encountered in even drier, more sparsely vegetated sites do not place a significant stress on the water balance of voles (Getz, 1970, 1971).

In mesic areas where standing water is not available, voles get water (preformed water) when eating green vegetation. Succulent vegetation associated with moist habitats is a likely reason for the positive responses of *Microtus* to soil moisture conditions. *M. pennsylvanicus* living in salt marshes obtain their water from the green sedges upon which they feed (Getz, 1966).

Responses to Habitat Features

In this section the various habitat types occupied by the genus *Microtus* are grouped according to those factors most important in determining local distributions. The species are placed in the habitat type with which they are most commonly associated; specific responses to the major features of each habitat type are discussed where appropriate.

Some species have very limited geographic ranges, such as *Microtus breweri, M. umbrosus, M. coronarius,* and *M. abbreviatus. Microtus nesophilus* and *M. ludovicianus* were also localized in distribution; both are now extinct. In addition, little habitat information has been presented for *M. quasiater, M. oaxacensis, M. guatemalensis,* and *M. canicaudus. M. canicaudus* has been separated only recently from *M. montanus* (Hsu and Johnson, 1970); I assume habitat requirements of *M. canicaudus* to be similar to those of *M. montanus* (given the potential habitat types within its range). I included the above species in the appropriate categories wherever possible; in most cases, however, little elaboration can be made in regard to their habitat requirements.

Vegetation Types

Species of *Microtus* occur from the Lower Sonoran (*M. montanus*) to the Arctic (*M. oeconomus, M. coronarius,* and *M. miurus*) life zones. Species associated with forested life zones (Hudsonian, Canadian, and Transition) are restricted for the most part to herbaceous forest clearings.

Graminoid habitats.—Grasslands and sedge marshes constitute the predominant *Microtus* habitats (Table 2); graminoid habitats utilized by species of *Microtus* range from relatively sparse, arid grasslands to densely vegetated salt and freshwater marshes. Temperature regimes of the grasslands inhabited by *Microtus* range from hot southern grasslands to the cold tundra.

Species associated with herbaceous vegetation consisting mainly of grasses or sedges include *Microtus pennsylvanicus, M. nesophilus, M. abbreviatus, M. miurus, M. oeconomus, M. montanus, M. ludovicianus, M. mexicanus,* and *M. townsendii.* Other species (*M. ochrogaster, M. californicus, M. longicaudus, M. quasiater,* and *M. breweri*) are abundant in grasslands which also may include considerable

TABLE 2
VEGETATION TYPES WITH WHICH SPECIES OF *Microtus* ARE COMMONLY ASSOCIATED

Graminoids	
M. abbreviatus	*M. miurus*
M. breweri	*M. montanus*
M. californicus	*M. nesophilus*†
M. canicaudus	*M. ochrogaster*
M. coronarius	*M. oeconomus*
M. longicaudus	*M. pennsylvanicus*
M. ludovicianus†	*M. quasiater*
M. mexicanus	*M. townsendii*
Forbs	
M. chrotorrhinus	*M. oregoni*
M. longicaudus	
Wooded	
Scrub or shrubs	
M. canicaudus	*M. montanus*
M. longicaudus	*M. parvulus*
M. mexicanus	
Deciduous (broadleaf) forests	
M. oaxacensis	*M. quasiater*
M. pinetorum	*M. umbrosus*
Coniferous forests	
M. coronarius	*M. richardsoni*
M. guatemalensis	*M. xanthognathus*
M. longicaudus	

† Extinct.

quantities of forbs or short woody shrubs. Although commonly associated with stream banks in forested areas, *M. richardsoni* is found most often in graminoid vegetation along streams or in grassy alpine meadows. *M. pennsylvanicus* appears to avoid habitats in which there are large numbers of woody plants in addition to graminoid vegetation.

Grassland sites do not necessarily have to be extensive or contiguous to be inhabited by some species of *Microtus* (see below). *M. mexicanus, M. montanus, M. longicaudus, M. quasiater, M. richardsoni,* and *M. pennsylvanicus* are commonly found in small, dispersed, grassy habitat patches or in small isolated alpine meadows within otherwise forested areas.

Other herbaceous habitats.—Few species occur exclusively in non-graminoid herbaceous habitats. *Microtus oregoni* occurs in redwood, fir, spruce, and hemlock forests where there is herbaceous vegetation (for example, in small clearings). *M. oregoni* is especially abundant in early successional clearcut timber sites where bracken fern and fireweed, as well as grasses, predominate. The species drops out 4 to 5 years after logging, when grasses and forbs are shaded out by woody sprouts of deciduous and coniferous trees (Sullivan, 1981). *M. chrotorrhinus* also is associated with clearcut forest areas in West Virginia (Kirkland, 1977*a*).

In Kentucky, *Microtus pinetorum* has been found in abandoned fields in which the dominant vegetation is a mixture of *Rubus* and *Andropogon*. *M. longicaudus* is less dependent upon the presence of grasses than are most other species, but the species normally is associated with graminoid habitats. *M. pennsylvanicus* may occur in *Sphagnum* mats, even where grasses or sedges are relatively scarce. *M. coronarius* extends into forested areas where there is a thick mossy mat, and few, if any, grasses or sedges.

Wooded habitats.—A few species inhabit grassy areas with an overstory of small trees and shrubs. In eastern Washington, *Microtus longicaudus* is abundant where *Crataegus* spp. and other shrubs are the dominant plants (Beck and Anthony, 1971; Randall and Johnson, 1979); elsewhere the species has been observed in scrub oak, sage brush, and in willow, alder, and aspen thickets (Borell and Ellis, 1934; Hall, 1946; Ingles, 1965). *M. montanus* has been captured in open aspen where the ground cover was sparse. At high population densities, *M. montanus* may extend from its characteristic grassy habitats out into shrub-dominated habitats (sometimes replacing *M. longicaudus* where the two species are sympatric; see below). *M. mexicanus* has been recorded from piñon, juniper, and yellow-pine habitats (Findley and Jones, 1962; Koestner, 1944). *M. parvulus* has been found in the ecotone between shrubby areas and pine stands. *M. quasiater* also occurs in wooded habitats.

The author trapped *Microtus pennsylvanicus* in isolated shrub-dominated deciduous forest clearings with a grass understory in New England. These appeared to represent remnants of populations of *M. pennsylvanicus* occupying once more extensive grassy clearings that were undergoing succession back to a forest.

Microtus pinetorum is characteristic of mature deciduous forests. Although it may occur in young pine plantations where grass is the dominant vegetation (Sartz, 1970), the species is not an inhabitant of mature pine forests. Forest types occupied by *M. pinetorum* range from mesic beech forests with well-developed litter and humus layers to scrub oaks where litter is scarce and the humus layer poorly developed (Jameson, 1949; Miller, 1964; Neill and Boyles, 1955). Other forests types commonly occupied by *M. pinetorum* include dry beech forests, spruce-yellow birch stands and red and white oak forests.

Microtus quasiater has been recorded from oak forests, but such sites most likely represent marginal habitats for this species. *M. oaxacensis* and *M. umbrosus* occur in high elevation evergreen broadleaf rainforests. *M. mexicanus* has also been recorded from cool wet oak forests in southern Mexico. *M. pennsylvanicus* may invade both deciduous and coniferous forests during peak density years (Cameron, 1964; Grant, 1971).

Microtus xanthognathus, M. coronarius, and *M. richardsoni* are characteristic of northern coniferous forests. However, all three are associated most often with sites where there is at least some graminoid vegetation. *M. xanthognathus* is found in black-spruce, white-spruce, birch, and aspen stands with a thick *Sphagnum* mat, horsetail (*Equisetum*), or clumps of sedges. Although usually associated with sites dominated by herbaceous vegetation, *M. oregoni* has been found in dry coniferous forests, as well as in damp mossy sites within such forests. *M. richardsoni* is found in marshy places alongside streams and in wet alpine and subalpine meadows within coniferous forest regions (Dalquest, 1948; Rasmussen and Chamberlain, 1959); infrequently it occurs in pure forest stands.

Microtus longicaudus has been recorded from yellow pine, lodgepole pine, hemlock, white fir, and spruce forests. *M. mexicanus* has been taken in pine forests, but usually where grasses are present in the understory. *M. guatemalenis* occurs in high-elevation pine cloud-forests where the understory is composed of low bushes, ferns, and bromeliads. *M. chrotorrhinus* is more abundant in rocky areas in coniferous forest than in similar rocky sites in deciduous forests (Kirkland, 1977*b*).

Rocky Habitats

The rock vole, *Microtus chrotorrhinus,* is associated primarily with broken rock outcrops, talus slopes and similar rocky situations. This species also has been found in sites where moss-covered rocks and logs are common (Hamilton and Whitaker, 1979; Kirkland and Knipe, 1979). *M. chrotorrhinus* usually is abundant where grasses are present among rocks, but it is frequently most common where there are dense stands of ferns.

Microtus oregoni and *M. longicaudus* also are found from time to time in rockslides. Both species are more abundant in herbaceous vegetation, however. *M. pinetorum* has been recorded from rocky areas in Oklahoma, but mainly where spaces between rocks were covered with dense herbaceous vegetation.

Moisture Regimes

Most species of *Microtus* are associated with mesic or wet places; none is found exclusively in arid habitats (Table 3). Those species commonly found in wet habitats include *M. pennsylvanicus, M. coronarius, M. xanthognathus, M. oeconomus, M. miurus, M. breweri, M. oaxacensis,* and *M. guatemalensis. Microtus oeconomus* is found in the wet swales throughout the vast flat tundra; where it occurs on mountain slopes, *M. oeconomus* is most abundant in wetter sites (Peterson, 1966). However, on Unalaska Island *M. oeconomus* was found to avoid very marshy sites. *M. miurus* also inhabits the wet tundra region, but avoids low swales; it is most abundant on peat mounds, terraces, raised polygons, and on stream and lake banks (Quay, 1951).

Microtus oaxacensis, M. umbrosus, and *M. guatemalensis* occur in high-elevation forests where the soil is cool and damp.

Although a number of species of *Microtus* occur in well-drained upland habitats, most also appear in wet marshes. *M. ochrogaster* appears to be relatively uncommon in sites with standing water; *M. abbreviatus* has not been taken in standing water. *M. ludovicianus* was recorded only from "damp" sites. Species commonly found in well-drained upland sites, but which also occur in wet marshy areas where standing water is present, include *M. californicus, M. oregoni, M. townsendii, M. longicaudus,* and the now extinct *M. nesophilus. M. xanthognathus* and *M. richardsoni* occur in wet areas adjacent to streams in forested areas; *M. longicaudus* also is adjacent to streams in some forested areas. Species occurring in coastal areas (*M. pennsylvanicus, M. californicus, M. townsendii, M. oregoni,* and *M. breweri*) commonly are found in salt marshes.

TABLE 3
SOIL MOISTURE CONDITIONS WITH WHICH SPECIES OF *Microtus* ARE COMMONLY ASSOCIATED

Semi-arid	
M. mexicanus	*M. pinetorum*
M. parvulus	*M. quasiater*
Mesic, well-drained	
M. abbreviatus	*M. montanus*
M. canicaudus	*M. ochrogaster*
M. chrotorrhinus	*M. pinetorum*
M. coronarius	*M. umbrosus*
M. ludovicianus†	
Wet, marshes	
M. breweri	*M. oeconomus*
M. coronarius	*M. pennsylvanicus*
M. guatemalensis	*M. richardsoni*
M. miurus	*M. xanthognathus*
M. oaxacensis	
Wide range of conditions, arid to marshes	
M. californicus	*M. oregoni*
M. longicaudus	*M. townsendii*
M. nesophilus†	

† Extinct.

Most species occupying wet areas readily enter water and swim; swimming behavior has been observed in *Microtus richardsoni, M. longicaudus, M. pennsylvanicus, M. californicus,* and *M. xanthognathus* (Blair, 1939; Dalquest, 1948; Ingles, 1965; Johnson, 1957; Lensink, 1954; Murie, 1960; Peterson, 1967). *M. californicus* and *M. longicaudus* dive and swim underwater. *M. pennsylvanicus* has been found in marshes where only clumps of vegetation extend above the water (Getz, 1961). Feeding platforms and nests are built above water in the sedges and cattails. Individuals living in such marshes resemble "small muskrats" (Murie, 1960) in their behavior.

Even though species occurring in wet areas appear to be strong swimmers, drowning may occur during extensive inundation of salt marshes, as during unusually high tides associated with storms. The combined effects of deeper water and strong wave action may cause mortality among "good" swimmers. *Microtus californicus* and *M.*

pennsylvanicus occasionally drown at such times (Hadaway and Newman, 1971; Harris, 1953).

In the southwestern regions of its range, *Microtus pennsylvanicus* is restricted mainly to the hydrosere, whereas in more northern areas of the west the species is an inhabitant of well-drained grasslands associated with deciduous and coniferous forests (Findley, 1954). When *M. pennsylvanicus* is found in well-drained upland habitats, it usually is restricted to sites with dense vegetation cover (Getz, 1971; Hodgson, 1972). However, such an association does not appear to be related to a more humid microclimate under vegetation (see above). Other species (*M. ochrogaster, M. californicus, M. montanus, M. coronarius,* and *M. chrotorrhinus*) occupying well-drained upland habitats are not so restricted to sites with dense vegetation cover. *M. chrotorrhinus* usually is found in crevices between and under rocks and boulders; this microhabitat is relatively mesic, even though well drained. The importance of microclimate upon the occurrence of *M. chrotorrhinus* in rocky habitats is not known.

Microtus mexicanus, M. pinetorum, and *M. parvulus* usually are associated with drier habitats than are other species of *Microtus. M. mexicanus* commonly is found in arid, sparsely vegetated habitats, including piñon, yellow pine, juniper, rabbit brush, and dry bunch grass. In other places, however, the species is abundant in mesic meadows within high-elevation coniferous forests. *M. mexicanus* also is found from time to time in marshy areas in desert regions, where runways may lead into water. And, *M. pinetorum* frequently is associated with deciduous forests where the substrate contains considerable humus and is relatively moist (Lowery, 1974; Peterson, 1966); however, the species is not abundant in swamps (Miller and Getz, 1969).

Species such as *Microtus californicus, M. oregoni, M. townsendii,* and *M. longicaudus,* although usually found in wet or mesic areas, also inhabit seasonally arid sites. Reproduction and population densities in these sites may decline during dry periods.

When they occur alone, some species frequently are found over a wide range of moisture conditions; but, when sympatric with other species of *Microtus,* there often is a segregation of species along the moisture gradient. Species with relatively wide moisture tolerances display more restricted distributions when sympatric with other species, as follows:

Microtus pennsylvanicus–M. ochrogaster: M. pennsylvanicus is in wetter areas, whereas *M. ochrogaster* occurs in well-drained sites (DeCoursey, 1957; Findley, 1954; Miller, 1969).

Microtus pennsylvanicus–M. montanus: *M. pennsylvanicus* is in moist sites, whereas *M. montanus* is more abundant in drier habitats (Hodgson, 1972; Murie, 1971).

Microtus mexicanus–M. longicaudus–M. montanus–M. pennsylvanicus: M. mexicanus is in the most arid places; *M. longicaudus* is in the next most arid sites; *M. montanus* often is restricted to mesic sites, *M. pennsylvanicus* is limited to grass-sedge meadows along streams (Findley and Jones, 1962).

Microtus montanus–M. longicaudus: M. montanus is in drier sites than is *M. longicaudus* in Eastern Washington, but in Nevada and Wyoming the reverse relationship was observed (Beck and Anthony, 1971; Borrel and Ellis, 1934; Findley, 1951; Vaughan, 1974).

Cover

Most species of *Microtus* display a positive response to vegetation cover; population densities are usually higher in sites with greater cover (Birney et al., 1976; Eadie, 1953; Grant et al., 1977).

Few species of *Microtus* occur in open habitats. Although usually more abundant in dense grasses, *M. mexicanus* may be found in relatively sparse grassy habitats. When sympatric with *M. montanus, M. mexicanus* is in more open sites while *M. montanus* is in densely vegetated habitats (Anderson, 1959; Findley and Jones, 1962). When sympatric with *M. pennsylvanicus,* however, *M. montanus* occurs in less-dense grassy habitats (Anderson, 1959; Hodgson, 1972).

Microtus ochrogaster commonly occurs in sparse grass habitats, even though it also occurs in dense vegetation. When sympatric with *M. pennsylvanicus, M. ochrogaster* is restricted to more sparsely vegetated sites; *M. pennsylvanicus* is in denser grass (Getz et al., 1978; Miller, 1969; Zimmerman, 1965). In central Illinois, *M. ochrogaster* is abundant in grassy sites that are mowed two to three times a year (for example, roadsides); *M. pennsylvanicus* is seldom found in such short grass habitats.

Microtus xanthognathus is more or less restricted to forested sites with a dense *Sphagnum* ground cover. *M. pinetorum* is frequently most abundant in deciduous forests with a thick leaf-litter layer, but it is not necessarily restricted to such habitats; it also is found commonly in areas with a sparse litter layer on the surface (Miller, 1964; Neill and Boyles, 1955).

Competitive Exclusion and Habitat Utilization

There is considerable evidence that competition between species of *Microtus* and with species of other genera influence both mammalian community structure and the habitat utilization of several species of *Microtus* (Rose and Birney, this volume). I summarize only the influence of competition upon habitat utilization in areas where given species appear to interact.

Where both *Microtus pennsylvanicus* and *M. montanus* are present (and when in approximately equal numbers), *M. pennsylvanicus* is restricted to wet or mesic areas, whereas *M. montanus* is prevalent in more arid sites (and occupies a wider range of habitat types than does *M. pennsylvanicus*). There are conflicting views as to why this occurs. Murie (1971) suggests *M. pennsylvanicus* is aggressively dominant over *M. montanus,* thus restricting *M. montanus* to the drier sites (wet areas are preferred habitat for *M. pennsylvanicus*). But, Stoecker (1972) indicates *M. montanus* is dominant over *M. pennsylvanicus* and that when *M. montanus* is removed from an area of possible competitive interaction, *M. pennsylvanicus* extends into more arid sites. This suggests *M. montanus* excludes *M. pennsylvanicus* from arid habitats.

When only one species is present, *Microtus longicaudus* and *M. montanus* may be found in shrub habitats and in grasslands. In areas where the two species are sympatric, however, *M. montanus* depresses *M. longicaudus* populations in shrub habitats, whereas *M. longicaudus* excludes *M. montanus* from grasslands (Randall and Johnson, 1979).

When it occurs alone, *Microtus ochrogaster* occurs in dense grassy habitats as well as in sparsely vegetated areas; in addition, *M. ochrogaster* occurs in both wet and well-drained areas when *M. pennsylvanicus* is not present. In areas where both species occur, *M. ochrogaster* usually is restricted to drier sites and to more sparsely vegetated habitats. When sympatric with *M. ochrogaster, M. pennsylvanicus* is most prevalent in low wet areas or in dense grasses. Krebs et al. (1969) indicated that both species cohabit the same study areas in central Indiana; however, there was evidence of higher densities of *M. ochrogaster* when *M. pennsylvanicus* was absent. Klatt and Getz (unpubl. observ.) have evidence of *M. pennsylvanicus* excluding *M. ochrogaster* from dense grassy habitats in central Illinois. The mechanism for such competitive exclusion is not known. Getz (1962) concluded that *M. ochrogaster* was aggressively dominant over *M. pennsylvanicus,* whereas Miller (1969) found the opposite.

Several studies have shown that *Microtus pennsylvanicus* is excluded from shrub or wooded areas by *Clethrionomys gapperi* (Cameron, 1964; Clough, 1964; Grant, 1971; Morris, 1969). Experimental removal studies indicate competitive interactions to be responsible for the exclusion of *M. pennsylvanicus* from wooded areas by *C. gapperi* (Cameron, 1964; Clough, 1964).

Sigmodon hispidus, a species which forms surface runways in dense grassy habitats, excludes *Microtus pinetorum* from such habitats, even though *M. pinetorum* is subfossorial (which reduces the potential for direct interaction) (Goertz, 1971). *M. pennsylvanicus,* a species which also uses surface runways and surface nests, and *M. pinetorum* commonly cohabit orchards with dense grass cover (Benton, 1955; Fisher and Anthony, 1980).

Habitat Utilization on Islands

Island populations of *Microtus pennsylvanicus* and *M. coronarius* have been found in wooded habitats as well as in grassland habitats, even though the apparent preferred habitat of these species is graminoid vegetation (Cameron, 1958; Grant, 1971). *M. coronarius* appears to be restricted to wooded island sites with mossy carpets (Swarth, 1911); *M. pennsylvanicus* has been taken in open woods, however.

In some instances occupancy of non-grassy habitats may involve "surplus" animals forced out of more favorable grassy habitats as a result of population pressure during peak periods of the population cycle. In other cases, absence of competitors (for example, *Clethrionomys gapperi*) may allow *Microtus pennsylvanicus* to occupy forested habitats on islands (Grant, 1971). When *C. gapperi* is present on islands, *M. pennsylvanicus* usually is restricted to grassy habitats (Cameron, 1958, 1964).

There is no indication of *Microtus townsendii* occurring in for-

TABLE 4
PRESUMED HABITAT-PATCH CONFIGURATION OCCUPIED BY *Microtus* SPECIES PRIOR TO HUMAN DISTURBANCE

Large, contiguous, relatively stable habitats	
M. californicus	*M. oeconomus*
M. miurus	*M. pinetorum*
M. ochrogaster	*M. townsendii*
Small, isolated, or ephemeral habitat patches	
M. canicaudus	*M. parvulus*
M. chrotorrhinus	*M. pennsylvanicus*
M. longicaudus	*M. quasiater*
M. mexicanus	*M. richardsoni*
M. montanus	*M. xanthognathus*
M. oregoni	
Entire species restricted to one or a very few small or localized areas	
M. abbreviatus	*M. ludovicianus*†
M. breweri	*M. nesophilus*†
M. coronarius	

† Extinct.

ested habitats when on islands. On islands, *M. townsendii* was recorded from under driftwood on sandy beaches and in rockpiles and dry grasslands as well as in wet marshes and "lush" vegetation, but not in forests (Cowan and Guiguet, 1965; Dalquest, 1940).

Habitat Configuration and Stability

It appears that there may be a relationship between patchiness or stability of habitat in which some species of *Microtus* arose and social structure displayed by the species (Getz, 1978; Getz and Carter, 1980; Lidicker, 1980; Madison, 1980; Wolff, 1980). Thus, it is of interest to identify those species that appear to have evolved in large contiguous permanent habitats as contrasted to species whose original habitat comprised small isolated or ephemeral patches. Such information can be used in explaining the similarities and differences in social organization and mating systems among different species.

As suggested previously, a species may occupy a variety of habitats under given population density conditions; in many instances populations are found in intervening marginal habitats at these times. This may give the impression of occupancy of larger contiguous habitat patches than occurs under lower density conditions. Thus, it is difficult to ascertain with a high degree of accuracy from published accounts the "normal" habitat in terms of patchiness. A study may have concentrated only on specific sites (and at a particular time), which biases the impression as to patch configuration of the habitat of the species. In addition, humans have disrupted the habitats of most species, thereby changing the original patch configuration; this further complicates determination of the configuration of the original species' habitat. As nearly as can be surmised from published accounts, Table 4 summarizes the general categorizations of habitat patch configuration. Insufficient data are available to estimate the habitat patch size and configuration of *Microtus oaxacensis, M. guatemalensis* and *M. umbrosus.*

Effects of Human Activities on Microtus *Habitats*

The original habitats of most species of *Microtus* have been altered greatly by a variety of human activities. Such changes include reduction in natural habitats and modification of patch size and dispersion. Those species whose habitats were altered by human activities include *M. ochrogaster, M. pennsylvanicus, M. californicus,* and *M. townsendii.*

Habitat reduction resulted primarily from conversion of grasslands for farming and grazing. The original prairie grassland habitats of *Microtus ochrogaster* especially were reduced by agriculture. Almost all the once extensive grasslands are now cultivated or grazed. *M. ochrogaster* does not occupy most agricultural croplands; thus, populations of *M. ochrogaster* now are relatively isolated in the few remnants of prairie areas or they occupy new habitats created by humans (see below). The original habitat of *M. californicus* also was reduced greatly by grazing and agriculture. Populations of *M. californicus* remain in ungrazed or less-disturbed grasslands; many of these grasslands now include a large number of exotic species of plants.

Species of *Microtus* occupying wet and marshy areas, including salt marshes (for example, *M. pennsylvanicus, M. californicus,* and *M. townsendii*) also experienced a reduction in available wetland habitats. Wet areas were drained for agriculture or filled in for industrial development (as in the case of salt marshes). Filling in of large areas of San Francisco Bay is a prime example of loss of salt-marsh habitats of *Microtus.*

The habitat of *Microtus nesophilus* on Great Gull and Little Gull Islands was completely destroyed by the construction of a military fort. The species declined rapidly in numbers from relatively high abundance to extinction. There is no indication of habitat disturbance being a factor in the extinction of *M. ludovicianus*; a relatively large area of apparently suitable habitat remains.

New habitats suitable for occupancy by *Microtus* also were created by humans. "New" habitats were formed for *M. pinetorum, M. ochrogaster, M. pennsylvanicus, M. californicus, M. montanus,* and perhaps *M. oregoni.* Some agricultural crops (alfalfa, wheat and timothy) provide at least a temporary habitat for *Microtus* (for example, *M. californicus, M. montanus,* and *M. ochrogaster*). Establishment of bluegrass pastures that are allowed to remain idle or are abandoned provides habitat for species such as *M. ochrogaster* and *M. pennsylvanicus.* Grassy roadsides along county roads, state highways, interstates, and railroads provide extensive habitats for *Microtus* (for example, *M. pennsylvanicus, M. ochrogaster*; Getz et al., 1978). Within the past decade financial constraints reduced mowing of many state and interstate roadsides creating considerable areas of dense grassy habitat. Such unmowed areas are especially important in providing grassy habitats otherwise scarce or absent in high-intensity agricultural and forested regions. There is evidence that such avenues of habitat were used by *M. pennsylvanicus* to effect a significant expansion of its range in the high intensity agricultural region of central Illinois.

Orchards with dense grassy ground cover provide a different, but suitable, habitat for *Microtus pinetorum,* as well as for species that normally make use of grassy habitats (especially *M. pennsylvanicus* and *M. ochrogaster*).

Clearcut forestry practices, and the resultant successional sequences, increase the available habitat for *Microtus oregoni.* Although similar successional sequences follow natural forest fires, clearcut logging operations provide extensive areas of suitable habitat for *M. oregoni* and *M. chrotorrhinus.*

Agricultural Habitats

Because of frequent disturbances (tillage, removal of vegetation at harvest, and grazing by livestock), *Microtus* species are seldom associated with agriculture in North America. Few agriculture systems provide adequate vegetation cover for a sufficient length of time to permit *Microtus* populations to become established in fields. Occasionally some species are found in crops, however; in a few instances there have been economically damaging vole outbreaks.

Microtus is associated most commonly with forage crops such as alfalfa, clover and timothy (Jameson, 1958; Lantz, 1905, 1907; Linduska, 1950; Morrison, 1953; White, 1965). When crops are cut and hay removed, cover is sufficiently disturbed to cause voles to disappear or decline to low densities. Only infrequently are voles able to achieve high densities in fields harvested at normal intervals. If such forage crops are not harvested, of course, voles may achieve high densities, depending upon the phase of the local population cycle.

Perhaps the most dramatic outbreak of *Microtus* in agricultural systems in the United States was that of the montane vole (*M. montanus*) in Nevada and California in 1906–1908 (Piper, 1909). In Humboldt County, Nevada, alone approximately 10,000 ha of alfalfa were completely destroyed; voles ate all parts of alfalfa plants, including roots. Estimated population densities were in excess of 25,000 voles/ha in areas with the most severe outbreaks. In 1957–1958 there was a more extensive outbreak of *M. montanus* in croplands throughout much of the western United States, including California, Oregon, Washington, northern Nevada, Utah, Idaho, southwestern Montana, and western Wyoming. Population densities of 5,000–7,500/ha were recorded locally; most densities were in the hundreds per ha, however (White, 1965). Predator increases, especially of owls, hawks, and gulls, were documented during this outbreak. Predator populations remained high following the decline of voles and served to drive vole densities to low levels (White, 1965).

Other species that have been recorded from forage crops include *Microtus ochrogaster, M. pennsylvanicus, M. coronarius,* and *M. californicus.* Both *M. ochrogaster* and *M. pennsylvanicus* occur in wheat fields in central Illinois (Getz, pers. observ.). There are only anecdotal data as to densities achieved before wheat is harvested in late June. In most cases wheat is combined before voles can achieve high densities. At least one field sustained losses of wheat of 25% in central Illinois (D. E. Kuhlman, pers. comm.).

During the growing season, corn does not provide suitable cover for *Microtus*. Formerly, both *M. pennsylvanicus* and *M. ochrogaster* were abundant in corn fields in winter when corn was placed in shocks rather than picked or combined in the field, as is now common practice in almost all regions (Getz, pers. observ.; Linduska, 1950). Voles undoubtedly moved from adjacent grassy habitats into shocks during winter; neither species was found in corn fields during summer.

Other crops in which *Microtus* have been observed include field beans (*M. pennsylvanicus*; Jackson, 1961); asparagus (*M. californicus*; Morrison, 1953); and potatoes (*M. californicus* and *M. coronarius*; Swarth, 1911; White, 1965).

Although they are not strictly agricultural habitats, orchards support populations of several species of *Microtus* (Holm, et al., 1959; Horsefall, 1953). *M. pinetorum, M. pennsylvanicus,* and *M. ochrogaster* commonly are found in apple, pear, and peach orchards; *M. californicus* has been recorded from citrus orchards (Morrison, 1953).

Literature Cited

ANDERSON, S. 1959. Distribution, variation, and relationships of the montane vole, *Microtus montanus*. Univ. Kansas Publ., Mus. Nat. Hist., 9:415–511.

BAKER, R. H., AND C. J. PHILLIPS. 1965. Mammals from El Nevado De Colima, Mexico. J. Mamm., 46:691–693.

BARBOUR, R. W., AND B. L. BAKER. 1950. Some mammals from Hart County, Kentucky. J. Mamm., 31:359–360.

BECK, L. R., AND R. G. ANTHONY. 1971. Metabolic and behavioral thermoregulation in the long-tailed vole, *Microtus longicaudus*. J. Mamm., 52:404–412.

BENTON, A. H. 1955. Observations of the life history of the northern pine vole. J. Mamm., 36:52–62.

BIRNEY, E. C., W. E. GRANT, AND D. D. BAIRD. 1976. Importance of vegetative cover to cycles of *Microtus* populations. Ecology, 57:1043–1051.

BLAIR, W. F. 1939. A swimming and diving vole. J. Mamm., 20:375.

BORELL, A. E., AND R. ELLIS. 1934. Mammals of the Ruby Mountain region of northeastern Nevada. J. Mamm., 15:12–44.

BROWN, L. N. 1968. Smallness of litter size in the Mexican vole. J. Mamm., 49:159.

CAMERON, A. W. 1958. Mammals of the islands in the Gulf of St. Lawrence. Bull. Natl. Mus. Canada, 154:1–165.

———. 1964. Competitive exclusion between rodent genera *Microtus* and *Clethrionomys*. Evolution, 18:630–634.

CLOUGH, G. C. 1964. Local distribution of two voles: evidence for interspecific interaction. Canadian Field-Nat., 78:80–89.
COLE, F. R., AND G. O. BATZLI. 1978. Influence of supplemental feeding on a vole population. J. Mamm., 59:809–819.
COWAN, I. MCT., AND C. J. GUIGUET. 1965. The mammals of British Columbia. Brit. Columbia Prov. Mus. Handbook II. Brit. Columbia Prov. Mus., Dept. Recreation Conserv., Victoria, B.C., 414 pp.
DALQUEST, W. W. 1940. New meadow mouse from the San Juan Islands, Washington. Murrelet, 21:7–8.
———. 1948. Mammals of Washington. Univ. Kansas Press, Lawrence, 444 pp.
DAVIS, W. B. 1944. Notes on Mexican mammals. J. Mamm., 25:370–403.
———. 1960. The mammals of Texas. Bull. Texas Fish and Game Commission, 41:1–252.
DAVIS, W. B., AND J. L. ROBERTSON, JR. 1944. The mammals of Culberson County, Texas. J. Mamm., 25:254–273.
DAVIS, W. B., AND R. J. RUSSELL. 1954. Mammals of the Mexican state of Morelos. J. Mamm., 35:63–80.
DECOURSEY, G. E. 1957. Identification, ecology and reproduction of *Microtus* in Ohio. J. Mamm., 38:44–52.
EADIE, W. R. 1953. Response of *Microtus* to vegetation cover. J. Mamm., 34:263–264.
FINDLEY, J. S. 1951. Habitat preferences of four species of *Microtus* in Jackson Hole, Wyoming. J. Mamm., 32:118–122.
———. 1954. Competition as a possible limiting factor in the distribution of *Microtus*. Ecology, 35:418–420.
FINDLEY, J. S., AND C. J. JONES. 1962. Distribution and variation of voles of the genus *Microtus* in New Mexico and adjacent areas. J. Mamm., 43:154–166.
FISHER, A. R., AND R. G. ANTHONY. 1980. The effect of soil texture on the distribution of pine voles in Pennsylvania orchards. Amer. Midland Nat., 104:39–46.
GASHWILER, J. S. 1972. Life-history notes on the Oregon vole, *Microtus oregoni*. J. Mamm., 53:558–569.
GETZ, L. L. 1961. Factors influencing the local distribution of *Microtus* and *Synaptomys* in southern Michigan. Ecology, 41:110–119.
———. 1962. Aggressive behavior of the meadow and prairie voles. J. Mamm., 43:351–358.
———. 1963. A comparison of the water balance of the prairie and meadow voles. Ecology, 44:202–207.
———. 1965. Humidities in vole runways. Ecology, 46:548–550.
———. 1966. Salt tolerances of salt marsh meadow voles. J. Mamm., 47:201–207.
———. 1970. Habitat of the meadow vole during a "population low." Amer. Midland Nat., 83:455–461.
———. 1971. Microclimate, vegetation cover, and local distribution of the meadow vole. Trans. Illinois Acad. Sci., 64:9–21.
———. 1978. Speculation on social structure and population cycles of microtine rodents. The Biologist, 60:134–147.
GETZ, L. L., AND C. S. CARTER. 1980. Social organization in *Microtus ochrogaster* populations. The Biologist, 62:56–69.
GETZ, L. L., F. R. COLE, AND D. GATES. 1978. Interstate roadsides as dispersal routes for *Microtus pennsylvanicus*. J. Mamm., 59:208–212.

GLASS, B. P., AND A. F. HALLORAN. 1961. The small mammals of the Wichita Mountain Wildlife Refuge, Oklahoma. J. Mamm., 42:234–239.

GOERTZ, J. W. 1971. An ecological study of *Microtus pinetorum* in Oklahoma. Amer. Midland Nat., 86:1–12.

GOODWIN, G. G. 1929. Mammals of the Cascapedia Valley, Quebec. J. Mamm., 10:239–246.

———. 1969. Mammals from the state of Oaxaca, Mexico, in the American Museum of Natural History. Bull. Amer. Mus. Nat. Hist., 141:1–269.

GRANT, P. R. 1971. The habitat preference of *Microtus pennsylvanicus,* and its relevance to the distribution of this species on islands. J. Mamm., 52:351–361.

GRANT, W. E., N. R. FRENCH, AND D. M. SWIFT. 1977. Response of a small mammal community to water and nitrogen treatments in a shortgrass prairie ecosystem. J. Mamm., 58:637–652.

HADAWAY, H. C., AND J. R. NEWMAN. 1971. Differential responses of five species of salt marsh mammals to inundation. J. Mamm., 52:818–820.

HALL, E. R. 1946. Mammals of Nevada. Univ. California Press, Berkeley, 710 pp.

HALL, E. R., AND W. W. DALQUEST. 1963. The mammals of Veracruz. Univ. Kansas Publ., Mus. Nat. Hist., 14:165–362.

HAMILTON, W. J., JR., AND J. O. WHITAKER. 1979. Mammals of the eastern United States. Second ed. Cornell Univ. Press, Ithaca, New York, 346 pp.

HANSON, H. C. 1944. Small mammal censuses near Prairie du Sac, Wisconsin. Trans. Wisconsin Acad. Sci. Arts Letters, 36:105–129.

HARRIS, V. T. 1953. Ecological relationships of meadow voles and rice rats in tidal marshes. J. Mamm., 34:479–487.

HODGSON, J. R. 1972. Local distribution of *Microtus montanus* and *M. pennsylvanicus* in southeastern Montana. J. Mamm., 53:487–499.

HOFFMANN, R. S., P. L. WRIGHT, AND F. E. NEWBY. 1969. The distribution of some mammals in Montana: I. Mammals other than bats. J. Mamm., 50: 579–604.

HOLM, L., F. A. GILBERT, AND E. H. HUICK. 1959. Elimination of rodent cover adjacent to apple trees. Weeds, 7:405–408.

HOOVEN, E. G. 1973. Notes on the water vole in Oregon. J. Mamm., 54:751–753.

HORSEFALL, F., JR. 1953. Mouse control in Virginia orchards. Virgin. Agric. Exp. Sta. Bull., 465:1–26.

HOWELL, A. B. 1916. Description of a new pine mouse from Florida. Proc. Biol. Soc. Washington, 29:83–84.

HSU, T. G., AND M. L. JOHNSON. 1970. Cytological distinction between *Microtus montanus* and *Microtus canicaudus.* J. Mamm., 51:824–826.

INGLES, L. G. 1954. Mammals in California and its coastal waters. Stanford Univ. Press, Stanford, California, 396 pp.

———. 1965. Mammals of the Pacific states. Stanford Univ. Press, Stanford, California, 506 pp.

IVEY, R. D. 1957. Ecological notes on the mammals of Bernalillo County, New Mexico. J. Mamm., 38:490–502.

JACKSON, H. H. T. 1961. Mammals of Wisconsin. Univ. Wisconsin Press, Madison, 504 pp.

JAMESON, E. W., JR. 1949. Some factors influencing the local distribution and abundance of woodland small mammals in central New York. J. Mamm., 30:221–235.

———. 1958. Consumption of alfalfa and wild oats by *Microtus californicus.* J. Wildl. Mgmt., 22:433–435.

JOHNSTON, R. F. 1957. Adaptations of salt marsh mammals to high tides. J. Mamm., 38:529–531.

JONES, J. K., JR., AND H. H. GENOWAYS. 1967. Notes on the Oaxacan vole, *Microtus oaxacensis.* J. Mamm., 48:320–321.

KIRKLAND, G. L. 1977*a.* Response of small mammals to the clearcutting of northern Appalachian forests. J. Mamm., 58:600–609.

———. 1977*b.* The rock vole, *Microtus chrotorrhinus* (Miller) (Mammalia: Rodentia) in West Virginia. Ann. Carnegie Mus. Nat. Hist., 46:45–53.

KIRKLAND, G. L., AND C. M. KNIPE. 1979. The rock vole (*Microtus chrotorrhinus*) as a Transition Zone species. Canadian Field-Nat., 93:319–321.

KOESTNER, E. J. 1944. Populations of small mammals on Cerro Potos, Nuevo Leon, Mexico. J. Mamm., 25:285–289.

KREBS, C. J. 1966. Demographic changes in fluctuating populations of *Microtus californicus.* Ecol. Monogr., 36:239–273.

KREBS, C. J., B. L. KELLER, AND R. H. TAMARIN. 1969. *Microtus* population biology: demographic changes in fluctuating populations of *M. ochrogaster* and *M. pennsylvanicus* in southern Indiana. Ecology, 50:587–607.

LANTZ, D. E. 1905. Meadow mice in relation to agriculture and horticulture. Yearb. U.S. Dept. Agric., 1905:362–376.

———. 1907. An economic study of field mice (genus *Microtus*). U.S. Dept. Agric. Biol. Survey Bull., 31:1–64.

LENSINK, C. J. 1954. Occurrence of *Microtus xanthognathus* in Alaska. J. Mamm., 36:259.

LIDICKER, W. Z., JR. 1980. The social biology of the California vole. The Biologist, 62:46–55.

LINDUSKA, J. P. 1950. Ecology and land-use relationships of small mammals on a Michigan farm. Michigan Dept. Conserv., Lansing, 144 pp.

LOWERY, G. H., JR. 1974. Mammals of Louisiana and its adjacent waters. Louisiana State Univ. Press, Baton Rouge, 565 pp.

MADISON, D. M. 1980. An integrated view of social biology of *Microtus pennsylvanicus.* The Biologist, 62:20–33.

MARTELL, A. M., AND A. RADVANYI. 1977. Changes in small mammal populations after clearcutting of northern Ontario black spruce forest. Canadian Field-Nat., 91:41–46.

MILLER, D. H. 1964. Northern records of the pine mouse in Vermont. J. Mamm., 45:627–628.

MILLER, D. H., AND L. L. GETZ. 1969. Life-history notes on *Microtus pinetorum* in central Connecticut. J. Mamm., 50:777–784.

MILLER, G. S. 1899. Preliminary list of the mammals of New York. Bull. New York State Mus., 6:271–390.

MILLER, W. C. 1969. Ecological and ethological isolating mechanisms between *Microtus pennsylvanicus* and *Microtus ochrogaster* at Terre Haute, Indiana. Amer. Midland Nat., 82:140–148.

MORRIS, R. D. 1969. Competitive exclusion between *Microtus* and *Clethrionomys* in the aspen parkland of Saskatchewan. J. Mamm., 50:291–301.

MORRISON, A. E. 1953. The meadow mouse (*Microtus californicus*) problem in Sacramento County. California Dept. Agric. Bull., 42:59–62.

MURIE, A. 1960. Aquatic voles. J. Mamm., 41:273–275.

MURIE, J. O. 1971. Behavioral relationships between two sympatric voles (*Microtus*): relevance to habitat segregation. J. Mamm., 52:181–186.

NEILL, W. T., AND J. M. BOYLES. 1955. Notes on the Florida pine mouse, *Pitymys parvulus.* J. Mamm., 36:138–139.

Osgood, W. H. 1901. Natural history of Queen Charlotte Island, British Columbia. N. Amer. Fauna, 21:1–87.

Peterson, R. L. 1966. The mammals of eastern Canada. Oxford Univ. Press, Toronto, 465 pp.

Peterson, R. S. 1967. The land mammals of Unalaska Island: present status and zoogeography. J. Mamm., 48:119–129.

Piper, S. E. 1909. The Nevada mouse plague of 1907–8. Farmers Bull., 352: 1–23.

Quay, W. B. 1951. Observations of mammals of the Seward Peninsula, Alaska. J. Mamm., 32:88–99.

Randall, J. A., and R. E. Johnson. 1979. Population densities and habitat occupancy by *Microtus longicaudus* and *M. montanus*. J. Mamm., 60:217–219.

Rasmussen, D. I., and N. V. Chamberlain. 1959. A new meadow mouse from Utah. J. Mamm., 40:53–56.

Rausch, R. L., and V. A. Rausch. 1968. On the biology and systematic position of *Microtus abbreviatus* Miller, a vole endemic to the St. Matthew Islands, Bering Sea. Z. Saugetierk., 33:65–99.

Sartz, R. S. 1970. Mouse damage to young plantations in southwestern Wisconsin. J. Forestry, 68:88–89.

Smith, J. D., and J. K. Jones, Jr. 1967. Additional records of the Guatemalan vole, *Microtus guatemalensis* Merriam. Southwestern Nat., 12:189–191.

Stoecker, R. E. 1972. Competitive relations between sympatric populations of voles (*Microtus montanus* and *M. pennsylvanicus*). J. Anim. Ecol., 41:311–329.

Sullivan, T. P. 1981. Comparative demography of *Peromyscus maniculatus* and *Microtus oregoni* populations after logging and burning of coastal forest habitat. Canadian J. Zool., 58:2252–2259.

Swarth, H. S. 1911. Birds and mammals of the 1909 Alexander Alaska Expedition. Univ. California Publ. Zool., 7:9–172.

Tamarin, R. H., and T. H. Kunz. 1974. *Microtus breweri.* Mamm. Species., 45: 1–3.

Timm, R. M., L. R. Heaney, and D. D. Baird. 1977. Natural history of rock voles (*Microtus chrotorrhinus*) in Minnesota. Canadian Field-Nat., 91:177–181.

Vaughan, T. A. 1974. Resource allocation in some sympatric subalpine rodents. J. Mamm., 55:764–795.

White, L. 1965. Biological and ecological considerations in meadow mouse population management. California Dept. Agric. Bull., 54(3):161–167.

Wolff, J. O. 1980. Social organization of the taiga vole (*Microtus xanthognathus*). The Biologist, 62:34–45.

Wolff, J. O., and W. Z. Lidicker. 1980. Population ecology of the taiga vole, *Microtus xanthognathus,* in interior Alaska. Canadian J. Zool., 58:1800–1812.

Woods, C. A., W. Post, and C. W. Kilpatrick. 1982. *Microtus pennsylvanicus* (Rodentia: Muridae) in Florida: a Pleistocene relict in a coastal saltmarsh. Bull. Florida State Mus., Biol. Sci., 28:25–52.

Wright, P. L. 1950. *Synaptomys borealis* from Glacier National Park, Montana. J. Mamm., 31:460.

Zimmerman, E. G. 1965. A comparison of habitat and food of two species of *Microtus.* J. Mamm., 46:605–612.

COMMUNITY ECOLOGY

ROBERT K. ROSE AND

ELMER C. BIRNEY*

Abstract

COMMUNITIES with *Microtus* tend to be structurally simple, usually grasslands or tundra, and to have no more than two species of *Microtus* and rarely more than six species of small mammals. *Microtus* often dominates both numerically and in total small mammal biomass, especially at higher latitudes. The small mammal community is most influenced by *Microtus* through its fluctuations in density, and thus also in biomass, by its relatively high level of diurnal activity, and by its year-round activity. Other species of small mammals may be adversely affected because *Microtus* usually is larger and behaviorally dominant and also because the mere presence of *Microtus* may focus predators on the area, especially during periods of high density. As generalized herbivores, primarily on grasses and herbs, *Microtus* has the potential to alter plant communities, either by selectively harvesting some species or through stimulating growth by grazing. Scarcely anything is known about the role *Microtus* plays in plant and small mammal communities, so both descriptive and experimental studies can make significant contributions to an understanding of the role and impact *Microtus* has on its communities.

Introduction

Microtus always lives with other small mammal associates, whether in combination with one or more shrews, or cricetine, sciurid, heteromyid, murid, or other microtine rodents. Because it occurs primarily in temperate grasslands and in tundra (Getz, this volume), we anticipate that *Microtus* will usually be a member of

* Order of authorship determined by flip of a coin.

structurally simple plant communities, regardless of latitude. In North America, grassland and tundra (and often *Microtus*) are found between 35 and 70°N, and also in isolated montane and plateau regions of southwestern U.S. and northern Mexico (Hoffmann and Koeppl, this volume). In these ecosystems, *Microtus* often contributes as much as 90% of the biomass of small mammals at the location. Consequently, an understanding of the role of *Microtus* is essential to an understanding of the ecology and dynamics of the ecosystem. *Microtus* has been evaluated in the context of primary consumers in grasslands, as in the IBP studies reported by Birney et al. (1976), French et al. (1976), and Grant and Birney (1979).

Microtus most frequently has been studied at the population level (Taitt and Krebs, this volume). Population studies have reported in great detail the patterns of density, population growth and survival, reproduction, behavior, dispersal, and changes in gene frequency, among others. Such studies have included only one or at most two species of *Microtus* or perhaps another microtine rodent, under the assumption that the common patterns underlying cycles could be detected in all microtines. The population dynamics and interactions of syntopic non-microtines have largely been ignored in the intensive study of *Microtus* population biology. As a result, we know very little about the role of *Microtus* in the small mammal community; that is, how *Microtus* affects other small mammals and how other small mammals affect *Microtus*. Some investigators, notably Lidicker (1973, 1978), have suggested that microtines should be studied in the community context, but this admonition has not been universally accepted. Indeed, we found that the majority of papers on *Microtus* population biology do not even list the small mammal associates in the community.

In sum, small mammal ecologists have looked at least coarsely at the role of *Microtus* in some grassland and tundra ecosystems, and in great detail at the population biology of *Microtus*. But there are no reported studies of the role of *Microtus* in the community of small mammals living at specific locations.

In a sense, a chapter on the community ecology of a genus is almost without precedent, especially a genus with 23 species living in a wide variety of environments from Guatemala to northern Alaska. Our goal in writing this chapter is to evaluate the role of *Microtus* in a range of successional, latitudinal, and altitudinal environments in the context of other small mammals living with them, and to explain the patterns of *Microtus* distribution and association in the context of evolutionary and historic events.

Communities of Small Mammals with Microtus

Patterns of Geographic Distribution

In general, mammals follow the biogeographic principle of having more species in the tropics and progressively fewer toward the poles (McCoy and Connor, 1980; Simpson, 1964; Wilson, 1974). Fleming's (1973) evaluation of forest-dwelling mammals at two locations at 65°N (15 and 16 species), 45 and 42°N (35 species each), and two locations at 9°N (70 species each) nicely illustrates this gradient of mammalian species in the New World. However, except at the extremes of latitude, small mammal communities do not follow this trend, for temperate and tropical grasslands, temperate forest, and tundra communities alike usually have six or fewer species (French, 1978). Instead of a gradient of numbers across the North American continent, numbers of small mammal species vary as much according to habitat type within climatic zones as across broad latitudinal zones. An even greater exception is the pattern of latitudinal gradients for the numbers of microtine, and, more specifically, *Microtus* species from the tundra to subtropical latitudes.

Numbers of species of *Microtus,* other microtines, and non-microtines for two north–south transects in North America are given in Table 1. Microtine species contribute more than 50% to the total rodent fauna north of 60°N in the western transect and north of 55°N in the eastern transect. South of 35°N, the number of *Microtus* species never exceeds one. Microtines other than *Microtus* are not found below 30°N along either transect. Thus, the trend of increasing numbers of species toward the tropics is strongly reversed for all microtine rodents, including *Microtus.*

Reasons for this reverse pattern of species diversity are many and varied, but originate in the biogeographic history of this exclusively Northern Hemisphere genus (Hoffmann and Koeppl, this volume). Given their northern origin, *Microtus* species tend to be well adapted physiologically, morphologically, and behaviorally to withstanding extreme cold and long winters, but are largely unable to with-

TABLE 1

NUMBER OF SPECIES OF *Microtus* COMPARED TO OTHER MICROTINES AND NON-MICROTINE RODENTS ALONG TWO NORTH-SOUTH TRANSECTS IN NORTH AMERICA (DATA FROM HALL, 1981)

	End points of transects					
	70°N, 14°W 15°N, 100°W			70°N, 110°W 15°N, 90°W		
Degrees N latitude	*Microtus*	Other microtines	Non-microtine rodents	*Microtus*	Other microtines	Non-microtine rodents
70	3	4	2	0	2	0
65	4	4	6	1	3	1
60	2	4	8	1	6	4
55	1	4	8	1	4	5
50	4	4	15	1	4	7
45	4	4	18	2	3	14
40	2	4	16	2	3	12
35	4	3	27	2	2	14
30	0	1	33	1	1	11
25	0	0	25		Gulf of Mexico	
20	1	0	25	0	0	16
15				1	0	16

stand hot, arid conditions. Consequently, summer heat more than winter cold seems to determine the locations at which *Microtus* can live. Only *M. ochrogaster, M. californicus,* and, at some localities, *M. montanus* are found in grasslands that are hot and dry.

Although such folivores (leaf-eaters) as *Sigmodon* are an important part of tropical grassland communities, they contribute relatively much less to the total small mammal community there compared to the importance of microtine folivores farther north, where vegetative structure and diversity are much reduced and many fewer mammalian species are found. It is in the grasslands, tundra, and taiga habitats that one or a few microtine rodents dominate and may occur with a few species of insectivores (mostly shrews), carnivores (mostly weasels), and omnivores (such as *Peromyscus maniculatus*).

When the geographic ranges of all North American *Microtus* are superimposed on a single map (Fig. 1), it can be seen that at many localities only a single species of the genus occurs. In addition to certain islands, these general regions include much of northeastern

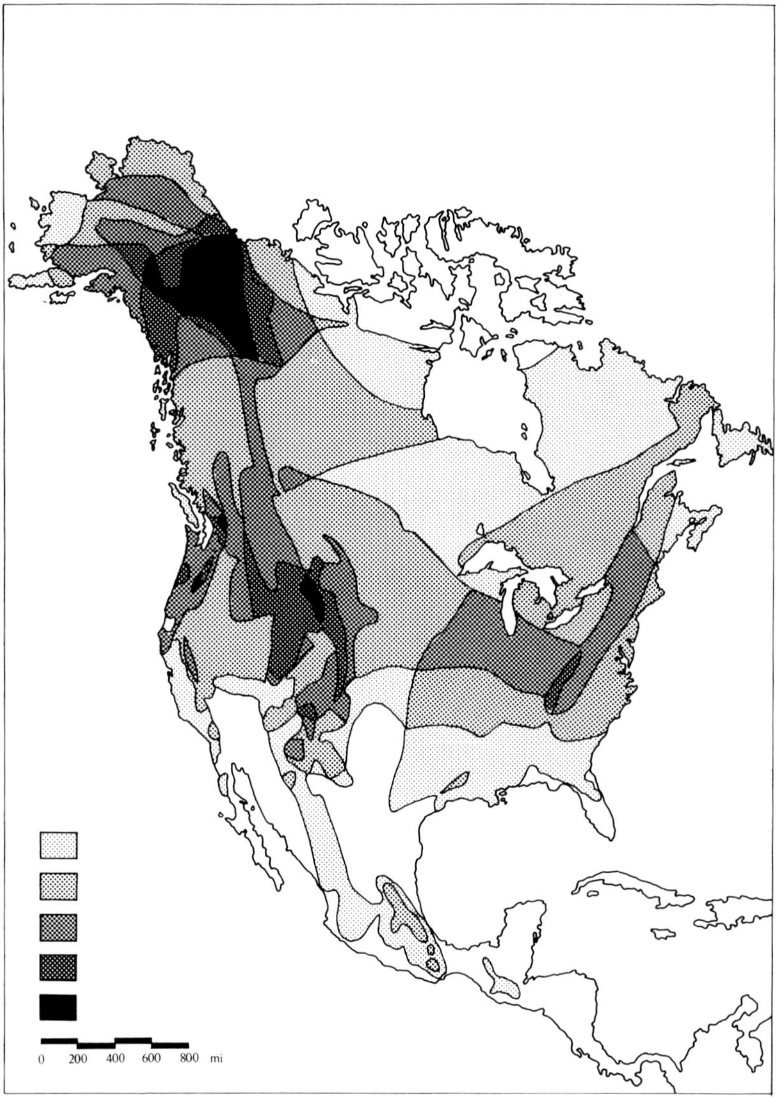

FIG. 1. Sketch map of North America showing approximate distributions of all species of *Microtus* in North America (compiled from Hall, 1981). Open areas indicate presence of no *Microtus* species. Stippling identifies areas that contain one (light stippling) to five (black) species of *Microtus*. Although as many as five or six species may overlap broadly, it is unusual for as many as three to co-occur in a single community.

Canada (*M. pennsylvanicus* being the only *Microtus*), southeastern U.S. (*M. pinetorum*), most of the range of the genus south of the U.S. (*M. mexicanus* and the relictual species *M. guatemalensis*; *M. quasiater, M. oaxacensis,* and *M. umbrosus* are sympatric and sometimes even syntopic with *M. mexicanus*), coastal areas of California and northern Baja California (*M. californicus*), and north-central Mackenzie Territory and sections of coastal Alaska (*M. oeconomus*). Other significant but small areas with only one *Microtus* species are western Kansas and adjacent Oklahoma (*M. ochrogaster*) and sections of New Mexico and Nevada (*M. longicaudus*). Two sympatric *Microtus* occur in much of the grasslands of the northern Great Plains and western Canada, where *M. pennsylvanicus* coexists with *M. ochrogaster, M. xanthognathus,* or *M. longicaudus.* Three and four broadly sympatric species tend to be limited to areas of considerable altitudinal relief and ecological diversity, including the Cascades, northern and southern Rockies, and parts of the Appalachians. The possibility of five *Microtus* species exists (on the basis of overlapping distributions only) for limited areas of the northern Rockies (mostly in Yukon) and the Cascades. Ranges of six species appear to approach each other closely in both the northern Cascades (*M. longicaudus, M. montanus, M. oregoni, M. pennsylvanicus, M. richardsoni,* and *M. townsendii*) and southern Cascades (*M. californicus* replaces *M. pennsylvanicus* as a possible sixth species). We know of no reports of more than three species of *Microtus* occurring together in a single small mammal community (see Getz, this volume). For example, even where Findley (1951, 1954) studied small mammal assemblages at Jackson Hole, Wyoming, no more than two of four species of *Microtus* were taken together in any of the 10 habitat types. Of the five *Microtus* in Colorado, Armstrong (1972) listed no more than three species for any of 14 community types. Possible triads were in yellow-pine woodland (*M. montanus, M. longicaudus,* and *M. mexicanus*), or montane subalpine meadow, highland streambank, and aspen woodland (*M. pennsylvanicus* replaces *M. mexicanus*). Steve West (pers. comm.) found three *Microtus* species together on only one of 25 study sites in central Alaska; that site, a recently burned black-spruce forest, also had three other microtine species. A total of six syntopic microtines is high, but non-*Microtus* species (for example, *Synaptomys* sp., *Clethrionomys* sp.) commonly occur with one or two species of *Microtus.*

The increase in small mammal species diversity in areas characterized by great altitudinal relief is well known, and the importance of this pattern to studies of latitudinal species diversity was reiterated recently by McCoy and Connor (1980). Its importance specifically to *Microtus* species was demonstrated for *M. longicaudus, M. pennsylvanicus, M. montanus,* and *M. mexicanus* in New Mexico by Findley (1954, 1969) and Findley and Jones (1962). Armstrong (1972:Fig. 121) illustrated the relationship between mammalian species density and mountainous regions in Colorado (see also Table 1).

In sum, communities with *Microtus* tend to be grasslands or tundra, and rarely to have more than two species of *Microtus* or six species of small mammals overall. Thus, their habitats tend to be structurally simple and the number of co-occurring species few. *Microtus* often dominates numerically and in its contribution to total small mammal biomass.

Environmental Parameters

Despite the fact that one or another species of *Microtus* can be found over most of North America, voles sometimes are restricted locally, and thus are not a ubiquitous component of North American grasslands and tundra. Many interrelated environmental parameters undoubtedly contribute to their presence or absence in a given community, including weather and climate, vegetative structure, food availability, competition, and predators.

Weather and climate.—Microtus is poorly adapted to conserve water or to thermoregulate at high ambient temperatures (Wunder, this volume). No *Microtus* species is found strictly in deserts or even desert grasslands. In southwestern Kansas, where *M. ochrogaster* reaches its southwestern distributional margin in relatively arid shortgrass prairie, this vole utilizes apparently self-dug burrows and is almost exclusively nocturnal during summer, presumably to avoid the extreme daytime heat and desiccating wind (Birney, pers. observ.). The short tail and ears and dense fur of *Microtus* serve well to conserve heat, but not to dissipate it.

In contrast, most or all species of *Microtus* are able to persist and even thrive in extremely cold climates. For example, *M. oeconomus* and *M. miurus* occur exclusively in the subarctic and tundra of northwestern Canada and Alaska. *M. xanthognathus, M. pennsylvanicus,* and *M. longicaudus* also extend their distributions inside the Arctic Circle. Although the air temperature may be as low as −70°C, the subnivean environment of the vole is close to 0°C. Winter survival of some species is enhanced in part by their habit of communal nesting. *M. xanthognathus* in central Alaska constructs large middens of stored food and insulation for winter survival of the five to 10 occupants (Wolff, 1980). Communal winter nesting is known for other species as well, including *M. pennsylvanicus* in New York (Madison, this volume) and *M. ochrogaster* in warmer eastern Kansas (Fitch, 1957).

Local weather conditions probably rarely affect the occurrence of voles in most small mammal communities, except indirectly through an effect on the vegetation. Martin (1960) reported that in the mixed prairie of western Kansas, *M. ochrogaster* was at low density during one drought and high density during another, indicating that even prolonged aridity does not invariably reduce the abundance of the species. However, on Martin's study area (a western wheatgrass community) the highest density recorded in two years was only 18.4 voles/ha, a much lower density than the 160 or more per ha reported for the same species in ungrazed tallgrass and in irrigated and fertilized shortgrass (Birney et al., 1976). Gaines and Rose (1976) reported densities of prairie voles of about 180/ha from brome oldfields in eastern Kansas. Thus, although vole populations can survive and apparently even thrive during temporary periods of drought, their role in the small mammal community of such areas may be relatively less than in areas of greater or more regular rainfall.

Flooding.—Flooding is a potentially serious short-term environmental factor that could affect small mammal communities. Voles are not adapted to climbing emergent vegetation, as has been observed for such rodents as *Peromyscus* and *Oryzomys* during floods. Wolff (1980) concluded that the flooding of old winter nests did not adversely affect *M. xanthognathus* because they dispersed at the time of snow melt. Similarly, Bee and Hall (1956) described the periodic flooding of the burrows of *M. miurus,* but the voles apparently were not excluded from the community by the temporary flooding. *M. pennsylvanicus* has been reported to avoid saturated substrates (Getz, 1967), but Lyon (1936) reported this vole living in grass tussocks surrounded by water in Indiana swamps. In peatland fens in northern Minnesota, Birney (pers. observ.) has studied breeding populations of *M. pennsylvanicus* living on sphagnum hummocks surrounded by standing water. Harper (1956) judged that a few hours of flooding during spring "break-up" in Keewatin had little effect on a population of *M. pennsylvanicus,* but that flooding and subsequent freezing on the same meadow in November greatly reduced their chances for winter survival.

Substrate.—Microtus species invariably use subterranean burrows to one degree or another. Soil richness and texture undoubtedly affect the local distribution and abundance of all species indirectly depending on their ability to burrow. Only for the fossorial species, *M. pinetorum,* has this been clearly demonstrated. Fisher and Anthony (1980), studying woodland voles in Pennsylvania orchards, failed to find them in one orchard with soils having relatively low percentages of gravel and sand and high percentages of fines and silts. They concluded that soil texture strongly influences the distribution of *M. pinetorum,* which requires more than 35% gravel and 20% clay, and less than 65% fines and 40% silt together with between 25 and 48% sand. In less-disturbed woodland habitats, this vole may burrow primarily in the duff and upper humus layers, and thus may be less rigidly tied to soil texture than to the surface covering.

Soil moisture may be of considerable importance, but how much of this is directly related to moisture and how much is indirect as moisture affects vegetation has not been determined. Murie (1969) showed that *M. pennsylvanicus* favored wet over dry substrates in the laboratory, but that *M. montanus* from the same area showed no preference. Getz (1967), on the other hand, found that *M. pennsylvanicus* avoided saturated substrates in the laboratory.

Microtus ochrogaster occupies burrows dug in hard, dry loam over much of its range, but most burrowing activities take place following autumnal rains that increase the friability of the soil (Rose, pers. observ.). Wolff and Lidicker (1980) noted that the complex, branching burrow systems of *M. xanthognathus* penetrated 15–25 cm, that is, to mineral soil or permafrost. Populations of *M. pennsylvanicus* on the Anoka Sand Plain of Minnesota reach high densities in the tall marsh grasses that grow there, but we know of no places where dry sand serves as a suitable substrate for *Microtus.* In Keewatin, Harper (1956) found *M. pennsylvanicus* in riverside meadows, sedge bogs, and on grass-covered sand dunes but never on the open summits of the gravelly ridges in the Barrens.

Rocky soils in mountainous areas serve as suitable substrates for voles of several species. For example, the usual habitat of *M. chrotorrhinus* seems to be the edges of boulder fields, although rock voles are sometimes found in unburned clearcuts (Kirkland, 1977), where limbs and brush piles may substitute for rocks.

Vegetation.—We believe that vegetation, more than any other single environmental factor, determines the presence or absence, as well as the relative role and importance of *Microtus,* in small mammal communities. Two field experiments on *M. ochrogaster* show the dramatic effect of increasing vegetative cover on this species. Birney et al. (1976) excluded cattle from grazing a 1-ha plot of tallgrass prairie in northeastern Oklahoma and observed the vole population increase dramatically during a single summer from none in May to 24 individuals/ha in October, while standing crop vegetation increased from 230 to 400 g dry weight/m^2. Only an occasional vole (1.0/ha) was trapped in an adjacent grazed control in October. Grant et al. (1977) provided irrigation water and nitrogen to two 1-ha plots of shortgrass prairie in eastern Colorado and compared the small mammal communities to those on initially similar controls. Over 4 years, *M. ochrogaster* located and became established on the experimental grids, showing a pattern of increasing from relatively low densities each spring to successively higher and earlier peak densities (over 100/ha in the fourth year) each summer or autumn. By comparison, no voles were trapped on the control grids until the third year of the study, and permanent populations never became established there. Cover levels on the experimental plots fluctuated between 600 and 1,200 g of dry weight/m^2, compared to 300–600 g/m^2 on the controls. Abramsky and Tracy (1979) speculated that shortgrass prairie is unsuitable for *M. ochrogaster* under conditions of normal rainfall and fertility; sparse vegetation and summer heat probably limit the distribution (Fig. 1) of these populations.

Birney et al. (1976; also see Elton, 1939; Frank, 1957; Getz, 1971) discussed several attributes of vegetative cover for *Microtus.* Of perhaps greatest importance is concealment and protection from predators. Getz (1970) concluded that heavy predation on a population of *M. pennsylvanicus* following mowing and baling of the vegetation accounted for the loss of most individuals, although his trapping results suggest that a few may have moved into an adjacent unmowed field.

Food provided by the vegetation obviously is also of great importance. Bee and Hall (1956), who studied the community association of five microtine species in northern Alaska, found that each species was associated with a particular vegetation type. Studies by Jung and Batzli (1981) demonstrated that secondary plant compounds differentially affected the growth rates of arctic microtines, and thus that the mere presence of green forage, even though it might provide adequate cover, is not synonymous with the presence of high-quality food for microtines. For most *Microtus* species, however, especially those that occur in vegetatively diverse habitats, a wide range of food is eaten (Zimmerman, 1965), and thus the species composition of grassy habitats is often of less importance to *Microtus* than is the presence of adequate cover (except see Batzli, this volume).

The presence of vegetative cover also must affect behavioral interactions among conspecifics. For example, Warnock (1965) demonstrated that cover reduced both fighting and mortality of crowded captive *M. pennsylvanicus.* Furthermore, the protection provided by dense cover undoubtedly permits daylight activity, which could be especially important for species living at high latitudes where daylight periods are long or even continuous during summer.

Hopkins (1954) measured the effects of a mulch layer in grassland habitat, and demonstrated its effect on the microhabitat. Such factors as surface-level humidity, temperature, penetration of light, and soil moisture all are affected by cover. Additionally, heavy cover prevents dense packing of snow at ground level, thus making the subnivean space more hospitable to the small mammals that live there.

Grant et al. (1982) demonstrated that cover levels on four grassland study areas had a greater effect on herbivorous rodents than on omnivorous or granivorous ones. Removal of cover by grazing ungulates affected the three most important herbivorous small mammals (*M. montanus, M. ochrogaster,* and *Sigmodon hispidus*) more adversely than any of the other eight common rodents. These results were interpreted as strong support for the hypothesis (French et al., 1976; Grant and Birney, 1979) that the general composition of grassland small mammal communities is determined primarily by structurally simple attributes (including cover) of the habitat. This hypothesis appears to be especially applicable to communities with one or more species of *Microtus.*

Not all species of *Microtus* are restricted to structurally simple grassland and tundra environments. Wolff and Lidicker (1980) pointed out that *M. xanthognathus* is restricted to the taiga. Within this broad habitat type, taiga voles appear to utilize a wide variety of forested and grassland areas from burned to unburned black-spruce forest to wet, grassy swamp. However, West (1979) found *M. xanthognathus* primarily in grass-sedge habitat associations with early successional stages, and considered *M. oeconomus* to have the widest habitat use pattern of Alaskan *Microtus*. Whitney (1976) also studied populations of *M. oeconomus* in vegetationally diverse taiga near Fairbanks, Alaska, but considered the species to have a narrower niche than sympatric *Clethrionomys rutilus*. Bee and Hall (1956) found *M. miurus* in a variety of wet and dry habitats, but usually associated with willows, on which it seemed to be partially dependent for winter food. *M. pinetorum,* commonly found in eastern deciduous forest, seems to reach high population densities only in grassy orchards (Benton, 1955), sometimes in the presence of *M. pennsylvanicus* (Fisher and Anthony, 1980). Additional evidence that grasses can enhance habitat quality of woodland voles was provided by Gentry (1968), who studied a population of *M. pinetorum* within enclosures in a *Lespedeza-Andropogon* oldfield in South Carolina, where trees were absent. Findley (1951) found *M. longicaudus* on forested rocky hillsides, in alder-willow swamps, and in grassy, open woods. Armstrong (1972) found long-tailed voles in a wide variety of habitats including sagebrush and pine woodland in Colorado. Other species that may be found in forested habitats include *M. pennsylvanicus,* especially in open woodlands with a grassy floor and on small islands (Cameron, 1958); *M. montanus,* but only if grass is available; *M. richardsoni,* in association with mountain streams and alpine marshes; *M. oeconomus,* present in all but the most mature black- and white-spruce forest in Alaska (West, 1979); and *M. oregoni,* which lives in a variety of habitats including damp areas within redwood, fir, spruce, and hemlock forests (Ingles, 1965).

Competition.—Despite the fact that there have been few studies of competition in *Microtus* (for example, Conley, 1976), we see competition as being very important in the shaping of communities with *Microtus.* There are many examples of *Microtus* numerically dominating other species, many of which have been given in this chapter. The most dramatic are those in which voles, such as *M.*

pennsylvanicus, outnumber all other small mammals combined, and may contribute more than 90% to total small mammal biomass (French, 1978; Pruitt, 1968). At some locations, two species share a prominent role in the community, such as in the central U.S. where *M. ochrogaster* and *M. pennsylvanicus* overlap in distribution (Krebs et al., 1969). At others, such as in eastern Kansas, *M. ochrogaster* shares the herbivore role with *Synaptomys cooperi,* another microtine rodent and a presumed ecological equivalent (Gaines et al., 1979) or with the larger cricetine, *Sigmodon hispidus* (Rose et al., 1977).

It is clear that *Microtus* is a dominant herbivore of northern origin and affinities and that *Sigmodon* is a dominant herbivore in grasslands from Mexico northward into the central plains. *S. hispidus* has moved progressively northward during historic times, and its movement across Kansas and into Nebraska has been documented by Genoways and Schlitter (1966). In part, this colonization northward was due to the ability of *Sigmodon* to use disturbed areas and perhaps cropland (Fleharty and Olson, 1969), but also to its ability to respond to semiarid conditions such as occurred during the 1930's "dustbowl" era. Droughts have a strongly adverse effect on *Microtus* (Martin, 1960; French et al., 1976), and this climatic factor may have contributed to the replacement of *M. ochrogaster* by *Sigmodon* as the dominant folivore in the grasslands of Kansas and perhaps of neighboring states as well. Some investigators (for example, Glass and Slade, 1980; Terman, 1974) have attempted to study competition between *Sigmodon* and *M. ochrogaster,* using combinations of field and laboratory experiments. *Sigmodon* tends to win under the conditions used in these studies. A counterbalancing force is high winter mortality in *Sigmodon,* which is poorly adapted to severe winters (Fleharty et al., 1972). There is good evidence that local populations of *Sigmodon* go extinct during severe winters (Slade, pers. comm.), at least in eastern Kansas. We imagine that such events would happen with greater frequency the farther north the populations. Thus, in this example of intergeneric competition of the dominant small herbivores in the central plains, it seems that *Microtus* contends better with the winters and *Sigmodon* with both summers and drought. Baker (1971) provided several examples of pairs of *Sigmodon* species that coexist in the Mexican grasslands in much the same way that pairs of *Microtus* do north of 35°N.

Competition has been proposed as the mechanism that tends to separate two or more coexisting *Microtus*. Findley (1951, 1954), in some of the earliest examples of possible biological competition in vertebrates, never found more than two of four *Microtus* species at the same location near Jackson Hole, Wyoming. The association between *M. montanus* and *M. pennsylvanicus* also has been studied by others, including Douglass (1976), Hodgson (1972), Koplin and Hoffmann (1968), and Murie (1969, 1971), using both laboratory and field experiments. Despite the numerous examples of possible competitive interactions of two *Microtus*, Krebs (1977) was unable to find any evidence that *M. ochrogaster* and *M. pennsylvanicus* had negative effects on one another. Nor could Gaines et al. (1979) find evidence that *M. ochrogaster* and *Synaptomys cooperi* adversely affected one another.

One of the most interesting examples of how competition may be important in shaping small mammal communities is found in the distributional patterns of *M. pennsylvanicus* and *Clethrionomys gapperi* in the islands of the St. Lawrence River and off the east coast of mainland Canada. In parts of the Maritime Provinces, *Clethrionomys* is absent, probably due to events of the post-Pleistocene period. There *M. pennsylvanicus* occupies a much wider range of habitats than is considered typical of that species, including interior forest habitats far removed from patches of grasses (Cameron, 1964). On islands in the St. Lawrence River, some of which have become connected with the mainland during historic times, some have *Microtus* and others have *Clethrionomys*. The species present lives in a wider range of habitats than would be characteristic on the nearby mainland where the two occur together. Cameron's explanation is that chance has played a role in determining which species colonized an island, but that once established the resident species was able to prevent successful colonizations by the other. Two later studies of this pair of microtines (Iverson and Turner, 1972; Turner et al., 1975) reported their winter coexistence, first in grassland habitat and then in spruce forest. In each case, when aggression levels increased with the onset of the reproductive season, the species that seemed to be in the "wrong" habitat left to return to its typical habitat. During the second study, Turner et al. (1975) used behavioral studies in the laboratory to determine that, although it dominated behaviorally throughout the winter, *Microtus* still was excluded by *Clethrionomys* from the forest habitat when breeding resumed. They interpreted these studies as competitive habitat exclusion related to reproduction-associated aggression. In a 10-year study of these two microtine rodents and *Peromyscus maniculatus* on islands in Maine, Crowell (1973) implicated competition as the principal reason for *Microtus* dominating the other two in nature.

Microtus pinetorum usually lives at low densities in disjunct populations in eastern deciduous forests. However, in orchards (Benton, 1955; Byers, this volume) or in enclosures where competitors are absent (Gentry, 1968), it can reach much higher densities. It is unclear how *M. pinetorum* responds to competition by *M. pennsylvanicus* but such studies are now in progress in orchards. *M. pinetorum* may be restricted mostly to forests because its poor competitive abilities prevent it from thriving elsewhere. If so, we would expect it to be displaced by *M. pennsylvanicus* in orchards.

Determining the role of competition in structuring communities with *Microtus* will require a combination of approaches including field experiments in which pairs of *Microtus* species coexist in some plots and live as separate species in others. Grant (1972) has conducted such studies with pairs of different species, including *Microtus,* in Ontario. Studies such as Getz (1963), of the renal efficiencies of *M. ochrogaster* and *M. pennsylvanicus,* and Zimmerman (1965), of the food habits of the same species, will be particularly useful in evaluating why species may be living syntopically in some places and not at others. Radiotelemetry and radio-isotopic techniques undoubtedly will be very useful in evaluating the microdistributions of individuals of the same and related species. We emphasize the need to have the non-*Microtus* rodents included as a part of these experiments because the evaluation of their role may be crucial to the proper interpretation of the results of all community studies.

Predation.—The importance of predation in population regulation and in determining the composition of small mammal communities has long been debated. Interactions between predators and *Microtus* species, considered in depth elsewhere (Pearson, this volume), may be relatively important under some circumstances in determining the magnitude of the impact of *Microtus* in the total small mammal community. Both mammalian (Pearson, 1971) and avian (Korschgen and Stuart, 1972) predators feed regularly and heavily on *Microtus* when they are available.

Pearson (1964:Fig. 2) clearly demonstrated the high percentage of a population of *M. californicus* that could be accounted for in predator scats as the vole population declined from August of one year until March of the next. Similarly, Maher (1967) observed evidence on Banks Island, Northwest Territories, that *Mustela erminea* had killed all but a few lemmings (both *Dicrostonyx* and *Lemmus*) on the island during winter after the lemming populations had been at least moderately high the previous autumn. Pearson (1971) concluded that predators have a major impact on microtine populations, especially following a "crash," when the presence of secondary prey species enables carnivores to exert heavy predation pressures on the remaining low population of voles. We concur with this conclusion, and suggest that such predator pressure may result in lower biomass and higher species diversity of the small mammal community than might otherwise exist. However, at moderate or high population densities, especially during periods of recruitment, we doubt that predators have much impact on the *Microtus* component of the community (see Golley, 1960).

The Influence of Microtus *on Communities*

Microtus influences its plant and animal communities because of frequently great density, relatively large size among small mammals, and indirectly because of high metabolic rates. In the extreme, these combine to produce denuded habitats during *Microtus* plagues, but more typically *Microtus* is a prominent, if not always dominant, member of the small mammal community. Its effects on plant communities are largely unmeasured but high differential consumption of some plant species may affect the relative success of plant species and thereby alter the habitat sufficiently to affect the animal component of the community.

The small mammal community with *Microtus* is often more variable than, for example, desert rodent or forest mammal communities, which typically lack *Microtus.* The latter communities have a high proportion of nocturnal species, and their numbers tend to fluctuate from season to season in a relatively predictable annual pattern. These communities may have some species that hibernate during the winter season, thereby affecting the seasonal dynamics of the community. Nevertheless, the year-to-year composition and biomass estimates of a desert or forest community of small mammals are likely to be more predictably constant than a community with *Microtus*.

By contrast, communities with *Microtus*: 1) often fluctuate greatly in numbers, not only from season to season but from year to year as well, mainly because of *Microtus*; 2) have proportionately more individuals active throughout the daylight hours as well as at night, which is largely due to the intermittent activity periods of *Microtus* (Madison, this volume; Shields, 1976); 3) have more predators focusing on them, because *Microtus* are relatively large among small mammals, often numerous, and available to diurnal as well as nocturnal predators; 4) have continuous activity because, although other community members such as *Zapus, Spermophilus,* and more rarely *Perognathus,* may hibernate, *Microtus* is active year-round; and 5) have relatively constant harvesting of vegetation because *Microtus,* with few exceptions, does not store food in caches. Communities with *Microtus,* then, often have high densities of small mammals that are active throughout the day, night, and year. Furthermore, during much of the year these small mammals tend to be dispersed more or less uniformly in the available habitat, in part because of spacing behavior described by Madison (this volume). In *M. xanthognathus* (Wolff, 1980) and *M. pennsylvanicus* (Madison, this volume), winter aggregations of voles conserve heat by communal nesting behavior but may suffer to a greater extent from predation because of it.

Effects of Density

Certainly the greatest influence of *Microtus* on the community is due to its great numbers when populations are near or at peak densities (see Taitt and Krebs, this volume). Densities of 100–300/ha are typical of peak periods in the multi-year cycle, and more than 1,000/ha have been reported. Only when the high densities persist for months or occur outside the growing season is there a significant depletion of the covering and edible vegetation. Rodent plagues can occur under these conditions, as reported for *M. oregoni* in 1957, when densities of 4,500–6,500/ha were estimated in agricultural fields in Oregon (Fed. Coop. Ext. Serv., 1959). Even at moderately high densities, it seems likely that the community of small mammals must be adversely affected, probably in many ways. As densities increase, suboptimal habitat is colonized by *Microtus*. The consequences of such habitat expansion rarely have been measured, except in the extreme case of house-mouse populations going to extinction as a result of successful colonization and subsequent population explosion of *M. californicus* on Brooks Island (Lidicker, 1966). Nevertheless, at high *Microtus* densities, most other small mammal species in the community will be affected somehow, either directly through interference competition for space or perhaps even for food, or indirectly through a physical alteration of the habitat as a result of partial denuding of vegetation, extensive digging of soil surface, and almost certainly by focusing predators on the large biomass of prey available in that habitat. It seems unlikely that a high biomass of *Microtus* would have a positive or beneficial impact on any species of small mammal, unless, as some have speculated, *Blarina* is a predator of nestling and young voles (Eadie, 1952).

Effects of Large Body Size

Not only is *Microtus* often abundant, but it is usually the largest small mammal species in the community, especially grasslands. Large body size accentuates the effects of numerical dominance and may help to promote the dominating influence of *Microtus* in many communities. For example, large body size in small mammals often is associated with large litter size, thereby contributing to species density and biomass. Also promoting the ability to produce large litters is their high metabolic rate, higher than predicted by the Kleiber curve (Kleiber, 1961). The high metabolic rates that promote rapid body growth, early maturity, and large litters, often in rapid succession, require the rapid conversion of grass into small mammal biomass. McNab (1980) speculated that because natural selection tends to favor as high a metabolic rate as the diet will permit, a species with a high metabolic rate potentially will be more successful than a competitor with a lower metabolic rate. In the community context, this may mean that *Microtus* has an edge over other species primarily because of its high metabolic rate. In sum, these factors combine to contribute to the influential position of *Microtus* in many small mammal communities.

Effects on Community Succession

Because high populations of *Microtus* often are associated with herbaceous vegetation of early stages of secondary plant succession, it might be expected that voles would influence the nature and rate of changes in plant communities. If that influence is real, then we would predict a concommitant secondary effect on succession of the small mammal community. Unfortunately, there is almost no information on the influence *Microtus* has on the dynamics of plant succession. Unless the climax vegetation is tundra or grassland, *Microtus* is a transitory species, present only in early to middle seral stages. For example, Wetzel (1958), who studied biological succession on abandoned strip mines in Illinois, found that *M. ochrogaster* was absent during the initial revegetation stages when annuals dominated the vegetation, but became the dominant element of the small mammal community after grasses and woody perennials achieved dominance of the plant community. Prairie voles were abundant only for about 20 years, and they disappeared from the area when the deciduous trees achieved approximately 65% of the plant coverage.

When forests are cut, significant and rapid changes in the vegetation composition occur. Herbaceous species tend to dominate for a few years, creating a habitat in which one or more species of *Microtus* often comes to dominate the small mammal community. Kirkland's (1977) study in the northern Appalachian forests demonstrated the transitory nature of *Microtus* in the deciduous and coniferous forests there. *M. pennsylvanicus* and *Synaptomys cooperi* were absent in both forest types that had not been cut for more than 25 years. After cutting, both microtines appeared, but they were absent after 5 years. *M. chrotorrhinus* was present at moderate densities in the 7- to 25-year-old forests, but increased significantly in both forest types after clearcutting and remained there for at least 15 years. Initial responses of the total small mammal community included increases in density and in community diversity as well as shifts in relative abundance of individual species and trophic groups. Krefting and Ahlgren (1974) reported similar responses by the small mammal communities following forest fires in Minnesota.

Gashwiler (1970) obtained similar results in a coniferous (mostly Douglas fir) forest in Oregon, where *M. oregoni* appeared in the clearcuts 1 year after cutting and increased to moderate densities by the fourth year, then decreased slightly but remained appreciably higher than populations in nearby virgin forest. *M. richardsoni* occasionally was taken on the clearcut but apparently did not establish a resident population there.

The ability of *Microtus* to colonize productive habitat quickly was demonstrated clearly by Grant et al. (1977), where only a single *M. ochrogaster* was trapped during 15,000 trap-nights in a grazed pasture and none was present on the nearby experimental grids prior to the application of irrigation water and nitrogen. Yet, within a few weeks a rapidly growing population of prairie voles was present in the dense vegetation that resulted from the experimental treatment. Although *Microtus* species can recolonize quickly after such disturbances as mowing (Getz, 1970) or grazing (Birney et al., 1976), succession of a small mammal community following the plowing of a prairie and its subsequent abandonment has not been studied adequately. In wetter tallgrass prairie, grasses undoubtedly would reappear more quickly than in drier mixed or shortgrass prairies, which would have a longer period of domination by annuals. Here, omnivores such as *Peromyscus maniculatus* probably would dominate for several years before *Microtus* would invade and come to dominate as the climax grasses reappeared. Succession in this case would lead to *Microtus* as the long-term dominant rather than as the transitory species it is when forest is the climax vegetation of the region.

Because the experiments excluding *Microtus* from some plots but not others have not been conducted, it is unknown whether *Microtus* influences the progression of plant succession at a given location. Although these exclosure studies would be long-term studies of plant and animal community dynamics, we believe that the influence of *Microtus* on the process can only be evaluated through such experimentation.

The Role of Microtus *in Small Mammal Communities*

The major role of *Microtus* in the small mammal community is as principal herbivore in almost all plant communities where it lives. As grazers, primarily of stems and leaves, *Microtus* has the potential to alter plant communities and indirectly to help determine the habitat structure and resources available to other syntopic small mammals.

Microtus is usually the dominant primary consumer among the small mammals living in grassland and tundra communities. Species of *Microtus* that have been studied for their dietary selection eat mostly vegetative plant parts. Zimmerman (1965), studying *Microtus* food and habitat in western Indiana, reported that *M. ochrogaster* ate proportionately more roots and seeds (18.8% of volume) than did *M. pennsylvanicus* (0.4% of volume). These two species ate insect material at the rate of 4.7 and 3.6%, respectively. Each species consumed a small amount of *Microtus* flesh and subterranean fungi, but about 93% of the volume of food was vascular plants, mostly stems and leaves. Zimmerman (1965) noted that *M. ochrogaster* took the most common plants in greatest frequency (also reported by Fleharty and Olson, 1969, and Martin, 1956, in Kansas), but some plants, especially the somewhat aromatic *Ambrosia, Aster,* and *Solidago,* generally were avoided. Meadow voles in Indiana (Zimmerman, 1965) ate fewer kinds of plants but were similar to prairie voles in relying heavily on the common species. M'Closkey and Fieldwick (1975), who evaluated the foods of coexisting *Peromyscus leucopus* and *M. pennsylvanicus,* found that the former ate 74% and the latter 8% insect material, the remainder being combinations of dicots, monocots, subterranean fungi and, for *Microtus* only, ferns (6%).

Food selection by *M. xanthognathus* in black-spruce forest has been studied by Wolff and Lidicker (1980) and West (1979), both in interior Alaska, and by Douglass (1976, 1977) in Northwest Territories. In Alaska, more than 85% of the diet was grasses and berries; in Wolff and Lidicker's (1980) study, a large proportion (37% of the volume) was *Equisetum* (horsetails). Douglass and Douglass (1977), who examined the summer foods of *M. xanthognathus,* reported the following composition of 629 piles of cuttings: 89% *Carex* spp., 5% *Rumex,* 3% *Calamogrostis,* 2% *Vaccinium,* and 1% *Equisetum.* Thus, despite their use of taiga as habitat, taiga voles ate little woody material but did rely heavily on the grasses and other herbs for food. This dietary selection possibly accounts for the fact that the densities of *M. xanthognathus* are much greater than have been reported for either *M. pinetorum* or *M. chrotorrhinus* in other forest environments.

Stomach content analyses, coupled with a census of the available foods, are badly needed to learn more of the details of the role of *Microtus* as consumers. Studies of food habits during periods of gradual community change may be especially revealing in explaining why *Microtus* often is present only for a relatively brief period in early seral stages. During biological succession, if *Microtus* persists in relying almost entirely on the ever-diminishing grasses and herbs, the replacement of *Microtus* by *Peromyscus leucopus, P. maniculatus* (woodland subspecies), or *Clethrionomys* spp. may be related more to diminishing food resources than to competition with these rodents. Although the water- and nitrogen-supplementation experiments of Grant et al. (1977) suggest a strong positive association between primary production of grasses on the Colorado shortgrass prairie and secondary production of *Microtus*, additional experimental studies are needed, including those of forest-dwelling *Microtus*, to demonstrate a link between the biomass of herbaceous vegetation and that of *Microtus*. The abundance of *M. pennsylvanicus*, *M. oeconomus*, and especially *M. xanthognathus* and vegetative cover values correlated positively in early successional stages of burned-over black-spruce forest in Alaska, but correlated negatively in advanced successional stages (West, 1979).

Relatively few attempts have been made to examine the biomass of small mammal communities, and to measure the changing role of the member species from year to year. Pruitt (1966) was unable to find synchrony between sample plots of either species or number of individuals. However, when he considered biomass per sample plot (Pruitt, 1968), he did detect synchrony among the biomasses of small mammals. Pruitt's studies, conducted over 8 years in different regions of Alaska, evaluated the differential contributions of two species of *Sorex*, two of *Microtus*, and those of three other microtine rodents. Pruitt (1968) interpreted these results to mean that ecosystem productivity "waxes and wanes in a regular progression." Chance, which he believed determined the "massive increase or decrease" of species, perhaps plays less of a role where the climatic extremes are not so severe. Martin (1956) looked at the relationship between plant production and the biomasses of *M. ochrogaster* and *Sigmodon hispidus*, but he only reported values for a single month; repeated values would have permitted an evaluation of the changing roles of the two herbivores to determine whether *Microtus* contributed relatively more during the cool months and *Sigmodon* more in the warm months.

Grant et al. (1982) compared the effects of habitat perturbation (grazing) on the small mammal biomass in different grassland types, using treatment and control grids. The detrimental effects were substantially greater in the tallgrass prairie (where *M. ochrogaster* and *Sigmodon hispidus* shared the herbivore role) than at the bunchgrass or shortgrass sites. Grant et al. (1982) suggested that seasonal and year-to-year fluctuations in the biomass of small mammal species cause a high variability in the community biomass of a site, and they argued that biomass changes are characteristic of many types of North American grasslands (French et al., 1976; Grant and

Birney, 1979). These variations are similar to what Pruitt (1968) called "fortuitous" events that determine the changing contributions of individual species from year to year at the same location. At the tallgrass site, Grant et al. (1982) found that grazing resulted in an increased contribution of *Spermophilus* and *Peromyscus maniculatus bairdii* to small mammal biomass; the contribution of *M. ochrogaster* and *Sigmodon* to biomass dropped by 90% on the grazed plots.

French et al. (1976) evaluated the energetics of small mammals of grassland ecosystems in the central U.S. Except for 1 year on a desert grassland, small mammals consumed less than 10% of the available herbage foods. By contrast, a high proportion of animal food was eaten at many sites in different years. These authors speculated that seed-eaters are more K-selected (they exhibit hibernation and torpor) and have social mechanisms and body-size differences to reduce competition. They argued that these adaptations contributed to their success relative to the grass-eaters in shortgrass prairie, where *Microtus* is abundant only on experimental plots in which water and nitrogen stimulated growth of grasses (Grant et al., 1977).

Golley (1960) measured energy flow in a grass-*Microtus*-*Mustela* system in Michigan. He estimated that *M. pennsylvanicus* consumed only 1.6% of the energy available to it, and that the weasel consumed 31% of energy available in the form of *Microtus*.

The presence of *Microtus* in a community often results in a significant physical alteration of the environment because they construct runways and burrows and extensively clip herbaceous vegetation. Pearson (1959), using photographs, showed that many other species of small mammals used runways built and maintained by *Microtus*. Digging activities of *Microtus* may create exposed soil substrates needed by seeds to germinate. Effects of grazing by *Microtus* are disputed and undoubtedly are variable; grazing may stimulate some plants to produce new vegetative growth but also may seriously or mortally wound other plants. Experiments to evaluate critically the role of *Microtus* in altering the habitat, using exclosures and measured densities of voles, have not been conducted at even a single location, to our knowledge. This is certainly an area of research where large contributions can be made in our understanding of the role of *Microtus* in the small mammal community and in the ecosystem.

Conclusions and Perspectives

Microtus is found in most grassland and tundra communities, and to a lesser extent in forest communities north of 35°N. As many as four to six species of *Microtus* may be broadly sympatric in some regions, such as in the western U.S. *Microtus* often is both the largest and the most numerous small mammal, and the genus may contribute 90% or more of the small mammal biomass per unit area. Exceptions to this trend can be found in marginal habitats, in the usually brief periods of low density in population cycles, in certain successional stages, and in forests. Predators may focus on *Microtus* where it is abundant, and *Microtus* influences the small mammal community in other ways. *Microtus* eats plant parts almost exclusively and is usually the dominant primary consumer.

Despite this prominent position in its community, *Microtus* rarely has been evaluated, and almost never studied, in the community context. Sometimes *Microtus* and one or two syntopic microtines are examined, either for evidence of competition or of synchrony of population cycles. In some instances, the composition and relative numbers of small mammals in the community are reported, permitting the reader to assess the potential effect of coexisting species on *Microtus*. Occasionally authors make it clear that non-microtines were or were not permanently removed from the study grids, but in many cases no statement is given about the occurrence of other species. Although it is understandable that microtine population ecologists may foresee little immediate benefit from the trapping, tagging, and handling during each trapping period of dozens of *Peromyscus, Sigmodon, Reithrodontomys,* or other species, an understanding of the dynamics of these species may be crucial to explaining microtine cycles, especially if Lidicker (1973, 1978) is correct in his assertion that many factors are involved in population regulation of *Microtus*. More importantly, neither the influence of *Microtus* on the small mammal community nor the role of *Microtus* in the ecosystem can be evaluated critically until all small mammals are examined together.

One thing we have learned, more than any other, from writing this chapter, is that the study of *Microtus* in the community context is a potentially fertile area of research. *Microtus* typically is not present in community studies of small mammals in desert (Brown,

1973, et seq.) nor in eastern decidious forest (Dueser and Shugart, 1978, 1979). Among those studying *Microtus,* only West (1979) has used Dueser and Shugart's technique of measuring vegetation structure and predicting which species will use which components of the physical habitats. Except for Grant's (1969, et seq.) experimental studies of competition with field populations of *M. pennsylvanicus* and one other species, planned experiments have not been conducted to learn more details of the respective roles of the four to six small mammal species in grassland and tundra communities. The study of mammalian community ecology in these plant communities will not be easy, in part because the number of *Microtus* often is much greater than that of all others. On the other hand, when numbers of *Microtus* are low, poor trapping success may cause the investigator to question whether or not to continue the study. Perhaps the best descriptive studies could be conducted in plant communities that are in transition; for example, large grasslands that grade into shrubby ecotones and then into young and old forest could be ideal. Here it would be possible to see the changing role of grassland *Microtus* as the woody elements increase to dominance. Leaps of insight will be possible using perturbation experiments, especially large and well-replicated ones in which more than two species can be evaluated simultaneously. Finally, some investigators, such as West (1979), have the necessary detailed information from fairly long-term studies to meld what may have been designed as multiple population studies into reports of small mammal communities with *Microtus.* Such reports would be extremely valuable in providing direction for the descriptive and experimental studies that are necessary if we are to learn the true influence and role of *Microtus* in small mammal communities.

Acknowledgments

We thank our wives, Aleene Rose and Marcia Birney, for their indulgence during the 10 days we devoted to writing the first draft of this chapter. Prassede Calabi, Ray Dueser, Roger Everton, Norm French, Lowell Getz, Gerda Nordquist, John Porter, and an anonymous reviewer all provided useful suggestions on earlier drafts. Steve West assisted us immeasurably by reviewing the manuscript, making a copy of his dissertation available to us, and especially by verifying our interpretation of statements about Alaskan mammals.

Neither of us has studied mammals in the tundra or taiga in North America and we thank Steve for contributing to the accuracy of several of our remarks. Full responsibility for all interpretations and conclusions, of course, rests with us.

Literature Cited

ABRAMSKY, Z., AND C. R. TRACY. 1979. Population biology of a "noncycling" population of prairie voles and a hypothesis on the role of migration in regulating microtine cycles. Ecology, 60:349–361.

ARMSTRONG, D. M. 1972. Distribution of mammals in Colorado. Monogr. Mus. Nat. Hist., Univ. Kansas, 3:1–415.

BAKER, R. H. 1971. Nutritional strategies of myomorph rodents in North American grasslands. J. Mamm., 52:800–805.

BEE, J. W., AND E. R. HALL. 1956. Mammals of northern Alaska. Misc. Publ. Mus. Nat. Hist., Univ. Kansas, 8:1–309.

BENTON, A. H. 1955. Observations on the life history of the northern pine mouse. J. Mamm., 36:52–62.

BIRNEY, E. C., W. E. GRANT, AND D. D. BAIRD. 1976. Importance of vegetative cover to cycles of *Microtus* populations. Ecology, 57:1043–1053.

BROWN, J. H. 1973. Species diversity of seed-eating desert rodents in sand dune habitats. Ecology, 54:775–787.

CAMERON, A. W. 1958. Mammals of the islands in the Gulf of St. Lawrence. Bull. Natl. Mus. Canada, 154:1–165.

———. 1964. Competitive exclusion between the rodent genera *Microtus* and *Clethrionomys*. Evolution, 18:630–634.

CONLEY, W. 1976. Competition between *Microtus*; a behavioral hypothesis. Ecology, 57:224–237.

CROWELL, K. L. 1973. Experimental zoogeography: introductions of mice to small islands. Amer. Nat., 107:535–558.

DOUGLASS, R. J. 1976. Spatial interactions and microhabitat selections of two locally sympatric voles, *Microtus montanus* and *M. pennsylvanicus*. Ecology, 57:346–352.

———. 1977. Population dynamics, home ranges, and habitat associations of the yellow-cheeked vole, *Microtus xanthognathus,* in the Northwest Territories. Canadian Field-Nat., 91:237–247.

DOUGLASS, R. J., AND K. S. DOUGLASS. 1977. Microhabitat selection of chestnut-cheeked voles (*Microtus xanthognathus*). Canadian Field-Nat., 91:72–74.

DUESER, R. D., AND H. H. SHUGART. 1978. Microhabitats in a forest-floor small mammal fauna. Ecology, 59:89–98.

———. 1979. Niche pattern in a forest-floor small-mammal fauna. Ecology, 60: 108–118.

EADIE, W. R. 1952. Shrew predation and vole populations on a limited area. J. Mamm., 33:185–189.

ELTON, C. 1939. On the nature of cover. J. Wildl. Mgmt., 3:332–338.

FEDERAL COOPERATIVE EXTENSION SERVICE. 1959. The Oregon meadow mouse irruption of 1957–1958. Oregon State Coll., Corvallis, 88 pp.

FINDLEY, J. S. 1951. Habitat preferences of four *Microtus* in Jackson Hole, Wyoming. J. Mamm., 32:118–120.

———. 1954. Competition as a possible limiting factor in the distribution of *Microtus*. Ecology, 35:418–420.

———. 1969. Biogeography of southwestern boreal and desert mammals. Misc. Publ. Mus. Nat. Hist., Univ. Kansas, 51:113–128.

FINDLEY, J. S., AND C. J. JONES. 1962. Distribution and variation of voles of the genus *Microtus* in New Mexico and adjacent areas. J. Mamm., 43:154–166.

FISHER, A. R., AND R. G. ANTHONY. 1980. The effect of soil texture on distribution of pine voles in Pennsylvania orchards. Amer. Midland Nat., 104:39–46.

FITCH, H. S. 1957. Aspects of reproduction and development in the prairie vole (*Microtus ochrogaster*). Univ. Kansas Publ., Mus. Nat. Hist., 10:129–161.

FLEHARTY, E. D., AND L. E. OLSON. 1969. Summer food habits of *Microtus ochrogaster* and *Sigmodon hispidus*. J. Mamm., 50:475–486.

FLEHARTY, E. D., J. R. CHOATE, AND M. A. MARES. 1972. Fluctuations in population density of the hispid cotton rat: factors influencing a "crash." Bull. So. California Acad. Sci., 71:132–138.

FLEMING, T. H. 1973. Numbers of mammal species in North and Central American forest communities. Ecology, 54:555–563.

FRANK, F. 1957. The causality of microtine cycles in Germany. J. Wildl. Mgmt., 21:113–121.

FRENCH, N. R. 1978. Small mammals as components of the consumer system. Pp. 61–67, *in* Populations of small mammals under natural conditions (D. P. Snyder, ed.). Spec. Publ. Ser., Pymatuning Lab. Ecol., Univ. Pittsburgh, 5:1–237.

FRENCH, N. R., W. E. GRANT, W. GRODZINSKI, AND D. M. SWIFT. 1976. Small mammal energetics in grassland ecosystems. Ecol. Monogr., 46:201–220.

GAINES, M. S., AND R. K. ROSE. 1976. Population dynamics of *Microtus ochrogaster* in eastern Kansas. Ecology, 57:1145–1161.

GAINES, M. S., C. L. BAKER, AND A. M. VIVAS. 1979. Demographic attributes of dispersing southern bog lemmings (*Synaptomys cooperi*) in eastern Kansas. Oecologia, 40:91–101.

GASHWILER, J. S. 1970. Plant and animal changes on a clearcut in west-central Oregon. Ecology, 51:1018–1026.

GENOWAYS, H. H., AND D. A. SCHLITTER. 1966. Northward dispersal of the hispid cotton rat in Nebraska and Missouri. Trans. Kansas Acad. Sci., 69:356–357.

GENTRY, J. B. 1968. Dynamics of an enclosed population of pine vole, *Microtus pinetorum*. Res. Population Ecol., 10:21–30.

GETZ, L. L. 1963. A comparison of water balance of the prairie and meadow voles. Ecology, 44:202–207.

———. 1967. Responses of selected small mammals to water. Occas. Papers Univ. Connecticut, Biol. Sci. Ser., 1:71–81.

———. 1970. Influence of vegetation on the local distribution of the meadow vole in southern Wisconsin. Occas. Papers Univ. Connecticut, Biol. Sci. Ser., 1:213–241.

———. 1971. Microclimate, vegetative cover, and local distribution of the meadow vole. Trans. Illinois Acad. Sci., 64:9–21.

GLASS, G. E., AND N. A. SLADE. 1980. Population structure as a predictor of spatial association between *Sigmodon hispidus* and *Microtus ochrogaster*. J. Mamm., 61:473–485.

GOLLEY, F. B. 1960. Energy dynamics of a food chain of an oldfield community. Ecol. Monogr., 30:187–205.

GRANT, P. R. 1969. Experimental studies of competitive interaction in a two-species system. I. *Microtus* and *Clethrionomys* species in enclosures. Canadian J. Zool., 47:1059–1082.

———. 1972. Interspecific competition among rodents. Ann. Rev. Ecol. Syst., 3: 79–106.

GRANT, W. E., AND E. C. BIRNEY. 1979. Small mammal community structure in North American grasslands. J. Mamm., 60:23–36.

GRANT, W. E., N. R. FRENCH, AND D. M. SWIFT. 1977. Response of a small mammal community to water and nitrogen treatments in a shortgrass prairie ecosystem. J. Mamm., 58:637–652.

GRANT, W. E., E. C. BIRNEY, N. R. FRENCH, AND D. M. SWIFT. 1982. Structure and productivity of grassland small mammal communities related to grazing-induced changes in vegetative cover. J. Mamm., 63:248–262.

HALL, E. R. 1981. The mammals of North America. Second ed. John Wiley and Sons, New York, 2:601–1181 + *90*.

HARPER, F. 1956. The mammals of Keewatin. Misc. Publ. Mus. Nat. Hist., Univ. Kansas, 12:1–96.

HODGSON, J. R. 1972. Local distribution of *Microtus montanus* and *Microtus pennsylvanicus* in southwestern Montana. J. Mamm., 53:487–499.

HOPKINS, H. H. 1954. Effect of mulch upon certain factors of the grassland environment. J. Range Mgmt., 7:255–258.

INGLES, L. G. 1965. Mammals of the Pacific states. Stanford Univ. Press, Stanford, California, 506 pp.

IVERSON, S. L., AND B. N. TURNER. 1972. Winter coexistence of *Clethrionomys gapperi* and *Microtus pennsylvanicus* in a grassland habitat. Amer. Midland Nat., 88:440–445.

JUNG, H. G., AND G. O. BATZLI. 1981. Nutritional ecology of microtine rodents: effects of plant extracts on the growth of arctic microtines. J. Mamm., 62: 286–292.

KIRKLAND, G. L., JR. 1977. Responses of small mammals to the clearcutting of northern Appalachian forests. J. Mamm., 58:600–609.

KLEIBER, M. 1961. The fire of life: an introduction to animal energetics. John Wiley and Sons, New York, 478 pp.

KOPLIN, J. R., AND R. S. HOFFMANN. 1968. Habitat overlap and competitive exclusion in voles (*Microtus*). Amer. Midland Nat., 80:494–507.

KORSCHGEN, L. J., AND H. B. STUART. 1972. Twenty years of avian predator-small mammal relationships in Missouri. J. Wildl. Mgmt., 36:269–282.

KREBS, C. J. 1977. Competition between *Microtus pennsylvanicus* and *Microtus ochrogaster*. Amer. Midland Nat., 97:42–49.

KREBS, C. J., B. L. KELLER, AND R. H. TAMARIN. 1969. *Microtus* population biology: demographic changes in fluctuating populations of *M. ochrogaster* and *M. pennsylvanicus* in southern Indiana. Ecology, 50:587–607.

KREFTING, L. W., AND C. E. AHLGREN. 1974. Small mammals and vegetation after fire in a mixed conifer-hardwood forest. Ecology, 55:1391–1398.

LIDICKER, W. Z., JR. 1966. Ecological observations on a feral house mouse population declining to extinction. Ecol. Monogr., 36:27–50.

———. 1973. Regulation of numbers in an island population of California voles, a problem in community dynamics. Ecol. Monogr., 43:271–302.

———. 1978. Regulation of numbers in small mammal populations—historical reflections and a synthesis. Pp. 122–141, *in* Populations of small mammals under natural conditions (D. P. Snyder, ed.). Spec. Publ. Ser., Pymatuning Lab. Ecol., Univ. Pittsburgh, 5:1–237.

LYON, M. W., JR. 1936. Mammals of Indiana. Amer. Midland Nat., 171–384.

MAHER, W. J. 1967. Predation by weasels on a winter population of lemmings, Banks Island, Northwest Territories. Canadian Field-Nat., 81:248–250.

MARTIN, E. P. 1956. A population study of the prairie vole (*Microtus ochrogaster*) in northeastern Kansas. Univ. Kansas Publ., Mus. Nat. Hist., 8:361–416.

———. 1960. Distribution of native mammals among the communities of the mixed prairie. Fort Hays Studies (new series), Sci. Ser., 1:1–26.

MCCOY, E. D., AND E. F. CONNOR. 1980. Latitudinal gradients in the species diversity of North American mammals. Evolution, 34:193–203.

M'CLOSKEY, R. T., AND B. FIELDWICK. 1975. Ecological separation of sympatric rodents (*Peromyscus* and *Microtus*). J. Mamm., 56:119–129.

MCNAB, B. K. 1980. Food habits, energetics, and the population biology of mammals. Amer. Nat., 116:106–123.

MURIE, J. O. 1969. An experimental study of substrate selection by two species of voles (*Microtus*). Amer. Midland Nat., 82:622–625.

———. 1971. Behavioral relationships between two sympatric voles (*Microtus*): relevance to habitat segregation. J. Mamm., 52:181–186.

PEARSON, O. P. 1959. A traffic survey of *Microtus-Reithrodontomys* runways. J. Mamm., 40:169–180.

———. 1964. Carnivore-mouse predation: an example of its intensity and bioenergetics. J. Mamm., 43:177–188.

———. 1971. Additional measurements of impact of carnivores on California voles (*Microtus californicus*). J. Mamm., 52:41–49.

PRUITT, W. O., JR. 1966. Ecology of terrestrial mammals. Pp. 519–564, *in* Environment of the Cape Thompson Region, Alaska (N. J. Wilimovsky and J. N. Wolfe, eds.). U.S. Atomic Energy Comm., 1,250 pp.

———. 1968. Synchronous biomass fluctuations of some northern mammals. Mammalia, 32:172–191.

ROSE, R. K., N. A. SLADE, AND J. H. HONACKI. 1977. Live trap preference among grassland mammals. Acta Theriol., 223:292–307.

SHIELDS, L. J. 1976. Telemetric determination of free-ranging rodent activities: the fine structure of *Microtus californicus* activity patterns. Unpubl. Ph.D. dissert., Univ. California, Los Angeles, 110 pp.

SIMPSON, G. G. 1964. Species density of North American Recent mammals. Syst. Zool., 13:57–73.

TERMAN, M. R. 1974. Behavioral interactions between *Microtus* and *Sigmodon*: a model for competitive exclusion. J. Mamm., 55:705–719.

TURNER, B. N., M. R. PERRIN, AND S. L. IVERSON. 1975. Winter coexistence of voles in spruce forest: the relevance of seasonal changes in aggression. Canadian J. Zool., 53:1004–1011.

WARNOCK, J. E. 1965. The effects of crowding on the survival of meadow voles (*Microtus pennsylvanicus*) deprived of cover and water. Ecology, 46:649–664.

WEST, S. D. 1979. Habitat response of microtine rodents to central Alaskan forest succession. Unpubl. Ph.D. dissert., Univ. California, Berkeley, 101 pp.

WETZEL, R. M. 1958. Mammalian succession in midwestern floodplains. Ecology, 39:262–271.

WHITNEY, P. 1976. Population ecology of two sympatric species of subarctic microtine rodents. Ecol. Monogr., 46:85–104.

WILSON, J. W., III. 1974. Analytical zoogeography of North American mammals. Evolution, 28:124–140.

WOLFF, J. O. 1980. Social organization of the taiga vole (*Microtus xanthognathus*). The Biologist, 62:34–45.

Wolff, J. O., and W. Z. Lidicker, Jr. 1980. Population ecology of the taiga vole, *Microtus xanthognathus,* in interior Alaska. Canadian J. Zool., 58: 1800–1812.
Zimmerman, E. G. 1965. A comparison of habitat and food of two species of *Microtus.* J. Mamm., 46:605–612.

BEHAVIOR

JERRY O. WOLFF

Abstract

BEHAVIOR of *Microtus* may be categorized as either non-social or social. Non-social behaviors such as locomotory, exploratory, body maintenance, swimming, and nest and runway construction are adapted to the two-dimensional grassland environment inhabited by these animals. The social organization of microtines is the result of behaviors associated with courtship and mating, parental care, social structure (spacing patterns), aggression, communication, and communal nesting. Mating systems of *Microtus* are commonly promiscuous (for example, *M. pennsylvanicus* and *M. richardsoni*), polygynous (for example, *M. xanthognathus, M. californicus,* and *M. montanus*), and rarely, but sometimes monogamous (for example, *M. ochrogaster*). Species-specific copulatory patterns are adapted to particular social organizations in specific habitats and may also be a reproductive isolating mechanism between similar sympatric species. Most social groupings consist of mother-young units and paternal care is minimal or non-existent. In some species territoriality occurs only in males (for example, *M. xanthognathus*), in females (for example, *M. pennsylvanicus* and *M. richardsoni*), or in both sexes (for example, *M. montanus, M. ochrogaster,* and *M. californicus*). Patterns of aggression may vary between species, but within a species they follow a predictable pattern that is correlated with a particular type of social system. If females are aggressive, they usually fight for space, whereas males fight for space and/or females. Scent-marking by the deposition of sebum from sebaceous glands located in the hip or flank region is described for several species and functions in individual recognition, territorial marking, and mate attraction. Communal winter nesting and food storing occur in several northern species and are adaptations for survival in severe boreal climates. An attempt is made to integrate the social structure and socio-ecology of *Microtus* within the life history framework of this mammal group.

Introduction

In North America, members of the genus *Microtus* are concentrated in grassland habitats between 40° and 70°N latitude. This range is characterized by a fluctuating environment which favors life history strategies adapted to seasonality and a variety of extrinsic variables. The adaptive zone of *Microtus* includes: 1) consumption of vegetation parts (primarily grasses); 2) r-selected reproductive features; 3) ability to colonize new habitats; and 4) a complex repertoire of behaviors associated with each of these features. These behaviors may be non-social, such as locomotory, exploratory, and foraging and food gathering behaviors, nest and runway construction, and body maintenance; or social, which include mating, parental, communicatory, agonistic, and other behaviors involving interactions between individuals. Social behavior is extremely complex and variable, and more difficult to observe, document, and interpret than non-social behavior, but it is essential to understanding the evolutionary significance of life history traits. In this chapter, I summarize the available literature on *Microtus* behavior and emphasize the evolutionary significance of social behavior and organization. An attempt also is made to compare behavioral patterns across species to show parallel adaptations to similar ecological regimes.

Non-social Behavior

A description and classification of behavioral components of locomotion, grooming, general body maintenance, and comfort movements have been described for several species of *Microtus* (Dewsbury et al., 1980; Jannett, 1977; Sloane et al., 1978; Webster et al., 1979; Wilson et al., 1976) (Table 1). Locomotor-exploratory behavior is the most prevalent behavior for all species. All species exhibit wall-seeking behavior, rearing at wall, grooming head moving, and freezing. Jumping is infrequent and climbing is not observed. Climbing does not appear to be an adaptive feature in *Microtus* species that inhabit a two-dimensional grassland habitat. In addition, depth perception is not apparent in *M. montanus* and is only slightly developed in *M. californicus* and *M. pennsylvanicus* (Sloane et al., 1978). In comparative studies between different taxa,

TABLE 1
NON-SOCIAL BEHAVIORS FOR NEW WORLD *Microtus*

	Locomotion, maintenance, and comfort movements[1]	Digging[2]	Swimming[3]	Runway construction[4]	Nest building[5]
M. californicus	X		X		X
M. canicaudus	X				X
M. montanus	X	X	X	X	X
M. ochrogaster	X	X	X	X	X
M. pennsylvanicus	X	X	X	X	X
M. richardsoni			X	X	X
M. xanthognathus			X	X	X

[1] Dewsbury et al. (1980); Jannett (1977); Sloane et al. (1978); Webster et al. (1979); Wilson et al. (1976).
[2] Webster et al. (1981).
[3] Evans et al. (1978); Getz (1967); Ludwig (1981); Wolff (pers. observ.).
[4] Fitzgerald and Madison (1983); Ludwig (1981); Thomas and Birney (1979); Wolff (1980); Wolff and Lidicker (1981).
[5] Ambrose (1973); Dalquest (1948); Hartung and Dewsbury (1979*a*); Jameson (1947); Jannett (1978*a*, 1981*a*); Ludwig (1981); Martin (1956); Maser and Storm (1970); Salt (1978); Thomas and Birney (1979); Wolff and Lidicker (1981).

field-dwelling species such as *Microtus* exhibit more boli deposition, freezing, and grooming compared to forest and desert dwelling genera (Wilson et al., 1976).

Apparently all *Microtus* species are capable of digging as evidenced by the extensive network of underground runways and tunnels; however, this behavior has not been analyzed and described for all species. Digging behaviors of three *Microtus* species (*M. montanus, M. ochrogaster,* and *M. pennsylvanicus*) have been observed on peat and sand substrates in the laboratory (Webster et al., 1981). The most prevalent digging pattern involved simultaneous use of the rear paws together with alternating use of the forepaws. The amount of digging for each species varied depending on substrate.

Swimming behavior has been documented and quantified in the laboratory for *M. pennsylvanicus, M. montanus, M. ochrogaster,* and *M. californicus* (Evans at al., 1978) (Table 1). Based on their tendency to enter the water and the amount of time spent swimming, Evans et al. (1978) concluded that *M. ochrogaster* was the best swimmer and *M. californicus* and *M. pennsylvanicus* were the worst.

Getz (1967) also found that *M. ochrogaster* avoided water more than *M. pennsylvanicus* and he correlated this with the dry grassland nature of *M. ochrogaster* in contrast to the more moist habitat characteristic of *M. pennsylvanicus. Microtus richardsoni* and *M. xanthognathus* occur along streams and in mesic habitats and both swim regularly (Ludwig, 1981; J. Wolff, pers. observ.).

Most *Microtus* species are active day and night (Madison, this volume) and use well-established runway systems. These systems consist of a complex network of above-ground runways and underground tunnels and burrows. *Microtus montanus* makes extensive use of tunnels, whereas *M. pennsylvanicus* is more active above ground. *Microtus pinetorum* is almost entirely fossorial, coming to the surface only occasionally to feed. About half of the runway systems of *M. xanthognathus* and *M. richardsoni* are above ground and the other half underground (Ludwig, 1981; Wolff and Lidicker, 1980). In *M. xanthognathus* and *M. richardsoni,* runway systems are concentrated along streams and frequently incorporate waterways into the runway system. Surface and subterranean runways of *Microtus* species in general are interconnected with numerous branches going to feeding areas, waterways, and dead ends which are apparently used for resting or temporary shelters. The number of underground versus above-ground runways is apparently related to friability of soils and accessibility of food. Several species are known to maintain runways to keep them clear of debris that may hinder movements (for example, *M. ochrogaster* [Thomas and Birney, 1979]; *M. xanthognathus* [Wolff, 1980]).

Nests usually are constructed of dried grass and may be located above or below ground. Exclusive use of grasses for nests has been reported for *M. canicaudus, M. montanus,* and *M. pennsylvanicus* (Maser and Storm, 1970), and *M. ochrogaster* (Jameson, 1947; Martin, 1956). *Microtus montanus* has surface and subsurface nests, but brood nests are always located underground (Jannett, 1978*a,* 1981*a*). Both male and female *M. ochrogaster* have been observed to construct nests in the laboratory, but males do most of the runway maintenance (Thomas and Birney, 1979). Ambrose (1973) found that most *M. pennsylvanicus* nests were located in slightly elevated dense tussocks of living grass.

Dalquest (1948) and Salt (1978) reported that water voles used subterranean nests in summer and subnivean nests on the soil surface in winter. Ludwig (1981), however, found that water voles used subterranean nests year-round. Nests ranged in size from 10 to 24 cm in diameter and were constructed of short segments of leaves and stems of grasses, sedges, and rushes (*Agropyron, Calamagrostis, Carex,* and *Juncus*) (Ludwig, 1981). Nest chambers were located beneath logs, stumps, or at the herbaceous/soil interface. Both summer and winter nests of *M. xanthognathus* are subterranean (Wolff and Lidicker, 1980). Eight summer nests examined by Wolff and Lidicker averaged 15 cm in diameter and were made of dried grass (*Calamagrostis*). Some nests were cup-shaped and others were round with an inner chamber. Most nests were situated at the moss-soil interface, but some were located on top of abandoned winter nests. Winter nests were larger than summer nests and were located in underground chambers, but above permafrost.

Hartung and Dewsbury (1979*a*) observed nest building behavior of *M. ochrogaster, M. montanus, M. californicus,* and *M. pennsylvanicus* in the laboratory. *Microtus ochrogaster* built few nests while the other three species built mostly cup-shaped nests and equal numbers of platform (pallet of cotton on floor but not shaped) and covered nests. Males and females built the same numbers of nests of each type.

Social Behavior

Mating Systems and Social Structure

Because of the secretive nature of voles, microtine social behavior has been difficult to study. Much of the information on *Microtus* behavior has been anecdotal or collected inadvertently in studies on demography. Several recent studies, using a variety of field and laboratory techniques, have provided insight into the social biology of a few select species of *Microtus*. The results of these studies have been discussed in detail (see The Biologist, Vol. 62, No. 1, 1980, Special Symposium Volume, Social Organization of Microtine Rodents).

Microtine behavioral systems are highly variable, but fall into four arrangements: 1) males occupy exclusive ranges and females mate polygynously or promiscuously within the range of a territorial male; 2) females occupy exclusive territories overlapped by home ranges of one or more males; 3) both males and females are territorial and intolerant of conspecific adults of the same sex, or of both sexes, except during courtship and mating; and 4) more than one male or female occupy exclusive communal territories. Various parameters of the social organization of several *Microtus* species are summarized in Table 2 and are discussed below.

*Meadow voles (*Microtus pennsylvanicus*)*.—The social biology of meadow voles has been studied most extensively by Madison (1978, 1979, 1980*a*, 1980*b*, 1980*c*, 1981, 1984), Madison et al. (1984), and Webster and Brooks (1981). With the aid of radiotelemetry, these studies have provided the most conclusive data on social organization in any microtine species. Meadow voles have a promiscuous mating system and socially are organized into territorial maternal-young units during the breeding season (Madison, 1980*a*) and communal mixed-sex and age groups during winter (Madison et al., 1984; Webster and Brooks, 1981; Table 2).

During the breeding season, reproductively active females maintain individual territories that are actively defended against other females. Madison (1980*a*) found that when overlap occurred between females, one female was usually 10–25 g larger than the other and only she bore young. Madison proposed that these females were mother-daughter units and the mother in some way inhibited the daughter from reproducing. Getz (1961) also found that subadults do not move from their home range before reaching sexual maturity. Other than these proposed mother-daughter units, territories remain exclusive with respect to other females during the breeding season. After reproductive shutdown in fall and winter, females will tolerate sons and other males in their nests (Madison, pers. comm.).

Home ranges of males may overlap those of several other males as well as those of several females (Getz, 1961; Madison 1980*c*; Webster and Brooks, 1981). Male ranges are three times larger than those of females (244 and 74 m^2, respectively; Madison, 1980*b*; see also Ambrose, 1969; Getz, 1961; Hamilton, 1937; Webster and Brooks, 1981). Home-range and territory sizes are inversely correlated with habitat quality and population density (Getz, 1961). Male home ranges are not well defined and may change daily; the greatest overlap occurs in the vicinity of estrous females (Getz, 1961; Madison, 1980*b*; Webster and Brooks, 1981).

The mating system of meadow voles appears to be promiscuous with males competing for access to females (Madison, 1980*a*, 1980*c*).

TABLE 2
DIFFERENT PARAMETERS OF THE SOCIAL ORGINIZATION OF SEVERAL *Microtus* SPECIES

	Mating system	Social system		Communal winter nesting	Food storing	References
		Males	Females			
M. californicus	Polygynous/facultative monogamy	Territorial	Territorial	?	Yes (lab)	Lidicker (1973, 1979, 1980; Pearson (1960)
M. montanus	Polygynous/facultative monogamy	Territorial	Territorial	?	?	Jannett (1977, 1978*a*, 1980, 1982)
M. ochrogaster	Monogamous	Territorial	Territorial	?	Yes	Getz and Carter (1980); Getz et al. (1981); Thomas and Birney (1979)
M. pennsylvanicus	Promiscuous	Home range	Territorial	Yes	Yes	Getz (1961, 1972, 1978); Madison (1978, 1980*a*, 1980*b*, 1980*c*, 1981); Madison et al. (1984); Webster and Brooks (1981)
M. pinetorum	Promiscuous within communal group	(Male, female, and offspring communal territories)		Yes	?	Fitzgerald and Madison (1981, 1983)
M. richardsoni	Promiscuous/polygynous	Home range	Territorial	?	?	Ludwig (1981)
M. xanthognathus	Polygynous	Territorial	Home range	Yes	Yes	Wolff (1980); Wolff and Lidicker (1980, 1981)

Based on spatial distribution and sequential use of live-traps, Reich and Tamarin (1980) found that female meadow voles avoided each other, and were indifferent towards males. Males, on the other hand, did not avoid each other, and were attracted to females. Webster and Brooks (1981) reported five male voles coming into the territory of an estrous female with four attempting to copulate with her. Using multiple-capture live-traps, Getz et al. (1981) caught male-female pairs in only 1.8% (128) out of 7,104 captures. No male-female pair was ever recaptured in the same trapping session or at other trap stations. Using radiotelemetry, Madison (1980*a*) located 100 voles over 14,000 times and had no instances of nest cohabitation or pair-bonding. Space use patterns of adults and lack of multiple captures of male-female pairs suggest a lack of external well-developed social grouping among adults during the summer breeding season.

Females appear to exhibit some choice in mate selection. Madison (1980*c*) proposed two possible strategies for mate selection by female meadow voles. One, supported by the observation of Webster and Brooks (1981), is that vocalization by a female may attract a known resident male who chases off "low quality" suitors. Thus, the female may assess male quality as a result of male-male competition. Secondly, Madison proposed that it may be advantageous for females to mate with all suitors to encourage their confidence of paternity. Males who are potentially sires of these offspring would be inhibited intrinsically from committing infanticide.

Multiple inseminations may also be a strategy to increase genetic variation and adaptation in littermates as suggested for ground squirrels (Hanken and Sherman, 1981). The benefits of secondary matings accruing to males as a result of sperm competition must also be considered (Dewsbury and Baumgardner, 1981).

*Montane voles (*Microtus montanus*)*.—The social organization of montane voles has been studied extensively in the laboratory and in fields of northwestern Wyoming by Jannett (1978*a,* 1978*b,* 1980, 1981*a,* 1981*b*). The social structure of montane voles is based on male and female territoriality and a variable mating system ranging from polygyny to facultative monogamy (Jannett, op. cit.) (Table 2).

Using a variety of field techniques including live-trapping, tracking animals implanted with irradiated tantalum (^{182}TA) wires, and manipulating populations in an enclosure, Jannett found that during the breeding season parous female montane voles were intrasexually territorial. Females maintained exclusive areas and drove away other females, but they did not drive away males or their own young. Adult males also maintained stable territories that were mutually exclusive of other territorial males, but that overlapped those of one or more females. Males shifted their activity within their territories to be in the vicinity of estrous females. Males and females are not known to co-nest (Jannett, 1982).

The use of space and territorial maintenance by females varies with population density (Jannett, 1980). In low-density areas where the chances of reestablishment are high, parous females abandon their young and maternal nest site and set up a new territory in a new area, while the young remain in the natal area. At high densities there is little vacant habitat available, and females continue to nest with juveniles from one or two litters; they do not desert their home site. Abandonment of the brood nest by the dam also may occur, as suggested by anecdotal observations, in *M. pennsylvanicus* (Getz, 1961; Hamilton, 1941; Madison, 1978; Myers and Krebs, 1971), *M. ochrogaster* (Myers and Krebs, 1971), *M. oeconomus* (Tast, 1966), and in two Old World species, *M. arvalis* (Frank, 1957) and *M. agrestis* (Myllymäki, 1977).

Female montane voles apparently mate with only one familiar male, but do not form a monogamous pair bond. Paternal behavior, such as sitting on the pups, licking pups, and manipulating nesting material, has been observed in the laboratory, but this is not necessarily indicative of monogamy in the wild (Hartung and Dewsbury, 1979*b*). Polygyny appears to be a common mating system in montane voles, although facultative monogamy obviously occurs at low densities.

*Prairie voles (*Microtus ochrogaster*).*—Although the mating system and social organization of prairie voles has not been documented in the field, the circumstantial evidence obtained from laboratory studies on parental care and mating behavior presents a strong case for monogamy. (Getz and Carter, 1980; Gray and Dewsbury, 1973; Thomas and Birney, 1979).

Thomas and Birney (1979) recorded monogamous mating in 26 of 27 groups observed in the laboratory. In only one case did they observe a polygynous mating. In this case, the two females nursed communally and co-nested with litters of different ages. Gray and Dewsbury (1973) and Dewsbury (1981) found that prairie voles failed to demonstrate the Coolidge effect (when a satiated male does not copulate with a new estrous female). This suggests that male prairie voles are not promiscuous by nature, but rather pair-bond with one female at a time.

In dyadic encounters in the laboratory, males and females from breeding pairs tended to show high levels of aggression toward unfamiliar animals of the opposite sex, but never toward each other (Getz et al., 1981). The male played the prominent role in attacking both male and female strangers (Getz and Carter, 1980). Introduction of a new male to caged females caused abortion in pregnant females (Stehn and Richmond, 1975). Females will accept a strange male only if the stud male is killed or removed (Getz et al., 1981).

Male and female prairie voles contribute equally to care of the young with the exception of lactation (Getz and Carter, 1980; Getz et al., 1981; Thomas and Birney, 1979). Paternal activities include nest and runway construction, food caching, and grooming, retrieving, and brooding the young. In eight out of 45 litters observed, males constructed a second nest and brooded part of the litter while the female brooded the remaining young in the primary nest (Thomas and Birney, 1979). In these cases, the litters that were separated into two nests were larger on average (3.5 pups/litter) than young kept in a single nest (2.5 pups/litter).

In *M. ochrogaster,* older pups frequently stay in the nest and groom, retrieve, and brood neonates from a succeeding litter (Getz and Carter, 1980; Getz et al., 1981; Thomas and Birney, 1979). Maternal care of the second litter is significantly less than that devoted to the first litter. Baby-sitting by the older litter, therefore, allows the breeding female more time for feeding and other activities away from the nest (Getz and Carter, 1980).

The only field study which examined the social structure of prairie voles was conducted by Getz et al. (1981). Using multiple-capture live-traps, Getz et al. captured male-female pairs together in 13.2% (1,664 out of 12,565) of their total captures. Multiple captures of males and females do not occur in a promiscuous species such as meadow voles. Getz and his colleagues found that these male-female associations persisted through the non-breeding season indicating a long-term pair bond.

*Taiga voles (*Microtus xanthognathus*).*—The only studies on the social system of taiga voles are those of Wolff (1980) and Wolff and Lidicker (1981). During the breeding season the social organization of taiga voles is based on male territoriality and a polygynous mating system (Table 2). The social system fits the model for resource-defense polygyny (Emlen and Oring, 1977). Based on a mark-recapture live-trapping study, Wolff (1980) found that males occupied well-defined territories. An average of two to four females had overlapping home ranges within the territory of each male. On two occasions, two pregnant females were caught together in the same trap. This does not occur in species in which females are territorial (for example, in *M. pennsylvanicus*; Getz et al., 1981).

Little evidence is available on mating behavior and paternal care in taiga voles. I have observed males in the laboratory mate with as many as three females in one day, indicating that multiple matings do occur. According to Dewsbury (1981), multiple matings are indicative of polygynous or promiscuous mating. I have observed males nesting with lactating females, but have not observed any paternal behaviors as described for prairie voles (Thomas and Birney, 1979). I have observed females retrieving young and tucking them under the male, but the male played no active role in retrieving or grooming the young.

*Pine voles (*Microtus pinetorum*).*—Anecdotal evidence by Paul (1970) and Boyette (1966) suggested that pine voles were "loosely colonial" or occurred in locally abundant aggregations (Benton, 1955; Hamilton, 1938). The most conclusive data on spacing, movements, and social organization of pine voles has been provided by a radiotelemetry and live-trapping study (Fitzgerald and Madison, 1981, 1983). Pine voles occur in apple orchards and their ecology and behavior are closely tied to the spacing of apple trees. Fitzgerald and Madison found that pine voles existed in discrete non-overlapping family units with an average of 4.2 individuals per unit (n = 20). Each family had a discrete non-overlapping territory with neighboring family units. The average family unit consisted of 1.9 adult scrotal males, 1.2 adult females, 0.7 subadult and juvenile males, and 0.4 subadult and juvenile females. Home ranges of family members overlapped extensively. All family members utilized one or two communal nests within the family territory and all of the members commonly used the same nest at the same time.

Fitzgerald and Madison (1981, 1983) found that home ranges of pine voles were linear with an average width for both males and females of 3 m (conforming to the approximate drip-line of the trees within a row). The average family unit occupied a territory

14.7 m long and 3.1 m wide. Home-range size averaged 44.7 m^2 for males and 41.7 m^2 for females. Fitzgerald and Madison (1981, 1983) concluded that each family was a discrete unit with little movement between family ranges. They recorded movement between territories in only 25 out of over 7,500 telemetry positions. Only six individuals moved permanently from one group to an adjacent group.

The mating system of pine voles has not been studied directly in the laboratory or in the field, but it has been inferred from radiotelemetry and live-trap data (Fitzgerald and Madison, 1981, 1983). The mating system of pine voles appears to be flexible, covering monogamy, polygyny, and even polyandry. The genetic relationships between and among breeding males and females in a family unit have not been determined. However, based on extensive trapping and radiotelemetry, the constituents of the group appear to be the founding pair and their mature (and immature) offspring.

*Water voles (*Microtus richardsoni*)*.—Several aspects of the social organization of water voles have recently been elucidated in a live-trapping and radio-tracking study conducted by Ludwig (1981) in west-central Alberta, Canada. Water voles have linear home ranges along streams (see also Anderson et al., 1976; Pattie, 1967). Home ranges of adult females are about 94 m long and 10 m wide and exhibit minimal or no overlap with other females. Mean home-range size for males is 332 m by 10 m and home ranges overlap those of other males and from one to four females. Female ranges are overlapped by one to three males. Home ranges for females are fairly stable throughout the breeding season and apparently are territories. Ludwig recorded one instance of male-female cohabitation which lasted a short time, but most voles nest singly. Based on male and female spacing patterns in the field, it appears as though water voles exhibit a promiscuous or polygynous mating system. The social organization of *M. richardsoni* is apparently very similar to that of *Arvicola terrestris* (Stoddart, 1970).

*California vole (*Microtus californicus*)*.—The social biology of the California vole has been reviewed by Lidicker (1980), who made reference to his earlier works (Lidicker, 1973, 1976, 1979) and those of Stark (1963), Pearson (1960), and Kenney et al. (1979). Lidicker concluded that the California vole is a "social moderate, avoiding the mongamous rigidity of *M. ochrogaster* on the one hand (Getz and Carter, 1980; Thomas and Birney, 1979) and the rampant polygyny or promiscuity of *M. xanthognathus* and *M. pennsylvanicus* on the other (Wolff, 1980; Madison, 1980*c*)."

Territorial behavior seems well developed in both sexes. Adult males have larger home ranges than do females (Batzli and Pitelka, 1971; Krebs, 1966; Lidicker, 1973), although both sexes have approximately the same size core areas where they spend over 85% of their time (Ford and Krumme, 1979). Unbalanced sex ratios in free-ranging populations suggest that one male may be mating with more than one female.

Lidicker (1976, 1979) introduced seven populations of California voles consisting of two or three pairs into 10 × 10-m enclosures. In five cases, fighting was intense; no reproduction occurred until a single pair remained. In one instance, one male and two females survived the initial fighting. Females divided up the enclosure, and both reproduced successfully while the male moved throughout. In the final case, two pairs persisted, dividing up the enclosure into two approximately equal territories. Six out of these seven cases resulted in monogamous matings. In a plastic runway system in the laboratory, adult males have been observed driving away and sometimes killing females that are not their mates (Lidicker, 1980).

Using automatic cameras placed in vole runways, Pearson (1960) found that: 1) individual runways were used by family groups ranging in number from 2 to 12 ($\bar{X} = 6$); 2) family groups consisted of an adult male and one or more females and their young; and 3) there was very little interchange of individuals among runway systems. This evidence further suggests that the mating system of California voles is bordering on monogamy-polygyny.

Only fragmentary information is available regarding paternal care of young. Brooding of young by fathers has been reported by Hatfield (1935) and Hartung and Dewsbury (1979*b*). In captivity, males gather nesting material and retrieve and manipulate nestlings; furthermore, lactating females are not antagonistic to their mates (Hartung and Dewsbury, 1979*b*; Lidicker, 1980). Given the opportunity, however, adult males will cannibalize nestlings which are not their own offspring (Lidicker, 1980).

Lidicker (1980) concluded that the basic social unit is the family group. Monogamy occurs at low densities and may be facultative as opposed to obligate (Kleiman, 1977). Polygyny occurs and may be the prevailing pattern at high densities. Weak pair-bonding occurs, but it is not the pair bond typical of monogamous species.

Dewsbury (1981) has proposed a "monogamy scale" by which rodent mating systems can be predicted by measuring a series of correlates derived from a variety of sources. Characteristics that appear to be correlated with monogamy include: sexual monomorphism (see also Dewsbury et al., 1980), latency to initiate copulation, allogrooming of female by the male, low number of ejaculations prior to satiety, lack of the Coolidge effect, lack of copulatory plugs, low reproductive potential, paternal behavior and pair-bonding, low rate of physical maturation, and delayed rate of sexual maturation. The converse of these characteristics are indicative of promiscuous or polygynous mating systems.

Based on the monogamy scale, Dewsbury predicted that *M. pinetorum, M. ochrogaster,* and *M. californicus* would be most likely to display monogamy and *M. montanus* and *M. pennsylvanicus* to be least likely. *Microtus xanthognathus, M. canicaudus, M. oeconomus,* and *M. montanus* fall somewhere between these two extremes on the scale. Evidence gathered from field studies is largely supportive of this model.

Copulatory Behavior

Descriptions of copulatory behavior and discussions on the adaptive significance of copulatory patterns in *Microtus* have been reported for *M. californicus* (Kenney et al., 1978), *M. montanus* (Dewsbury, 1973), *M. ochrogaster* (Gray and Dewsbury, 1973), *M. pennsylvanicus* (Gray and Dewsbury, 1975; Gray et al., 1977), *M. pinetorum* (Dewsbury, 1976), and *M. canicaudus, M. oeconomus,* and *M. xanthognathus* (Dewsbury, 1982). The basic motor pattern of copulation in all *Microtus* species includes the following. The male mounts the female from behind, grasping her flanks with his forepaws. Concommitantly, the female assumes a lordotic posture. On mounting, the male executes a series of short, rapid pelvic movements and vigorously palpates the females flanks. Extra-vaginal thrusting usually occurs before intromission, which is then followed by intra-vaginal thrusting. Ejaculation occurs at the terminal portion of certain intromissions, usually following several intra-vaginal thrusts. Non-copulatory behaviors such as running, sniffing partner, nuzzling, sparring, genital grooming, general grooming, and locomotory-exploratory behavior commonly occur between copulatory bouts.

The number of ejaculations, mounts, intromissions, thrusts per intromission, and time intervals between each behavior vary considerably between species. For instance, *M. montanus* and *M. ochrogaster* exhibit multiple intromissions followed by multiple ejaculations, whereas *M. pennsylvanicus, M. californicus,* and *M. pinetorum* exhibit a single intromission followed by multiple ejaculations. The mean number of ejaculations prior to satiety range from 2.0 in *M. ochrogaster* (Gray and Dewsbury, 1973) to 5.0 in *M. montanus* (Dewsbury, 1973) and 5.9 in *M. pennsylvanicus* (Gray and Dewsbury, 1975). The mean time interval between intromissions within a given ejaculatory series was 14.8 s in *M. montanus* (Dewsbury, 1973) and 32.9 s in *M. pennsylvanicus* (Gray and Dewsbury, 1975). *Microtus montanus* and *M. pennsylvanicus* exhibit the Coolidge effect, whereas *M. ochrogaster* does not (Dewsbury, 1981).

Communal Winter Nesting and Food Storing

Communal winter nesting and storing food in the vicinity of the nest occur in several species of *Microtus* (Table 2). These behaviors, which appear to be more common at northern than at southern latitudes, are apparent adaptations for overwintering in cold environments. The energetic gains from communal nesting have been well documented (Beck and Anthony, 1971; Gebczynska and Gebczynski, 1971; Wiegert, 1961; Wrabetz, 1980). West and Dublin (1984) and Madison et al. (1984) provide reviews on communal nesting in small mammals. Communal nesting consists of group living in which 5–10 or more individuals co-nest during part of the year. Communal nesting does not normally occur during the reproductive season (except in pine voles; Fitzgerald and Madison, 1981, 1983), but is rather common during the non-reproductive season, usually winter. Food storage consists of collecting and storing food in a food cache which is then eaten during the subsequent inclement period.

Communal winter nesting of non-reproductive individuals of mixed sex and age groups has been reported in meadow voles (Madison et al., 1984; Webster and Brooks, 1981). Madison et al. (1984) found that winter communes of *M. pennsylvanicus* consisted of non-overlapping maternal families in early winter and shifted to mixed non-lineage groups during late winter. They found that winter communal nesting did not always occur, but was dependent on ambient temperature and snowfall. Communal nesting was not found during the summer breeding season, but females tolerate sons and fathers in their nests in late fall.

Winter food caching by meadow voles (*M. pennsylvanicus*) has been reported on a number of occasions (Bailey, 1920; Gates and Gates, 1980; Hatt, 1930; Lantz, 1907; Riewe, 1973). Caches contained fruits of *Falcata comosa,* and tubers of *Helianthus tuberosus* (Bailey, 1920), roots of *Convolvulus sepium* (Lantz, 1907), and leaves and roots of *Leontodon autumnalis* and *Trifolium* spp. (Riewe, 1973). Gates and Gates (1980) described a meadow-vole food cache consisting of underground parts of *Potentilla canadensis, Viola papilionacea,* and *Ranunculus bulbosa.* Food hoarding and communal nesting in non-reproductive individuals is probably the typical behavior pattern of *M. pennsylvanicus* in winter, and no doubt occurs in many other species of *Microtus* as well.

Communal winter nesting in groups of 5–10 individuals also occurs in taiga voles (Wolff, 1980; Wolff and Lidicker, 1981). An underground food cache that contains rhizomes of *Equisetum* and *Epilobium* is located adjacent to the nest. The nest and food cache are frequently located about 30 cm under the ground, often under a tangled mass of branches, roots, or a fallen log. Nests have up to five entrances, whereas the food cache has a single access from the nest. Food is collected and stored from mid-August to mid-September. Taiga voles remain active all winter, but over 90% of their food consists of rhizomes stored in the food cache and the remainder is obtained from foraging under snow (Wolff and Lidicker, 1980).

Each communal group consists of an average of 7.1 individuals of mixed sex and age groups (Wolff and Lidicker, 1981). Communal groups may contain sisters but most group members do not appear to be siblings or parent-offspring groups. Wolff and Lidicker (1981) concluded that communal winter nesting was a thermoregulatory behavior adapted to survival in severe boreal climates. Communal nesting with non-relatives may be a mechanism to reduce predation on family units or to reduce the chance of inbreeding (Wolff, 1980; Wolff and Lidicker, 1981).

The singing vole (*M. miurus*) is also known to nest communally and store food (Murie, 1961). Singing voles build haypiles which consist of fireweed (*Epilobium*), horsetail (*Equisetum*), coltsfoot (*Petasites*), willow leaves (*Salix*), mountain avens (*Dryas*), lupine (*Lupinus*), sage (*Artemesia*), pyrola (*Pyrola*), and grass (*Calamagrostis*).

These plant parts are clipped and layered over rocks or in lower branches of willow clumps to dry before being cached underground. The size of these haypiles may range from a handful to over a bushel (Murie, 1961).

Communal groups of prairie voles are known to occur in field populations (Criddle, 1926; Fitch, 1957), but they have not been studied in detail. Prairie voles are known to store food in the field (Hamilton and Whitaker, 1979; Jameson, 1947) and in the laboratory (Lanier et al., 1974). Thomas and Birney (1979) observed reproductively active prairie voles of both sexes and all age groups caching food in the laboratory. Food was stored both before and after the birth of a litter.

Food caches are not known for *M. californicus* (Stark, 1963), but food and nesting material are sometimes hoarded in captivity (Lidicker, 1980). Pearson (1960) observed California voles carrying blades and stems of grass, herbs (*Rumex*), and wild oats (*Avena*) at all times of the year. Whitaker and Martin (1977) have some field and laboratory evidence for food storing in *M. chrotorrhinus*. *Microtus oeconomus* stores rhizomes of *Equisetum* (Wolff, 1984). *Microtus brandti,* an apparent colonial species from the Old World, also stores food (Naumov, 1972, *in* Anderson, 1980).

Olfactory Communication

Many species of *Microtus* possess enlarged modified sebaceous glands on the posterolateral portion of the body which are used for scent-marking. In *Microtus,* these glands are present either on the flanks or hips, or do not occur at all (Quay, 1968; Table 3). Although scent glands do not normally occur in *M. pennsylvanicus* and *M. longicaudus,* Jannett (1975) was able to induce their development by administering testosterone to mature males. Tamarin (1981) reported one incidence of gland development in a 73-g scrotal male *M. pennsylvanicus* from an outdoor enclosure and Jannett (1975) caught one adult scrotal male *M. longicaudus* that had visible hip glands. However, Boonstra and Youson (1982) reported the regular occurrence of hip glands in *M. pennsylvanicus* in Ontario.

In species that have them, scent glands are more prevalent in males than females. Glands begin to develop at the time of sexual maturity and regress during the non-breeding season (Howell, 1924; MacIsaac, 1977; Wolff and Lidicker, 1980).

Scent-marking (the deposition of glandular secretions) has been

TABLE 3

SUMMARY OF SCENT-GLAND INFORMATION FOR NEW WORLD *Microtus* SPECIES WHERE ADEQUATE DATA ARE AVAILABLE. GLAND LOCATION IS ACCORDING TO QUAY (1968)

	Gland location			Scent marking described	Reference for scent marking
	Hip	Flank	Sex		
M. abbreviatus		X	M		
M. californicus	X		M	X	Lidicker (1980)
M. chrotorrhinus	X		M, ?		
M. miurus		X	M, F	X	Youngman (1975)
M. montanus	X		M	X	Jannett and Jannett (1974)
M. oeconomus	X		M, F		
M. richardsoni		X	M, F	X	Jannett and Jannett (1974, 1981)
M. townsendii	X		M, F	X	MacIsaac (1977)
M. xanthognathus		X	M, F	X	Wolff and Johnson (1979)

described for a few select species. Taiga voles scent-mark by scratching the flank glands with their hindfeet, which stimulates the flow of sebum from the gland (Wolff and Johnson, 1979). The gland is then rubbed on the surface of objects in the environment. Males mark more frequently than do females and marking occurs more in strange environments than in home cages. Scent-marking in taiga voles is apparently used for individual recognition, to indicate reproductive condition, and for marking territorial boundaries (Wolff and Johnson, 1979).

In *M. richardsoni,* glands begin to develop in young as small as 19 g and reach a peak in July (males) or July–August (females) (Jannett and Jannett, 1974; Ludwig, 1981). Glands in males are 2–3 times larger than in females and are positively correlated with body weight. When glands are functional, the hair covering the raised gland is greasy and matted down. At the end of the breeding season the gland regresses and becomes nonfunctional.

Jannett and Jannett (1974, 1981) described two distinct marking patterns in which the flank gland secretions were deposited. Drum-marking involved raking the feet over the glands; flank-rubbing involved rubbing the flank gland against objects in the environment. Both behaviors are more common in males than in females and do not occur in juveniles. The behaviors and the context in which they are used are similar to those described for *M. xanthognathus* (Wolff and Johnson, 1979) and *Arvicola terrestris* (Stoddart, 1970).

Flank glands, similar to those described for *M. xanthognathus* and *M. richardsoni,* also occur in singing voles, *M. miurus* (Youngman, 1975). Sexually excited males scratch these glands with their hindfeet when the gland becomes hypertrophied during the breeding season. Females apparently recognize males and assess their reproductive condition by smelling these glands (Youngman, 1975).

MacIsaac (1977) also showed a correlation between hip-gland development and reproductive condition in male Townsend's voles (*M. townsendii*). He found a positive correlation between testes weight and hip-gland size. MacIsaac also noted that a greater proportion of breeding females possessed hip glands than did non-breeding females. MacIsaac described scent-marking behavior in Townsend's voles: "marking action consists of three distinct figure-eight motions of the hips. In each instance, the hips touched the upper sides of the plexiglas tube," presumably depositing sebum on the walls of the tube. A similar form of marking behavior has been recorded for montane voles, *M. montanus* (Jannett and Jannett, 1974).

Hip glands are present in some male California voles (*M. californicus*) and their activity is correlated with reproduction (Lidicker, 1980). Lidicker assumed hip glands had a social function though he was not able to discern its exact nature. California voles have been observed swaggering from side to side in plastic tunnels apparently rubbing their hips on the walls of the tube. *Microtus montanus* has also been observed raising its hips in a tunnel (Jannett and Jannett, 1974).

Jannett (1981*b*) discussed the evolutionary significance of scent glands of *M. montanus* in a social context. He found that agonistic attacks between males were directed more at glands than other parts of the body. More wounding in glandular than non-glandular areas also has been reported in *M. townsendii* (MacIsaac, 1977), *M. californicus* (Lidicker, 1980), and *M. oeconomus* (Quay, 1968). Jannett (1981*b*) concluded that scent glands are indicative of a type of social organization and are used in territorial defense. Males of both *M. xanthognathus* (Wolff, 1980; Wolff and Johnson, 1979) and *M. montanus* have well-developed posterolateral scent glands and marking behaviors and both species are territorial and polygynous

(Jannett, 1981*b*). Neither *M. ochrogaster* nor *M. pennsylvanicus* appear to have well-developed posterolateral scent glands and their other glands are relatively small (Jannett, 1980; but see Boonstra and Youson, 1982); neither has stable polygynous relationships (Getz and Carter, 1980; Madison, 1980*c*). In non-territorial species, or during non-breeding seasons, glands may be a "behavioral load" (Jannett, 1981*b*) and either have been selected against or regress as a mechanism to reduce aggression and promote sociality (Clarke and Frearson, 1972; Jannett, 1981*b*; Wolff, 1980, 1984; Wolff and Lidicker, 1981).

Scent-marking by dragging the anogenital region on the substrate has been reported for male taiga voles, *M. xanthognathus* (Wolff and Johnson, 1979) and montane voles, *M. montanus* (Jannett, 1981*b*). Reich and Tamarin (1980) found that male *M. pennsylvanicus* and *M. breweri* were attracted to the scent of females, but not the reverse. Deposition of droppings into scat piles or latrine sites also seems to have a communicatory significance. Wolff (1980) reported that taiga voles deposited scat piles at junctions of runways and along borders of territories. He also noted that in the laboratory, dominant males had 2–3 scat piles in a 2 × 3-m enclosure. They also were used by pregnant or lactating females, but not by non-reproductive females or subordinate males. Jannett (1981*b*) found that scat piles of adult male *M. montanus* were concentrated in the vicinities of brood nests of females in their territories. He also found that non-territorial adult males do not scent-mark during the non-breeding season. Scat piles or latrine sites also have been reported for *M. richardsoni* (Ludwig, 1981), *M. miurus* (Murie, 1961), *Arvicola terrestris* (Stoddart, 1970), *M. chrotorrhinus* (Martin, 1971), *M. pennsylvanicus, M. oeconomus,* (Wolff, pers. observ.); they probably occur in most other *Microtus* species as well.

Vocalization

Several types of vocalizations have been reported for *Microtus*; they serve a variety of communicatory functions. D. Colvin (1973) recorded vocalizations by free-ranging *M. montanus* and *M. longicaudus* that were engaged in an agonistic encounter. He also recorded vocalizations of each species in both offensive and defensive behaviors during dyadic aggressive encounters in the laboratory. Caplis (1977, *in* Madison, 1980*c*) found that *M. pennsylvanicus* was more apt to vocalize in defensive than in offensive displays. Vocalizations during agonistic encounters also have been recorded for *M. montanus* (Jannett, 1981*b*), *M. californicus, M. ochrogaster* (D. Colvin, 1973; Househecht, 1968), *M. oeconomus,* and *M. xanthognathus* (pers. observ.). These vocalization patterns, which are qualitatively similar and occur under similar conditions, probably characterize most, if not all, *Microtus* species.

Wolff (1980) described a high-pitched vocalization by taiga voles (*M. xanthognathus*) which he has interpreted as an alarm call. The call is ventriloquial, making it hard to locate in the field. The calls are given by males and females of all age groups and are most common during the breeding season and again in fall, primarily around nesting areas. Similar calls have been reported for the singing vole (*M. miurus*), and the context in which they are given appears similar to *M. xanthognathus* (Youngman, 1975).

M. Colvin (1973) discussed the structure and function of ultrasound production in neonates of five *Microtus* species (*M. pennsylvanicus, M. montanus, M. californicus, M. longicaudus,* and *M. ochrogaster*). She concluded that stressed neonates used ultrasounds to elicit parental care. Neonates subjected to stress (for example, cold) produced ultrasounds that elicited a warming response by their mother. The intensity and frequency of calling were most pronounced during early development and decreased with age of neonates (DeGhett, 1976).

Agonistic Behavior

Agonistic behavior consists of a set of behavioral acts occurring in aggressive interactions which include all acts of aggression and submission (Wittenberger, 1981). Aggression, the most conspicuous and most studied component of agonistic behavior, includes a repertoire of behaviors in which one individual displays a physical act of fighting or threat of fighting toward an opponent to obtain dominance or access to females, food, space, or some other resource. The basic components of an encounter between two voles have been described by Banks and Fox (1968), Clarke (1956), D. Colvin (1973), Skirrow (1969), Tamura (1966), and Turner and Iverson (1973).

Clarke (1956) described and illustrated agonistic behavior in the Old World short-tailed vole (*M. agrestis*), which is probably similar for most if not all vole species. The basic dominant display involves raising the body off the ground, tail extended straight and parallel to the ground, and ears cocked forward. This position is often accompanied by a raising of one or both forefeet and gnashing of the teeth. The typical submissive posture consists of lowering the body, sometimes rolling over in a supine position, ears flattened against the body or flopped downward, and tail raised slightly or sometimes in a sigmoid shape when the animal is in a defensive or retaliatory position. Jannett (1977) described a subordinate behavior of a *M. montanus* in which the animal remains quiet, with head held low, eyes partly closed, and ears somewhat flat. Clarke (1956) also described several other behaviors associated with aggressive encounters. These include: *digging,* simulated digging or tunneling activity in the sawdust or substrate; *marking time,* movement of legs while the body remains in place; *fidgeting,* general body movements; *waltzing,* rotating in place up to 360° while marking time; and *dancing,* rapid movements of feet with a sudden change in direction of the body. Autogrooming and toilet behaviors were also commonly observed during agonistic encounters, especially by subordinate animals.

D. Colvin (1973) classified the basic components of an encounter into nine functional categories: approach, offense, attack, chase, defense, retreat, vocalization, box, and wrestle. This classification is similar to that described for collared lemmings, *Dicrostonyx torquatus* (Allin and Banks, 1968). Turner and Iverson (1973) added several behavioral components to this list, some of which were not aggressive behaviors: time together, naso-anal, grooming self, following, mutual upright, threat, fighting, and submissive. Rothstein (1976) and Skirrow (1969) presented more detailed descriptions of microtine behaviors.

These behaviors have been observed in the laboratory, but are quite stereotyped and are likely to occur in a similar pattern in a natural setting. Aggressive encounters have been observed in the field on several occasions. D. Colvin (1973) recorded five of these behaviors in an agonistic encounter that he observed in the field between an adult male *M. montanus* and an adult male *M. longicaudus.* These behaviors included vocalization, chase, retreat, attack, and wrestle. Madison (1980*c*) documented 35 behavioral interactions between adult *M. pennsylvanicus* in natural populations. Nine of these interactions were between females, one between males, and seven involved females rejecting the advances of males. Madison concluded that behavioral interactions involving defense of space were most common among females, whereas aggression involving males was usually associated with competition for mates. Similar results have been found by Webster (1979).

Caplis (1977, *in* Madison, 1980*c*) studied aggressive behavior of reproductively active male and female meadow voles in dyadic encounters in the laboratory. She found that males and females exhibited the same level of aggressive activity, but males exhibited more open conflict than females, and females exhibited more noncontact threat displays than males. Both males and females exhibited less aggression when paired with neighbors than when paired with strangers. Neighbor recognition implies a form of "social order" or "kin recognition" among free-ranging voles (Madison, 1980*c*).

Wounding patterns have been used on various occasions as an indirect measure of aggression (Christian, 1971; Getz, 1972; Rose, 1979; Rose and Gaines, 1976; Turner and Iverson, 1973). Madison (1980*c*) summarized the results of several studies on *M. pennsylvanicus* as follows. Christian (1971) found that wounding in meadow voles is 1) frequent among males and almost non-existent among females, 2) linked to sexual activity among males (immature males were rarely attacked), and 3) dependent on density among sexually mature males. Rose (1979), on the other hand, found 1) considerable wounding among females as well as males, 2) wounding during breeding and non-breeding seasons, and 3) no density dependence in wounding among males or females. Turner and Iverson (1973) found that 1) aggressive acts (primarily threats, vocalizations, mutual uprights, and tail wounding) increased in frequency as males became reproductively active and decreased in frequency as the breeding season ended, 2) submissive behaviors were most common early in the reproductive period, 3) allogrooming was most common when juveniles were in the population, 4) adult males were more aggressive than young of the year, and 5) residents were more aggressive than nonresidents. Getz (1972) found 1) no indication of greater antagonism between adult males than between adult females or between males and females, 2) no significant antagonism between adult and immature males, and 3) no indication of lasting male-female pair formation. Miller (1969) found that males were more aggressive than females.

In *M. ochrogaster,* wounding is more frequent in males (32.6%)

than in females (18.3%) and is the most intense during the reproductive period (Rose and Gaines, 1976). Wounding was more common in medium-sized males and large females than in small nonreproductive males or females. In *M. richardsoni,* adult males also show more signs of wounding than females (64% versus 20%, respectively) (Ludwig, 1981). In *M. montanus,* fighting is most intense in adult males following snowmelt just prior to the breeding season and establishment of territories (Jannett, 1981*a*).

Rose and Hueston (1978) documented some of the problems in using wounding as a measure of aggression. They found that 90% of wounds heal by 2–4 weeks and are undetectable, and by 8 weeks, all wounds are totally healed. Field measurements are therefore conservative and may vary seasonally; there is little wounding during the non-breeding season in winter when population densities are usually lower. Aggression also may vary with density, phase of population cycles, and between residents and dispersers (Krebs, 1970; Reich et al., 1982; Turner and Iverson, 1973). Although there are conflicting results in data on wounding and aggression, the points about which all studies agree is that wounding is more common among males than females and that this wounding reflects physical conflict associated with breeding activity (Madison, 1980*c*).

Patterns of aggression may vary between species, but within a species they follow a predictable pattern that is correlated with a particular type of social system. The social system, in turn, is based on several factors such as defensibility of resources (Emlen and Oring, 1977), polygyny-threshold models (Orians, 1969), and parental investment (Trivers, 1972). Within a species, if females are aggressive, they usually fight for space, whereas males may fight for space or females. In *M. pennsylvanicus,* a promiscuous species, females are territorial and males have large overlapping home ranges (Madison, 1980*c*). Females are aggressive toward other females in defense of territories and males are aggressive toward other males in the presence of estrous females. Estrous females are also aggressive toward males and may reject certain "low quality" males (Madison, 1980*c*). Aggression is reduced during winter when the animals are communally nesting (Webster, 1979). In a polygynous species such as *M. xanthognathus,* males are extremely aggressive and fight for territories (Wolff, 1980). Females, on the other hand, are aggressive toward strange males and strange females, but are amicable with other familiar females in the male's territory. During the non-breeding season, all animals are less aggressive and nest communally (Wolff and Lidicker, 1981).

The social system of California voles (*M. californicus*) ranges from monogamy to polygyny; both sexes are territorial (Lidicker, 1980). During the breeding season, adult male California voles are antagonistic toward each other, and females are amiable unless an adult male is present, in which case they fight (Lidicker, 1980). Adult males are sometimes aggressive toward (and may even kill) females that are not their mates. In *M. montanus,* patterns of aggression are apparently similar to those of California voles (Jannett, 1980, 1981*b*; Randall, 1978), and both species have a similar social system. In *M. ochrogaster,* which is monogamous and territorial, paired males and females are aggressive toward strangers of either sex (Getz, 1962; Getz et al., 1981; Miller, 1969; Thomas and Birney, 1979). Aggression in other species of voles has not been evaluated with regard to the species social system, but it is likely that predictable patterns will emerge that fit these models.

Summary of Social Organization

The social organization of microtines is the result of behaviors associated with courtship and mating, parental care, social structure (spacing patterns), aggression, and communication. Mating systems are commonly promiscuous (for example, *M. pennsylvanicus* and *M. richardsoni*), polygynous (for example, *M. xanthognathus, M. californicus,* and *M. montanus*), and rarely, but sometimes monogamous (*M. ochrogaster*). Mating systems may be facultative (*M. californicus* and *M. montanus*) or obligate (*M. ochrogaster*); some species exhibit one, two, or all three mating patterns, depending on the social environment. Species-specific copulatory patterns are apparently adaptive to particular social organization in specific habitats and also may be a reproductive isolating mechanism between similar sympatric species (Kenney et al., 1978). Paternal care may be an important component of monogamous species, but in most microtines it is minimal or non-existent. Most social groupings are mother-young units, but some species have extended families that include two or more generations in one nest (for example, *M. montanus, M. ochrogaster,* and *M. pinetorum*).

In some species only males are territorial (for example, *M. xanthognathus* and *M. agrestis*), only females (for example, *M. penn-*

sylvanicus and *M. richardsoni*) or both sexes are territorial (for example, *M. montanus, M. ochrogaster,* and *M. californicus*). *Microtus xanthognathus* and *M. richardsoni* live in patchy riparian habitats but exhibit different behavioral systems. The relationship between habitat and social structure of *M. montanus, M. californicus,* and *M. pennsylvanicus* is not clear, but see Jannett (1980), Lidicker (1980), and Madison (1980*c*) for interpretations. *Microtus ochrogaster* lives in a stable, relatively uniform habitat in which food is a limiting resource. These ecological conditions apparently select for monogamy, a strong pair bond, paternal care, and dispersal of young to reduce competition (Getz and Carter, 1980).

These behavioral systems are maintained by agonistic behavior. Aggression may be for defense of territories or for access to estrous females. Aggression and territoriality may also regulate population numbers (Getz, 1978; Jannett, 1981*b*; Madison, 1980*a*). Webster and Brooks (1981) suggest that social behavior and demography are closely integrated and it is essential to know the social-behavior characteristics of the species to understand its population dynamics. They concluded that "population dynamics of microtine rodents may be better understood by combining sociobiological investigation with the traditional demographic manipulation of 'black box' populations of voles."

Dispersal is another important aspect of microtine social biology (Lidicker, this volume). Dispersal following weaning may include all offspring, just male or just female offspring, or in some cases the dam may abandon her nest and leave it for her offspring. Communication, which is an essential component of maintaining social organization, may include scent-marking and production of pheromones associated with reproduction (Seabloom, this volume), establishment of dominance relations, or individual recognition. Vocalizations are used by neonates to elicit maternal care, as a threat or defensive behavior in agonistic encounters, or as an alarm signal to warn conspecifics.

In seasonal environments, overwintering behavioral strategies, such as communal nesting and food storing, are adaptations for survival in severe boreal climates. Communal nesting requires a different suite of behaviors than those used during the reproductive season, or by a social or territorial species. Although mammal social behavior is extremely labile (Wilson, 1975) and is subject to differential expression resulting from learning, developmental processes, and the social environment, predictable patterns do emerge in microtine socio-ecology. Because of these influences, social systems may vary between populations within a species, or between years within the same population. Relationships between social structure and ecological parameters have been postulated for several groups of mammals (Bradbury, 1980; Clutton-Brock and Harvey, 1977; Crook et al., 1976) and undoubtedly are relevant to microtine social organization (Anderson, 1980; Getz, 1978; Webster and Brooks, 1981). An understanding of microtine behavior is in its infancy, but is recognized as an essential and integral component of the life-history strategies of this mammal group.

Literature Cited

ALLIN, J. T., AND E. M. BANKS. 1968. The behavioral biology of the collared lemming *Dicrostonyx groenlandicus* (Traill): I. Agonistic behavior. Anim. Behav., 16:245–262.

AMBROSE, H. W., III. 1969. A comparison of *Microtus pennsylvanicus* home ranges as determined by isotope and live trap methods. Amer. Midland Nat., 81:535–555.

———. 1973. An experimental study of some factors affecting the spatial and temporal activity of *Microtus pennsylvanicus*. J. Mamm., 54:79–100.

ANDERSON, P. K. 1980. Evolutionary implications of microtine behavioral systems on the ecological stage. The Biologist, 62:70–88.

ANDERSON, P. K., P. H. WHITNEY, AND J. P. HUANG. 1976. *Arvicola richardsoni:* ecology and biochemical polymorphism in the front ranges of southern Alberta. Acta. Theriol., 21:425–468.

BAILEY, V. 1920. Identity of the bean mouse of Lewis and Clark. J. Mamm., 1:70–72.

BANKS, E. M., AND S. F. FOX. 1968. Relative aggression of two sympatric rodents: a preliminary report. Comm. Behav. Biol., 2:51–58.

BATZLI, G. O., AND F. A. PITELKA. 1971. Condition and diet of cycling populations of the California vole, *Microtus californicus*. J. Mamm., 52:141–163.

BECK, L. R., AND R. G. ANTHONY. 1971. Metabolic and behavioral thermoregulation in the long-tailed vole, *Microtus longicaudus*. J. Mamm., 52:404–412.

BENTON, A. I. 1955. Observations on the life history of the northern pine mouse. J. Mamm., 36:52–62.

BOONSTRA, R., AND J. YOUSON. 1982. Hip glands in a field population of *Microtus pennsylvanicus*. Canadian J. Zool., 60:2155–2958.

BOYETTE, J. G. 1966. A behavioral study of the pine mouse, *Pitymys pinetorum pinetorum* (LeConte). Unpubl. Ph.D. dissert., North Carolina State Univ., Raleigh, 134 pp.

BRADBURY, J. W. 1980. Foraging, social dispersion and mating systems. Pp. 189–208, *in* Sociobiology: beyond nature/nurture (G. W. Barlow and J. Silverberg, eds.). Westview Press, Boulder, Colorado, 627 pp.

CHRISTIAN, J. J. 1971. Fighting, maturity, and population density in *Microtus pennsylvanicus*. J. Mamm., 52:556–567.

Clarke, J. R. 1956. The aggressive behavior of the vole. Behaviour, 9:1–23.
Clarke, J. R., and S. Frearson. 1972. Sebaceous glands on the hindquarters of the vole, *Microtus agrestis*. J. Reprod. Fert., 31:477–481.
Clutton-Brock, T. H., and P. H. Harvey. 1977. Primate ecology and social organization. J. Zool., 183:1–39.
Colvin, D. V. 1973. Agonistic behavior in males of five species of voles *Microtus*. Anim. Behav., 21:471–480.
Colvin, M. A. 1973. Analysis of acoustic structure and function in ultrasounds of neonatal *Microtus*. Behaviour, 44:234–263.
Criddle, S. 1926. The habits of *Microtus minor* in Manitoba. J. Mamm., 7:193–200.
Crook, J. H., J. E. Ellis, and J. D. Goss-Custard. 1976. Mammalian social systems: structure and function. Anim. Behav., 24:261–274.
Dalquest, W. W. 1948. Mammals of Washington. Univ. Kansas Publ., Mus. Nat. Hist., 2:1–444.
DeGhett, V. J. 1976. The ontogeny of ultrasonic vocalization in *Microtus montanus*. Behaviour, 60:115–121.
Dewsbury, D. A. 1973. Copulatory behavior of montane voles (*Microtus montanus*). Behaviour, 44:186–202.
———. 1976. Copulatory behavior of pine voles (*Microtus pinetorum*). Perceptual and Motor Skills, 43:91–94.
———. 1981. An exercise in the prediction of monogamy in the field from laboratory data on 42 species of muroid rodents. The Biologist, 63:128–162.
———. 1982. Copulatory behavior of three species of *Microtus*. J. Mamm., 63: 306–309.
Dewsbury, D. A., and D. J. Baumgardner. 1981. Studies of sperm competition in two species of muroid rodents. Behav. Ecol. Sociobiol., 9:121–133.
Dewsbury, D. A., D. J. Baumgardner, R. L. Evans, and D. G. Webster. 1980. Sexual dimorphism for body mass in 13 taxa of muroid rodents under laboratory conditions. J. Mamm., 61:146–149.
Dewsbury, D. A., D. L. Lanier, and A. Miglietta. 1980. A laboratory study in climbing behavior in 11 species of muroid rodents. Amer. Midland Nat., 103:66–72.
Emlen, S. T., and L. W. Oring. 1977. Ecology, sexual selection, and the evolution of mating systems. Science, 197:215–223.
Evans, R. L., E. M. Katz, N. L. Olson, and D. A. Dewsbury. 1978. A comparative study of swimming behavior in eight species of muroid rodents. Bull. Psychonomic Soc., 11:168–170.
Fitch, H. S. 1957. Aspects of reproduction and development in the prairie vole (*Microtus ochrogaster*). Univ. Kansas Publ., Mus. Nat. Hist., 10:131–161.
Fitzgerald, R. W., and D. M. Madison. 1981. Spacing, movements, and social organization of a free-ranging population of pine voles *Microtus pinetorum*. Pp. 54–59, *in* Proceedings of the fifth eastern pine and meadow vole symposium (R. E. Byers, ed.). Gettysburg, Pennsylvania, 144 pp.
———. 1983. Social organization of a free-ranging population of pine voles, *Microtus pinetorum*. Behav. Ecol. Sociobiol., 13:183–187.
Ford, R. G., and D. W. Krumme. 1979. The analysis of space use patterns. J. Theor. Biol., 76:125–155.
Frank, F. 1957. The causality of microtine cycles in Germany. J. Wildl. Mgmt., 21:113–121.
Gates, J. D., and D. M. Gates. 1980. A winter food cache of *Microtus pennsylvanicus*. Am. Midland Nat., 103:407–408.
Gebczynska, Z., and M. Gebczynski. 1971. Insulating properties of the nest and

social temperature regulation in *Clethrionomys glareolus* (Schreber). Ann. Zool. Fennica, 8:104–108.

GETZ, L. L. 1961. Home ranges, territory and movement of the meadow vole. J. Mamm., 42:24–36.

———. 1962. Aggressive behavior of the meadow and prairie voles. J. Mamm., 43:351–358.

———. 1967. Responses of selected small mammals to water. Univ. Connecticut Occas. Papers, Biol. Sci. Ser., 1:71–81.

———. 1972. Social structure and aggressive behavior in a population of *Microtus pennsylvanicus*. J. Mamm., 53:310–317.

———. 1978. Speculation on social structure and population cycles of microtine rodents. Biologist, 60:134–147.

GETZ, L. L., AND C. S. CARTER. 1980. Social organization in *Microtus ochrogaster* populations. The Biologist, 62:56–69.

GETZ, L. L., C. S. CARTER, AND L. GAVISH. 1981. The mating system of the prairie vole, *Microtus ochrogaster:* field and laboratory evidence for pair-bonding. Behav. Ecol. Sociobiol., 8:189–194.

GRAY, G. D., AND D. A. DEWSBURY. 1973. A quantitative description of copulatory behavior in prairie voles (*Microtus ochrogaster*). Brain Behav. Evol., 43: 351–358.

———. 1975. A quantitative description of copulatory behavior in meadow voles (*Microtus pennsylvanicus*). Anim. Behav., 23:261–267.

GRAY, G. D., A. M. KENNEY, AND D. A. DEWSBURY. 1977. Adaptive significance of the copulatory behavior pattern of male meadow voles (*Microtus pennsylvanicus*) in relation to induction of ovulation and implantation in females. J. Comp. Physiol. Psych., 91:1308–1319.

HAMILTON, W. J., JR. 1937. Growth and life span of the field mouse. Amer. Nat., 71:500–507.

———. 1938. Life history notes on the northern pine mouse. J. Mamm., 19:163–170.

———. 1941. Reproduction of the field mouse *Microtus pennsylvanicus* (Ord.). Cornell Univ. Agric. Exp. Sta., Mem., 237:1–23.

HAMILTON, W. J., JR., AND J. O. WHITAKER, JR. 1979. Mammals of the eastern United States. Cornell Univ. Press, Ithaca, New York, 368 pp.

HANKEN, J., AND P. W. SHERMAN. 1981. Multiple paternity in Belding's ground squirrel litters. Science, 212:351–353.

HARTUNG, T. G., AND D. A. DEWSBURY. 1979*a*. Nest-building behavior in seven species of muroid rodents. Behav. Neural Biol., 27:532–539.

———. 1979*b*. Paternal behavior in six species of muroid rodents. Behav. Neural Biol., 26:466–478.

HATFIELD, D. M. 1935. A natural history study of *Microtus californicus*. J. Mamm., 16:261–271.

HATT, R. T. 1930. The biology of the voles of New York. Roosevelt Wild Life Bull., 5:513–623.

HOUSEHECHT, C. R. 1968. Sonographic analysis of vocalizations of three species of mice. J. Mamm., 49:555–560.

HOWELL, A. B. 1924. Individual and age variation in *Microtus montanus yosemite*. J. Agric. Res., 28:977–1015.

JAMESON, W. E., JR. 1947. Natural history of the prairie vole (mammalian genus *Microtus*). Univ. Kansas Publ., Mus. Nat. Hist., 1:125–151.

JANNETT, F. J., JR., 1975. The "hip glands" of *Microtus pennsylvanicus* and *M. longicaudus* (Rodentia: Muridae), voles "without" hip glands. Syst. Zool., 24:171–175.

———. 1977. On the sociobiology of the montane vole, *Microtus montanus nanus*

(Rodentia: Muridae). Unpubl. Ph.D. dissert., Cornell Univ., Ithaca, New York, 167 pp.
———. 1978*a*. The density-dependent formation of extended maternal families of the montane vole, *Microtus montanus nanus*. Behav. Ecol. Sociobiol., 3:245–263.
———. 1978*b*. Dosage response of the vesicular, preputial, anal, and hip glands of the male vole, *Microtus montanus* (Rodentia: Muridae), to testosterone propionate. J. Mamm., 59:772–779.
———. 1980. Social dynamics of the montane vole, *Microtus montanus,* as a paradigm. The Biologist, 62:3–19.
———. 1981*a*. Sex ratios in high-density populations of the montane vole, *Microtus montanus,* and the behavior of territorial males. Behav. Ecol. Sociobiol., 8:297–307.
———. 1981*b*. Scent mediation of intraspecific, interspecific, and intergeneric agonistic behavior among sympatric species of voles (Microtinae). Behav. Ecol. Sociobiol., 8:293–296.
———. 1982. Nesting patterns of adult voles, *Microtus montanus,* in field populations. J. Mamm., 63:495–498.
JANNETT, F. J., JR., AND J. JANNETT. 1974. *Drum-marking* by *Arvicola richardsoni* and its taxonomic significance. Amer. Midland Nat., 92:230–234.
———. 1981. Convergent evolution in the flank gland marking behavior of a rodent and a shrew. Mammalia, 45:45–52.
KENNEY, A. M., T. G. HARTUNG, AND D. A. DEWSBURY. 1979. Copulatory behavior and the initiation of pregnancy in California voles (*Microtus californicus*). Brain Behav. Evol., 16:176–191.
KENNEY, A. M., ET AL. 1978. Male copulatory behavior and the induction of ovulation in female voles: a quest for species specificity. Hormones Behav., 11:123–130.
KLEIMAN, D. G. 1977. Monogamy in mammals. Quart. Rev. Biol., 52:39–69.
KREBS, C. J. 1966. Demographic changes in fluctuating populations of *Microtus californicus*. Ecol. Monogr., 36:239–273.
———. 1970. *Microtus* population biology: behavioral changes associated with the population cycle in *M. ochrogaster* and *M. pennsylvanicus*. Ecology, 51: 34–52.
LANIER, D. L., D. Q. ESTEP, AND D. A. DEWSBURY. 1974. Food hoarding in muroid rodents. Behav. Biol., 11:177–187.
LANTZ, D. E. 1907. An economic study of field mice (Genus *Microtus*). U.S. Dept. Agric. Biol. Surv. Bull., 31:1–64.
LIDICKER, W. Z., JR. 1973. Regulation of numbers in an island population of the California vole, a problem in community dynamics. Ecol. Monogr., 43: 271–302.
———. 1976. Experimental manipulation of the timing of reproduction in the California vole. Res. Population Ecol., 18:14–27.
———. 1979. Analysis of two freely-growing enclosed populations of the California vole. J. Mamm., 60:447–466.
———. 1980. The social biology of the California vole. The Biologist, 62:46–55.
LUDWIG, D. R. 1981. The population biology and life history of the water vole (*Microtus richardsoni*). Unpubl. Ph.D. dissert., Univ. Calgary, Calgary, Alberta, 274 pp.
MACISAAC, G. L. 1977. Reproductive correlates of the hip gland in voles (*Microtus townsendii*). Canadian J. Zool., 55:939–941.
MADISON, D. M. 1978. Movement indicators of reproductive events among female meadow voles as revealed by radiotelemetry. J. Mamm., 59:835–843.
———. 1979. Impact of spacing behavior and predation on population growth in

meadow voles. Pp. 20–29, *in* Proceedings of the third eastern pine and meadow vole symposium (R. E. Byers, ed.). New Paltz, New York, 86 pp.

———. 1980*a*. Space use and social structure in meadow voles, *Microtus pennsylvanicus*. Behav. Ecol. Sociobiol., 7:65–71.

———. 1980*b*. Movement types and weather correlates in free-ranging meadow voles. Pp. 34–42, *in* Proceedings of the fourth eastern pine and meadow vole symposium (R. E. Byers, ed.). Hendersonville, North Carolina, 91 pp.

———. 1980*c*. An integrated view of the social biology of *Microtus pennsylvanicus*. The Biologist, 62:20–33.

———. 1981. Time patterning of nest visitation by lactating meadow voles. J. Mamm., 62:389–391.

———. 1984. Group nesting and its ecological and evolutionary significance in overwintering microtine rodents. Pp. 267–274, *in* Winter ecology of small mammals (J. F. Merritt, ed.). Spec. Publ., Carnegie Mus. Nat. Hist. 10: 1–380.

Madison, D. M., R. Fitzgerald, and W. McShea. 1984. Dynamics of social nesting in overwintering meadow voles (*Microtus pennsylvanicus*): possible consequences for population cycles. Behav. Ecol. Sociobiol., 15:9–17.

Martin, E. P. 1956. A population study of the prairie vole (*Microtus ochrogaster*) in northeastern Kansas. Univ. Kansas Publ., Mus. Nat. Hist., 8:361–416.

Martin, R. L. 1971. The natural history and taxonomy of the rock vole, (*Microtus chrotorrhinus*). Unpubl. Ph.D. dissert., Univ. Connecticut, Storrs, 164 pp.

Maser, C., and R. M. Storm. 1970. A key to the Microtinae of the Pacific Northwest. Oregon State Univ. Book Stores, Corvallis, 86 pp.

Miller, W. C. 1969. Ecological and ethological isolating mechanisms between *Microtus pennsylvanicus* and *Microtus ochrogaster* at Terre Haute, Indiana. Amer. Midland Nat., 82:140–148.

Murie, A. 1961. A naturalist in Alaska. Devin-Adair, Old Greenwich, Connecticut, 302 pp.

Myers, J. H., and C. J. Krebs. 1971. Genetic, behavioral and reproductive attributes of dispersing field voles *Microtus pennsylvanicus* and *Microtus ochrogaster*. Ecol. Monogr., 41:53–78.

Myllymäki, A. 1977. Intraspecific competition and home range dynamics in the field vole *Microtus agrestis*. Oikos, 29:553–569.

Orians, G. H. 1969. On the evolution of mating systems in birds and mammals. Amer. Nat., 103:589–603.

Pattie, D. L. 1967. Dynamics of alpine small mammal populations. Unpubl. Ph.D. dissert., Univ. Montana, Missoula, 103 pp.

Paul, J. R. 1970. Observations on the ecology, populations, and reproductive biology of the pine vole, *Microtus pinetorum*, in North Carolina. Rept. Invest., Illinois State Mus., Springfield, Illinois, 20:1–28.

Pearson, O. P. 1960. Habits of *Microtus californicus* revealed by automatic photographic records. Ecol. Monogr., 30:231–249.

Quay, W. B. 1968. The specialized posterolateral sebaceous glandular regions in microtine rodents. J. Mamm., 49:427–445.

Randall, J. A. 1978. Behavioral mechanisms of habitat segregation between sympatric species of *Microtus*: habitat preference and interspecific dominance. Behav. Ecol. Sociobiol., 3:187–202.

Reich, L. M., and R. H. Tamarin. 1980. Trap use as an indicator of social behavior in mainland and island voles. Acta Theriol., 25:295–307.

Reich, L. M., K. M. Wood, B. E. Rothstein, and R. H. Tamarin. 1982. Aggressive behavior in male *Microtus breweri* and its demographic implications. Anim. Behav., 30:117–122.

Riewe, R. R. 1973. Food habits of insular meadow voles, *Microtus pennsylvanicus terraenovae* (Rodentia: Cricetidae), in Notre Dame Bay, Newfoundland. Canadian Field-Nat., 87:5-13.

ROSE, R. K. 1979. Levels of wounding in the meadow vole, *Microtus pennsylvanicus*. J. Mamm., 60:37-45.

ROSE, R. K., AND M. S. GAINES. 1976. Levels of aggression in fluctuating populations of the prairie vole, *Microtus ochrogaster*, in eastern Kansas. J. Mamm., 57:43-57.

ROSE, R. K., AND W. D. HUESTON. 1978. Wound healing in meadow voles. J. Mamm., 59:186-188.

ROTHSTEIN, B. 1976. Selected aspects of the behavioral ecology of *Microtus breweri*. Unpubl. Ph.D. dissert., Boston Univ., Boston, 172 pp.

SALT, J. R. 1978. Notes on the status and life-history of Richardson's vole in Alberta. Alberta Nat., 8:160-169.

SKIRROW, M. 1969. Behavioural studies of five microtine rodents. Unpubl. Ph.D. dissert., Univ. of Calgary, Alberta, 211 pp.

SLOANE, S. A., S. L. SHEA, M. M. PROCTER, AND D. A. DEWSBURY. 1978. Visual cliff performance in 10 species of muroid rodents. Anim. Learn. Behav., 6:244-248.

STARK, H. E. 1963. Nesting habits of the California vole, *Microtus californicus*, and microclimatic factors affecting its nests. Ecology, 44:663-669.

STEHN, R., AND M. E. RICHMOND. 1975. Male-induced pregnancy termination in the prairie vole, *Microtus ochrogaster*. Science, 187:1211-1213.

STODDART, D. M. 1970. Individual range, dispersion and dispersal in a population of water voles (*Arvicola terrestris*, L.). J. Anim. Ecol., 39:403-425.

TAMARIN, R. H. 1981. Hip glands in wild-caught *Microtus pennsylvanicus*. J. Mamm., 62:421.

TAMURA, M. 1966. Aggressive behavior in the California meadow mouse (*Microtus californicus*). Unpubl. M.S. thesis, Univ. California, Berkeley, 71 pp.

TAST, J. 1966. The root vole, *Microtus oeconomus* (Pallas), as an inhabitant of seasonally flooded land. Ann. Zool. Fennica, 3:127-171.

THOMAS, J. A., AND E. C. BIRNEY. 1979. Parental care and mating system of the prairie vole, *Microtus ochrogaster*. Behav. Ecol. Sociobiol., 5:171-186.

TRIVERS, R. L. 1972. Parental investment and sexual selection. Pp. 136-179 *in* Sexual selection and the descent of man, 1871-1971 (B. Campbell, ed.). Aldine, Chicago, 378 pp.

TURNER, B. N., AND S. L. IVERSON. 1973. The annual cycle of aggression in male *Microtus pennsylvanicus* and its relation to population parameters. Ecology, 54:967-981.

WEBSTER, A. B. 1979. A radiotelemetry study of social behavior and activity of free-ranging meadow voles, *Microtus pennsylvanicus*. Unpubl. M.S. thesis, Univ. Guelph, Guelph, Ontario, 110 pp.

WEBSTER, A. B., AND R. J. BROOKS. 1981. Social behavior of *Microtus pennsylvanicus* in relation to seasonal changes in demography. J. Mamm., 62:738-751.

WEBSTER, D. G., D. J. BAUMGARDNER, AND D. A. DEWSBURY. 1979. Open-field behavior in eight taxa of muroid rodents. Bull. Psychonomic Soc., 13: 90-92.

WEBSTER, D. G., M. H. WILLIAMS, R. D. OWENS, V. B. GEIGER, AND D. A. DEWSBURY. 1981. Digging behavior in 12 taxa of muroid rodents. Anim. Learn. Behav., 9:173-177.

WEST, S. D., AND H. T. DUBLIN. 1984. Behavioral strategies of small mammals under winter conditions: solitary or social? Pp. 293-299, *in* Winter ecology of small mammals (J. F. Merritt, ed.). Spec. Publ., Carnegie Mus. Nat. Hist., 10:1-380.

WHITAKER, J. O., JR., AND R. L. MARTIN. 1977. Food habits of *Microtus chrotor-*

rhinus from New Hampshire, New York, Labrador, and Quebec. J. Mamm., 58:99–100.

WIEGERT, R. G. 1961. Respiratory energy loss and activity patterns in the meadow vole, *Microtus pennsylvanicus pennsylvanicus*. Ecology, 42:245–253.

WILSON, E. O. 1975. Sociobiology. Belknap Press, Cambridge, Massachusetts, 697 pp.

WILSON, R. C., T. VACEK, D. L. LANIER, AND D. A. DEWSBURY. 1976. Open-field behavior in muroid rodents. Behav. Biol., 17:495–506.

WITTENBERGER, J. F. 1981. Animal social behavior. Duxbury Press, Boston, 722 pp.

WOLFF, J. O. 1980. Social organization of the taiga vole (*Microtus xanthognathus*). The Biologist, 62:34–45.

———. 1984. Overwintering behavioral strategies in taiga voles (*Microtus xanthognathus*). Pp. 315–318, *in* Winter ecology of small mammals (J. F. Merritt, ed.). Spec. Publ., Carnegie Mus. Nat. Hist., 10:1–380.

WOLFF, J. O., AND M. F. JOHNSON. 1979. Scent marking in taiga voles. J. Mamm., 60:400–403.

WOLFF, J. O., AND W. Z. LIDICKER, JR. 1980. Population ecology of the taiga vole, *Microtus xanthognathus*, in interior Alaska. Canadian J. Zool., 48: 1800–1812.

———. 1981. Communal winter nesting and food sharing in taiga voles. Behav. Ecol. Sociobiol., 9:237–240.

WRABETZ, M. J. 1980. Nest insulation: a method of evolution. Canadian J. Zool., 58:938–940.

YOUNGMAN, P. M. 1975. Mammals of the Yukon Territory. Natl. Mus. Nat. Sci., Ottawa, 192 pp.

ACTIVITY RHYTHMS AND SPACING

DALE M. MADISON

Abstract

MICROTINE rodents have different behavioral and physiological rhythms, but the 2–6 h ultradian rhythm of activity is a dominant feature in the day-to-day existence of these species. Variability in the timing of this rhythm with maintenance activities, growth, reproduction, and a complex of other social and environmental stimuli frequently make the characterization of these rhythms difficult, but no less significant, under field conditions. The ultradian rhythm is essentially a feeding rhythm, and the periodicity is linked closely to food quality and energy needs. Circadian rhythms occur in microtines, but infradian rhythms need further study. Recent technical advances combined with adjustments or controls for the shortcomings of traditional laboratory studies give promise of significant advances in the understanding of the mechanisms and adaptive significance of microtine activity rhythms. This review identifies six generalities or hypotheses for future study.

Studies of spacing in microtines have been concerned primarily with home-range size, but despite rather sophisticated analytical approaches in these studies, little insight has been gained beyond that expressed by Burt over 40 years ago. In this review, the home-range concept of Burt (1943) is applied to microtine rodents, and a 24-h home-range model, based on radiotelemetry data from *Microtus pennsylvanicus,* is developed. Home ranges are classified into stable, variable, and shifting types. General categories of movement are also defined: local, distant reconnaissance, and dispersal. These types of home range and movement vary in their frequency of occurrence in the order presented above, the most frequent listed first. Variability in space use is discussed with respect to energetics, diet, gender differences, reproductive condition, social factors, interspecific interactions, and weather and seasonal factors. Six generalities or hypotheses relative to space use are presented for future study and testing.

Introduction

Concern for patterns of movement in microtine rodents in time and space is fundamental to a consideration of a host of behavioral and ecological issues. Emphasis in this chapter is placed on descriptions of movement patterns in time and space and on questions of adaptive significance. The meadow vole, *Microtus pennsylvanicus*, receives the most emphasis, because it is the most thoroughly studied and widely distributed species of the genus *Microtus* in North America. I also include information on some Old World species for comparison. Finally, the chapter is not so much a review as it is 1) an appeal for greater awareness among investigators of the natural patterns of movement of microtine rodents, and 2) a statement of the flexibility that at least certain microtine rodents have in adjusting to their environment.

Activity Rhythms

Rhythms of behavior among voles include those less than 24 h (ultradian rhythms), those of approximately 24 h (circadian rhythms), and possibly those greater than 24 h (infradian rhythms) (Aschoff, 1981). Terms such as nocturnal, diurnal, and crepuscular refer to circadian rhythms in which the active phase of the organism occurs at night, during the day, or at dawn and dusk, respectively. Where activity is distributed randomly throughout the diel (24-h) period, the organism is said to be arrhythmic (Daan, 1981). A strict ultradian pattern has no nocturnal, diurnal, or crepuscular emphasis, but ultradian rhythms in *Microtus* commonly have these emphases because of the concurrent presence of circadian rhythms. Thus, for example, a nocturnal-ultradian rhythm is one in which the regular, short term pulses of activity occur at night, either exclusively or with greater amplitude or duration (that is, the active phase of the ultradian period is elongated but the period remains the same). The information on rhythms to follow complements the more physiological discussions of endogenicity and cueing in *Mammal Review* (1972, Vol. 1, nos. 7–8), Aschoff (1981), Aschoff et al. (1982), Pinter and Negus (1965), Rowsemitt (1981), and Seabloom (this volume). Most of the rhythms referred to in this review have not been rigorously quantified and verified, such as by time-series analyses (Broom, 1979; Rowsemitt et al., 1982; Sollberger, 1965), and thus most of the conclusions reached should be interpreted as first approximations for the genus *Microtus*.

Methods

A large array of techniques have been used to record the activity rhythms of voles (Table 1). Generally, different methods show different types of activity (for example, nesting, feeding, reconnaissance and exploration, nursing, defecation, and reingestion), and the activities often show different temporal patterning. For example, activity wheels typically measure movements that are naturally expressed during the night, but omit foraging and nesting activity that commonly occur in the same organisms in the same cage throughout the diel cycle (Calhoun, 1945; Daan and Slopsema, 1978; Dewsbury, 1980; Lehmann, 1976; Lehmann and Sommersberg, 1980; Mather, 1981). Wheel-running itself may vary with cage size, for Lehmann (1976) observed Old World *M. agrestis* to change from a nocturnal-ultradian pattern, to a strict nocturnal pattern, and then to a strict ultradian pattern in successively smaller cages. Nest monitors in the field do not discriminate between foraging, social or other activities (Barbour, 1963; Madison, 1981). Multiple monitors in the same cage were used by Daan and Slopsema (1978) to distinguish between ultradian feeding (photocell and food hopper), nesting (treadle), and nocturnal wheel-running, but whether these devices reveal natural patterns is subject to criticism. For example, Graham (1968) showed that free-ranging meadow voles, *Microtus pennsylvanicus,* were diurnal, but caged individuals in the field were crepuscular, and caged voles in the laboratory were nocturnal. Also, Kavanau (1962) showed that photoperiods with abrupt light-on, light-off transitions in the laboratory affect rodents differently than the same photoperiod with gradual intensity transitions (for example, dawn and dusk).

Although studies relying on mechanical devices in the laboratory can be criticized for their lack of natural relevance, studies of free-ranging voles relying on radiotelemetry or radioisotopes can also be criticized. Hamley and Falls (1975) demonstrated that radiotransmitter collars with 10-cm whip antennas affect activity levels in caged meadow voles, and Webster and Brooks (1980) showed that meadow voles in winter typically lose 2–3 g after being tagged with transmitters. Isotopes, instead of imposing a weight burden on the

TABLE 1
TYPES OF ACTIVITY RHYTHMS AND THE TECHNIQUES USED IN STUDIES OF *Microtus*

Species	Study conditions*	Activity rhythms†			Technique	Source
		Ultradian	Circadian	Other		
New World						
M. californicus	F, Su, A, W, Sp	None	Crepuscular (Su)	Variable	Photography	Pearson (1960)
	Su, W	2.0–6.0	Nocturnal (Su)		Radiotelemetery	Shields (1976)
M. canicaudus	L	—	—	Arrhythmic?	Observed	Baumgardner et al. (1980)
	L	—	Nocturnal		Activity wheel	Dewsbury (1980)
M. miurus	Su, F	—	Nocturnal (Su)		Activity wheel	Swade and Pittendrigh (1967)
M. montanus	L	—	Nocturnal		Observed	Baumgardner et al. (1980)
	L	—	Nocturnal		Activity wheel	Dewsbury (1980)
	L	Variable	Nocturnal	Variable	Activity wheel	Seed and Khalili (1971)
	L	3.0	Nocturnal (Su) Diurnal (W)	Variable	Activity wheel	Rowsemitt (1981)
M. ochrogaster	W, F	Variable	Diurnal		Radioisotopes	Barbour (1963)
	L	—	—	Arrhythmic?	Observed	Baumgardner et al. (1980)
	L	—	Nocturnal		Activity wheel	Calhoun (1945)
	A, F	—	Crepuscular		Photography	Carley et al. (1970)

TABLE 1
CONTINUED

Species	Study conditions*	Activity rhythms† Ultradian	Circadian	Other	Technique	Source
	L	—	Nocturnal		Activity wheel	Dewsbury (1980)
	W, F	—	Nocturnal		Trapping	Glass and Slade (1980)
	Su, W, F	—	Diurnal		Trapping	Martin (1956)
M. pennsylvanicus	Su, F	3.0	—		Radioisotopes	Ambrose (1973)
	L	—	—	Arrhythmic?	Observed	Baumgardner et al. (1980)
	L	—	Nocturnal		Activity wheel	Dewsbury (1980)
	Su, A, W, Sp, F, L	2.0–6.0	Diurnal (W, F) Crepuscular (W, C) Crepuscular (S, F) Nocturnal (L)		Radioisotopes, treadle	Graham (1968)
	Su, A, W, Sp, F	—	Crepuscular (W, F) Diurnal (Su, F)		Trapping	Hamilton (1937)
	L	2.0–4.0	—		Treadle	Hatfield (1940)
	Su, F	—	Crepuscular		Magnetic tagging	Heidt (1971)
	Su, F	4.0–6.5	—		Radiotelemetry	Madison (1981)

TABLE 1
CONTINUED

Species	Study conditions*	Activity rhythms† Ultradian	Circadian	Other	Technique	Source
	W, F	4.0	—		Radioisotopes	This paper (Fig. 1)
	W, G	2.0–4.0	Nocturnal		Passage counter	This paper (Fig. 2)
	Sp, F	2.0–3.0	—		Radiotelemetry	McShea and Madison (1984)
	Su, F	—	Nocturnal		Photography	Osterberg (1962)
	L	0.3–3.0	—		Treadle	Ouellette and Heisinger (1980)
	L	1.0–5.0	—		Activity wheel	Seabloom (1965)
	A, F, C	2.0–4.0	—	Variable	Treadle	Stebbins (pers. comm.)
	Su, A, W, F	2.0–5.0	—	Variable	Radiotelemetry	Webster and Brooks (1981*a*)
	L	2.0–3.6	Nocturnal	Variable	O_2 consumption	Wiegert (1961)
M. pinetorum	Su, F	—	Nocturnal	Variable	Radiotelemetry	Gettle (1975)
	W, Sp, Su, A, F	—	Nocturnal (Su)	Arrhythmic (W)?	Trapping	Paul (1970)
	Sp, Su, F	—	Arrhythmic		Trapping	Wolff and Lidicker (1980)
M. xanthognathus	L	3.5–6.0			Thermistor	Wolff and Lidicker (1981)
Old World						
M. agrestis	W, Su, F	—	Nocturnal (Su) Diurnal (W)	Variable	Trapping	Baumler (1975)

TABLE 1
CONTINUED

Species	Study conditions*	Activity rhythms† Ultradian	Circadian	Other	Technique	Source
	A, F, C	2.0–4.0	Nocturnal		Treadle	Davis (1933)
	Su, A, W, Sp, F, C	None?	Nocturnal (Su) Diurnal (W)	Arrhythmic (A, Sp)?	Treadle	Erkinaro (1961, 1970)
	Su, F, C, L	1.5–3.0	Nocturnal		Treadle Activity wheel	Lehmann (1976)
	L	4.0	—		Passage counter	Mossing (1975)
	Sp, G	—	Nocturnal		Activity wheel	Nygren (1978)
	L	4.0	—		Treadle	Rasmuson et al. (1977)
M. arvalis	L	2.0–4.0	Nocturnal	Variable	Activity wheel Treadle Light beam	Daan and Slopsema (1978)
	L	3.0	—		Treadle	Durup (1956)
	Su, A, W, Sp, F, C	—	Nocturnal (Su) Diurnal (W)	Variable	Treadle	Erkinaro (1970)
	L	—	Late day, early evening		Physiological measures	Kossut et al. (1974)

TABLE 1
CONTINUED

Species	Study conditions*	Activity rhythms† Ultradian	Circadian	Other	Technique	Source
	Su, A, W, Sp, F	2.0	Diurnal (W)	Arrhythmic (Su, A, Sp)?	Passage counter	Lehmann and Sommersberg (1980)
	Su, F	1.0–5.0	—		Radioisotopes	Nikitina et al. (1972)
	Su, A, W, Sp, F, C	2.0	Diurnal (W) Nocturnal (Su)		Treadle	Ostermann (1956)
	Su, A, W, Sp, F	2.0	Crepuscular (Su) Diurnal (W)		Trapping	Rijnsdorp et al. (1981)
M. oeconomus	Su, A, W, Sp, F, C	2.0	Variable		Treadle	Erkinaro (1970)
	Su, F	2.4–4.8	—		Radioisotopes	Karulin et al. (1976)
	Su, F	—	Nocturnal (Su)		Activity wheel	Swade and Pittendrigh (1967)

* Abbreviations: Su, summer; A, autumn; W, winter; Sp, spring; F, field; G, greenhouse; C, cage; L, laboratory cage.

† Ultradian rhythm (in h) and circadian patterns are approximations by the author if the original investigator(s) did not state the period or pattern. Circadian patterns are highly variable, ranging from only a slight emphasis in activity during the active phase to confinement of activity to the active phase (usually in laboratory studies). The term "variable" was used if patterns could not be characterized or if individual patterns varied considerably.

free-ranging vole, expose the organism to very high gamma emission that could easily have detrimental effects (Mihok, pers. comm.).

Despite the wide variety of potential biases inherent in the different methods, a little common sense and "natural-mindedness" during interpretation reduces much of the apparent contradiction and allows laboratory data to be used, at least as a first reading of natural rhythms of behavior.

Ultradian Rhythms

The short-term activity rhythm, typically varying from 2 to 4 h, is common for vole species when study methods allow it to be measured (Table 1). The more common findings are that: 1) the period varies within and between individuals; 2) the activity pulses are more prominent at certain times of the 24-h cycle; 3) the ultradian peaks shift with season; and 4) the peaks appear to synchronize with dawn or dusk, but gradually drift out of phase because of individual variation until resynchronization 24 h later. Figure 1 shows one example for *M. pennsylvanicus* of a natural winter ultradian rhythm with a 4-h period. The vole was carrying a 50 μCi Ta-182 collar, and the vole's movement was monitored every 15 min for 24 h with a portable scintillation meter and probe. During tracking the vole was in a meadow under 1 m of snow. The data suggest that there is a free-running rhythm under snow, as observed for beavers (Potvin and Bovet, 1975). Figure 2 shows the shifting of this rhythm to a nocturnal-ultradian pattern under the same photoperiod but with no snow cover and at moderate temperatures in a greenhouse. The records give a clear indication of the variability, and the periodicity, typical of ultradian rhythms.

Circadian Rhythms

The available literature on rhythms in microtines leaves little doubt that most, if not all, microtines are flexible in their activity scheduling through the diel period, and that circadian rhythms exist, as evidenced by free-running rhythms slightly shorter or longer than 24 h in voles held under constant light or darkness (Calhoun, 1945; Daan and Slopsema, 1978; Lehmann, 1976; Mossing, 1975; Seed and Khalili, 1971; Swade and Pittendrigh, 1967). Under laboratory conditions, voles are active at night, yet under natural con-

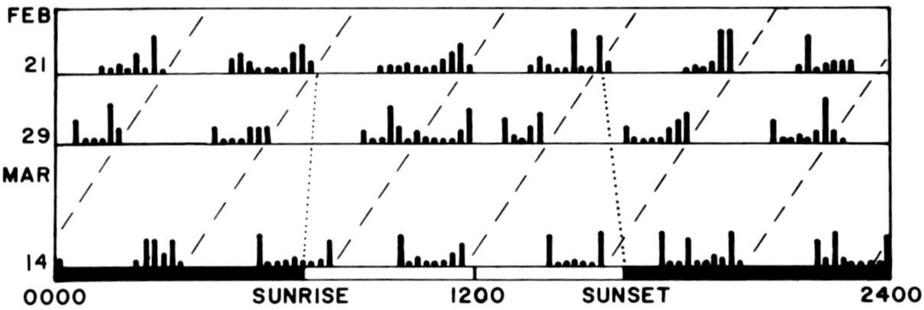

FIG. 1. Activity rhythm of a 30-g female meadow vole (*M. pennsylvanicus*) wearing a Ta-182 collar in a field covered with 1 m of snow in Quebec, Canada, 1975. The vertical axis is movement (m) between 15-min detection points. The smallest vertical unit indicates any movement up to 1 m, or the stationary position of a vole away from the nest. The spacing between the 3 days for which data were obtained reflects the time elapsed between these days. Dashed lines represent ultradian periods of about 4 h that have an underlying, free-running circadian periodicity of 23.85 h/day. The dotted line represents time of sunrise and sunset.

ditions voles are commonly found to be more diurnal or crepuscular (Calhoun, 1945; Graham, 1968; Heidt, 1971; Seed and Khalili, 1971). There is also a seasonal shift, to be discussed later, from a nocturnal or crepuscular pattern during summer to a diurnal emphasis during winter (for example, see Baumler, 1975; Carley et al., 1970; Erkinaro, 1961; Lehmann, 1976). But whatever the emphasis is in activity (nocturnal or diurnal), some activity outside the nest usually occurs in nature during the "inactive" phase, unlike the condition for strictly nocturnal or diurnal rodents (for example, *Peromyscus* and *Tamias*).

The patterns above are generalizations and therefore should not be considered rules, for some circadian periods can vary considerably. For example, Erkinaro (1970) noticed during one January that *M. oeconomus* was conspicuously nocturnal, but observed during the following January an obvious diurnal pattern. Pearson (1960) observed distinct diurnal and nocturnal patterns among *M. californicus* in the same population at the same time in comparable habitats only 9.5 m apart.

Infradian Rhythms

Behavioral rhythms in *Microtus* with period lengths greater than 24 h are not clearly described. Behavioral estrus with a period

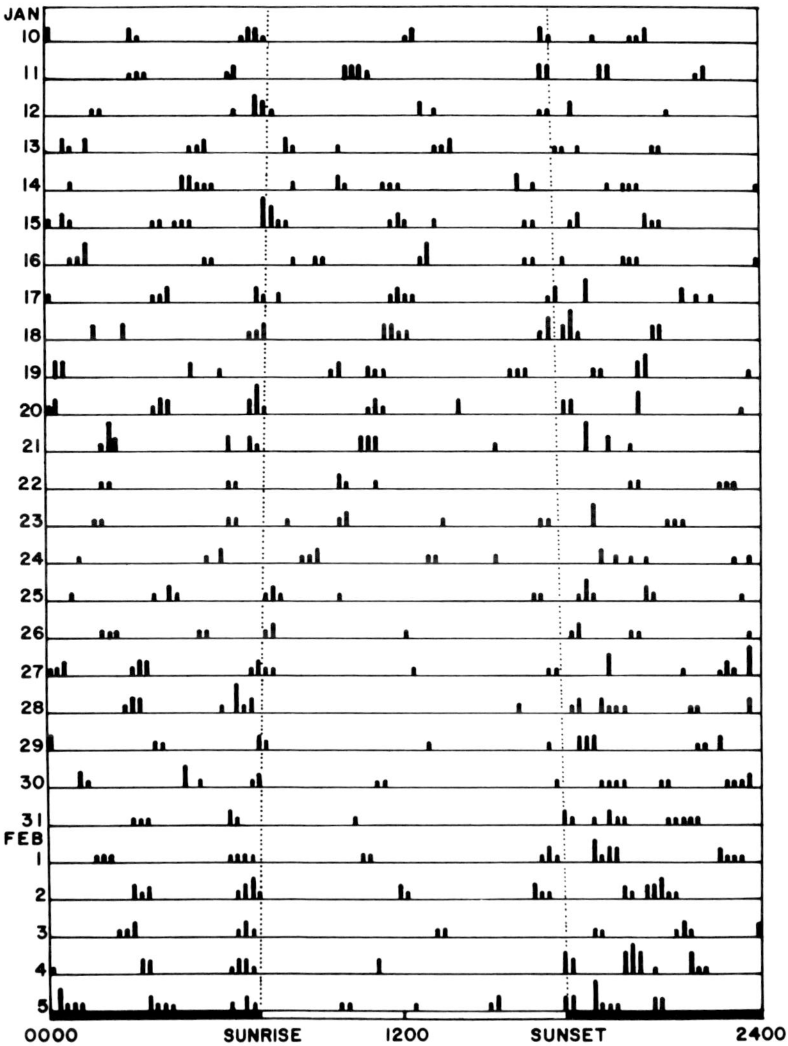

FIG. 2. Activity rhythm of a solitary, 45-g female meadow vole (*M. pennsylvanicus*) for 27 days in a 3 × 3-m grass enclosure wired with passage counters inside a greenhouse in Montreal, Quebec, 1975. The number of passages used each 15 min is shown. The vertical axis is in units of 0–4, 5–9, 10–14, 15–19, and 20+ passages (the shortest vertical bar indicates 0–4 passages; the tallest, 20+ passages). Dotted lines give sunrise and sunset.

length of several days occurs (Hutchinson, 1972), but female voles have not been observed in isolation for behavioral changes during these cycles. No clear behavioral "circarhythms" (*sensu* Aschoff, 1981) greater than 24 h are known for *Microtus*; ground squirrels (*Spermophilus lateralis*) are the closest relatives with demonstrated circannual behavioral rhythms (Pengelley and Fisher, 1957).

Factors Correlated with Activity Rhythms

Genetic factors.—The only study of *Microtus* showing a genetic basis for intraspecific differences in rhythmic behavior is by Rasmuson et al. (1977). *M. agrestis* from northern populations of Sweden showed 4-h ultradian rhythms, whereas southern populations showed very low levels of activity and no ultradian periodicity. Hybrids showed intermediate activity levels but ultradian rhythms similar to the northern populations. Both sexes gave the same result.

Energetics, diet, and food.—Energetic considerations involving weight, metabolic rate, and diet have been linked with the existence and period of ultradian rhythms. In eutherian mammals, ultradian periods are common among species feeding on high bulk diets (Ashby, 1972), and the short-term rhythms are specifically associated with foraging and food intake (Daan and Aschoff, 1981, 1982). The herbivorous diet of *Microtus,* consisting of large amounts of low-quality food, necessitates frequent feeding through the 24-h cycle with brief rest periods for efficient digestive processing (Daan and Aschoff, 1981). Granivorus rodents, such as *Peromyscus,* do not exhibit comparable ultradian rhythms, nor are they active throughout the diel cycle as are the herbivorus microtines (Hansson, 1971). Since bulk feeding also entails frequent defecation, the necessity of leaving the nest intermittently to avoid fouling the nest has been suggested as another reason for the ultradian rhythm (Lehmann, 1976). The habit of fecal reingestion during the inactive phase of the ultradian cycle is consistent with the fouling-avoidance explanation (Ouellette and Heisinger, 1980). The period length of the ultradian rhythm has been shown to be directly proportional to body weight, and inversely proportional to metabolic rate (Daan and Aschoff, 1981, 1982; Daan and Slopsema, 1978; Lehmann, 1976). Hence, the smaller the vole, the greater will be the energy needs per gram body weight, and the shorter will be the length of the ultradian period.

Gender and reproduction.—An examination of the literature for gender and reproductive differences in behavioral rhythms reveals several correlations. Evans (1970) and Madison (pers. observ.) show female meadow voles to be more diurnal than males, but other workers report no gender differences for *M. pennsylvanicus* (Graham, 1968; Stebbins, pers. comm.), *M. californicus* (Pearson, 1960), or *M. agrestis* (Rasmuson et al., 1977). Webster and Brooks (1981*a*) showed that reproductively active female meadow voles are about 180 degrees out of phase with the rest of the population in the dawn ultradian period of activity. This difference might be linked with the greater energy demands of these females. For example, Madison (1981) found that the period of the ultradian rhythm decreases during lactation from 6.5 to 4.0 h, and Kaczmarski (1966) and Migula (1969) showed that the energy needs of lactating voles increase rapidly during lactation to their highest levels near weaning. This inverse relationship between period length and energy needs in lactating voles correlates with the findings discussed in the previous section. The relationship even occurs for communally nursing females with different size young in the same nest (McShea and Madison, 1984). Finally, Rowsemitt (1981) showed that castrated male *M. montanus* are diurnal and that intact and sham-castrated males are nocturnal, suggesting that non-reproductives in nature may be more diurnal.

Social factors.—The influence of social behavior on rhythmic activity is demonstrated by the synchronization of the ultradian rhythms of some voles (Daan and Slopsema, 1978; Graham, 1968; Lehmann and Sommersberg, 1980; Madison, 1984; Madison et al., 1984; Rasmuson et al., 1977; Rijnsdorp et al., 1981; Webster and Brooks, 1981*a*), but not others (McShea and Madison, 1984). Evans (1970) showed that a male *M. pennsylvanicus* in the presence of a female is more active, especially during the day, than when alone. Since an isolated male is equally active both day and night, and since an isolated female is more active during the day, the results indicate the effect of the female on the male. Juvenile voles have rhythms that differ from those of adults. They are more nocturnal in *M. agrestis* (Baumler, 1975) and *M. pennsylvanicus* (Webster, 1979). In *M. arvalis,* the juveniles do not synchronize with the adults until at least a week after emergence from the natal nest (Lehmann and Sommersberg, 1980). The small size of juvenile voles relegates them to subordinate social status in the population

(Turner and Iverson, 1973), and direct competition between adults and young would be reduced substantially if these animals were active at times different from the adults. The absence of apparent differences in activity rhythms of adult and juvenile *M. californicus* (Pearson, 1960) and *M. pinetorum* (FitzGerald, pers. comm.) suggests that these species may live in cohesive family groups where competition and the need for temporal isolation is reduced. Such social organization is known for *M. pinetorum* (FitzGerald and Madison, 1983). Since both social status and energy requirements vary with body size, any final statement regarding the reason for rhythm differences in voles of various sizes must await further study.

Interspecific interactions.—Three different kinds of interspecific interactions, specifically predation, parasitism, and competition, appear to be correlated with behavioral rhythms in voles. Predation was implicated as a causal agent in the diurnal synchrony of ultradian rhythms in Old World *M. arvalis* (Daan and Slopsema, 1978; Rijnsdorp et al., 1981). In this case, kestrels preyed intensively on voles, and any vole that was out of phase with the activity of other voles in the population stood a much greater chance of being taken by a kestrel. Lehmann and Sommersberg (1980) questioned this "safety-in-numbers" hypothesis for *M. arvalis* and suggested instead that the synchronous ultradian rhythmicity is for the purposes of social signalling and territorial defense, the advantage of strong defense being the inheritance of the family territory by kin. However, in revealing that the daytime activity is within grass runways, and that the night activity is outside these tunnels on the surface, Lehmann and Sommersberg gave further evidence of apparent predation pressure during the day. Voles may also avoid the active periods of predators. Hamilton (1937) indicated that the activity peak of *M. pennsylvanicus* just before dusk corresponds to, and results from, a lull in activity of a wide range of predators, and the same is true during the secondary peak at dawn. Fulk (1972) suggested that *M. pennsylvanicus* decreases the chances of shrew predation by becoming more diurnal in areas of overlap with this predator.

Parasitism is also a type of interspecific interaction, and one case has been reported in which a trypanosome parasite actually induced a change in the rhythmic behavior of *M. montanus* (Seed and Khalili, 1971). In this case, the change was the result of neurological damage caused by the parasite.

Temporal avoidance of interspecific competition is suggested for prairie voles. *M. ochrogaster* has non-overlapping activity peaks with sympatric *Peromyscus maniculatus* and *Reithrodontomys megalotis* (Carley et al., 1970) and with *Sigmodon hispidus* (Glass and Slade, 1980).

Weather and seasonal factors.—The effects of weather variables and seasonal changes on the activity rhythms of voles have been studied by many investigators. Temperature extremes emerge as a potentially important factor in several ways. In the summer, high daytime temperatures depress daytime activity in *M. pennsylvanicus* (Getz, 1961) and *M. californicus* (Pearson, 1960), and this may account for the depression of summer daytime activity observed in *M. ochrogaster* (Martin, 1956), *M. agrestis* (Davis, 1933; Erkinaro, 1961; Lehmann, 1976), *M. californicus* (Shields, 1976), *M. xanthognathus* (Wolff and Lidicker, 1980), and *M. arvalis* (Erkinaro, 1970; Ostermann, 1956; Rijnsdorp et al., 1981). Cold temperatures during winter, especially at night, correlate with the more diurnal activity of overwintering *M. ochrogaster* (Barbour, 1963; Carley et al., 1970; Martin, 1956), *M. agrestis* (Baumler, 1975; Erkinaro, 1961), and *M. arvalis* (Erkinaro, 1970; Lehmann and Sommersberg, 1980). With a temperature increase but no change in photoperiod during winter, meadow voles (*M. pennsylvanicus*) shift from an ultradian to a nocturnal-ultradian pattern of movement (Fig. 1). The link between temperature extremes and altered behavioral or seasonal rhythms in *M. pennsylvanicus* (and probably other species) may be confounded by other factors, because several studies on this species show no major seasonal or temperature effects on activity rhythms (Madison, pers. observ.; Osterberg, 1962; Stebbins, pers. comm.; Webster and Brooks, 1981*a*), and one study shows longer ultradian periods of activity at high temperatures (20 to 35°C) than at low temperatures (0°C) (Hatfield, 1940). The appearance of synchronous communal nesting and huddling during winter in *M. pennsylvanicus* and other species (Madison, 1984); Webster and Brooks, 1981*a*; Wolff, 1980; Wolff and Lidicker, 1981), and the increased movement during winter on warm days or on days following heavy snow strongly suggests that low temperature stimulates synchronous nest use and inhibits activity during the winter (Madison et al., 1984).

No clear effects of precipitation on activity rhythms are reported in the literature, although Pearson (1960) felt that the summer activity pattern of *M. californicus* is determined by the availability of dew early in the morning. Activity levels were reported to increase during rainfall and overcast conditions for *M. pennsylvanicus* (Bider, 1968), *M. californicus* (Pearson, 1960), and *M. agrestis* (Baumler, 1975). Other investigators found the opposite to be true for *M. pennsylvanicus*. Madison (1980*a*) observed increased activity on warm, dry days with high barometric pressure and low relative humidity, especially following days of wet weather. Graham (1968) noticed positive correlations with light and temperature, and negative correlations with humidity. Lehmann and Sommersberg (1980) showed that when precipitation was combined with cold temperatures during late autumn, the combination markedly reduced activity in *M. agrestis*.

Lighting conditions may affect behavioral rhythms as a result of changes in both photoperiod and intensity of illumination. The seasonal shift from an emphasis on nocturnal-crepuscular behavior during summer to diurnal behavior during winter, as reported earlier for several species, may depend on seasonal changes in photoperiod rather than on temperature changes. Rowsemitt (1981) showed that male *M. montanus* under constant temperature conditions shift from a nocturnal pattern under 16L:8D to diurnal pattern under 8L:16D. The fact that five *Microtus* species show free-running rhythms under constant light or dark is firm evidence of photoperiodic events acting as zeitgebers (Calhoun, 1945; Daan and Slopsema, 1978; Lehmann, 1976; Mossing, 1975; Seed and Khalili, 1971; Swade and Pittendrigh, 1967). In Fig. 1, the ultradian rhythm of a meadow vole under 1 m of snow suggests the possibility of a free-running system under constant darkness. The ultradian pulse at dawn, which often synchronizes with dawn (see Fig. 2), loses about 8 min/day over the 29 days of Ta-182 tracking. A partial day of tracking 1 week later (not included in Fig. 1) agrees with the explanation of a free-running rhythm. Light penetration through the snow is essentially extinguished at a 50-cm snow depth (Evernden and Fuller, 1972). Light intensity effects are demonstrated: 1) by the preference of *M. californicus* and *M. agrestis* for low intensity light (Erkinaro, 1973; Kavanau and Havenhill, 1976); 2) by the disappearance of wheel-running activity for *M. agrestis* during the subjective night under high-intensity light, but not low-intensity light (Lehmann, 1976); 3) by the depressed activity of *M. pennsyl-*

vanicus on bright moon-lit nights (Doucet and Bider, 1969); and 4) by the increased activity of *M. californicus* on moonless nights (Pearson, 1960). The rate of change of light intensity, sudden in the laboratory but gradual in the field, also appears to have an effect (Kavanau, 1962).

Spacing

Few other subjects have been given as much attention among microtine rodents as has spacing, which subsumes home range, density, territoriality, and dispersal, to mention a few. And few other subjects in this volume overlap as broadly with the others as does spacing. Space use is the product of movement through time, and any understanding of why this movement takes place must include a consideration of factors relating to competition (intraspecific and interspecific), resource needs (food, habitat), reproduction, and so forth. Obviously, the treatment here must be limited; and as with activity rhythms, the emphasis is mainly on description and on direct correlations between area use or use intensity and ecological and social variables. The concepts of home range, territory, and dispersion are reviewed, but the emphasis is on an examination of extensive and intensive radiotelemetry data for free-ranging *M. pennsylvanicus* not yet published.

Methods

A wide variety of techniques have been used to record home range and movement in microtines, and many analytical methods have been employed (Table 2). Both the techniques and analytical methods have received ample review (Brown, 1966; Ford and Krumme, 1979; Hayne, 1950; Koeppl et al., 1975; Meserve, 1971; Sanderson, 1966; Schoener, 1981; Van Vleck, 1969; Van Winkle, 1975), so no further review is attempted here. Basically, as was mentioned by Sanderson (1966), no single analytical method gives measures of space use suitable for all potential uses. And it is apparent that techniques of analysis have in most cases gone far beyond the practical or meaningful limits of the data set. Too little is known about where voles go, why they go there, and what happens there, and too much time is spent analyzing data on capture points that are at

TABLE 2
HOME RANGE, MOVEMENTS, AND SPACE USE CORRELATIONS IN *Microtus*

Species	Method	Analysis*	Approximate area (m²), distance (m) **	Correlations: Repro-duction	Den-sity	Food	Season	Sex	Hab-itat	Source
New World:										
M. pennsyl-vanicus	^{182}Ta	See ref.	♂ 52 (Su) ♀ 40		+			♂ > ♀		Ambrose (1973)
	^{198}Au	*AMAM,* IBS EBS, RL	♂ 312 (Su) ♀ 136					♂ > ♀		Ambrose (1969)
	Trapping	IBS	♂ 1,619 (Sp, Su) ♀ 1,012					♂ > ♀	X	Blair (1940)
	^{182}Ta	MMAM	♂ 139 (Su) ♂ 2 (W)				Su > W			Douglass (1976)
	Trapping	EBS	♂ 550 (X) ♀ 300		X		X Su > W	X ♂ > ♀	X	Getz (1961)
	Trapping	EBS	♂ 650 (X) ♀ 400				Su > W, ♂ Su < W, ♀	♂ > ♀	0	Getz (1970)
	Trapping	V	?					♂ > ♀		Hamilton (1937)

TABLE 2
CONTINUED

Species	Method	Analysis*	Approximate area (m^2), distance (m) **	Correlations: Repro-duction	Den-sity	Food	Season	Sex	Hab-itat	Source
	Trapping	*MAM*, IBS	♂ 364 (Su) ♀ 162					♂ > ♀		Hayne (1950)
	Radiotelemetry	MAM	♀ 100 (Su)	−♀, lact.						Madison (1978)
	Radiotelemetry	MAM	♂ 192 (Su) ♀ 68					♂ > ♀		Madison (1980*b*)
	Radiotelemetry	MAM	52 (comb., A, W)	−♀, lact.						Madison et al. (1984)
	Trapping	MAM	♂ 1,416 (Su) ♀ 526	+♂, RA				♂ > ♀		McCann (1976)
	^{32}P	V, *RL*	♂ 120 (Su)							Miller (1957)
	Dyes	GDM	200 (comb., pooled)							New (1958)
	Radiotelemetry	MAM	♀ 40 (Su) ♀ 19 (W)				Su > W		X	Pagano and Madison (1981)

TABLE 2
CONTINUED

Species	Method	Analysis*	Approximate area (m^2), distance (m) **	Correlations: Reproduction	Correlations: Density	Correlations: Food	Correlations: Season	Correlations: Sex	Correlations: Habitat	Source
	Trapping	GDM	60 (comb.)							Stickel and Warbach (1960)
	Trapping	ADM	♂ 10, ♀ 7 (Su, W)					♂ > ♀?		Tamarin (1977)
	Trapping	BVN	♂ 12,964 (RA) ♂ 1,387 (NR)	+♂, RA	–		Su > W			Turner and Iverson (1973)
	Trapping	*IBS*, NS	♂ 1,943, ♀ 1,619 (Su)		–♂ 0, ♀			♂ > ♀?		Van Vleck (1969)
	Radiotelemetry	AA (X)	♂ 102, ♀ 57 (Su, A)	+♂, RA			0, ♂	♂ > ♀		Webster and Brooks (1981*b*)
M. breweri	Trapping	ADM	♂ 13, ♀ 10 (Su, W)					♂ > ♀?		Tamarin (1977)
M. californicus	Isotope	PUD/MAP	♂ 45, ♀ 32 (pooled)							Ford and Krumme (1979)

TABLE 2
CONTINUED

				Correlations						
Species	Method	Analysis*	Approximate area (m^2), distance (m) **	Repro-duction	Den-sity	Food	Season	Sex	Hab-itat	Source
	Trapping	ADM	♂ 40 (comb.) ♀ 20	+♂, RA	–	+	Su > W	♂ > ♀ (RA) ♂ = ♀ (NR)		Krebs (1966)
	Photo-graphy	V DM (X)	15 (comb.)							Pearson (1960)
M. montanus	^{182}Ta	MMAM	♂ 77 (Su) ♂ 7 (W)				Su > W, ♂			Douglass (1976)
	^{182}Ta	MAM	♀ 10 (lact.)							Jannett (1978)
M. ochrogas-ter	Trapping	RL	12 (pooled)		–	0				Abramsky and Tracy (1980)
	^{60}Co	*MAM*, MMAM	♂ 850 (Sp, Su) ♀ 162					♂ > ♀		Harvey and Barbour (1965)
	Trapping	IBS	♂ 567 (comb.) ♀ 486				0	♂ = ♀		Martin (1956)
	Trapping	IBS, *MAM*	♂ 162 (Su) ♀ 283		–			♂ = ♀		Meserve (1971)

TABLE 2
CONTINUED

Species	Method	Analysis*	Approximate area (m^2), distance (m) **	Correlations: Repro-duction	Den-sity	Food	Season	Sex	Hab-itat	Source
M. oregoni	Trapping	*EBS*, RL	♂ 907 (Sp, Su) ♀ 575				Sp > Su, ♂ Sp = Su, ♀	♂ > ♀ (Sp) ♂ = ♀ (Su)		Gashwiler (1972)
M. pinetorum	Radiote-lemetry	RL	♂ 19 (A) ♀ 14					♂ = ♀		FitzGerald and Madison (1981)
	Radiote-lemetry	RL, *MAM*	♂ 45 (comb.) ♀ 42					♂ = ♀		FitzGerald and Madison (1983)
	Radiote-lemetry	*MAM*, ADM	♂ 23 (Su) ♀ 22		–					Gettle (1975)
	Trapping	IBS	♂ 2,024 (A) ♀ 1,821					♂ = ♀		Goertz (1971)
	Radiote-lemetry	MAM	♀ 40 (Su) ♀ 19 (W)				Su > W			Pagano and Madison (1981)

TABLE 2
CONTINUED

Species	Method	Analysis*	Approximate area (m^2), distance (m) **	Correlations: Reproduction	Correlations: Density	Correlations: Food	Correlations: Season	Correlations: Sex	Correlations: Habitat	Source
	Trapping	RL	19 (comb.)							Paul (1970)
	Trapping	GDM	60 (comb.)							Stickel and Warbach (1960)
M. richardsoni	Radiotelemetry	RL	♂ 3♂22 (Su) ♀ 94	+♂, RA				♂ > ♀		Ludwig (1981)
M. townsendii	Trapping	BVN	♂ 900 (comb.) ♀ 500		–	–				Taitt and Krebs (1981)
M. xanthognathus	Trapping	*MAM*, RL	♂ 1,100 (Su, A) ♀ 2,000							Douglass (1977)
	Trapping	PUD/MAP	♂ 650 (pooled) ♀ 583							Wolff and Lidicker (1980)
Old World:										
M. agrestis	^{160}Co	MAM	♀ 196 (Sp, Su)	0			0			Godfrey (1954)
	^{32}P	V								Myllymäki et al. (1971)
	^{131}I ^{51}Cr									

TABLE 2
CONTINUED

Species	Method	Analysis*	Approximate area (m^2), distance (m) **	Correlations: Reproduction	Density	Food	Season	Sex	Habitat	Source
	Trapping	UVN	♂ 600 (comb.) ♀ 300		−♀	−♀		♂ > ♀		Myllymäki (1977)
M. arvalis	Trapping	ADM	♂ 13 (X) ♀ 6	+♂, RA			Su > A, ♂			Dub (1971)
	^{60}Co	MMAM	♂ 300 (Su) ♀ 400							Nikitina et al. (1977)
	Trapping	MAM	♂ 900 (Sp, Su) ♀ 375							Nikitina et al. (1972)
M. montebelli	Trapping	MAM	♂ 364 (Su) ♀ 162					♂ > ♀		Tanaka (1972)
M. oeconomus	^{60}Co	MMAM	♂ 3,000 (Su) ♀ 900					♂ > ♀		Karulin et al. (1976)

TABLE 2
CONTINUED

				Correlations						
Species	Method	Analysis*	Approximate area (m²), distance (m) **	Repro-duction	Den-sity	Food	Season	Sex	Hab-itat	Source
	^{60}Co	MMAM	♂ 5,200 (Su) ♀ 1,300					♂ > ♀		Nikitina et al. (1977)
	Trapping	*EBS*, ADM	♂ 2,500 (Su) ♀ 530	+♂, RA			Su > W, ♂	♂ > ♀ (Su) ♂ = ♀ (W)		Tast (1966)

* Abbreviations: AA, activity area; ADM, average distance moved; AMAM, adjusted minimum area method; BVN, bivariate normal; DM, distance moved; EBS, exclusive boundary strip; GDM, greatest distance moved; IBS, inclusive boundary strip; MAM, minimum area method; MMAM, modified minimum area method; NS, number of different stations at which animal was captured; PUD/MAP, population utilization distribution and probability of location; RL, range length; UVN, univariate normal; V, verbal description of range size. Where two or more analyses are listed, the analysis giving the area or distance in the next column is in italics. The letter X appears wherever the actual results could not be reduced to tabular form because of their complexity.

** Abbreviations and symbols: ♂, male; ♀, female; Su, summer; A, autumn; W, winter; Sp, spring; RA, reproductively active; NR, not reproductively active; comb., combined data for sexes or seasons; pooled, value for each sex is a composite for all voles of the same sex; lact., lactating; +, increase in size; −, decrease in size; 0, no change in size.

best a small and abstract sampling of vole movement and behavior (see Hayne, 1950). But few alternatives exist, and the reward for meaningful explanations concerning vole space and resource utilization, no matter how tentative, is considerable. And so the attempts continue.

More recent technology permits the collection of many positions on free-ranging voles per unit time, and this is at least an advance in the right direction. When monitoring the minute-to-minute or hour-to-hour movements of many voles over many days, certain patterns of area use and movement emerge that can be defined and used as a framework for further, especially comparative, studies. A classification of types of home range and movement in *Microtus pennsylvanicus* accompanies the different facets of space use reviewed below.

Home Range

A home range according to Burt (1943) is "that area traversed by the individual in its normal activities of food gathering, mating, and caring for young." The subsequent discussion by Burt (1943) implies a short-term range, one whose value would change with age, season, reproductive condition, density, and so on. Burt clearly did not imply that there is a typical home-range value for a species that encompasses a single area within which all these activities occur, yet many investigators apparently seek and publish such values. Burt's home range would include all the routine travels occurring over just a few days, and the value would require recalculation with each major change in environmental or individual condition. Since voles have small home ranges relative to their mobility (that is, a vole can move across its entire range with a few seconds, certainly in less than 1 min), and since voles typically have four to six activity periods every 24 h (see section on Activity Rhythms), I use the one-day-range as a home-range unit for voles, and classify types of ranges based on how these daily values vary through time. Each daily range is composed of 24 positions, one per h, or of 144 positions, one per 10 min. A convex polygon (formed by a line connecting the positions around the perimeter) is used to represent the daily range (Fig. 3).

The convex-polygon or minimum-area method (Dalke, 1942) is used in the present study because it is the easiest way of identifying and enclosing the actual positions recorded for an animal that is active in essentially two dimensions. Until more is known about the motivation and manifestation of space use in nature, any model is quite arbitrary, and so the simplest was chosen. The frequency of peripheral and multiple areas of high-use intensity and the occurrence of both sharp and gradual border segments for the same individual must eventually be recognized. The study of these fine-grained patterns may answer basic questions regarding the determinants of space use. Exact location information, especially for locations visited less frequently, is essentially lost when probability models are used.

The important features of the daily range estimates in this study are the short duration (24 h) of the estimates and the fixed time interval between positions. As such, the estimates are sensitive to, and representative of, day-to-day changes in vole movement. No matter how sophisticated the mathematical manipulations applied to position information (for example, to capture data), as the time span over which the data are collected increases, the estimates of range use and overlap (and therefore estimates of social interactions) become exaggerated. This bias would occur for *M. pennsylvanicus* because: 1) the daily ranges of males expand or shift with the occurrence of estrus in neighboring females; 2) the daily ranges of females contract at parturition and expand during weaning (Madison, 1978); 3) the cumulative area, but not the daily range, continues to expand over long periods of study, especially for males; and 4) fluctuating densities and high mortality rates for microtines (Madison, 1979; Pearson, 1971) create chronic instability in space ownership, such that range values pooled for several days or more would likely indicate overlap between two individuals whose actual periods of residence did not overlap. The daily range values minimize the above problems.

Based on long sequences of daily ranges for over 100 meadow voles to date, three general types of home ranges emerge. The *stable home range* is one where the center of activity varies little from one day to the next, and where the convex polygons of the successive daily ranges overlap considerably (Fig. 3A). The *variable home range* may be either *disjunctive* or *floating*. The disjunctive range is one in which two or more areas of intense utilization are separated by areas used only in transit. The center of activity is stable, although it rarely marks an area of intense utilization (Fig. 3B). The floating

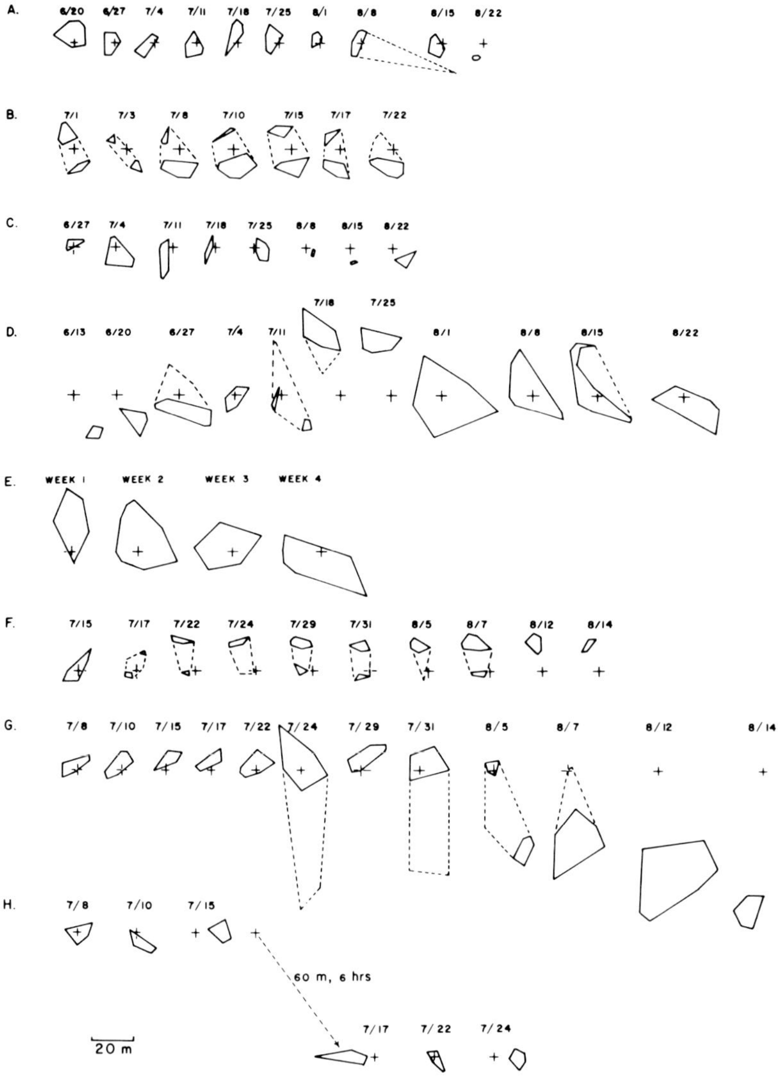

FIG. 3. Types of home range and movement for meadow voles (*M. pennsylvanicus*). All home ranges are composed of 24 radiotelemetry positions, one each h for 24 consecutive h. Dashed lines enclose areas that are 40% or more of the home-range size but contain no telemetry positions (other than the one or two peripheral positions indicated. A, stable: female, 40 g, New York, 1978; B, variable disjunctive: male, 52 g, Virginia, 1975; C, variable floating: female, 35 g, New York, 1978; D, variable

range is one in which the center of activity may shift noticeably on a daily basis, but does not change much over the long term. The successive polygons of the floating range may at times fail to overlap (Fig. 3C, D). The third home-range type is the *shifting home range.* Unlike the stable and variable home ranges, the shifting range shows a significant net change in center of activity. The shifting range may be *conjunctive* or *disjunctive.* The conjunctive shift in home range is a gradual, unidirectional displacement of the successive daily ranges, with each subsequent range overlapping the previous range (Fig. 3E). A disjunctive shift in home range occurs when a vole passes back and forth between two separate areas but eventually shifts all of its activity from one area to the other (Fig. 3F, G). The shifting home range is a transient state of area use, and perhaps shouldn't be classified as a home-range type; but because the organism still remains in the same general region, the shifting home range is still considered a form of local area utilization, hence a type of home range. Burt (1943) also included the shifting range as a home-range type.

The stable and variable home-range types are much more common than the shifting type. They are shown by 69% of adult male and 89% of adult female meadow voles under summer breeding conditions in good habitat (Madison, 1980*a*), but the percentages are bound to vary under a wide variety of environmental and social conditions. Tanaka (1972) reported stable home ranges in about 56% of the *M. montebelli* studied. Shifting home ranges occur in about 31% of male and 11% of female *M. pennsylvanicus* (Madison, 1980*a*), and these values agree with those of 12 to 19% reported by Getz (1961).

Territory

Another type of space-use pattern frequently mentioned in the literature for voles is territoriality. The territory may include the entire home range (all-purpose territory), or a smaller space unit

---

←

floating: male, 63 g, New York, 1978; E, conjunctive shifting: male, 37 g, Quebec, 1974; F, disjunctive shifting: female, 40 g, Virginia, 1975; G, disjunctive shifting: male, 40 g, Virginia, 1975; H, dispersal: male, 37 g, Virginia, 1975.

within the home range (feeding territory, nesting territory; Nice, 1937). Definitions vary but a common definition is the sole occupation of an area (at least with respect to others of the same sex during breeding activity) in a region where the density conditions lead to expectations of overlap. Such a situation exists for reproductive female meadow voles, but not for males (Madison, 1980*b*, 1980*c*).

Territoriality among *Microtus* varies from individual territories for males (*M. xanthognathus*; Wolff, 1980) or females (*M. pennsylvanicus*; Madison, 1980*b*) or both (*M. montanus*; Jannett, 1980), to pair territories (*M. ochrogaster*; Getz and Carter, 1980; *M. californicus*; Lidicker, 1980), and finally to communal territories (*M. pinetorum*; FitzGerald and Madison, 1983). These territorial patterns may vary with reproductive activity, density, and season. For example, *M. ochrogaster* shifts from pair territories to loose polygynous or promiscuous groups with an increase in population density (Getz and Carter, 1980), and *M. pennsylvanicus* shifts from female territories during the summer breeding period to communal groups during the winter (Madison, 1984; Madison et al., 1984).

Figure 4 shows the maintenance of exclusivity by female meadow voles during breeding in October, and the existence of communal groups in December. The communal groups had non-overlapping membership in November and December, but by January meadow voles moved freely between the groups. In October, the one female with the largest home range that "overlapped" the ranges of the others did not normally occupy the area of overlap, and was only located in the overlap area twice during one "distant reconnaissance" trip (see next section).

Movement Types

A close examination of the sequence of positions of free-ranging *M. pennsylvanicus*, coupled with notes on what the voles are doing at each check, allows an evaluation of movement and space use in connection with home range. The first category of movement is *local* movement. These movements are either *maintenance* or *reconnaissance.* Maintenance movements are often localized around the nest, and the vole is frequently seen chewing on grass blades or in the act of grooming. Usually no more than 0–3 m of movement occurs between successive 10-min or 60-min position checks (Fig. 5, positions 1–4, 10–14). The local reconnaissance is characterized by

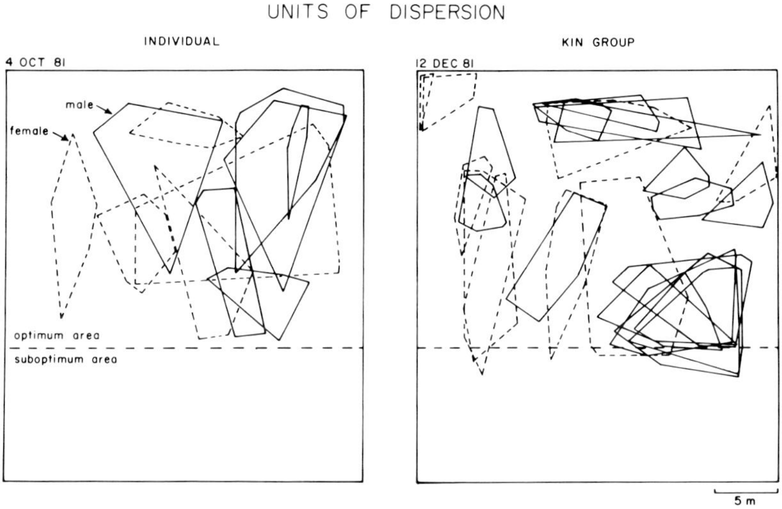

FIG. 4. Individual and group units of dispersion in meadow voles (*M. pennsylvanicus*) radiotracked in field enclosures in New York. Each vole is represented by a polygon enclosing 10 positions collected hourly from 0700 h to 1600 h. The suboptimum area was created by repeated mowing and the collection of cuttings during the summer. Only six males and five females, all of adult size, were present on 4 October; four adults of each sex plus 17 offspring from the original five females made up the kin groups on 12 December.

loops of movement during which the vole is usually seen in alert postures or moving. Although some nibbling on grass may be seen occasionally, no sustained grazing is observed (Fig. 5, positions 5–9). The distinction between maintenance and local reconnaissance is more clear at night. During the night, the sleeping location is well defined. Maintenance activities occur near the nest, and local reconnaissance occurs away from the night nest about once every bout of activity (Figs. 5, 6). The local reconnaissance loops are thought to involve scent-marking or be surveys for other voles, since little feeding or shelter seeking is apparent during these runs.

The second category of movement is the *distant reconnaissance.* This type is also called "wandering," "sallies," or "excursions" in the literature (Ambrose, 1969; Burt, 1943; Jannett, 1978; Lidicker, this volume; Madison, 1978, 1980*a*; Martin, 1956; Myllymäki, 1977; Stickel and Warbach, 1960). This movement is quite similar to

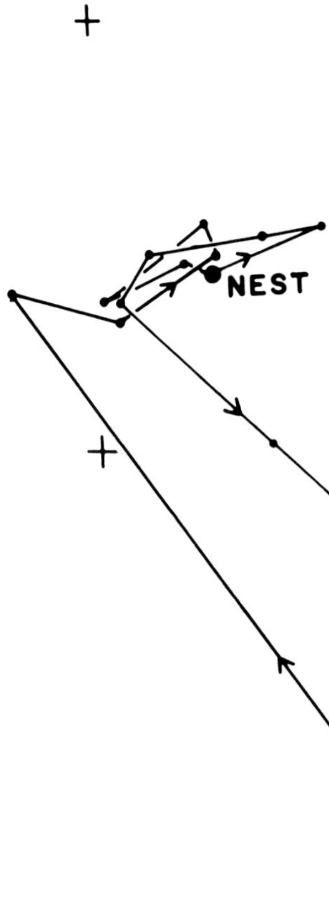

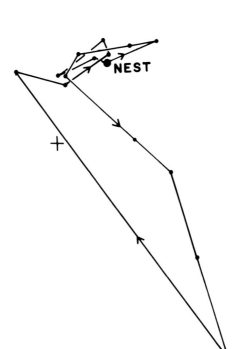

FIG. 5. Local movements for a 52 g male meadow vole (*M. pennsylvanicus*) from 2150 h to 0200 h on 17 and 18 August 1975 in Virginia (see Fig. 6, male 2). Positions (•) were recorded using radiotelemetry every 10 min; 14 such positions are represented between nest (●) departure at 2150 and nest return at 0200 h (position 1 is first dot after leaving nest, position 2 is second dot, etc.). Approximate course is indicated by straight lines. Distance between reference markers (+) is 15 m.

local reconnaissance in that the vole is typically "on the move." It differs in occurring at least one range length beyond the normal daily range. Such trips may last up to 12 h, but 2 to 5-h journeys are most common. Considerable distances are sometimes reached, not atypically of 50 m or more. The trips begin and end suddenly; there is no change in behavior either before or after the trip that might suggest the occurrence of this behavior (Fig. 3A [8/8], G [7/24, 7/31]). Distant reconnaissance has many potential reproductive advantages to both sexes (Madison, 1978, 1980*b*, 1980*c*), but it also may be a means of assessing food and shelter resources in adjacent areas at times when these are declining in the immediate home area. That distant reconnaissance in males is about twice as frequent as that for females in both meadow voles (Madison, 1980*a*) and prairie voles (Martin, 1956) suggests that males use these trips at least in part to maximize paternity.

The third general category of movement is *dispersal*. It is similar to wandering in its suddenness and long distance nature, but the vole in this case does not return to its former home range (Fig. 3H [7/17]). The incidence and significance of dispersal is discussed by Lidicker (this volume).

Of all these types of movement during the reproductive season, the local-maintenance and reconnaissance types are the most common, occurring essentially during each of the 4–6 activity periods each day. Distant reconnaissance occurs at least once every 20 days for females, and at least once every 12 days for males. Dispersal is relatively rare for *M. pennsylvanicus* under the conditions studied, having occurred in three out of the 56 voles tracked for 3 or more weeks (Madison, 1980*a*, 1980*c*).

Dispersion

An understanding of factors influencing space use must include a clear definition of the unit of dispersion (Brown and Orians, 1970). Specifically, do individuals move about more or less independently of other individuals, or do pairs or larger assemblages move about together, occupy the same range and nest, and use the same basic resource base? Individual and social units of dispersion demand different sets of analytical precautions during studies of resource preference and space use.

For *M. pennsylvanicus*, the unit of dispersion changes seasonally, although the dispersion pattern (uniform vs. random vs. clumped) does not. From spring to mid-fall, individual units of dispersion appear (Fig. 4). The females involved in breeding have uniform (territorial) distributions; the males are more variable and range from random to clumped (for example, around estrous females) (Madison, 1980*a*, 1980*c*). From mid-fall to early winter, the unit of dispersion changes to communal (kin) groups; these groups show little overlap, suggesting territorial female families (Madison, 1984; Madison et al., 1984). Figure 4 shows the territories of five females in December that had terminated breeding for the year. Each of these females shared their nest and home range with a group composed of the female's offspring and from 0 to 2 adult males. This kin group gradually gives way to mixed lineage groups for the rest of winter. Mixed lineage groups arise when, as a result of winter mortality among many kin groups, the voles redistribute themselves in space in order to stay above the minimum "huddle" density necessary for overwinter survival (Madison et al., 1984). Home-range size and overlap is similar within the kin and mixed lineage groups, but the latter group is more permeable to changing membership, and hence is not territorial. In addition, since the total population density gradually decreases with winter, and since group size necessarily remains about the same, the mixed groups become more separated as the winter progresses. The transition from group to solitary living with the onset of breeding in spring includes some communal nesting and even communal nursing among females, but these groups disappear by May (McShea and Madison, 1984).

Besides meadow voles, *M. arvalis* also changes from a female territorial system in summer to a group unit in winter (Chelkowska, 1978; Mackin-Rogalska, 1979). *M. xanthognathus* shifts from a male territorial organization to non-kin communal groups from summer to winter (Wolff, 1980). There are no known microtine species that exhibit individual units of dispersion throughout the year; however, several microtines, such as *M. pinetorum,* live in cohesive social units year-round (FitzGerald and Madison, 1981, 1983; Madison, 1984). The unit of dispersion varies with density from more or less stable pairs to largely individual units associated with polygyny and promiscuity in *M. ochrogaster* (Getz and Carter, 1980) and *M. californicus* (Lidicker, 1980).

Factors Correlated with Space Use

Energetics, diet, and food.—Despite the large amount of general literature concerning the effect of food on density and movement, not much is known concerning voles in the genus *Microtus* (Table 2). McNab's (1963) prediction that home-range size should increase with decreased food resources is supported by Taitt and Krebs (1981) and Taitt et al. (1981) for *M. townsendii,* and by

Myllymäki (1977) for *M. agrestis*. However, no such relation was found between home-range length and biomass of preferred food for *M. ochrogaster* (Abramsky and Tracy, 1980), and a positive relation between food availability and movement was noted for *M. californicus* (Krebs, 1966). Since density was not controlled in the above studies, and since density typically increases with extra food, the changes in movement and home-range size above may result from social factors and not be due to the changes in available food. Thus, the issue remains to be resolved.

Gender and reproduction.—Considerable information shows that at least for certain species the size of the home range is larger for males than females, and that the degree of difference is a function of reproductive activity (Table 2). Recent radiotelemetric studies have confirmed the above relations for *M. pennsylvanicus* (Gaulin and FitzGerald, in press; Madison, 1980*b*; Webster and Brooks, 1981*b*). In this species, the range of the female decreases during early lactation, but returns to normal values with weaning (Madison, 1978). If many females are breeding in a population, the average short-term home range for the females is smaller because of the home-range reduction during lactation. However, the reduction may be offset under natural conditions by the tendency of females of some species to shift home ranges (Myers and Krebs, 1971; Tast, 1966) or show distant reconnaissance (Madison, 1978) just before parturition. The range of breeding male meadow voles (*M. pennsylvanicus*) is typically much larger during the reproductive season, but once the communal groups form during mid- to late fall (see section on Dispersion), the range size of males decreases to about the size of female home ranges, which change little from summer to winter. The large size of the male range during the breeding period is primarily the result of distant reconnaissance movements and floating and shifting home ranges, all likely the result of mating activity (Madison, 1980*a*, 1980*b*, 1980*c*; see section on Home Range).

The above pattern for meadow voles is probably also characteristic of most other microtines. Exceptions arise in those species that live in social groups year-round. In *M. pinetorum*, the male and female home ranges of each exclusive social group essentially coincide during all seasons (FitzGerald and Madison, 1981, 1983). Similar isometry is predicted during the breeding season in situations in which monogamy often occurs, such as in *M. ochrogaster* (Getz and Carter, 1980) and *M. californicus* (Lidicker, 1980). Isometry is predicted to be the basic condition for all microtines outside the breeding season, and it may even prevail among adult non-reproductives during the breeding period (Webster and Brooks, 1981*b*).

Social factors.—The influence of social factors on space use is suggested by non-random patterns of spacing in homogeneous habitat, by differences in the space use of voles of different social status, and by differences in spacing and movements of voles at different population densities. The overdispersion of breeding female meadow voles strongly suggests mutual antagonism and female avoidance (Madison, 1980*b*, 1980*c*). That these exclusive areas between females are not strictly necessary for, nor determined by, individual food needs is suggested by the cohabitation of these same areas by extended family units of up to seven subadult and adult voles during the late fall and winter (Madison, 1984; Madison et al., 1984). Other species of voles also exhibit territoriality (see Wolff, this volume; Madison, 1980*b*). The only study to date to determine the effects of social status on space use in *Microtus* concerns meadow voles (Ambrose, 1973). Dominant *M. pennsylvanicus,* as determined in dyadic encounters, were much less likely to change home ranges in the field than were subordinate voles. The effect of social variables on spacing also should be apparent under conditions of different population density. This relation assumes that as density increases, so should competition for spatially distributed resources. The cost of utilization or defense of widely dispersed resources should increase, and so it is expected that home-range size should decrease with increased density, at least to some minimal level necessary for survival. The general pattern among voles is a negative relationship between density and home range (see Table 2). For *M. oeconomus,* this relationship is parabolic and is expressed as:

$$S = 0.11 + \left(\frac{3.55}{d}\right)$$

where S is the home range size in ha and d is the density in voles/ha (Okulova et al., 1971). Ambrose (1973) found that meadow voles (*M. pennsylvanicus*) didn't change home-range size with increased density, but rather increased the intensity of utilization within the home range. In this study, the home ranges already may have been at the minimum levels tolerated. Van Vleck (1969) observed a negative relationship only for males, but his measure of space use (the number of different traps visited) was not very refined, especially for female voles with small home ranges relative to the trap spacing (14 m). Other aspects of spacing relating to social behavior are discussed by Wolff (this volume).

Interspecific interactions.—Very little is known regarding the effects of predation, parasitism, or interspecific competition on space use in *Microtus*. In some circumstances shrews are known to kill voles, but Barbehenn (1958) found no negative effect of the presence of *Blarina* or *Sorex* on meadow-vole distribution. However, Fulk (1972) showed that *M. pennsylvanicus* tended to avoid areas occupied by *Blarina brevicauda*. Recently, Madison et al. (1984) showed that predation by foxes and weasels on overwintering meadow voles appeared to stimulate spatial avoidance and smaller nesting groups in the voles. Interspecific competition as measured by spatial avoidance has been demonstrated for *M. ochrogaster,* which avoids cohabitation with *Sigmodon* (Glass and Slade, 1980), and *M. montanus* appears to exclude *M. pennsylvanicus* from certain habitats (Stoecker, 1972). That such relationships may be complex is suggested by Douglass (1976), who found the opposite relationship between *M. montanus* and *M. pennsylvanicus.*

Weather and seasonal factors.—The time required for the collection of information in most studies of space use precludes the measurement of day-night shifts in home-range use as well as responses to daily weather variations. Radiotelemetry permits the measurement of these local changes in spacing, and most information of this kind is available only for *M. pennsylvanicus.* During summer, meadow voles appear to vary their movements between day and night. Figure 6 shows four voles whose positions were determined every 10 min for 24 h, thus giving 24 positions every 4 h (the same number of positions that constitute all the daily ranges in Fig. 3). The 4-h ranges show that the nest used during the night is different from the nest or refuges used during most of the day for all four voles. The space use at night is reduced for females, but not for males, and this agrees with the lower activity of females at night (Evans, 1970; Fig. 6). The space-use patterns of these voles, which were selected for study because of their close proximity, vary from no overlap between the females and between the males during the 0400–0750 period, to generally higher levels of overlap or proximity during the day. Why there appears to be a nighttime reduction in space use for females is not known, but the fact that lactating fe-

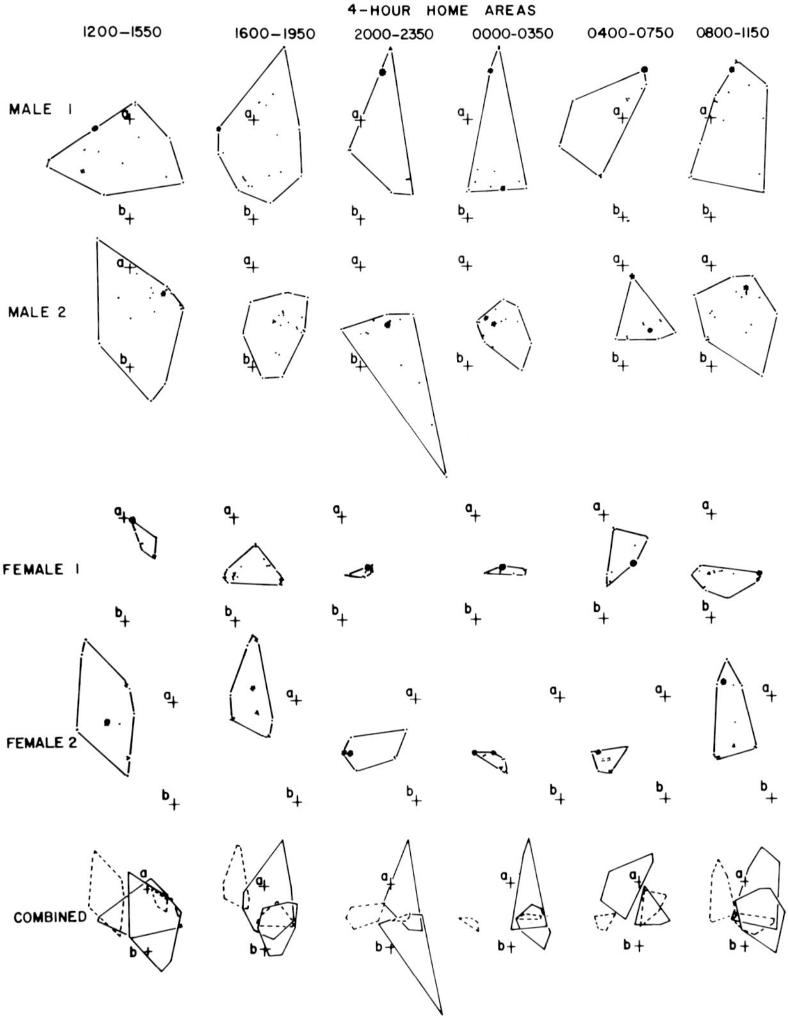

FIG. 6. Space use for four free-ranging meadow voles (*M. pennsylvanicus*) during a 24-h period on 17 and 18 August 1975 in Virginia. Positions were recorded by radiotelemetry every 10 min for all four voles. The space use for each vole is shown for each 4-h period, first separately, then combined. Reference markers (ᵃ+, ᵇ+) are the same for all voles and are 15 m apart. Note that the scale was changed for combined plots. Males 1 and 2 were 50 g each; female 1 was 41 g; female 2 was 43 g.

males show this reduction throughout the 24-h period suggests that energetic demands peculiar to females may be a factor (Madison, 1978).

Day-to-day changes in space use in response to weather conditions have been recorded only for *M. pennsylvanicus* (Madison, 1980*a*; Madison et al., 1984). The home ranges of both males and females significantly increase with environmental temperature. Male home ranges also significantly increase with time since precipitation and with higher barometric pressures. Blair's (1940) finding that meadow voles have larger home ranges in dry habitats than in wet habitats generally agrees with the above observation. Why meadow voles, and males in particular, show larger home ranges under "good" weather conditions is not known. Madison (1980*a*) speculated that reduced ability to detect inhibitory pheromonal signals on dry days may be an important factor.

Seasonal changes in space use are relatively well known for microtines. Two patterns appear to be common. The first is a reduction in home-range size of males during the non-breeding season (see section on Gender and Reproduction). The second is a shift in home range during periods of habitat flooding in fall and spring (Hansson, 1977; Ludwig, 1981; Tast, 1966; Webster, 1979). Two other patterns that are hypothesized to be common are: 1) local shifts in home range during winter as a result of vole efforts to locate larger huddling groups for thermal benefit or to escape predation (Madison, 1984; Madison et al., 1984); and 2) shifts in home range during spring from overwintering groups to dispersed, individual ranges for purposes of maximizing reproductive success.

Generalities and Predictions for Future Testing

Day-night patterns of activity and home-range size in microtine rodents have been studied for many years, but generalizations concerning activity and spacing have been slow in coming. Insights from recent radiotelemetric studies of rhythms and space use combined with information from laboratory and mark-recapture studies permit certain tentative generalizations that can be used to form hypotheses for future experimental studies, as follows.

Activity Rhythms

1) A recurring ultradian rhythm with a 2- to 6-h period, each entailing 1–3 h of rest and 1–3 h of activity, is typical for microtine rodents.
2) The period of the ultradian rhythm is inversely related to energy demand; thus, reproductively active males, late gestating or lactating females, and small-sized voles should show shorter periods.
3) The period of the ultradian rhythm can be modified by conserving energy; thus, if social synchrony is critical to survival, small-sized voles may "huddle" more and breeding voles may temporarily forego reproduction to maintain synchrony.
4) Rhythm synchrony between voles is most conspicuous in the morning, and sunrise appears to be the timing event for circadian periodicities.
5) Some voles in a population may adjust the phasing of their ultradian rhythm to reduce social confrontation or competition for resources.
6) Microtines tend to be more day-active in winter and more night-active in summer.

Spacing

1) Most microtine species exhibit individual units of dispersion during most of the breeding season, especially those members of each species that are reproductively active.
2) Most microtine species are promiscuous or polygynous and, during the breeding season, males of these species have larger home ranges than females.
3) Microtine species that live throughout the year in cohesive social groups tend toward monogamy, and the home-range size for males and females of these species approach isometry.
4) Whether voles live alone or in social groups during the breeding season, group living and home-range isometry between the sexes appears to be the general rule during the non-breeding or winter season.
5) Absolute home-range size for adult male voles during the non-breeding season or winter period is equivalent to, or only slightly smaller than, that of females of the same species in comparable habitat during the summer.

6) Non-breeding, winter groups are composed of kin early in the winter, but by late winter usually are composed of voles of mixed lineage.

Acknowledgments

I thank Brad Davis, Melissa Ditton, Randy FitzGerald, Bill McShea, Bruce Webster, and many other field assistants who helped collect the data presented and discussed here. The chapter considerably benefited from discussions with, or the editorial criticisms and general help of, Pat DeCoursey, Bill Lidicker, Norm Negus, Carol Rowsemitt, Frank Sulzman, Bob Tamarin, Jerry Wolff, and Irv Zucker. The research was supported by the National Research Council of Canada, McGill University, the Research Foundation of the State University of New York, the National Science Foundation (DEB-22821), and the U.S. Fish and Wildlife Service (Contract No. 14-16-0009-79-066).

Literature Cited

Abramsky, Z., and C. R. Tracy. 1980. Relation between home range size and regulation of population size in *Microtus ochrogaster*. Oikos, 34:347–355.

Ambrose, H. W., III. 1969. A comparison of *Microtus pennsylvanicus* home ranges as determined by isotope and live trap methods. Amer. Midland Nat., 81: 535–555.

———. 1973. An experimental study of some factors affecting the spatial and temporal activity of *Microtus pennsylvanicus*. J. Mamm., 54:79–110.

Aschoff, J. 1981. A survey on biological rhythms. Pp. 3–10, *in* Handbook of neurobiology (J. Aschoff, ed.). Plenum, New York, 563 pp.

Aschoff, J., S. Daan, and G. A. Groos (eds.). 1982. Vertebrate circadian systems. Springer-Verlag, New York, 363 pp.

Ashby, K. R. 1972. Patterns of daily activity in mammals. Mamm. Rev., 1:171–185.

Barbehenn, K. R. 1958. Spatial and population relationships between *Microtus* and *Blarina*. Ecology, 39:293–304.

Barbour, R. W. 1963. *Microtus*: a simple method of recording time spent in the nest. Science, 141:41.

Baumgardner, D. J., S. E. Ward, and D. A. Dewsbury. 1980. Diurnal patterning of eight activities in 14 species of muroid rodents. Anim. Learn. Behav., 8:322–330.

Baumler, W. 1975. Activity of some small mammals in the field. Acta Theriol., 20:365–377.

Bider, J. R. 1968. Animal activity in uncontrolled terrestrial communities as determined by a sand transect technique. Ecol. Monogr., 38:269–308.

Blair, W. F. 1940. Home ranges and populations of the meadow vole in southern Michigan. J. Wildl. Mgmt., 4:149–161.

Broom, D. M. 1979. Methods of detecting and analyzing activity rhythms. Biol. Behav., 4:3–18.

Brown, J. L., and G. H. Orians. 1970. Spacing patterns in mobile animals. Ann. Rev. Ecol. Syst., 1:239–262.

Brown, L. E. 1966. Home range and movement of small mammals. Pp. 111–142, *in* Play exploration and territory in mammals (P. A. Jewell and C. Loizos, eds.). Academic Press, New York, 280 pp.

Burt, W. H. 1943. Territoriality and home range concepts as applied to mammals. J. Mamm., 24:346–352.

Calhoun, J. B. 1945. Diel activity rhythms of the rodents, *Microtus ochrogaster* and *Sigmodon hispidus hispidus*. Ecology, 26:251–273.

Carley, C. J., E. D. Fleharty, and M. A. Mares. 1970. Occurrence and activity of *Reithrodontomys megalotis, Microtus ochrogaster* and *Peromyscus maniculatus* as recorded by a photographic device. Southwestern Nat., 15:209–216.

Chelkowska, H. 1978. Variations in numbers and social factors in a population of field voles. Acta Theriol., 23:213–238.

Daan, S. 1981. Adaptive daily strategies in behavior. Pp. 275–298, *in* Handbook of neurobiology (J. Aschoff, ed.). Plenum, New York, 563 pp.

Daan, S., and J. Aschoff. 1981. Short-term rhythms in activity. Pp. 491–498, *in* Handbook of neurobiology (J. Aschoff, ed.). Plenum, New York, 563 pp.

———. 1982. Circadian contributions to survival. Pp. 305–321, *in* Vertebrate circadian systems (J. Aschoff, S. Daan, and G. A. Groos, eds.). Springer-Verlag, New York, 363 pp.

Daan, S., and S. Slopsema. 1978. Short-term rhythms in foraging behavior of the common vole, *Microtus arvalis*. J. Comp. Physiol., 127:215–227.

Dalke, P. D. 1942. The cottontail rabbits in Connecticut. Connecticut State Geol. Nat. Hist. Surv. Bull., 65:197.

Davis, D. H. S. 1933. Rhythmic activity in the short-tailed vole, *Microtus*. J. Anim. Ecol., 2:232–238.

Dewsbury, D. A. 1980. Wheel-running behavior in 12 species of muroid rodents. Behav. Proc., 5:271–282.

Doucet, G. J., and J. R. Bider. 1969. Activity of *Microtus pennsylvanicus* related to moon phase and moonlight revealed by the sand transect technique. Canadian J. Zool., 47:1183–1186.

Douglass, R. J. 1976. Spatial interactions and microhabitat selections of two locally sympatric voles, *Microtus montanus* and *Microtus pennsylvanicus*. Ecology, 57:346–352.

———. 1977. Population dynamics, home ranges, and habitat associations of the yellow-cheeked vole, *Microtus xanthognathus*, in the Northwest Territories. Canadian Field-Nat., 91:237–247.

Dub, M. 1971. Movements of *Microtus arvalis* Pall. and a method of estimating its numbers. Zool. Listy, 20:1–14.

Durup, H. 1956. Observations on the activity rhythm of captive voles (*Microtus arvalis* Pallas.). Mammalia, 20:390–404.

Erkinaro, E. 1961. The seasonal change of the activity of *Microtus agrestis*. Oikos, 12:157–163.

———. 1970. The phasing of locomotory activity of *M. agrestis* (L), *M. arvalis* (Pall) and *M. oeconomus* (Pall). Aquilo, Ser. Zool., 8:1–29.

———. 1973. Activity optimum in *Microtus agrestis, Arvicola terrestris* and *Apodemus flavicollis* (Rodentia) dependent on the intensity of illumination. Aquilo, Ser. Zool., 14:89–92.

EVANS, F. 1970. Seasonal effects of light, temperature, and radiation on activity patterns of the meadow vole (*Microtus pennsylvanicus*). Final Rept., U.S. Atomic Energy Comm. Contract No. AT(11-1)-1486, Chicago, Illinois, 20 pp.

EVERNDEN, L. N., AND W. A. FULLER. 1972. Light alteration caused by snow and its importance to subnivean rodents. Canadian J. Zool., 50:1023–1032.

FITZGERALD, R., AND D. MADISON. 1981. Spacing, movements and social organization of a free-ranging population of pine voles, *Microtus pinetorum*. Pp. 54–59, *in* Proceedings of the fifth eastern pine and meadow vole symposium (R. E. Byers, ed.). Gettysburg, Pennsylvania, 144 pp.

———. 1983. Social organization of a free-ranging population of pine voles, *Microtus pinetorum*. Behav. Ecol. Sociobiol., 13:183–187.

FORD, R. G., AND D. W. KRUMME. 1979. The analysis of space use patterns. J. Theor. Biol., 76:125–155.

FULK, G. W. 1972. The effect of shrews on the space utilization of voles. J. Mamm., 53:461–478.

GASHWILER, J. S. 1972. Life history notes on the Oregon vole, *Microtus oregoni*. J. Mamm., 53:558–569.

GAULIN, S. J. C. In press. Sex differences in spatial ability: an evolutionary hypothesis and test. Amer. Nat.

GETTLE, A. S. 1975. Densities, movements and activities of pine voles (*Microtus pinetorum*) in Pennsylvania. Unpubl. M.S. thesis, Pennsylvania State Univ., State College, 66 pp.

GETZ, L. L. 1961. Responses of small mammals to live-traps and weather conditions. Amer. Midland Nat., 66:160–170.

———. 1970. Influence of vegetation on the local distribution of the meadow vole in southern Wisconsin. Occas. Papers Univ. Connecticut, 1:213–241.

GETZ, L. L., AND C. S. CARTER. 1980. Social organization in *Microtus ochrogaster* populations. The Biologist, 62:56–59.

GLASS, G. E., AND N. A. SLADE. 1980. The effect of *Sigmodon hispidus* on spatial and temporal activity of *Microtus ochrogaster*: evidence for competition. Ecology, 60:358–370.

GODFREY, G. K. 1954. Tracing field voles (*Microtus agrestis*) with a Geiger-Müller counter. Ecology, 35:5–10.

GOERTZ, J. W. 1971. An ecological study of *Microtus pinetorum* in Oklahoma. Amer. Midland Nat., 86:1–12.

GRAHAM, W. 1968. Daily activity patterns in the meadow vole, *M. pennsylvanicus*. Unpubl. Ph.D. dissert., Univ. Michigan, Ann Arbor, 98 pp.

HAMILTON, W. J., JR. 1937. Activity and home range of the field mouse, *Microtus pennsylvanicus pennsylvanicus*. Ecology, 18:255–263.

HAMLEY, J. M., AND J. B. FALLS. 1975. Reduced activity in transmitter-carrying voles. Canadian J. Zool., 53:1476–1478.

HANSSON, L. 1971. Small rodent food, feeding and population dynamics. Oikos, 22:183–198.

———. 1977. Spatial dynamics of field voles, *Microtus agrestis* in heterogeneous landscapes. Oikos, 29:539–544.

HARVEY, M. J., AND R. W. BARBOUR. 1965. Home range of *Microtus ochrogaster* as determined by a modified minimum area method. J. Mamm., 46:398–402.

HATFIELD, D. M. 1940. Activity and food consumption in *Microtus* and *Peromyscus*. J. Mamm., 21:29–36.

HAYNE, D. W. 1950. Apparent home range of *Microtus* in relation to distance between traps. J. Mamm., 31:26–39.

HEIDT, G. A. 1971. Daily summer activity of the meadow vole, *Microtus pennsylvanicus*. Michigan Academician, 3:31–39.

HUTCHINSON, J. S. M. 1972. The oestrous cycle with particular reference to the neural control of the ovary. Mamm. Rev., 1:209–216.

JANNETT, F. J., JR. 1978. The density-dependent formation of extended maternal families of the montane vole, *Microtus montanus nanus*. Behav. Ecol. Sociobiol., 3:245–263.

———. 1980. Social dynamics of the montane vole, *Microtus montanus,* as a paradigm. The Biologist, 62:3–19.

KACZMARSKI, F. 1966. Bioenergetics of pregnancy and lactation in the bank vole. Acta Theriol., 19:409–417.

KARULIN, B. E., V. Y. LITVIN, N. A. NIKITINA, L. A. KHLYAP, AND V. YU OKHOTSKII. 1976. A study of activity, mobility and diurnal range in *Microtus oeconomus* on the Yamal Penninsula by means of marking with radioactive cobalt. Zool. Zhur., 55:1052–1060.

KAVANAU, J. L. 1962. Twilight transitions and biological rhythmicity. Nature, 194:1293–1295.

KAVANAU, J. L., AND R. M. HAVENHILL. 1976. Compulsory regime and control of environment in animal behavior. III. Light level preferences of small nocturnal mammals. Behaviour, 59:203–225.

KOEPPL, J. W., N. A. SLADE, AND R. S. HOFFMANN. 1975. A bivariate home range model with possible application to ethological data analysis. J. Mamm., 56:81–90.

KOSSUT, M., A. ZIEMBA, AND J. GILL. 1974. Diurnal rhythm of blood lactic acid and tissue glycogen in the common vole (*Microtus arvalis* Pall). Bull. de l'Acad. Pol. des Sci., 22:725–729.

KREBS, C. J. 1966. Demographic changes in fluctuating populations of *Microtus californicus*. Ecol. Monogr., 36:239–273.

LEHMANN, U. 1976. Short-term and circadian rhythms in the behavior of the vole, *Microtus agrestis* (L). Oecologia, 23:185–199.

LEHMANN, U., AND C. W. SOMMERSBERG. 1980. Activity patterns of the common vole, *Microtus arvalis*—automatic recording of behavior in an enclosure. Oecologia, 47:61–75.

LIDICKER, W. Z., JR. 1980. The social biology of the California vole. The Biologist, 62:46–55.

LUDWIG, D. R. 1981. The population biology and life history of the water vole, *Microtus richardsoni*. Unpubl. Ph.D. dissert., Univ. of Calgary, Calgary, Alberta, 266 pp.

MACKIN-ROGALSKA, R. 1979. Elements of the spatial organization of a common vole population. Acta Theriol., 24:171–199.

MADISON, D. 1978. Movement indicators of reproductive events among female meadow voles as revealed by radiotelemetry. J. Mamm., 59:835–843.

———. 1979. Impact of spacing behavior and predation on population growth in meadow voles. Pp. 20–29, *in* Proceedings of the third eastern pine and meadow vole symposium (R. E. Byers, ed.). New Paltz, New York, 86 pp.

———. 1980*a*. Movement types and weather correlates in free-ranging meadow voles. Pp. 34–42, *in* Proceedings of the fourth eastern pine and meadow vole symposium (R. E. Byers, ed.). Hendersonville, North Carolina, 91 pp.

———. 1980*b*. Space use and social structure in meadow voles, *Microtus pennsylvanicus*. Behav. Ecol. Sociobiol., 7:65–71.

———. 1980*c*. An integrated view of the social biology of *Microtus pennsylvanicus*. The Biologist, 62:20–33.

———. 1981. Time patterning of nest visitation by lactating meadow voles. J. Mamm., 62:389–391.

———. 1984. Group nesting and its ecological and evolutionary significance in overwintering microtine rodents. Pp. 267–274, *in* Winter ecology of small mammals (J. F. Merritt, ed.). Spec. Publ., Carnegie Mus. Nat. Hist., 10: 1–380.

MADISON, D. M., R. W. FITZGERALD, AND W. J. MCSHEA. 1984. Dynamics of social nesting in overwintering meadow voles (*Microtus pennsylvanicus*): possible consequences for population cycling. Behav. Ecol. Sociobiol., 15: 9–17.

MARTIN, E. P. 1956. A population study of the prairie vole (*Microtus ochrogaster*) in northeastern Kansas. Univ. Kansas Publ., Mus. Nat. Hist., 8:361–416.

MATHER, J. G. 1981. Wheel-running activity: a new interpretation. Mamm. Rev., 11:41–51.

MCCANN, S. A. 1976. Home ranges of the meadow vole and deer mouse (on a reclamation test pit in eastern Montana). Proc. Montana Acad. Sci., 36: 11–17.

MCNAB, B. K. 1963. Bioenergetics and the determination of home range size. Amer. Nat., 47:133–140.

MCSHEA, W. J., AND D. M. MADISON. 1984. Communal nesting by reproductively active females in a spring population of *Microtus pennsylvanicus*. Canadian J. Zool., 62:344–346.

MESERVE, P. L. 1971. Population ecology of the prairie vole, *Microtus ochrogaster* in the western mixed prairie of Nebraska. Amer. Midland Nat., 86:417–433.

MIGULA, P. 1969. Bioenergetics of pregnancy and lactation in European common vole. Acta Theriol., 13:167–179.

MILLER, L. S. 1957. Tracing vole movements by radioactive excretory products. Ecology, 38:132–136.

MOSSING, T. 1975. Measuring small mammal locomotory activity with passage counters. Oikos, 26:237–239.

MYERS, J. H., AND C. J. KREBS. 1971. Genetic, behavioral, and reproductive attributes of dispersing field voles, *Microtus pennsylvanicus* and *Microtus ochrogaster*. Ecol. Monogr., 41:53–78.

MYLLYMÄKI, A. 1977. Intraspecific competition and home range dynamics in the field vole, *Microtus agrestis*. Oikos, 29:553–569.

MYLLYMÄKI, A., A. PAASIKALLIO, AND U. HÄKKINEN. 1971. Analysis of a "standard trapping" of *Microtus agrestis* (L.) with triple isotope marking outside the quadrat. Ann. Zool. Fennica, 8:22–34.

NEW, J. G. 1958. Dyes for studying the movements of small mammals. J. Mamm., 39:416–429.

NICE, M. M. 1937. Studies in the life history of the song sparrow. Trans. Linn. Soc. New York, 4:1–247.

NIKITINA, N. A., B. E. KARULIN, AND N. S. ZEN'KOVICH. 1972. The activity and territory of the common vole (*Microtus arvalis* Pall). Byull. Mosk. o-va. Ispyt. Prir. Otd. Biol., 77:55–64.

NIKITINA, N. A., ET AL. 1977. On the size of daily territory and probable structure of individual ranges in some species of rodents. Zool. Zhur., 56:1860–1869.

NYGREN, J. 1978. Interindividual influence on diurnal rhythms of activity in cycling and noncycling populations of the field vole, *Microtus agrestis* L. Oecologia, 35:231–239.

OKULOVA, M. M., V. A. ARISTOVA, AND T. V. KOSHKINA. 1971. Influence of population density upon size of home range of small rodents in the west Siberian taiga. Zool. Zhur., 50:908–915.
OSTERBERG, D. M. 1962. Activity of small mammals as recorded by a photographic device. J. Mamm., 43:219–229.
OSTERMANN, K. 1956. On the activity of native Muridae and Glividen. Zool. Jahrb., Physiol., 66:355–388.
OUELLETTE, P. E., AND J. F. HEISINGER. 1980. Reingestion of feces by *Microtus pennsylvanicus*. J. Mamm., 61:366–368.
PAGANO, R., AND D. MADISON. 1981. Seasonal variations in movements and habitat use by pine and meadow voles. Pp. 35–44, *in* Proceedings of the fifth eastern pine and meadow vole symposium (R. E. Byers, ed.). Gettysburg, Pennsylvania, 144 pp.
PAUL, J. R. 1970. Observations on the ecology, populations and reproductive biology of the pine vole, *Microtus pinetorum,* in North Carolina. Rept. Invest., Illinois State Mus., 20:1–28.
PEARSON, O. P. 1960. Habits of *Microtus californicus* revealed by automatic photographic records. Ecol. Monogr., 30:231–249.
———. 1971. Additional measurements of the impact of carnivores on California voles (*Microtus californicus*). J. Mamm., 52:41–49.
PENGELLEY, E. T., AND K. C. FISHER. 1957. Onset and cessation of hibernation under constant temperature and light in the golden-mantled ground squirrel, *Citellus lateralis*. Nature, 180:1371–1372.
PINTER, A. J., AND N. C. NEGUS. 1965. Effects of nutrition and photoperiod on reproductive physiology of *Microtus montanus*. Amer. J. Physiol., 208:633–638.
POTVIN, C. L., AND J. BOVET. 1975. Annual cycle of patterns of activity rhythms in beaver colonies (*Castor canadensis*). J. Comp. Physiol., 98:243–256.
RASMUSON, B., M. RASMUSON, AND J. NYGREN. 1977. Genetically controlled differences in behavior between cycling and noncycling populations of field vole (*Microtus agrestis*). Hereditas, 87:33–42.
RIJNSDORP, A., S. DAAN, AND C. DIJKSTRA. 1981. Hunting in the kestrel, *Falco tinnunculus,* and the adaptive significance of daily habits. Oecologia, 50: 391–406.
ROWSEMITT, C. N. 1981. Hormonal regulation of activity patterns in *Microtus montanus,* the montane vole. Unpubl. Ph.D. dissert., Univ. Utah, Salt Lake City, 109 pp.
ROWESMITT, C. N., ET AL. 1982. Photoperiodic induction of diurnal locomotor activity in *Microtus montanus,* the montane vole. Canadian J. Zool., 60: 2798–2803.
SANDERSON, G. C. 1966. The study of mammal movements—a review. J. Wildl. Mgmt., 30:215–235.
SCHOENER, T. W. 1981. An empirically based estimate of home range. Theor. Population Biol., 20:281–325.
SEABLOOM, R. W. 1965. Daily motor activity and corticosterone secretion in the meadow vole. J. Mamm., 46:286–295.
SEED, J. R., AND N. KHALILI. 1971. The changes in locomotor rhythms of *Microtus montanus* infected with *Trypanosoma gambiense*. J. Interdiscip. Cycle Res., 2:91–99.
SHIELDS, L. J. 1976. Telemetric determination of the activity of free-ranging rodents; the fine structure of *Microtus californicus* activity patterns. Unpubl. Ph.D. dissert., Univ. California, Los Angeles, 109 pp.
SOLLBERGER, A. 1965. Biological rhythm research. Elsevier, New York, 461 pp.

STICKEL, L. F., AND O. WARBACH. 1960. Small mammal populations of a Maryland woodlot 1949–1954. Ecology, 42:269–286.

STOECKER, R. E. 1972. Competitive relations between sympatric populations of voles (*Microtus montanus* and *M. pennsylvanicus*). J. Anim. Ecol., 41:311–329.

SWADE, R. H., AND C. S. PITTENDRIGH. 1967. Circadian locomotor rhythms of rodents in the Arctic. Amer. Nat., 101:431–466.

TAITT, M. J., AND C. J. KREBS. 1981. The effect of extra food on small rodent populations: II. Voles (*Microtus townsendii*). J. Anim. Ecol., 50:125–137.

TAITT, M. J., J. H. W. GIPPS, C. J. KREBS, AND Z. DUNDJERSKI. 1981. The effect of extra food and cover on declining populations of *Microtus townsendii*. Canadian J. Zool., 59:1593–1599.

TAMARIN, R. H. 1977. Dispersal in island and mainland voles. Ecology, 58:1044–1054.

TANAKA, R. 1972. Investigation into the edge effect by use of capture-recapture data in a vole population. Res. Population Ecol., 13:127–151.

TAST, J. 1966. The root vole, *Microtus oeconomus* (Pallas), as an inhabitant of seasonally flooded land. Ann. Zool. Fennica, 3:127–171.

TURNER, B. N., AND S. L. IVERSON. 1973. The annual cycle of aggression in male *Microtus pennsylvanicus,* and its relation to population parameters. Ecology, 54:967–981.

VAN VLECK, D. B. 1969. Standardization of *Microtus* home range calculations. J. Mamm., 50:69–80.

VAN WINKLE, W. 1975. Comparison of several probabilistic home-range models. J. Wildl. Mgmt., 39:118–123.

WEBSTER, A. B. 1979. A radiotelemetry study of social behavior and activity of free-ranging meadow voles, *Microtus pennsylvanicus*. Unpubl. M.S. thesis, Univ. Guelph, Guelph, Ontario, 110 pp.

WEBSTER, A. B., AND R. J. BROOKS. 1980. Effects of radiotransmitters on the meadow vole, *Microtus pennsylvanicus*. Canadian J. Zool., 58:997–1001.

———. 1981*a*. Daily movements and short activity periods of free-ranging meadow voles, *Microtus pennsylvanicus*. Oikos, 37:80–87.

———. 1981*b*. Social behavior of *Microtus pennsylvanicus* in relation to seasonal changes in demography. J. Mamm., 62:738–751.

WIEGERT, R. G. 1961. Respiratory energy loss and activity patterns in the meadow vole, *Microtus pennsylvanicus pennsylvanicus*. Ecology, 42:245–253.

WOLFF, J. O. 1980. Social organization of the taiga vole (*Microtus xanthognathus*). The Biologist, 62:34–45.

WOLFF, J. O., AND W. Z. LIDICKER, JR. 1980. Population ecology of the taiga vole, *Microtus xanthognathus* in interior Alaska. Canadian J. Zool., 58:1800–1812.

———. 1981. Communal winter nesting and food sharing in taiga voles. Behav. Ecol. Sociobiol., 9:237–240.

DISPERSAL

WILLIAM Z. LIDICKER, JR.

Abstract

DISPERSAL is a major factor in the life history of voles. Moreover, it is a heterogeneous phenomenon encompassing a variety of timings, motivations, and consequences. The study of dispersal will, therefore, be more effective if this variety of movement patterns is acknowledged. A preliminary and heuristic classification of dispersal for the genus *Microtus* is proposed. Among 10 North American species, only the pine vole fails to show definite evidence of pre-saturation types of dispersal.

Attempts to characterize dispersers are hampered by the inherent heterogeneity of the behavior. With respect to sex, age, and reproductive status, the following generalizations can be made: 1) males predominate slightly overall, but saturation dispersers are unbiased sexually or even female dominated; 2) subadults dispersing during the breeding season typically are coming rapidly into breeding condition and often reach sexual maturity at a younger age than residents; 3) adult males moving at the beginning of the breeding season are reproductively active; and 4) pregnant females have been found dispersing in at least four species. Behaviorally, dispersers tend to be less aggressive than residents. A phenotypic-plasticity model is proposed to explain this relationship. The possibility that dispersers as a class may be genetically distinct from residents is explored. The evidence fails to support such a conclusion, although in some cases dispersers are not a genetically random subset of residents and heterozygous genotypes are sometimes in excess among dispersers.

Dispersal is increasingly viewed as having significant demographic causes and consequences. These impacts stem from the quantity of dispersal, the differential nature of dispersers, the success rate of dispersers in reestablishing themselves, and the spatial structuring of populations. These effects are reviewed, and it is concluded that pre-saturation dispersal is a key element in many of the observed processes. Of particular interest is the question of the role of dispersal in population regulation, and especially in our understanding of the enigmatic multi-annual cycles often exhibited by voles. The best evidence that vole populations can be regulated by dispersal comes from the "fence effect." This has been demonstrated for at least six species of *Microtus*. This evidence and the widespread occurrence of pre-saturation dispersal combine to suggest a model of regulation in which dispersal prevents or slows population growth as long as a dispersal sink is available. With the filling of the sink, populations grow to peak densities. Conditions suitable for multi-annual cycling occur when habitat patchiness provides a limited availability of survival habitat relative to colonizing habitat during the poorest time of the annual cycle. The recently proposed hypothesis that immigration is required for multi-annual cycles is found to be unnecessary and without significant support.

Lastly, dispersal is discussed in terms of the evolutionary issues upon which it impinges. Voles offer considerable potential for contributing to general theory in this area. For species exhibiting multi-annual cycles, selection should favor the evolution of pre-saturation dispersal from low-density populations. This pattern should be more characteristic of species inhabiting patchy rather than more continuous habitat. Other areas of inquiry include life-history correlates of dispersal types, heritabilities of dispersal, dispersal polymorphisms, demic differentiation and species cohesion, and the possible role of group selection.

Introduction

Movements of voles away from their home ranges have profound and pervasive influences on many aspects of vole biology. There are consequences for individual fitness, social structure, demography, and evolution. Moreover, such dispersal movements are extremely common, impinging regularly on the lives of nearly every individual vole. Not only may individual voles themselves become dispersers one or more times during their relatively brief lives, but they also are very likely to have to contend with other dispersing voles intruding upon their home ranges.

It would be a serious mistake, however, to assume that the phenomenon of dispersal is homogenous throughout the genus *Micro-*

tus, or even within a single species. Just as there is a multitude of causes and consequences of mortality within the genus, so too we should anticipate that dispersal will have a variety of motivations, timings, and consequences. It is surely a heterogeneous phenomenon with many explanations.

In this discussion dispersal is defined as any movement in which an individual leaves its home range without returning. If such movements result in individuals entering or leaving the demographic unit (population) under study, they become immigration and emigration, respectively (Lidicker, 1975; Lidicker and Caldwell, 1982; Tamarin, 1980). Other related phenomena are excursions, in which individuals leave their home ranges but return after a brief exploratory episode, and nomadism, in which there is no established home range. The study of dispersal is a relatively new aspect of *Microtus* biology and has received detailed attention only in recent years. Data are therefore few and unevenly distributed among North American species. I organized this chapter around the techniques used, the kinds of dispersal found in *Microtus,* the characterization of dispersers, the demographic causes and consequences, and the evolutionary implications of dispersal.

Review of Techniques

A major problem in the study of dispersal among small, cryptic, and short-lived members of the genus *Microtus* is the technique used to identify dispersing individuals. The problem is exacerbated by the near certainty that dispersal is heterogeneous with respect to its causal factors, average distance moved, and quality of voles involved. Hence, a particular technique likely will be biased toward identifying only a particular subset of dispersers. For example, traps set to intercept dispersers at a considerable distance from a source population will underestimate dispersal if most movements are short, if dispersers suffer high mortality, or if dispersers are relatively untrappable.

Traditionally, dispersal was an indistinguishable component of "gross mortality." It did not really matter if an individual dispersed or fell prey to a predator. The demographic, social, and genetic consequences were assumed to be the same. Recently, some authors caught up in the enthusiasm for the importance of dispersal, have gone to the other extreme and assumed that all losses were due to dispersal unless proven otherwise (for example, Hilborn, 1975; Hilborn and Krebs, 1976).

Attempts to measure dispersal in voles directly have met with varied success. A widely used technique is to trap out an area and then assume that individuals caught subsequently are dispersers (Baird and Birney, 1982; Gaines et al., 1979; Hilborn and Krebs, 1976; Keith and Tamarin, 1981; Krebs et al., 1976; Myers and Krebs, 1971; Staples and Terman, 1977; Tamarin, 1977). This poses several sources of error. Because *Microtus* tend to have relatively low trappabilities (Boonstra and Krebs, 1978; Hilborn et al., 1976; Stoddart, 1982), it is extremely difficult to trap out an area. Thus some residents will almost surely remain, possibly to be caught later as "dispersers." Additionally, residents on the edge of such low-density areas will be very likely to expand their home ranges into it. Thirdly, low-density areas may induce some individuals to colonize, such as those on an excursion, who otherwise might not become dispersers. Finally, the subsequent history of colonizers to a trapped-out area may be significantly different from those that disperse into undisturbed areas.

Some workers (Beacham, 1979*a*, 1980, 1981; Hestbeck, 1982; Tamarin, 1980) have attempted to minimize these biases by providing barriers or poor habitat strips around their trapped-out areas ("sinks"; see Lidicker, 1975). This was intended to discourage nearby residents and others not highly motivated to move from reaching the low-density patches. Hestbeck's (1982) experiments included social as well as physical barriers. A variant of this was Tamarin et al.'s (1984) use of partial enclosures, opening only into nonhabitat (forest in this case). To minimize the magnetic effect of low-density patches, Krebs et al. (1978) tried "pulsed removals." By regular but infrequent trapping episodes, more normal densities were maintained on experimental plots. However, this complicated further the problem of distinguishing residents from immigrants. Dueser et al. (1981) tried a single trapping-out of residents followed by no further manipulations. They then assumed that all individuals first caught above a certain body weight were immigrants while those caught first at a lower weight were born on the plot. This is a credible way to circumvent some of the difficulties mentioned above, but fails to avoid the serious problem of incomplete trapping. Almost surely, some individuals born on the area will escape capture until they are above the arbitrary weight level and will be classified as dispersers. Likewise, some individuals may disperse before they reach that critical weight, and be classed incorrectly as resident recruits. The magnitude of these errors is unknown.

Another approach is to use leaky enclosures. If the exits are difficult to transgress, then it can be assumed that successful voles are highly motivated to disperse. If the escape routes are then monitored, dispersing individuals can be identified. For example, Riggs (1979) used long exit tubes leading from the corners of large enclosures. These tubes were guarded by an earth barrier, a bare area, and sometimes a pool of water. Gaines et al. (1979) employed exit traps placed at 15.2-m intervals around three 0.8-ha enclosures. Entrance to the traps was via a pipe opening into the center of a 1-m buffer strip of suboptimal habitat maintained around the edges of the enclosures. Verner (1979) also used dispersal exits in his study. This approach does not absolutely exclude residents from exploring the exit paths and also carries the artificial conditions associated with enclosed populations.

Garsd and Howard (1981, 1982) reported on a long-term study in which drift fences equipped with drop-bottles filled with alcohol were used. This requires a minimum of effort, but unless the drift fences are placed beyond a substantial strip of non-habitat, it is very difficult to distinguish residents from dispersers.

Finally, there is the long-standing technique of trapping at various distances from a marked source population (Stoddart, 1970; Wolff and Lidicker, 1980). This can be done with assessment lines extending from the source population or by sampling at various distances away. This technique gives reliable data when a marked animal is caught and can even distinguish excursions if live-traps are used. However, because of the geometry of area-distance effects this approach is extremely inefficient and unlikely to provide quantifiable results.

Radioactive isotopes have been used occasionally to relocate adult voles. Godfrey (1954) used ^{60}Co on leg rings to determine home-range size in 23 *M. agrestis.* Hilborn and Krebs (1976) glued ^{182}Ta wires to the ear tags of 219 *M. townsendii,* and assessed dispersal rates by whether or not the radioactive tags remained on their grids. They found that tags could be detected as much as two feet underground, permitting the location of dead voles. The method, however, fails to distinguish between losses from predation and dispersal. Wolff and Holleman (1978) marked three pregnant females (*M. xanthognathus*) with ^{65}Zn and then were able to follow movements of the radioactively tagged juveniles. This approach was expanded by Tamarin et al. (1983) who used eight different radionuclides, sometimes in combinations, to greatly increase the number of pregnant females in a single population that could be marked simultaneously. The use of radioactive materials clearly has some potential in dispersal studies. However, there are severe limitations on the number of animals that can be marked in this way, on the distances over which movements can be detected, and on the appropriateness of using this approach in populated areas.

The use of radio transmitters to track vole movements is in its infancy, and promises to be a much more widely used technique in the future. Madison (1978, 1980*a*, 1980*b*, 1981) pioneered this approach on voles, greatly increasing our understanding of spacing behavior and social dynamics in *M. pennsylvanicus.*

As always, each technique offers certain advantages and liabilities. With increased knowledge, we should be able to design techniques that improve resolution. In part this will be abetted by focussing our attention on specific types of dispersal rather than by trying to measure a general class of behavior that may defy simplistic evaluations.

A Classification of Dispersal

Within the genus *Microtus* it is already clear that dispersal behavior is generally not independent of season, density, and life-history events. Moreover, a variety of proximal motivating circumstances can be invoked. This variety tempts one to erect different categories of dispersal behavior that will be helpful in organizing our thinking about dispersal and in designing research programs for its further elucidation. I therefore propose the following tentative classification of dispersal for members of the genus *Microtus.*

A) Saturation
B) Pre-saturation
  1) Seasonal
  2) Ontogenetic
  3) Colonizing
  4) Interference

I do not imply that all categories will apply to all species in the genus, but only that evidence exists for these five types of dispersal in at least one species. These categories also are not discrete nor mutually exclusive. Ambiguous cases and combinations of types are to be anticipated. The value of such a classification is intended to be heuristic, not operational.

Saturation dispersal refers to the classic situation in which essential resources (food, water, shelter) are limiting numbers; that is, the population is at its carrying capacity, and individuals leave because to stay would result in their prompt demise. For a more complete discussion of this phenomenon, see Lidicker (1975). This is the kind of dispersal most logically incorporated into "gross mortality." By contrast, pre-saturation dispersal occurs when individuals leave home before carrying capacity is reached. In some cases these movements are correlated with regularly recurring seasonal events (B-1) such as reproduction or preparation for over-wintering. They may also occur (B-2) at a certain life stage (many species), or when empty habitat becomes available (B-3), such as following a population crash. Caution is required in identifying individual cases, because some instances of saturation dispersal may also occur regularly at particular seasons or perhaps result in colonization.

I know of only one case of interference dispersal, which is characterized by movements motivated by predators, parasites, or superior competitors. Fulk (1972) reported that movements of *M. pennyslvanicus* were responsive to the presence of the predatory shrew, *Blarina brevicauda.*

Table 1 summarizes available information on dispersal organized into the four common categories. Saturation dispersal is surely not as rare as implied by the table. It must occur in all unconfined populations at least occasionally (when densities reach carrying capacity). The European species *M. agrestis* and *M. arvalis* also have been shown to exhibit all four types of dispersal (Hansson [1977], Myllymäki [1977], and Pokki [1981] for *M. agrestis*; and Frank [1954], Mackin-Rogalska [1979], and Pelikán [1959] for *M. arvalis*).

One type of movement not included in Table 1, but that could be considered a form of ontogenetic dispersal because it involves a particular sex and age group, is that which occurs when a reproductive female abandons her nest to her weaned young. Sometimes this merely involves changing nests within the same home range and in other cases the home range is shifted as well. Only in the latter case should this phenomenon be considered dispersal. Apparently, this interesting and important behavior is widespread in *Microtus,* occurring in at least five species (data summarized in Jannett, 1980).

There have been at least two other attempts to classify movements among voles. Madison (1980*a*) distinguished "shifters" and "wanderers" from "dispersers" based on patterns revealed by telemetry. Shifters seem closest to residents in that they progressively occupied different sections of a composite home range, or gradually moved their home range in some direction. Wanderers, on the other hand, either returned to a previous home range, and hence were on an excursion, or did not establish home ranges and were the same as nomads. Baird and Birney (1982) differentiated moving voles into true dispersers, which colonize trapped-out areas, and "movers," which travel long distances within a trapping grid. The latter category was dominated by adult males, and may have been composed largely of individuals on excursions. In neither of these papers was dispersal as defined here explictly viewed as a heterogeneous phenomenon.

Characterization of Dispersers

The attributes of dispersers can only be documented when dispersers can be reliably distinguished from other individuals. Some of the difficulties encountered in such identifications were pointed out above. A second difficulty stems from the presumed heterogeneity of dispersal behavior among voles. If dispersal varies in its causes, timing, and consequences, we should anticipate that dispersers will be a correspondingly heterogeneous assemblage. Hopefully, in the future we will be able to characterize dispersers in relation to specific sorts of dispersal behavior. Only a beginning toward a realization of this goal can be made at present.

Following the review by Gaines and McClenaghan (1980), I will discuss the characteristics of dispersers in three categories: demographic, behavioral, and genetic.

Demographic Features

It is a common feature among mammals that males tend to be the more dispersive sex (Greenwood, 1980). Among species of *Microtus* this tendency is true mainly for subadults, and then not to a

TABLE 1
EVIDENCE FOR FOUR KINDS OF DISPERSAL AMONG SPECIES OF NORTH AMERICAN *Microtus*. ASSIGNMENT TO CATEGORY IS SOMETIMES SUBJECTIVE BECAUSE CRITICAL INFORMATION IS NOT PROVIDED BY AUTHORS

Species	Dispersal categories			
	Saturation	Seasonal	Ontogenic	Colonizing
M. breweri	Tamarin (1977)		Keith and Tamarin (1981) (males only)	Keith and Tamarin (1981)
M. californicus	Lidicker (1980)	Lidicker (1973, 1980)	Lidicker (1975, 1980)	Lidicker and Anderson (1962)
M. montanus		Jannett (1980)		
M. ochrogaster			Gaines et al. (1979); Getz and Carter, (1980)	Abramsky and Tracy (1979); Gaines et al. (1979)
M. oeconomus				Buchalczyk and Pucek (1978); Tast (1966)
M. pennsylvanicus	Grant (1971); Madison (1980*c*) (predicted); Tamarin (1977)	Baird and Birney (1982); Getz (1961, 1972); Madison (1978, 1980*c*, 1984); Morris (1969); Myers and Krebs (1971); Riewe (1973); Turner et al. (1975); Webster and Brooks (1981)	Baird and Birney (1982); Dueser et al. (1981)	Baird and Birney (1982); Dueser, et al. (1981); Getz, et al. (1978); Keith and Tamarin (1981); Van Vleck (1968)

TABLE 1
CONTINUED

Species	Dispersal categories			
	Saturation	Seasonal	Ontogenic	Colonizing
M. pinetorum	Benton (1955) (predicted); Gentry (1968); Staples and Terman (1977)	? Gentry (1968)		
M. richardsoni			Ludwig (1984)	Ludwig (1984)
M. townsendii	Beacham (1980, 1981)	Beacham (1979*a*, 1979*b*, 1980, 1981)	Beacham (1979*a*, 1979*b*, 1980)	Hilborn and Krebs (1976)
M. xanthognathus		Wolff (1980); Wolff and Lidicker (1980, 1981)	Wolff and Lidicker (1980, 1981)	Wolff and Lidicker (1980)

marked degree. For example, only 58% of dispersers in *M. pennsylvanicus* are males (Dueser et al., 1981). In some cases a slight plurality of males among dispersers is correlated with an excess of males in the source population as well (Krebs et al., 1976; Riggs, 1979; Tamarin, 1977). Adult males may predominate among dispersers moving at the beginning of the breeding season (Beacham, 1981; Lidicker, 1973; Pearson, 1960; Wolff and Lidicker, 1980), which is caused by a social reorganization that typically occurs at this time. Dispersal that occurs during summer lulls in reproduction or at unfavorable times of the year (probably saturation dispersal) tends to involve random samples of the population with respect to sex and age. In two such cases (Tamarin [1977] for *M. pennsylvanicus,* and Riggs [1979] for *M. californicus*), adult females were found to disperse in excess of the their proportions in the population. Generally, when numbers are summed over all seasons, many of these interesting details are obscured, and little sex or age bias in dispersals emerges. For example, in *M. agrestis* the overall sex ratio among dispersers is 54% males to 46% females (Pokki, 1981). Gaines et al. (1979) found that *M. ochrogaster* dispersing into removal grids were male-biased, but those colonizing burned areas or leaving enclosures were not. This result cautions against lumping results from different conditions of dispersal as well as over seasons.

One interesting behavioral attribute that tends to equalize dispersal between sexes among subadults is the tendency of litter mates to disperse as a group. Evidence was provided by Hilborn (1975) for four species of *Microtus,* and his conclusions were supported independently by Beacham (1979*b*) for *M. townsendii.*

The reproductive status of dispersers is a complex and controversial matter. Clearly, adults that disperse at the start of breeding (mainly males) are reproductively active. Saturation dispersers generally are non-reproductive as are subadults moving after the end of the breeding season (for example, *M. xanthognathus,* Wolff and Lidicker, 1980). Subadults dispersing during the breeding season are typically coming rapidly into breeding condition so that they can breed without delay upon establishing a new home range. Thus, such dispersers intercepted while leaving tend to be pre-reproductive and those caught upon arrival, for example in a trapped-out area, are reproductively active. Probably consistent with this, Tamarin (1977) reported that on the average dispersers in both *M. breweri* and *M. pennsylvanicus* were in reproductive condition to a greater extent than residents. Baird and Birney (1982) reported the same finding in *M. pennsylvanicus*. Probably the act of dispersal serves to release subadults, especially females, from reproductive inhibition perpetrated by their home social environment (Lidicker, 1975). Thus, sexual maturity may be reached sooner in dispersers than in residents. Evidence for this is available for *M. pennsylvanicus* (Myers and Krebs, 1971; but see Baird and Birney, 1982), *M. ochrogaster* (Gaines et al., 1979; Myers and Krebs, 1971; Richmond and Conaway, 1969), and *M. townsendii* (Beacham, 1981; Krebs et al. 1976). In *M. townsendii,* however, Beacham (1981) found that at least some subadults became reproductively mature before they dispersed.

Dueser et al. (1981) made the interesting claim that dispersers (*M. pennsylvanicus*), once reestablished, continue to have a greater reproductive potential than non-dispersers. Lifespans were comparable between the two groups. Pregnant females were found dispersing in *M. oeconomus* (Tast, 1966), *M. xanthognathus* (Wolff and Lidicker, 1980), *M. montanus* (Jannett, 1980), and *M. pennsylvanicus* (Dueser et al. 1981). Additional examples of this probably will be found in those species in which adult females sometimes leave their home range to their weaned young (Jannett, 1980). An explanation for this curious finding may lie in the observation by Madison (1978) that female *M. pennsylvanicus* have a tendency to make excursions (distance reconnaissance) just before parturition. Myers and Krebs (1971) reported considerable dispersal among lactating females of *M. pennsylvanicus* and *M. ochrogaster*. Lastly, Myllymäki (1977) suggested that breeding female *M. agrestis* are the most efficient colonizers, as Mackin-Rogalska (1979) suggested for *M. arvalis*. Collectively this evidence adds to a surprisingly large role for reproductively active females in dispersal, a group traditionally thought to be least likely to leave home.

Correlations between dispersal and body weight are of limited value unless controlled for age and season. Further confusion is sometimes built into studies where the operational definition of disperser involves body weight. Generally, body weight is assumed to measure age. Therefore, the results usually are concordant with the age correlations given above. It would clearly be of great importance to know if dispersers as a group were in better or worse condition than residents. But I know of no study that examines this question by controlling for age effects on body weight. On average, pre-saturation dispersers should be in better condition than those fleeing saturated conditions (Lidicker, 1975).

Behavioral Features

Considerable attention has been directed to the possibility that dispersers are behaviorally divergent from residents in ways other than the dispersal act itself. In particular, aggressive behavior has been examined because of its connection to the Chitty-Krebs hypothesis of density regulation in multi-annual cycles (Krebs, 1978*a*). At first a genetic polymorphism in aggressive behavior was hypothesized to be the key element in determing this cycle. Later, aggression was coupled with dispersal. The hypothesis predicts that during population increases, aggressive morphs will tend to make dispersers out of non-aggressive individuals, thus slowing local population growth and increasing the population of aggressive types in the source population. Under unfavorable conditions such dense and highly aggressive populations will decline rapidly with almost all losses being due to mortality. During the subsequent low-density period, the non-aggressive, dispersal morph is favored. This model predicts that dispersers are largely of the pre-saturation type and relatively non-aggressive. It further predicts that in populations that do not show multi-annual cycles, aggression will be independent of dispersal and undifferentiated between residents and dispersers. This last prediction is strongly supported by data for *M. breweri* on Muskeget Island, Masschusetts (Reich et al., 1982).

Krebs (1970) found changes in aggressiveness (males) associated with different phases of the density cycle in *M. ochrogaster* and *M. pennsylvanicus*. He did not, at that time, correlate these differences with dispersal, but did suggest that emigration might be the mechanism selecting for increased aggression in growing populations. In 1971, Myers and Krebs reported that dispersing males of both *M. ochrogaster* and *M. pennsylvanicus* showed less exploratory behavior in a maze than did males from control populations. On the other hand, male *M. pennsylvanicus* from removal grids (dispersers) were more aggressive than control males, at least during periods of high density. Male *M. ochrogaster* from removal grids, however, tended to be behaviorally subordinate. Turner and Iverson (1973) reported that resident *M. pennsylvanicus* were more aggressive than nonresidents, and they did not find any consistent relation between aggression and density. In the case of *M. breweri,* which does not show multi-annual cycles, Reich and Tamarin (1980) concluded that dispersers had higher levels of avoidance behavior as compared to residents. Thus, dispersers were likely to be subordinates as was the case for *M. ochrogaster.* Krebs et al. (1978) compared the behavior of dispersers and residents in *M. townsendii.* Generally dispersers showed less wounding, were more submissive in staged diadic encounters, and vocalized more. For most species tested, therefore, dispersers seemed to be less aggressive than residents. This finding is concordant with the Chitty-Krebs model.

Christian (1970) and Anderson (1980) also predicted that dispersers will be social subordinates, but for different reasons. Rather than suggesting that a behavioral polymorphism is involved, they argued that young are subordinate to parents and it is in the parents' best interest to have the young disperse. Dispersal is thus involuntary. Anderson (1980) further predicted that fathers will drive off their sons, mothers will expel offspring only when resources become scarce, and sex ratio of dispersers will be strongly biased toward males early in the breeding season and tend toward equality later, and males will move farther than females. This model fails to account for the high proportion of adults that disperse in *Microtus* and for the relatively high proportion of females among dispersing subadults. It also tends to negate selection for dispersal through individual advantage to the dispersers. Anderson's (1980) model, however, could apply to ontogenetic dispersal; its predictions should be tested.

The tendency for dispersers to be relatively non-aggressive can support still other explanations of dispersal behavior. It is my suspicion that dispersers are non-aggressive because they are not residents. That is, they are deficient in the well-known "territorial imperative" of property owners. This model predicts that if and when dispersers reestablish home ranges, they will become more aggressive. Aggressive behavior should in this case also have low heritability (in contrast to the Chitty-Krebs model). It is therefore of interest that Anderson (1975) reported zero heritability for agonistic behavior in *M. townsendii.* Socially mediated proximate motivations are not ruled out by the model, but are presumed to interact with age, reproductive condition, and local density. In fact, this phenotypic-plasticity model also explains the reproductive stunting that occurs in high density populations (Batzli et al., 1977;

Lidicker, 1979, 1980). If reproductive maturation is an invitation for aggression, as seems likely, it should be advantageous for subadults to delay maturity under high-density situations if the chances of finding a suitable place for reestablishment are greatly reduced. As peak numbers are approached, average aggressiveness should fall rather than reach a maximum; mature adults, however, should remain aggressive and in fact some could be induced thereby to become dispersers. This possibility could explain the high level of aggression among male dispersers found in peak populations of *M. pennsylvanicus* by Myers and Krebs (1971). The phenotypic-plasticity model shares some features with Anderson's (1980) model but is more comprehensive in its incorporation of 1) adult dispersal, 2) greater emphasis on female movements, and 3) non-forced dispersal. It applies particularly to pre-saturation dispersal because there probably is no controversy about saturation dispersers being behaviorally subordinate for economic and social reasons.

Bekoff suggested (Bekoff, 1977; Gaines and McClenaghan, 1980) that social interactions occurring prior to dispersal are most critical in determining who is going to disperse and when; the predominant social behavior around the time of dispersal is avoidance. Bekoff's (1977) idea is compatible with either phenotypic-variation or behavioral-polymorphism models, and would seem to apply most specifically to ontogenetic dispersal. Data to test his model are not available for *Microtus*. A final behavioral trait of dispersers is the apparent tendency for littermates to disperse or not disperse as a unit (Beacham, 1979*b*; Hilborn, 1975). This trait supports either the Chitty-Krebs polymorphism model or my phenotypic-plasticity model, but is inconsistent with the Christian-Anderson social-subordination model.

Genetic Features

The possibility that dispersers may be genetically distinct from residents has been the subject of widespread speculation and investigation. The idea of a dispersal morph is central to recent versions of the Chitty-Krebs hypothesis of population regulation. Evolutionary and behavioral ecologists also have been fascinated by the possibility of a genetic polymorphism for dispersal behavior. As early as 1949 Burt suggested that some individuals were programmed genetically for dispersal while others were not. The idea was developed more rigorously by Howard (1960), Johnston (1961), Lidicker (1962), and others (see Lidicker and Caldwell, 1982: Part I, for review).

With the widespread availability of electrophoretic techniques, a search was made for biochemical markers that might be associated in some way with dispersal behavior. The available data are summarized in Table 2. The two loci most frequently investigated are transferrin and leucine aminopeptidase (both from plasma). In addition, Pickering et al. (1974) found differences in allele frequency at an esterase locus in a very small sample of *M. pennsylvanicus.* The results reported from Baird and Birney (1982) are summaries of a complex data set involving comparisions among sex and age groups, summer and autumn cohorts, and "movers" as well as dispersers and residents.

My conclusions from these data are that no consistent pattern has emerged, and that this approach has failed to support the hypothesis of a genetic polymorphism for dispersal. Interpretation of the LAP data is especially difficult since allelic frequencies at this locus are known to show shifts with season and density. Of course, the Chitty-Krebs model is not refuted by the biochemical data because no functional connection between these biochemical traits and dispersal has been suggested, and indeed it would be surprising if they were found to be correlated in some way. LeDuc and Krebs (1975) experimentally manipulated LAP genotypes in populations of *M. townsendii* but could not produce any alteration of overall demography. This result thus fails to support a possible connection between LAP genotypes and dispersal in this species (Krebs et al., 1976). The most that can be extracted from the biochemical data at this time is that dispersers are sometimes non-random samples of source populations.

An intriguing finding was reported by Tamarin (1977) for *M. breweri.* He reported that the frequency of a white blaze on the forehead occurs more frequently among dispersers. Perhaps it is worth mentioning that Garten (1977) found an association between exploratory activity and overall heterozygosity at a series of biochemical loci in *Peromyscus polionotus.* Contrary conclusions were drawn by Blackwell and Ramsey (1972), although their study was limited to three loci. Some possible support for Garten's notion could be gleaned from Table 2; heterozygote genotypes are sometimes found in excess among dispersers. This is an area that would warrant further careful work in the future.

TABLE 2
BIOCHEMICAL TRAITS FOUND TO BE PRESENT IN GREATER FREQUENCY IN DISPERSERS AS COMPARED TO RESIDENTS

Species	Sex		LAP	Tf	References
M. breweri	♂		—	Tf^C/Tf^E†	Keith and Tamarin (1981)
M. californicus	♂, ♀		—	Not polymorphic	Riggs (1979)
M. ochrogaster	♂, ♀		—	Tf^F/Tf^F	Meyers and Krebs (1971)
				—	Gaines et al. (1979)
M. pennsylvanicus	♂		SS*	Tf^E/Tf^E*	Myers and Krebs (1971)
	♀		SS*	Tf^C/Tf^E**	
	♂, ♀		—	Tf^C/Tf^C***	Verner (1979)
	♂	(subadult, summer)	F		
	♂, ♀	(summer)		FS[1]	Baird and Birney (1982)
M. townsendi	♂, ♀		F and S††		Krebs et al. (1976)
	♀		FS††	—	

Abbreviations: F, fast moving allele; LAP, leucine aminopeptidase; S, slow moving allele; TF, transferrin; —, no difference between colonizers and residents.

* During late population peak and decline.

** Periods of population increase.

*** Significant for only one month; and among males for subadults only.

† Two month period only; adults.

†† Different alleles predominant among colonizers in different areas; FS in excess in one summer only.

[1] Only two alleles were distinguished in this study.

Demographic Causes and Consequences

With the recognition that dispersal is more than a safety valve for saturated habitats and that it can be high, investigators have inquired increasingly into its relationship to other demographic processes, including the regulation of numbers. This last relationship is particularly significant for *Microtus* in view of the enigmatic multi-annual cycles of abundance often seen in this group. The demographic role of dispersal was reviewed by Lidicker (1975) and

Gaines and McClenaghan (1980) for small mammals in general and (with respect to density regulation) by Tamarin (1980) for rodents, and by Tamarin (1978) and Taitt and Krebs (this volume) for *Microtus*.

A corollary of this increasing focus on the demographic aspects of dispersal has been the growing realization of the importance of spatial structuring in understanding microtine population dynamics. Dispersal is studied most meaningfully in the context of the spatial and temporal discontinuities in numbers; empirical documentation of such patterns of distribution is being accumulated at an accelerating rate. This area of investigation is reviewed for *Microtus* by Lidicker (in press).

The demographic implications of dispersal have to do both with the quantity of dispersal and with the probability that dispersers are qualitatively non-random subsets of source populations. They further concern the success rate of dispersers both in travelling through unfamiliar and often hostile terrain and in establishing new home sites.

Evidence already summarized on the nature of dispersers strongly suggests that in *Microtus* dispersers are generally a non-random subset of source populations. We can therefore anticipate that dispersal will have an impact on age structure, natality and mortality rates, and sex ratios through the differential loss or gain of dispersers. The particular effect of course will depend on the kind of biases that characterize dispersal in any given instance. Myllymäki (1977), for example, claims that in *M. agrestis* the female-biased sex ratios he observed during the breeding season, and especially at peak densities, were caused by differential dispersal. Dueser et al. (1981) found that in populations of *M. pennsylvanicus* that were dominated by dispersers, reproductive rates were higher than in other populations. Differences in age structure between populations dominated by residents on the one hand, or by immigrants on the other, can also be anticipated, but they have not been documented for *Microtus*.

Quantitative information on the success rate of dispersers is not available for species of *Microtus*. It generally is assumed that dispersers suffer higher mortality rates than residents. They often must cross regions of marginal or unsuitable habitat and confront physical barriers of various kinds. Encounter rates with predators, parasites, and competitors may be greatly enhanced. Ambrose (1972) reported higher predation rates for *M. pennsylvanicus* unfamiliar with an artificial environment than for voles given 4 days to familiarize themselves with the experimental habitat. And, finally, dispersers can expect to traverse socially hostile neighborhoods as well. In all of this potential adversity, dispersers that begin their journeys in good physical condition are surely more likely to succeed. We can therefore predict that the success rate of pre-saturation dispersers generally will be much greater than for saturation dispersers (Lidicker, 1975). It is satisfying to note that pre-saturation dispersal has been found to characterize unequivocally all species of *Microtus* for which dispersal data are available (see Table 1), with the exception of *M. pinetorum*. Population density and the availability of empty habitat also will be critically important in affecting success rates. For populations exhibiting multi-annual cycles of abundance, we can therefore anticipate that average success will vary tremendously with stage of the density cycle.

The final step in successful dispersal is the establishment of a new home range. If empty habitat is available, this should pose minimal risks associated with establishing a system of burrows and runways and finding a mate. On the other hand, if the disperser attempts to immigrate into an existing population, social antagonisms may have to be overcome and possibly complex problems of mate choice confronted. This is an important but virtually unexplored area of microtine research.

The aspect of dispersal and demography which has received the greatest attention is that relating to the quantity rather than the quality of dispersers. Gaines and McClenaghan (1980) reviewed the data relating dispersal and population density, much of which is on *Microtus*. They concluded that: 1) the number of dispersers is correlated positively with population density; 2) a less consistent positive relationship can be found between density and rates of population increase; and 3) more dispersal consistently occurs during periods of increasing density than during phases of decline. This last point emphasizes the prevalence of pre-saturation dispersal in voles, and sets the stage for an examination of dispersal and population growth rates.

A potentially important relationship between dispersal and population growth rates is predicted from the basic growth equation in which additions are derived from reproduction and immigration while losses are composed of deaths plus emigration (for general treatment, see Lidicker and Caldwell, 1982). If there is a positive net emigration rate and densities are below carrying capacity, a suppressing effect of dispersal on growth rates will occur. The best documented case in *Microtus* for suppressed growth rates because of dispersal is that for *M. californicus* (Lidicker, 1975, 1980). Some evidence is also available for *M. pennsylvanicus* and *M. ochrogaster* (Krebs et al., 1969).

Just as emigration can suppress population growth rate, immigration can enhance it. Clearly, where refugial populations are expanding into uninhabited or low-density areas, the densities in such non-refugial habitats will be determined largely by immigration. Tast (1966) described how *M. oeconomus* seasonally re-invades flooded areas. Dueser et al. (1981), in their studies of *M. pennsylvanicus,* described grid populations that were more than 75% dispersers, and claimed further that for some populations dispersal may continue to be a greater source of recruits than reproduction. Similarly, Ostfeld and Klosterman (pers. comm.) studied *M. californicus* in patchy habitats and reported that some habitats are chronically inhabited largely by immigrants.

The intriguing and important question of the potential role of dispersal in population regulation was reviewed by Lidicker (1975), Tamarin (1978, 1980), Krebs (1978*a,* 1978*b*), and Taitt and Krebs (this volume). Certainly dispersal could serve as a regulating factor if net losses to emigration increased proportionally as density increased (Lidicker, 1978; Nakano, 1981). Gaines and McClenaghan (1980), however, claimed that there is no evidence of such a proportional increase in dispersal with density. This statement was based on an analysis of "recovery ratios" (number of colonizers in removal areas divided by population size on control areas) in six species of rodents (including four species of *Microtus*). They also failed to find any proportional increase in dispersal with density in *Sigmodon hispidus* (McClenaghan and Gaines, 1976). What would be critical, however, is an analysis of how dispersal proportion changes as the population approaches zero growth rate (from positive or negative directions). A regulating influence by dispersal is not incompatible with the possibility that at times the population may be regulated by other factors or even sometimes behave as if non-regulated.

The best evidence that *Microtus* populations are in fact sometimes regulated by dispersal is the "fence effect" phenomenon. When dispersal is prevented in growing populations by enclosing them in a fence or on a small island, densities characteristically increase dramatically. This has been demonstrated for at least six species of *Microtus* (Boonstra and Krebs, 1977; Clarke, 1955; Gentry, 1968; Hatt, 1930; Houlihan, 1963; Krebs, 1979; Krebs et al., 1969, 1973; Lidicker, 1979; Lousch, 1956; Tamarin and Krebs, 1969; van Wijngaarden, 1960; Wiegert, 1972). This impressive evidence, and that for extensive and widespread pre-saturation dispersal (mentioned above) suggests that numbers in unenclosed populations are ordinarily regulated by dispersal, but that when dispersal is prevented by the filling of the dispersal sink, peak densities result (Lidicker, 1973, 1975). Hestbeck (1982) modified this model slightly by suggesting that what is proximally important is not the filling of usable habitat but the erection of social barriers to dispersal.

The above view of dispersal in vole populations implies that dispersal plays a density regulating role in two classes of circumstances: 1) when a population is surrounded by a permanent dispersal sink; and 2) when a population exhibiting multi-annual cycles undergoes the long growth phase. An example of the former was described by Abramsky and Tracy (1979). They studied populations of *M. ochrogaster* living in artificially fertilized and watered plots surrounded by shortgrass prairie, which is very poor habitat for this species. In multi-annual cycles, dispersal should act in a regulating fashion during most of the low phase. This should be followed by a rapid increase in numbers when dispersal fails to keep up with reproduction because of a nearly filled dispersal sink and the longer breeding seasons and reduced mortality rates often associated with "pre-high" situations. Under peak and initially declining conditions, saturation dispersal should occur followed by a period of little or no dispersal.

Recently, the curious idea was advanced that not only is emigration important in determining population numbers, but immigration is critical for generating multi-annual cycles (Abramsky and Tracy, 1979; Dueser et al., 1981; Gaines et al., 1979; Rosenzweig and Abramsky, 1980). Such a role for immigration has been attributed to: 1) disruption of stability by influx of inappropriate genotypes to a habitat patch (Abramsky and Tracy, 1979; Rosenzweig and Abramsky, 1980); 2) prevention of local extinction (Gaines et al., 1979); and 3) a source of vigorous recruits to the populations

(Dueser et al., 1981). In addition, Smith et al. (1975) implied that high densities are encouraged by immigration through outbreeding, which leads to increased heterozygosity levels with consequent improvements in vigor and reproductive performance. Only the first of these would seem to relate directly to multi-annual cycles. Moreover, such genetic perturbations seem unnecessarily complex, and may require an inappropriate time scale.

The factual basis for this immigration hypothesis seems to be the findings of Abramsky and Tracy (1979) and Gaines et al. (1979), who showed that enclosed populations of *M. ochrogaster* in which emigration is permitted do not develop multi-annual cycles. They came to the unnecessary conclusion that what is critically lacking in these cases is immigration. In my view, their results are more easily interpreted as instances of unfilled dispersal sinks preventing density buildup. Moreover, Tamarin et al. (1984) found that normal cycles occurred in *M. pennsylvanicus* housed in enclosures in which emigration but not immigration was permitted. According to my model, these results are expected because the emigration filter (forest in this case) was sufficient to extend the period of population growth but was inadequate to prevent peak densities from developing eventually. What is therefore lacking in the non-cyclic examples is not immigration but sufficient frustrated dispersal to generate a peak density and subsequent crash.

In recent years considerable attention has been directed toward connecting an explanation of multi-annual cycles in microtines to micro-spatial structuring of populations (Abramsky and Van Dyne, 1980; Anderson, 1980; Bowen, 1982; Charnov and Finerty, 1980; Cockburn and Lidicker, 1983; Hansson, 1977; Hestbeck, 1982; Mackin-Rogalska, 1979; Rosenzweig and Abramsky, 1980; Stenseth, 1977; Stenseth et al., 1977). This approach is clearly a correlate of the potential importance of dispersal in microtine population dynamics. Discontinuities in distribution (structuring) become interesting when they are variously connected and modified by dispersal. The role of population structuring in understanding multi-annual cycles was reviewed by Lidicker (in press).

Up to this point my model of the role of dispersal in multi-annual cycles has two components. First, pre-saturation dispersal must occur so that population growth can be suppressed for long periods, even at low densities. In addition to evidence already cited, a general relationship between pre-saturation dispersal and multi-annual cyclicity is supported by Gliwicz (1980), Krebs and Myers (1974), Rasmuson et al. (1977), Stenseth (1978), and Tamarin (1978). Possibly correlated with this evidence is the contention by Gaines and McClenaghan (1980) that males predominate among dispersers in cycling species but not in non-cyclers. Second, large dispersal sinks must exist which become periodically filled, causing frustration of dispersal. In my recent review (Lidicker, in press) a third component is added. It seems characteristic of cycling populations that there is a limited availability of good survival habitats during the most stressful times of the year. Survival habitat (sensu Anderson, 1980) is strongly limited relative to "colonizing habitat." This feature is important in that densities are caused to periodically decline to levels several orders of magnitude below carrying capacities characteristic of favorable times. If severe declines don't occur, recovery of densities from seasonal lows is rapid enough for annual peaks to be produced. Charnov and Finerty (1980) also predicted that patchy habitats are required for multi-annual cycles to occur. If any one of these components is missing, multi-annual cycles will not result. Of course, variations in the size of annually occurring peaks is to be expected, and occasional irruptions also may occur in non-cycling species because of some unusually favorable circumstance. These latter variations should not be construed as multi-annual cycles in the sense intended here.

Evolutionary Issues

The evolution of dispersal behavior and the influence of dispersal on evolutionary processes constitute two enormous areas of inquiry. For brief overviews, see Gaines and McClenaghan (1980:186–189) and Lidicker and Caldwell (1982: Part V). With respect to *Microtus,* these subjects mostly raise questions for future investigation.

In my view, however, research on microtine rodents will likely make a significant contribution to our understanding of these evolutionary issues. This is not only because microtines are relatively well known, but also because they exhibit a rich variety of dispersal behaviors, temporal density patterns, habitat relationships, social habits, and spatial structuring configurations. Moreover, these variations can be studied in the same population (temporally), intraspecifically, interspecifically, and intergenerically. Thus, the evolutionary biologist should find a substrate for answering a variety of questions relating to dispersal.

Studies on species of *Microtus* have been, or should be in the future, addressed to the following general questions relating to dispersal and evolution.

1) How does environmental heterogeneity in space and time contribute to the evolution of various kinds of dispersal?

2) Are there particular life history features or social systems that are conducive to, or inhibiting to, the evolution of dispersal?

3) What is the nature of the genetic substrate for dispersal behavior, and how does this vary across different kinds of dispersal?

4) Are there circumstances in which polymorphisms for dispersal occur?

5) What are the consequences of dispersal for demic differentiation and species cohesion?

6) Is group selection involved in the evolution of dispersal?

Environmental heterogeneity as a factor in the evolution of dispersal has been treated extensively in the theoretical literature. There seems no doubt that a positive relationship exists. On the other hand, Hamilton and May (1977) argued that dispersal can evolve even in stable habitats. Applications of this body of theory directly to *Microtus* have been limited (but see Hansson, 1977; Stenseth, 1980; Tamarin, 1978). The nearly ubiquitous occurrences of pre-saturation types of dispersal in this genus strongly argues for some sort of selective advantage for it. We can predict that pre-saturation dispersal of some kind will be more prevalent in species inhabiting small patches of non-permanent habitat, such as *M. xanthognathus,* than in those occurring (at least historically) in more continuous habitat, such as *M. ochrogaster.*

Although at least some kinds of dispersal seem to be important components of the life history of all species of *Microtus,* much remains to be learned regarding correlations between particular kinds of dispersal and life-history details (including social behavior). A few authors have concluded that dispersal is quantitatively low (Madison, 1980*c*; Tamarin et al., 1984; Verner, 1979), but these views are atypical among *Microtus* biologists. Recent attention has been directed at elucidating the possible role of dispersal in multi-annual cycles exhibited by many populations (see review by Lidicker, in press). In the model outlined, a prominent but not exclusive role for dispersal is proposed to explain this interesting pattern of density fluctuation.

Little progress has been made in illuminating the genetic basis for dispersal in *Microtus*. As pointed out above, such behaviors are almost certainly heterogeneous, greatly complicating such an analysis. Moreover, the inheritance of even one type of dispersal is likely to be complex. Ontogenetic and seasonal types of dispersal imply a strong genetic basis. Colonizing dispersal may not be rooted firmly in the genotype, and saturation dispersal should be least influenced by genetic constitution. The only attempt to measure heritability has been by Anderson (1975; see also Krebs, 1979), who reported that *M. townsendii* exhibited moderate heritability on the basis of comparisions between residency length within and between groups of siblings. Although a higher correlation in length of residency among sibs suggests a strong genetic basis for dispersal, this result is confounded by non-genetic factors that may affect littermates collectively, such as maternal influences. To a large extent these non-genetic influences were factored out by Anderson's findings that the correlation with residency was significantly higher on unfenced grids (where dispersal was possible) than on fenced grids. Concordant with this result is the evidence that sibling groups either disperse or don't disperse as units (Beacham, 1979*b*; Hilborn, 1975).

High heritabilities and genetic polymorphisms for dispersal behavior are predicted by the Chitty-Krebs model of population regulation in multi-annually cycling microtines (Krebs, 1978*a*). As pointed out above, the evidence so far fails to support the prediction of dispersal polymorphisms. However, the subject is sufficiently difficult and important that it warrants further investigation.

The role of dispersal in demic differentiation is a major area of inquiry in population genetics (see also Gaines, this volume, for related discussion). The availability of electrophoretic techniques has permitted an empirical approach to this issue on a fine temporal and spatial scale. In *M. californicus,* Bowen (1982) and Lidicker (unpubl. observ.) demonstrated that genetic heterogeneity among small demes persisting at low densities is high relative to a more general panmixia prevailing at high densities. Moreover, stochastic processes are critical in determining the genetic composition of refugial demes. The approach needs to be expanded to larger geographical arenas and to other species. Voles should contribute substantially to future advances in this area.

Finally, and perhaps most intriguing of all, investigations on dispersal in voles has the potential for contributing to one of the current major philosophical issues now raging in evolutionary biology. I refer to the general issue of levels of natural selection, and in particular to whether or not group selection has played a significant role in evolution. Van Valen (1971) gave us a general model that suggested (under a rather robust set of conditions) that group selection can indeed lead to the evolution of dispersal (including polymorphisms). Charnov and Finerty (1980) have suggested that kin selection and dispersal may interact to explain low levels of aggression at low densities (when voles mostly interact with relatives) and rapidly increasing aggression in growing populations (when dispersal brings non-relatives into frequent contact).

Of course, it is difficult to make critical observations or do experiments on such relatively long-lived animals as voles to directly test a particular evolutionary hypothesis. We can, however, discover whether or not the appropriate substrate for a given selection model exists in nature. This at least allows us to support the claim that a particular model can or cannot be operating, even if it is extremely difficult to establish that it actually does. By analogy with individual-level selection, we observe differential reproduction and survival among individuals, and feel comfortable about natural selection occurring at this level even though we may not be able to show a direct connection between observed fitness differences and some actual change in genetic composition of a population. In this regard, Wilson's (1975, 1977) trait-group model of group selection seems particularly relevant to voles. In at least two species of *Microtus*, populations alternate, seasonally or multi-annually, through phases characterized by small isolated trait groups and large panmictic assemblages (Bowen, 1982; Lidicker, in press; Wolff and Lidicker, 1981). In my view, this is an area that warrants additional attention.

Summary and Conclusions

Dispersal is a major factor in the lives of voles. It also is definitely not a homogenous phenomenon, varying importantly in its timing, proximal motivations, demographic consequences, and in the nature of the dispersers themselves. This heterogeneity adds complexity to the inherent difficulty of studying dispersal in such small, cryptic, short-lived, and secretive animals. Techniques of study should be designed specifically for a particular kind of dispersal in order to maximize effectiveness. Useful, if not always satisfying, results have been obtained with trapped-out grids, with and without barriers of poor habitat, and with and without "pulsed removals." Another approach has been to use leaky enclosures. This gives more secure identification of dispersers, but also incorporates the artifacts of confinement. Assessment trap-lines provide accuracy but low resolution. Radioactive isotopes have been used with some success, and radio transmitters have considerable potential for making important contributions.

A classification for dispersal as found in the genus *Microtus* is proposed. This includes saturation dispersal and four categories of pre-saturation dispersal: seasonal, ontogenetic, colonizing, and interference. With the interesting exception of the pine vole (*M. pinetorum*), at least some type of pre-saturation dispersal is found in all species for which data are available (nine North American and two European species). Undoubtedly saturation dispersal is ubiquitous as well, but it has not been so widely documented.

The characterization of dispersers has been confused by the general failure to distinguish among the different kinds of dispersal. Some tentative generalizations are possible, however, based on available data. Males predominate only slightly among dispersers. The strongest male biases are present during seasonal dispersal that occurs in association with the beginning of the breeding season, and among juvenile emigrants. Saturation dispersal tends to be unbiased for sex or is female dominated. Subadults dispersing during the breeding season are typically coming rapidly into breeding condition and on average seem to reach sexual maturity at a younger age than residents. Adult males moving at the beginning of the breeding season are reproductively active; adult females may be the most adept colonizers. In at least three species, pregnant females have been found dispersing. Saturation dispersers are generally non-reproductive. Little is known about the general physiological condition of dispersers.

Dispersers tend to be less aggressive than residents. This generalization fits the Chitty-Krebs model of population regulation, the Christian-Anderson social-subordination model, and a new phenotypic-plasticity model proposed here. Testable predictions differentiate the three models relating dispersal and aggressive behavior.

The data available so far on *Microtus* best support the third model, which incorporates adult as well as subadult movements, low heritabilities for dispersal, voluntary as well as forced movements, and a greater emphasis on female dispersal.

The possibility that dispersers as a class may be genetically distinct from residents has been explored extensively. The strongest support for this proposition comes from evidence (four species) that litters tend to disperse, or not disperse, as units. Biochemical genetic data suggest that at least in some cases, dispersers are not a random subset of residents. However, no consistent association of dispersal with particular genotypes has been found, and there is no evidence at all for a genetic polymorphism for dispersal. In some cases heterozygote genotypes have been found in excess among dispersers.

The demographic causes and consequences of dispersal have received increasing attention. There is a growing realization of the importance of spatial structuring in understanding vole population dynamics. Demographic implications of dispersal stem from: 1) the nature of dispersers relative to residents; 2) the success rate of dispersers in reestablishing home ranges; and 3) the quantity of emigration versus immigration. Because dispersers are generally a nonrandom subset of residents (at least for pre-saturation dispersal), they should have (and some evidence exists for) impacts on age structure, natality and mortality rates, and sex ratios. Little information is available on survival rates of dispersers and on reestablishment effectiveness. I assume that pre-saturation dispersers are more successful than saturation dispersers, and that colonization of empty habitat is less risky than immigration. If true, selection should strongly favor pre-saturation dispersal from low density populations during favorable seasons of the year. Quantitative data on these processes are needed badly. The quantative component of dispersal has received the greatest attention. Clear impacts on population growth rates, both by emigration and immigration, have been demonstrated for a few species.

Research on *Microtus* has pioneered investigations into the role of dispersal in density regulation. Although it is theoretically feasible that dispersal can perform such a role, good evidence is difficult to obtain. The "fence effect" phenomenon, known for six species of *Microtus,* is the best evidence that densities reach supra-normal levels when dispersal is prevented. This evidence, in addition to the existence of pre-saturation dispersal, has led to a model in which dispersal plays an important role in regulating numbers when densities are low. With the filling of the dispersal sink and the frustration of dispersal that follows, densities rise to peak levels. A second circumstance in which dispersal plays such a critical regulating role is when a population of voles is surrounded by a permanent dispersal sink. These early models have now been expanded to describe the role of dispersal in the multi-annual cycle. In addition to pre-saturation dispersal and a large dispersal sink being consistent features of multi-annual cycles, a third feature has been added, namely the condition that survival habitat is strongly limited periodically compared to colonizing habitat. This last condition assures that populations will go regularly through bottlenecks of very low densities. This three-part model, of course, does not purport to explain multi-annual cycles, but emphasizes that dispersal is an important component of this demographic pattern.

Finally, dispersal in *Microtus* is discussed in terms of the evolutionary issues with which it impinges. Because of the importance of dispersal to evolutionary processes and because of the complex spatial and temporal structuring exhibited by at least some species, dispersal inevitably will be central to any discussion of evolution in this group. Six general questions relating dispersal and evolution in voles are proposed, and the status of research in each of these areas is reviewed. Areas of inquiry include the role of environmental heterogeneity, life-history correlates of dispersal types, heritabilities of kinds of dispersal, dispersal polymorphisms, demic differentiation and species cohesion, and the possible role of group selection. I predict that, on these general topics, research with voles will make substantial contributions to our understanding of evolutionary processes.

Literature Cited

ABRAMSKY, Z., AND C. R. TRACY. 1979. Population biology of a "noncycling" population of prairie voles and a hypothesis on the role of migration in regulating microtine cycles. Ecology, 60:349–361.

ABRAMSKY, Z., AND G. VAN DYNE. 1980. Field studies and a simulation model of small mammals inhabiting a patchy environment. Oikos, 35:90–92.

AMBROSE, H. W., III. 1972. Effect of habitat familiarity and toe-clipping on rate of owl predation in *Microtus pennsylvanicus.* J. Mamm., 53:909–912.

ANDERSON, J. L. 1975. Phenotypic correlations among relatives and variability in reproductive performance in populations of the vole *Microtus townsendii.* Unpubl. Ph.D. dissert., Univ. British Columbia, Vancouver, 207 pp.

ANDERSON, P. K. 1980. Evolutionary implications of microtine behavioral systems on the ecological stage. The Biologist, 62:70–88.
BAIRD, D. D., AND E. C. BIRNEY. 1982. Characteristics of dispersing meadow voles Microtus pennsylvanicus. Amer. Midland Nat., 107:262–283.
BATZLI, G. O., L. L. GETZ, AND S. S. HURLEY. 1977. Suppression of growth and reproduction of microtine rodents by social factors. J. Mamm., 58:583–591.
BEACHAM, T. D. 1979*a*. Size and growth characteristics of dispersing voles, *Microtus townsendii*. Oecologia, 42:1–10.
———. 1979*b*. Dispersal tendency and duration of life of littermates during population fluctuations of the vole *Microtus townsendii*. Oecologia, 42:11–21.
———. 1980. Dispersal during population fluctuations of the vole, *Microtus townsendii*. J. Anim. Ecol., 49:867–877.
———. 1981. Some demographic aspects of dispersers in fluctuating populations of the vole Microtus townsendii. Oikos, 36:272–280.
BEKOFF, M. 1977. Mammalian dispersal and the ontogeny of individual behavioral phenotypes. Amer. Nat., 111:715–732.
BENTON, A. H. 1955. Observations on the life history of the northern pine mouse. J. Mamm., 36:52–62.
BLACKWELL, T. L., AND P. R. RAMSEY. 1972. Exploratory activity and lack of genotypic correlates in *Peromyscus polionotus*. J. Mamm., 53:401–403.
BOONSTRA, R., AND C. J. KREBS. 1977. A fencing experiment on a high-density population of *Microtus townsendii*. Canadian J. Zool., 55:1166–1175.
———. 1978. Pitfall trapping of *Microtus townsendii*. J. Mamm., 59:136–148.
BOWEN, B. S. 1982. Temporal dynamics of microgeographic structure of genetic variation in *Microtus californicus*. J. Mamm., 63:625–638.
BUCHALCZYK, T., AND Z. PUCEK. 1978. The succession of small mammals in a drained peat-bog. P. 193, *in* Abst. Papers, Second Congr. Theriol. Internatl., Brno, Czechoslovakia, 469 pp.
BURT, W. H. 1949. Territoriality. J. Mamm., 30:25–27.
CHARNOV, E. L., AND J. P. FINERTY. 1980. Vole population cycles; a case for kin-selection? Oecologia, 45:1–2.
CHRISTIAN, J. J. 1970. Social subordination, population density, and mammalian evolution. Science, 168:84–90.
CLARKE, J. R. 1955. Influence of numbers on reproduction and survival in two experimental vole populations. Proc. Royal Soc. London, Ser. B, 144: 68–85.
COCKBURN, A., AND W. Z. LIDICKER, JR. 1983. Microhabitat heterogeneity and population ecology of an herbivorous rodent, *Microtus californicus*. Oecologia, 59:167–177.
DUESER, R. D., M. L. WILSON, AND R. K. ROSE. 1981. Attributes of dispersing meadow voles in open-grid populations. Acta Theriol., 26:139–162.
FRANK, F. 1954. Beiträge zur Biologie der Feldmaus, *Microtus arvalis* (Pallas). I. Gehegeversuche. Zool. Jahrb. (Abteil. Syst., Ökol. u. Geog. der Tiere), 82:354–404.
FULK, G. W. 1972. The effect of shrews on the space utilization of voles. J. Mamm., 53:461–478.
GAINES, M. S., AND L. R. MCCLENAGHAN, JR. 1980. Dispersal in small mammals. Ann. Rev. Ecol. Syst., 11:163–196.
GAINES, M. S., A. M. VIVAS, AND C. L. BAKER. 1979. An experimental analysis of dispersal in fluctuating vole populations: demographic parameters. Ecology, 60:814–828.
GARSD, A., AND W. E. HOWARD. 1981. A 19-year study of microtine population fluctuations using time-series analysis. Ecology, 62:930–937.

———. 1982. Microtine population fluctuations: an ecosystem approach based on time-series analysis. J. Anim. Ecol., 51:225–234.

GARTEN, C. T., JR. 1977. Relationships between exploratory behaviour and genic heterozygosity in the oldfield mouse. Anim. Behav., 25:328–332.

GENTRY, J. B. 1968. Dynamics of an enclosed population of pine mice, *Microtus pinetorum*. Res. Population Ecol., 10:21–30.

GETZ, L. L. 1961. Home ranges, territoriality, and movements of the meadow vole. J. Mamm., 42:24–36.

———. 1972. Social structure and aggressive behavior in a population of *Microtus pennsylvanicus*. J. Mamm., 53:310–317.

GETZ, L. L., AND C. S. CARTER. 1980. Social organization in *Microtus ochrogaster* populations. The Biologist, 62:56–69.

GETZ, L. L., F. R. COLE, AND D. L. GATES. 1978. Use of interstate roadsides as dispersal routes by *Microtus pennsylvanicus*. J. Mamm., 50:208–212.

GLIWICZ, J. 1980. Island populations of rodents: their organization and functioning. Biol. Rev., 55:109–138.

GODFREY, G. K. 1954. Tracing field voles (*Microtus agrestis*) with a Geiger-Muller counter. Ecology, 35:5–10.

GRANT, P. R. 1971. The habitat preference of *Microtus pennsylvanicus,* and its relevance to the distribution of this species on islands. J. Mamm., 52:351–361.

GREENWOOD, P. J. 1980. Mating systems, philopatry and dispersal in birds and mammals. Anim. Behav., 28:1140–1162.

HAMILTON, W. D., AND R. M. MAY. 1977. Dispersal in stable habitats. Nature, 269:578–581.

HANSSON, L. 1977. Spatial dynamics of field voles Microtus agrestis in heterogeneous landscapes. Oikos, 29:539–544.

HATT, R. T. 1930. The biology of the voles of New York. Roosevelt Wildl. Bull., 5:505–623.

HESTBECK, J. B. 1982. Population regulation of cyclic mammals: the social fence hypothesis. Oikos, 39:157–163.

HILBORN, R. 1975. Similarities in dispersal tendency among siblings in four species of voles (*Microtus*). Ecology, 56:1221–1225.

HILBORN, R., AND C. J. KREBS. 1976. Fates of disappearing individuals in fluctuating populations of *Microtus townsendii*. Canadian J. Zool., 54:1507–1518.

HILBORN, R., J. A. REDFIELD, AND C. J. KREBS. 1976. On the reliability of enumeration for mark and recapture census of voles. Canadian J. Zool., 54:1019–1024.

HOULIHAN, R. T. 1963. The relationship of population density to endocrine and metabolic changes in the California vole Microtus californicus. Univ. California Publ. Zool., 65:327–362.

HOWARD, W. E. 1960. Innate and environmental dispersal of individual vertebrates. Amer. Midland Nat., 63:152–161.

JANNETT, F. J., JR. 1980. Social dynamics of the montane vole, *Microtus montanus,* as a paradigm. The Biologist, 62:3–19.

JOHNSTON, R. F. 1961. Population movements of birds. Condor, 63:386–389.

KEITH, T. P., AND R. H. TAMARIN. 1981. Genetic and demographic differences between dispersers and residents in cycling and noncycling vole populations. J. Mamm., 62:713–725.

KREBS, C. J. 1970. *Microtus* population biology: behavioral changes associated with the population cycle in *M. ochrogaster* and *M. pennsylvanicus*. Ecology, 51: 34–52.

———. 1978*a*. A review of the Chitty hypothesis of population regulation. Canadian J. Zool., 56:2463–2480.

———. 1978*b*. Aggression, dispersal, and cyclic changes in populations of small mammals. Pp. 49–60, *in* Aggression, dominance, and individual spacing (L. Krames, P. Pliner, and T. Alloway, eds.). Plenum Publ., New York, 173 pp.

———. 1979. Dispersal, spacing behaviour, and genetics in relation to population fluctuations in the vole *Microtus townsendii*. Fortschr. Zool., 25:61–77.

KREBS, C. J., AND J. H. MYERS. 1974. Population cycles in small mammals. Adv. Ecol. Res., 8:267–399.

KREBS, C. J., J. A. REDFIELD, AND M. J. TAITT. 1978. A pulsed-removal experiment on the vole *Microtus townsendii*. Canadian J. Zool., 56:2253–2262.

KREBS, C. J., B. L. KELLER, AND R. H. TAMARIN. 1969. *Microtus* population biology: demographic changes in fluctuating populations of *M. ochrogaster* and *M. pennsylvanicus* in southern Indiana. Ecology, 50:587–607.

KREBS, C. J., M. S. GAINES, B. L. KELLER, J. H. MYERS, AND R. H. TAMARIN. 1973. Population cycles in small rodents. Science, 179:35–41.

KREBS, C. J., ET AL. 1976. *Microtus* population biology: dispersal in fluctuating populations of *M. townsendii*. Canadian J. Zool., 54:79–95.

LEDUC, J., AND C. J. KREBS. 1975. Demographic consequences of artificial selection at the LAP locus in voles (*Microtus townsendii*). Canadian J. Zool, 53:1825–1840.

LIDICKER, W. Z., JR. 1962. Emigration as a possible mechanism permitting the regulation of population density below carrying capacity. Amer. Nat., 96: 29–33.

———. 1973. Regulation of numbers in an island population of the California vole, a problem in community dynamics. Ecol. Monogr., 43:271–302.

———. 1975. The role of dispersal in the demography of small mammals. Pp. 103–128, *in* Small mammals: their production and population dynamics (F. B. Golley, K. Petrusewicz, and L. Ryszkowski, eds.). Cambridge Univ. Press, London, 451 pp.

———. 1978. Regulation of numbers in small mammal populations, historical reflections and a synthesis. Pp. 122–141, *in* Populations of small mammals under natural conditions (D. P. Snyder, ed.). Spec. Publ. Ser., Pymatuning Lab. Ecol., Univ. Pittsburgh, 5:1–237.

———. 1979. Analysis of two freely-growing enclosed populations of the California vole. J. Mamm., 60:447–466.

———. 1980. The social biology of the California vole. The Biologist, 62:46–55.

———. In press. Population structuring as a factor in understanding microtine cycles. Acta Zool. Fennica.

LIDICKER, W. Z., JR., AND P. K. ANDERSON. 1962. Colonization of an island by *Microtus californicus*, analyzed on the basis of runway transects. J. Anim. Ecol., 31:503–517.

LIDICKER, W. Z., JR., AND R. L. CALDWELL. 1982. Dispersal and migration. Benchmark papers in ecology, Vol. 11 (F. B. Golley, ed.). Hutchinson and Ross Publ. Co., Stroudsburg, Pennsylvania, 311 pp.

LOUSCH, C. D. 1956. Adrenocortical activity in relation to the density and dynamics of three confined populations of *Microtus pennsylvanicus*. Ecology, 37:701–713.

LUDWIG, D. 1984. *Microtus richardsoni* microhabitat and life history. Pp. 319–331, *in* Winter ecology of small mammals (J. F. Merritt, ed.). Spec. Publ. Carnegie Mus. Nat. Hist., 10:1–380.

MACKIN-ROGALSKA, R. 1979. Elements of the spatial organization of a common vole population. Acta Theriol., 24:171–199.

MADISON, D. M. 1978. Movement indicators of reproductive events among female meadow voles as revealed by radiotelemetry. J. Mamm., 59:835–843.

———. 1980*a*. Movement types and weather correlates in free-ranging meadow voles. Pp. 34–42, *in* Proc. fourth eastern pine and meadow vole symp. (R. E. Byers, ed.). Hendersonville, North Carolina, 91 pp.

———. 1980*b*. Space use and social structure in meadow voles, *Microtus pennsylvanicus*. Behav. Ecol. Sociobiol., 7:65–71.

———. 1980*c*. An integrated view of the social biology of *Microtus pennsylvanicus*. The Biologist, 62:20–33.

———. 1981. The patterning of nest visitation by lactating meadow voles. J. Mamm., 62:389–391.

———. 1984. Group nesting and its ecological and evolutionary significance in overwintering microtine rodents. Pp. 267–274, *in* Winter ecology of small mammals (J. F. Merritt, ed.). Spec. Publ. Carnegie Mus. Nat. Hist., 10: 1–380.

McClenaghan, L. R., Jr., and M. S. Gaines. 1976. Density-dependent dispersal in *Sigmodon*: a critique. J. Mamm., 57:758–759.

Morris, R. D. 1969. Competitive exclusion between *Microtus* and *Clethrionomys* in the aspen parkland of Saskatchewan. J. Mamm., 50:291–301.

Myers, J. H., and C. J. Krebs. 1971. Genetic, behavioral, and reproductive attributes of dispersing field voles *Microtus pennsylvanicus* and *Microtus ochrogaster*. Ecol. Monogr., 41:53–78.

Myllymäki, A. 1977. Demographic mechanisms in the fluctuating populations of the field vole Microtus agrestis. Oikos, 29:468–493.

Nakano, T. 1981. Population regulation by dispersal over patchy environment. I. Regulation by the threshold dispersal. Res. Population Ecol., 23:1–18.

Pearson, O. P. 1960. Habits of *Microtus californicus* revealed by automatic photographic recorders. Ecol. Monogr., 30:231–249.

Pelikán, J. 1959. Bionomie hraboše polního. A. Stanoviště, sídliště a etologie. Pp. 80–100, *in* Hraboš polní, *Microtus arvalis* (J. Kratochvíl, ed.). Naklad., Cesk. Akad., Věd., Praha, 359 pp.

Pickering, J., L. L. Getz, and G. S. Whitt. 1974. An esterase phenotype correlated with dispersal in *Microtus*. Trans. Illinois State Acad. Sci., 67: 471–475.

Pokki, J. 1981. Distribution, demography and dispersal of the field vole, Microtus agrestis (L.), in the Tvarminne archipelago, Finland. Acta Zool. Fennica 164:1–48.

Rasmuson, B., M. Rasmuson, and J. Nygren. 1977. Genetically controlled differences between cycling and recycling populations of field vole (*Microtus agrestis*). Hereditas, 87:33–41.

Reich, L. M., and R. H. Tamarin. 1980. Trap use as an indicator of social behavior in mainland and island voles. Acta Theriol., 25:295–307.

Reich, L. M., K. M. Wood, B. E. Rothstein, and R. H. Tamarin. 1982. Aggressive behaviour of male *Microtus breweri* and its demographic implications. Anim. Behav., 30:117–122.

Richmond, M., and C. H. Conaway. 1969. Induced ovulation and oestrus in *Microtus ochrogaster*. J. Reprod. Fert., Suppl., 6:357–376.

Riewe, R. R. 1973. Habitat utilization by meadow voles, Microtus pennsylvanicus terranovae (Bangs, 1884) (Mammalia, Rodentia, Cricetidae), on the islands in Notre Dame Bay, Newfoundland, Canada. Saugetierk. Mitt., 21: 340–348.

Riggs, L. A. 1979. Experimental studies of dispersal in the California vole, *Microtus californicus*. Unpubl. Ph.D. dissert., Univ. California, Berkeley, 236 pp.

Rosenzweig, M. L., and Z. Abramsky. 1980. Microtine cycles: the role of habitat heterogeneity. Oikos, 34:141–146.

Smith, M. H., C. T. Garten, Jr., and P. R. Ramsey. 1975. Genic heterozygosity and population dynamics in small mammals. Pp. 85–102, *in* Isozymes, IV.

Genetics and evolution (C. L. Markert, ed.). Academic Press, New York, 965 pp.

Staples, P. P., and C. R. Terman. 1977. An experimental study of movement in natural populations of *Mus musculus, Microtus pennsylvanicus,* and *Microtus pinetorum.* Res. Population Ecol., 18:267–283.

Stenseth, N. C. 1977. On the importance of spatio-temporal heterogeneity for the population dynamics of rodents: towards a theoretical foundation of rodent control. Oikos, 29:545–552.

———. 1978. Demographic strategies in fluctuating populations of small rodents. Oecologia, 33:149–172.

———. 1980. Spatial heterogeneity and population stability: some evolutionary consequences. Oikos, 35:165–184.

Stenseth, N. C., L. Hansson, and A. Myllymäki. 1977. Population dynamics of the field vole (*Microtus agrestis* (L.)): a model. EPPO Bull., 7:371–384.

Stoddart, D. M. 1970. Individual range, dispersion and dispersal in a population of water voles (*Arvicola terrestris,* L.). J. Anim. Ecol., 39:403–425.

———. 1982. Does trap odour influence estimation of population size of the short-tailed vole, *Microtus agrestis*? J. Anim. Ecol., 51:375–386.

Tamarin, R. H. 1977. Dispersal in island and mainland voles. Ecology, 58:1044–1054.

———. 1978. Dispersal, population regulation, and K-selection in field mice. Amer. Nat., 112:545–555.

———. 1980. Dispersal and population regulation in rodents. Pp. 117–133, *in* Biosocial mechanisms of population regulation (M. N. Cohen, R. S. Malpass, and H. G. Klein, eds.). Yale Univ. Press, New Haven, Connecticut, 406 pp.

Tamarin, R. H, and C. J. Krebs. 1969. *Microtus* population biology: II. Genetic changes at the transferrin locus in fluctuating populations of two vole species. Evolution, 23:183–211.

Tamarin, R. H., L. M. Reich, and C. A. Moyer. 1984. Meadow vole cycles within fences. Canadian J. Zool., 62:1796–1804.

Tamarin, R. H., M. Sheridan, and C. K. Levy. 1983. Determining matrilineal kinship in natural populations of rodents using radionuclides. Canadian J. Zool., 61:271–274.

Tast, J. 1966. The root vole, *Microtus oeconomus* (Pallas), as an inhabitant of seasonally flooded land. Ann. Zool. Fennica, 3:127–171.

Turner, B. N., and S. L. Iverson. 1973. The annual cycle of aggression in male *Microtus pennyslvanicus,* and its relation to population parameters. Ecology, 54:967–981.

Turner, B. N., M. R. Perrin, and S. L. Iverson. 1975. Winter coexistence of voles in spruce forest: relevance of seasonal changes in aggression. Canadian J. Zool., 53:1004–1011.

Van Valen, L. 1971. Group selection and the evolution of dispersal. Evolution, 25:591–598.

Van Vleck, D. B. 1968. Movements of *Microtus pennsylvanicus* in relation to depopulated areas. J. Mamm., 49:92–103.

van Wijngaarden, A. 1960. The population dynamics of four confined populations of the continental vole *Microtus arvalis* (Pallas). R.I.V.O.N. Mededeling, 84:1–28.

Verner, L. 1979. The significance of dispersal in fluctuating populations of *Microtus ochrogaster* and *M. pennsylvanicus.* Unpubl. Ph.D. dissert., Univ. Illinois, Urbana, 86 pp.

Webster, A. B., and R. J. Brooks. 1981. Social behavior of *Microtus pennsylvanicus* in relation to seasonal changes in demography. J. Mamm., 62:738–751.

WIEGERT, R. G. 1972. Population dynamics of cotton rats (*Sigmodon hispidus*) and meadow voles (*Microtus pennsylvanicus*) in field enclosures in South Carolina. Bull. Georgia Acad. Sci., 30:103–110.

WILSON, D. S. 1975. A theory of group selection. Proc. Natl. Acad. Sci., 72:143–146.

———. 1977. Structured demes and the evolution of group-advantageous traits. Amer. Nat., 111:157–185.

WOLFF, J. O. 1980. Social organization of the taiga vole (*Microtus xanthognathus*). The Biologist, 62:34–45.

WOLFF, J. O., AND D. F. HOLLEMAN. 1978. Use of radioisotope labels to establish genetic relationships in free-ranging small mammals. J. Mamm., 59:859–860.

WOLFF, J. O., AND W. Z. LIDICKER, JR. 1980. Population ecology of the taiga vole, *Microtus xanthognathus,* in interior Alaska. Canadian J. Zool., 58: 1800–1812.

———. 1981. Communal winter nesting and food sharing in taiga voles. Behav. Ecol. Sociobiol., 9:237–240.

PARASITES

ROBERT M. TIMM

Abstract

THE objective of this review is to bring together and summarize the diverse literature on parasites of New World *Microtus,* to summarize life cycles of the ectoparasitic fauna, and to put the different groups of parasites into a biological perspective. The literature on parasites of *Microtus* contains over 485 primary references covering the 91-year period from 1894 to 1984. However, of the 26 species of New World *Microtus* now recognized, parasite data exist for only 16 species. Most of the data available are for six of the most widely distributed species, *Microtus californicus, M. longicaudus, M. montanus, M. ochrogaster, M. pennsylvanicus,* and *M. pinetorum.*

The ectoparasites on *Microtus* belong to the orders Acari (mites and ticks), Anoplura (suckling lice), Coleoptera (beetles), Diptera (flies), and Siphonaptera (fleas). Twelve families of mites are known from *Microtus.* These range in size from minute demodicids that live within hair follicles and sebaceous glands to the large, active laelapids. Very little work has been done on any of the mites with the exception of chiggers (family Trombiculidae). Most groups are in need of taxonomic revision. Chiggers have been intensively studied, both taxonomically and biologically, as they are of direct medical importance to man. Eighteen species of ticks have been reported from *Microtus.* Several species of ticks carried by *Microtus* are responsible for diseases that affect man, and the systematics and ecology of these vectors have received much attention. Only two species of sucking lice are true parasites of *Microtus,* although a few other species have been reported in the literature as being found on *Microtus.* The systematic relationships of the lice are well understood; however, little work has been done on their biology. Lice have been reported on only 12 species of *Microtus*; the absence of lice on several species (for example, *M. chrotorrhinus*) has not been explained. Parasitic beetles belonging to two families have been found only occasionally on *Microtus.* It is likely that they are regularly associated with *Microtus,* living primarily within the nest and hence seldom encountered. Two families of parasitic flies are known from *Microtus.* Both bot flies and flesh flies are uncommon parasites of *Microtus,* and if found in high numbers may have an adverse affect upon the host. Seventeen genera of fleas regularly parasitize *Microtus* in North America, and 26 other genera are reported as of accidental occurrence. A tremendous body of literature exists on the systematics and ecology of fleas, especially with respect to bubonic plague. However, little work has been undertaken on the effects of fleas or the diseases they transmit on *Microtus.* Most species of *Microtus* have several species of fleas; more than one species may be present on an individual host with additional species being restricted to the nest.

Endoparasites belong to the Acanthocephala, Cestoda, Nematoda, and Trematoda. Only two species of acanthocephalan have been found parasitizing *Microtus.* Several species of cestodes, nematodes, and trematodes have been reported from *Microtus,* and it is certain that this list will increase with additional study. A briefly annotated list of the endoparasites on New World *Microtus* is appended.

Introduction

Voles of the genus *Microtus* constitute one of the most widespread and intensively studied groups of mammals. However, of the species of *Microtus* now recognized from North America, parasites have been reported from only 16 species. This is not due to an absence of parasites, but rather reflects lack of study. Undoubtedly a diverse parasite fauna will be found on the remaining species of voles. Of the 16 species for which some parasite data exist, the vast majority of records are from six species, *M. californicus, M. longicaudus, M. montanus, M. ochrogaster, M. pennsylvanicus,* and *M. pinetorum.* The number of species of parasites recorded from a given vole species is a direct reflection of how well studied the host is. The extent of the host's geographic range can also affect the total number of parasite species as different parasites will occur in various habitats. Thus, widely distributed species like *M. pennsylvanicus* can be expected to have more species of parasites than a more restricted species. It is also possible that a single individual vole of a widely distributed species may harbor more species of parasites than an individual from a geographically restricted species. However, this remains to be tested. In spite of the volume of literature available on *Microtus,* we actually know very little about the biology of the parasites, and even less of the effects on their hosts.

The objective of this chapter is to bring together the literature on ectoparasites of New World *Microtus,* and to put the various groups of parasites into a biological perspective, rather than just provide a list of names. A list of endoparasite records is presented in Appendix A. Because more is known about the distribution and systematics of North American ticks, lice, and fleas parasitizing *Microtus,* each genus and species is discussed briefly. Since the systematics and ecology of the mites are less well known and there are so many more of them, mites are discussed by family. The discussions of each group of parasites vary considerably in content, reflecting the current state of knowledge of that particular parasite on *Microtus.* Brief, informative summaries of all the ectoparasites reported from *Microtus* are presented, with an emphasis on what is known about the biology of those species on *Microtus.* This chapter should also guide the reader to the primary literature and point out interesting and fruitful areas for future research.

References included are those to the primary literature; secondary listings of parasites from the various species of *Microtus* are generally not mentioned. No human-created experimental infections are included. Current scientific names for all species of parasites are used throughout. Synonymies are included within species lists for ticks, lice, and fleas. For synonymies of mites see the review paper of North American mites parasitizing mammals by Whitaker and Wilson (1974). Whitaker's (1968) review of parasites on *Peromyscus* provides an excellent summary on collecting and preserving parasites, and his (Whitaker, 1982) "Ectoparasites of mammals of Indiana" provides keys to many of the species dealt with here.

Mites

The largest group of ectoparasites of *Microtus* are the mites and ticks of the order Acari. At least 12 families of mites and dozens of species are known to parasitize New World *Microtus* and undoubtedly more will be found. The life cycle of a typical parasitic mite includes the following stages: egg, larva (a relatively inactive stage that often does not feed), protonymph (usually an active feeding stage), deutonymph (an active feeding stage), and adult. Some mites are ovoviviparous so that the egg stage and perhaps the larval stage are bypassed. Considerable morphological diversity is found within parasitic mites, ranging from the large active laelapids (about 1 mm in length) to the minute follicle-inhabiting mites with reduced or highly modified legs. There are numerous reports of mites on *Microtus*, but surprisingly little work has been done on the effects of these mites on their hosts. An excellent list, including synonymies, of North American mites found on mammals was published by Whitaker and Wilson (1974). Because of the diversity and complexity of parasitic mites, a brief summary is presented of the families known to be parasitic on *Microtus*.

Cheyletidae.—Cheyletids are a diverse group of mites including both parasitic species living in fur of the host and free-living predatory species. Parasitic forms feed on tissue fluids and usually occur in low numbers. They seldom cause much damage to the host although they can cause dermatitis. The group is in need of revision.

Demodicidae.—Demodicid mites are minute (0.1 to 0.4 mm in length), vermiform, and live within hair follicles, lymph nodes, and sebaceous glands. They are thought to be rigidly host specific. *Demodex* is often found within the meibomian glands of the eyelids. Severe infestations of *Demodex* cause the eyelids to be sealed shut in mice, a disease known as pseudoblepharitis simplex (lid sealing).

Ereynetidae.—Nasal mites are widely distributed in birds, but few species are known from mammals. Within the genus *Speleorodens* there is no active nymphal stage; the larva gives rise directly to the adult. They reside within the nasal mucosa and apparently ingest whole blood. The only transfer between hosts apparently occurs between parents and offspring. Three adult females and a single larva of *S. michigensis* were taken by Ford (1962) from a single *Microtus pennsylvanicus* in Michigan. A review of what little is known about the biology of these nasal mites is found in OConnor (1978). It is likely that nasal mites will be found on other species and populations of *Microtus*.

Glycyphagidae.—Adult glycyphagids are free-living inhabitants within nests of mammals where they probably feed on fungi. The deutonymphs are usually found only on the mammalian host, either as a parasite in hair follicles or externally phoretic. Spicka and OConnor (1980:474) reported 500–1,000 *Glycyphagus microti* on *Microtus pinetorum*, and stated that the deutonymphs "may serve two purposes: 1) to disperse the species by transferral from host to host and nest to nest, and 2) to relieve pressures of overpopulation in the nest."

Laelapidae.—Laelapids are a large group of both parasitic and free-living mites. Most of the large, active mites commonly observed on small mammals belong to this family, with both *Androlaelaps* and *Laelaps* being especially abundant on *Microtus*. Timm (1972*a*) reported 61 *Laelaps kochi* from an apparently healthy adult *M. pennsylvanicus* in Nebraska, which is an unusually high parasite load. Not all laelapids found on mammals are obligate parasites; many of the free-living forms are found as predators of other mites in mammal nests. *Haemogamasus ambulans,* a common parasitic mite on *Microtus,* is known to feed on a variety of substances in addition to blood. Some of the nominal species actually represent species complexes that have yet to be investigated adequately (i.e. *Androlaelaps fahrenholzi* and *Eulaelaps stabularis*). Several species of laelapids are known to transmit tularemia.

Listrophoridae.—Fur mites feed in hair follicles, and are often abundant on rodents. They cause loss of hair, dermatitis, and skin inflammation from scratching.

Macronyssidae.—Mesostigmatic mites of the genus *Ornithonyssus* are large obligatory blood feeders. In laboratory colonies they cause severe exsanguination in sucklings; however, they apparently cause little damage to healthy adult animals when found in moderate numbers. *Ornithonyssus bacoti* has been shown to transmit murine typhus. *O. bursa* is commonly known as the tropical fowl mite; the single report from *Microtus* may be accidental.

Myobiidae.—Fur mites live in the pelage of their hosts, feeding on interstitial fluids, and may be found in high numbers, but they apparently cause little damage. Adults, larval stages, and eggs are found attached to the base of hairs; the entire life cycle is spent on the host.

Myocoptidae.—Myocoptid fur mites feed on the surface of the skin by attaching to the proximal portion of the hair shaft, and may be very abundant. Damage to the host includes dermatitis, pruritus, and hair loss.

Psorergatidae.—Psorergatic mange mites are cutaneous and subcutaneous parasites on a wide variety of mammals. *Psorergates canadensis* was found on *Microtus pennsylvanicus* by Kok et al. (1971: 1243) "within the epidermis of the ear concha, causing hyperceratosis. In the hosts observed they seem to be a low-grade pathogen."

Psorergates simplex is known to cause subcutaneous cysts and ulcerous nodules in its hosts, and is an important parasite in laboratory colonies of mice.

Sarcoptidae.—Sarcoptic itch mites or scabies mites live in the skin and burrow in the upper layers. Sarcoptids usually do not cause pathologies. In a severe infestation in *Microtus californicus*, *Notoedres muris* was found to "invade the ears, eyelids, and nose as well as the feet, tail, and anal region" (Lavoipierre, 1964:10); Lidicker (1973) reported that the highest incidence on Brooks Island (California) occurred during the winter months.

Trombiculidae.—Larval trombiculid mites are known as chiggers, and are parasites on mammals, birds, reptiles, and amphibians. They are parasitic only in the larval stage; all post-larval stages are free-living. Chiggers show a broad range of host specificity, with many occurring on a large number of hosts, whereas others are restricted to very few hosts. They are often associated with particular soil or habitat types rather than specific hosts. The larvae inject saliva into the host and feed on partly digested fluids; nymphs and adults are predaceous on small arthropods or arthropod eggs. Trombiculid mites have a complex life cycle that includes four major stages: the egg, larva, nymph, and adult; there are three intervening inactive stages (see Table 1). Population levels of chiggers on rodents vary considerably, but there is seldom much damage to the host. The site of attachment is often clustered, especially on the ears and genitalia. Attached larvae are generally orange or red in color, and usually feed on a host for just a few days. Within the north temperate zone most species have one generation per year and a distinct seasonal pattern of abundance, with late summer and fall peaks being typical. *Eutrombicula alfreddugesi*, a common chigger on both man and *Microtus*, is known to have a single generation per year in the northern part of its range, and several generations per year in the south. Chiggers are responsible for the transmission of several rickettsial diseases, including scrub typhus. Additionally, dermatitis may be produced as a result of the salivary secretions of the feeding mite. A tremendous body of literature exists on the ecology and systematics of chiggers since they are of direct medical importance to humans. Keys and synopses to the various groups of North American chiggers were provided by Brennan and Goff (1977), Brennan and Jones (1959), Gould (1956), Jenkins (1949), Kardos (1954), Loomis (1956), and Wharton and Fuller (1952).

TABLE 1
LIFE CYCLE OF *Eutrombicula alfreddugesi* (AFTER WOLFENBARGER, 1952)

Major stages	Intervening stages	Characteristic features	Duration (days)
Egg		Spherical, laid singly	15–20
	Deutovum	Quiescent, within broken egg shell, unsegmented appendages	(minimum 13)
Larva		Active, six segmented legs	Up to 24 before feeding (over 30) 1–4 on host (1–48) 1–8 after leaving host (average 2)
	Prenympha	Quiescent, within dead larval integument	9–10 (about 6)
Nymph		Active with eight legs, two pairs of genital suckers	12–32 (minimum 7)
	Preadult	Quiescent, within nymphal integument	5–10 (minimum 7)
Adult		Active, with eight legs, three pairs of genital suckers	Up to 52 (over 20 months) Eggs laid within 14 (12)

Ecological studies of chiggers in the midwest were conducted by Kardos (1954) and Loomis (1956).

The records of mites parasitizing *Microtus* are as follows:

Microtus abbreviatus
Laelapidae
Haemogamasus ambulans (Thorell, 1872) (Rausch and Rausch, 1968 [reported as *H. alaskensis* Ewing])
Laelaps clethrionomydis Lange, 1955 (Rausch and Rausch, 1968)
Laelaps kochi Oudemans, 1836 (Rausch and Rausch, 1968)
Microtus breweri
Laelapidae
Androlaelaps fahrenholzi (Berlese, 1911) (Strandtmann, 1949)
Laelaps kochi Oudemans, 1836 (Winchell, 1977)
Microtus californicus
Laelapidae
Androlaelaps fahrenholzi (Berlese, 1911) (Holdenried et al., 1951; Jameson, 1947; Strandtmann, 1949)

Haemogamasus ambulans (Thorell, 1872) (Furman, 1959*a*, 1959*b*; Holdenried et al., 1951; Keegan, 1951)
Haemogamasus liponyssoides Ewing, 1925 (Furman, 1959*a*; Holdenried et al., 1951; Radovsky, 1960*a*, 1960*b*)
Haemogamasus reidi Ewing, 1925 (Keegan, 1951; Redington, 1971)
Laelaps kochi Oudemans, 1836 (Evans and Till, 1966; Ewing, 1933; Grant, 1947; Holdenried et al., 1951; Jameson, 1947)
Sarcoptidae
Notoedres muris Mégnin, 1877 (Lavoipierre, 1964; Lidicker, 1973)
Trombiculidae
Acomatacarus hirsutus (Ewing, 1931) (Brennan and Jones, 1954)
Euschoengastia ambocalis Wrenn and Loomis, 1973 (original description)
Euschoengastia criceticola Brennan, 1948 (Brennan and Jones, 1954; Gould, 1956)
Euschoengastia oregonensis (Ewing, 1929) (Gould, 1956)
Euschoengastia peromysci (Ewing, 1929) (Gould, 1956)
Euschoengastia pomerantzi Brennan and Jones, 1954 (original description)
Euschoengastia radfordi Brennan and Jones, 1954 (original description)
Neotrombicula californica (Ewing, 1942) (Brennan and Jones, 1954; Ewing, 1942; Gould, 1956; Holdenried et al., 1951)
Neotrombicula cavicola (Ewing, 1931) (Gould, 1956)
Neotrombicula dinehartae (Brennan and Wharton, 1950) (Brennan and Jones, 1954)
Neotrombicula jewetti (Brennan and Wharton, 1950) (Brennan and Jones, 1954)
Odontacarus hirsutus (Ewing, 1931) (Brennan and Jones, 1954)
Walchia americana (Ewing, 1942) (Brennan and Jones, 1954)

Microtus chrotorrhinus
Glycyphagidae
Glycyphagus hypudaei (Koch, 1841) (Whitaker and French, 1982)
Glycyphagus sp. (*hypudaei* group) (Kirkland and Jannett, 1982)
Orycteroxenus canadensis Fain, Kok, Lukoschus, and Clulow, 1971 (Whitaker and French, 1982)
Orycteroxenus soricis (Oudemans, 1915) (Whitaker and French, 1982)
Laelapidae
Androlaelaps fahrenholzi (Berlese, 1911) (Timm, pers. observ.; Whitaker and French, 1982)
Echinonyssus isabellinus (Oudemans, 1913) (Whitaker and French, 1982)
Eulaelaps stabularis (Koch, 1836) (Whitaker and French, 1982)
Haemogamasus ambulans (Thorell, 1872) (Martin, 1972; Timm et al., 1977; Whitaker and French, 1982)
Haemogamasus liponyssoides Ewing, 1925 (Whitaker and French, 1982)
Laelaps alaskensis Grant, 1947 (Kirkland and Jannett, 1982; Martin, 1972; Timm, 1974, 1975; Tipton, 1960; Whitaker and French, 1982)
Laelaps kochi Oudemans, 1836 (Kirkland and Jannett, 1982; Komarek and Komarek, 1938; Linzey and Linzey, 1973; Timm, 1974, 1975; Timm et al., 1977; Tipton, 1960; Whitaker and French, 1982)
Listrophoridae
Listrophorus mexicanus Fain and Hyland, 1972 (Whitaker and French, 1982)
Listrophorus squamiferus Fain and Hyland, 1972 (Kirkland and Jannett, 1982)

Myobiidae
Radfordia hylandi Fain and Lukoschus, 1977 (Whitaker and French, 1982)
Radfordia sp. (Kirkland and Jannett, 1982; Whitaker and French, 1982)
Myocoptidae
Myocoptes canadensis Radford, 1955 (Kirkland and Jannett, 1982)
Myocoptes japonensis Radford, 1955 (Whitaker and French, 1982)
Myocoptes squamosus Fain, Munting, and Lukoschus, 1969 (Whitaker and French, 1982)
Trichoecius tenax (Michael, 1889) (Whitaker and French, 1982)
Trichoecius sp. (Kirkland and Jannett, 1982; Whitaker and French, 1982)
Trombiculidae
Euschoengastia blarinae (Ewing, 1931) (Whitaker and French, 1982)
Euschoengastia peromysci (Ewing, 1929) (Farrell, 1956; Komarek and Komarek, 1938)
Euschoengastia setosa (Ewing, 1937) (Whitaker and French, 1982)
Miyatrombicula esoensis (Sasa and Ogata, 1953) (Whitaker and French, 1982)
Neotromibucla harperi (Ewing, 1928) (Kirkland and Jannett, 1982; Martin, 1972?; Timm et al., 1977; Whitaker and French, 1982)
Neotrombicula microti (Ewing, 1928) (Buech et al., 1977; Timm et al., 1977)

Microtus longicaudus
Laelapidae
Androlaelaps fahrenholzi (Berlese, 1911) (Allred and Beck, 1966; Augustson, 1941*b*; Hansen, 1964; Whitaker and Maser, 1984)
Echinonyssus incomptis (Eads and Hightower, 1952) (Allred and Beck, 1966)
Echinonyssus isabellinus (Oudemans, 1913) (Allred and Beck, 1966; Hansen, 1964; Herrin, 1970; Jameson and Brennan, 1957; Kinsella and Pattie, 1967)
Eubrachylaelaps debilis Jameson, 1950 (Allred and Beck, 1966; Furman, 1955)
Eulaelaps stabularis (Koch, 1836) (Whitaker and Maser, 1984)
Haemogamasus ambulans (Thorell, 1872) (Allred and Beck, 1966; Hansen, 1964; Jameson and Brennan, 1957)
Haemogamasus liponyssoides Ewing, 1925 (Allred and Beck, 1966; Augustson, 1941*b*; Hansen, 1964; Jameson and Brennan, 1957)
Haemogamasus longitarsus (Banks, 1910) (Allred and Beck, 1966)
Haemogamasus occidentalis (Keegan, 1951) (Allred and Beck, 1966; Whitaker and Maser, 1984)
Haemogamasus reidi Ewing, 1925 (Allred and Beck, 1966; Hansen, 1964; Jameson and Brennan, 1957; Redington, 1971; Whitaker and Maser, 1984)
Laelaps alaskensis Grant, 1947 (Jameson and Brennan, 1957)
Laelaps incilis Allred and Beck, 1966 (original description)
Laelaps kochi Oudemans, 1836 (Allred and Beck, 1966; Augustson, 1941*b*; Hansen, 1964; Jameson and Brennan, 1957; Whitaker and Maser, 1984)
Trombiculidae
Chatia ochotona (Radford, 1942) (Gould, 1956; Traub and Nadchatram, 1966)
Euschoengastia oregonensis (Ewing, 1929) (Allred and Beck, 1966)
Euschoengastia peromysci (Ewing, 1929) (Jameson and Brennan, 1957)

Euschoengastia radfordi Brennan and Jones, 1954 (Jameson and Brennan, 1957)
Leptotrombidium potosina Hoffmann, 1950 (Brennan and Beck, 1955)
Neotrombicula browni (Brennan and Wharton, 1950) (Brennan and Wharton, 1950 [original description]; Kardos, 1954; Radford, 1954; Wharton and Fuller, 1952)
Neotrombicula californica (Ewing, 1942) (Brennan and Beck, 1955)
Neotrombicula harperi (Ewing, 1928) (Allred and Beck, 1966; Brennan and Beck, 1955; Brennan and Wharton, 1950; Kardos, 1954; Wharton and Fuller, 1952)
Neotrombicula jewetti (Brennan and Wharton, 1950) (Brennan and Wharton, 1950 [original description]; Jameson and Brennan, 1957; Radford, 1954; Wharton and Fuller, 1952)
Neotrombicula microti (Ewing, 1928) (Brennan and Beck, 1955; Kardos, 1954)

Microtus mexicanus
Laelapidae
Androlaelaps fahrenholzi (Berlese, 1911) (Allred and Beck, 1966; Bassols, 1981)
Echinonyssus breviseta Strandtmann and Morlan, 1953 (Bassols, 1981)
Echinonyssus utahensis Allred and Beck, 1966 (Hoffman et al., 1972)
Haemogamasus ambulans (Thorell, 1872) (Bassols, 1981)
Haemogamasus reidi Ewing, 1925 (Redington, 1971)
Laelaps kochi Oudemans, 1836 (Bassols, 1981)
Listrophoridae
Listrophorus mexicanus Fain, 1970 (Fain and Hyland, 1974)
Myobiidae
Radfordia hylandi Fain and Lukoschus, 1977 (original description)
Trombiculidae
Neotrombicula microti (Ewing, 1928) (Brennan and Wharton, 1950; Wharton and Fuller, 1952)

Microtus montanus
Glycyphagidae
Glycyphagus hypudaei (Koch, 1841) (Whitaker and Maser, 1984)
Laelapidae
Androlaelaps fahrenholzi (Berlese, 1911) (Allred, 1970; Allred and Beck, 1966; Augustson, 1941*b*; Hansen, 1964; Kartman et al., 1958*b*; Strandtmann, 1949; Whitaker and Maser, 1984)
Brevisterna utahensis (Ewing, 1933) (Kartman et al., 1958*b*)
Echinonyssus isabellinus (Oudemans, 1913) (Allred, 1970; Allred and Beck, 1966; Hansen, 1964; Herrin, 1970; Kinsella and Pattie, 1967; Whitaker and Maser, 1984)
Echinonyssus occidentalis (Ewing, 1923) (Augustson, 1941*b*)
Eubrachylaelaps croweri Jameson, 1947 (Hansen, 1964)
Eubrachylaelaps debilis Jameson, 1950 (Whitaker and Maser, 1984)
Eulaelaps stabularis (Koch, 1836) (Hansen, 1964; Whitaker and Maser, 1984)
Haemogamasus ambulans (Thorell, 1872) (Allred and Beck, 1966; Hansen, 1964; Keegan, 1951)
Haemogamasus liponyssoides Ewing, 1925 (Augustson, 1941*b*; Hansen, 1964)
Haemogamasus occidentalis (Keegan, 1951) (Whitaker and Maser, 1984)

Haemogamasus reidi Ewing, 1925 (Augustson, 1941*b*; Whitaker and Maser, 1984)
Ischyropoda armatus Keegan, 1951 (Allred, 1970)
Laelaps alaskensis Grant, 1947 (Hansen, 1964; Kartman et al., 1958*b*; Kinsella and Pattie, 1967; Whitaker and Maser, 1984)
Laelaps incilis Allred and Beck, 1966 (original description)
Laelaps kochi Oudemans, 1836 (Allred and Beck, 1966; Augustson, 1941*b*; Hansen, 1964; Kartman et al., 1958*b*; Kinsella and Pattie, 1967; Tipton, 1960; Whitaker and Maser, 1984)

Listrophoridae
Listrophorus mexicanus Fain, 1970 (Whitaker and Maser, 1984)

Psorergatidae
Psorergates townsendi Giesen, Lukoschus, Whitaker, and Gettinger, 1983 (original description and type-host)

Trombiculidae
Comatacarus americanus Ewing, 1942 (Easton, 1975)
Neotrombicula californica (Ewing, 1942) (Gould, 1956)
Neotrombicula cavicola (Ewing, 1931) (Easton, 1975)
Neotrombicula harperi (Ewing, 1928) (Allred and Beck, 1966; Easton, 1975; Kardos, 1954)
Neotrombicula microti (Ewing, 1928) (Kardos, 1954; Kinsella and Pattie, 1967)

Microtus ochrogaster

Glycyphagidae
Glycyphagus hypudaei (Koch, 1841) (Basolo and Funk, 1974; Buckner and Gleason, 1974; Fain and Whitaker, 1973; McDaniel, 1979; Mumford and Whitaker, 1982; Rupes and Whitaker, 1968; Turner, 1974; Whitaker and Wilson, 1968)
Orycteroxenus soricis (Oudemans, 1915) (Mumford and Whitaker, 1982)

Laelapidae
Androlaelaps fahrenholzi (Berlese, 1911) (Amin, 1973, 1976*b*; Basolo and Funk, 1974; Batson, 1965; Buckner and Gleason, 1974; Jameson, 1947; Mumford and Whitaker, 1982; Rapp, 1962; Strandtmann, 1949; Timm, 1972*b*; Turner, 1974; Whitaker and Wilson, 1968)
Echinonyssus utahensis Allred and Beck, 1966 (Timm, 1972*b*)
Eulaelaps stabularis (Koch, 1836) (Batson, 1965; Jameson, 1947; Mumford and Whitaker, 1982; Whitaker and Wilson, 1968)
Haemogamasus ambulans (Thorell, 1872) (Turner, 1974)
Haemogamasus liponyssoides Ewing, 1925 (Keegan, 1951; Mumford and Whitaker, 1982; Whitaker and Wilson, 1968; Wilson, 1957 [reported as *H. barberi* Ewing])
Laelaps alaskensis Grant, 1947 (Mumford and Whitaker, 1982; Whitaker and Wilson, 1968)
Laelaps kochi Oudemans, 1836 (Basolo and Funk, 1974; Buckner and Gleason, 1974; Jameson, 1947; Mumford and Whitaker, 1982; Rapp, 1962; Timm, 1972*b*; Tipton, 1960; Turner, 1974; Whitaker and Wilson, 1968; Wilson, 1957)

Listrophoridae
Listrophorus mexicanus Fain, 1970 (Basolo and Funk, 1974; Buckner and Gleason, 1974 [reported as *L. leuckarti*]; Mumford and Whitaker, 1982)
Listrophorus sp. (Jameson, 1947)

Macronyssidae

Ornithonyssus bacoti (Hirst, 1913) (Buckner and Gleason, 1974; Mumford and Whitaker, 1982; Turner, 1974)

Myobiidae

Radfordia ensifera (Poppe, 1896) (Manischewitz, 1966)

Radfordia hylandi Fain and Lukoschus, 1977 (Mumford and Whitaker, 1982)

Radfordia lemnina (Koch, 1841) (Basolo and Funk, 1974; Buckner and Gleason, 1974; Whitaker and Wilson, 1968)

Myocoptidae

Myocoptes japonensis Radford, 1955 (Basolo and Funk, 1974)

Myocoptes musculinus (Koch, 1844) (Basolo and Funk, 1974; McDaniel, 1979; Mumford and Whitaker, 1982; Turner, 1974; Whitaker and Wilson, 1968)

Myocoptes sp. (Basolo and Funk, 1974; Buckner and Gleason, 1974; Jameson, 1947)

Trichoecius tenax (Michael, 1889) (Mumford and Whitaker, 1982)

Trombiculidae

Euschoengastia diversa Farrell, 1956 (Farrell, 1956 [original description]; Loomis, 1956)

Euschoengastia peromysci (Ewing, 1929) (Basolo and Funk, 1974; Jameson, 1947 [reported as *Ascoschöngastia breviceps*]; Loomis, 1956)

Euschoengastia setosa (Ewing, 1937) (Lampe et al., 1974; Mumford and Whitaker, 1982; Turner, 1974; Whitaker and Loomis, 1979)

Euschoengastia trigenuala Farrell, 1956 (Loomis, 1956)

Eutrombicula alfreddugesi (Oudemans, 1910) (Loomis, 1956; Mumford and Whitaker, 1982; Turner, 1974; Whitaker and Loomis, 1979; Wolfenbarger, 1952)

Eutrombicula lipovskyana Wolfenbarger, 1952 (Loomis, 1956; Wolfenbarger, 1952 [original description])

Eutrombicula lipovskyi (Brennan and Wharton, 1950) (Kardos, 1954; Loomis, 1956)

Neotrombicula autumnalis (Shaw, 1790) (Kardos, 1954; Loomis, 1956)

Neotrombicula sylvilagi (Brennan and Wharton, 1950) (Kardos, 1954; Loomis, 1956)

Neotrombicula whartoni (Ewing, 1929) (Basolo and Funk, 1974; Kardos, 1954; Loomis, 1956; Mumford and Whitaker, 1982; Whitaker and Loomis, 1979)

Pseudoschongastia hungerfordi Lipovsky, 1951 (Loomis, 1956)

Microtus oeconomus

Laelapidae

Androlaelaps fahrenholzi (Berlese, 1911) (Strandtmann and Wharton, 1958)

Echinonyssus isabellinus (Oudemans, 1913) (Strandtmann and Wharton, 1958)

Eulaelaps stabularis (Koch, 1836) (Strandtmann and Wharton, 1958)

Haemogamasus reidi Ewing, 1925 (Keegan, 1951)

Laelaps kochi Oudemans, 1836 (Strandtmann and Wharton, 1958)

Myobiidae

Radfordia lemnina (Koch, 1841) (Fain and Lukoschus, 1977)

Microtus oregoni
Glycyphagidae
Dermacarus ondatrae Rupes and Whitaker, 1968 (Whitaker and Maser, 1984)
Glycyphagus hypudaei (Koch, 1841) (Whitaker and Maser, 1984)
Laelapidae
Androlaelaps fahrenholzi (Berlese, 1911) (Strandtmann, 1949; Whitaker and Maser, 1984)
Eulaelaps stabularis (Koch, 1836) (Whitaker and Maser, 1984)
Haemogamasus ambulans (Thorell, 1872) (Keegan, 1951)
Haemogamasus occidentalis (Keegan, 1951) (Whitaker and Maser, 1984)
Laelaps kochi Oudemans, 1836 (Whitaker and Maser, 1984)
Listrophoridae
Listrophorus mexicanus Fain, 1970 (Whitaker and Maser, 1984)
Myobiidae
Radfordia hylandi Fain and Lukoschus, 1977 (Whitaker and Maser, 1984)
Trombiculidae
Euschoengastia oregonensis (Ewing, 1929) (Easton, 1975)
Neotrombicula cavicola (Ewing, 1931) (Brennan and Wharton, 1950; Easton, 1975; Wharton and Fuller, 1952)
Neotrombicula harperi (Ewing, 1928) (Easton, 1975)
Microtus pennsylvanicus
Demodicidae
Demodex sp. (Nutting and Desch, 1979)
Dermanyssidae
Dermanyssus sp. (Drummond, 1957)
Ereynetidae
Speleorodens michigensis Ford, 1962 (original description and type-host)
Glycyphagidae
Dermacarus newyorkensis Fain, 1969 (Fain, 1969*a* [original description and type-host], 1969*b*; Rupes and Whitaker, 1968)
Glycyphagus hypudaei (Koch, 1841) (Fain, 1969*b*; Mumford and Whitaker, 1982; Rupes and Whitaker, 1968; Whitaker and French, 1982; Whitaker and Wilson, 1968)
Glycyphagus microti Spicka and OConnor, 1980 (original description)
Orycteroxenus soricis (Oudemans, 1915) (Fain, 1969*b*)
Laelapidae
Androlaelaps fahrenholzi (Berlese, 1911) (Allred and Beck, 1966; Amin, 1973, 1976*b*; Baker, 1946; Drummond, 1957; Florschutz and Darsie, 1960; Genoways and Jones, 1972; Harper, 1961; Jameson, 1947; Judd, 1950, 1953; Lawrence et al., 1965; MacCreary, 1945*a*; Mellott and Connell, 1965; Mumford and Whitaker, 1982; Strandtmann, 1949; Timm, 1972*a*, 1972*b*, 1975; Turner, 1974; Whitaker and French, 1982; Whitaker and Wilson, 1968; Wilson, 1967)
Androlaelaps sp. (Wright, 1979)
Echinonyssus carnifex Koch, 1839 (Lawrence et al., 1965)
Echinonyssus isabellinus (Oudemans, 1913) (Allred and Beck, 1966; Harper, 1961; Herrin, 1970; Timm, 1972*a*, 1972*b*, 1975; Whitaker and French, 1982)

Echinonyssus sp. (Amin, 1976*b*; Genoways and Jones, 1972; Scholten et al., 1962; Wright, 1979)
Eulaelaps stabularis (Koch, 1836) (Drummond, 1957; Genoways and Jones, 1972; Lawrence et al., 1965; Timm, 1975; Wilson, 1967; Wright, 1979)
Haemogamasus ambulans (Thorell, 1872) (Drummond, 1957; Harper, 1956, 1961; Keegan, 1951; Lawrence et al., 1965; Timm, 1975; Whitaker and French, 1982)
Haemogamasus liponyssoides Ewing, 1925 (Drummond, 1957; Keegan, 1951; Lawrence et al., 1965; MacCreary, 1945*a*; Mellott and Connell, 1965; Mumford and Whitaker, 1982; Timm, 1975)
Haemogamasus longitarsus (Banks, 1910) (Ewing, 1925 [described as *H. microti*]; Keegan, 1951)
Laelaps alaskensis Grant, 1947 (Amin, 1973, 1976*b*; Drummond, 1957; Florschutz and Darsie, 1960; Harper, 1956, 1961; Lawrence et al., 1965; Mellott and Connell, 1965; Mumford and Whitaker, 1982; Timm, 1975; Whitaker and French, 1982; Whitaker and Wilson, 1968; Wilson, 1967)
Laelaps kochi Oudemans, 1836 (Allred and Beck, 1966; Amin, 1973, 1976*b*; Baker, 1946; Drummond, 1957; Florschutz and Darsie, 1960; Genoways and Jones, 1972; Harper, 1956, 1961; Jameson, 1947; Judd, 1950, 1953, 1954; Lampe et al., 1974; Lawrence et al., 1965; MacCreary, 1945*a*; Mellott and Connell, 1965; Mumford and Whitaker, 1982; Scholten et al., 1962; Shoemaker and Joy, 1967; Timm, 1972*a*, 1972*b*, 1975; Tipton, 1960; Turner, 1974; Whitaker and French, 1982; Whitaker and Wilson, 1968)
Laelaps multispinosa (Banks, 1910) (Lawrence et al., 1965)
Laelaps muris (Ljungh, 1799) (Judd, 1950, 1953, 1954)

Listrophoridae
Listrophorus mexicanus Fain, 1970 (McDaniel et al., 1967; Mumford and Whitaker, 1982; Whitaker and French, 1982; Whitaker and Wilson, 1968 [reported as *L. leuckarti*])
Listrophorus pitymys Fain and Hyland, 1972 (Fain and Hyland, 1974)
Listrophorus squamiferus Fain and Hyland, 1972 (Fain and Hyland, 1974; McDaniel et al., 1967 [reported as *L. leuckarti*])
Listrophorus sp. (Drummond, 1957)

Macronyssidae
Ornithonyssus bacoti (Hirst, 1913) (Drummond, 1957; Mumford and Whitaker, 1982)
Ornithonyssus bursa (Berlese, 1888) (Drummond, 1957)

Myobiidae
Protomyobia brevisetosa Jameson, 1948 (Whitaker and French, 1982)
Protomyobia claparedei (Poppe, 1896) (Manischewitz, 1966)
Radfordia ensifera (Poppe, 1896) (Manischewitz, 1966)
Radfordia hylandi Fain and Lukoschus, 1977 (Fain and Lukoschus, 1977 [original description]; Mumford and Whitaker, 1982; Whitaker and French, 1982)
Radfordia lemnina (Koch, 1841) (Drummond, 1957; Ewing, 1938; Manischewitz, 1966)

Myocoptidae

Myocoptes japonensis Radford, 1955 (Fain and Hyland, 1970; Fain et al., 1970; Mumford and Whitaker, 1982; Radford, 1955 [originally described as *M. jamesoni*]; Whitaker and French, 1982)

Myocoptes musculinus (Koch, 1844) (Harper, 1956; McDaniel, 1979)

Myocoptes squamosus Fain, Munting, and Lukoschus, 1969 (Fain and Hyland, 1970; Whitaker and French, 1982)

Myocoptes sp. (Drummond, 1957)

Trichoecius tenax (Michael, 1889) (Fain and Hyland, 1970; Fain et al., 1970; Whitaker and French, 1982)

Psorergatidae

Psorergates canadensis Kok, Lukoschus, and Clulow, 1971 (original description and type-host)

Psorergates simplex Tyrrell, 1883 (Lee and Horvath, 1969)

Trombiculidae

Euschoengastia diversa Farrell, 1956 (original description)

Euschoengastia peromysci (Ewing, 1929) (Farrell, 1956; MacCreary, 1945*a* [reported as *Neoschöngastia breviceps*]; Manischewitz, 1966; Mumford and Whitaker, 1982; Whitaker and Loomis, 1979)

Euschoengastia setosa (Ewing, 1937) (Turner, 1974)

Euschoengastia sp. (Drummond, 1957; Wilson, 1967)

Eutrombicula alfreddugesi (Oudemans, 1910) (Ewing, 1944; Jenkins, 1949; MacCreary, 1945*a* [reported as *E. tropica*]; Mumford and Whitaker, 1982; Wharton and Fuller, 1952; Whitaker and Loomis, 1979)

Eutrombicula splendens (Ewing, 1913) (Wharton and Fuller, 1952)

Eutrombicula sp. (Wright, 1979)

Miyatrombicula esoensis (Sasa and Ogata, 1953) (Whitaker and French, 1982)

Neotrombicula autumnalis (Shaw, 1790) (Kardos, 1954; Loomis, 1956)

Neotrombicula bisignata (Ewing, 1929) (Brennan and Wharton, 1950; Ewing, 1929*a* [original description and type-host]; Radford, 1954; Wharton and Fuller, 1952)

Neotrombicula goodpasteri (Brennan and Wharton, 1950) (Brennan and Wharton, 1950 [original description]; Radford, 1954; Wharton and Fuller, 1952)

Neotrombicula harperi (Ewing, 1928) (Brennan and Wharton, 1950; Harper, 1929; Lawrence et al., 1965; Manville, 1949; Timm, pers. observ.; Wharton and Fuller, 1952; Whitaker and French, 1982)

Neotrombicula lipovskyi (Brennan and Wharton, 1950) (Mumford and Whitaker, 1982; Whitaker and Loomis, 1979)

Neotrombicula microti (Ewing, 1928) (Baker, 1946; Brennan and Wharton, 1950; Ewing, 1928; Lawrence et al., 1965; Timm, pers. observ.; Wharton and Fuller, 1952)

Neotrombicula richmondi (Brennan and Wharton, 1950) (Brennan and Wharton, 1950 [original description]; Radford, 1954; Wharton and Fuller, 1952)

Neotrombicula subsignata (Brennan and Wharton, 1950) (Brennan and Wharton, 1950 [original description and type-host]; Genoways and Jones, 1972; Kardos, 1954; Radford, 1954; Wharton and Fuller, 1952)

Neotrombicula whartoni (Ewing, 1929) (Brennan and Wharton, 1950; Drummond, 1957; Farrell, 1956; Kardos, 1954; MacCreary, 1945*a*; Manischewitz, 1966; Mumford and Whitaker, 1982; Wharton and Fuller, 1952; Whitaker and Loomis, 1979)
Neotrombicula sp. (Manville, 1949)

Microtus pinetorum

Cheyletidae

Eucheyletia bishoppi Baker, 1949 (original description)

Glycyphagidae

Dermacarus sp. (Benton, 1955*a*)
Glycyphagus hypudaei (Koch, 1841) (Fain, 1969*b*; Fain and Whitaker, 1973; Mumford and Whitaker, 1982)
Glycyphagus microti Spicka and OConnor, 1980 (original description and type-host)
Orycteroxenus soricis (Oudemans, 1915) (Fain and Whitaker, 1973)

Laelapidae

Androlaelaps fahrenholzi (Berlese, 1911) (Benton, 1955*a*; Drummond, 1957; Ellis, 1955; Hays and Guyton, 1958; Jameson, 1947; Judd, 1950; MacCreary, 1945*a*; Mellott and Connell, 1965; Morlan, 1952; Mumford and Whitaker, 1982; Strandtmann, 1949; Whitaker and Wilson, 1968)
Eulaelaps stabularis (Koch, 1836) (Jameson, 1947; Mumford and Whitaker, 1982; Whitaker and Wilson, 1968)
Haemogamasus ambulans (Thorell, 1872) (Keegan, 1951; Whitaker and Wilson, 1968)
Haemogamasus liponyssoides Ewing, 1925 (Drummond, 1957; Keegan, 1951; Morlan, 1952)
Haemogamasus longitarsus (Banks, 1910) (Drummond, 1957; Keegan, 1951; MacCreary, 1945*a*; Mellott and Connell, 1965; Mumford and Whitaker, 1982; Whitaker and Wilson, 1968; Wilson, 1957)
Laelaps alaskensis Grant, 1947 (Benton, 1955*a*; Mumford and Whitaker, 1982; Whitaker and Wilson, 1968)
Laelaps kochi Oudemans, 1836 (Drummond, 1957; Hamilton, 1938; Hays and Guyton, 1958; Mumford and Whitaker, 1982; Whitaker and Wilson, 1968)

Listrophoridae

Listrophorus pitymys Fain and Hyland, 1972 (Fain and Hyland, 1972 [original description], 1974)
Listrophorus sp. (Drummond, 1957)

Macronyssidae

Ornithonyssus bacoti (Hirst, 1913) (Mumford and Whitaker, 1982)

Myobiidae

Radfordia ensifera (Poppe, 1896) (Manischewitz, 1966)
Radfordia hylandi Fain and Lukoschus, 1977 (Fain and Lukoschus, 1977 [original description]; Mumford and Whitaker, 1982)
Radfordia lemnina (Koch, 1841) (Drummond, 1957; Manischewitz, 1966)

Myocoptidae

Myocoptes canadensis Radford, 1955 (Mumford and Whitaker, 1982)
Myocoptes musculinus (Koch, 1844) (Mumford and Whitaker, 1982)
Myocoptes sp. (Benton, 1955*a*; Drummond, 1957)

Psorergatidae
Psorergates pinetorum Giesen, Lukoschus, Whitaker, and Gettinger, 1983 (original description and type-host)
Trombiculidae
Euschoengastia carolinensis Farrell, 1956 (original description)
Euschoengastia diversa Farrell, 1956 (Loomis, 1956)
Euschoengastia ohioensis Farrell, 1956 (Farrell, 1956 [original description]; Mumford and Whitaker, 1982; Whitaker and Loomis, 1979)
Euschoengastia peromysci (Ewing, 1929) (Farrell, 1956; Manischewitz, 1966; Mumford and Whitaker, 1982; Whitaker and Loomis, 1979)
Eutrombicula alfreddugesi (Oudemans, 1910) (Wolfenbarger, 1952)
Leptotrombidium myotis (Ewing, 1929) (Loomis, 1956; Manischewitz, 1966)
Neotrombicula goodpasteri (Brennan and Wharton, 1950) (Brennan and Wharton, 1950 [original description]; Radford, 1954; Wharton and Fuller, 1952)
Neotrombicula lipovskyi (Brennan and Wharton, 1950) (Kardos, 1954; Loomis, 1956; Mumford and Whitaker, 1982; Whitaker and Loomis, 1979)
Neotrombicula microti (Ewing, 1928) (Kardos, 1954)
Neotrombicula whartoni (Ewing, 1929) (MacCreary, 1945*a*; Manischewitz, 1966)

Microtus richardsoni
Glycyphagidae
Glycyphagus hypudaei (Koch, 1841) (Whitaker and Maser, 1984)
Laelapidae
Androlaelaps fahrenholzi (Berlese, 1911) (Whitaker and Maser, 1984)
Echinonyssus isabellinus (Oudemans, 1913) (Kinsella and Pattie, 1967; Ludwig, 1984; Whitaker and Maser, 1984)
Haemogamasus ambulans (Thorell, 1872) (Kinsella and Pattie, 1967)
Haemogamasus liponyssoides Ewing, 1925 (Kinsella and Pattie, 1967)
Haemogamasus occidentalis (Keegan, 1951) (Whitaker and Maser, 1984)
Haemogamasus reidi Ewing, 1925 (Whitaker and Maser, 1984)
Laelaps alaskensis Grant, 1947 (Kinsella and Pattie, 1967; Ludwig, 1984; Whitaker and Maser, 1984)
Laelaps kochi Oudemans, 1836 (Kinsella and Pattie, 1967)
Listrophoridae
Listrophorus mexicanus Fain, 1970 (Whitaker and Maser, 1984)
Myocoptidae
Myocoptes japonensis Radford, 1955 (Whitaker and Maser, 1984)
Trombiculidae
Neotrombicula microti (Ewing, 1928) (Brennan and Wharton, 1950; Ewing, 1928 [original description and type-host]; Radford, 1954; Wharton and Fuller, 1952)

Microtus townsendii
Glycyphagidae
Glycyphagus hypudaei (Koch, 1841) (Whitaker and Maser, 1984)
Laelapidae
Androlaelaps fahrenholzi (Berlese, 1911) (Whitaker and Maser, 1984)
Echinonyssus isabellinus (Oudemans, 1913) (Whitaker and Maser, 1984)
Echinonyssus obsoletus Jameson, 1950 (Whitaker and Maser, 1984)

Eubrachylaelaps debilis Jameson, 1950 (Whitaker and Maser, 1984)
Eulaelaps stabularis (Koch, 1836) (Whitaker and Maser, 1984)
Haemogamasus occidentalis (Keegan, 1951) (Keegan, 1951 [original description and type-host]; Whitaker and Maser, 1984)
Haemogamasus reidi Ewing, 1925 (Whitaker and Maser, 1984)
Laelaps kochi Oudemans, 1836 (Whitaker and Maser, 1984)
Listrophoridae
Listrophorus mexicanus Fain, 1970 (Whitaker and Maser, 1984)
Psorergatidae
Psorergates townsendi Giesen, Lukoschus, Whitaker, and Gettinger, 1983 (original description and type-host)
Trombiculidae
Neotrombicula jewetti (Brennan and Wharton, 1950) (Brennan and Wharton, 1950 [original description]; Radford, 1954; Wharton and Fuller, 1952)
Microtus sp. (Mexico)
Laelapidae
Eulaelaps stabularis (Koch, 1836) (de Barrera, 1979)
Echinonyssus breviseta Strandtmann and Morlan, 1953 (de Barrera, 1979)
Echinonyssus utahensis Allred and Beck, 1966 (de Barrera, 1979)
Haemogamasus ambulans (Thorell, 1872) (de Barrera, 1979)
Laelaps kochi Oudemans, 1836 (de Barrera, 1979)

Ticks

All ticks known from *Microtus* belong to the family Ixodidae (hard ticks). The life cycle of a typical ixodid tick includes four stages: egg, nymph, larva, and adult. For the most part, ticks are not strongly host specific, although nymphs and larvae generally feed on small mammals, birds, or reptiles, and adults feed on larger mammals. Larvae, nymphs, and adults all require blood meals for metamorphosis. The entire life cycle may require 1–3 years. The life cycle and natural history of *Dermacentor variabilis,* the American dog tick, is perhaps the best known of all ticks, and is summarized as follows. Eggs hatch in 30–35 days. Newly hatched larvae, called seed ticks, feed on small mammals for 5–12 days, drop from the host, and metamorphose into the nymphal stage. Nymphs feed 6–10 days and drop off to metamorphose into adults. Copulation takes place on the host. Males may copulate with several different females. Females die soon after egglaying. Nymphs and adults can withstand long periods (hundreds of days) without feeding. Unfed adults and larvae are the main overwintering stage. In

Novia Scotia, larvae are active from April through September, nymphs are active from May through August, and adult activity extends from April to mid-August. Also, Garvie et al. (1978:28) found that "The voles *Microtus pennsylvanicus* and *Clethrionomys gapperi* sustained almost 80% of all larvae [*Dermacentor variabilis*] and over 85% of all nymphs collected from mammal hosts."

Ticks are responsible for the transmission of numerous diseases including babesiosis (*Babesia*), Colorado tick-fever virus, relapsing fever, several *Rickettsia* diseases (for example, Q fever and Rocky Mountain spotted fever), tick paralysis, and tularemia. Additionally, exsanguination by a heavy load of ticks may be significant to a mouse. A recent review of tickborne disease is found in Hoogstraal (1981).

Keys for the identification of North American ticks were provided by Clifford et al. (1961), Cooley and Kohls (1945), Gregson (1956), Keirans and Clifford (1978), and Sonenshine (1979). An excellent and comprehensive bibliography to the ticks was provided by Hoogstraal (see *Bibliography of ticks and tickborne diseases from Homer (about 800 B.C.) to 31 December 1981,* NAMRU-3, Cairo; seven volumes have been published as of 1983).

Amblyomma maculatum, the Gulf Coast tick, ranges from southeastern U.S. through Central and South America. The larvae and nymphs are found on small mammals and ground-dwelling birds. The adults generally are found on larger mammals, especially livestock.

Dermacentor andersoni is known as the Rocky Mountain spotted fever tick because it is one of the primary vectors of the *Rickettsia* causing the disease; it is also a vector of tick paralysis, Colorado tick fever, tularemia, and American Q fever. It is one of the most abundant ticks found in the western half of the U.S. and Canada. Small mammals, especially chipmunks, are the primary hosts; larvae, nymphs, and adults are most common on hosts in spring and summer.

Dermacentor occidentalis, the Pacific Coast tick, is common in western California and Oregon. Small mammals are typical hosts for larvae and nymphs, whereas adults are common on deer, cattle, and horses. It is present on hosts during all seasons of the year, but adults generally are most abundant during the rainy season.

Dermacentor variabilis, the American dog tick, is the most abundant tick in the eastern two-thirds of North America, east of the

Rocky Mountains. Larvae and nymphs have been recovered from most species of small mammals, but are especially abundant on cricetines; adults generally feed on dogs, foxes, and other medium-sized carnivores. It is the eastern U.S. counterpart of *D. andersoni.* In southern U.S. it breeds throughout the year; in northern states a distinct seasonality is found. It is the main vector of Rocky Mountain spotted fever in the eastern U.S. Ecological studies on *D. variabilis* were provided by Campbell (1979), Garvie et al. (1978), and Sonenshine (1979). See references in those papers.

Haemaphysalis leporispalustris, the rabbit tick, is found throughout North, Central, and South America. Lagomorphs (both *Lepus* and *Sylvilagus*) are preferred hosts; however, larvae and nymphs are often found on other small mammals and ground-feeding birds. This species is an important vector of Rocky Mountain spotted fever and tularemia.

Ixodes angustus is found throughout North America, and is one of the most common ticks on small mammals. In the Pacific Northwest, Bishopp and Trembley (1945) reported finding adult ticks on small mammals throughout the year, but immatures not later than the end of October. In northeastern Minnesota, Timm (1975) found larvae and nymphs of *I. angustus* on all species of shrews, moles, and cricetines.

Ixodes auritulus is an uncommon species that has been collected primarily from birds along the coast of northwestern North America.

Ixodes californicus is a poorly known and rarely collected species from the far western U.S. It has been taken from both birds and small mammals.

Ixodes cookei is a widely distributed species, although it appears to be most abundant in the east. It has been found on a variety of small mammals and birds. Sonenshine (1979:30) reported that "larvae and nymphs are most abundant on hosts during winter months," and that medium-sized carnivores, especially skunks, raccoons, and foxes, appeared to be preferred hosts.

Ixodes dammini is a widely distributed tick in the eastern U.S. that was described only recently (see Spielman et al., 1979). Adults appear most frequently on white-tailed deer and larvae and nymphs on a wide variety of small mammals. This species was confused for decades with *I. scapularis* and many of the older records of *scapularis* actually refer to *dammini*. *I. dammini* is the major vector of human babesia, a parasitic protozoan, in the northeastern U.S. Main et al. (1982) reported that both larvae and nymphs were abundant on small mammals in Connecticut from April through October, with peaks of abundance in early and late summer.

Ixodes dentatus is found in the northcentral and eastern U.S., with cottontail rabbits of the genus *Sylvilagus* being the most common hosts. Larvae and nymphs are occasionally found on birds and rodents. Larvae appear to be most abundant on hosts in fall whereas adults are most abundant in spring. This species is a known vector of Rocky Mountain spotted fever.

Ixodes eastoni is a recently recognized species from the Black Hills area of South Dakota and adjacent Wyoming. It has been reported on several species of small mammals, including the genera *Clethrionomys, Eutamias, Microtus, Neotoma, Peromyscus,* and *Zapus*. Adults of *I. eastoni* were confused previously with *I. ochotonae* and immature stages with *I. angustus* (Keirans and Clifford, 1983).

Ixodes kingi is called the rotund tick, and is found in the western U.S. and northern Mexico on a variety of mammals. Carnivores seem to be preferred hosts.

Ixodes muris is called the mouse tick, and is restricted to northeastern U.S.; it is generally found on cricetine rodents, although it is found occasionally on shrews. Smith (1944:231) reported that *Microtus* is the most important host and that "adults of the mouse tick do not mate on the host, but on the ground before the females have attached."

Ixodes ochotonae is aptly named the pika tick; most of the records are from *Ochotona*. It is found in the far western U.S. and British Columbia.

Ixodes pacificus is restricted to the Pacific coastal regions of California, Oregon, and Washington. Adults feed primarily on mammals and are most active from fall to spring; larvae and nymphs feed primarily on lizards. Adults are considered a serious pest on dogs, livestock, and man.

Ixodes sculptus is called the black-legged tick and is common in the midwest and western North America. Ground squirrels are the primary hosts, although it has been collected from a wide variety of small mammals and may be a pest on cattle.

Ixodes spinipalpis is an uncommon tick found in northwestern U.S. and adjacent Canada. Lagomorphs seem to be preferred hosts, although it has been collected on other mammals.

The records of ticks parasitizing *Microtus* are as follows:

Microtus breweri
- *Dermacentor variabilis* (Say, 1821) (Spielman and Piesman, 1979)
- *Ixodes dammini* Spielman, Clifford, Piesman, and Corwin, 1979 (original description)
- *Ixodes muris* Bishopp and Smith (Spielman et al., 1979; Winchell, 1977)

Microtus californicus
- *Dermacentor occidentalis* Marx, 1892 (Furman and Loomis, 1984; Holdenried et al., 1951; Mohr et al., 1964)
- *Dermacentor variabilis* (Say, 1821) (Coultrip et al., 1973; Furman and Loomis, 1984)
- *Ixodes angustus* Neumann, 1899 (Cooley and Kohls, 1945; Furman and Loomis, 1984; Holdenried et al., 1951; Mohr et al., 1964)
- *Ixodes pacificus* Cooley and Kohls, 1943 (Arthur and Snow, 1968; Furman and Loomis, 1984; Mohr et al., 1964)
- *Ixodes spinipalpis* Hadwen and Nuttall, 1916 (Furman and Loomis, 1984; Mohr et al., 1964)
- *Ixodes* sp. (Holdenried et al., 1951)

Microtus canicaudus
- *Ixodes angustus* Neumann, 1899 (Easton and Goulding, 1974)

Microtus chrotorrhinus
- *Ixodes angustus* Neumann, 1899 (Kirkland and Jannett, 1982; Timm, 1974, 1975; Timm et al., 1977; Whitaker and French, 1982)
- *Ixodes* sp. (Komarek and Komarek, 1938)

Microtus longicaudus
- *Dermacentor andersoni* Stiles, 1908 (Augustson, 1941*b*; Bacon, 1953; Beck, 1955; Chamberlin, 1937; Clark et al., 1970; Hansen, 1964; Johnson, 1966; Stout, 1979)
- *Dermacentor variabilis* (Say, 1821) (Stout, 1979; Stout et al., 1971)
- *Dermacentor* sp. (Beck, 1955)
- *Ixodes angustus* Neumann, 1899 (Chamberlin, 1937; Cooley and Kohls, 1945; Easton and Goulding, 1974; Furman and Loomis, 1984; Stout, 1979)
- *Ixodes californicus* Banks, 1904 (Chamberlin, 1937)
- *Ixodes eastoni* Keirans and Clifford, 1983 (original description)
- *Ixodes sculptus* Neumann, 1904 (Allred et al., 1960)
- *Ixodes spinipalpis* Hadwen and Nuttall, 1916 (Stout, 1979)
- *Ixodes* sp. (Allred et al., 1960)

Microtus miurus
- *Ixodes angustus* Neumann, 1899 (Rausch, 1964)

Microtus montanus
- *Dermacentor andersoni* Stiles, 1908 (Allred, 1968*b*; Bacon, 1953; Bacon et al., 1959; Bishopp and Trembley, 1945; Hansen, 1964; Harkema, 1936; Hooker et al., 1912 [reported as *D. venustus*])
- *Dermacentor* sp. (Beck, 1955)
- *Ixodes angustus* Neumann, 1899 (Allred et al., 1960; Furman and Loomis, 1984; Seidel and Booth, 1960)

Ixodes kingi Bishopp, 1911 (Allred, 1968*b*)
Ixodes muris Bishopp and Smith, 1937 (Johnson, 1966)
Ixodes sculptus Neumann, 1904 (Allred et al., 1960)
Ixodes sp. (Allred, 1968*b*)

Microtus ochrogaster
Dermacentor andersoni Stiles, 1908 (Cooley, 1938; Parker and Wells, 1917 [reported as *D. venustus*])
Dermacentor variabilis (Say, 1821) (Basolo and Funk, 1974; Buckner and Gleason, 1974; Cooney and Burgdorfer, 1974; Jameson, 1947; Mumford and Whitaker, 1982)
Ixodes sculptus Neumann, 1904 (Jameson, 1947)
Ixodes spinipalpis Hadwen and Nuttall, 1916 (Turner, 1974)

Microtus oeconomus
Ixodes angustus Neumann, 1899 (Fay and Rausch, 1969; Schiller and Rausch, 1956)

Microtus pennsylvanicus
Dermacentor andersoni Stiles, 1908 (Cooley, 1938; Gregson, 1956; Harkema, 1936; Hooker et al., 1912 [reported as *venustus*]; Hunter and Bishopp, 1911 [reported as *D. venustus*]; Turner, 1974)
Dermacentor variabilis (Say, 1821) (Anastos, 1947; Anderson and Magnarelli, 1980; Bequaert, 1945; Bishopp and Smith, 1938; Campbell, 1979; Carey et al., 1980; Clifford et al., 1961; Coher and Shaw, 1951; Cooley, 1938; Dodds et al., 1969; Drummond, 1957; Eddy and Joyce, 1944; Garvie et al., 1978; Gould and Miesse, 1954; Hertig and Smiley, 1937; Knipping et al., 1950*a*; Larrouse et al., 1928; Lawrence et al., 1965; MacCreary, 1945*b*; Magnarelli et al., 1983; McEnroe, 1983; Mellott and Connell, 1965; Mumford and Whitaker, 1982; Parker et al., 1933; Smith et al., 1946; Sonenshine, 1972, 1979; Sonenshine and Atwood, 1967; Sonenshine and Levy, 1972; Sonenshine and Stout, 1968; Sonenshine et al., 1965, 1966; Spielman and Piesman, 1979; Timm, 1972*b*; Wilkinson, 1979; Wilson, 1943; Wilson and Baker, 1972; Wright, 1979)
Haemaphysalis leporispalustris (Packard, 1869) (Lawrence et al., 1965; Martell et al., 1969; Wright, 1979)
Ixodes angustus Neumann, 1899 (Burroughs et al., 1945; Gregson, 1956; Martell et al., 1969; Timm, 1975; Wright, 1979)
Ixodes cookei Packard, 1869 (Clifford et al., 1961)
Ixodes dammini Spielman, Clifford, Piesman, and Corwin, 1979 (Anderson and Magnarelli, 1980; Carey et al., 1980; Main et al., 1982; Spielman and Piesman, 1979; Spielman et al., 1979 [original description]; White and White, 1981)
Ixodes dentatus Marx, 1899 (Bequaert, 1945; MacCreary, 1945*b*; Sonenshine et al., 1965, 1966)
Ixodes eastoni Keirans and Clifford, 1983 (original description)
Ixodes muris Bishopp and Smith, 1937 (Anastos, 1947; Bequaert, 1945; Bishopp and Smith, 1937 [original description and type-host]; Bishopp and Trembley, 1945; Clifford et al., 1961; Cooley and Kohls, 1945; Easton, 1983*b*; Jones and Thomas, 1980; Martell et al., 1969; Smith, 1944; Spielman et al., 1979; Timm, 1975; Wright, 1979)

Ixodes scapularis Say, 1821 (Bequaert, 1945; Cooley and Kohls, 1945)
Ixodes spinipalpis Hadwen and Nuttall, 1916 (Turner, 1974)

Microtus pinetorum

Amblyomma maculatum Koch, 1844 (Bishopp and Hixson, 1936)
Dermacentor variabilis (Say, 1821) (Bequaert, 1945; Bishopp and Smith, 1938; Bishopp and Trembley, 1945; Carey et al., 1980; Clifford et al., 1961; Cooley, 1938; MacCreary, 1940, 1945*b*; Mellott and Connell, 1965; Mumford and Whitaker, 1982; Smith et al., 1946; Sonenshine, 1972, 1979; Sonenshine and Levy, 1972; Sonenshine et al., 1965, 1966; Tugwell and Lancaster, 1962; Wilson and Baker, 1972)
Ixodes dammini Spielman, Clifford, Piesman, and Corwin, 1979 (Carey et al., 1980; Main et al., 1982)

Microtus townsendii

Ixodes angustus Neumann, 1899 (Bishopp and Trembley, 1945; Cooley and Kohls, 1945; Easton and Goulding, 1974)

Microtus sp.

Ixodes auritulus Neumann, 1904 (Gregson, 1956)
Ixodes ochotonae Gregson, 1941 (Gregson, 1956)

Lice

Lice (Anoplura: Hoplopleuridae) of three genera (*Hoplopleura, Neohaematopinus,* and *Polyplax*) are known from North American *Microtus.* American workers commonly recognize two orders of lice, the Anoplura or sucking lice, and the Mallophaga or chewing lice; Europeans generally recognize a single order, Phthiraptera. The Mallophaga are found primarily on birds, although a few genera parasitize mammals; the Anoplura are exclusively parasites of mammals. Anoplurans feed exclusively on blood and have complex, highly specialized mouthparts modified to pierce the skin of the host.

The entire life cycle of lice is spent on the host, and transmission occurs only when hosts are in direct contact, for the lice cannot live independently of the host. Each individual egg, called a nit, is glued to a single hair. There are three nymphal instars and the duration of the life cycle is about a month. The number of lice on an individual host varies greatly; Cook and Beer (1958) reported a range of 1–748 *Hoplopleura acanthopus* per host on *Microtus pennsylvanicus,* with a mean infestation rate for male voles of 25.1 and for females 10.1 lice per infested host. They (1958:651) found a "positive correlation between age and rate of infestation in male meadow voles with the older animals having higher rates than the younger";

no corresponding correlation was found in female voles. Also (p. 649), "over the whole year . . . 72.6% of the male meadow voles harbored lice as opposed to only 60.9% of the females." Rates of infestation varied with the year and season, with peak rates found in December and April. Female lice are more numerous than males on *M. pennsylvanicus,* which Cook and Beer attributed to a shorter life span of males. The main factor controlling louse populations may be the efficiency of the host at mutual and self grooming; molting of hair on the host may be significant in egg loss. Cook and Beer (1958:419) also stated that ". . . in general higher infestations were found on host populations which were stable or declining, and the lower rates were on hosts which were increasing." On *M. arvalis* in the U.S.S.R., Vysotskaia (1950) reported that *H. acanthopus* occurred all over the host's body in spring and summer, but in fall was concentrated anteriorly, especially in the region of the neck and chest up to the ears. In winter, lice were concentrated in the region of the neck. These changes in position on the host's body were attributed to changes in nest temperature. In cold periods, the lice congregated on the warmest parts of the body. Cook and Beer (1955, 1958) provided detailed studies of population dynamics of *Hoplopleura acanthopus* on *Microtus pennsylvanicus* in Minnesota.

It seems probable that reproduction in these lice may be cued to the reproductive cycle of their hosts, as has been demonstrated in the rabbit flea, *Cediopsylla simplex* (Rothschild and Ford, 1964, 1966, 1969). The reproductive steroids of the host presumably trigger the reproductive steroids of the parasite. This remains to be tested in lice, but may prove to be a fruitful area of research. Anoplurans may prove to be important in the transmission of tularemia (*Francisella tularensis*).

Hoplopleura is a worldwide genus of some 117 species that parasitizes rodents. *H. acanthopus* is a true parasite of microtine rodents; it is found on *Clethrionomys, Lemmus, Microtus,* and *Synaptomys.* The species as now defined is Holarctic; however, in reality the microtine *Hoplopleura* is most likely a complex of several closely related species. *H. hesperomydis* is a true parasite of *Peromyscus,* the few records from *Microtus* being either natural transfers or contamination.

Neohaematopinus is a worldwide genus of about 41 species that parasitizes rodents and insectivores. *N. sciurinus* is a true parasite of tree squirrels of the genus *Sciurus*; the single report from *M. longicaudus* is probably a contaminate.

Polyplax is a worldwide genus of about 76 species, most of which parasitize murid rodents. *P. alaskensis* is a Holarctic species on microtine rodents, especially *Clethrionomys* and *Microtus*. *P. serrata* and *P. spinulosa* are worldwide species whose normal hosts are murid rodents, *Mus* and *Rattus,* respectively.

The records of lice parasitizing *Microtus* are as follows:

Microtus breweri
Polyplax alaskensis Ewing, 1927 (Scanlon and Johnson, 1957; Winchell, 1977)
Microtus californicus
Hoplopleura acanthopus (Burmeister, 1838) (Ferris, 1921; Holdenried et al., 1951; Jameson, 1947; Jellison et al., 1958; Kellogg and Ferris, 1915; Mohr and Stumpf, 1964; Ryckman and Lee, 1958)
Polyplax alaskensis Ewing, 1927 (Ferris, 1916, 1923 [reported as *P. abscisa* and *P. spinulosa*]; Holdenried et al., 1951 [reported as *P. abscisa*]; Mohr and Stumpf, 1964 [reported as *P. abscisa*]; Ryckman and Lee, 1958 [reported as *P. abscisa*]; Scanlon and Johnson, 1957)
Microtus longicaudus
Hoplopleura acanthopus (Burmeister, 1838) (Augustson, 1941*b*; Emerson et al., 1984; Hansen, 1964; Ignoffo, 1956; Morlan and Hoff, 1957; Spencer, 1966)
Hoplopleura hesperomydis (Osborn, 1891) (Morlan and Hoff, 1957)
Neohaematopinus sciurinus (Mjoberg, 1910) (Augustson, 1941*b*)
Polyplax alaskensis Ewing, 1927 (Ignoffo, 1956 [reported as *P. abscisa*]; Kellogg and Ferris, 1915 [reported as *P. spinulosa*])
Microtus mexicanus
Hoplopleura acanthopus (Burmeister, 1838) (Emerson, 1971)
Polyplax alaskensis Ewing, 1927 (Emerson, 1971)
Microtus miurus
Polyplax alaskensis Ewing, 1927 (Quay, 1951)
Microtus montanus
Hoplopleura acanthopus (Burmeister, 1838) (Allred, 1970; Augustson, 1941*b*; Emerson et al., 1984; Hansen, 1964; Jellison et al., 1958, 1959; Kartman et al., 1958*b*; Seidel and Booth, 1960; Spencer, 1966; Stanford, 1934)
Polyplax alaskensis Ewing, 1927 (Allred, 1970 [reported as *P. spinulosa*]; Hansen, 1964 [reported as *P. spinulosa*]; Scanlon and Johnson, 1957)
Polyplax serrata (Burmeister, 1839) (Augustson, 1941*b*)
Polyplax spinulosa (Burmeister, 1839) (Hansen, 1964)
Microtus ochrogaster
Hoplopleura acanthopus (Burmeister, 1838) (Basolo and Funk, 1974; Batson, 1965; Buckner and Gleason, 1974; Ferris, 1951; Jameson, 1947; Mumford and Whitaker, 1982; Turner, 1974)
Hoplopleura hesperomydis (Osborn, 1891) (Buckner and Gleason, 1974)
Microtus oeconomus
Polyplax alaskensis Ewing, 1927 (Quay, 1949, 1951; Scanlon and Johnson, 1957)

Microtus oregoni
Hoplopleura acanthopus (Burmeister, 1838) (Emerson et al., 1984; Spencer, 1966)
Polyplax spinulosa (Burmeister, 1839) (Spencer, 1966)
Microtus pennsylvanicus
Hoplopleura acanthopus (Burmeister, 1838) (Amin, 1976*b*; Cook and Beer, 1955, 1958, 1959; Florschutz and Darsie, 1960; Genoways and Jones, 1972; Harper, 1956, 1961; Ignoffo, 1959; Jameson, 1947; Judd, 1953, 1954; Lampe et al., 1974; Lawrence et al., 1965; MacCreary, 1945*a*; Mathewson and Hyland, 1962; Mumford and Whitaker, 1982; Race, 1956; Scholten et al., 1962; Spencer, 1966; Timm, 1972*b*, 1975; Wilson, 1967)
Hoplopleura erraticus (Osborn, 1896) (original description; probably a misidentification)
Hoplopleura hesperomydis (Osborn, 1891) (Cook and Beer, 1958; Race, 1956)
Neohaematopinus sciurinus (Mjoberg, 1910) (Gyorkos and Hilton, 1982*a*, 1982*b*)
Polyplax alaskensis Ewing, 1927 (Baker, 1946; Ferris, 1942 [reported as *P. abscisa*]; Florschutz and Darsie, 1960; Ignoffo, 1959 [reported as *P. abscisa*]; Mathewson and Hyland, 1962; Race, 1956 [reported as *P. abscisa*]; Scanlon and Johnson, 1957; Whitaker and French, 1982; Wilson, 1943 [reported as *P. spinulosa*])
Polyplax serrata (Burmeister, 1839) (Race, 1956)
Microtus pinetorum
Hoplopleura acanthopus (Burmeister, 1838) (Benton, 1955*a*; Ferris, 1921, 1951; Hamilton, 1938; Mumford and Whitaker, 1982; Race, 1956)
Hoplopleura hesperomydis (Osborn, 1891) (Race, 1956)
Polyplax alaskensis Ewing, 1927 (Morlan, 1952 [reported as *P. spinulosa*]; Race, 1956 [reported as *P. abscisa*])
Microtus townsendii
Hoplopleura acanthopus (Burmeister, 1838) (Spencer, 1966)

Beetles

Leptinidae.—Beetles of the genus *Leptinus* represent one of the few groups of parasitic Coleoptera. *Leptinus* is a Holarctic genus, with three species in the Nearctic and six species in the Palearctic. They are small beetles, usually only 2–3 mm in length, and have greatly reduced or no eyes, and hindwings reduced or absent. All members of the family Leptinidae are parasitic on mammals. In North America two genera are found in addition to *Leptinus: Leptinillus* with one species on beaver (*Castor canadensis*) and one on mountain beaver (*Aplodontia rufa*), and *Platypsyllus* with one species on beaver.

Adults of *Leptinus* are found either on the mammalian host or in the host's nest. Small mammals, especially cricetines, shrews, and moles are typical hosts. Both adults and larvae probably feed on "dead organic matter, such as skin debris, hair fragments, skin-gland secretions, and excreta" rather than live tissue (Peck, 1982: 1518). Eggs, larvae, and pupae are found in the nest. Adults are more abundant on mammals during winter months. There may be up to three generations per year; adult and larval stages overlap. Little is known about the biology of the North American species and the effect of beetles on their hosts. The absence of *Leptinus* on ground squirrels, pocket gophers, pocket mice, and woodrats is of interest considering its wide distribution on shrews, moles, voles, and deer mice.

A recent revision, including an excellent key, of the *Leptinus* of North America was provided by Peck (1982), who concluded that there are three species in North America: *Leptinus americanus,* restricted to the central United States; *Leptinus occidentamericanus,* found in western North America from California to Alaska; and *Leptinus orientamericanus,* widespread east of the Mississippi River.

The records of *Leptinus* parasitizing *Microtus* are as follows:

Microtus oregoni
Leptinus occidentamericanus Peck, 1982 (Maser and Hooven, 1971 [reported as *L. testaceus*; Peck, 1982 [original description]; Spencer, 1956 [reported as *L. testaceus*])
Microtus pennsylvanicus
Leptinus americanus LeConte, 1866 (Peck, 1982)
Leptinus orientamericanus Peck, 1982 (original description)
Microtus pinetorum
Leptinus orientamericanus Peck, 1982 (original description)
Microtus townsendii
Leptinus occidentamericanus Peck, 1982 (original description)

Cryptophagidae.—A single species of cryptophagid or silken fungus beetle, *Cryptophagus bolivari,* has been collected on *Microtus mexicanus* and *Peromyscus melanotis* in México (Barrera and Martinez, 1968). Although little is known of the diet of these beetles, the genus *Cryptophagus* has been found associated with mammals on several occasions; it is likely that they feed on dead skin and scrapings from the hair which might include grains of pollen and smaller soft-bodied arthropods. Nothing is known of the effects of these beetles on their hosts.

Flies

The dipteran family Cuterebridae (bot flies or warbles) is found only in the New World; larvae in all species are subcutaneous, obligate parasites of mammals. The genus *Cuterebra* includes approximately 36 species, and is distributed widely throughout North America. The primary hosts are sciuromorph and myomorph rodents and lagomorphs. Adults are short-lived and apparently do not feed; they are typical winged flies that resemble bumblebees.

Cuterebrids are not common on *Microtus,* even in areas where they heavily infest *Peromyscus* and sciurids. The highest incidence of *Cuterebra* infestation reported in *Microtus* was on *M. chrotorrhinus* in the Great Smokey Mountains, with 65% of the animals captured carrying one or more bots (Komarek and Komarek, 1938); more typical infestation rates range from 6 to 45% (Maurer and Skaley, 1968). The following discussion of a generalized life cycle for *Cuterebra* is based on other hosts because little has been done to date on *Microtus* parasitized by bots.

Although rarely observed in the field, adult bots emerge, mate, and oviposit during mid-summer. Females probably oviposit along runways and burrows of the hosts, with no direct contact between the gravid female bot fly and the host. Egg-hatching is triggered by a sudden rise in environmental temperature as would occur near a potential host. After hatching, the first-instar larvae assume a "questing position," standing on their caudal ends. They then attach to any object coming in contact with them. It is believed that the larvae crawl over the body of the host and are only able to enter through a natural body orifice. For 7–10 days after entering through the nose or mouth, the larvae migrate dorsally and medially between the skin and muscle layers until the breathing hole is cut, marking the site of warble formation. Larvae are typically located in the posterior third of the abdomen, although they are occasionally found on the neck, back, flank, and between the forelegs. Commonly, one to three larvae are found per host, with similar infestation rates for male and female hosts. Peak infestations occur from mid-August through mid-September. Larval development is completed in 3½ weeks, when the third-instar larvae emerge through the breathing hole, burrow into the soil and pupate, overwintering in the puparium.

The effect of bot flies on their hosts has been a matter of debate for some time. The popular notion in the literature is that bot flies live in the testis and castrate their hosts. In recent reviews of the subject, Timm and Lee (1981, 1982) demonstrated that bot flies are found exclusively in the subcutaneous region between the skin and underlying muscle. They do not consume muscle or reproductive tissue, but rather feed on the tissue debris and exudate produced. The site of larval development is usually in the posterior third of the host's body, but is unrelated to the gonads. Upon emergence of the mature third-instar larvae, the wound heals rapidly, with few apparent aftereffects. Bot-fly larvae can have a physiological effect upon their hosts. In *Peromyscus,* significantly lower erythrocyte counts, hematocrit percentages, albumin–globulin ratios, and hemoglobin concentrations have been found, whereas the leucocyte number, spleen size, and thymus size were significantly larger (Clough, 1965; see Timm and Cook, 1979, for a review). Timm and Cook (1979) found no significant reduction in reproduction in adult *Peromyscus leucopus* parasitized by *Cuterebra fontinella.* In adult females there was no significant decrease in the number of embryos, corpora lutea, or placental scars; in adult male mice the presence of one or two larvae had no effect on the size of the reproductive organs.

An excellent and recent review of cuterebrid biology was provided by Catts (1982).

The records of bot flies parasitizing *Microtus* are as follows:

Microtus chrotorrhinus
- *Cuterebra* sp. (Komarek and Komarek, 1938; Martin, 1972)

Microtus oregoni
- *Cuterebra* sp. (Hunter et al., 1972)

Microtus pennsylvanicus
- *Cuterebra fontinella* Clark, 1827 (Getz, 1970 [listed as *C. angustifrons*]; Timm, pers. observ.)
- *Cuterebra grisea* Coquillett, 1904 (Buckner, 1958)
- *Cuterebra* sp. (Amin, 1973; Clough, 1965; Hensley, 1976; Iverson and Turner, 1968; Jacobsen, 1966; Lawrence et al., 1965; Manville, 1961; Maurer and Skaley, 1968; Seton, 1909; White and White, 1981)

Microtus pinetorum
- *Cuterebra* sp. (Hamilton, 1930)

Microtus townsendii
- *Cuterebra grisea* Coquillett, 1904 (Beacham and Krebs, 1980; Boonstra, 1977; Boonstra and Krebs, 1978; Boonstra et al., 1980)
- *Wohlfahrtia vigil* (Walker, 1849) (Boonstra, 1977; Boonstra and Krebs, 1978)

Microtus sp.
- *Cuterebra grisea* Coquillett, 1904 (Buckner, 1958)

Fleas

Fleas (Siphonaptera) are obligate parasites that are found on most species of mammals and on a few species of birds. Adults are active and may be found either on the host or in the nest or burrow. Eggs are generally laid in the nest. The larvae are active and maggot-like, but are not parasitic. They feed on a variety of organic materials, often including the feces of the adults. After two larval molts, the mature larva pupates in a cocoon spun from secretions from the salivary glands. Adult fleas may live for several hundred days and move between various hosts; they feed only on blood. An excellent series on the systematics and distribution of Siphonaptera worldwide was provided by Lewis (1975 and references therein).

Amphipsylla is a genus of approximately 27 species centered mainly in the Siberian subregion of the Palaearctic; most parasitize rodents, especially microtines. Two species are found on microtines in the northern Nearctic. *A. marikovskii* is a Holarctic species with New World populations recognized as a separate subspecies (*A. m. ewingi*); it is marginally separable from the Siberian populations and is known only from Alaska off *Microtus oeconomus*. *A. sibirica* also is a Holarctic species with several recognized subspecies, two of which occur in North America. *A. s. pollionis* is known from Alaska and northern Canada and is a parasite of microtines, especially *M. pennsylvanicus*.

Atyphloceras is a Holarctic genus containing six species; of these, four are found in the Nearctic. Microtine and cricetine rodents are the primary hosts. *A. bishopi* is found in the eastern U.S. and adjacent Canada, with *Microtus* and *Clethrionomys* being the primary hosts. *A. echis* is found in the western U.S. and is a true parasite of *Neotoma*; the few records from *Microtus californicus* can be considered accidental. *A. multidentatus* is a common winter nest flea found in the western U.S. and British Columbia; the genera *Microtus* and *Peromyscus* are probably the primary hosts, although this species has been taken from *Clethrionomys, Lagurus, Mus, Neotoma, Reithrodontomys, Rattus,* and *Tamiasciurus*. *A. tancitari* is known only from a few higher elevation localities in southcentral Mexico; it has been recorded from *Microtus mexicanus, Peromyscus,* and *Reithrodontomys*.

Catallagia is a genus of 15 species occurring mainly in the Nearctic, but a few representatives occur in the eastern Palaearctic. Microtine rodents appear to be the normal hosts, but accidental hosts often include carnivores and insectivores. *C. borealis* is a winter flea found in the northeastern U.S. and adjacent Canada; *Clethrionomys gapperi* is the normal host, although records from *M. chrotorrhinus* and *M. pennsylvanicus* are not uncommon. *C. charlottensis* is a common nest flea of *Microtus* and *Peromyscus* found in the late winter and spring in the Pacific Northwest. *C. dacenkoi* is a Holarctic species; the Nearctic populations represent a subspecies (*C. d. fulleri*) distinct from Siberian populations. It has been found only in Alaska, Northwest Territories, and the Yukon, on both *Clethrionomys* and *Microtus*. *C. decipiens* is a widespread and common flea in western North America and is known from a variety of small mammals, including *Clethrionomys, Microtus, Neotoma, Peromyscus, Reithrodontomys,* and sciurids. *C. jellisoni* is known only from Alberta and British Columbia from *Clethrionomys gapperi, Microtus pennsylvanicus,* and *Neotoma cinerea*. *C. mathesoni* is known only from the west coast of the U.S.; most records are from *Peromyscus*. *C. sculleni* occurs in coastal British Columbia, California, Oregon, and Washington on a variety of small mammals, including *Clethrionomys, Microtus, Neotoma,* and *Peromyscus*.

Ctenophthalmus is a genus of approximately 116 species found in all zoogeographic regions, although it is most abundant in the Palaearctic and Ethiopian regions; it includes about 10% of all known fleas. Most are parasites of rodents, although a few are found exclusively on Insectivora. *C. caballeroi* was described from the nest of *Microtus mexicanus mexicanus* and is only known from a few specimens collected in southcentral Mexico. *C. haagi* is known only from a few specimens collected in south-central Mexico; most records are from *M. mexicanus*. *C. pseudagyrtes* is an abundant flea that occurs throughout the year in eastern North America; it has been collected on numerous species of small mammals including most rodents, insectivores, and smaller carnivores.

Delotelis is a northern and western Nearctic genus of two species; their apparent rarity is due to their occurrence in nests. *D. hollandi* is known only from northern California, Oregon, and British Columbia; *Microtus* and *Peromyscus* are the most common hosts. *D. telegoni* appears to be widespread in northwestern North America; *Clethrionomys* and *Microtus* appear to be the most common hosts.

Epitedia is an exclusively Nearctic genus of seven species which primarily parasitize cricetids and insectivores. *E. scapani* is found in the Pacific coastal lowlands of northern California, Oregon, Washington, and adjacent British Columbia; *Microtus* and *Peromyscus* appear to be the most common hosts. *E. stanfordi* is a winter flea found in the Rocky Mountain region of the U.S.; various species of *Peromyscus* appear to be the primary hosts, although it has been collected on a variety of small mammals. *E. stewarti* is known only from northern California and Oregon; it has been collected on *Microtus californicus, Peromyscus maniculatus,* and *Sorex trowbridgei. E. wenmanni,* a common, transcontinental species throughout North America to northern Mexico, has two recognizable subspecies that intergrade over a broad area of the U.S. (Benton, 1955*b*). *Peromyscus* is the most common host, although it is likely that this species can complete its life cycle on a wide variety of small mammals, including *Microtus.*

Hystrichopsylla is a Holarctic genus of 15 species; six species are found in the Nearctic; most appear to be weakly host specific. *H. dippiei* is a widely distributed and common flea in the midwestern and western Nearctic with four distinctive subspecies; it usually is not abundant on the host itself, suggesting that it is a nest flea. Adults are most commonly collected during fall, winter, and spring. *H. occidentalis* is restricted to far-western North America, from Alaska south to Arizona and California. Campos and Stark (1979) recognized three distinctive subspecies; *Microtus* and *Peromyscus* are the most common hosts. *H. orophila* is known only from southcentral Mexico; the type host is *Microtus mexicanus*; it also has been collected on *Peromyscus maniculatus. H. tahavuana* is restricted to eastern North America; the true hosts are *Condylura cristata, Parascalops breweri,* and *Blarina brevicauda.*

Jellisonia is a poorly known genus of nine species distributed from southwestern U.S. through Mexico and Central America. Most records are from *Peromyscus. J. hayesi* is known only from a few specimens from central Mexico, although Traub (1950) recognized two distinct subspecies. *J. h. breviloba* was described from *M. mexicanus.*

Malaraeus is a Holarctic genus of roughly 12 species; most are parasites of cricetine and microtine rodents. *M. bitterrootensis* is a rare flea found in northwestern U.S. and adjacent Canada; *Ochotona* appears to be the primary host. *M. dobbsi* is known by several specimens, all from only one locality in Oregon off *Microtus oregoni*; repeated attempts to obtain additional specimens of this species have failed. *M. euphorbi* is a poorly known flea found in northwestern U.S. and southwestern Canada; most records are from early spring off *Peromyscus. M. penicilliger* is a widespread and abundant Holarctic species with several described subspecies, two of which occur in northwestern North America. Microtines are the primary hosts. This species is generally the most abundant flea on the far-northern *Microtus, M. abbreviatus* and *M. oeconomus* (Haas et al., 1978). *M. penicilliger* is often placed in a separate genus, *Amalaraeus,* by Eurasian workers. *M. telchinus* is a widespread and common flea in western North America. *Peromyscus* appears to be the most common host, although it has been collected from numerous mammal species; adults can be collected during all seasons of the year.

Megabothris is a Holarctic genus of 18 species, most of which parasitize microtines. *M. abantis* ranges in western North America from New Mexico north to Alaska; it is found on most species of western and northern microtines. *M. acerbus* is a chipmunk flea found in the northeastern U.S. and adjacent Canada; *Tamias striatus* is the primary host, and the single record from *M. pennsylvanicus* must be considered an accidental occurrence. Two subspecies of *M. asio* are recognized in northern North America, and a single intergrade has been described from southeastern Wisconsin (Amin, 1976*a*). *M. asio asio* is widespread and common in the east and is a true parasite of *Microtus*; it is usually more abundant in the nest than on the host. *M. a. megacolpus* is a western flea parasitizing *Microtus* primarily. *M. calcarifer* is a Holarctic species; Alaskan populations are recognized as a distinct subspecies, *M. c. gregsoni. Microtus* and *Clethrionomys* are the primary hosts. Three subspecies of *M. clantoni* are found in a restricted area of western U.S., and are true parasites of *Lagurus. M. groenlandicus* is a transcontinental Nearctic species occurring only in northern Alaska and Canada; lemmings (both *Dicrostonyx* and *Lemmus*) and *Microtus* are the primary hosts. *M. lucifer* is a rarely collected parasite of *Microtus* from the Rocky Mountain region of Alberta, British Columbia, and western U.S. *M. quirini* is a transcontinental vole flea found throughout the northern tier of states in the U.S. and in adjacent Canada; *Microtus* is the primary host, although *M. quirini* frequently is collected on *Clethrionomys* and *Zapus.*

Monopsyllus is a Holarctic genus of 22 species, 13 of which occur in North America; most species parasitize squirrels, but two species are known only from *Ochotona,* and a few are found on a variety of hosts. Johnson (1961) provided the most recent revision of this group, although now that additional specimens are available, the specific and generic status of several members should be reexamined. *M. ciliatus* has four recognizable subspecies, and occurs throughout western North America west of the 100th meridian, from Alaska south to Arizona. It is primarily a squirrel flea, with the majority of records coming from *Eutamias, Sciurus, Spermophilus,* and *Tamiasciurus*; the one record from *Microtus longicaudus* can be considered an accidental occurrence. *M. eumolpi* is a true parasite of *Eutamias* with two subspecies found throughout the range of *Eutamias* in the northern midwest and western portions of North America; it has been collected also from a wide variety of small mammals. *M. vison* is a common, northern sciurid flea, but has been collected on a variety of hosts. *M. wagneri* is found from the upper midwest to the west coast of the U.S. and Canada; *Peromyscus* appears to be the primary host although it is taken occasionally from microtines.

Orchopeas is a Nearctic genus of nine species in need of revision. Most of the species are parasites of squirrels; however, a few infest cricetids, especially *Peromyscus* and *Neotoma. O. caedens* is a northern squirrel flea, especially abundant on *Tamiasciurus*; the single record from *Microtus oeconomus* can be considered accidental. *O. howardii* is a true parasite of tree squirrels (*Glaucomys, Sciurus,* and *Tamiasciurus*), and is found from southern Canada south to Venezuela, with three recognized subspecies. It is an abundant flea; adults are present during all months of the year, and are found occasionally on a variety of small mammals. *O. leucopus* is one of the most abundant species of fleas found in North America; it is perhaps a true parasite of *Peromyscus,* although it frequently is found on many other species of mammals, suggesting that it is not an obligate parasite of *Peromyscus. O. sexdentatus* is a true parasite of woodrats and is found throughout North America wherever *Neotoma* occurs; the few records from *Microtus* can be considered accidental.

Peromyscopsylla is a Holarctic genus of 17 species; most are parasites of microtines and murids. Johnson and Traub (1954) provided an excellent revision of the genus. *P. catatina* is found in the northeastern U.S. and adjacent Canada; *Microtus* and *Clethrionomys* are the primary hosts, although it has been recovered from numerous other species during all seasons of the year. *P. ebrighti* is a poorly known species from southern California. *P. hamifer,* a Holarctic species, is widely distributed throughout the northern half of this continent, and is generally most abundant in fall and winter. North American populations are all referred to *P. h. hamifer. P.*

hesperomys is an abundant flea throughout the U.S. and Canada, and extends south to central Mexico; adults occur throughout the year and cricetines, especially *Peromyscus* and *Neotoma,* are the primary hosts. *P. ostsibirica* is a Holarctic species in which both Siberian populations and those in Alaska and adjacent Canada are little differentiated; *Microtus* is the primary host of this summer flea. *P. scotti* is a poorly collected flea from the eastern U.S.; it is apparently a fall and winter flea with *Peromyscus* as the primary host. *P. selenis* is a fall and winter flea parasitizing microtines in the western U.S. and adjacent Canada.

Pleochaetis is a New World genus of 16 species restricted to southwestern U.S., Central America, and northern South America. Most are parasites of cricetid rodents although much remains to be learned about the systematics and host relationships of this group. *P. asetus* is known from the Mogollon Mountains of New Mexico and Cerro Potosi, Nuevo Leon; *Microtus mexicanus* is probably the true host, although this flea also has been collected on *Peromyscus* and *Neotoma. P. sibynus* has a wide distribution in Mexico with two recognized subspecies; specimens are known from *Microtus mexicanus, Neotoma, Peromyscus,* and *Reithrodontomys. P. aztecus, P. mathesoni, P. mundus, P. paramundus,* and *P. parus* are all poorly known species that have been collected on only a few occasions in central Mexico, primarily from *Microtus* and *Peromyscus.*

Rhadinopsylla is a Holarctic complex genus of some 55 species; ten species are known from the Nearctic. Most are found as adults exclusively during winter months, and are nest fleas; they seldom occur on the host per se, but seem to be associated with a wide variety of rodents. Prior to Smit's (1957) revision, all eastern North American specimens of the genus were included within *R. fraterna.* Smit recognized several species within that complex; thus, all older records of *R. fraterna* must now be considered in doubt. *R. fraterna* (sensu stricto) is found in the Rocky Mountain region of the U.S. and adjacent Canada, and is generally considered a true parasite of *Cynomys* and *Spermophilus. R. mexicana* is known only from Mexico and has been collected primarily on *Neotoma* and *Peromyscus. R. orama* is known only from the eastern U.S., and is probably a true parasite of microtines, especially *Microtus. R. sectilis* is a widely distributed flea in western North America, and has been associated with a wide variety of rodents.

Stenoponia is a Holarctic genus of 14 species of which only two are found in North America. The vast majority of taxa are Palaearctic; they occur primarily on murid rodents, usually are nest fleas, and occur as adults mainly in winter months. *S. americana* is a widely distributed and common flea in eastern North America; it has been collected on a wide variety of small mammals, including both rodents and insectivores, and lacks host specificity. *S. ponera* is known only from Mexico and, in addition to *Microtus mexicanus*, has been collected on *Peromyscus* and *Eutamias*; most records are from fall and from elevations of 3,050–3,350 m.

Strepsylla is a poorly known Nearctic genus of eight recognized species ranging from Guatemala north to central Mexico. Most records are from *Peromyscus*, but very little is known of the biology of this group. *S. mina* was described from *Microtus mexicanus phaeus*; it is known only from a few higher-elevation localities in southcentral Mexico; it also has been taken on *Neotomodon alstoni* and *Peromyscus melanotis*.

Many other species of fleas have been taken from *Microtus*, which in our present state of knowledge are assumed to be accidental. These include: *Anomiopsyllus falsicalifornicus, A. nudatus-princei* (complex), *Callistopsyllus deuterus, Carteretta carteri, Cediopsylla inaequalis, Ceratophyllus niger, Corrodopsylla curvata, Corypsylla kohlsi, C. ornata, Dactylopsylla bluei, D. rara, Dasypsullus gallinulae, Diamanus montanus, Doratopsylla blarinae, Echidnophaga gallinacea, Foxella ignota, Hoplopsylla anomalus, Leptopsylla segnis, Megarthroglossus bisetis, M. divisus, Meringis cummingi, M. hubbardi, M. parkeri, M. shannoni, Nearctopsylla hyrtaci, Neopsylla inopina, Nosopsyllus fasciatus, Opisocrostis bruneri, Opisodasys keeni, O. pseudarctomys, Oropsylla arctomys, O. idahoensis, Pulex irritans, P. simulans, Thrassis spenceri, T. bacchi,* and *Xenopsylla cheopis*.

The records of fleas parasitizing *Microtus* are as follows:

Microtus abbreviatus

Malaraeus penicilliger (Grube, 1851) (Holland, 1963; Rausch and Rausch, 1968)

Megabothris groenlandicus (Wahlgren, 1903) (Rausch and Rausch, 1968)

Microtus breweri

Epitedia wenmanni (Rothschild, 1904) (Fox, 1940*a*; Main, 1970; Winchell, 1977)

Microtus californicus

Anomiopsyllus falsicalifornicus C. Fox, 1929 (Barnes et al., 1977; Linsdale and Davis, 1956 [reported as *A. congruens*])

Atyphloceras echis Jordan and Rothschild, 1915 (Jellison and Senger, 1976; Linsdale and Davis, 1956 [reported as *A. longipalpus*])

Atyphloceras multidentatus (C. Fox, 1909*b*) (Augustson, 1943 [reported as *A. artius*]; Augustson and Wood, 1953; Burroughs, 1944; Coultrip et al., 1973; Fox, 1909*b* [original description]; Hopkins and Rothschild, 1962; Hubbard, 1947 [reported as *A. felix*]; Jellison and Senger, 1976; Kartman,

1958, 1960; Kartman and Prince, 1956; Kartman et al., 1958*a*, 1958*d*; Linsdale and Davis, 1956; Macchiavello, 1954; Miles et al., 1957; Mitzmain, 1909; Murray, 1957; Stark and Miles, 1962; Stewart, 1940 [reported as *A. felix*])

Carteretta carteri Fox, 1927 (Augustson, 1943; Macchiavello, 1954)

Catallagia charlottensis (Baker, 1898) (Fox, 1909*a*; Macchiavello, 1954)

Catallagia sculleni Hubbard, 1940 (Burroughs, 1944 [reported as *C. vonbloekeri*])

Catallagia wymani (Fox, 1909) (Fox, 1909*c* [original description and type-host]; Kartman, 1958, 1960; Kartman et al., 1958*a*, 1958*d*; Macchiavello, 1954; Miles et al., 1957; Murray, 1957; Stark and Miles, 1962)

Cediopsylla inaequalis (Baker, 1895) (Linsdale and Davis, 1956)

Ceratophyllus niger C. Fox, 1908 (Murray, 1957)

Corrodopsylla curvata (Rothschild, 1915) (Miles et al., 1957)

Corypsylla ornata C. Fox, 1908 (Murray, 1957)

Dactylopsylla bluei C. Fox, 1909 (Hubbard, 1947; Macchiavello, 1954)

Diamanus montanus (Baker, 1895) (Kartman et al., 1958*d*; Linsdale and Davis, 1956; Miles et al., 1957)

Echidnophaga gallinacea (Westwood, 1875) (Augustson, 1943; Linsdale and Davis, 1956)

Epitedia stewarti Hubbard, 1940 (Hopkins and Rothschild, 1962)

Foxella ignota (Baker, 1895) (Murray, 1957)

Hoplopsyllus anomalus (Baker, 1904) (Holdenried et al., 1951; Linsdale and Davis, 1956; Rutledge et al., 1979)

Hystrichopsylla dippiei (Rothschild, 1902) (Burroughs, 1944; Macchiavello, 1954; Mitzmain, 1909)

Hystrichopsylla gigas (Kirby, 1837) (Holdenried et al., 1951) (questionable identification)

Hystrichopsylla occidentalis Holland, 1949 (Campos and Stark, 1979; Coultrip et al., 1973; Holland, 1957; Hopkins and Rothschild, 1962; Kartman et al., 1958*a*, 1958*c*, 1958*d*, 1960; Miles et al., 1957; Quan et al., 1960*a*, 1960*b*; Schwan, 1975; Stark and Kinney, 1962; Stark and Miles, 1962)

Leptopsylla segnis (Schonherr, 1811) (Fox, 1909*a* [reported as *Ctenopsyllus musculi* (Duges)]; Hardy et al., 1974; Kartman et al., 1958*d*; Macchiavello, 1954; Miles et al., 1957; Mitzmain, 1909 [reported as *C. musculi*]; Murray, 1957; Schwan, 1975)

Malareus telchinus (Rothschild, 1905) (Augustson, 1943; Augustson and Wood, 1953; Burroughs, 1944; Burroughs et al., 1945; Coultrip et al., 1973; Fox, 1909*a*; Jellison and Senger, 1976; Kartman et al., 1958*a*, 1958*d*, 1960; Lidicker, 1973; Linsdale and Davis, 1956; Macchiavello, 1954; Miles et al., 1957; Mitzmain, 1909; Murray, 1957; Quan et al., 1960*a*; Rutledge et al., 1979; Schwan, 1975; Stark and Kinney, 1962; Stark and Miles, 1962; Wagner, 1936*b*)

Meringis cummingi (C. Fox, 1926) (Holdenried et al., 1951)

Monopsyllus wagneri (Baker, 1904) (Kartman et al., 1958*d*; Linsdale and Davis, 1956; Miles et al., 1957; Rutledge et al., 1979)

Nosopsyllus fasciatus (Bosc, 1801) (Adams et al., 1970; Doane, 1908; Kartman et al., 1958*a*, 1958*d*; Lidicker, 1973; Macchiavello, 1954; Miles et al., 1957; Stark and Miles, 1962)

Opisodasys keeni (Baker, 1896) (Augustson, 1955; Holdenried et al., 1951 [reported as *O. nesiotus*]; Kartman et al., 1958*a,* 1958*d;* Miles et al., 1957; Murray, 1957; Quan et al., 1960*a;* Stark and Miles, 1962)

Orchopeas sexdentatus (Baker, 1904) (Holdenried et al., 1951; Linsdale and Davis, 1956; Macchiavello, 1954)

Peromyscopsylla ebrighti (C. Fox, 1926) (Burroughs, 1944)

Peromyscopsylla hesperomys (Baker, 1904) (Linsdale and Davis, 1956; Macchiavello, 1954; Stewart, 1940)

Peromyscopsylla selenis (Rothschild, 1906) (Hubbard, 1947; Jellison and Senger, 1976; Johnson and Traub, 1954)

Xenopsylla cheopis (Rothschild, 1903) (Kartman et al., 1958*d;* Miles et al., 1957)

Microtus canicaudus

Atyphloceras multidentatus (C. Fox, 1909) (Easton, 1983*a;* Faulkenberry and Robbins, 1980; Hubbard, 1941*a,* 1947; Robbins, 1983; Robbins and Faulkenberry, 1982)

Catallagia charlottensis (Baker, 1898) (Faulkenberry and Robbins, 1980; Hubbard, 1941*a,* 1947; Robbins, 1983; Robbins and Faulkenberry, 1982)

Catallagia sculleni Hubbard, 1940 (Easton, 1983*a;* Hubbard, 1941*a,* 1947 [reported as *C. chamberlini*])

Corrodopsylla curvata (Rothschild, 1915) (Faulkenberry and Robbins, 1980; Robbins, 1983)

Epitedia scapani (Wagner, 1936) (Hubbard, 1941*a,* 1947 [reported as *E. jordani*])

Hystrichopsylla dippiei Rothschild, 1902 (Hubbard, 1941*a,* 1947)

Hystrichopsylla occidentalis Holland, 1949 (Faulkenberry and Robbins, 1980; Robbins, 1983)

Megabothris abantis (Rothschild, 1905) (Hubbard, 1947)

Monopsyllus wagneri (Baker, 1904) (Faulkenberry and Robbins, 1980; Robbins, 1983)

Nosopsyllus fasciatus (Bosc, 1801) (Faulkenberry and Robbins, 1980; Robbins, 1983)

Opisodasys keeni (Baker, 1896) (Hubbard, 1941*a*)

Peromyscopsylla selenis (Rothschild, 1906) (Faulkenberry and Robbins, 1980; Hubbard, 1941*a,* 1947; Robbins, 1983)

Rhadinopsylla sectilis (Jordan and Rothschild, 1923) (Hubbard, 1941*a,* 1941*b,* 1947 [reported as *Micropsylla goodi*])

Microtus chrotorrhinus

Atyphloceras bishopi Jordan, 1933 (Benton and Kelly, 1975; Benton and Smiley, 1963; Martin, 1972)

Catallagia borealis Ewing, 1929 (Benton and Kelly, 1975; Benton and Smiley, 1963; Martin, 1972; Whitaker and French, 1982)

Ctenophthalmus pseudagyrtes Baker, 1904 (Benton and Cerwonka, 1964; Benton and Kelly, 1975; Benton et al., 1969; Brown, 1968; Geary, 1959; Jameson, 1943*a;* Linzey and Linzey, 1973; Lovejoy and Gaughan, 1975; Martin, 1972; Whitaker and French, 1982)

Epitedia wenmanni (Rothschild, 1904) (Benton and Kelly, 1975; Martin, 1972; Whitaker and French, 1982)

Megabothris asio (Baker, 1904) (Benton, 1980; Benton and Cerwonka, 1964; Benton and Kelly, 1975; Benton et al., 1969; Martin, 1972)

Megabothris quirini (Rothschild, 1905) (Benton, 1980; Benton and Cerwonka,

1964; Benton and Kelly, 1975; Benton and Timm, 1980; Benton et al., 1969; Brown, 1968; Main, 1970; Martin, 1972; Osgood, 1964; Timm, 1974, 1975; Whitaker and French, 1982)

Orchopeas leucopus (Baker, 1904) (Martin, 1972)

Peromyscopsylla catatina (Jordan, 1928) (Benton, 1980; Benton and Cerwonka, 1964; Benton and Kelly, 1975; Benton and Smiley, 1963; Benton and Timm, 1980; Benton et al., 1969; Brown, 1968; Johnson and Traub, 1954; Martin, 1972; Timm, 1974, 1975; Whitaker and French, 1982)

Peromyscopsylla hesperomys (Baker, 1904) (Benton and Kelly, 1975)

Microtus longicaudus

Anomiopsyllus nudatus-A. princei complex (Haas et al., 1973)

Atyphloceras multidentatus (C. Fox, 1909) (Hopkins and Rothschild, 1962; Hubbard, 1941*a*)

Callistopsyllus deuterus Jordan, 1937 (Augustson, 1941*b*)

Catallagia charlottensis (Baker, 1898) (Holland, 1949*b*; Hubbard, 1947 [reported as *C. motei*])

Catallagia decipiens Rothschild, 1915 (Beck, 1955; Egoscue, 1966, 1976; Haas et al., 1973; Hansen, 1964; Holland, 1949*b*; Hopkins and Rothschild, 1962; Hubbard, 1947; Morlan, 1955)

Catallagia sculleni Hubbard, 1940 (Jameson and Brennan, 1957)

Corrodopsylla curvata (Rothschild, 1915) (Hopkins and Rothschild, 1966)

Delotelis hollandi Smit, 1952 (Jameson and Brennan, 1957; Smit, 1952)

Delotelis telegoni (Rothschild, 1905) (Holland, 1949*b*; Jellison and Senger, 1973; Morlan, 1955; Stark, 1959)

Epitedia scapani (Wagner, 1936) (Hopkins and Rothschild, 1962; Hubbard, 1941*a*, 1947 [reported as *E. jordani*])

Epitedia stanfordi Traub, 1944 (Egoscue, 1966, 1976)

Epitedia wenmanni (Rothschild, 1904) (Easton, 1982; Jameson and Brennan, 1957)

Hystrichopsylla dippiei Rothschild, 1902 (Egoscue, 1966; Haas et al., 1973; Hansen, 1964; Holland, 1949*a*, 1949*b*, 1957; Hopkins and Rothschild, 1962; Hubbard, 1947; Morlan, 1955)

Hystrichopsylla occidentalis Holland, 1949 (Campos and Stark, 1979; Holland, 1957)

Malaraeus telchinus (Rothschild, 1905) (Dunn and Parker, 1923; Egoscue 1966, 1976; Haas, 1973; Hansen, 1964; Holland, 1949*b*; Hubbard, 1947; Jameson and Brennan, 1957; Morlan, 1955; Wagner, 1936*a*)

Megabothris abantis (Rothschild, 1905) (Allred, 1952; Augustson, 1941*b*; Beck, 1955; Burroughs, 1947, 1953; Egoscue, 1966, 1976; Haas et al., 1973; Hansen, 1964; Holland, 1949*b*, 1958; Hubbard, 1941*a*, 1947; Jellison and Senger, 1973; Morlan, 1955; Tipton, 1950)

Megabothris asio (Baker, 1904) (Hubbard, 1940*a*, 1947)

Megabothris quirini (Rothschild, 1905) (Hubbard, 1947; Wiseman, 1955)

Megarthroglossus bisetis Jordan and Rothschild, 1915 (Haas et al., 1973)

Megarthroglossus divisus (Baker, 1895) (Holland, 1949*b*)

Meringis hubbardi Kohls, 1938 (Egoscue, 1966)

Meringis parkeri Jordan, 1937 (Stark, 1959)

Monopsyllus ciliatus Baker, 1904 (Hubbard, 1941*a*, 1947)

Monopsyllus eumolpi (Rothschild, 1905) (Egoscue, 1966; Morlan, 1955)
Monopsyllus wagneri (Baker, 1904) (Augustson, 1941*b*; Beck, 1955; Egoscue, 1966, 1976; Haas et al., 1973; Hansen, 1964; Holland, 1949*b*; Hubbard, 1947; Jameson and Brennan, 1957; Morlan, 1955)
Neopsylla inopina Rothschild, 1915 (Hansen, 1964; Svihla, 1941)
Opisodasys keeni (Baker, 1896) (Egoscue, 1976; Hubbard, 1947)
Orchopeas leucopus (Baker, 1904) (Egoscue, 1976)
Oropsylla idahoensis (Baker, 1904) (Haas et al., 1973; Hubbard, 1947)
Peromyscopsylla hamifer (Rothschild, 1906) (Egoscue, 1976; Haas, 1973; Haas et al., 1973; Holdenried and Morlan, 1956; Hopkins and Rothschild, 1971; Morlan, 1955)
Peromyscopsylla hesperomys (Baker, 1904) (Haas et al., 1973; Hubbard, 1947)
Peromyscopsylla selenis (Rothschild, 1906) (Augustson, 1941*b*; Egoscue, 1966, 1976; Haas, 1973; Haas et al., 1973; Hansen, 1964; Holland, 1949*b*; Hopkins and Rothschild, 1971; Jameson and Brennan, 1957; Jellison and Senger, 1973; Johnson and Traub, 1954; Morlan, 1955; Tipton, 1950)
Rhadinopsylla sectilis Jordan and Rothschild, 1923 (Hubbard, 1947)

Microtus mexicanus
Atyphloceras tancitari Traub and Johnson, 1952 (Traub and Johnson, 1952)
Catallagia sp. (Barrera, 1968)
Ctenophthalmus caballeroi Barrera and Machado, 1960 (Barrera, 1968; Barrera and Machado, 1960 [original description])
Ctenophthalmus haagi Traub, 1950 (Hopkins and Rothschild, 1966; Traub, 1950 [original description; from *M. mexicanus phaeus*])
Ctenophthalmus pseudagyrtes Baker, 1904 (Barrera, 1968; Tipton and Mendez, 1968)
Epitedia wenmanni (Rothschild, 1904) (Tipton and Mendez, 1968)
Hystrichopsylla orophila Barrera, 1952 (Barrera, 1952 [original description], 1968)
Jellisonia hayesi Traub, 1950 (Barrera, 1968; Traub, 1950 [original description])
Pleochaetis asetus Traub, 1950 (Barrera, 1968; Tipton and Machado-Allison, 1972; Tipton and Mendez, 1968; Traub, 1950 [original description])
Pleochaetis aztecus Barrera, 1954 (Barrera, 1968)
Pleochaetis mathesoni Traub, 1950 (Barrera, 1968)
Pleochaetis mundus (Jordan and Rothschild, 1922) (Barrera, 1968)
Pleochaetis paramundus Traub, 1950 (Barrera, 1968)
Pleochaetis parus Traub, 1950 (Barrera, 1968)
Pleochaetis sibynus Jordan, 1925 (Barrera, 1968; Fox, 1939*b*; Tipton and Mendez, 1968; Traub, 1950)
Pulex simulans Baker, 1895 (Tipton and Mendez, 1968)
Rhadinopsylla mexicana (Barrera, 1952) (Barrera, 1968; Tipton and Mendez, 1968)
Stenoponia ponera Traub and Johnson, 1952 (Tipton and Mendez, 1968)
Strepsylla mina Traub, 1950 (Hopkins and Rothschild, 1962; Traub, 1950 [original description; from *M. mexicanus phaeus*])

Microtus miurus
Corrodopsylla curvata (Rothschild, 1915) (Hopla, 1965*b*)
Malaraeus penicilliger (Grube, 1851) (Hopla, 1965*b*; Rausch, 1964)

Megabothris calcarifer (Wagner, 1913) (Hopla, 1965*b*; Hubbard, 1960; Rausch, 1964)
Megabothris groenlandicus (Wahlgren, 1903) (Hopla, 1965*b*; Hubbard, 1960; Jellison and Senger, 1976; Rausch, 1964)
Megabothris quirini (Rothschild, 1905) (Hopla, 1965*b*)
Peromyscopsylla ostsibirica (Scalon, 1936) (Rausch, 1964)

Microtus montanus

Amphipsylla sibirica (Wagner, 1898) (Allred, 1968*a*; Eads et al., 1979)
Callistopsyllus deuterus Jordan, 1937 (Augustson, 1941*b*)
Catallagia decipiens Rothschild, 1915 (Allred, 1952; Beck, 1955; Haas et al., 1973; Hansen, 1964; Holland, 1949*b*; Hopkins and Rothschild, 1962; Stark, 1959)
Catallagia mathesoni Jameson, 1950 (original description)
Catallagia sculleni Hubbard, 1940 (Augustson, 1941*a* [described as *C. rutherfordi* from *M. montanus dutcheri*]; Stark and Kinney, 1969)
Corrodopsylla curvata (Rothschild, 1915) (Haas et al., 1973; Hansen, 1964)
Dactylopsylla rara I. Fox, 1940 (Haas et al., 1973)
Delotelis hollandi Smit, 1952 (original description)
Epitedia stanfordi Traub, 1944 (Stark, 1959)
Epitedia wenmanni (Rothschild, 1904) (Allred, 1952; Beck, 1955; Stark, 1959; Tipton, 1950)
Hoplopsyllus anomalus (Baker, 1904) (Allred, 1952; Beck, 1955)
Hystrichopsylla dippiei Rothschild, 1902 (Beck, 1955, Haas et al., 1973; Holland, 1949*b*, 1957; Tipton, 1950)
Malaraeus bitterrootensis (Dunn, 1923) (Wiseman, 1955)
Malaraeus euphorbi (Rothschild, 1905) (Allred, 1968*a*)
Malaraeus telchinus (Rothschild, 1905) (Allred, 1952, 1968*a*; Beck, 1955; Haas et al., 1973; Hansen, 1964; Hartwell et al., 1958; Seidel and Booth, 1960; Stark, 1959; Tipton, 1950)
Megabothris abantis (Rothschild, 1905) (Allred, 1952; Augustson, 1941*b*; Beck, 1955; Haas et al., 1973; Hansen, 1964; Hubbard, 1947, 1949*c*; Jellison and Senger, 1973; Kartman and Prince, 1956; Kinsella and Pattie, 1967; Stark, 1959)
Megabothris asio (Baker, 1904) (Hansen, 1964; Holland, 1950; Hubbard, 1949*c*)
Megabothris clantoni Hubbard, 1949 (Hansen, 1964; Hubbard, 1949*b*)
Megabothris lucifer (Rothschild, 1905) (Holland, 1941, 1949*a*, 1949*b*; Jellison and Senger, 1976; Wagner, 1936*b*)
Meringis hubbardi Kohls, 1938 (Hansen, 1964)
Meringis parkeri Jordan, 1937 (Allred, 1968*a*)
Meringis shannoni (Jordan, 1929) (Bacon, 1953)
Monopsyllus eumolpi (Rothschild, 1905) (Allred, 1952; Beck, 1955; Hansen, 1964; Stark, 1959)
Monopsyllus wagneri (Baker, 1904) (Allred, 1952, 1968*a*; Bacon, 1953; Beck, 1955; Haas et al., 1973; Hansen, 1964; Stark, 1959)
Nosopsyllus fasciatus (Bosc, 1801) (Allred, 1952; Beck, 1955)
Opisodasys keeni (Baker, 1896) (Stark, 1959; Stark and Kinney, 1969)
Oropsylla idahoensis (Baker, 1904) (Haas et al., 1973)

Peromyscopsylla hamifer (Rothschild, 1906) (Haas et al., 1973; Johnson and Traub, 1954; Stark, 1959)
Peromyscopsylla selenis (Rothschild, 1906) (Augustson, 1941*b*; Haas, 1973; Haas et al., 1973; Hansen, 1964; Hopkins and Rothschild, 1971; Hubbard, 1947, 1949*c*; Johnson and Traub, 1954; Stark, 1959; Stark and Kinney, 1969)
Thrassis bacchi (Rothschild, 1905) (Allred, 1968*a*)

Microtus ochrogaster
Ctenophthalmus pseudagyrtes Baker, 1904 (Basolo and Funk, 1974; Batson, 1965; Buckner and Gleason, 1974; Hopkins and Rothschild, 1966; Jameson, 1947; Jellison and Senger, 1973; Layne, 1958; Mumford and Whitaker, 1982; Poorbaugh and Gier, 1961; Senger, 1966; Verts, 1961; Whitaker and Corthum, 1967)
Epitedia wenmanni (Rothschild, 1904) (Basolo and Funk, 1974; Buckner and Gleason, 1974; Hopkins and Rothschild, 1962; Jameson, 1947; Poorbaugh and Gier, 1961; Verts, 1961; Whitaker and Corthum, 1967; Wilson, 1957)
Hystrichopsylla dippiei Rothschild, 1902 (Hopkins and Rothschild, 1962)
Malaraeus euphorbi (Rothschild, 1905) (Senger, 1966)
Megabothris asio (Baker, 1904) (Verts, 1961)
Monopsyllus wagneri (Baker, 1904) (Turner, 1974)
Nearctopsylla hyrtaci (Rothschild, 1904) (Jellison and Senger, 1973; Senger, 1966)
Nosopsyllus fasciatus (Bosc, 1801) (El-Wailly, 1967; Jameson, 1947)
Orchopeas howardii (Baker, 1895) (Jameson, 1947)
Orchopeas leucopus (Baker, 1904) (Buckner and Gleason, 1974; Easton, 1982; El-Wailly, 1967; Jameson, 1947; Jellison and Senger, 1973; Lampe et al., 1974; Poorbaugh and Gier, 1961; Rapp and Gates, 1957; Turner, 1974; Verts, 1961)
Orchopeas sexdentatus (Baker, 1904) (Rapp and Gates, 1957)
Peromyscopsylla scotti I. Fox, 1939 (Buckner and Gleason, 1974)
Rhadinopsylla sectilis Jordan and Rothschild, 1923 (Senger, 1966)
Stenoponia americana (Baker, 1899) (Buckner and Gleason, 1974; Hopkins and Rothschild, 1962; Poorbaugh and Gier, 1961; Verts, 1961; Whitaker and Corthum, 1967; Wilson, 1957)

Microtus oeconomus
Amphipsylla marikovskii Ioff and Tiflov, 1939 (Fox, 1940*b* [reported as *A. ewingi*]; Holland, 1963; Hopkins and Rothschild, 1971; Hopla, 1965*a*, 1965*b*)
Catallagia dacenkoi Ioff, 1940 (Hopkins and Rothschild, 1962; Hopla, 1965*a*, 1965*b*; Hubbard, 1960; Jellison and Senger, 1976)
Ceratophyllus garei Rothschild, 1902 (Hopla, 1965*b*)
Corrodopsylla curvata (Rothschild, 1915) (Haas et al., 1982; Hopla, 1965*b*)
Epitedia wenmanni (Rothschild, 1904)(Haas et al., 1979; Hubbard, 1960)
Hystrichopsylla occidentalis Holland, 1949 (Campos and Stark, 1979; Haas et al., 1979; Holland, 1957)
Malaraeus penicilliger (Grube, 1851) (Haas et al., 1979, Haas et al., 1982; Holland, 1958, 1963; Hopla, 1965*a*, 1965*b*, 1980; Hubbard, 1960; Rausch et al., 1969)

Megabothris abantis (Rothschild, 1905) (Haas et al., 1979, 1982; Rausch et al., 1969; Schiller and Rausch, 1956)
Megabothris calcarifer (Wagner, 1913) (Haas et al., 1979, 1982; Holland, 1958, 1963; Hopla, 1965*a*, 1965*b*, 1980; Hubbard, 1960)
Megabothris groenlandicus (Wahlgren, 1903) (Hubbard, 1960)
Megabothris quirini (Rothschild, 1905) (Hopla, 1965*a*, 1965*b*, 1980)
Monopsyllus vison (Baker, 1904) (Hopla, 1965*b*)
Orchopeas caedens (Jordan, 1925) (Hopla, 1965*b*)
Peromyscopsylla hamifer (Rothschild, 1906) (Quay, 1951)
Peromyscopsylla ostsibirica (Scalon, 1936) (Haas et al., 1982; Holland, 1958, 1963; Hopkins and Rothschild, 1971; Hopla, 1965*a*, 1965*b*, 1980; Hubbard, 1960; Jellison and Senger, 1976; Rausch et al., 1969)

Microtus oregoni
Atyphloceras multidentatus (C. Fox, 1909) (Holland, 1949*b*,; Hopkins and Rothschild, 1962; Hubbard, 1941*a*, 1947)
Catallagia charlottensis (Baker, 1898) (Holland, 1949*b*; Hubbard, 1941*a*, 1947)
Corrodopsylla curvata (Rothschild, 1915) (Holland, 1949*b*; Hubbard, 1941*a*, 1947 [reported as *Doratopsylla jellisoni* Hubbard])
Corypsylla ornata C. Fox, 1908 (Holland, 1949*b*; Hopkins and Rothschild, 1962)
Delotelis hollandi Smit, 1952 (Hopkins and Rothschild, 1962; Smit, 1952)
Delotelis telegoni (Rothschild, 1905) (Holland, 1949*b*)
Epitedia scapani (Wagner, 1936) (Hopkins and Rothschild, 1962; Hubbard, 1941*a*, 1947 [reported as *E. jordani*])
Hystrichopsylla dippiei Rothschild, 1902 (Hubbard, 1941*a*, 1947)
Hystrichopsylla occidentalis Holland, 1949 (Campos and Stark, 1979; Holland, 1957; Hopkins and Rothschild, 1962)
Malaraeus dobbsi Hubbard, 1940 (Hubbard, 1940*b* [original description], 1941*a*; Jellison and Senger, 1976)
Megabothris abantis (Rothschild, 1905) (Holland, 1949*b*, Hubbard, 1941*a*, 1947; Wagner, 1936*a*)
Megabothris quirini (Rothschild, 1905) (Hubbard, 1947)
Opisodasys keeni (Baker, 1896) (Holland, 1949*b*)
Peromyscopsylla hesperomys (Baker, 1904) (Hubbard, 1947; Johnson and Traub, 1954)
Peromyscopsylla selenis (Rothschild, 1906) (Holland, 1949*b*; Hubbard, 1941*a*)
Rhadinopsylla sectilis (Jordan and Rothschild, 1923) (Holland, 1949*b*)

Microtus pennsylvanicus
Amphipsylla marikovskii Ioff and Tiflov, 1939 (Hopla, 1965*a*)
Amphipsylla sibirica (Wagner, 1898) (Brown, 1944; Hopkins and Rothschild, 1971; Jordan and Rothschild, 1913; Rothschild, 1905 [reported as *Ceratophyllus pollionis*]; Wagner, 1936*a*)
Atyphloceras bishopi Jordan, 1933 (Baker, 1946; Benton, 1980; Benton and Cerwonka, 1960; Benton and Kelly, 1971, 1975; Benton and Smiley, 1963; Buckner and Blasko, 1969; Burbutis, 1956; Cressey, 1961; Fox, 1940*a*; Geary, 1959; Holland, 1949*a*, 1958; Holland and Benton, 1968; Hopkins and Rothschild, 1962; Jameson, 1943*a*; Jordan, 1933; Lawrence et al., 1965; Main, 1970; Mathewson and Hyland, 1964; Miller and Benton, 1973; Scharf and Stewart, 1980)

Catallagia borealis Ewing, 1929 (Benton, 1980; Ewing, 1929*b* [original description and type-host]; Fox, 1940*a*; Fuller, 1943*a*, 1943*b*; Holland and Benton, 1968; Hopkins and Rothschild, 1962; Main, 1970)

Catallagia charlottensis (Baker, 1898) (Holland, 1949*b*)

Catallagia dacenkoi Ioff, 1940 (Holland, 1951; Hopkins and Rothschild, 1962; Hopla, 1965*a*)

Catallagia decipiens Rothschild, 1915 (Easton, 1982; Holland, 1949*b*; Hopkins and Rothschild, 1962)

Catallagia jellisoni Holland, 1954 (Hopkins and Rothschild, 1962)

Corrodopsylla curvata (Rothschild, 1915) (Robert and Bergeron, 1977; Verts, 1961)

Ctenophthalmus pseudagyrtes Baker, 1904 (Amin, 1973, 1976*a*; Baker, 1946; Batson, 1965; Bell and Chalgren, 1943, Benton, 1966; Benton and Kelly, 1969, 1975; Benton and Krug, 1956; Benton and Timm, 1980; Benton et al., 1969; Brimley, 1938; Brown, 1944; Brown, 1968; Burbutis, 1956; Connor, 1960; Cressey, 1961; Cummings, 1954; Erickson, 1938*a*; Fox, 1940*a*; Fuller, 1943*a*, 1943*b*; Gates, 1945; Geary, 1959; Gyorkos and Hilton, 1982*b*; Holland and Benton, 1968; Hopkins and Rothschild, 1966; Hubbard, 1949*a*; Jameson, 1943*b*; Jordan, 1928; Joyce and Eddy, 1944; Judd, 1950; Knipping et al., 1950*b*; Lawrence et al., 1965; Lovejoy and Gaughan, 1975; MacCreary, 1945*a*; Main, 1970, 1983; Main et al., 1979; Mathewson and Hyland, 1964; Miller and Benton, 1973; Osgood, 1964; Quackenbush, 1971; Rapp and Gates, 1957; Robert, 1962; Robert and Bergeron, 1977; Rothschild, 1904; Scharf and Stewart, 1980; Stewart, 1928, 1933; Timm, 1975; Tindall and Darsie, 1961; Verts, 1961; Whitaker and Corthum, 1967; White and White, 1981; Woods and Larson, 1971; Wright, 1979)

Delotelis telegoni (Rothschild, 1905) (Brown, 1944; Holland, 1949*b*, Hopkins and Rothschild, 1962; Rothschild, 1905 [original description and cotype host]; Tiraboschi, 1907)

Doratopsylla blarinae C. Fox, 1914 (Benton, 1966; Fox, 1940*a*; Main, 1970)

Epitedia stanfordi Traub, 1944 (Hopkins and Rothschild, 1962)

Epitedia wenmanni (Rothschild, 1904) (Allred, 1952; Baker, 1946; Beck, 1955; Benton and Kelly, 1971, 1975; Benton and Timm, 1980; Burbutis, 1956; Connor, 1960; Cressey, 1961; Fox, 1940*a*; Fuller, 1943*a*; Gabbutt, 1961; Geary, 1959; Holland, 1949*b*; Holland and Benton, 1968; Hopkins and Rothschild, 1962; Joyce and Eddy, 1944; Knipping et al., 1950*b*; Lawrence et al., 1965; Main, 1970, 1983; Main et al., 1979; Mathewson and Hyland, 1964; Mumford and Whitaker, 1982; Osgood, 1964; Stark, 1959; Timm, 1972*b*; Tindall and Darsie, 1961; Verts, 1961; Whitaker and Corthum, 1967; Wright, 1979)

Hoplopsyllus anomalus (Baker, 1904) (Allred, 1952; Beck, 1955)

Hystrichopsylla dippiei Rothschild, 1902 (Easton, 1981; Fox, 1940*a*; Holland, 1957; Jordan, 1929; Timm, 1975)

Hystrichopsylla occidentalis Holland, 1949 (Campos and Stark, 1979; Egoscue, 1966)

Hystrichopsylla tahavuana Jordan, 1929 (Benton, 1966; Benton and Kelly, 1975; Benton et al., 1969; Geary, 1959; Hopkins and Rothschild, 1962; Jordan,

1929 [original description]; Main, 1970; Osgood, 1964; Quackenbush, 1971)

Malaraeus penicilliger (Grube, 1851) (Holland, 1952b; Hopla, 1965*a*)

Megabothris abantis (Rothschild, 1905) (Holland, 1949*b*; Rothschild, 1905 [original description and type host])

Megabothris acerbus (Jordan, 1925) (Benton and Kelly, 1975)

Megabothris asio (Baker, 1904) (Amin, 1976*a*; Baker, 1946; Benton, 1966, 1980; Benton and Kelly, 1975; Benton and Krug, 1956; Benton and Timm, 1980; Benton et al., 1969, 1971; Brown, 1968; Burbutis, 1956; Connor, 1960; Cressey, 1961; Cummings, 1954; Florschutz and Darsie, 1960; Fox, 1939*a*, 1940*a*; Fuller, 1943*a*; Gabbutt, 1961; Geary, 1959; Gyorkos and Hilton, 1982*b*; Harper, 1956, 1961; Holland, 1949*a*, 1949*b*, 1950, 1958; Holland and Benton, 1968; Jellison and Senger, 1973; Jordan, 1929 [described as *Ceratophyllus megacolpus*, 1933]; Knipping et al., 1950*b*; Lawrence et al., 1965; Lovejoy and Gaughan, 1975; MacCreary, 1945*a*; Main, 1970; Main et al., 1979; Mathewson and Hyland, 1964; Miller and Benton, 1973; Mumford and Whitaker, 1982; Osgood, 1964; Quackenbush, 1971; Robert, 1962; Robert and Bergeron, 1977; Scharf and Stewart, 1980; Scholten et al., 1962; Timm, 1975; Tindall and Darsie, 1961; Verts, 1961; Wagner, 1936*a* [reported as *M. megacolpus*]; Woods and Larson, 1969; Wright, 1979)

Megabothris calcarifer (Wagner, 1913) (Holland, 1950, 1958; Hopla, 1965*a*)

Megabothris groenlandicus (Wahlgren, 1903) (Holland, 1952*a*)

Megabothris lucifer (Rothschild, 1905) (Brown, 1944; Genoways and Jones, 1972; Holland, 1949*b*; Rothschild, 1905 [original description and cotype-host]; Woods and Larson, 1971)

Megabothris quirini (Rothschild, 1905) (Benton, 1966; Benton and Kelly, 1975; Benton and Timm, 1980; Benton et al., 1969, 1971; Buckner, 1964; Fox, 1940*a*; Fuller, 1943*a*; Gabbutt, 1961; Geary, 1959; Gyorkos and Hilton, 1982*b*; Harper, 1956; Holland, 1949*b*; Hopla, 1965*a*, 1980; Hubbard, 1947; Jordan, 1932; Knipping et al., 1950*b*; Lawrence et al., 1965; Lovejoy and Gaughan, 1975; Quackenbush, 1971; Robert, 1962; Timm, 1975; Wagner, 1936*a*; Whitaker and French, 1982; Woods and Larson, 1969; Wright, 1979)

Monopsyllus eumolopi (Rothschild, 1905) (Jordan, 1932)

Monopsyllus vison (Baker, 1904) (Robert, 1962)

Monopsyllus wagneri (Baker, 1904) (Beck, 1955; Benton and Timm, 1980; Easton, 1982; Genoways and Jones, 1972; Timm, 1972*b*; Verts, 1961)

Nosopsyllus fasciatus (Bosc, 1801) (Allred, 1952; Baker, 1946; Beck, 1955; Fuller, 1943*a*; Geary, 1959; Holland and Benton, 1968; Jameson, 1943*a*)

Opisocrostis bruneri (Baker, 1895) (Amin, 1973, 1976*a*; Benton et al., 1971; Benton and Timm, 1980; Woods and Larson, 1969)

Opisodasys pseudarctomys (Baker, 1904) (Holland and Benton, 1968)

Orchopeas howardii (Baker, 1895) (Main et al., 1979; Mathewson and Hyland, 1964; White and White, 1981)

Orchopeas leucopus (Baker, 1904) (Amin, 1973, 1976*a*; Benton and Kelly, 1975; Buckner, 1964; Cressey, 1961; Fox, 1940*a*; Fuller, 1943*a*; Gates, 1945; Geary, 1959; Genoways and Jones, 1972; Holland and Benton, 1968;

Joyce and Eddy, 1944; Knipping et al., 1950*b*; Lawrence et al., 1965; Main, 1970; Main et al., 1979; Mathewson and Hyland, 1964; Robert, 1962; Timm, 1975; Verts, 1961; Whitaker and Corthum, 1967)

Oropsylla arctomys (Baker, 1904) (Verts, 1961)

Peromyscopsylla catatina (Jordan, 1928) (Baker, 1946; Benton and Kelly, 1975; Benton and Krug, 1956; Benton and Timm, 1980; Benton et al., 1969; Buckner, 1964; Buckner and Blasko, 1969; Easton, 1981, 1982; Fox, 1940*a*; Fuller, 1943*a*; Geary, 1959; Harper, 1956; Holland and Benton, 1968; Hopkins and Rothschild, 1971; Jordan, 1929; Lawrence et al., 1965; Lovejoy and Gaughan, 1975; Mathewson and Hyland, 1964; Stewart, 1933; Timm, 1975)

Peromyscopsylla hamifer (Rothschild, 1906) (Benton, 1980; Benton and Miller, 1970; Benton and Timm, 1980; Cressey, 1961; Haas and Wilson, 1973; Holland, 1958; Holland and Benton, 1968; Hopkins and Rothschild, 1971; Hubbard, 1949*a*; Johnson and Traub, 1954; Knipping et al., 1950*b* [originally reported as *P. catatina*]; Lawrence et al., 1965; Lovejoy and Gaughan, 1975; Main, 1970, 1983; Main et al., 1979; Miller and Benton, 1973; Mumford and Whitaker, 1982; Timm, 1975; Whitaker and Corthum, 1967)

Peromyscopsylla hesperomys (Baker, 1904) (Benton and Kelly, 1975; Johnson and Traub, 1954)

Peromyscopsylla ostsibirica (Scalon, 1936) (Haas et al., 1982; Hopla, 1965*a*)

Peromyscopsylla scotti I. Fox, 1939 (Benton and Kelly, 1975)

Peromyscopsylla selenis (Rothschild, 1906) (Hopkins and Rothschild, 1971; Johnson and Traub, 1954; Rothschild, 1906; Wagner, 1936*a* [reported as *Ctenopsylla selenis*])

Rhadinopsylla fraterna (Baker, 1895) (Hopkins and Rothschild, 1962; Smit, 1957)

Rhadinopsylla orama Smit, 1957 (Benton, 1980; Fox 1940*a* [questionable identification]; Fuller, 1943*a*; Miller and Benton, 1973; Smit, 1957 [original description; type collected in nest])

Stenoponia americana (Baker, 1899) (Benton and Kelly, 1971, 1975; Fox, 1940*a*; Fuller, 1943*a*; Hopkins and Rothschild, 1962; MacCreary, 1945*a*; Main, 1983; Main et al., 1979; Miller and Benton, 1973; Quackenbush, 1971; Tindall and Darsie, 1961)

Thrassis bacchi (Rothschild, 1905) (Easton, 1982)

Microtus pinetorum

Atyphloceras bishopi Jordan, 1933 (Benton and Kelly, 1975; Main et al., 1979)

Ctenophthalmus pseudagyrtes Baker, 1904 (Benton, 1955*a*; Benton and Kelly, 1969, 1975; Benton and Krug, 1956; Benton et al., 1969; Burbutis, 1956; Cressey, 1961; Fox, 1940*a*; Harlan and Palmer, 1974; Holland and Benton, 1968; Hopkins and Rothschild, 1966; Jameson, 1943*b*, 1947; Jordan, 1928; Layne, 1958; MacCreary, 1945*a*; Main, 1970, 1983; Main et al., 1979; Mathewson and Hyland, 1964; Miller and Benton, 1973; Morlan, 1952; Mumford and Whitaker, 1982; Palmer and Wingo, 1972; Sanford and Hays, 1974; Schiefer and Lancaster, 1970; Tindall and Darsie, 1961; Whitaker and Corthum, 1967)

Doratopsylla blarinae C. Fox, 1914 (Benton, 1955*a*; Benton and Kelly, 1975; Burbutis, 1956; Miller and Benton, 1973)

Epitedia wenmanni (Rothschild, 1904) (Burbutis, 1956)
Hystrichopsylla tahavuana Jordan, 1929 (Benton and Kelly, 1975; Benton and Smiley, 1963; Holland, 1949*a*, 1957)
Megabothris asio (Baker, 1904) (Miller and Benton, 1973)
Opisodasys pseudarctomys (Baker, 1904) (Holland and Benton, 1968)
Orchopeas howardii (Baker, 1895) (Morlan, 1952)
Orchopeas leucopus (Baker, 1904) (Benton and Kelly, 1975; Benton et al., 1969; Ellis, 1955; Holland and Benton, 1968; Jameson, 1947; MacCreary, 1945*a*; Main et al., 1979; Tindall and Darsie, 1961)
Peromyscopsylla catatina (Jordan, 1928) (Benton et al., 1969; Holland and Benton, 1968)
Peromyscopsylla hamifer (Rothschild, 1906) (Main et al., 1979)
Peromyscopsylla hesperomys (Baker, 1904) (Main, 1983)
Rhadinopsylla orama Smit, 1957 (Benton, 1980; Benton and Kelly, 1975; Holland and Benton, 1968; Hopkins and Rothschild, 1962; Miller and Benton, 1973; Smit, 1957)
Stenoponia americana (Baker, 1899) (Benton and Kelly, 1975; Benton and Smiley, 1963; Burbutis, 1956; Hopkins and Rothschild, 1962; MacCreary, 1945*a*; Main et al., 1979; Palmer and Wingo, 1972; Sanford and Hays, 1974; Tindall and Darsie, 1961; Wilson, 1957)

Microtus richardsoni
Catallagia charlottensis (Baker, 1898) (Hubbard, 1947)
Catallagia sculleni Hubbard, 1940 (Holland, 1949*b*)
Hystrichopsylla dippiei Rothschild, 1902 (Hubbard, 1947; Jellison and Senger, 1973; Senger, 1966)
Megabothris abantis (Rothschild, 1905) (Egoscue, 1966; Hubbard, 1947; Jellison and Senger, 1973; Kinsella and Pattie, 1967; Ludwig, 1984)
Megabothris asio (Baker, 1904) (Ludwig, 1984)
Monopsyllus eumolpi (Rothschild, 1905) (Ludwig, 1984)
Monopsyllus wagneri (Baker, 1904) (Allred, 1952)
Nearctopsylla hyrtaci (Rothschild, 1904) (Ludwig, 1984)
Opisodasys keeni (Baker, 1896) (Stark, 1959)
Peromyscopsylla hamifer (Rothschild, 1906) (Ludwig, 1984)
Peromyscopsylla hesperomys (Baker, 1904) (Hubbard, 1947)
Peromyscopsylla selenis (Rothschild, 1906) (Gresbrink and Hopkins, 1982; Hopkins and Rothschild, 1971; Hubbard, 1947; Ludwig, 1984)
Stenoponia americana (Baker, 1899) (Hopkins and Rothschild, 1962)
Thrassis alpinus Stark, 1957 (Senger, 1966)

Microtus townsendii
Atyphloceras multidentatus (C. Fox, 1909) (Holland, 1949*b*; Hoplins and Rothschild, 1962; Hubbard, 1947; Macchiavello, 1954)
Catallagia charlottensis (Baker, 1898) (Holland, 1949*b*; Hopkins and Rothschild, 1962; Hubbard, 1947; Macchiavello, 1954; Svihla, 1941)
Catallagia sculleni Hubbard, 1940 (Hopkins and Rothschild, 1962)
Corrodopsylla curvata (Rothschild, 1915) (Hubbard, 1947; Macchiavello, 1954)
Corypsylla ornata C. Fox, 1908 (Holland, 1949*b*)
Corypsylla kohlsi Hubbard, 1940 (Fox, 1940*c* [described as *Corypsylloides spinata*]; Macchiavello, 1954)

Delotelis hollandi Smit, 1952 (Hopkins and Rothschild, 1962; Smit, 1952 [original description and type-host])
Delotelis telegoni (Rothschild, 1905) (Holland, 1949*b*; Hubbard, 1947; Jellison and Senger, 1976; Macchiavello, 1954)
Epitedia scapani (Wagner, 1936) (Hopkins and Rothschild, 1962; Hubbard, 1947; Macchiavello, 1954)
Hystrichopsylla dippiei Rothschild, 1902 (Hubbard, 1947; Macchiavello, 1954; Svihla, 1941)
Hystrichopsylla occidentalis Holland, 1949 (Holland, 1957; Hopkins and Rothschild, 1962)
Megabothris abantis (Rothschild, 1905) (Hubbard, 1947; Macchiavello, 1954; Svihla, 1941; Wagner, 1936*a*)
Megabothris quirini (Rothschild, 1905) (Hubbard, 1947)
Monopsyllus wagneri (Baker, 1904) (Hubbard, 1947; Macchiavello, 1954)
Opisodasys keeni (Baker, 1896) (Holland, 1949*b*; Macchiavello, 1954)
Peromyscopsylla hesperomys (Baker, 1904) (Hubbard, 1947; Macchiavello, 1954)
Peromyscopsylla selenis (Rothschild, 1906) (Hopkins and Rothschild, 1971; Svihla, 1941)
Rhadinopsylla sectilis Jordan and Rothschild, 1923 (Hopkins and Rothschild, 1962; Hubbard, 1941*b*, 1947 [reported as *Micropsylla goodi*]; Macchiavello, 1954)

Directions for Future Research

A review of the literature on parasites of North American *Microtus* contains over 485 primary references covering the 91-year period from 1894 to 1984. Most of these papers deal with the taxonomy of the various groups of parasites and their distribution on the hosts. Surprisingly, with this wealth of literature, we actually know very little about the biology of parasites on *Microtus*. Future research on systematic problems of many of the groups of parasites is needed, most especially of the mites, the most diverse and poorly known of the parasitic groups.

One of the most productive areas for future research will be exploring aspects of the biology of hosts and parasites from an evolutionary perspective. Future research should address co-evolution in the broadest sense between hosts and parasites, including co-accommodation, co-adaptation, and co-speciation. One of the most challenging, yet most fruitful directions will be in statistical quantification of the cost of parasitism. Hopefully, future studies will be able to directly or indirectly measure increased or decreased reproductive success by both host and parasites. Such questions might include: 1) What are the selective forces exerted by the host on the parasites, and conversely, what are the selective forces exerted by the parasites on the host? 2) What is the cost of parasitism to the host? 3) How are the reproductive cycles of the parasites cued to the reproductive cycle of the host? 4) What is the role of parasites in the epidemiology of diseases among hosts? 5) Can parasites affect the behavior of the host? 6) Is there a genetic basis for resistance to parasitic infections by the host, and can this be selected for? 7) Can parasites play a role in regulating host populations? and 8) Can parasites or the diseases transmitted by them be responsible for delineating geographic ranges of species? Certainly we would expect massive infestations of parasites to alter the behavior or reproductive cycle of the host, but given lower "normal" levels of infestation, can the host be altered in more subtle ways through hormonal imbalance, odors, etc? The rapidly expanding field of biogeography has provided interesting and potentially productive directions for future studies in parasitology. The application of island biogeography theory to host–parasite systems leads to questions such as: Can an individual host, a population, or entire species be viewed as an island for parasites?

The study of parasites has been a part of both our basic and applied sciences for decades, yet it is still an extremely fruitful area of future research. There remains much to learn about the biology of *Microtus* with respect to its parasites and about the biology of those parasites.

Acknowledgments

I thank A. H. Benton, J. B. Kethley, B. M. OConnor, R. L. Wenzel, and J. O. Whitaker for freely sharing with me their knowledge of and literature on parasites. B. L. Clauson, R. H. Tamarin, and J. O. Whitaker reviewed, in detail, the entire manuscript; R. L. Rausch reviewed the section on endoparasites and provided numerous references. J. S. Ashe reviewed the section on parasitic beetles. J. Shaw provided much assistance in locating obscure references.

Literature Cited

ADAMS, W. H., R. W. EMMONS, AND J. E. BROOKS. 1970. The changing ecology of murine (endemic) typhus in southern California. Amer. J. Tropical Med. Hyg., 19:311–318.

ALLRED, D. M. 1952. Plague important fleas and mammals in Utah and the western United States. Great Basin Nat., 12:67–75.

———. 1968*a*. Fleas of the national reactor testing station. Great Basin Nat., 28: 73–87.

———. 1968*b*. Ticks of the national reactor testing station. Brigham Young Univ. Sci. Bull., Biol. Ser., 10(1):1–29.

———. 1970. Mites and lice of the national reactor testing station. Brigham Young Univ. Sci. Bull., Biol. Ser., 12(1):1–17.

ALLRED, D. M., AND D E. BECK. 1966. Mites of Utah mammals. Brigham Young Univ. Sci. Bull., Biol. Ser., 8:1–123.

ALLRED, D. M., D E. BECK, AND L. D. WHITE. 1960. Ticks of the genus *Ixodes* in Utah. Brigham Young Univ. Sci. Bull., Biol. Ser., 1(4):1–42.

AMIN, O. M. 1973. A preliminary survey of vertebrate ectoparasites in southeastern Wisconsin. J. Med. Entomol., 10:110–111.

———. 1976*a*. Host associations and seasonal occurrence of fleas from southeastern Wisconsin mammals, with observations on morphologic variations. J. Med. Entomol., 13:179–192.

———. 1976*b*. Lice, mites, and ticks of southeastern Wisconsin mammals. Great Lakes Entomol., 9:195–198.

ANASTOS, G. 1947. Hosts of certain New York ticks. Psyche, 54:178–180.

ANDERSON, J. F., AND L. A. MAGNARELLI. 1980. Vertebrate host relationships and distribution of ixodid ticks (Acari: Ixodidae) in Connecticut, USA. J. Med. Entomol., 17:314–323.

ARTHUR, D. R., AND K. R. SNOW. 1968. *Ixodes pacificus* Cooley and Kohls, 1943: its life-history and occurrence. Parasitology, 58:893–906.

AUGUSTSON, G. F. [1941*a*] 1942. Some new California Siphonaptera. Bull. S. California Acad. Sci., 40:140–146.

———. [1941*b*] 1942. Ectoparasite-host records from the Sierran region of east-central California. Bull. S. California Acad. Sci., 40:147–157.

———. 1943. Preliminary records and discussion of some species of Siphonaptera from the Pacific Southwest. Bull. S. California Acad. Sci., 42:69–89.

———. 1955. Records of fleas from the Pacific South-west. Bull. S. California Acad. Sci., 54:36–39.

AUGUSTSON, G. F., AND S. F. WOOD. 1953. Notes on California mammal ectoparasites from the Sierra Nevada foothills of Madera County. Bull. S. California Acad. Sci., 52:48–56.

BACON, M. 1953. A study of the arthropods of medical and veterinary importance in the Columbia Basin. Tech. Bull. Washington Agric. Exp. Sta., 11: 1–40.

BACON, M., C. H. DRAKE, AND N. G. MILLER. 1959. Ticks (Acarina: Ixodoidea) on rabbits and rodents of eastern and central Washington. J. Parasitol., 45:281–286.

BAKER, E. W. 1949. A review of the mites of the family Cheyletidae in the United States National Museum. Proc. U.S. Natl. Mus., 99:267–320.

BAKER, J. A. 1946. A rickettsial infection in Canadian voles. J. Exp. Med., 84: 37–50.

BARNES, A. M., V. J. TIPTON, AND J. A. WILDIE. 1977. The subfamily Anomiopsyllinae (Hystrichopsyllidae: Siphonaptera). I. A revision of the genus *Anomiopsyllus* Baker. Great Basin Nat., 37:138–206.

BARON, R. W. 1971. The occurrence of *Paruterina candelabraria* (Goeze, 1782) and *Cladotaenia globifera* (Batsch, 1786) in Manitoba. Canadian J. Zool., 49: 1399–1400.

BARRERA, A. 1952. Notas sobre sifonapteros. IV. Descripcion de *Hystrichopsylla orophila* nov. sp. (Siph., Hystichops.). Ciencia, 12:39–42.

———. 1968. Distribución cliserial de los Siphonaptera del Volcán Popocatépetl, su interpretación biogeográfica. Anal. Inst. Biol., Univ. Nac. Autó. México, Ser. Zool., 39:35–100.

BARRERA, A., AND C. MACHADO. 1960. Un nuevo ectoparásito de *Microtus m. mexicanus* Saussure: *Ctenophthalmus caballeroi* sp. nov. y claves para las especies americanas hasta ahora conocidas (Insecta: Siphonaptera). Pp. 549–553, *in* Libro Homenaje al Dr. Eduardo Caballero y Caballero. Inst. Polit. Nac., México, D.F., 602 pp.

BARRERA, A., AND A. MARTINEZ. [1968] 1970. Nuevo criptofágido mexicano: *Cryptophagus bolivari* nov. sp. (Ins.: Col.). An. Esc. Nac. Cienc. Biol., México, 17:151–156.

BASOLO, F., JR., AND R. C. FUNK. 1974. Ectoparasites from *Microtus ochrogaster, Peromyscus leucopus,* and *Cryptotis parva* in Coles County, Illinois. Trans. Illinois State Acad. Sci., 67:211–221.

BASSOLS B., I. 1981. Catálogo de los ácaros Mesostigmata de mamíferos de México. An. Esc. Nac. Cienc. Biol., México, 24:9–49.

BATSON, J. 1965. Studies on the prairie vole, *Microtus ochrogaster,* in central Kentucky. Trans. Kentucky Acad. Sci., 25:129–137.

BEACHAM, T. D., AND C. J. KREBS. 1980. Pitfall versus live-trap enumeration of fluctuating populations of Microtus townsendii. J. Mamm., 61:486–499.

BECK, D E. 1955. Distributional studies of parasitic arthropods in Utah, determined as actual and potential vectors of Rocky Mountain spotted fever and plague, with notes on vector-host relationships. Brigham Young Univ. Sci. Bull., Biol. Ser., 1(1):1–64.

BELL, J. F., AND W. S. CHALGREN. 1943. Some wildlife diseases in the eastern United States. J. Wildl. Mgmt., 7:270–278.

BENTON, A. H. 1954. Notes on *Moniliformis clarki* (Ward) in eastern New York (Moniliformidae: Acanthocephala). J. Parasitol., 40:102–103.

———. 1955*a*. Observations on the life history of the northern pine mouse. J. Mamm., 36:52–62.

———. 1955*b*. The taxonomy and biology of *Epitedia wenmanni* (Rothschild, 1904) and *E. testor* (Rothschild, 1915) (Hystrichopsyllidae: Siphonaptera). J. Parasitol., 41:491–495.

———. 1966. Siphonaptera collected on Tug Hill, Lewis County, New York. Pp. 76–78, *in* The mammals of the Tug Hill Plateau, New York (P. F. Connor, ed.). Bull. New York State Mus., Sci. Ser., 406:1–82.

———. 1980. An atlas of the fleas of the eastern United States. Marginal Media Press, Fredonia, New York, 177 pp.

BENTON, A. H., AND R. H. CERWONKA. 1960. Host relationships of some eastern Siphonaptera. Amer. Midland Nat., 63:383–391.

———. 1964. The Siphonaptera of Whiteface Mountain. Atmospheric Sci. Res. Center, State Univ. New York, 21:4–14.

BENTON, A. H., AND D. L. KELLY. 1969. Notes on the biology of *Ctenophthalmus p. pseudagyrtes* Baker in the northeast (Siphonaptera: Hystrichopsyllidae). J. New York Entomol. Soc., 77:70–74.

———. 1971. Siphonaptera from Long Island, New York. Pp. 77–78, *in* The mammals of Long Island, New York (P. F. Connor, ed.). Bull. New York State Mus., Sci. Ser., 416:1–78.

———. 1975. An annotated list of New York Siphonaptera. J. New York Entomol. Soc., 83:142–156.

BENTON, A. H., AND R. F. KRUG. 1956. Mammals and siphonapterous parasites of Rensselaer County, New York. Bull. New York State Mus., Sci. Ser., 353:1–21.

BENTON, A. H., AND D. H. MILLER. 1970. Ecological factors in the distribution of the flea Peromyscopsylla hamifer hamifer (Rothschild). Amer. Midland Nat., 83:301-303.

BENTON, A. H., AND D. SMILEY. 1963. The fleas of Ulster County, New York. Bull. John Burroughs Nat. Hist. Soc., 6:1-7.

BENTON, A. H., AND R. M. TIMM. 1980. Siphonaptera of Minnesota. Pp. 158-177, *in* An atlas of the fleas of the eastern United States (A. H. Benton, ed.). Marginal Media Press, Fredonia, New York, 177 pp.

BENTON, A. H., O. R. LARSON, AND B. A. VEN HUIZEN. 1971. Siphonaptera from Itasca State Park. J. Minnesota Acad. Sci., 37:91-92.

BENTON, A. H., H. H. TUCKER, JR., AND D. L. KELLY. 1969. Siphonaptera from northern New York. J. New York Entomol. Soc., 77:193-198.

BEQUAERT, J. C. 1945. The ticks, or Ixodoidea, of the northeastern United States and eastern Canada. Entomol. Amer., 25:73-232.

BISHOPP, F. C., AND H. HIXSON. 1936. Biology and economic importance of the Gulf coast tick. J. Econ. Entomol., 29:1068-1076.

BISHOPP, F. C., AND C. N. SMITH. 1937. A new species of Ixodes from Massachusetts. Proc. Entomol. Soc. Washington, 39:133-138.

———. 1938. The American dog tick, eastern carrier of Rocky Mountain spotted fever. Circ. U.S. Dept. Agric., 478:1-25.

BISHOPP, F. C., AND H. L. TREMBLEY. 1945. Distribution and hosts of certain North American ticks. J. Parasitol., 31:1-54.

BOONSTRA, R. 1977. Effect of the parasite *Wohlfahrtia vigil* on *Microtus townsendii* populations. Canadian J. Zool., 55:1057-1060.

BOONSTRA, R., AND C. J. KREBS. 1978. Pitfall trapping of *Microtus townsendii*. J. Mamm., 59:136-148.

BOONSTRA, R., C. J. KREBS, AND T. D. BEACHAM. 1980. Impact of botfly parasitism on *Microtus townsendii* populations. Canadian J. Zool., 58:1683-1692.

BRENNAN, J. M., AND D E. BECK. 1955. The chiggers of Utah (Acarina: Trombiculidae). Great Basin Nat., 15:1-26.

BRENNAN, J. M., AND M. L. GOFF. 1977. Keys to the genera of chiggers of the Western Hemisphere (Acarina: Trombiculidae). J. Parasitol., 63:554-566.

BRENNAN, J. M., AND E. K. JONES. 1954. A report on the chiggers (Acarina: Trombiculidae) of the Frances Simes Hastings Natural History Reservation, Monterey County, California. Wasmann J. Biol., 12:155-194.

———. 1959. Keys to the chiggers of North America with synonymic notes and descriptions of two new genera (Acarina: Trombiculidae). Ann. Entomol. Soc. America, 52:7-16.

BRENNAN, J. M., AND G. W. WHARTON. 1950. Studies on North American chiggers. No. 3. The subgenus Neotrombicula. Amer. Midland Nat., 44:153-197.

BRIMLEY, C. S. 1938. The insects of North Carolina. North Carolina Dept. Agric., Div. Entomol., Raleigh, 560 pp.

BROWN, J. H. 1944. The fleas (Siphonaptera) of Alberta, with a list of the known vectors of sylvatic plague. Ann. Entomol. Soc. America, 37:207-213.

BROWN, N. R. 1968. Notes on the Siphonaptera of New Brunswick. Canadian Entomol., 100:486-498.

BUCKNER, C. H. 1958. Cuterebrids (*Cuterebra grisea* Coq.) attacking small mammals. Bimonthly Prog. Rept., Forest Biol. Div., Canadian Dept. Agric., 14:2-3.

———. 1964. Fleas (Siphonaptera) of Manitoba mammals. Canadian Entomol., 96:850-856.

BUCKNER, C. H., AND G. G. BLASKO. 1969. Additional range and host records of the fleas (Siphonaptera) of Manitoba. Manitoba Entomol., 3:65–69.

BUCKNER, R. L., AND L. N. GLEASON. 1974. Arthropod ectoparasites and their seasonal occurrences on *Microtus ochrogaster* and *Peromyscus leucopus* from Warren County, Kentucky. Trans. Kentucky Acad. Sci., 35:70–75.

BUECH, R. R., R. M. TIMM, AND K. SIDERITS. 1977. A second population of rock voles, *Microtus chrotorrhinus,* in Minnesota with comments on habitat. Canadian Field-Nat., 91:413–414.

BURBUTIS, P. P. 1956. The Siphonaptera of New Jersey. Bull. New Jersey Agric. Exp. Sta., 782:1–36.

BURROUGHS, A. L. 1944. The flea *Malaraeus telchinum* a vector of *P. pestis.* Proc. Soc. Exp. Biol. Med., 55:10–11.

———. 1947. Sylvatic plague studies. The vector efficiency of nine species of fleas compared with *Xenopsylla cheopis.* J. Hyg., 45:371–396.

———. 1953. Sylvatic plague studies. X. Survival of rodent fleas in the laboratory. Parasitology, 43:35–48.

BURROUGHS, A. L., R. HOLDENRIED, D. S. LONGANECKER, AND K. F. MEYER. 1945. A field study of latent tularemia in rodents with a list of all known naturally infected vertebrates. J. Infect. Dis., 70:115–119.

CAMPBELL, A. 1979. Ecology of the American dog tick, *Dermacentor variabilis* in southwestern Nova Scotia. Pp. 135–143, *in* Recent advances in acarology, Vol. II (J. G. Rodriguez, ed.). Academic Press, New York, 569 pp.

CAMPOS, E. G., AND H. E. STARK. 1979. A revaluation of the *Hystrichopsylla occidentalis* group, with description of a new subspecies (Siphonaptera: Hystrichopsyllidae). J. Med. Entomol., 15:431–444.

CAREY, A. B., W. L. KRINSKY, AND A. J. MAIN. 1980. *Ixodes dammini* (Acari: Ixodidae) and associated ixodid ticks in south-central Connecticut, USA. J. Med. Entomol., 17:89–99.

CATTS, E. P. 1982. Biology of New World bot flies: Cuterebridae. Ann. Rev. Entomol., 27:313–338.

CHAMBERLIN, W. J. 1937. The ticks of Oregon. Bull. Oregon State College Agric. Exp. Sta. 349:1–34.

CHANDLER, A. C., AND D. M. MELVIN. 1951. A new cestode, *Oochoristica pennsylvanica,* and some new or rare helminth host records from Pennsylvania mammals. J. Parasitol., 37:106–109.

CLARK, G. M., C. M. CLIFFORD, L. V. FADNESS, AND E. K. JONES. 1970. Contributions to the ecology of Colorado tick fever virus. J. Med. Entomol., 7:189–197.

CLIFFORD, C. M., G. ANASTOS, AND A. ELBL. 1961. The larval ixodid ticks of the eastern United States (Acarina–Ixodidae). Misc. Publ., Entomol. Soc. Amer., 2:213–237.

CLOUGH, G. C. 1965. Physiological effect of botfly parasitism on meadow voles. Ecology, 46:344–346.

COHER, E. I., AND F. R. SHAW. 1951. The distribution of *Dermacentor variabilis.* J. Econ. Entomol., 44:998.

CONNOR, P. F. 1960. The small mammals of Otsego and Schoharie counties, New York. Bull. New York State Mus., Sci. Ser., 382:1–84.

COOK, E. F., AND J. R. BEER. 1955. The louse populations of some cricetid rodents. Parasitology, 45:409–420.

———. 1958. A study of louse populations on the meadow vole and deer mouse. Ecology, 39:645–659.

———. 1959. The immature stages of the genus *Hoplopleura* (Anoplura: Hoplopleuridae) in North America, with descriptions of two new species. J. Parasitol., 45:405–416.

COOLEY, R. A. 1938. The genera *Dermacentor* and *Otocentor* (Ixodidae) in the United States, with studies in variation. U.S. Natl. Inst. Health Bull., 171: 1–89.

COOLEY, R. A., AND G. M. KOHLS. 1945. The genus *Ixodes* in North America. U.S. Natl. Inst. Health Bull., 184:1–246.

COONEY, J. C., AND W. BURGDORFER. 1974. Zoonotic potential (Rocky Mountain spotted fever and tularemia) in the Tennessee Valley region. I. Ecologic studies of ticks infesting mammals in Land Between the Lakes. Amer. J. Trop. Med. Hyg., 23:99–108.

COULTRIP, R. L., ET AL. 1973. Survey for the arthropod vectors and mammalian hosts of Rocky Mountain spotted fever and plague at Fort Ord, California. J. Med. Entomol., 10:303–309.

CRESSEY, R. F. 1961. Additional records of New England Siphonaptera. J. New York Entomol. Soc., 69:1–4.

CUMMINGS, E. D. 1954. Notes on some Siphonaptera from Albany County, New York. J. New York Entomol. Soc., 62:161–165.

DE BARRERA, I. B. 1979. Mesostigmatid ectoparasites of mammals in Mexico. Pp. 475–480, *in* Recent advances in acarology, Vol. II (J. G. Rodriguez, ed.). Academic Press, New York, 569 pp.

DIKMANS, G. 1935. New nematodes of the genus *Longistriata* in rodents. J. Washington Acad. Sci., 25:72–81.

DOANE, R. W. 1908. Notes on fleas collected on rat and human hosts in San Francisco and elsewhere. Canadian Entomol., 40:303–304.

DODDS, D. G., A. M. MARTELL, AND R. E. YESCOTT. 1969. Ecology of the American dog tick, *Dermacentor variabilis* (Say), in Nova Scotia. Canadian J. Zool., 47:171–181.

DOUTHITT, H. 1915. Studies on the cestode family Anoplocephalidae. Illinois Biol. Monogr., 1:1–97.

DRUMMOND, R. O. 1957. Ectoparasitic Acarina from small mammals of the Patuxent Refuge, Bowie, Maryland. J. Parasitol., 43:50.

DUNN, L. H., AND R. R. PARKER. 1923. Fleas found on wild animals in the Bitteroot Valley, Mont. Publ. Health Rept., 38:2763–2775.

DURETTE-DESSET, M.-C. 1967. Evolution des nématodes héligmosomes en rapport avec celle de leurs hôtes fondamentaux, les Microtidae. C. R. Acad. Sc. Paris, 265:1500–1503.

———. 1968. Les systèmes d'arêtes cuticulaires chez lez nématodes heligmosomes. III. Étude de sept espèces parasites de rongeurs néarctiques et rétablissement du genre *Heligmosomoides* Hall, 1916. Bull. Mus. Nat. Hist. Naturelle, 2e ser., 40:186–209.

———. 1974. Nippostrongylinae (Nematoda:Heligmosomidae) néarctiques. Ann. Parasitol. Hum. Comp., 49:435–450.

DURETTE-DESSET, M.-C., J. M. KINSELLA, AND D. J. FORRESTER. 1972. Arguments en faveur de la double origine des nématodes néarctiques du genre *Heligmosomoides* Hall, 1916. Ann. Parasitol. Hum. Comp., 47:365–382.

EADS, R. B., E. G. CAMPOS, AND A. M. BARNES. 1979. New records for several flea (Siphonaptera) species in the United States, with observations on species parasitizing carnivores in the Rocky Mountain region. Proc. Entomol. Soc. Washington, 81:38–42.

EASTON, E. R. 1975. Ectoparasites in two diverse habitats in western Oregon. II Chiggers (Acari: Trombiculidae). J. Med. Entomol., 12:295–298.

———. 1981. New geographical records for some fleas (Siphonaptera) from the Black Hills of South Dakota. Entomol. News, 92:45–47.

———. 1982. An annotated checklist of the fleas of South Dakota (Siphonaptera). Entomol. News, 93:155–158.

———. 1983*a*. Ectoparasites in two diverse habitats in western Oregon. III. Interrelationship of fleas (Siphonaptera) and their hosts. J. Med. Entomol., 20:216–219.

———. 1983*b*. The ticks of South Dakota: an annotated checklist (Acari: Ixodoidea). Entomol. News, 94:191–195.

EASTON, E. R., AND R. L. GOULDING. 1974. Ectoparasites in two diverse habitats in western Oregon. I. *Ixodes* (Acarina: Ixodidae). J. Med. Entomol., 11: 413–418.

EDDY, G. W., AND C. R. JOYCE. 1944. The seasonal history and hosts of the American dog tick, Dermacentor variabilis, in Iowa. Iowa State College, J. Sci., 18:313–324.

EDWARDS, R. L. 1949. Internal parasites of central New York muskrats (*Ondatra z. zibethica* L.). J. Parasitol., 35:547–548.

EGOSCUE, H. J. 1966. New and additional host-flea associations and distributional records of fleas from Utah. Great Basin Nat., 26:71–75.

———. 1976. Flea exchange between deer mice and some associated small mammals in western Utah. Great Basin Nat., 36:475–480.

ELLIS, L. L., JR. 1955. A survey of the ectoparasites of certain mammals in Oklahoma. Ecology, 36:12–18.

EL-WAILLY, A. 1967. Fleas of mammals in Douglas County, Kansas. Bull. Biol. Res. Center, 3:42–53.

EMERSON, K. C. 1971. New records of Anoplura from Mexico. J. Kansas Entomol. Soc., 44:374–377.

EMERSON, K. C., C. MASER, AND J. O. WHITAKER, JR. 1984. Lice (Mallophaga and Anoplura) from mammals of Oregon. Northwest Sci., 58:153–161.

ERICKSON, A. B. 1938*a*. Parasites of some Minnesota rodents. J. Mamm., 19:252–253.

———. 1938*b*. Parasites of some Minnesota Cricetidae and Zapodidae, and a host catalogue of helminth parasites of native American mice. Amer. Midland Nat., 20:575–589.

EVANS, G. O., AND W. M. TILL. 1966. Studies on the British Dermanyssidae (Acari: Mesostigmata). Part II. Classification. Bull. British Mus. (Nat. Hist.), Zool., 14:107–370.

EWING, H. E. 1925. New mites of the parasitic genus Haemogamasus Berlese. Proc. Biol. Soc. Washington, 38:137–143.

———. 1928. A preliminary key to the larvae of fifteen species of the mite genus Trombicula, with descriptions of four new species. Proc. Entomol. Soc. Washington, 30:77–80.

———. 1929*a*. Four new species of chiggers (Acarina–Trombidiidae). Entomol. News, 40:294–297.

———. 1929*b*. Notes on the siphonapteran genus Catallagia Rothschild, including the description of a new species. Proc. Biol. Soc. Washington, 42:125–128.

———. 1933. New genera and species of parasitic mites of the superfamily Parasitoidea. Proc. U.S. Natl. Mus., 82:1–14.

———. 1938. North American mites of the subfamily Myobiinae, new subfamily (Arachnida). Proc. Entomol. Soc. Washington, 40:180–197.

———. 1942. Remarks on the taxonomy of some American chiggers (Trombicu-

linae), including the descriptions of new genera and species. J. Parasitol., 28:485–493.
———. 1944. The trombiculid mites (chigger mites) and their relation to disease. J. Parasitol., 30:339–365.
FAIN, A. 1969*a*. Diagnoses de nouveaux hypopes pilicoles ou endofolliculaires (Acarina: Sarcoptiformes). Rev. Zool. Bot. Africaines, 79:409–412.
———. 1969*b*. Les deutonymphes hypopiales vivant en association phoretique sur les mammiferes (Acarina: Sarcoptiformes). Bull. Inst. Royal Sci. Nat. Belgium, 45(33):1–262.
FAIN, A., AND K. HYLAND. 1970. Notes on the Myocoptidae of North America with description of a new species on the eastern chipmunk, *Tamias striatus* Linnaeus. J. New York Entomol. Soc., 78:80–87.
———. 1972. Description of new parasitic mites from North-American mammals (Acarina: Sarcoptiformes). Rev. Zool. Bot. Africaines, 85:174–176.
———. 1974. The listrophoroid mites in North America. II. The family Listrophoridae Megnin and Trouessart (Acarina: Sarcoptiformes). Bull. Inst. Royal Sci. Nat. Belgium, 50(1):1–69.
FAIN, A., AND F. S. LUKOSCHUS. 1977. Nouvelles observations sur les Myobiidae parasites des rongeurs (Acarina: Prostigmates). Acta Zool. Pathol. Antverpiensia, 69:11–98.
FAIN, A., AND J. O. WHITAKER, JR. 1973. Phoretic hypopi of North American mammals (Acarina: Sarcoptiformes, Glycyphagidae). Acarologia, 15:144–170.
FAIN, A., A. J. MUNTING, AND F. LUKOSCHUS. 1970. Les Myocoptidae parasites des rongeurs en Hollande et en Belgique (Acarina: Sarcoptiformes). Acta Zool. Pathol. Antverpiensia, 50:67–172.
FARRELL, C. E. 1956. Chiggers of the genus Euschongastia (Acarina: Trombiculidae) in North America. Proc. U.S. Natl. Mus., 106:85–235.
FAULKENBERRY, G. D., AND R. G. ROBBINS. 1980. Statistical measures of interspecific association between the fleas of the gray-tailed vole, *Microtus canicaudus* Miller. Entomol. News, 91:93–101.
FAY, F. H., AND R. L. RAUSCH. 1969. Parasitic organisms in the blood of arvicoline rodents in Alaska. J. Parasitol., 55:1258–1265.
FERRIS, G. F. 1916. A catalogue and host list of the Anoplura. Proc. California Acad. Sci., 6:129–213.
———. 1921. Contributions toward a monograph of the sucking lice, Part II. Stanford Univ. Publ., Univ. Ser. Biol. Sci., 2:57–133.
———. 1923. Contributions toward a monograph of the sucking lice, Part IV. Stanford Univ. Publ., Univ. Ser. Biol. Sci., 2:179–270.
———. 1942. Some North American, rodent-infesting lice (Insecta: Anoplura). Microentomology, 7:84–90.
———. 1951. The sucking lice. Mem. Pacific Coast Entomol. Soc., 1:1–320.
FISH, P. G. 1972. Notes on *Moniliformis clarki* (Ward) (Acanthocephala: Moniliformidae) in west central Indiana. J. Parasitol., 58:147.
FISHER, R. L. 1963. *Capillaria hepatica* from the rock vole in New York. J. Parasitol., 49:450.
FLORSCHUTZ, O., JR., AND R. F. DARSIE, JR. 1960. Additional records of ectoparasites on Delaware mammals. Entomol. News, 71:45–52.
FORD, H. G. 1962. *Speleognathopsis michigensis* (Acarina: Speleognathidae), a new species of nasal mite from the meadow mouse, *Microtus pennsylvanicus* (Ord). Trans. Amer. Microscopical Soc., 81:104–105.

Fox, C. 1909*a*. A report on the species of the Siphonaptera found within the boundaries of the city and county of San Francisco, Cal. Entomol. News, 20:10–11.

———. 1909*b*. A new species of Ceratophyllus: a genus of the Siphonaptera. Entomol. News, 20:107–110.

———. 1909*c*. A new species of Odontopsyllus—a genus of the Siphonaptera. Entomol. News, 20:241–243.

Fox, I. 1939*a*. New species and a new genus of Nearctic Siphonaptera. Proc. Entomol. Soc. Washington, 41:45–50.

———. 1939*b*. New species and records of Siphonaptera from Mexico. Iowa State College, J. Sci., 13:335–339.

———. 1940*a*. Fleas of eastern United States. Iowa State College Press, Ames, 191 pp.

———. 1940*b*. Notes on North American dolichopsyllid Siphonaptera. Proc. Entomol. Soc. Washington, 42:64–69.

———. 1940*c*. Siphonaptera from western United States. J. Washington Acad. Sci., 30:272–276.

Freeman, R. S. 1954. Studies on the biology of *Taenia crassiceps* (Zeder, 1800) Rudolphi, 1810. J. Parasitol., Suppl., 40:41.

———. 1962. Studies on the biology of Taenia crassiceps (Zeder, 1800) Rudolphi, 1810 (Cestoda). Canadian J. Zool., 40:969–990.

Freeman, R. S., and K. A. Wright. 1960. Factors concerned with the epizootiology of *Capillaria hepatica* (Bancroft, 1893) (Nematoda) in a population of *Peromyscus maniculatus* in Algonquin Park, Canada. J. Parasitol., 46: 373–382.

Fuller, H. S. 1943*a*. Fleas of New England. J. New York Entomol. Soc., 51: 1–12.

———. 1943*b*. Studies on Siphonaptera of eastern North America. Bull. Brooklyn Entomol. Soc., 38:18–23.

Furman, D. P. 1955. Revision of the genus Eubrachylaelaps (Acarina: Laelaptidae) with the descriptions of two new species from Mexico. Ann. Entomol. Soc. Amer., 48:51–59.

———. 1959*a*. Feeding habits of symbiotic mesostigmatid mites of mammals in relation to pathogen-vector potentials. Amer. J. Trop. Med. Hyg., 8: 5–12.

———. 1959*b*. Observations on the biology and morphology of *Haemogamasus ambulans* (Thorell) (Acarina: Haemogamasidae). J. Parasitol., 45:274–280.

Furman, D. P., and E. C. Loomis. 1984. The ticks of California (Acari: Ixodida). Bull. California Insect Surv., 25:1–239.

Gabbutt, P. D. 1961. The distribution of some small mammals and their associated fleas from central Labrador. Ecology, 42:518–525.

Garvie, M. B., J. A. McKiel, D. E. Sonenshine, and A. Campbell. 1978. Seasonal dynamics of American dog tick, *Dermacentor variabilis* (Say), populations in southwestern Nova Scotia. Canadian J. Zool., 56:28–39.

Gates, D. B. 1945. Notes on fleas (Siphonaptera) in Nebraska. Entomol. News, 56:10–13.

Geary, J. M. 1959. The fleas of New York. Mem. Cornell Univ. Agric. Exp. Sta., 355:1–104.

Genoways, H. H., and J. K. Jones, Jr. 1972. Mammals from southwestern North Dakota. Occas. Papers Mus., Texas Tech Univ., 6:1–36.

Getz, L. L. 1970. Botfly infestations in Microtus pennsylvanicus in southern Wisconsin. Amer. Midland Nat., 84:187–197.

GIESEN, K. M. T., F. S. LUKOSCHUS, J. O. WHITAKER, JR., AND D. GETTINGER. 1983. Four new species of itch mites (Acari: Psorergatidae: Prostigmata) from small mammals in North America. J. Med. Entomol., 20:164–173.

GOULD, D. J., AND M. L. MIESSE. 1954. Recovery of a *Rickettsia* of the spotted fever group from *Microtus pennslyvanicus* from Virginia. Proc. Soc. Exp. Biol. Med., 85:558–561.

GOULD, O. J. 1956. The larval trombiculid mites of California (Acarina: Trombiculidae). Univ. California Publ. Entomol., 11:1–116.

GRANT, C. D. 1947. North American mites of the genus Laelaps (Arachnida: Acarina: Parasitidae). Microentomology, 12:2–21.

GREGSON, J. D. 1956. The Ixodoidea of Canada. Publ. Canada Dept. Agric., Sci. Ser., Entomol. Div., 930:1–92.

GRESBRINK, R. A., AND D. D. HOPKINS. 1982. Siphonaptera: host records from Crater Lake National Park, Oregon. Northwest Sci., 56:176–179.

GYORKOS, T. W., AND D. F. J. HILTON. 1982*a*. Range extensions for some ectoparasites from rodents of southeastern Quebec. Canadian J. Zool., 60: 486–488.

———. 1982*b*. The prevalence and distribution patterns of ectoparasites from wild rodents in southeastern Québec. Nat. Canadien (Rev. Écol. Syst.), 109: 139–145.

HAAS, G. E. 1973. Morphological notes on some Siphonaptera (Leptopsyllidae and Ceratophyllidae) of New Mexico. Amer. Midland Nat., 90:246–252.

HAAS, G. E., AND N. WILSON. 1973. Siphonaptera of Wisconsin. Proc. Entomol. Soc. Washington, 75:302–314.

HAAS, G. E., R. E. BARRETT, AND N. WILSON. 1978. Siphonaptera from mammals in Alaska. Canadian J. Zool., 56:333–338.

HAAS, G. E., R. P. MARTIN, M. SWICKARD, AND B. E. MILLER. 1973. Siphonaptera-mammal relationships in northcentral New Mexico. J. Med. Entomol., 10:281–289.

HAAS, G. E., T. RUMFELT, L. JOHNSON, AND N. WILSON. 1979. Siphonaptera from mammals in Alaska. Supplement I. Canadian J. Zool., 57:1822–1825.

HAAS, G. E., N. WILSON, R. L. ZARNKE, R. E. BARRETT, AND T. RUMFELT. 1982. Siphonaptera from mammals in Alaska. Supplement III. Western Alaska. Canadian J. Zool., 60:729–732.

HALL, J. E., AND B. SONNENBERG. 1955. Some helminth parasites of rodents from localities in Maryland and Kentucky. J. Parasitol., 41:640–641.

HAMILTON, W. J., JR. 1930. Notes on the mammals of Breathitt County, Kentucky. J. Mamm., 11:306–311.

———. 1938. Life history notes on the northern pine mouse. J. Mamm., 19:163–170.

HANSEN, C. G. 1964. Ectoparasites of mammals from Oregon. Great Basin Nat., 24:75–81.

HANSEN, M. F. 1947. Three anoplocephalid cestodes from the prairie meadow vole, with description of *Andrya microti* n. sp. Trans. Amer. Microscopical Soc., 66:279–282.

———. 1950. A new dilepidid tapeworm and notes on other tapeworms of rodents. Amer. Midland Nat., 43:471–479.

HARDY, J. L., W. C. REEVES, R. P. SCRIVANI, AND D. R. ROBERTS. 1974. Wild mammals as hosts of group A and group B arboviruses in Kern County, California: a five-year serologic and virologic survey. Amer. J. Trop. Med. Hyg., 23:1165–1177.

HARKEMA, R. 1936. The parasites of some North Carolina rodents. Ecol. Monogr., 6:153–232.

HARLAN, H. J., AND D. B. PALMER, JR. 1974. Ectoparasites of mammals and birds from Fort Bragg, North Carolina. J. Elisha Mitchell Sci. Soc., 90: 141–144.

HARPER, F. 1929. Notes on the mammals of the Adirondacks. New York State Mus. Handb., 8:51–118.

———. 1956. The mammals of Keewatin. Misc. Publ. Mus. Nat. Hist., Univ. Kansas, 12:1–94.

———. 1961. Land and fresh-water mammals of the Ungava Peninsula. Misc. Publ. Mus. Nat. Hist., Univ. Kansas, 27:1–178.

HARRAH, E. C. 1922. North American monostomes, primarily from fresh water hosts. Illinois Biol. Monogr., 7:1–106.

HARTWELL, W. V., S. F. QUAN, K. G. SCOTT, AND L. KARTMAN. 1958. Observations on flea transfer between hosts; a mechanism in the spread of bubonic plague. Science, 127:814.

HARWOOD, P. D. 1939. Notes on Tennessee helminths. IV. North American trematodes of the subfamily Notocotylinae. J. Tennessee Acad. Sci., 14:421–437.

HAYS, K. L., AND F. E. GUYTON. 1958. Parasitic mites (Acarina: Mesostigmata) from Alabama mammals. J. Econ. Entomol., 51:259–260.

HENSLEY, M. S. 1976. Prevalence of cuterebrid parasitism among woodmice in Virginia. J. Wildl. Dis., 12:172–179.

HERRIN, C. S. 1970. A systematic revision of the genus *Hirstionyssus* (Acari: Mesostigmata) of the Nearctic region. J. Med. Entomol., 7:391–437.

HERTIG, M., AND C. SMILEY. 1937. The problem of controlling woodticks on Martha's Vineyard. Vineyard Gaz., 15 Jan., pp. 1–7.

HNATIUK, J. M. 1966. First occurrence of Echinococcus multilocularis Leuckart, 1863 in Microtus pennsylvanicus in Saskatchewan. Canadian J. Zool., 44: 493.

HOFFMANN, A., I. B. DE BARRERA, AND C. MÉNDEZ. 1972. Nuevos hallazgos de ácaros en México. Rev. Soc. Mex. Hist. Nat., 33:151–159.

HOLDENRIED, R., AND H. B. MORLAN. 1956. A field study of wild mammals and fleas of Santa Fe County, New Mexico. Amer. Midland Nat., 55:369–381.

HOLDENRIED, R., F. C. EVANS, AND D. S. LONGANECKER. 1951. Host-parasite-disease relationships in a mammalian community in the central coast range of California. Ecol. Monogr., 21:1–18.

HOLLAND, G. P. 1941. Further records of Siphonaptera for British Columbia. Proc. Entomol. Soc. British Columbia, 37:10–14.

———. 1949*a*. The Siphonaptera of Canada. Tech. Bull., Canadian Dept. Agric., Ottawa, 817:1–306.

———. 1949*b*. A revised check list of the fleas of British Columbia. Proc. Entomol. Soc. British Columbia., 45:7–14.

———. 1950. Notes on *Megabothris asio* (Baker) and *M. calcarifer* (Wagner) with the description of a new subspecies (Siphonaptera: Ceratophyllidae). Canadian Entomol., 82:126–133.

———. 1951. A note on the occurrence of *Catallagia dacenkoi* Ioff in North America, with the description of a Nearctic subspecies (Siphonaptera: Neopsyllidae). Canadian Entomol., 83:156–160.

———. 1952*a*. Notes on some Siphonaptera from Canada. Canadian Entomol., 84:65–73.

———. 1952*b*. Descriptions of fleas from northern Canada (Siphonaptera). Canadian Entomol., 84:297–308.

———. 1957. Notes on the genus *Hystrichopsylla* Rothschild in the New World, with descriptions of one new species and two new subspecies (Siphonaptera: Hystrichopsyllidae). Canadian Entomol., 89:309–324.

———. 1958. Distribution patterns of northern fleas (Siphonaptera). Proc. Tenth Internatl. Congr. Entomol., 1:645–658.

———. 1963. Faunal affinities of the fleas (Siphonaptera) of Alaska: with an annotated list of species. Pp. 45–63, *in* Pacific basin biogeography (J. L. Gressitt, ed.). Bishop Mus. Press, Honolulu, Hawaii, 563 pp.

HOLLAND, G. P., AND A. H. BENTON. 1968. Siphonaptera from Pennsylvania mammals. Amer. Midland Nat., 80:252–261.

HOLLIMAN, R. B., AND B. J. MEADE. 1980. Native trichinosis in wild rodents in Henrico County, Virginia. J. Wildl. Dis., 16:205–207.

HOOGSTRAAL, H. 1981. Changing patterns of tickborne diseases in modern society. Ann. Rev. Entomol., 26:75–99.

HOOKER, W. A., F. C. BISHOPP, AND H. P. WOOD. 1912. The life history and bionomics of some North American ticks. Bull. U.S. Dept. Agric. Bur. Entomol., 106:1–239.

HOPKINS, G. H. E., AND M. ROTHSCHILD. 1962. An illustrated catalogue of the Rothschild collection of fleas (Siphonaptera) in the British Museum (Natural History) with keys and short descriptions for the identification of families, genera, species and subspecies of the order. III. Hystrichopsyllidae (Acedestiinae, Anomiopsyllinae, Hystrichopsyllinae, Neopsyllinae, Rhadinopsyllinae and Stenoponiinae). British Mus. (Nat. Hist.) Publ., 410:1–560.

———. 1966. An illustrated catalogue. . . . IV. Hystrichopsyllidae (Ctenophthalminae, Dinopsyllinae, Doratopsyllinae and Listropsyllinae). British Mus. (Nat. Hist.) Publ., 652:1–549.

———. 1971. An illustrated catalogue. . . . V. Leptopsyllidae and Ancistropsyllidae. British Mus. (Nat. Hist.) Publ., 706:1–530.

HOPLA, C. E. 1965*a*. Alaskan hematophagous insects, their feeding habits and potential as vectors of pathogenic organisms. I: The Siphonaptera of Alaska. Arctic Aeromed. Tech. Rept., 64(12):1–344.

———. 1965*b*. Ecology and epidemiology research studies in Alaska: a report of field collections and laboratory diagnostic assay. Univ. Oklahoma Res. Inst., 1471:1–242.

———. 1980. Fleas as vectors of tularemia in Alaska. Pp. 287–300, *in* Fleas (R. Traub and H. Starcke, eds.). Proc. Internatl. Conf. Fleas. A. A. Balkema, Rotterdam, 420 pp.

HUBBARD, C. A. 1940*a*. American mole and shrew fleas (a new genus, three new species). Pacific Univ. Bull., 37(2):1–12.

———. 1940*b*. A review of the western fleas of the genus Malaraeus with one new species and the description of a new Thrassis from Nevada. Pacific Univ. Bull., 37(6):1–4.

———. 1941*a*. The fleas of rare western mice. Pacific Univ. Bull., 37(9A):1–4.

———. 1941*b*. History of the flea genus Micropsylla. Pacific Univ. Bull., 37(10): 1–4.

———. 1947. Fleas of western North America. Iowa State College Press, Ames, 533 pp.

———. 1949*a*. Fleas in the collection of the Royal Ontario Museum of Zoology. Canadian Entomol., 81:11–12.

———. 1949*b*. Additional data upon the fleas of the sagebrush vole. Entomol. News, 60:169–174.

———. 1949*c*. Fleas of the State of Nevada. Bull. S. California Acad. Sci., 48: 115–128.

———. 1960. A packet of fleas from Alaska. Entomol. News, 71:245–247.

HUNTER, D. M., R. M. F. S. SADLEIR, AND J. M. WEBSTER. 1972. Studies on the ecology of cuterebrid parasitism in deermice. Canadian J. Zool., 50: 25–29.

HUNTER, W. D., AND F. C. BISHOPP. 1911. The Rocky Mountain spotted-fever tick, with special reference to the problem of its control in the Bitter Root Valley in Montana. Bull. U.S. Dept. Agric. Bur. Entomol., 105:1–47.

IGNOFFO, C. M. 1956. Notes on louse-host associations of the Great Salt Lake Desert with keys to the lice. Great Basin Nat., 16:9–17.

———. 1959. Key and notes to the Anoplura of Minnesota. Amer. Midland Nat., 61:470–479.

IVERSON, S. L., AND B. N. TURNER. 1968. The effect of *Cuterebra* spp. on weight, survival and reproduction in *Microtus pennsylvanicus*. Manitoba Entomol., 2:70–75.

JACOBSEN, B. 1966. Unidentified *Cuterebra* in mice and voles. Proc. Entomol. Soc. Manitoba, 22:29.

JAMESON, E. W., JR. 1943*a*. Notes on some fleas of New York state. Canadian Entomol., 75:177.

———. 1943*b*. Notes on the habits and siphonapterous parasites of the mammals of Welland County, Ontario. J. Mamm., 24:194–197.

———. 1947. Natural history of the prairie vole (mammalian genus *Microtus*). Univ. Kansas Publ., Mus. Nat. Hist., 1:125–151.

———. 1950. Catallagia mathesoni, a new hystrichopsyllid flea (Siphonaptera) from California. J. Kansas Entomol. Soc., 23:94–96.

JAMESON, E. W., JR., AND J. M. BRENNAN. 1957. An environmental analysis of some ectoparasites of small forest mammals in the Sierra Nevada, California. Ecol. Monogr., 27:45–54.

JELLISON, W. L., AND C. M. SENGER. 1973. Fleas of Montana. Res. Rept., Montana Agric. Exp. Sta., 29:1–79.

———. 1976. Fleas of western North America except Montana in the Rocky Mountain Laboratory collection. Pp. 55–136, *in* Papers in honor of Jerry Flora (H. C. Taylor, Jr. and J. Clark, eds.). Western Washington State College, Bellingham, 281 pp.

JELLISON, W. L., J. F. BELL, AND C. R. OWEN. 1959. Mouse disease studies. Pp. 71–80, *in* The Oregon meadow mouse irruption of 1957–1958. Bull. Oregon State College, Corvallis, 88 pp.

JELLISON, W. L., ET AL. 1958. Preliminary observations on diseases in the 1957–58 outbreak of Microtus in western United States. Trans. Twenty-third N. Amer. Wildl. Conf., 137–145.

JENKINS, D. W. 1949. Trombiculid mites affecting man IV. Revision of Eutrombicula in the American hemisphere. Ann. Entomol. Soc. Amer., 42:289–318.

JOHNSON, D. E. 1966. Ticks of Dugway Proving Ground and vicinity and their host associations. Proc. Utah Acad. Sci. Arts Letters, 43:49–66.

JOHNSON, P. T. 1961. A revision of the species of *Monopsyllus* Kolenati in North America (Siphonaptera, Ceratophyllidae). Tech. Bull., U.S. Dept. Agric., 1227:1–69.

JOHNSON, P. T., AND R. TRAUB. 1954. Revision of the flea genus Peromyscopsylla. Smithsonian Misc. Coll., 123(4):1–68.

JONES, G. S., AND H. H. THOMAS. 1980. Ticks from mammals from Prince Edward Island, New Brunswick, northern Nova Scotia, and Gaspé Peninsula, Quebec. Canadian J. Zool., 58:1394–1397.

JORDAN, K. 1928. Siphonaptera collected during a visit to the eastern United States of North America in 1927. Novitates Zool., 34:178–188.

———. 1929. On a small collection of Siphonaptera from the Adirondacks, with a list of the species known from the state of New York. Novitates Zool., 35:168–177.

———. 1932. Siphonaptera collected by Mr. Harry S. Swarth at Atlin in British Columbia. Novitates Zool., 38:253–255.

———. 1933. Records of Siphonaptera from the state of New York. Novitates Zool., 39:62–65.

JORDAN, K., AND N. C. ROTHSCHILD. 1913. On the genus *Amphipsylla,* Wagn. (1909). Zoologist, 17:401–410.

JOYCE, C. R., AND G. W. EDDY. 1944. A list of fleas (Siphonaptera) collected at Tama, Iowa. Iowa State College J. Sci., 18:209–215.

JUDD, W. W. 1950. Mammal host records of Acarina and Insecta from the vicinity of Hamilton, Ontario. J. Mamm., 31:357–358.

———. 1953. Mammal host records of Acarina and Insecta from the vicinity of London, Ontario. J. Mamm., 34:137–139.

———. 1954. Some records of ectoparasitic Acarina and Insecta from mammals in Ontario. J. Parasitol., 40:483–484.

KARDOS, E. H. 1954. Biological and systematic studies on the subgenus *Neotrombicula* (genus *Trombicula*) in the central United States (Acarina, Trombiculidae). Univ. Kansas Sci. Bull., 36:69–123.

KARTMAN, L. 1958. An insecticide-bait-box method for the control of sylvatic plague vectors. J. Hyg., 56:455–465.

———. 1960. Further observations on an insecticide-bait-box meth DDT powder. J. Hyg., 58:119–124.

KARTMAN, L., AND F. M. PRINCE. 1956. Studies on *Pasteurella pestis* in fleas. V. The experimental plague-vector efficiency of wild rodent fleas compared with *Xenopsylla cheopis,* together with observations on the influence of temperature. Amer. J. Trop. Med. Hyg., 5:1058–1070.

KARTMAN, L., V. I. MILES, AND F. M. PRINCE. 1958*a*. Ecological studies of wild rodent plague in the San Francisco Bay area of California. Amer. J. Trop. Med. Hyg., 7:112–124.

KARTMAN, L., F. M. PRINCE, AND S. F. QUAN. 1958*c*. Studies on *Pasteurella pestis* in fleas. VII. The plague-vector efficiency of *Hystrichopsylla linsdalei* compared with *Xenopsylla cheopis* under experimental conditions. Amer. J. Trop. Med. Hyg., 7:317–322.

KARTMAN, L., S. F. QUAN, AND V. I. MILES. 1960. Ecological studies of wild rodent plague in the San Francisco Bay area of California. V. The distribution of naturally infected fleas during an epizootic in relation to their infection rates. Amer. J. Trop. Med. Hyg., 9:96–100.

KARTMAN, L., F. M. PRINCE, S. F. QUAN, AND H. E. STARK. 1958*d*. New knowledge on the ecology of sylvatic plague. Ann. New York Acad. Sci., 70:668–711.

KARTMAN, L., K. F. MURRAY, F. M. PRINCE, S. F. QUAN, AND M. A. HOLMES. 1958*b*. Public health implications of the Microtus outbreak in Oregon and California during 1957–1958. California Vector News, 5:19–24.

KEEGAN, H. L. 1951. The mites of the subfamily Haemogamasinae (Acari: Laelaptidae). Proc. U.S. Natl. Mus., 101:203–268.

KEIRANS, J. E., AND C. M. CLIFFORD. 1978. The genus *Ixodes* in the United

States: A scanning election microscope study and key to the adults. J. Med. Entomol. Suppl., 2:1–149.

———. 1983. *Ixodes (Pholeoixodes) eastoni* n. sp. (Acari: Ixodidae), a parasite of rodents and insectivores in the Black Hills of South Dakota, USA. J. Med. Entomol., 20:90–98.

KELLOGG, V. L., AND G. F. FERRIS. 1915. The Anoplura and Mallophaga of North American mammals. Leland Stanford Junior Univ. Publ., Univ. Ser., 20:1–74.

KINSELLA, J. M. 1967. Helminths of Microtinae in western Montana. Canadian J. Zool., 45:269–274.

KINSELLA, J. M., AND D. L. PATTIE. 1967. Ectoparasites of small mammals of the alpine Beartooth Plateau, Wyoming. Canadian J. Zool., 45:233–235.

KIRKLAND, G. L., JR., AND F. J. JANNETT, JR. 1982. *Microtus chrotorrhinus*. Mamm. Species, 180:1–5.

KNIPPING, P. A., B. B. MORGAN, AND R. J. DICKE. 1950*a*. Notes on the distribution of Wisconsin ticks. Trans. Wisconsin Acad. Sci. Arts Letters, 40:185–197.

———. 1950*b*. Preliminary list of some fleas from Wisconsin. Trans. Wisconsin Acad. Sci. Arts Letters, 40:199–206.

KOK, N. J. J., F. S. LUKOSCHUS, AND F. V. CLULOW. 1971. Three new itch mites from Canadian small mammals (Acarina: Psorergatidae). Canadian J. Zool., 49:1239–1248.

KOMAREK, E. V., AND R. KOMAREK. 1938. Mammals of the Great Smoky Mountains. Bull. Chicago Acad. Sci., 5:137–162.

KUNS, M. L., AND R. RAUSCH. 1950. An ecological study of helminths of some Wyoming voles (*Microtus* spp.) with a description of a new species of *Nematospiroides* (Heligmosomidae: Nematoda). Zoologica, 35:181–188.

LAMPE, R. P., J. K. JONES, JR., R. S. HOFFMANN, AND E. C. BIRNEY. 1974. The mammals of Carter County, southeastern Montana. Occas. Papers Mus. Nat. Hist., Univ. Kansas, 25:1–39.

LARROUSE, F., A. G. KING, AND S. B. WOLBACH. 1928. The overwintering in Massachusetts of Ixodiphagus caucurtei. Science, 67:351–353.

LAVOIPIERRE, M. M. J. 1964. Mange mites of the genus *Notoedres* (Acari: Sarcoptidae) with descriptions of two new species and remarks on notoedric mange in the squirrel and the vole. J. Med. Entomol., 1:5–17.

LAWRENCE, W. H., K. L. HAYS, AND S. A. GRAHAM. 1965. Arthropodous ectoparasites from some northern Michigan mammals. Occas. Papers Mus. Zool., Univ. Michigan, 639:1–7.

LAYNE, J. N. 1958. Records of fleas (Siphonaptera) from Illinois mammals. Nat. Hist. Misc., Chicago Acad. Sci., 162:1–7.

LEE, C., AND D. J. HORVATH. 1969. Management of the meadow vole (*Microtus pennsylvanicus*). Lab. Anim. Care, 19:88–91.

LEIBY, P. D. 1962. Helminth parasites recovered from some rodents in southeastern Idaho. Amer. Midland Nat., 67:250.

———. 1965. Cestode in North Dakota: Echinococcus in field mice. Science, 150: 763.

LEIBY, P. D., AND F. H. WHITTAKER. 1966. Occurrence of *Taenia crassiceps* in the conterminous United States. J. Parasitol., 52:786.

LEIBY, P. D., W. P. CARNEY, AND C. E. WOODS. 1970. Studies on sylvatic echinococcosis. III. Host occurrence and geographic distribution of *Echinococcus multilocularis* in the north central United States. J. Parasitol., 56:1141–1150.

LEWIS, R. E. 1975. Notes on the geographical distribution and host preferences in the order Siphonaptera. Part 6. Ceratophyllidae. J. Med. Entomol., 11: 658–676.

LICHTENFELS, J. R., AND A. J. HALEY. 1968. New host records of intestinal nematodes of Maryland rodents and suppression of *Capillaria bonnevillei* Grundmann and Frandsen, 1960 as a synonym of *C. americana* Read, 1949. Proc. Helminthol. Soc. Washington, 35:206–211.

LIDICKER, W. Z., JR. 1973. Regulation of numbers in an island population of the California vole, a problem in community dynamics. Ecol. Monogr., 43: 271–302.

LINSDALE, J. M., AND B. S. DAVIS. 1956. Taxonomic appraisal and occurrence of fleas at the Hastings Reservation in central California. Univ. California Publ. Zool., 54:293–370.

LINZEY, D. W., AND A. V. LINZEY. 1973. Notes on parasites of small mammals from Great Smoky Mountains National Park, Tennessee-North Carolina. J. Elisha Mitchell Sci. Soc., 89:120.

LOCHMILLER, R. L., R. M. ROBINSON, AND R. L. KIRKPATRICK. 1982*a*. Infection of *Microtus pinetorum* with the nematode *Capillaria gastrica* (Baylis, 1926) Baylis, 1931. Proc. Helminthol. Soc. Washington, 49:321–323.

LOCHMILLER, R. L., E. J. JONES, J. B. WHELAN, AND R. L. KIRKPATRICK. 1982*b*. The occurrence of *Taenia taeniaeformis* strobilocerci in *Microtus pinetorum*. J. Parasitol., 68:975–976.

LOOMIS, R. B. 1956. The chigger mites of Kansas (Acarina, Trombiculidae). Univ. Kansas Sci. Bull., 37:1195–1443.

LOVEJOY, D. A., AND P. J. GAUGHAN. 1975. Notes on a collection of mammal-fleas from New Hampshire. Entomol. News, 86:145–149.

LUBINSKY, G. 1957. List of helminths from Alberta rodents. Canadian J. Zool., 35:623–627.

LUBINSKY, G., B. R. JACOBSEN, AND R. W. BARON. 1971. Wildlife foci of *Capillaria hepatica* infections in Manitoba. Canadian J. Zool., 49:1201–1202.

LUDWIG, D. R. 1984. *Microtus richardsoni*. Mamm. Species, 223:1–6.

MACCHIAVELLO, A. 1954. Reservoirs and vectors of plague. B. Plague reservoirs and other animals susceptible to plague infection either spontaneously or experimentally. Trop. Med. Hyg., 57:158–171.

MACCREARY, D. 1940. Meadow mouse is the preferred host of the spotted fever tick in Delaware. Delaware Agric. Exp. Sta. Bull., 227:229–230.

———. 1945*a*. Some ectoparasites, excluding Ixodoidea, of Delaware mammals. J. Econ. Entomol., 38:126–127.

———. 1945*b*. Ticks of Delaware, with special reference to *Dermacentor variabilis* (Say) vector of Rocky Mountain spotted fever. Delaware Agric. Exp. Sta. Bull., 252:1–22.

MAGNARELLI, L. A., ET AL. 1983. Rickettsiae-infected ticks (Acari: Ixodidae) and seropositive mammals at a focus for Rocky Mountain spotted fever in Connecticut, USA. J. Med. Entomol., 20:151–156.

MAIN, A. J. 1970. Distribution, seasonal abundance and host preference of fleas in New England. Proc. Entomol. Soc. Washington, 72:73–89.

———. 1983. Fleas (Siphonaptera) on small mammals in Connecticut, USA. J. Med. Entomol., 20:33–39.

MAIN, A. J., A. B. CAREY, M. G. CAREY, AND R. H. GOODWIN. 1982. Immature *Ixodes dammini* (Acari: Ixodidae) on small animals in Connecticut, USA. J. Med. Entomol., 19:655–664.

MAIN, A. J., A. B. CAREY, M. G. CAREY, AND V. A. NELSON. 1979. Additional records of Siphonaptera in southern New England. Entomol. News, 90: 135–140.

MANISCHEWITZ, J. R. 1966. Studies on parasitic mites of New Jersey. J. New York Entomol. Soc., 74:189–197.

MANVILLE, R. H. 1949. A study of small mammal populations in northern Michigan. Misc. Publ. Mus. Zool., Univ. Michigan, 73:1–83.

———. 1961. Cutaneous myiasis in small mammals. J. Parasitol., 47:646.

MARTELL, A. M., R. E. YESCOTT, D. G. DODDS. 1969. Some records for Ixodidae of Nova Scotia. Canadian J. Zool., 47:183–184.

MARTIN, R. L. 1972. Parasites and diseases of the rock vole. Occas. Papers, Biol. Sci. Ser., Univ. Connecticut, 2:107–113.

MASER, C., AND E. F. HOOVEN. 1971. New host and locality records for *Leptinus testaceus* Muller in western Oregon (Coleoptera: Leptinidae). Coleopterists Bull., 25:119–120.

MATHEWSON, J. A., AND K. E. HYLAND. 1962. The ectoparasites of Rhode Island mammals. II. A collection of Anoplura from non-domestic hosts (Anoplura). J. New York Entomol. Soc., 70:167–174.

———. 1964. The ectoparasites of Rhode Island mammals. III. A collection of fleas from nondomestic hosts (Siphonaptera). J. Kansas Entomol. Soc., 37: 157–163.

MAURER, F. W., JR., AND J. E. SKALEY. 1968. Cuterebrid infestation of *Microtus* in eastern North Dakota, Pennsylvania, and New York. J. Mamm., 49: 773–774.

MCBEE, R. H., JR. 1977. Varying prevalence of *Taenia taeniaeformis* strobilocerci in *Microtus pennsylvanicus* of Montana. Great Basin Nat., 37:252.

MCDANIEL, B. 1979. Host records of ectoparasites from small mammals of South Dakota. Southwestern Nat., 24:689–691.

MCDANIEL, B., J. P. SHOEMAKER, AND S. J. JOY. 1967. The discovery of Listrophorus leuckarti Pagenstecher on Microtus pennsylvanicus pennsylvanicus from North America (Acarina: Listrophoridae). Proc. Entomol. Soc. Washington, 69:340–343.

MCENROE, W. D. 1983. The role of the summer cohort in the population regulation of the two cohort cycle of Dermacentor variabilis (Say). Folia Parasitol., 30:163–168.

MCINTOSH, A., AND G. E. MCINTOSH. 1934. A new trematode, *Notocotylus bassalli* n. sp. (Notocotylidae), from a meadow mouse. Proc. Helminthol. Soc. Washington, 2:80.

MCPHERSON, S. E., AND J. D. TINER. 1952. A new nematode (*Rictularia microti*) from a vole on St. Lawrence Island, Alaska. Nat. Hist. Misc., Chicago Acad. Sci., 108:1–7.

MEGGITT, F. J. 1924. The cestodes of mammals. Frommannsche Buchdr. (H. Pohle), Jena, D.D.R., 282 pp.

MELLOTT, J. L., AND W. A. CONNELL. 1965. A preliminary list of Delaware Acarina. Trans. Amer. Entomol. Soc., 91:85–94.

MILES, V. I., A. R. KINNEY, AND H. E. STARK. 1957. Flea-host relationships of associated *Rattus* and native wild rodents in the San Francisco Bay area of California, with special reference to plague. Amer. J. Trop. Med. Hyg., 6:752–760.

MILLER, D. H., AND A. H. BENTON. 1973. An annotated list of the Siphonaptera of Connecticut. J. New York Entomol. Soc., 81:210–213.

MITZMAIN, M. B. 1909. List of the Siphonaptera of California. Canadian Entomol., 41:197–204.

MOHR, C. O., AND W. A. STUMPF. 1964. Louse and chigger infestations as related to host size and home ranges of small mammals. Trans. Twenty-ninth N. Amer. Wildl. Nat. Res. Conf., 29:181–195.

MOHR, C. O., D E. BECK, AND E. P. BRINTON. 1964. Observations on host-parasite relationships and seasonal history of ticks in San Mateo County, California. Great Basin Nat., 24:1–6.

MORLAN, H. B. 1952. Host relationships and seasonal abundance of some southwest Georgia ectoparasites. Amer. Midland Nat., 48:74–93.

———. 1955. Mammal fleas of Santa Fe County, New Mexico. Texas Rept. Biol. Med., 13:93–125.

MORLAN, H. B., AND C. C. HOFF. 1957. Notes on some Anoplura from New Mexico and Mexico. J. Parasitol., 43:347–351.

MUMFORD, R. E., AND J. O. WHITAKER, JR. 1982. Mammals of Indiana. Indiana Univ. Press, Bloomington, 537 pp.

MURRAY, K. F. 1957. An ecological appraisal of host-ectoparasite relationships in a zone of epizootic plague in central California. Amer. J. Trop. Med. Hyg., 6:1068–1086.

NUTTING, W. B., AND C. E. DESCH, JR. 1979. Relationships between mammalian and demodicid phylogeny. Pp. 339–345, *in* Recent advances in acarology, Vol. II (J. G. Rodriguez, ed.). Academic Press, New York, 569 pp.

OCONNOR, B. M. 1978. A redescription of *Speleorodens michigenesis* (Ford) n. comb. (Acari: Ereynetidae), a nasal mite of microtine rodents, with comments on generic relationships in the Speleognathinae. J. New York Entomol. Soc., 86:123–129.

OHBAYASHI, M. 1971. *Hepatozoon sp.* in northern voles, *Microtus oeconomus,* on St. Lawrence Island, Alaska. J. Wildl. Dis., 7:49–51.

OSBORN, H. 1896. Insects affecting domestic animals: an account of the species of importance in North America, with mention of related forms occurring on other animals. U.S. Dept. Agric. Div. Entomol. Bull. 5:1–302.

OSGOOD, F. L., JR. 1964. Fleas of Vermont. J. New York Entomol. Soc., 72: 29–33.

PALMER, D. B., JR., AND C. W. WINGO. 1972. Siphonaptera occurring on Missouri mammals. Trans. Missouri Acad. Sci., 6:43–55.

PARKER, R. R., AND R. W. WELLS. 1917. Some facts of importance concerning the Rocky Mountain spotted fever tick, (*Dermacentor venustus* Banks) in eastern Montana. Bienn. Rept. Montana State Bd. Entomol., 1915–1916: 45–56.

PARKER, R. R., C. B. PHILIP, AND W. L. JELLISON. 1933. Rocky Mountain spotted fever. Potentialities of tick transmission in relation to geographical occurrence in the United States. Amer. J. Trop. Med., 13:341–380.

PECK, S. B. 1982. A review of the ectoparasitic *Leptinus* beetles of North America (Coleoptera: Leptinidae). Canadian J. Zool., 60:1517–1527.

PLATT, T. R. 1978. A report of *Polymorphus paradoxus* (Acanthocephala) in *Microtus pennsylvanicus* from Hastings Lake, Alberta (Canada). Proc. Helminthol. Soc. Washington, 45:255.

POINAR, G. O., JR. 1965. Life history of *Pelodera strongyloides* (Schneider) in the orbits of murid rodents in Great Britain. Proc. Helminthol. Soc. Washington, 32:148–151.

POORBAUGH, J. H., AND H. T. GIER. 1961. Fleas (Siphonaptera) of small mammals in Kansas. J. Kansas Entomol. Soc., 34:198–204.

PRICE, H. F. 1931. Life-history of *Schistosomatium douthitti* (Cort). Amer. J. Hyg., 13:685–727.

QUACKENBUSH, R. E. 1971. Fleas from Windham County, Vermont (Siphonaptera). J. New York Entomol. Soc., 79:15–18.

QUAN, S. F., V. I. MILES, AND L. KARTMAN. 1960*a*. Ecological studies of wild rodent plague in the San Francisco Bay area of California. III. The natural infection rates with *Pasteurella pestis* in five flea species during an epizootic. Amer. J. Trop. Med. Hyg., 9:85–90.

QUAN, S. F., L. KARTMAN, F. M. PRINCE, AND V. I. MILES. 1960*b*. Ecological studies of wild rodent plague in the San Francisco Bay area of California. IV. The fluctuation and intensity of natural infection with *Pasteurella pestis* in fleas during an epizootic. Amer. J. Trop. Med. Hyg., 9:91–95.

QUAY, W. B. 1949. Further description of *Polyplax alaskensis* Ewing (Anoplura). Psyche, 56:180–183.

———. 1951. Observations on mammals of the Seward Peninsula, Alaska. J. Mamm., 32:88–99.

QUENTIN, J.-C. 1971. Sur les modalités d'évolution chez quelques lignées d'Helminthes de rongeuers Muroidea. Cah. O.R.S.T.O.M., Ser. Entomol. Med. Parasitol. IX, 2:103–176.

RACE, S. R. 1956. The Anoplura of New Jersey. J. New York Entomol. Soc., 64: 173–184.

RADFORD, C. D. 1954. The larval genera and species of "harvest mites" (Acarina: Trombiculidae). Parasitology, 44:247–276.

———. 1955. Some new and little-known mites of the genus *Myocoptes* (Claparede (Acarina: Listrophoridae). Parasitology, 45:275–286.

RADOVSKY, F. J. 1960*a*. *Haemogamasus liponyssoides hesperus,* n. ssp., with a discussion of the *H. liponyssoides* complex (Acarina: Haemogamasidae). J. Parasitol., 46:401–409.

———. 1960*b*. Biological studies on *Haemogamasus liponyssoides* Ewing (Acarina: Haemogamasidae). J. Parasitol., 46:410–417.

RANKIN, J. S., JR. 1945. Ecology of the helminth parasites of small mammals collected from Northrup Canyon, upper Grand Coulee, Washington. Murrelet, 26:11–14.

RAPP, W. F., JR. 1962. Distributional notes on parasitic mites. Acarologia, 4: 31–33.

RAPP, W. F., JR. AND D. B. GATES. 1957. A distributional check-list of the fleas of Nebraska. J. Kansas Entomol. Soc., 30:50–53.

RAUSCH, R. L. 1946. *Paranoplocephala troeschi,* new species of cestode from the meadow vole, *Microtus p. pennsylvanicus* Ord. Trans. Amer. Microscopical Soc., 65:354–356.

———. 1952*a*. Studies on the helminth fauna of Alaska. XI. Helminth parasites of microtine rodents—taxonomic considerations. J. Parasitol., 38:415–444.

———. 1952*b*. Helminths from the round-tailed muskrat, *Neofiber alleni nigrescens* Howell, with descriptions of two new species. J. Parasitol., 38:151–156.

———. 1957. Distribution and specificity of helminths in microtine rodents: evolutionary implications. Evolution, 11:361–368.

———. 1964. The specific status of the narrow-skulled vole (subgenus *Stenocranius* Kashchenko) in North America. Z. Saugetierk., 29:343–358.

———. 1976. The genera *Paranoplocephala* Lühe, 1910 and *Anoplocephaloides* Baer, 1923 (Cestoda: Anoplocephalidae), with particular reference to species in rodents. Ann. Parasitol. Human Comp., 51:513–562.

———. 1977. The specific distinction of *Taenia twitchelli* Schwartz, 1924 from *T. martis* (Zeder, 1803) (Cestoda: Taeniidae). Pp. 357–366, *in* Excerta parasitológica en memoria del Dr. Eduardo Caballero y Caballero (B. Villa-R., ed.). Univ. Nac. Autó. México, Inst. Biol., Pub. Espec., 4:1–553.

———. 1980. Redescription of *Diandrya composita* Darrah, 1930 (Cestoda: Anoplocephalidae) from Nearctic marmots (Rodentia: Sciuridae) and the relationships of the genus *Diandrya* emend. Proc. Helminthol. Soc. Washington, 47:157–164.

RAUSCH, R. L., AND V. R. RAUSCH. 1968. On the biology and systematic position of *Microtus abbreviatus* Miller, a vole endemic to the St. Matthew Islands, Bering Sea. Z. Saugetierk., 33:65–99.

———. 1969. Studies on the helminth fauna of Alaska. XLVII. *Sobolevingylus microti* sp. nov. (Nematoda: Pseudaliidae), a lungworm of rodents. Canadian J. Zool., 47:443–447.

RAUSCH, R. L., AND S. H. RICHARDS. 1971. Observations on parasite-host relationships of *Echinococcus multilocularis* Leuckart, 1893, in North Dakota. Canadian J. Zool., 49:1317–1330.

RAUSCH, R. L., AND E. L. SCHILLER. 1949. Some observations on cestodes of the genus *Paranoplocephala* Luehe, parasitic in North American voles (*Microtus* spp.). Proc. Helminthol. Soc. Washington, 16:23–31.

———. 1951. Hydatid disease (*Echinococcosis*) in Alaska and the importance of rodent intermediate hosts. Science, 113:57–58.

———. 1954. Studies on the helminth fauna of Alaska. XXIV. *Echinococcus sibiricensis* n. sp., from St. Lawrence Island. J. Parasitol., 40:659–662.

———. 1956. Studies on the helminth fauna of Alaska. XXV. The ecology and public health significance of *Echinococcus sibiricensis* Rausch and Schiller, 1954, on St Lawrence Island. Parasitology, 46:395–419.

RAUSCH, R. L., AND J. D. TINER. 1949. Studies on the parasitic helminths of the north central states. II. Helminths of voles (*Microtus* spp.). Amer. Midland Nat., 41:665–694.

RAUSCH, R. L., B. E. HUNTLEY, AND J. G. BRIDGENS. 1969. Notes on *Pasteurella tularensis* from a vole, *Microtus oeconomus* Pallas, in Alaska. Canadian J. Microbiol., 15:47–55.

RAUSCH, R. L., B. B. BABERO, V. R. RAUSCH, AND E. L. SCHILLER. 1956. Studies on the helminth fauna of Alaska. XXVII. The occurrence of larvae of *Trichinella spiralis* in Alaskan mammals. J. Parasitol., 42:259–271.

REDINGTON, B. C. 1971. Studies on the morphology and taxonomy of *Haemogamasus reidi* Ewing, 1925 (Acari: Mesostigmata). Acarologia, 12:643–667.

ROBBINS, R. G. 1983. Seasonal dynamics of fleas associated with the gray-tailed vole, *Microtus canicaudus* Miller, in western Oregon. J. New York Entomol. Soc., 91:348–354.

ROBBINS, R. G., AND G. D. FAULKENBERRY. 1982. A population model for fleas of the gray-tailed vole, *Microtus canicaudus* Miller. Entomol. News, 93: 70–74.

ROBERT, A. 1962. Siphonapteres recoltes sur les petits rongeurs du Parc du Mont Tremblant et leurs relations avec leurs hotes. Ann. Entomol. Soc. Quebec, 7:3–18.

ROBERT, S., AND J.-M. BERGERON. 1977. Les Siphonapteres de la region de Sherbrooke, Quebec. Canadian Entomol., 109:1571–1582.

ROTHSCHILD, M., AND R. FORD. 1964. Breeding of the rabbit flea (*Spilopsyllus cuniculi*) (Dale)) controlled by the reproductive hormones of the host. Nature, 201:103–104.

———. 1966. Hormones of the vertebrate host controlling ovarian regression and copulation of the rabbit flea. Nature, 211:261–266.

———. 1969. Does a pheromone-like factor from the nestling rabbit stimulate impregnation and maturation in the rabbit flea? Nature, 221:1169–1170.

ROTHSCHILD, N. C. 1904. Further contributions to the knowledge of the Siphonaptera. Novitates Zool., 11:602–653.

———. 1905. On North American *Ceratophyllus,* a genus of Siphonaptera. Novitates Zool., 12:153–174.

———. 1906. Three new Canadian fleas. Canadian Entomol., 38:321–325.

RUPES, V., AND J. O. WHITAKER, JR. 1968. Mites of the subfamily Labidophorinae (Acaridae, Acarina) in North America. Acarologia, 10:493–499.

RUTLEDGE, L. C., M. A. MOUSSA, B. L. ZELLER, AND M. A. LAWSON. 1979. Field studies of reservoirs and vectors of sylvatic plague at Fort Hunter Liggett, California. J. Med. Entomol., 15:452–458.

RYCKMAN, R. E., AND R. D. LEE. 1958. Recent collections of Mallophaga and Anoplura from southern California. Pan-Pacific Entomol., 34:35–40.

SANFORD, L. G., AND K. L. HAYS. 1974. Fleas (Siphonaptera) of Alabama and their host relationships. Bull. Alabama Agric. Exp. Sta., Auburn Univ., 458:1–42.

SCANLON, J. E., AND P. T. JOHNSON. 1957. On some microtine-infesting Polyplax (Anoplura). Proc. Entomol. Soc. Washington, 59:279–283.

SCHAD, G. A. 1954. Helminth parasites of mice in northeastern Quebec and the coast of Labrador. Canadian J. Zool., 32:215–224.

SCHARF, W. C., AND K. R. STEWART. 1980. New records of Siphonaptera from northern Michigan. Great Lakes Entomol., 13:165–167.

SCHIEFER, B. A., AND J. L. LANCASTER, JR. 1970. Some Siphonaptera from Arkansas. J. Kansas Entomol. Soc., 43:177–181.

SCHILLER, E. L. 1952*a*. Studies on the helminth fauna of Alaska. X. Morphological variation in *Hymenolepis horrida* (von Linstow, 1901) (Cestoda: Hymenolepididae). J. Parasitol., 38:554–568.

———. 1952*b*. *Hymenolepis johnsoni,* n. sp., a cestode from the vole *Microtus pennsylvanicus drummondii.* J. Washington Acad. Sci., 42:53–55.

———. 1953. Studies on the helminth fauna of Alaska. XV. Some notes on the cysticercus of *Taenia polyacantha* Leuckart, 1856, from a vole (*Microtus oeconomus operarius* Nelson). J. Parasitol., 39:344–347.

SCHILLER, E. L., AND R. RAUSCH. 1956. Mammals of the Katmai National Monument, Alaska. Arctic, 9:191–201.

SCHOLTEN, T. H., K. RONALD, AND D. M. MCLEAN. 1962. Parasite fauna of the Manitoulin Island region. I. Arthropoda parasitica. Canadian J. Zool., 40:605–606.

SCHWAN, T. G. 1975. Flea reinfestation on the California meadow vole (*Microtus californicus*). J. Med. Entomol., 11:760.

SEIDEL, D. R., AND E. S. BOOTH. 1960. Biology and breeding habits of the meadow mouse, *Microtus montanus,* in eastern Washington. Walla Walla College Publ., 29:1–12.

SENGER, C. M. 1966. Notes of fleas (Siphonaptera) from Montana. J. Kansas Entomol. Soc., 39:105–109.

SETON, E. T. 1909. Life-histories of northern animals. Vol. I. Charles Scribner's Sons, New York, 673 pp.

SHOEMAKER, J. P., AND S. J. JOY. 1967. Some ectoparasites from West Virginia mammals, II. Proc. West Virginia Acad. Sci., 39:78–80.

SMIT, F. G. A. M. 1952. A new flea from western North America (Siphonaptera, Hystrichopsyllidae, Neopsyllinae). Proc. Entomol. Soc. Washington, 54: 269–273.

———. 1957. New hystrichopsyllid Siphonaptera. Bull. British Mus. (Nat. Hist.), Entomol., 6(2):1–76.

SMITH, C. N. 1944. Biology of *Ixodes muris* Bishopp and Smith (Ixodidae). Ann. Entomol. Soc. Amer., 37:221–234.

SMITH, C. N., M. M. COLE, AND H. K. GOUCK. 1946. Biology and control of the American dog tick. U.S. Dept. Agric. Tech. Bull., 905:1–74.

SONENSHINE, D. E. 1972. Ecology of the American dog tick, *Dermacentor variabilis,* in a study area in Virginia. 1. Studies on population dynamics using radioecological methods. Ann. Entomol. Soc. Amer., 65:1164–1175.

———. 1979. Ticks of Virginia (Acari: Metastigmata). Res. Div. Bull., Virginia Polytechnic Inst. State Univ., 139:1–42.

SONENSHINE, D. E., AND E. L. ATWOOD. 1967. Dynamics of feeding of the American dog tick, *Dermacentor variabilis* (Acarina: Ixodidae). Ann. Entomol. Soc. Amer., 60:362–373.

SONENSHINE, D. E., AND G. F. LEVY. 1972. Ecology of the American dog tick, *Dermacentor variabilis,* in a study area in Virginia. 2. Distribution in relation to vegetative types. Ann. Entomol. Soc. Amer., 65:1175–1182.

SONENSHINE, D. E., AND I. J. STOUT. 1968. Use of old-field habitats by the American dog tick, *Dermacentor variabilis*. Ann. Entomol. Soc. Amer., 61:679–686.

SONENSHINE, D. E., E. L. ATWOOD, AND J. T. LAMB, JR. 1966. The ecology of ticks transmitting Rocky Mountain spotted fever in a study area in Virginia. Ann. Entomol. Soc. Amer., 59:1234–1262.

SONENSHINE, D. E., J. T. LAMB, JR., AND G. ANASTOS. 1965. The distribution, hosts and seasonal activity of Virginia ticks. Virginia J. Sci., 16:26–91.

SPENCER, G. J. 1956. North American beetles infesting mammals. Proc. Entomol. Soc. British Columbia, 53:21–22.

———. 1966. Anoplura from British Columbia and some adjacent areas. J. Entomol. Soc. British Columbia, 63:23–30.

SPICKA, E. J., AND B. M. OCONNOR. 1980. Description and life-cycle of *Glycyphagus (Myacarus) microti* sp. n. (Acarina: Sarcoptiformes: Glycyphagidae) from *Microtus pinetorum* from New York, U.S.A. Acarologia, 21:451–476.

SPIELMAN, A., AND J. PIESMAN. 1979. Transmission of human babesiosis on Nantucket. Pp. 257–262, *in* Recent advances in acarology, Vol. II (J. G. Rodriguez, ed.). Academic Press, New York, 569 pp.

SPIELMAN, A., C. M. CLIFFORD, J. PIESMAN, AND M. D. CORWIN. 1979. Human babesiosis on Nantucket Island, USA: description of the vector, *Ixodes (Ixodes) dammini,* n. sp. (Acarina: Ixodidae). J. Med. Entomol., 15:218–234.

STANFORD, J. S. 1934. Some ectoparasites of Utah birds and mammals. Proc. Utah Acad. Sci., 11:247.

STARK, H. E. 1959. The Siphonaptera of Utah. Their taxonomy, distribution, host relations, and medical importance. U.S. Dept. Health Ed. Welfare, Publ. Health Serv., Atlanta, Georgia, 239 pp.

STARK, H. E., AND A. R. KINNEY. 1962. Abandonment of disturbed hosts by their fleas. Pan-Pacific Entomol., 38:249–251.

———. 1969. Abundance of rodents and fleas as related to plague in Lava Beds National Monument, California. J. Med. Entomol., 6:287–294.

STARK, H. E., AND V. I. MILES. 1962. Ecological studies of wild rodent plague in the San Francisco Bay area of California. VI. The relative abundance of certain flea species and their host relationships on coexisting wild and domestic rodents. Amer. J. Trop. Med. Hyg., 11:525–534.

STEWART, M. A. 1928. Siphonaptera. Pp. 868–869, *in* A list of the insects of New York with a list of the spiders and certain other allied groups (M. D. Leonard, ed.). Mem. Cornell Univ. Agric. Exp. Sta., 101:1–1121.

———. 1933. Revision of the list of Siphonaptera from New York state. J. New York Entomol. Soc., 41:253–262.

———. 1940. New Siphonaptera from California. Pan-Pacific Entomol., 16: 17–28.

STILES, C. W., AND A. HASSALL. 1894. A preliminary catalogue of the parasites contained in the collection of the U.S. Bureau of Animal Industry. Vet. Mag., Philadelphia, 1894:245–253, 331–354.

STOUT, I. J. 1979. Ecology of spotted fever ticks in eastern Washington. Pp. 113–121, *in* Recent advances in acarology, Vol. II (J. G. Rodriguez, ed.). Academic Press, New York, 569 pp.

STOUT, I. J., ET AL. 1971. *Dermacentor variabilis* (Say) (Acarina: Ixodidae) established in southeastern Washington and northern Idaho. J. Med. Entomol., 8:143–147.

STRANDTMANN, R. W. 1949. The blood-sucking mites of the genus *Haemolaelaps* (Acarina: Laelaptidae) in the United States. J. Parasitol., 35:325–352.

STRANDTMANN, R. W., AND G. W. WHARTON. 1958. A manual of mesostigmatid mites parasitic on vertebrates. Inst. Acarology Contrib., 4:1–330.

SVIHLA, R. D. 1941. A list of the fleas of Washington. Univ. Washington Publ. Biol., 12:9–20.

TIMM, R. M. 1972*a*. Mites (Acari: Laelapidae) parasitic on the meadow vole, *Microtus pennsylvanicus*. Acarologia, 14:18–20.

———. [1972*b*] 1973. Comments on ectoparasites of two species of Microtus in Nebraska. Trans. Kansas Acad. Sci., 75:41–46.

———. 1974. Rediscovery of the rock vole (*Microtus chrotorrhinus*) in Minnesota. Canadian Field-Nat., 88:82.

———. 1975. Distribution, natural history, and parasites of mammals of Cook County, Minnesota. Occas. Papers Bell Mus. Nat. Hist., Univ. Minnesota, 14:1–56.

TIMM, R. M., AND E. F. COOK. 1979. The effect of bot fly larvae on reproduction in white-footed mice, Peromyscus leucopus. Amer. Midland Nat., 101: 211–217.

TIMM, R. M., AND R. E. LEE, JR. 1981. Do bot flies, *Cuterebra* (Diptera: Cuterebridae), emasculate their hosts? J. Med. Entomol., 18:333–336.

———. 1982. Is host castration an evolutionary strategy of bot flies? Evolution, 36:416–417.

TIMM, R. M., L. R. HEANEY, AND D. D. BAIRD. 1977. Natural history of rock voles (*Microtus chrotorrhinus*) in Minnesota. Canadian Field-Nat., 91:177–181.

TINDALL, E. E., AND R. F. DARSIE, JR. 1961. New Delaware records for mammalian ectoparasites, including Siphonaptera host list. Bull. Brooklyn Entomol. Soc., 56:89–99.

TIPTON, V. J. 1950. New distributional records for Utah Siphonaptera. Great Basin Nat., 10:62–65.

———. 1960. The genus Laelaps with a review of the Laelaptinae and a new subfamily Alphalaelaptinae (Acarina: Laelaptidae). Univ. California Publ. Entomol., 16:233–356.

TIPTON, V. J., AND C. E. MACHADO-ALLISON. 1972. Fleas of Venezuela. Brigham Young Univ. Sci. Bull., Biol. Ser., 17(6):1–115.

TIPTON, V. J., AND E. MENDEZ. 1968. New species of fleas (Siphonaptera) from Cerro Potosi, Mexico, with notes on ecology and host parasite relationships. Pacific Insects, 10:177–214.

TIRABOSCHI, C. 1907. État actuel de la question du véhicule de la peste. Arch. Parasitol., 11:545–620.

TRAUB, R. 1950. Siphonaptera from Central America and Mexico: A morphological study of the aedeagus with descriptions of new genera and species. Fieldiana Zool. Mem., Chicago Nat. Hist. Mus., 1:1–235.

TRAUB, R., AND P. T. JOHNSON. 1952. *Atyphloceras tancitari* and *Jellisonia bonia,* new species of fleas from Mexico (Siphonaptera). Amer. Mus. Novitates, 1558:1–19.

TRAUB, R., AND M. NADCHATRAM. 1966. A revision of the genus *Chatia* Brennan, with synonymic notes and descriptions of two new species from Pakistan (Acarina: Trombiculidae). J. Med. Entomol., 2:373–383.

TUGWELL, P., AND J. L. LANCASTER, JR. 1962. Results of a tick-host study in northwest Arkansas. J. Kansas Entomol. Soc., 35:202–211.

TURNER, R. W. 1974. Mammals of the Black Hills of South Dakota and Wyoming. Misc. Publ. Mus. Nat. Hist., Univ. Kansas, 60:1–178.

VAN CLEAVE, H. J. 1953. Acanthocephala of North American mammals. Illinois Biol. Monogr., 23(1–2):1–179.

VERTS, B. J. 1961. Observations on the fleas (Siphonaptera) of some small mammals in northwestern Illinois. Amer. Midland Nat., 66:471–476.

VOGE, M. 1948. A new anoplocephalid cestode, *Paranoplocephala kirbyi,* from *Microtus californicus californicus.* Trans. Amer. Microscopical Soc., 67:299–303.

VOGEL, H. 1957. Über den *Echinococcus multilocularis* Süddeutschlands. I. Das Bandwurmstadium von Stämmen menschlicher und tierischer Herkunft. Z. Tropenmed. Parasitol., 8:404–456.

VYSOTSKAIA, S. O. 1950. Seasonal changes in the infestation of the grey vole with lice. (In Russian) Parizibol. Sborn., Zool. Inst. Akad. Nauk SSSR, Leningrad, 12:73–79.

WAGNER, J. 1936*a*. The fleas of British Columbia. Canadian Entomol., 68:193–207.

———. 1936*b*. Neue nordamerikanische Floharten. Z. Parasitenk., 8:654–658.

WALTON, A. C. 1923. Some new and little known nematodes. J. Parasitol., 10:59–70.

WHARTON, G. W., AND H. S. FULLER. 1952. A manual of the chiggers: the biology, classification, distribution, and importance to man of the larvae of the family Trombiculidae (Acarina). Mem. Entomol. Soc. Washington, 4:1–185.

WHITAKER, J. O., JR. 1968. Parasites. Pp. 254–311, *in* Biology of *Peromyscus* (Rodentia) (J. A. King, ed.). Spec. Publ., Amer. Soc. Mamm., 2:1–593.

———. 1982. Ectoparasites of mammals of Indiana. Monogr. Indiana Acad. Sci., 4:1–240.

WHITAKER, J. O., JR., AND D. ADALIS. 1971. Trematodes and cestodes from the digestive tracts of *Synaptomys cooperi* and 3 species of *Microtus* from Indiana. Proc. Indiana Acad. Sci., 80:489–494.

WHITAKER, J. O., JR., AND K. W. CORTHUM, JR. 1967. Fleas of Vigo County, Indiana. Proc. Indiana Acad. Sci., 76:431–440.

WHITAKER, J. O., JR., AND T. W. FRENCH. 1982. Ectoparasites and other associates of some insectivores and rodents from New Brunswick. Canadian J. Zool., 60:2787–2797.

WHITAKER, J. O., JR., AND R. B. LOOMIS. 1979. Chiggers (Acarina: Trombiculidae) from the mammals of Indiana. Proc. Indiana Acad. Sci., 88:426–433.

WHITAKER, J. O., JR., AND C. MASER. 1984. Parasitic mites of voles of the genera *Microtus* and *Clethrionomys* from Oregon. Northwest Sci., 58:142–150.

WHITAKER, J. O., JR., AND N. WILSON. 1968. Mites of small mammals of Vigo County, Indiana. Amer. Midland Nat., 80:537–542.

———. 1974. Host and distribution lists of mites (Acari), parasitic and phoretic, in the hair of wild mammals of North America, north of Mexico. Amer. Midland Nat., 91:1–67.

WHITE, D. J., AND C. P. WHITE. 1981. The occurrence and relevance of arthropods

of medical and veterinary importance captured during a survey on Plum Island, New York. J. New York Entomol. Soc., 89:2–15.
WILKINSON, P. R. 1979. Early achievements, recent advances, and future prospects in the ecology of the Rocky Mountain wood tick. Pp. 105–112, *in* Recent advances in acarology, Vol. II (J. G. Rodriguez, ed.). Academic Press, New York, 569 pp.
WILSON, L. W. 1943. Some mammalian ectoparasites from West Virginia. J. Mamm., 24:102.
WILSON, N. 1957. Some ectoparasites from Indiana mammals. J. Mamm., 38:281–282.
———. 1967. Ectoparasites of Canadian birds and mammals. Proc. Entomol. Soc. Washington, 69:349–353.
WILSON, N., AND W. W. BAKER. 1972. Ticks of Georgia (Acarina: Metastigmata). Bull. Tall Timbers Res. Sta., 10:1–29.
WINCHELL, E. J. 1977. Parasites of the beach vole, *Microtus breweri* Baird 1858. J. Parasitol., 63:756–757.
WISEMAN, J. S. 1955. The Siphonaptera (fleas) of Wyoming. Univ. Wyoming Publ., 19:1–28.
WOLFENBARGER, K. A. 1952. Systematic and biological studies on North American chiggers of the genus *Trombicula,* subgenus *Eutrombicula* (Acarina, Trombiculidae). Ann. Entomol. Soc. Amer., 45:645–677.
WOODHEAD, A. E., AND H. MALEWITZ. 1936. *Mediogonimus ovilacus,* n. g., n. sp. J. Parasitol., 22:273–275.
WOODS, C. E., AND O. R. LARSON. [1969] 1970. North Dakota fleas. II. Records from man and other mammals. Proc. North Dakota Acad. Sci., 23:31–40.
———. 1971. North Dakota fleas. III. Additional records from mammals. Proc. North Dakota Acad. Sci., 24:36–39.
WRENN, W. J., AND R. B. LOOMIS. 1973. A new species of *Euschoengastia* (Acarina: Trombiculidae) from western North America, and the status of *E. californica* (Ewing). J. Med. Entomol., 10:97–100.
WRIGHT, B. 1979. Mites, ticks, fleas, and lice in the Nova Scotia Museum and Acadia University Museum collections. Proc. Nova Scotia Inst. Sci., 29: 185–196.
ZAJAC, A. M., AND J. F. WILLIAMS. 1980. Infection with *Schistosomatium douthitti* (Schistosomatidae) in the meadow vole (*Microtus pennsylvanicus*) in Michigan. J. Parasitol., 66:366–367.
———. 1981. The pathology of infection with *Schistosomatium douthitti* in the laboratory mouse and the meadow vole, *Microtus pennsylvanicus.* J. Comp. Pathol., 91:1–10.
ZIMMERMAN, W. J. 1971. Trichinosis. Pp. 127–139, *in* Parasitic diseases of wild mammals (J. W. Davis and R. C. Anderson, eds.). Iowa State Univ. Press, Ames, 364 pp.

Appendix A. Endoparasites

Acanthocephalans

Microtus ochrogaster
Moniliformis clarki (Ward, 1917) (Fish, 1972)

Microtus pennslyvanicus
Moniliformis clarki (Ward, 1917) (Benton, 1954; Fish, 1972)
Polymorphus paradoxus Connell and Corner, 1957 (Platt, 1978)
Microtus pinetorum
Moniliformis clarki (Ward, 1917) (Benton, 1954, 1955*a*; Fish, 1972; Van Cleave, 1953)

Cestodes

Microtus abbreviatus
Andrya arctica Rausch, 1952 (Rausch and Rausch, 1968)
Andrya macrocephala Douthitt, 1915 (Rausch and Rausch, 1968)
Paranoplocephala infrequens (Douthitt, 1915) (Rausch and Rausch, 1968) (=*Anoplocephaloides* sp.; *A. infrequens* as presently understood is restricted to pocket gophers; at least two species of morphologically similar cestodes of the genus *Anoplocephaloides* occur in voles in the Arctic [R. L. Rausch, pers. comm.])
Paranoplocephala omphalodes (Hermann, 1783) (Rausch, 1976; Rausch and Rausch, 1968)
Taenia crassiceps (Zeder, 1800) (Rausch and Rausch, 1968) (larval stage)
Microtus breweri
Andrya macrocephala Douthitt, 1915 (Winchell, 1977)
Microtus californicus
Andrya macrocephala Douthitt, 1915 (Rausch, 1952*b*; Voge, 1948 [reported as *A. kirbyi*])
Microtus chrotorrhinus
Andrya macrocephala Douthitt, 1915 (Martin, 1972; Schad, 1954)
Hymenolepis horrida (von Linstow, 1901) (Schiller, 1952a)
Taenia crassiceps (Zeder, 1800) (Martin, 1972) (larval stage)
Microtus longicaudus
Andrya communis Douthitt, 1915 (Rankin, 1945) (=*A. primordialis* Douthitt, 1915)
Hymenolepis diminuta (Rudolphi, 1819) (Rankin, 1945)
Hymenolepis horrida (von Linstow, 1901) (Kinsella, 1967; Kuns and Rausch, 1950; Schiller, 1952*a*)
Paranoplocephala infrequens (Douthitt, 1915) (Kinsella, 1967; Kuns and Rausch, 1950) (=*Anoplocephaloides troeschi* Rausch, 1946)
Taenia mustelae Gmelin, 1790 (Kinsella, 1967) (larval stage)
Microtus mexicanus
Paranoplocephala infrequens (Douthitt, 1915) (Rausch, 1952*a*)(=*A. troeschi*)
Microtus miurus
Andrya arctica Rausch, 1952 (Rausch, 1952a [original description])
Hymenolepis horrida (von Linstow, 1901) (Schiller, 1952*a*)
Paranoplocephala infrequens (Douthitt, 1915) (Rausch, 1952*a*) (=*Anoplocephaloides* sp.)
Paranoplocephala omphalodes (Hermann, 1783) (Rausch, 1952*a,* 1976)
Taenia tenuicollis Rudolphi, 1809 (Rausch, 1952*a*) (=*T. mustelae*) (larval stage)
Microtus montanus
Andrya communis Douthitt, 1915 (Rankin, 1945) (=*A. primordialis* Douthitt, 1915)
Andrya macrocephala Douthitt, 1915 (Kinsella, 1967; Kuns and Rausch, 1950)

Andrya primordialis Douthitt, 1915 (Kuns and Rausch, 1950)
Hymenolepis horrida (von Linstow, 1901) (Kuns and Rausch, 1950; Schiller, 1952*a*)
Paranoplocephala infrequens (Douthitt, 1915) (Kinsella, 1967; Kuns and Rausch, 1950; Rausch, 1952*a,* 1976) (=*A. troeschi*)

Microtus ochrogaster
Andrya macrocephala Douthitt, 1915 (Hansen, 1947 [reported as *A. microti,* 1950]; Lubinsky, 1957)
Choanotaenia nebraskensis Hansen, 1950 (original description)
Choanotaenia sp. (Rausch and Tiner, 1949)
Hymenolepis horrida (von Linstow, 1901) (Schiller, 1952*a*)
Hymenolepis sp. (Rausch and Tiner, 1949)
Paranoplocephala borealis (Douthitt, 1915) (Rausch, 1952*a*) (=*Anoplocephaloides* sp.)
Paranoplocephala infrequens (Douthitt, 1915) (Hansen, 1950; Whitaker and Adalis, 1971) (=*A. troeschi*)
Paranoplocephala troeschi Rausch, 1946 (Whitaker and Adalis, 1971) (=*A. troeschi*)
Paranoplocephala sp. (Rausch and Tiner, 1949) (=*Anoplocephaloides* sp.)
Taenia mustelae Gmelin, 1790 (Lubinsky, 1957 (larval stage)
Taenia taeniaeformis (Batsch, 1786) (Rausch and Tiner, 1949; Whitaker and Adalis, 1971) (larval stage)

Microtus oeconomus
Andrya macrocephala Douthitt, 1915 (Rausch, 1952*a*)
Echinococcus granulosus (Batsch, 1786) (Rausch and Schiller, 1951) (=*E. multilocularis*; larval stage)
Echinococcus multilocularis Leuckart, 1863 (Ohbayashi, 1971; Vogel, 1957) (larval stage)
Echinococcus sibiricensis Rausch and Schiller, 1954 (Rausch and Schiller, 1954 [original description], 1956) (=*E. multilocularis*; larval stage)
Echinococcus sp. (Rausch, 1952*a*; Rausch and Schiller, 1951) (=*E. multilocularis*; larval stage)
Paranoplocephala infrequens (Douthitt, 1915) (Rausch, 1952*a,* 1957) (=*Anoplocephaloides* sp.)
Paranoplocephala omphalodes (Hermann, 1783) (Rausch, 1976)
Taenia polyacantha Leuckart, 1856 (Schiller, 1953) (larval stage)
Taenia twitchelli Schwartz, 1924 (Rausch, 1977) (larval stage)

Microtus pennsylvanicus
Andrya communis Douthitt, 1915 (Douthitt, 1915 [original description]; Lubinsky, 1957) (=*A. primordialis*)
Andrya macrocephala Douthitt, 1915 (Hall and Sonnenberg, 1955; Kuns and Rausch, 1950; Lubinsky, 1957; Mumford and Whitaker, 1982; Schad, 1954; Whitaker and Adalis, 1971)
Andrya primordialis Douthitt, 1915 (Kuns and Rausch, 1950; Meggitt, 1924)
Andrya sp. (Erickson, 1938*b*; Hall and Sonnenberg, 1955)
Cladotaenia globifera (Batsch, 1786) (Baron, 1971) (larval stage)
Cladotaenia sp. (Whitaker and Adalis, 1971)
Echinococcus multilocularis Leuckart, 1863 (Hnatiuk, 1966; Leiby, 1965; Leiby et al., 1970; Rausch and Richards, 1971) (larval stage)

Hymenolepis evaginata Barker and Andrews, 1915 (Rausch and Tiner, 1949)
Hymenolepis fraterna Stiles, 1906 (Rausch and Tiner, 1949)
Hymenolepis horrida (von Linstow, 1901) (Kinsella, 1967; Lubinsky, 1957; Schiller, 1952*a*)
Hymenolepis johnsoni Schiller, 1952 (Rausch, 1952*a*; Schiller, 1952*b* [original description and type-host])
Paranoplocephala borealis (Douthitt, 1915) (Rausch, 1952*a*) (=*Anoplocephaloides* sp.)
Paranoplocephala infrequens (Douthitt, 1915) (Hall and Sonnenberg, 1955; Kinsella, 1967; Kuns and Rausch, 1950; Lubinsky, 1957; Mumford and Whitaker, 1982; Rausch, 1946, 1952*a*; Rausch and Schiller, 1949; Schad, 1954) (=*A. troeschi*)
Paranoplocephala troeschi Rausch, 1946 (Mumford and Whitaker, 1982; Rausch, 1946 [original description and type-host], 1976; Rausch and Tiner, 1949) (=*A. troeschi*)
Paranoplocephala variabilis (Douthitt, 1915) (Kinsella, 1967; Lubinsky, 1957; Schad, 1954) (=*A. variabilis*)
Paranoplocephala sp. (Erickson, 1938*a*; Rausch and Tiner, 1949) (=*Anoplocephaloides*)
Paruterina candelabraria (Goeze, 1782) (Baron, 1971) (larval stage)
Taenia crassiceps (Zeder, 1800) (Freeman, 1954, 1962; Leiby and Whittaker, 1966) (larval stage)
Taenia mustelae Gmelin, 1790 (Lubinsky, 1957) (larval stage)
Taenia taeniaeformis (Batsch, 1786) (Erickson, 1938*b*; Kinsella, 1967; McBee, 1977; Rausch and Tiner, 1949) (larval stage)
Taenia tenuicollis Rudolphi, 1809 (Schad, 1954) (=*T. mustelae*)

Microtus pinetorum
Hymenolepis pitymi Yarkinsky, 1952 (original description)
Taenia taeniaeformis (Batsch, 1786) (Lochmiller et al., 1982*b*) (larval stage)
Taenia sp. (Erickson, 1938*b*; Lochmiller et al., 1982*b*; Whitaker and Adalis, 1971) (larval stage)

Microtus richardsoni
Andrya macrocephala Douthitt, 1915 (Kuns and Rausch, 1950)
Andrya primordialis Douthitt, 1915 (Kuns and Rausch, 1950)
Andrya sp. (Kuns and Rausch, 1950)
Hymenolepis horrida (von Linstow, 1901) (Kuns and Rausch, 1950; Schiller, 1952*a*)
Paranoplocephala infrequens (Douthitt, 1915) (Kuns and Rausch, 1950; Rausch, 1952*a*) (=*A. troeschi*)

Microtus xanthognathus
Taenia martis americana Wahl, 1967 (Rausch, 1977) (larval stage)

Nematodes

Microtus abbreviatus
Heligmosomoides bullosus matthewensis Durette-Desset, 1967 (Durette-Desset, 1968)
Heligmosomum nearcticum Durette-Desset, 1967 (Durette-Desset, 1968)
Heligmosomum sp. (Rausch and Rausch, 1968)

Microtus californicus
Heligmosomoides montanus Durette-Desset, 1967 (Durette-Desset et al., 1972)
Pelodera sp. (Poinar, 1965) (larval stage in eyes)
Microtus chrotorrhinus
Capillaria hepatica (Bancroft, 1893) (Fisher, 1963)
Cheiropteranema sp. (Komarek and Komarek, 1938)
Nematospiroides dubius Baylis, 1926 (Schad, 1954)
Microtus longicaudus
Aspiculuris tetraptera (Nitzsch, 1821) (Kinsella, 1967)
Heligmosomoides microti (Kuns and Rausch, 1950) (Kinsella, 1967)
Heligmosomoides montanus Durette-Desset, 1967 (Durette-Desset, 1968)
Heligmosomum costellatum (Dujardin, 1845) (Kinsella, 1967)
Mastophorus sp. (Kinsella, 1967) (=*Protospirura* sp.)
Nematospiroides longispiculatus Dikmans, 1940 (Rausch, 1952*a*) (=*Heligmosomoides longispiculatus*)
Pelodera sp. (Kinsella, 1967) (larval stage in eyes)
Syphacia obvelata (Rudolphi, 1802) (Kinsella, 1967; Rankin, 1945) (Quentin [1971] concluded that *Syphacia nigeriana* Baylis, 1928, is the only species of *Syphacia* parasitizing *Microtus* in North America; *S. obvelata* is restricted in occurrence to *Rattus* and perhaps other murids.)
Microtus mexicanus
Syphacia nigeriana Baylis, 1928 (Quentin, 1971)
Microtus miurus
Heligmosomum nearcticum Durette-Desset, 1967 (Durette-Desset, 1968)
Rictularia microti McPherson and Tiner, 1952 (McPherson and Tiner, 1952 [original description]; Quentin, 1971) (=*Pterygodermatites microti*)
Rictularia sp. (Rausch, 1952*a*)
Trichinella spiralis (Owen, 1835) (Rausch et al., 1956) (=*T. nativa* Britov and Boev, 1972)
Microtus montanus
Nematospiroides microti Kuns and Rausch, 1950 (Kinsella, 1967; Kuns and Rausch, 1950 [original description]) (=*Heligmosomoides microti*)
Syphacia obvelata (Rudolphi, 1802) (Kinsella, 1967; Kuns and Rausch, 1950; Leiby, 1962; Rankin, 1945) (=*S. nigeriana* ?)
Microtus ochrogaster
Boreostrongylus dikmansi Durette-Desset, 1974 (original description)
Capillaria sp. (Dunaway et al., 1968)
Longistriata carolinensis Dikmans, 1935 (original description) (=*B. carolinensis*)
Syphacia obvelata (Rudolphi, 1802) (Rausch and Tiner, 1949) (=*S. nigeriana* ?)
Trichuris sp. (Rausch and Tiner, 1949)
Microtus oeconomus
Heligmosomoides bullosus bullosus Durette-Desset, 1967 (Durette-Desset, 1968)
Heligmosomum nearcticum Durette-Desset, 1967 (Durette-Desset, 1968)
Pterygodermatites microti (McPherson and Tiner, 1952) (Quentin, 1971)
Rictularia microti McPherson and Tiner, 1952 (original description) (=*P. microti*)
Sobolevingylus microti Rausch and Rausch, 1969 (original description and type-host)
Syphacia nigeriana Baylis, 1928 (Quentin, 1971)

Microtus pennsylvanicus
- *Capillaria hepatica* (Bancroft, 1893) (Freeman and Wright, 1960; Lubinsky et al., 1971)
- *Capillaria muris-sylvatici* (Diesing, 1851) (Rausch and Tiner, 1949)
- *Dictyocaulus viviparus* (Bloch, 1782) (Rausch and Tiner, 1949)
- *Heligmosomoides longispiculatus* (Dikmans, 1940) (Durette-Desset et al., 1972)
- *Heligmosomoides wisconsinensis* Durette-Desset, 1967 (Durette-Desset, 1968; Durette-Desset et al., 1972)
- *Heligmosomum costellatum* (Dujardin, 1845) (Kinsella, 1967)
- *Heligmosomum microti* (Kuns and Rausch, 1950) (Kinsella, 1967; Kuns and Rausch, 1950) (=*Heligmosomoides microti*)
- *Heligmosomum nearcticum* Durette-Desset, 1967 (Durette-Desset, 1968)
- *Longistriata dalrympei* Dikmans, 1935 (Dikmans, 1935 [original description]; Lichtenfels and Haley, 1968; Rausch and Tiner, 1949)
- *Mastophorus muris* (Gmelin, 1790) (Rausch and Tiner, 1949) (=*Protospirura muris*)
- *Nematospira turgida* Walton, 1923 (original description and type-host)
- *Nematospiroides longispiculatus* Dikmans, 1940 (original description) (=*Heligmosomoides longispiculatus*)
- *Nematospiroides* sp. (Hall and Sonnenberg, 1955; Rausch and Tiner, 1949) (=*Heligmosomoides* sp.)
- *Oxyuris* sp. (Stiles and Hassall, 1894)
- *Rictularia coloradensis* Hall, 1916 (Lubinsky, 1957) (=*Pterygodermatites coloradensis*)
- *Syphacia nigeriana* Baylis, 1928 (Quentin, 1971)
- *Syphacia obvelata* (Rudolphi, 1802) (Erickson, 1938*a*, 1938*b*; Kinsella, 1967; Kuns and Rausch, 1950; Rausch and Tiner, 1949; Schad, 1954) (=*S. nigeriana* ?)
- *Syphacia* sp. (Hall and Sonnenberg, 1955; Lichtenfels and Haley, 1968)
- *Trichinella spiralis* (Owen, 1835) (Holliman and Meade, 1980)
- *Trichuris opaca* Barker and Noyes, 1915 (Hall and Sonnenberg, 1955; Lichtenfels and Haley, 1968; Rausch and Tiner, 1949)
- *Trichuris* sp. (Hall and Sonnenberg, 1955)

Microtus pinetorum
- *Capillaria gastrica* (Baylis, 1926) (Lochmiller et al., 1982*a*)
- *Oxyuris* sp. (Stiles and Hassall, 1894)
- *Trichinella spiralis* (Owen, 1835) (Zimmermann, 1971)
- *Trichuris opaca* Barker and Noyes, 1915 (Hall and Sonnenberg, 1955)
- *Trichuris* sp. (Benton, 1955*a*)

Microtus richardsoni
- *Nematospiroides microti* Kuns and Rausch, 1950 (original description)
- *Syphacia obvelata* (Rudolphi, 1802) (Kuns and Rausch, 1950) (=*S. nigeriana* ?)
- *Trichuris opaca* Barker and Noyes, 1915 (Kuns and Rausch, 1950)

Trematodes

Microtus miurus
- *Brachylaima rauschi* McIntosh, 1951 (Rausch, 1952*a*)

Microtus montanus
- *Quinqueserialis hassalli* (McIntosh and McIntosh, 1934) (Kuns and Rausch, 1950) (=*Q. quinqueserialis*; Barker and Laughlin, 1911)

Microtus oeconomus
- *Quinqueserialis quinqueserialis* (Barker and Laughlin, 1911) (Rausch, 1952*a*)

Microtus pennsylvanicus
- *Brachylaima* sp. (Rausch, 1952*a*)
- *Entosiphonus thompsoni* Sinitsin, 1931 (Rausch and Tiner, 1949)
- *Mediogonimus ovilacus* Woodhead and Malewitz, 1936 (Rausch and Tiner, 1949; Woodhead and Malewitz, 1936 [original description])
- *Monostomum* sp. (Stiles and Hassall, 1894)
- *Plagiorchis muris* Tanabe, 1922 (Kinsella, 1967; Schad, 1954)
- *Quinqueserialis hassalli* (McIntosh and McIntosh, 1934) (Harwood, 1939; Kuns and Rausch, 1950; McIntosh and McIntosh, 1934 [original description and type-host]; Rausch, 1952*a*; Rausch and Tiner, 1949) (=*Q. quinqueserialis*)
- *Quinqueserialis quinqueserialis* (Barker and Laughlin, 1911) (Edwards, 1949; Harrah, 1922; Kinsella, 1967; Rausch, 1952*a*; Schad, 1954)
- *Schistosomatium douthitti* (Cort, 1915) (Price, 1931; Zajac and Williams, 1980, 1981)

PREDATION

OLIVER P. PEARSON

Abstract

MICROTUS is killed and eaten by an enormous variety of vertebrates of every class and of every size from shrews to bears. Some of its predators are generalists that consume numerous other kinds of prey, and some specialize on *Microtus. Microtus* is palatable to generalists and specialists alike, and, since it chooses to live in relatively open habitats, each individual is so vulnerable that the entire population is at risk.

Most hawks are generalists, but several species of owls and kites are specialists on *Microtus.* One specialist (a male white-tailed kite) needed to hunt only an average of 8 min to catch a mouse. By hunting less than 20% of the daylight hours, he caught 21 mice in one day.

Raptors frequently establish themselves in regions where *Microtus* is abundant; in such places raptor assemblages may reach densities as high as one raptor to each 1,300 *Microtus.* The impact of an individual raptor on a *Microtus* population can be estimated by the following relationship between body weight of the raptor and number of 35-g *Microtus* consumed/raptor/km^2 per day:

$$\text{Impact} = \frac{121}{\text{Wt}^{0.69}}$$

Populations of raptors respond to changes in abundance of *Microtus* by adjusting their use of alternative prey (functional response) or by a numerical response achieved by immigration-emigration or by changes in nesting attempts and nesting success.

Among mammalian predators, ermines (*Mustela erminea*) are *Microtus* specialists. In one study, 99% of their diet consisted of *Microtus,* which precluded a functional response; the numerical response resulted in ratios of as few as 42 voles/ermine to as many as 800. In another study of the impact of an assemblage of middle-sized, generalist carnivores during three cycles of *Microtus* abundance, the numerical response of the carnivores was between 6 and

47-fold and the functional response between 2.7- and 5.2-fold. The numbers of mice per carnivore varied from 5,400 during the increase phase of the vole cycle (very low predation pressure) to 24 near the end of a crash (very high predation pressure). The destabilizing effect of such shifts in predation pressure suggests that carnivore predation may actually cause the multi-year *Microtus* cycles of abundance.

Fishes, amphibians, and reptiles all prey on *Microtus,* but the intensity of this predation has been measured only for a few species of snakes. In one study, copperheads (*Ancistridon*) ate about 20 30-g *Microtus*/ha/year. Two of 14 other species of snakes in the same area were important predators on *Microtus* also.

The summed effort of the numerous predators removes enormous numbers of *Microtus* from the population, but we are only beginning to measure the demographic results and to speculate about what strategies *Microtus* is using to minimize the impact of predators.

Introduction

It is possible to find in nature an array of predator-prey systems that range from clumsy to deadly efficient. One end of the spectrum might be the predation of rats on humans. Every year, a few neglected babies or incapacitated adults are attacked by rats. Near the middle of the spectrum lies the mink-muskrat system in which mink capture primarily surplus muskrats, described by Errington (1946) as "a harassed and battered lot congregating about the fringes of areas dominated by muskrats already in residence." At the deadly efficient end of the spectrum lie several systems involving *Microtus,* such as kite-*Microtus* and short-tailed weasel-*Microtus* systems. In fact, *Microtus* is sometimes so easy to capture that some species of predators catch not just the homeless and maladjusted but practically every one. No terrestrial or avian predator is too large to prey on *Microtus,* and almost every predator large enough to subdue a *Microtus* does so occasionally, from 10-g shrews (Hamilton, 1940) to ospreys (Proctor, 1977) to grizzly bears (Sheldon, 1930). I do not try to document all of this carnage but mention a few of the interesting extremes and concentrate on examples that give exceptional insight into the interaction between predator and prey, examples in which an attempt was made to measure the intensity of predation, and examples that contain information on the functional and numerical responses of a predator species. By functional response I mean change in the number of *Microtus* killed per unit time per individual predator, and by numerical response I mean change in the density of a population of predators in response to change in the density of *Microtus* (Holling, 1959).

The reader will note that studies of predation on *Microtus* have not reached a sophisticated level. We are emerging from a century of reports on the contents of owl pellets (in which *Microtus* is frequently dominant), but we have barely begun to learn what segments of vole populations are most vulnerable to which predators, what is the impact of different predators on vole densities in different habitats or different seasons, and how voles have adapted their individual life styles and their social systems in response to what appears to be a vulnerability unusually high among mammals. Progress has been slow because of the difficulty of measuring the abundance and the hunting range of different predators, and of measuring the demographics of the *Microtus* populations themselves. Such difficulties have not even permitted us to reach agreement on one of the central themes of microtine biology: the causation of the multi-annual cycle of abundance observed in many populations of microtines.

Predation by Birds

An assortment of non-raptors is known to catch and eat *Microtus*, such as jays, crows, ravens, shrikes, gulls, and herons, but rarely does *Microtus* make up a large proportion of their diet. Shrikes, for example, seem to attack unselectively almost anything that moves, provided it is within a reasonable (but great) size range (Miller, 1931). Under special circumstances some of these raptors may even consume a lot of mice, such as when gulls and crows follow the cutters in fields of artichokes infested with 1,000 or more *Microtus californicus* per ha (Gordon, 1977), or when large flocks of ravens select *Microtus* out of a mixed plague of *Mus* and *Microtus* (Hall, 1927), but rarely do these non-raptor generalists have an important impact on *Microtus* populations. Even among the raptors themselves (hawks, owls, and kites) only a handful of species specialize year-round in the capture of mice. Snyder and Wiley (1976) listed the categories of prey captured by 44 species of raptors. More than 90%

of the captures of eight of them consisted of mammals, usually mice, frequently *Microtus*. These eight species were the barn owl, great grey owl, hawk owl, long-eared owl, short-eared owl, saw-whet owl, boreal owl, and white-tailed kite. The diet of four other species of raptors was more than 50% mammal (ferruginous hawk, 85%; golden eagle, 72%; rough-legged hawk, 62%; and red-tailed hawk, 51%), but the *Microtus* content of some of these would not be expected to be high. I describe below a predator-prey system in which an entire assemblage of species of raptors seems to concentrate on *Microtus*, and another system in which the existence of one of the raptor species seems to depend completely on *Microtus* even though the diet is not entirely *Microtus*.

Raptor Assemblages

The most ambitious and most convincing measurement of the impact of avian predators on microtine populations were made in Michigan on a 93-km^2 township devoted primarily to dairy farming (Craighead and Craighead, 1956). The township consisted of woodland (11% of the area), fields, and wet areas. An overwintering assemblage of raptors fed primarily on *Microtus* and was then largely replaced by a nesting assemblage. Raptors were censused visually while they were hunting or at their roosting or nesting sites. *Microtus* was censused on sample areas, then the population of the entire area was calculated taking into account the extent of the different qualities of *Microtus* habitat and the relative abundance of voles in each kind. During the autumn and winter of 1941, a year of *Microtus* abundance, good habitat was estimated to support 343 *Microtus pennsylvanicus*/ha and the entire 93-km^2 study area a total of 303,000 *Microtus*. Six species of hawks and four species of owls preyed on this population.

Table 1 illuminates some of the details of this unusually well-documented predation. During winter of 1942, 159 raptors preyed heavily on the abundant vole population, and *Microtus* made up 87% of their diet. During the ensuing summer, voles made up only 28% of the diet of the 63 pairs of breeding raptors. During winter of 1948, when voles were only one-quarter as abundant as before, the much-reduced raptor population (59 birds) included only 55% *Microtus* in its diet. This indicates both a numerical response and a functional response to *Microtus* abundance that resulted in a five-fold difference in the total number of *Microtus* eaten. In summer

TABLE 1

PREDATION BY HAWKS AND OWLS ON *Microtus* ON A 93-KM^2 STUDY AREA IN MICHIGAN. THE DATA WERE ASSEMBLED FROM DIFFERENT CHAPTERS OF CRAIGHEAD AND CRAIGHEAD (1956)

	Microtus population	Percent representation of *Microtus* in collective raptor diet	No. of raptors	*Microtus*-raptor ratio	No. of *Microtus* eaten	Percent of *Microtus* population eaten
1942 Winter	303,000	87	96 hawks 63 owls	1,905:1	79,437	26
1942 Summer		28	42 pairs hawks 21 pairs owls		8,127	
1948 Winter	75,000	55	27 hawks 32 owls	1,271:1	16,341	22
1948 Summer		32	44 pairs hawks 22 pairs owls		8,211	

of 1948 a raptor assemblage of about the same size as that in 1942 included about the same proportion of *Microtus* in its diet. Since each individual and each species of the winter assemblage of raptors was feeding heavily on *Microtus*, the most timely information for every *Microtus* when it left its safe retreat was: how many of "us" are there and how many of "them"? This *Microtus*-raptor ratio during the winter of mouse abundance was about 2000:1. During the winter of lower *Microtus* density, the ratio was about 1300:1. Note that this lower number represents a moderately higher predation pressure. In other words, predation pressure measured in this way (numerical ratio of mice to raptors) was greater in the winter of 1948 in spite of the fact that the raptors ate only one-fifth as many *Microtus*. In both winters they ate roughly the same proportion of the *Microtus* crop (26% in 1942 and 22% in 1948).

The Craigheads emphasized the around-the-clock danger to *Microtus* from the diurnal hawk assemblage and the nocturnal owl assemblage. They also estimated the abundance of seven species of mammalian carnivores (fox, opossum, raccoon, skunk, badger, weasel, and mink), totalling between 277 and 346 individuals in the 93-km^2 township, and stated that during winter of 1941–1942 these carnivores were feeding largely on *Microtus*. They did not attempt to calculate the impact of these carnivores, but from metabolic considerations it is obvious that the carnivores were probably consuming as many *Microtus* as were the raptors. Their report did not include house cats, whose impact also may be considerable (see below).

The data of Baker and Brooks (1981, 1982) in a study of overwintering rough-legged and red-tailed hawks near the Toronto airport confirm that the abundance of raptors reported by the Craigheads is not unique. *Microtus pennsylvanicus* was present at measured densities about the same as on the best *Microtus* habitat on the Craigheads' study area in Michigan during the winter of 1942, and the two species of hawks had established themselves at Toronto at densities (0.33 to 0.72/ha) three to five times as great as the hawk assemblages on the study area in Michigan, or two to four times as dense as the entire raptor assemblage in Michigan. The greater density at Toronto was presumably made possible by the fact that three-fourths of the 827-ha study area consisted of good *Microtus* habitat undiluted by woodlots. My calculations of the predation pressure of these two species of hawks at Toronto fall between 1,300 and 3,000 voles/hawk, which brackets the total pressure (1,905/raptor) in Michigan. The overwinter raptor catch accounted for 19% of the population loss during that period. The authors stated that diurnal raptor predation of this magnitude is not important in vole declines.

There are many other reports of winter concentrations of avian predators on *Microtus*-rich areas. Many of these concern species that breed in the north and congregate farther south in winters following peak population of voles and lemmings. Davis (1937), for example, reported conspicuous 3- or 4-year peaks in the number of northern shrikes reported on Christmas bird counts in New England, and noted that this cycle agreed exactly with maxima in the number of arctic fox pelts marketed. The fox population presumably was reflecting vole or lemming abundance in northern Canada. Snowy owl "invasions" during winter frequently have been related to the collapse of microtine populations in the north (Gross, 1947). These emigrant owls frequently establish themselves in regions where *Microtus* is available. An especially impressive winter assemblage of owls was noted during the winter of 1978–1979 on 60-km^2 Amherst Island in Lake Ontario (Sayr, 1980). The meadow vole population had exploded in the autumn, and owls were abundant throughout the winter. In March a census revealed 34 great gray owls, 22 long-eared owls, 20 short-eared owls, 13 snowy owls, and a dozen other owls of six different species, giving a total of .017 owls/ha (one owl/59 ha). During the same winter great gray owls appeared on Neebish Island in Michigan, where they readily captured *Microtus* through a considerable snow cover (Master, 1979). Pellets indicated a diet of 96% *Microtus pennsylvanicus* and 4% short-tailed shrews (*Blarina brevicauda*).

Kites

White-tailed kites (*Elanus leucurus*) prey almost entirely on small mammals, primarily *Microtus,* and are noted for being responsive to the abundance of *Microtus* (Waian and Stendell, 1970). They frequently remain at the same place all year long. Stendell (1972) took advantage of the relative ease of observing and censusing kites to provide many insights into the machinery of predation by this species. The kites studied were living on three islands in an area of rotational agriculture. The two most vulnerable and probably most abundant prey species, estimated from nearly 6,000 mice in pellets, were *Microtus californicus* (75% by frequency and 89% by biomass) and *Mus musculus* (21% frequency and 9% biomass). Relative numbers of *Microtus* in the fields over which the kites were hunting were estimated during a 2½-year period by a combination of counts of active runways, live-trapping, and grid-trapping, and were related to the abundance of kites. Fluctuations in the number of *Microtus* tended to be approximately synchronous, but local highs of *Mus* could always be found. On Grizzly Island the numbers of mice trapped were 1,010 *Microtus,* 1,614 *Mus,* 22 *Reithrodontomys,* and 3 *Sorex*. *Mus* may be the most abundant species but it apparently is not the preferred prey. The number of kites preying on these mice on Grizzly Island, which has a total area of 3,500 ha of which 1,400 ha are suitable *Microtus* habitat, varied from three nesting pairs one year to 20 nesting pairs the next. The peak population was 72 kites, which then dropped to 10. The numerical interaction can be traced in Fig. 1 (top). While the *Microtus* population increased about five- or six-fold, the kite population increased by the same amount, initially by immigration, then by reproduction. During the decline of the vole population, kite numbers remained surprisingly stable until the *Microtus* density became very low. At this time the kite population decreased rapidly as a result of emigration and mortality. Note (Fig. 1, top) the important role that was played at this time by *Mus* serving as an alternative prey. They probably kept the kites from leaving the area until the *Microtus* had declined to a very low density.

Figure 1 (bottom) shows that *Microtus* made up at least 40% of the kite diet throughout the vole cycle, that it increased to about 80–85% when *Microtus* was at its peak, and that it remained above

---

→

FIG. 1. Top: numerical response of a population of white-tailed kites to one cycle of abundance of *Microtus californicus*. The solid line and closed circles indicate response during the increase phase of the vole cycle; dashed line and open circles represent response during the decline phase; circled points indicate periods when large numbers of house mice (*Mus musculus*) were taken by kites. Bottom: functional response of a population of white-tailed kites to one cycle of abundance of *Microtus californicus*. The percentage differences between the indicated values and 100% were made up almost entirely by *Mus musculus*. Graphs are modified slightly from Stendell (1972).

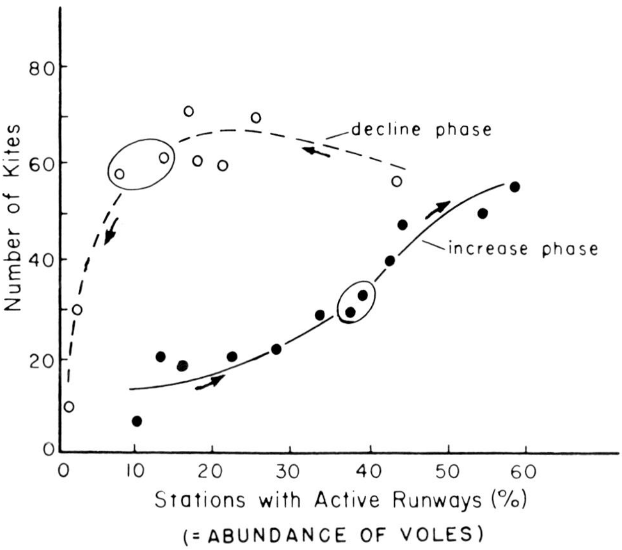
Number of Kites
decline phase
increase phase
Stations with Active Runways (%)
(= ABUNDANCE OF VOLES)

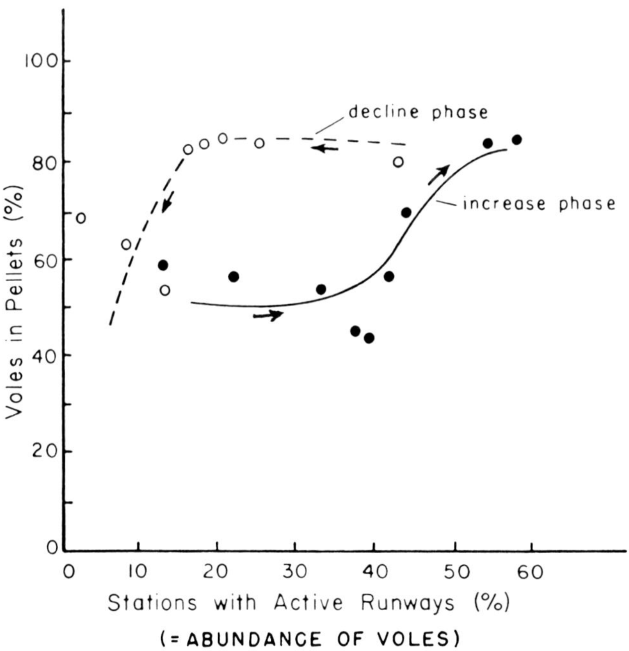
Voles in Pellets (%)
decline phase
increase phase
Stations with Active Runways (%)
(= ABUNDANCE OF VOLES)

80% of the diet throughout much of the collapse of the vole population. Because the number of kites remained high during much of the decline of *Microtus,* and because the percentage of *Microtus* in the diet remained high also, it is obvious that as the *Microtus* population collapsed the intensity of kite predation increased to about five times as much as it was when the vole population was beginning to increase. Other species of predators were present also, of course. For example, at dusk on a summer evening on 1,400-ha Jersey Island about 30 kites were hunting over a large field that contained an abundant population of *Microtus* but no *Mus.* Immediately after dusk, at least 10 barn owls were observed in the same area. These two species of raptors together must have been taking about 120 *Microtus*/day, which would be the equivalent of the standing crop of a dense *Microtus* population on 0.5 ha.

When *Microtus* was abundant on Grizzly Island in the summer of 1970, Stendell (1972) counted 50 kites, between 50 and 60 marsh hawks, between 35 and 40 short-eared owls, and as many as 8 barn owls. Although the island is not effectively isolated from the mainland, and therefore one cannot assume that all of the raptors were obtaining all of their food from the 1,400 ha of suitable *Microtus* habitat on the island, there can be no doubt that every *Microtus* had reason for concern because roughly 150 very competent raptors were hunting over 1,400 ha of mouse habitat—one raptor for each 9 ha.

The effectiveness of kites as *Microtus* hunters is documented by the performance of a male kite that was watched all day. He was hunting over a field that supported approximately 346 *Microtus*/ha. He supplied almost all of the food for himself, his mate, and five 4-week-old nestlings. During his 899-min day he made 38 hunting flights, 21 of which were successful (17 *Microtus* and four *Mus*). He needed an average of only 8 min to catch a mouse. One mouse was taken from him by a marsh hawk. Note that he was able to catch this many mice by hunting less than 20% of his total time during daylight hours (Table 2). Other species of raptors also find mouse-catching easy. A pair of barn owls brought an average of 1.8 mice/h to the nest (Smith et al., 1974).

Stendell showed that most of the changes in density of kites occurred immediately prior to or during their breeding season. Numbers at other times of the year were relatively stationary. Vole density during the initial stages of the kite nesting season deter-

TABLE 2

Activity Budget of a Male Kite throughout a Day in Which He Made 38 Hunting Flights and Caught 17 *Microtus* and 4 *Mus* (from Stendell, 1972)

Activity	Time (min)	Percent of total time
Perched	681	75.8
Flight (total)	(218)	24.2
Hunting	168	18.8
Near nest	22	2.4
Aggressive	6	0.6
Courtship	3	0.3
Miscellany*	19	2.1
Total	899	100.0

* Mostly flights between perches.

mined whether the kites remained in an area. In a year of diminishing *Microtus* density, a population of 68 kites in late January decreased to 24 in mid-February and to less than 12 after April 1. Nesting success, however, was not lower in low vole years, but during vole abundance many pairs of kites fledged two broods. It is apparent, therefore, that the numerical response of kites to the highly fluctuating abundance of *Microtus* stems from both immigration–emigration and reproduction, and that the kite strategy is one of nomadism rather than site faithfulness. Long-term survival of kite populations depends upon asynchrony of the vole population over extensive areas and the kite's ability to find local vole highs.

In a quite different habitat at the Hastings Natural History Reservation in California, a small number of kites hunted over grassy fields in which censuses of *Microtus* were being carried out (Stendell and Myers, 1973). During three successive summers in which densities of *Microtus* were 62/ha, 11/ha, and less than 2/ha, the proportion of *Microtus* in kite pellets remained above 83%. No *Mus* were present, but alternative prey were gophers, harvest mice, kangaroo rats, pocket mice, birds, and insects. The kites persisted in hunting over the fields with *Microtus* densities lower than 2/ha and apparently survived by spending more time hunting for each mouse captured.

Warner and Rudd (1975) studied kites hunting over agricultural land in central California and confirmed the ease with which captures are made. During April and May when a male was supplying food for his mate and nestlings, he spent 15% of the day hunting, but later when males and females were hunting independently, they each spent only 5% of the day hunting. Thirty-nine percent of the hunting forays, which lasted an average of 6.1 ± *SE* 0.7 min each, ended in a successful strike, and 63% of all strikes were successful. Half of the hunts were within 0.1 km of the nest tree, and 96% were within 1 km.

Other Birds

Boonstra (1977) gave information on the minimum amount of predation on a population of *Microtus townsendii* living on an island near Vancouver. He marked almost all of the *Microtus* on three study grids with metal ear tags and looked for the tags in the pellets and feces of predators. He listed short-eared owls, great-horned owls, snowy owls, barn owls, marsh hawks, rough-legged hawks, red-tailed hawks, northern shrikes, great blue herons, cats, and raccoons. The latter two were destroyed on sight. His Table 2 shows recovery of 3.1%, 5.9%, and 7.4% of the ear tags from mice that disappeared from the three grids during winter of 1972–1973, 30.3% of those disappearing between October and December, 1973, and 19% of those disappearing between December of 1973 and April of 1974. Beacham (1979) carried out a similar study on a nearby island in 1977 and reported that the proportion of loss accounted for tended to be between 10 and 15% (10 to 15% of the tags were actually recovered). The intensity of predation was directly proportional to the size of the *Microtus* population. He also supplied some of the best evidence concerning what segments of the *Microtus* population suffered the most severe predation. Small males tended to be the animals most likely to be caught by avian predators, whereas large females were least likely. The average duration of life, measured as the time between first and last capture, was higher in females (21.1 weeks) than in males (18.0 weeks). This is consistent with the predator selection of smaller and presumably younger males. He attributed most of the predation to great blue herons and marsh hawks. On one occasion he saw seven herons on his 0.84-ha trapping area.

I have cited a number of studies that document a numerical response of raptors to changes in vole numbers, but none of them illuminates the role played by nesting in the numerical response as effectively as a 16-year study by Hamerstrom (1979). She measured relative abundance of *Microtus pennsylvanicus* as it went through a series of population cycles. In spite of the fact that marsh hawks have a widely varied diet, the number of their nests increased dramatically (2.7-fold) in years when vole numbers were high, and only in those years. The actual number of marsh hawks varied less (1.4-fold), probably because a smaller proportion of them nested during *Microtus* lows than at highs. Nesting success of the hawks was 62.1% at vole lows and 83.1% at highs, but the number of young per successful nest remained at 3.1 during highs and lows. Nevertheless, the total production of young hawks per unit area increased about 3.6-fold during *Microtus* highs. Some other species, such as kites (Stendell, 1972) and barn owls (Wallace, 1948), increased production of young during *Microtus* highs by repeat nesting.

Owls locate their prey by sight when light is adequate—and it usually is. Great-horned owls and barn owls can see a dead mouse at light intensity of 13×10^{-6} foot candles (Marti, 1974), which is about half as bright as a clear starlit night without any moon. A long-eared owl can see a dead mouse at 70×10^{-8} foot candles (Marti, 1974), which is about as bright as in a forest on a hazy, moonless night. Burrowing owls, which are rather crepuscular, need about six times as much light as barn owls. All four of these species can also locate and capture live mice in total darkness. Payne (1962) and Konishi (1973) described the remarkable skill of barn owls in this kind of passive acoustical localization. Owls also are equipped with plumage that muffles their flight. This presumably prevents their prey from hearing their approach and at the same time may prevent interference with their own acoustical detection of noises made by the prey.

Raptor Impact

I noted above various examples of the pressure of raptors on *Microtus* populations. As a result of the fact that home ranges of raptors and food consumption are both closely related to body weight, it becomes possible to make a useful estimate of the impact of each individual raptor on a population of *Microtus*. Using the data in Newton's (1979) Fig. 10 of home ranges of pairs of hawks plotted against body weight (in g), I calculated a relationship:

$$\frac{\text{Home range per}}{\text{individual bird in km}^2} = .00026 \times \text{Wt}^{1.39} \quad (1)$$

The slope of this curve is very close to that calculated by Schoener (1968) for predatory birds and by Harestad and Bunnell for mammals (1979). See also Jenkins (1981).

From data given by Brown and Amadon (1968), Craighead and Craighead (1956), and Graber (1962), I calculated that for 17 species of raptors ranging in size from saw-whet owl to eagle:

$$\frac{\text{Number of } \textit{Microtus} \text{ consumed}}{\text{per bird per day}} = .0315 \times \text{Wt}^{0.70} \quad (2)$$

I assumed an average body weight of 35 g/*Microtus,* and where appropriate have allowed for discard of stomach and intestines of each *Microtus* (12% of body weight according to Stendell, 1972).

Combining equations (1) and (2):

$$\frac{\text{Impact (number of } \textit{Microtus} \text{ consumed}}{\text{per bird per km}^2 \text{ per day)}} = \frac{121}{\text{Wt}^{0.69}} \quad (3)$$

The number emerging from this equation is based on the assumption that the raptor is living entirely on *Microtus.* If *Microtus* provides only 80% by weight of the diet, then the impact must be reduced by 20%. If only 20% of the home range of the raptor is *Microtus* habitat, then the impact figure could be refined by multiplying by five to arrive at a figure for impact per bird per square km of *Microtus* habitat. Different average body weights of *Microtus* can be accommodated also by scaling up or down from 35 g.

Note that the slope of the line representing this relationship is negative: the larger the raptor, the less its impact per km^2 of raptor home range (Fig. 2). For example, if a 1,500-g great-horned owl and a 245-g long-eared owl were living in the same region and were subsisting entirely on 35-g *Microtus,* the impact of the horned owl would be expected to be 0.79 *Microtus*/km^2/day (from equation 3), and the long-eared owl would be expected to eat 3½ times as many per km^2 (2.74 from equation 3).

The impact of predation of the intensity calculated for a single long-eared owl on a non-breeding *Microtus* population of 1,000/km^2 (=10/ha) amounts to about 2% of the population per week. I cited above an observation of a kite hunting persistently over a field with a *Microtus* density less than 200/km^2 (less than 2/ha). The

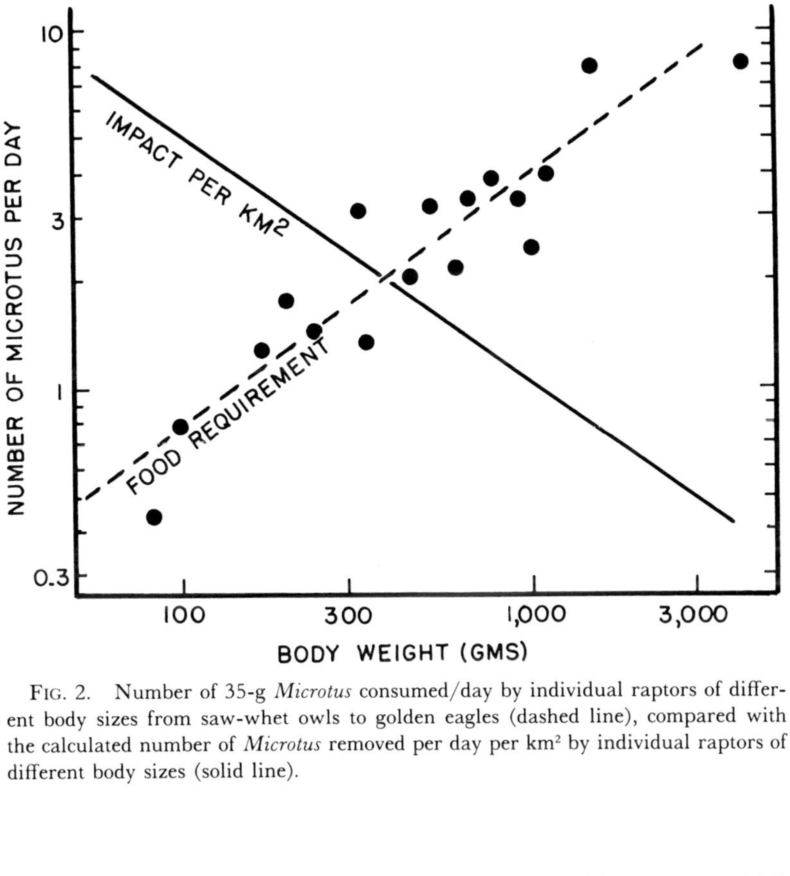

FIG. 2. Number of 35-g *Microtus* consumed/day by individual raptors of different body sizes from saw-whet owls to golden eagles (dashed line), compared with the calculated number of *Microtus* removed per day per km² by individual raptors of different body sizes (solid line).

impact of this one individual in this example would amount to 10% of the *Microtus* population per week. Levels of predation such as this are probably appropriate for the raptor nesting season during which territories such as those presented by Newton (1979) are maintained. At other seasons, however, raptors may gather at much greater densities, attracted by abundant and vulnerable prey. When one realizes that a *Microtus* specialist such as the white-tailed kite can support itself by hunting only 5% of the day (see above) or that a pair of barn owls can deliver an average of 1.8 mice/h to the nest (Smith et al., 1974), that a pair of barn owls may accumulate at a nest 67 uneaten mice in 8 days (Wallace, 1948), and that as many as 14 barn owls may roost in a single tree (Reed, 1897) or 300 along 4.8 km of cliff (Dixon and Bond, 1937), then one marvels at the ability of *Microtus* to survive at all. It must be assumed that before the last *Microtus* is caught, the *Microtus* specialists either starve or move away in search of denser *Microtus* populations, and the generalists either emigrate or switch to other prey. The *Microtus* population survives by becoming sparse.

Predation by Mammals

Mammalian predators of *Microtus* hunt them with almost all the physical and sensory equipment of the avian hunters and resort to two additional skills: sense of smell and ability to dig. It is possible that mammalian vision and hearing are not as acute as in some raptors, but when combined with a sense of smell they enable even relatively clumsy carnivores such as badgers and skunks to catch voles. Pearson (1959) showed that there is enough traffic in *Microtus* runways so that a carnivore the size of a fox could, if it was as clever at detecting active runways as are osmatically dull humans, catch its daily food requirements just by sitting and waiting beside runways. Most mammalian predators either sit and wait or cruise slowly through suitable habitat looking, listening, and sniffing for clues to *Microtus* presence. When a mouse is detected, wolves, coyotes, dogs, foxes, and cats use a characteristic high pounce, the purpose of which may be to force the mouse into making a commitment to its direction of escape and thereby decrease the number of variables that the predator must compute. Cats use this high, curved jump only in tall grass, but foxes use it even when the grass is short (Leyhausen, 1978).

The mobility imparted by the power of flight would seem to give raptors a great advantage by enabling them to skim the easy catches off of a larger area. To the contrary, the home ranges of avian raptors are much smaller than the home ranges of mammalian carnivores of similar body size (based on a comparison of equation (1) above with the equation for mammalian carnivores given by Harestad and Bunnell, 1979).

Shrews

Because of their small size shrews are able to follow *Microtus* down its runways into its nests. Even small species of *Sorex* probably eat newborn voles when they encounter them. *Blarina*, the short-tailed shrew, is a more effective killer and can kill *Microtus* that are twice its size (Martinsen, 1969). Its venomous bite and pugnacious personality undoubtedly help to compensate for its small size, but it is uncertain how effectively it uses its venom to kill or to paralyze mice in nature (Pearson, 1942; Tomasi, 1978). Indeed, there are conflicting reports about how effective a *Microtus* predator it is in the wild. Hahn (1908) saw a successful attack by *Blarina* on a *Microtus pinetorum* that was larger than the shrew, and Maurer (1970) interrupted an attack on *M. pennsylvanicus*. Shull (1907) found a *Blarina* nest with the remains of about 23 voles in and around it. Eadie (1952) identified the contents of hundreds of *Blarina* scats collected in *Microtus* habitat during five autumns and winters near Ithaca, New York. He found that voles formed a significant portion of the fall and winter diet in every year. Up to 56% of the scats contained *Microtus* remains in some seasons. Shrews maintained a fairly high population density even after a prolonged depression in vole numbers. In fact, shrew densities seemed to approximate or even exceed vole densities. Invertebrates served as alternative prey and permitted such a low *Microtus*/predator ratio during periods of *Microtus* scarcity.

In contrast, Whitaker and Ferraro (1963) made a careful analysis of the contents of 221 stomachs of *Blarina* taken at Ithaca in the summer and found no mammal remains at all. Whitaker and Mumford (1972) found mouse remains in only one of 125 *Blarina* stomachs collected in Indiana, none in 109 *Cryptotis* stomachs, none in 50 *Sorex cinereus,* and none in seven *S. longirostris.* The low vole content in these extensive samples of *Blarina,* in contrast to Eadie's scat samples, was probably due to a difference in habitats sampled (*Blarina* lives in both forests and fields) and a difference in seasons of collection. Platt (1976), studying *Microtus* and *Blarina* in large outdoor enclosures at Ithaca, found that *Blarina* foraged for *Microtus* in winter and switched to invertebrates in the spring. Barbehenn (1958) acknowledged that *Blarina* was an effective predator on *Microtus,* but noted that populations of the two species appear to fluctuate independently. They do not constitute, therefore, a closely coupled predator-prey system.

Weasels

Weasels are traditional enemies of *Microtus,* and even the smaller species such as *Mustela nivalis* (40 to 90 g) kill mice with great ease

(Heidt, 1972). They kill and stockpile numerous mice in the wild but prefer to eat only *Microtus* (Ryszkowski et al., 1973). The small species seem to be vole specialists.

An especially favorable field situation for studying weasels was exploited by Fitzgerald (1977). He studied a number of mountain meadows in California isolated by pine forests. The meadows were buried under 1–3 meters of snow throughout each of the four winters of his study. *Microtus montanus* were censused on mark-and-recapture grids in the autumn and spring, and their subnivean nests were censused each spring when the snow melted. There was an average of slightly less than one nest for each vole censused in the autumn. At the spring census of nests, many of them had been occupied by ermines (*Mustela erminea*) and a few by long-tailed weasels (*M. frenata*). The ermine occupant would line the nest with the fur of his victims and leave skulls, feet, and other parts lying about. Fitzgerald found on the average the remains of 54 voles at the nests occupied by each ermine. Ermines were censused by tracking in the snow. Average territories covered about 3.5 ha of meadow. Counts of the number of ermines were confirmed calorically: since 99% of the diet consisted of *Microtus,* the number of *Microtus* needed for over-winter survival of one ermine could be calculated, and this number was in good agreement with the tracking information and with the body-count of *Microtus* eaten during the winter.

In some meadows population densities of *Microtus* varied as much as 100-fold during the study. The density was low in winter of 1966–1967, moderate in winter of 1967–1968, and high in 1968–1969. Table 3 summarizes, during the three winters, the pressure of ermine predation on *Microtus* in a cluster of six meadows totalling 14 ha. A relatively low *Microtus* population of 292 individuals entered the winter of 1966–1967 at a ratio of 97 voles/ermine and emerged in the spring with a population of 126 *Microtus* at a ratio of 42/ermine. This high predation pressure then apparently relaxed, through the loss of two ermines, and the population was able to build up to 783 *Microtus* in autumn, at which time only one ermine was present, and the pressure was reduced to 783:1. This pressure was enough to reduce the population only slightly to 722 in the spring. The population entered the winter of 1968–1969 at a high density, but an increase in the number of ermine to a ratio of 198:1 was then associated with a reduction in the population to

TABLE 3

ERMINE PREDATION AT THE ONSET AND END OF WINTER, BASED ON THE NUMBER OF VOLES AND ERMINE AND ON KNOWN VOLE MORTALITY (FROM FITZGERALD, 1977)

	Winter		
	1966–67	1967–68	1968–69
Number of vole nests	292	783	793
Number of ermine present	3	1	4
Vole : ermine ratio in autumn	97:1	783:1	198:1
Maximum voles surviving in spring	126	722	386
Estimated vole : ermine ratio in spring	42:1	722:1	96:1

386 in the spring. The spring ratio of 96:1 was followed by a depression of the *Microtus* population throughout the breeding season of 1969. Minimum estimates of the percent of the vole population eaten by ermine during the four winters varied from 5.9% to 54.3%. Predation was most severe when voles were at lowest density. In two of the meadows during the winter of 1966–1967, at least 81% and 83% of the voles present in the autumn were eaten by ermines.

Since such a high percentage of the diet of these ermines consisted of *Microtus,* the response of these predators to changes in *Microtus* density was almost entirely a numerical response. It had a magnitude of about four-fold. Raymond and Bergeron (1982), studying an ermine–*Microtus pennsylvanicus* system in Quebec, found that a numerical response appeared within 12 months and could be attributed to both reproduction and immigration. However, this numerical response occurred only among male ermines.

Tapper (1979) studied the little European weasel, *Mustela nivalis,* on a 25-km^2 area in southern England. The *Microtus arvalis* in the area went through a 4-year cycle with densities 14 times greater at the peak than at the low. Weasel numbers varied by a factor of two, with females failing to reproduce during the year of lowest vole numbers. The weasel population seemed to be quite mobile, however, so that failure of reproduction was soon adjusted by immigration. The proportion of voles in the weasel diet increased 3.4-fold from the lowest *Microtus* years to the highest. The combined numerical and functional response of this weasel population gives them a potential $2 \times 3.4 = 6.8$-fold range in amount of predation on the *Microtus* population.

Large Carnivores

The larger carnivores usually have a varied diet and, although they may specialize on *Microtus* for a few weeks or months, usually switch, as do shrews, to other foods at other seasons. Nevertheless, large carnivores may be efficient mouse-catchers. *Microtus,* along with pocket gophers, was the staple food item in the diet of coyotes in Yellowstone Park from April to November (Murie, 1940). Murie watched a coyote for 1½ h, hunting on a snowfield in a meadow. It pounced 30 times without success, but also in the same interval caught and swallowed 11 animals, all of which appeared to be *Microtus.* By following trails of red foxes in the snow, Murie (1936) showed that location and capture of mice was easy, even under the snow. Rabbits, mice, and shrews were caught in excess and merely cached uneaten. At Mount McKinley in Alaska during a series of years when hares were scarce, voles made up nearly two-thirds of the red fox diet in summer and three-fourths in winter (Murie, 1944). Even in a year when voles were scarce, they were dominant in the diet. Mullen and Pitelka (1972) reported on the uncanny ability of arctic foxes and red foxes to detect mouse carcasses under as much as 0.75 m of snow. Scott (1943) showed that red foxes preferred to eat *Microtus* and were more likely to cache or discard *Peromyscus,* shrews, weasels, and other prey. Their diet in Iowa (primarily rabbits and *Microtus*) was surprisingly similar to that of horned owls in the same area (Scott and Klimstra, 1955).

Wolves frequently eat *Microtus.* Murie (1944) found as many as six mice in one wolf scat at Mount McKinley and saw as many as 17 pounces in one h. He once fed up to 19 mice and two shrews in quick succession to a captive wolf pup. Mowat (1963) saw a wolf catch and eat six voles in 10 min, 23 in one feeding bout.

Sheldon (1930) found mice in two of 10 stomachs of grizzly bears and described a grizzly hunting them in the snow, using its nose as a plow, then digging the mouse out and catching it with a paw. Murie (1944) found only one vole in 201 grizzly scats from the Mount McKinley area.

Lynx canadensis in Newfoundland fed primarily on hares, but

14% of the stomachs and scats contained *Microtus pennsylvanicus*. The frequency was low in winter and higher in years of *Microtus* abundance (Saunders, 1963).

Many domestic cats, in spite of gratuitous alternative "prey" in the form of table scraps and cat food, cannot resist the hunting urge. Capture of two to three voles/day is not unusual (Bradt, 1949; Toner, 1956). George (1974) tabulated the number of prey items brought home during 3 years by three cats living in his home in southern Illinois. *Microtus ochrogaster* and *M. pinetorum* were the most frequent of the 18 species of prey. Diurnal predation yielded half of the prey, crepuscular predation 20%, and nocturnal predation 30%. The sex ratio of captured voles of each species was approximately equal. Captures were much less frequent in winter, which George attributed to the fact that the cats had already captured a considerable proportion of the voles on their hunting area. He estimated that the combined predation by domestic cats on farms in the midwest seriously reduces the carrying capacity of the environment for overwintering raptors.

Christian (1975) marked a population of *Microtus pennsylvanicus* with metal ear tags and then looked for the tags in the droppings of 10 to 12 domestic cats that lived on a farm across a road from the study area and that were fed commercial cat food and table scraps by the owners. Losses due to predation by the cats accounted for at least 16% of those voles disappearing from the study area. Voles of different sex and age were preyed upon in the same proportion as they appeared in the trapped sample, indicating either that the predation by cats was non-selective or that its bias was the same as the trapping bias.

Carnivore Assemblages

Madison (1979) marked a total of 93 *Microtus pennsylvanicus* with radiotransmitters during three different summers in three different areas. Thirty (32%) of the marked individuals were killed by predators. Domestic cats, snakes, and weasels were the three dominant predators. Another 11 telemetered voles disappeared. If all of these had been removed by predators, the rate would have been 44%, which is an upper limit for the intensity of predation during these 3-month periods. Predation was most intense on individuals living close to suboptimal habitats.

TABLE 4
IMPACT OF CARNIVORES DURING THREE *Microtus* DECLINES ON 14 HA IN CALIFORNIA (FROM PEARSON 1964, 1966, 1971)

	1961	1963	1965
Number of *Microtus*/ha (high–low)	312–<2	540–30	>25–<2
Number of carnivores on 14 ha (high–low)	8–0.17	4.4–0.4	2.16–0.35
Numerical response of carnivores	47×	11×	6×
Functional response of carnivores[1]	—	5.2×	2.7×
Greatest monthly impact[2]	>90%	20%	33%
Percent of vole standing crop eaten	88%	25%	33%
Mouse-carnivore ratio (min., max.)	±550:1, 72:1	5,400:1, ±500:1	880:1, 24:1

[1] Greatest monthly average number of *Microtus* eaten/day/carnivore divided by the corresponding lowest monthly average.
[2] Number of *Microtus* recovered in scats divided by the number existing at the beginning of the month, ×100.

Pearson (1964, 1966, 1971) censused *Microtus californicus* on 14 ha of annual grassland during part of two population declines and during all of a third. The population density reached peaks of 314/ha, 540/ha, and more than 25/ha with lows of less than 2/ha between (Table 4). Carnivores were censused by their droppings. The species present were feral cats, raccoons, striped skunks, spotted skunks, and gray foxes, approximately in that order of abundance. For the calculations, the carnivores were treated as a single species of 3-kg carnivore, since the source of each dropping was not determined. As many as 88% of one of the peak populations was eaten before the beginning of the next breeding season. The numerical response of the carnivores varied from 47-fold to six-fold in the three cycles and lagged behind the *Microtus* numbers by a few months. It took many months for the carnivore numbers to recover after their prey started to recover. The functional response, to the contrary, was rapid. As soon as the *Microtus* population began to increase, the carnivores switched promptly back to a high-*Microtus* diet. The functional response varied from 2.7-fold during one decline to 5.2-fold during another. Intensity of predation, as measured by numbers of *Microtus*/carnivore, was lowest during the buildup of the *Microtus* population (5,000) and greatest (72, 500, 224) late in the three declines. One morning when the 1961 peak had dropped to 18 voles/ha, none of them breeding, and the average carnivore was still eating three *Microtus*/day, I (Pearson, 1964) saw six feral cats hunting on the 14-ha study area. It would have required the standing crop of *Microtus* on 1 ha every day to support these cats, not mentioning the other predators. By March, no *Microtus* could be trapped on the census grid. Study of these three cycles led Pearson (1971) to speculate that mouse–carnivore ratios of less than 100 would prevent growth of even maximally reproducing *Microtus* populations, ratios between 200 and 1,000 would slow the growth of breeding populations and cause abrupt declines in non-breeding populations, and ratios higher than 1,000 would be relatively ineffective in preventing increases of breeding populations.

The considerable variation of measurements in the three cycles (Table 4) arises from sources such as: the measuring period was not the same in the three cycles; the carnivore population was reduced by park officials beginning in 1963; and no effort was made to estimate the impact of snakes and raptors, an impact that may have been unequal in the three cycles. Nevertheless, it is clear that through numerical and functional responses the carnivores had the potential to bring 16 (in 1965) and more than 200 (in 1961) times as much predation pressure to bear on the *Microtus* population at one stage of the cycle as at another. However, the carnivores used their reserve predatory power at an inappropriate time to "control" the vole population. The most intense predatory pressure was always at the end of the vole decline, thereby depressing the population even farther. The presence of a limited supply of alternative prey, especially harvest mice and pocket gophers, enabled the carnivores to persist in their search for the last *Microtus*. The fact that *Microtus* is the preferred prey is shown in that the population density of *Reithrodontomys megalotis* frequently was greater than that of *Microtus californicus*, but *Reithrodontomys* was relatively ignored by the carnivores except when *Microtus* was scarce. The intense and persistent predation during and following the collapse of the *Microtus* populations showed that the carnivores were catching more than just "surplus" *Microtus*. This persistence, made possible by the presence of a limited amount of alternative prey, kept the carnivores on the scene long enough to prevent a resurgence of the *Microtus* population for one or more breeding seasons and led me (Pearson, 1966) to suggest that carnivore predation is an essential component of the multi-annual microtine cycle. Raptors, in contrast to carnivores, tend to leave the scene when *Microtus* becomes scarce.

Many people have resisted accepting the importance of predation in driving the microtine cycle because they have expected predators to have their influence at the peak of the cycle. In reality, other factors must help the predators stop a vigorously growing microtine population. The carnivores play their role during and following the decline by depressing the population to extremely low levels and delaying its recovery. The role of alternative prey may also be misunderstood if they are thought of as "buffer species." If they are present in limited supply they increase rather than buffer the amplitude of the microtine cycle.

Predation by Fish, Amphibians, and Reptiles

Microtus enters water voluntarily and swims competently (Blair, 1939; Murie, 1960; Peterson, 1947). Consequently, it is exposed to predation by fish, turtles, and alligators. This predation surely has negligible population consequences. Bullfrogs are predation generalists and have a reputation for eating any moving object that they can swallow or partially swallow. Korschgen and Baskett (1963) found that *M. ochrogaster* made up an average of 15.3% by volume of the stomach contents of bullfrogs, and during one summer month as much as 43.9%. Even salamanders eat *Microtus.* Wilson (1970) found a 98-g *Dicamptodon ensatus* that had swallowed a 27-g *Microtus longicaudatus.* Bury (1971) found two *Microtus* in 12 *Dicamptodon* stomachs examined.

A microtine Pyrrhic victory has been called to my attention by my colleague Harry Greene. He found a large red-legged frog (*Rana aurora*) lying dead at the edge of a pond. A young-adult *Microtus californicus* had been half-swallowed, head first, the posterior half still protruding from the frog's mouth. The partially decomposed and pickled frog, without mouse, weighed 48 g.

Snakes are traditional enemies of mice, but their impact has rarely been quantified. Fitch (1960) provided data for three of 15 species of snakes on the University of Kansas Natural History Reservation. The diet of copperheads (*Ancistridon contortix*) was 39% by weight *Microtus ochrogaster,* which makes this vole by far the most important food for this snake. Population density of copperheads on the reservation in the autumn, after birth of the young, exceeds 12/ha, and Fitch estimated that a typical copperhead consumes eight meals totalling approximately twice its own body weight in the course of a growing season. I have calculated that the impact of copperheads in this habitat would be about 20 30-g *M. ochrogaster*/ha/year.

In the same habitat racers (*Coluber constrictor*) occupy grasslands at densities of 2.5–7.5/ha. Sixty-six percent of their diet by weight consists of small mammals, mostly *Microtus* (Fitch, 1963*a*). The pilot black snakes (*Elaphe obsoleta*) on the same reservation ate primarily small mammals, and the most frequent of these was *M. ochrogaster* (Fitch, 1963*b*). Blacksnake densities varied between an annual minimum of 2.1/ha and an annual maximum of 4.2/ha. The combined population density of these three species of snakes averages about 11 individuals/ha; all of them are deadly *Microtus* predators. The density of *Microtus* during a 2-year census in the same fields varied between 360/ha and 62/ha (Martin, 1956) and dropped much lower in the following year. It is probable that in some seasons these three predators outnumber the voles.

In another study, racers and pilot black snakes preyed on a population of *Microtus pennsylvanicus,* 36 of which were equipped with radiotransmitters (Madison, 1978). During a 1-month interval, six of these *Microtus* were eaten and recovered from snakes. The snakes preyed selectively on lactating females and their litters and on large males. Madison (1978) suggested that boldness in the presence of a predator, or perhaps chemical signals, make these subgroups of vole populations especially vulnerable to predation by snakes.

Discussion

The preceding documentation demonstrates that many species of predators can and do catch *Microtus* with great ease and that in many situations a single species of avian or mammalian or reptilian predator catches a lot of *Microtus.* An assemblage of predators has an even greater impact. Capture of more than 20% of a vole population per month is not uncommon. After a long non-breeding season, attrition of this severity sometimes places *Microtus* in the awkward position of starting the breeding season surrounded by persisting predators that can eat the offspring produced by the surviving *Microtus* faster than they can be produced. In spite of the quantities of *Microtus* harvested by predators, many people doubt that predation has any marked effect on *Microtus* numbers. Martin (1956), for example, censused *Microtus ochrogaster* on the University of Kansas Natural History Reservation for 2 years and concluded: "Although voles were a common item of prey for many species of predators on the Reservation, no marked effect on the density of the population of this vole could be attributed to predation pressure. Only when densities reached a point that caused many voles to expose themselves abnormally could they be heavily preyed upon. Their normally secretive habits, keeping them more or less out of sight, suggest that they are an especially obvious illustration of the concept that predation is an expression of population vulnerability, rising to high levels only when a population is ecologically insecure, rather than a major factor regulating population levels."

In the same report he lists the following *Microtus* predators living on the Reservation: four species of snakes, 15 species of birds, and nine species of mammals. He gives no support for his disbelief in an effective pressure on the *Microtus* population. I believe that when measurements are available they will show that here, as elsewhere, many species of snakes and raptors and carnivores do not wait until the meadows are overflowing with insecure or maladjusted *Microtus*: they kill *Microtus* with great ease even when populations are low. If a particular predator is a resident generalist with access to alternative prey, or is a nomadic specialist (for example, kites or short-eared owls), its effect would be expected to stabilize vole density, as pointed out by Andersson and Erlinge (1977). The effect of stabilizing predation on a prey population is not easily detected because its greatest expression leads to an absence of any change in the density of the prey. If, however, a predator is a resident specialist, such as an ermine, its predatory effect would be to destabilize vole densities. Amplitude of change would be increased, and the period of the microtine cycle of abundance would be increased. Martin's (1956) voles, which in 2 years underwent a five-fold change of density, were responding to predation from a mixture of specialist–generalist and resident–nomadic species, as well as to other complex influences such as weather.

Most of the adaptations of *Microtus* seem to equip it for life in grasslands rather than for defense against predators. Its size is convenient for a host of predators from shrews to grizzly bears. Speed, acceleration, and agility are relatively poor. Senses are probably less acute than in most of the other species of small mammals living nearby. It possesses scent glands that function for intraspecific communication but that are ineffective in masking its basic delicious flavor. It is primarily a grass-eater, so the more it eats the more it becomes exposed to its enemies. It does not hibernate or estivate to avoid difficult or dangerous seasons of the year, and it is active both day and night, so it exposes itself to risk from both nocturnal and diurnal predators. Few *Microtus* store food and so they must venture out of their nests at frequent intervals. *M. californicus* in the wild is equally active day and night in winter but is primarily active early in the morning during summer. This change seems to be driven by moisture requirements rather than by predation (Pearson, 1960). Males of *M. californicus* make more excursions out into the runways than do females, but the average male excursion is briefer. Daytime excursions last much longer than nighttime excursions. These and other differences in behavior affect the vulnerability of different subgroups of the population. The catch by still-hunters such as copperheads should show a bias toward males; sweeping hunters such as barn owls and marsh hawks should encounter a less-biased sex ratio. Field data on the vulnerability of different subsets of the *Microtus* population are needed urgently.

A frequently mentioned stratagem against predators, one that is effective at the population level if not at the level of the individual, is a high rate of reproduction. Most species of *Microtus* have high (and elastic) reproductive potential. Litter size is not notably large, but post-partum breeding is common, and early sexual maturity, which through compounding is most important for rapid population growth, may be spectacular. I have caught 15-g *M. californicus* carrying conspicuous embryos. These females must have become pregnant at not more than two weeks of age. Most individuals of a *Microtus* population also initiate breeding in synchrony so that a pulse of young emerge at a presumably favorable season and overwhelm the appetites of the available predators. No predators are able to outbreed *Microtus,* so a numerical response of the carnivores usually lags behind an increasing vole population.

The grassland in which most *Microtus* live is a relatively simple habitat that does not promote species diversity (Cody, 1966). Consequently, two or more species of *Microtus* rarely live in the same meadow and share the reproductive costs of saturating the predators. In fact, the simplicity of grassland is probably a necessary condition for the microtine cycle of abundance. There are no multiannual cycles of rodents in rainforest, a habitat so complex, with alternative prey so varied and abundant, that predators presumably are supported for long periods at a more constant density than in grasslands.

Various social strategies found in *Microtus* restrict population growth and thereby tend to keep population density below a level that attracts nomadic predators. Cannibalism is one of these (Fitch, 1957). Dispersal is another (Lidicker, 1975). Dispersal may occur at various stages in the cycle of abundance, at various seasons, and may involve different classes of the population. They may disperse into good, or marginal, or even submarginal habitat. All of these kinds of dispersers will have increased their vulnerability to predation and can be thought of as dispersing into a sink that is the collective maw of their predators (Tamarin, 1978).

Conclusions

It will be many years before we fully understand the populational consequences of predation on microtines. We already know that predation is a vital concern at the level of the individual. A sophisticated *Microtus,* cowering in its retreat contemplating an excursion out into the grassland, could best calculate the probability of its survival for one more day in a dangerous world if it knew: How many of "us" are there? What is our sex ratio and age composition? How many of "them" are there? How many of them are generalists or specialists? How many resident or nomadic? How many nocturnal or diurnal? How many are still-hunters? What is this week's rate of change of their numbers and ours? How many alternative prey are there? He could then optimize the time, duration, and direction of his excursion. Leopold (1933) called attention to almost all of these variables that affect prey mortality, but in the ensuing 50 years we have failed to provide more than the sparsest of field data. We are ready to document which predator catches which mouse, but not yet can we predict how that event will alter the course of the predator and prey populations.

Future research probably will focus on the complex effects of predation on the demographies of predator and prey. Progress may be slow because we are still waiting for mammalogists to provide us with a good method of measuring densities of *Microtus,* a good method of defining and measuring meaningful subcategories of the populations, a good method of anticipating future reproductive performance of populations and, consequently, an adequate method of predicting potential growth of a population. Achievement of these goals would simplify the design and interpretation of much-needed experimental manipulations of predator–*Microtus* systems. Meanwhile, many "natural experiments" wait to be exploited. Islands with and without various predators could be investigated profitably and could be manipulated with the expectation of getting interpretable results.

In view of the many marvelous interactions that have been described in other animal groups, it is not unreasonable to expect that coevolution, driven by the selective force of the intense predation documented in this review, has provided some fascinating predator-prey interactions waiting to be revealed.

Literature Cited

ANDERSSON, M., AND S. ERLINGE. 1977. Influence of predation on rodent populations. Oikos, 29:591–597.

BAKER, J. A., AND R. J. BROOKS. 1981. Distribution patterns of raptors in relation to density of meadow voles. Condor, 83:42–47.

———. 1982. Impact of raptor predation on a declining vole population. J. Mamm., 63:297–300.

BARBEHENN, K. R. 1958. Spatial and population relationships between *Microtus* and *Blarina.* Ecology, 39:293–304.

BEACHAM, T. D. 1979. Selectivity of avian predation in declining populations of the vole *Microtus townsendii.* Canadian J. Zool., 57:1767–1772.

BLAIR, W. F. 1939. A swimming and diving meadow vole. J. Mamm., 20:375–376.

BOONSTRA, R. 1977. Predation on *Microtus townsendii* populations: impact and vulnerability. Canadian J. Zool., 55:1631–1643.

BRADT, G. W. 1949. Farm cat as a predator. Michigan Conserv., 18:23–25.

BROWN, L., AND D. AMADON. 1968. Eagles, hawks and falcons of the world. 2 vols. Country Life Books, McGraw Hill, New York, 945 pp.

BURY, R. B. 1971. Small mammals and other prey in the diet of the Pacific giant salamander (Dicamptodon ensatus). Amer. Midland Nat., 87:524–526.

CHRISTIAN, D. P. 1975. Vulnerability of meadow voles, *Microtus pennsylvanicus,* to predation by domestic cats. Amer. Midland Nat., 93:498–502.

CODY, M. L. 1966. The consistency of intra-and inter-continental grassland bird species counts. Amer. Nat., 100:371–376.

Craighead, J. J., and F. C. Craighead, Jr. 1956. Hawks, owls and wildlife. Wildl. Mgt. Inst., Washington, 443 pp.

Davis, D. E. 1937. A cycle in northern shrike emigrations. Auk, 54:43–49.

Dixon, J. S., and R. M. Bond. 1937. Raptorial birds in the cliff areas of Lava Beds National Monument, California. Condor, 39:97–102.

Eadie, W. R. 1952. Shrew predation and vole populations on a localized area. J. Mamm., 33:185–189.

Errington, P. L. 1946. Predation and vertebrate populations. Quart. Rev. Biol., 21:144–177, 221–245.

Fitch, H. S. 1957. Aspects of reproduction and development in the prairie vole (Microtus ochrogaster). Univ. Kansas Publ., Mus. Nat. Hist., 10:129–161.

———. 1960. Autecology of the copperhead. Univ. Kansas Publ., Mus. Nat. Hist., 13:85–288.

———. 1963*a*. Natural history of the racer Coluber constrictor. Univ. Kansas Publ., Mus. Nat. Hist., 15:351–468.

———. 1963*b*. Natural history of the black rat snake (*Elaphe o. obsoleta*) in Kansas. Copeia, 1963:649–658.

Fitzgerald, B. M. 1977. Weasel predation on a cyclic population of the montane vole (*Microtus montanus*) in California. J. Anim. Ecol., 46:367–397.

George, W. G. 1974. Domestic cats as predators and factors in winter shortages of raptor prey. Wilson Bull., 86:384–396.

Gordon, B. L. 1977. Monterey Bay area: natural history and cultural imprints. Second ed. Boxwood Press, Pacific Grove, California, 321 pp.

Graber, R. R. 1962. Food and oxygen consumption in three species of owls (Strigidae). Condor, 64:473–487.

Gross, A. O. 1947. Cyclic invasions of the snowy owl and the migration of 1945–1946. Auk, 64:584–601.

Hahn, W. L. 1908. Notes on the mammals and cold-blooded vertebrates of the Indiana University Farm, Mitchell, Indiana. Proc. U.S. Natl. Mus., 35: 545–581.

Hall, E. R. 1927. An outbreak of house mice in Kern County, California. Univ. California Publ. Zool., 30:189–203.

Hamerstrom, F. 1979. Effect of prey on predator: voles and harriers. Auk, 96: 370–374.

Hamilton, W. J., Jr. 1940. The biology of the smoky shrew (*Sorex fumeus fumeus* Miller). Zoologica, 25:473–492.

Harestad, A. S., and F. L. Bunnell. 1979. Home range and body weight—a reevaluation. Ecology, 60:389–402.

Heidt, G. A. 1972. Anatomical and behavioral aspects of killing and feeding by the least weasel, *Mustela nivalis* L. Arkansas Acad. Sci. Proc., 26:53–54.

Holling, C. S. 1959. The components of predation as revealed by a study of small mammal predation of the European pine sawfly. Canadian Entomol., 91: 293–320.

Jenkins, S. H. 1981. Common patterns in home range-body size relationship of birds and mammals. Amer. Nat., 118:126–128.

Konishi, M. 1973. How the owl tracks its prey. Amer. Scientist, 61:414–424.

Korschgen, L. J., and T. S. Baskett. 1963. Food of impoundment- and stream-dwelling bullfrogs in Missouri. Herpetologica, 19:89–99.

Leopold, A. 1933. Game management. Scribner's, New York, 481 pp.

Leyhausen, P. 1978. Cat behavior: the predatory and social behavior of domestic and wild cats. Garland, New York, 340 pp.

LIDICKER, W. Z., JR. 1975. The role of dispersal in the demography of small mammals. Pp. 103–134, *in* Small mammals: their productivity and population dynamics (F. B. Golley, K. Petrusewicz, and L. Ryszkowski, eds.). Internatl. Biol. Prog., Cambridge Univ. Press, London, 5:1–451.

MADISON, D. M. 1978. Behavioral and sociochemical susceptibility of meadow voles (Microtus pennsylvanicus) to snake predators. Amer. Midland Nat., 100:23–28.

———. 1979. Impact of spacing behavior and predation on population growth in meadow voles. Pp. 20–29, *in* Proceedings of the third eastern pine and meadow vole symposium (R. E. Byers, ed.). New Paltz, New York, 86 pp.

MARTI, C. D. 1974. Feeding ecology of four sympatric owls. Condor, 76:45–61.

MARTIN, E. P. 1956. A population study of the prairie vole (Microtus ochrogaster) in northeastern Kansas. Univ. Kansas Publ., Mus. Nat. Hist., 8:361–416.

MARTINSEN, D. L. 1969. Energetics and activity patterns of short-tailed shrews (*Blarina*) on restricted diets. Ecology, 50:505–510.

MASTER, L. L. 1979. Some observations on great gray owls and their prey in Michigan. Jack-Pine Warbler, 57:215–217.

MAURER, F. W., JR., 1970. Observation of fighting between a vole and a shrew. Amer. Midland Nat., 84:549.

MILLER, A. H. 1931. Systematic revision and natural history of the American shrikes (Lanius). Univ. California Publ. Zool., 38:11–242.

MOWAT, F. 1963. Never cry wolf. Little, Brown and Co., Boston, 247 pp.

MULLEN, D. A., AND F. A. PITELKA. 1972. Efficiency of winter scavengers in the Arctic. Arctic, 25:225–231.

MURIE, A. 1936. Following fox trails. Misc. Publ. Mus. Zool., Univ. Michigan, 32:1–45.

———. 1940. Ecology of the coyote in the Yellowstone. Fauna of the National Parks of the United States. Bull. U.S. Dept. Interior, 4:1–206.

———. 1944. The wolves of Mount McKinley. Fauna of the National Parks of the United States, Fauna Series No. 5, 238 pp.

———. 1960. Aquatic voles. J. Mamm., 41:273–275.

NEWTON, I. 1979. Population ecology of raptors. Buteo, Vermillion, South Dakota, 399 pp.

PAYNE, R. S. 1962. How the barn owl locates prey by hearing. Living Bird, 1:151–159.

PEARSON, O. P. 1942. On the cause and nature of a poisonous action produced by the bite of a shrew (*Blarina brevicauda*). J. Mamm., 23:159–166.

———. 1959. A traffic survey of *Microtus-Reithrodontomys* runways. J. Mamm., 40:169–180.

———. 1960. Habits of Microtus californicus revealed by automatic photographic recorders. Ecol. Monogr., 30:231–249.

———. 1964. Carnivore-mouse predation: an example of its intensity and bioenergetics. J. Mamm., 45:177–188.

———. 1966. The prey of carnivores during one cycle of mouse abundance. J. Anim. Ecol., 35:217–233.

———. 1971. Additional measurements of the impact of carnivores on California voles (*Microtus californicus*). J. Mamm., 52:41–49.

PETERSON, R. L. 1947. Further observations on swimming and diving of meadow voles. J. Mamm., 297–298.

PLATT, W. J. 1976. The social organization and territoriality of short-tailed shrew (*Blarina brevicauda*) populations in old-field habitats. Anim. Behav., 24: 305–318.

PROCTOR, N. S. 1977. Osprey catches vole. Wilson Bull., 89:625.
RAYMOND, M., AND J-M. BERGERON. 1982. Réponse numérique de l'hermine aux fluctuations d'abondance de *Microtus pennsylvanicus*. Canadian J. Zool., 60:542–549.
REED, J. H. 1897. Notes on the American barn owl in eastern Pennsylvania. Auk, 14:374–383.
RYSZKOWSKI, L., J. GOSZCZYNSKI, AND J. TRUSZKOWSKI. 1973. Trophic relationships of the common vole in cultivated fields. Acta Theriol., 18:125–165.
SAUNDERS, J. K. 1963. Food habits of the lynx in Newfoundland. J. Wildl. Mgmt., 27:384–390.
SAYR, R. 1980. An invasion to remember. Audubon, 82:52–55.
SCHOENER, T. W. 1968. Sizes of feeding territories among birds. Ecology, 49:123–141.
SCOTT, T. G. 1943. Some food coactions of the northern plains red fox. Ecol. Monogr., 13:427–479.
SCOTT, T. G., AND W. D. KLIMSTRA. 1955. Red foxes and a declining prey population. Southern Illinois Univ., Monogr. Ser., 1:1–123.
SHELDON, C. 1930. The wilderness of Denali: explorations of a hunter-naturalist in northern Alaska. Scribner's, New York, 412 pp.
SHULL, A. F. 1907. Habits of the short-tailed shrew *Blarina brevicauda* (Say). Amer. Nat., 41:495–522.
SMITH, D. G., C. R. WILSON, AND H. H. FROST. 1974. History and ecology of a colony of barn owls in Utah. Condor, 76:131–136.
SNYDER, N. F. R., AND J. W. WILEY. 1976. Sexual size dimorphism in hawks and owls of North America. Ornithol. Monogr., 20:1–96.
STENDELL, R. 1972. The occurrence, food habits, and nesting strategy of white-tailed kites in relation to a fluctuating vole population. Unpubl. Ph.D. dissert., Univ. California, Berkeley, 224 pp.
STENDELL, R., AND P. MYERS. 1973. White-tailed kite predation on a fluctuating vole population. Condor, 75:359–360.
TAMARIN, R. H. 1978. Dispersal, population regulation, and K-selection in field mice. Amer. Nat., 112:545–555.
TAPPER, S. 1979. The effect of fluctuating vole numbers (*Microtus agrestis*) on a population of weasels (*Mustela nivalis*) on farmland. J. Anim. Ecol., 48: 603–617.
TOMASI, T. E. 1978. Function of venom in the short-tailed shrew, *Blarina brevicauda*. J. Mamm., 59:852–854.
TONER, G. C. 1956. House cat predation on small mammals. J. Mamm., 37:119.
WAIAN, L. B., AND R. STENDALL [STENDELL]. 1970. The white-tailed kite in California with observation of the Santa Barbara population. California Fish and Game, 56:188–198.
WALLACE, G. J. 1948. The barn owl in Michigan. Its distribution, natural history and food habits. Michigan State Coll., Agric. Exp. Sta. Tech. Bull., 208: 1–61.
WARNER, J. S., AND R. L. RUDD. 1975. Hunting by the white-tailed kite (*Elanus leucurus*). Condor, 77:226–230.
WHITAKER, J. O., JR., AND M. G. FERRARO. 1963. Summer food of 220 short-tailed shrews from Ithaca, New York. J. Mamm., 44:419.
WHITAKER, J. O., JR., AND R. E. MUMFORD. 1972. Food and ectoparasites of Indiana shrews. J. Mamm., 53:329–335.
WILSON, R. L. 1970. *Dicamptodon ensatus* feeding on a microtine. J. Herpetol., 4:93.

POPULATION DYNAMICS AND CYCLES

MARY J. TAITT AND CHARLES J. KREBS

Abstract

WE address two questions about North American *Microtus*: 1) what type of numerical changes occur in their populations? and 2) what factors must be invoked to explain these population changes?

Historically, studies of *Microtus* population dynamics have centered around descriptions of multi-annual cycles in abundance. Examination of field data collected over the last two decades on species of *Microtus* in North America reveals three demographic patterns: annual fluctuations, multi-annual cycles, and both, in sequence. Out of a total of 106 years of data, we estimated 59% were years of annual fluctuations and 41% were cyclic. In two species exhibiting both patterns in sequence there were 9 years of annual fluctuations and three multi-annual cycles. It appears that annual fluctuations in density are more common than multi-annual cycles in some *Microtus* populations.

If we compare annual fluctuations and cycles, we find that the amplitude of numerical change is always less than five-fold for annual fluctuations and usually over 10-fold for cycles. Peak cyclic densities are typically three times greater than the maximum densities of annual fluctuations. Substantial spring declines in density are characteristic of annual fluctuations, whereas little or no spring decline (particularly in female numbers) occurs in years of cyclic peak densities.

There are still problems associated with obtaining reliable estimates of population parameters for *Microtus* species. The use of more than one trapping technique, especially in high density populations, is strongly recommended.

Microtus numbers increase when extra food is provided experimentally to field populations, but no one yet has prevented a cyclic decline by food addition. It is not yet certain whether plant secondary compounds play any role in vole cycles. Predation interacts with cover to affect vole numbers, and predators can take large numbers of voles under certain conditions. Predators may prolong the phase of low vole densities but it is not clear that they can generate cycles.

Spacing behavior operating through differential dispersal may be a key element in the adjustment of *Microtus* densities to available resources. Surplus voles exist in some populations, but we do not know what role such voles play in generating the population dynamics observed. Spacing behavior could be under both genotypic and phenotypic control, which suggests a multi-factor component in vole population dynamics. There is renewed interest in physiological responses of voles and lemmings to stress, and speculations about its effect on suppression of the immune-inflammatory system, especially at high population densities.

A brief consideration of two phenomena suggests how multi-factor explanations could be associated with population cycles in *Microtus*. Body weight may be heritable, but the expression of the trait could be modified by, for example, food conditions in the increase phase or population density at the peak. Mature female voles should perhaps be considered analogous to territorial male birds in maintaining space for production of offspring. The size of territories, and hence the number of mature females, may be determined partly by genetic predisposition and partly by behavioral adjustments to environmental conditions and to local vole density.

Future modeling and research on *Microtus* population dynamics should address the two patterns of fluctuation described. Heritability of growth, reproduction, dominance, and dispersal should be investigated in populations exhibiting both patterns of fluctuation in sequence as well as in predominantly cyclic and non-cyclic populations. Realistic multi-factor hypotheses must be formulated. These should assign factors in a hierarchy over time to predict the patterns observed and be testable by field experiments. There is still much to do.

Introduction

Population dynamics of species in the genus *Microtus* have been, with other small rodents, the subject of several reviews. Historical descriptions of outbreaks and plagues were compiled by Charles Elton (1942) in his book "Voles, Mice and Lemmings." The economic consequences of rodent population irruptions, curiosity about mechanisms of population regulation, and a desire to predict abundance have stimulated much research into rodent population dynamics since Elton's book. Most of the research done up to the early 1970s was reviewed extensively by Krebs and Myers (1974).

In the present review, we evaluate field studies that, for the most part, were conducted since the review by Krebs and Myers (1974), and are restricted to rodents of the genus *Microtus* in North America. We attempt to answer two major questions in this chapter: 1) What type of population changes occur in *Microtus* species in North America? and 2) What factors must be invoked to explain these population changes? By a critical evaluation of past work we hope to provide a paradigm for future studies on these rodents.

Methods of Study

Voles of the genus *Microtus* typically live in underground burrow systems in grasslands. Where grass cover is dense, they develop extensive surface runways. Direct observation of individual voles in the field is, therefore, virtually impossible. Most population data are collected as a result of trapping individuals.

Researchers in North America use snap-traps for census work and live-traps for continuous mark-recapture monitoring of vole populations. Most of the live-traps in use are Longworths (Chitty and Kempson, 1949), or Shermans (Morris, 1968), although pitfalls (Boonstra and Krebs, 1978; Kott, 1965) and multiple-catch traps are also used.

Live-traps are usually placed in square grids with a specific distance (often 25 ft, 7.62 m) between stations. One or two traps are put at each point on the grid, and positioned in active surface runways. In order to catch voles of some species, it is necessary to pre-bait for a period before commencing with a regular trapping program (for example, *M. townsendii* has to be pre-baited for four weeks before appreciable numbers are caught). In the pre-baiting period, food is put in each trap, which is then locked open and placed in position on the grid. Many studies over the last decade have used the field technique suggested by Krebs (1966). In this technique the traps are set with food and bedding (usually a handful of oats and cotton batting). A typical trapping session involves setting traps in the afternoon, checking them for voles the next morning, re-setting, and checking that afternoon, re-setting and checking for the last time the next morning. The traps are then locked open with a handful of oats as pre-bait over the interval until the next trapping session, normally two weeks later. In summer, the daytime trapping period is abandoned to avoid death from overheating of surface metal traps. This is not a problem with pitfall traps.

When a vole is first caught, it is individually marked for future identification. This is most often done by placing a numbered fingerling fish-tag in one ear; alternatively, a system of toe-clipping is used. On first capture within a trapping session, individuals are sexed and weighed to the nearest g. Males are classified according to the position of the testes, either abdominal or scrotal. Females are checked for vaginal perforation: open or closed (estrus or anestrus); size of nipples and amount of lactation tissue: small, medium or large (not lactating, beginning or end of lactation, mid-lactation); separation of the pubic bones: closed (immature), slightly open (previously littered), or open (has just or is about to deliver). All pregnancies and trap litters are recorded. In some studies the number of wounds is recorded; recent wounds are easily identified by blowing the fur and looking for small, usually paired, incisions which indicate the bite of another vole. Every time an individual is caught its number and grid location is recorded.

There is a large literature on the problems of estimating population size in small mammals; we do not review it here (Seber, 1982). The studies that we review are based on live-trapping with a single type of trap. There is now a suggestion in at least one species (*M. townsendii* at high density in summer when daytime trapping is not possible) that pitfall trapping is needed in addition to Longworth trapping to census adult populations (Beacham and Krebs, 1980; Boonstra and Krebs, 1978). In these two studies of peak populations, 40–45% of the adult voles were captured only in pitfall traps. We do not know if these adults could have been caught in Longworth traps if the number of Longworths had been doubled or quadrupled. Nor do we know whether this problem is specific to *M. townsendii,* but it is clear that future studies should use two different trapping techniques whenever possible. Alternatively, multiple-capture traps could be used.

Details of trapping methods might be less critical in vole population studies if we could use mark-recapture methods such as the Jolly-Seber model (Jolly, 1965; Seber, 1982). Because of early indications that *Microtus* does not respond randomly to traps (Krebs, 1966; Leslie et al., 1953) many workers have used enumeration to provide an estimate of abundance. Enumerated densities (minimum number alive) have a negative bias. Hilborn et al. (1976) estimated at least a 10–20% bias in enumerated densities of five species of *Microtus* but pointed out that if unmarked animals had very low probabilities of capture, the minimum-number-alive estimator would seriously underestimate the true number. This is another way of emphasizing the need for pitfall trapping or additional techniques for sampling voles which might not be caught in normal live-traps.

Jolly and Dickson (1983) argued for the use of Jolly-Seber estimates in populations whose individuals show unequal catchability. The Jolly-Seber estimates will have a negative bias under these conditions, but less of a bias than enumeration techniques. Carothers (1973, 1979) showed that unequal catchability has only a very small effect on Jolly-Seber estimates of numbers and survival, if the probability of capture is above 0.5 in each trapping session. These studies suggest that small mammal ecologists should use Jolly-Seber estimates to estimate numbers rather than enumeration methods, but it is important to qualify this recommendation with the reminder that no statistical method can provide accurate estimates of abundance when a large fraction of the population does not enter the traps at all.

Many factors can affect trapping success in small rodents and odors associated with traps is one possibly important factor (Boonstra and Krebs, 1976; Stoddart, 1982). In *M. townsendii,* individuals entered dirty Longworth traps more than clean traps during the breeding season. Voles also may avoid traps visited by other species. Boonstra et al. (1982) showed that *M. pennsylvanicus* was much less likely to be caught in a Longworth trap previously occupied by *Blarina, Mus, Zapus,* or *Peromyscus.* Stoddart (1982) claimed that unmarked *M. agrestis* was more readily caught in clean traps than in dirty ones, but his conclusions cannot be accepted because of faulty experimental design (no pre-baiting) and no suitable controls to measure late summer recruitment of young (cf. Chitty and Phipps, 1966:323). Further work on the effects of odor on trapping success in *Microtus* will be useful particularly if it addresses how present trapping techniques could be improved.

We assume in this chapter that population data obtained by live-trapping is a reliable index of actual changes in numbers if sampling is done at least monthly with an excess of live-traps and a probability of capture above 50% for adult animals. Attempts to sample at a lower intensity have so far proven unreliable at providing a detailed picture of population dynamics, although they may reveal large-scale trends.

Observed Population Patterns

In the last decade, field studies have been conducted on populations of *Microtus* in North America at locations shown in Fig. 1. These empirical studies tend to be short-term and are usually conducted in man-made grasslands where grass cover is dense and the number of voles can be substantial in a 2–3 year period (average workspan of a graduate student). This raises an important general question: are the population dynamics observed in these habitats typical? Bearing this in mind, and trying to allow for differences in trapping regime, sampling periods, and grid size, we ask what population patterns have been observed in the North American species of *Microtus*.

In Tables 1–6, we summarize the demographic patterns observed on control areas in studies of North American *Microtus* populations. We calculated densities of voles by adding a boundary strip one-half the inter-trap distance to each edge of the live-trapping area. In some cases authors have already presented population data as densities and we used these when given. In all cases we rounded densities to the nearest 5/ha because of the error in estimating numbers from published graphs, so the density estimates we give should be viewed as approximations only. We divided demographic patterns into two classes: 1) annual fluctuations, and 2) multi-annual cycles. Annual fluctuations generally have an autumn or winter, end-of-breeding season maximum, and a spring, or onset-of-breeding, minimum. Cycles are defined by a low-peak-decline sequence over at least two years, and by additional demographic criteria defined by Krebs and Myers (1974) when such data are available. When long-term, detailed data are available (Figs. 2, 3), the classification of annual versus cyclic patterns is usually clear. Problems arise in classifying some studies, particularly short-term ones. We think that these two patterns could be quantified by analyzing the variance of spring breeding densities, or more precisely the variance of the natural logarithms of spring densities. For an-

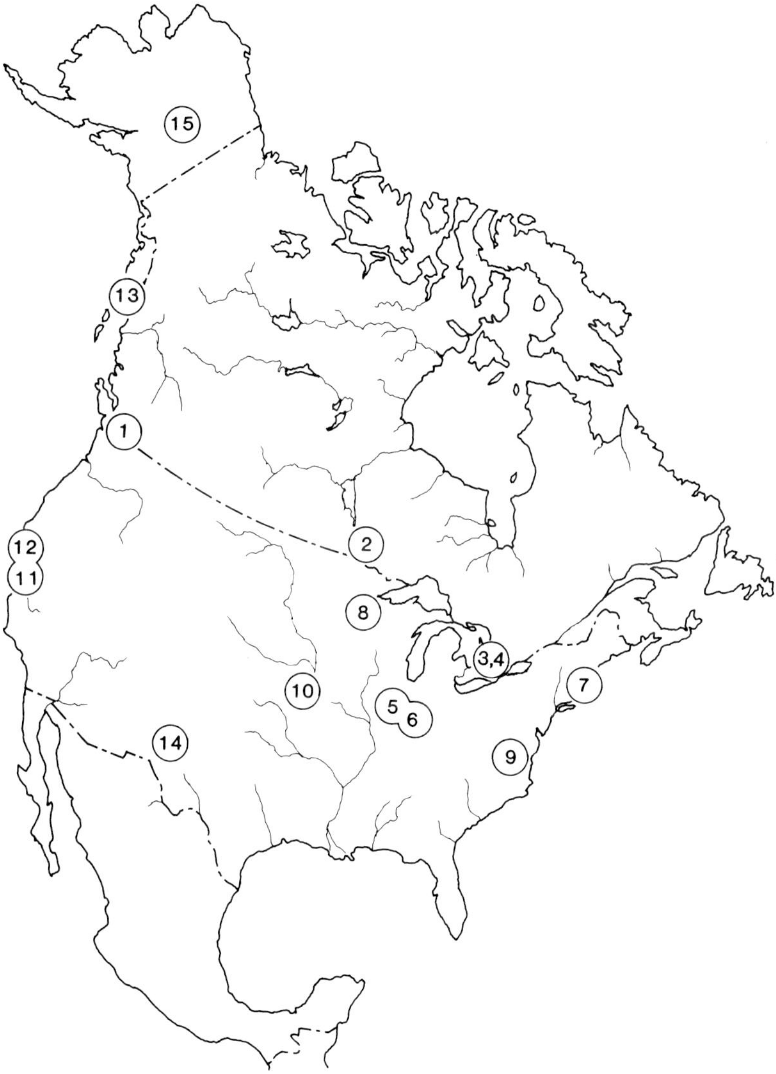

FIG. 1. Population study sites of *Microtus* in North America. Numbers refer to studies identified in Tables 1–6.

TABLE 1
POPULATION DENSITIES FROM LIVE-TRAPPING STUDIES OF *Microtus townsendii* IN BRITISH COLUMBIA

		Density/ha			Spring dynamics				
Grid	Years	High	Low	Pattern	Density[1]	Sex[2]	Notes[3]	Map location (Fig. 1)	References
I	1971–76	285	150	Annual	Low	Both	Perennial grassland;	1	Krebs (1979)
		385	85	Annual	Low	Both	no competitors;		
		385	75	Annual	Low	Both	Westham Island		
		625	40	Cycle	435	♂ only			
C1	1980	260	85	Annual	Low	Both	Winter–spring study	1	Taitt et al. (1981)
C2	1980	150	30	Annual	Low	Both	Winter–spring study		Taitt et al. (1981)
C1	1981	375	125	Annual	Low	Both	Winter–spring study		Taitt and Krebs (1982)
C2	1981	175	145	Annual	Low	Both	Winter–spring study		Taitt and Krebs
C	1982	345	265	Annual?	Low	Both	Winter–spring study		Taitt and Krebs (1983)
A	1976–78	800	65	Cycle	365	♂ only	Perennial grassland;	1	Beacham (1979*a*)
D	1976–78	665	40	Cycle	430	♂ only	no competitors;		
							Reifel Island		
C	1971–75	400?	50	Cycle?					
		210	150	Annual	Low	Both	Perennial grassland;	1	Krebs (1979)
		360	115	Annual	Low	Both	no competitors;		
		210	150	Annual	Low	Both	Mainland		
E	1971–76	50	15	Annual	Low	Both	Perennial grassland;	1	Krebs (1979)
		100	65	Annual	Low	Both	*M. oregoni* and		
		100	85	Annual	Low	Both	*Peromyscus mani-*		
		525	150?	Cycle?	185?	♂ only	*culatus*; Mainland		

[1] Density in number/ha at the end of the spring decline. Low means equal to the low density given in previous column.
[2] Sex indicates whether the spring decline occurred in both sexes or only in one sex primarily.
[3] Species listed here were present on the grid; they may or may not have been competitors.

nual fluctuations we expect this variance to be less than 0.5, and for cycles, greater than 1.0. Note that spring densities are critical, not autumn densities (Krebs and Myers, 1974). We do not know whether the dichotomy between annual and cyclic populations is real, or whether there is a continuum between the two extremes. In the following, we discuss demographic patterns for each species.

M. townsendii

All of the long-term population data on this species come from the Vancouver area of British Columbia. We identified (Table 1) four probable cycles in four populations of this species and 13 annual fluctuations in three populations. Figure 2 illustrates population changes on one area that was monitored for 11 years. A cyclic peak is evident in 1975 but in most years annual fluctuations occur. Cyclic peaks in this species ranged from 525 to 800/ha, averaging 697 voles/ha (Longworth-trapped population only). Annual fluctuations had average maximums of 239 voles/ha and minimums of 94 voles/ha. Most of the communities studied consisted only of this vole species. One area (grid E; see Krebs, 1979:Fig. 3) contained *Peromyscus maniculatus* and *M. oregoni* when *M. townsendii* was at low numbers, but both these potential competitors disappeared when *M. townsendii* increased above 100/ha.

M. pennsylvanicus

Studies on *M. pennsylvanicus* have been conducted over a broad geographic range (Fig. 1) and an array of demographic patterns has been described. There are large differences in average density of this species in different areas and these regional differences cannot be due simply to techniques (Table 2). In Ontario, recent work indicates that annual fluctuations are common with maximum densities averaging 410/ha and minima averaging 120/ha. Boonstra and Rodd (1983) provided 3 years of data from Toronto showing annual fluctuations at high densities. A striking population pattern was observed by Iverson, Turner and Mihok in Manitoba (Fig. 3; Mihok, in press). This population exhibited a cycle, a cyclic low density followed by another cycle, then three annual fluctuations. In Manitoba, densities were very low, averaging 90/ha at cyclic peaks and 10/ha at cyclic lows; annual fluctuations averaged 55/ha at maximum and 30/ha at minimum.

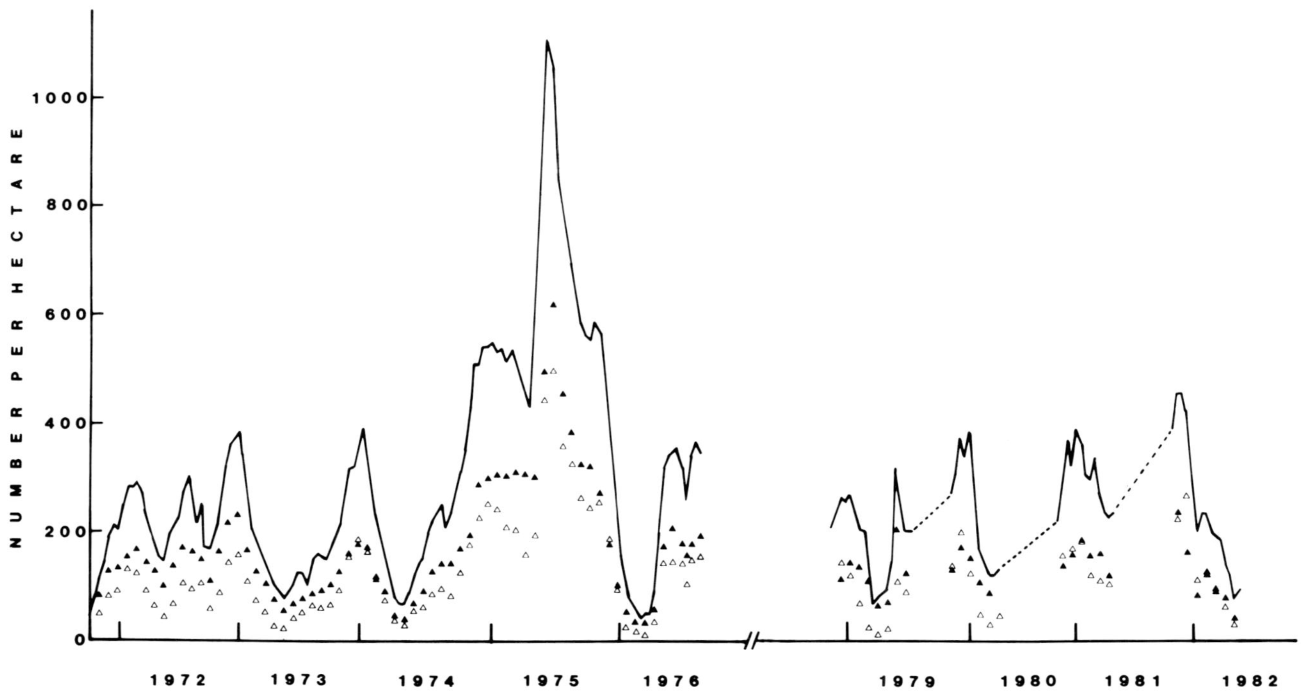

FIG. 2. Population densities of *Microtus townsendii* on control grids on Westham Island, British Columbia. Pitfall trap data are included for summers 1975, 1976, and 1979. Symbols are: △, males; ▲, females.

Indiana data on *M. pennsylvanicus* are almost intermediate between cyclic and annual fluctuations and we interpret them as 2-year cycles. The cyclic maxima averaged 180/ha and the minima averaged 40/ha. These figures are similar to those obtained by Tamarin (1977) in Massachusetts. Virginia data on this species seem to show the end of one cycle and then 2 years of annual fluctuations averaging 85/ha maximum and 35/ha minimum. In Minnesota, 2 years of annual fluctuations averaged 85/ha maximum and 10/ha minimum. In Illinois, *M. pennsylvanicus* invaded habitats formerly occupied by *M. ochrogaster*; to date, populations are sparse, with maxima averaging only 30/ha. From these studies we estimate that, for 33 years of data, 17 years showed annual fluctuations and 16 years were cyclic. There is no clear evidence of a competitive density reduction in those areas in which a second *Microtus* species occurred.

M. ochrogaster

Populations of *M. ochrogaster* have been studied extensively in Kansas, Illinois, and Indiana. Most populations studied in Illinois and Indiana showed 2–4 year cycles in numbers, averaging 130 voles/ha at the peak and often falling to local extinction during cyclic lows (average 4/ha). In Indiana and, since 1975 in Illinois, there was potential competition from *M. pennsylvanicus*. Krebs (1977) could find no clear evidence of competition between these two species in Indiana. But in Illinois the 1975 *M. ochrogaster* peak (*M. pennsylvanicus* present) was only half that of the 1972 peak when *M. pennsylvanicus* was absent (Getz et al., 1979:fig. 1). In Kansas after an initial 3-year cycle (Gaines and Rose, 1976), *M. ochrogaster* populations exhibited a series of annual fluctuations averaging 55/ha at the maximum and 15/ha at the minimum (Gaines et al., 1979). Densities in Kansas were higher in the one cyclic peak observed (120/ha), and fell to less than 5/ha in the cyclic low. Other studies in Kansas (Martin, 1956) reported an absence of cycling in *M. ochrogaster* during 4 years. For the studies that are included in Table 3 we tallied 13 years of cyclic populations out of 20 total years of data.

M. californicus

The California vole (Table 4) has a restricted geographical distribution but has been studied extensively by the research group at

TABLE 2

POPULATION DENSITIES FROM LIVE-TRAPPING FOR *M. pennsylvanicus*. SEE FOOTNOTES OF TABLE 1

		Density/ha			Spring dynamics				
Grid	Years	High	Low	Pattern	Density	Sex	Notes	Map location (Fig. 1)	References
C	1968–78	85	5	Cycle	75				
		90	15	Cycle	40		Mainland, Manitoba;	2	Mihok (in press)
		50	30	Annual	Low		no competitors		
		60	30	Annual	Low				
		55	35	Annual	Low				
	1977–78	400	80	Annual?	Low		Mainland, Ontario; no competitors	3	Webster and Brooks (1981)
SG	1974–76	265	15	Annual	Low		Mainland, Ontario;		Baker and Brooks
OF	1974–76	200	50	Annual	Low		no competitors; SG, short grass; OF, old field		(1981)
C	1978–81	500	115	Annual	Low				
		415	265	Annual	Low		Mainland, Ontario;	4	Boonstra and Rudd (1983)
		665	215	Annual	Low		no competitors		
A	1975–76	10	0	Annual			Mainland, Illinois;	5	Getz et al. (1979)
B	1976–76	50	10	Cycle	30		*M. ochrogaster*		
P	1975–76	15	5	Annual	Low		A, alfalfa;		
		30	?	Annual			B, bluegrass; P, prairie colonizing		

TABLE 2
CONTINUED

		Density/ha			Spring dynamics				
Grid	Years	High	Low	Pattern	Density	Sex	Notes	Map location (Fig. 1)	References
A	1965–70	190	55	Cycle	95	♂ > ♀			
		155	30	Cycle	95	♂ > ♀	Mainland, Indiana; *M. ochrogaster*	6	Myers and Krebs (1971)
F	1967–70	75	5	Cycle	45	♂ only			
I	1967–70	210	35	Cycle	80	♂ > ♀			
D	1972–75	220	0	Cycle	135	♂ only	Mainland, Massachusetts; *P. leucopus*	7	Tamarin (1977)
F	1972–75	255	30	Cycle	75	♂ only			
WL	1973–75	80	10	Annual	Low		Mainland, Minnesota; no competitors; WL, wetland	8	Birney et al. (1976)
		95	10	Annual	Low				
1	1974–78	225	40	Cycle			Mainland, Virginia; *Peromyscus maniculatus*	9	Dueser et al. (1981)
		115	40	Annual	Low				
		115	40	Annual	Low				
		15	0	Annual	Low				
5	1976–77	90	55	Annual	Low				

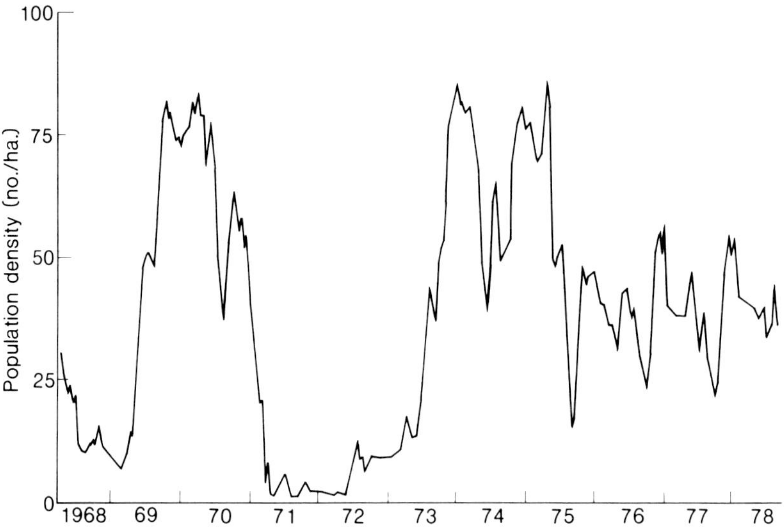

FIG. 3. Population densities of *Microtus pennsylvanicus* on a control oldfield at Pinawa, Manitoba (reproduced, with permission, from Mihok, in press).

Berkeley led by Pearson, Lidicker, and Pitelka. Unfortunately, like most vole population studies, techniques have not been standardized and we can only hope that results are comparable, as Pearson (1971) demonstrated for two studies. Lidicker (1973) reported the longest time series for this species (13 years), but we consider only the first 5 years to be sufficiently accurate for this analysis. Lidicker (1973) found annual fluctuations to be common on Brooks Island and Krebs (1966) reported cases of annual fluctuations on the mainland. Krohne (1982) recently reported annual fluctuations in perennial grasslands in northern California. Densities varied greatly in different areas. Lidicker's (1973) Brooks Island densities were 3–10 times those reported in areas on the mainland. This difference may be due to an island effect or a difference in techniques. For mainland sites, cyclic peak densities averaged 570 voles/ha, and cyclic lows average 15/ha. Annual fluctuations on the mainland reached average maxima of 85/ha and average minima of 20/ha. We do not know if *M. californicus* cycles in southern California. Blaustein (1980) reported declines that could be either cyclic or the result of an irregular annual fluctuation with frequent extinctions. For the studies summarized in Table 4, we suggest that there were 7 years

TABLE 3

POPULATION DENSITIES FROM LIVE-TRAPPING FOR *M. ochrogaster*. SEE FOOTNOTES OF TABLE 1

Grid	Years	Density/ha High	Density/ha Low	Pattern	Spring dynamics Density	Spring dynamics Sex	Notes	Map location (Fig. 1)	References
C	1975–76	90	20	Annual?			Mainland, Illinois; *M. pennsylvanicus* removed; predation—cats	5	Cole and Batzli (1978)
		70	5	Annual?					
A	1972–76	240	0	Cycle			Mainland, Illinois; A, alfalfa; no competitors	5	Getz et al. (1979)
		100	5	Cycle?	60				
B	1972–76	130	0	Cycle			*M. pennsylvanicus*; B, bluegrass		
		60	5	Cycle?	10				
A	1965–70	140	0	Cycle	35	♂ only	Mainland, Indiana; *M. pennsylvanicus* spring influx	6	Myers and Krebs (1971)
		35	0	Annual?	3				
H	1967–79	135	0	Cycle?	25	Both			Krebs (1970)
A	1970–73	155	0	Cycle	Low		Mainland, Kansas; no competitors	10	Gaines and Rose (1976)
B	1970–73	120	10	Cycle	Low				
C	1970–73	125	0	Cycle?	Low				
D	1970–73	85	5	Cycle?	Low				
B	1973–76	55	10	Annual	28				
		50	0	Annual?			Mainland, Kansas; no competitors	10	Gaines et al. (1979)
D	1973–77	60	30	Annual	Low				
		60	20	Annual	Low				
		45	15	Annual	Low				
I	1975–76	65	5	Annual	Low				

TABLE 4

POPULATION DENSITIES FROM LIVE-TRAPPING FOR *M. californicus*. SEE FOOTNOTES OF TABLE 1

Grid	Years	Density/ha		Pattern	Spring dynamics		Notes	Map location (Fig. 1)	References
		High	Low		Density	Sex			
BI	1959–63	1,580	50	Cycle?	952		Brooks Island, California; *Mus musculus*, rats; annual grassland	11	Lidicker (1973)
		1,250	450	Annual?	Low				
		650	150	Annual	Low				
		1,000	?	Annual?	Low				
TC	1962–64	640	25	Cycle					
RFS3	1962–64	300	0	Cycle	60		Mainland, California; annual grassland	12	Krebs (1966)
PARR	1962–64	1,150	20	Cycle?					
RFS4	1962–64	160	10	Annual					
RFS5	1962–64	50	2	Annual					
Richmond	1966–68	395	10	Cycle	100		Mainland, California; annual grassland	12	Batzli and Pitelka (1971)
Russell	1966–68	370	?	Cycle	105				
A	1977–79	100	25	Annual	Low				
		125	35	Annual	Low		Mainland, California; perennial grasslands	12	Krohne (1982)
B	1977–79	45	25	Annual	Low				
		40	20	Annual	Low				

of cycles and 7 years of annual fluctuations reported in this species. There are no apparent competitors of *M. californicus,* which seems to dominate all other rodents in its grassland habitat (Blaustein, 1980; DeLong, 1966; Lidicker, 1966). We did not include Garsd and Howard's (1982) analysis of pit-trap data; we do not know whether their pitfall technique adequately measures vole population densities.

M. oregoni

The Oregon vole is unusual for *Microtus* species because it lives in a variety of habitats from virgin conifer forests to clearcut areas in forests and grasslands (Hawes, 1975). It has never been recorded at high densities (Table 5), so it illustrates the difficulty of trying to determine if cycles are present. There is no clear evidence for cycles except for two cases reported in Sullivan and Krebs (1981). Gashwiler (1972) reported some fluctuations in *M. oregoni* in clear-cut habitats but little fluctuation in virgin timber areas. Hawes (1975) found only annual fluctuations in *M. oregoni* and showed that this species was reduced in density when it came into competition with *M. townsendii.* Petticrew and Sadleir (1974) reported a possible cycle of *M. oregoni* in a Douglas-fir plantation; Taitt (1978) found *M. oregoni* invading a forest trapping area in 1 of 3 years of study. We conclude that *M. oregoni* populations may cycle, but they most frequently have annual fluctuations that average 32/ha at maximum and 7/ha at minimum density. Cyclic populations are suggested to have peak densities 2–3 times the annual maxima (Table 5).

M. breweri

This island species was shown to have annual fluctuations on Muskeget Island (Tamarin, 1977); the average peak was 170 voles/ha and the average minimum was 68/ha (Table 6).

M. longicaudus

Few studies of *M. longicaudus* have been carried out (Table 6). In Alaska, an annual cycle at low density seemed to occur in logged areas (Van Horne, 1982). Densities averaged 33/ha at maximum and 11/ha at minimum. Conley (1976) reported a possible cyclic peak of this species at 105/ha in a New Mexico grassland. In the

TABLE 5
POPULATION DENSITIES FROM LIVE-TRAPPING FOR *M. oregoni*. SEE FOOTNOTES OF TABLE 1

		Density/ha			Spring dynamics			Map location	
Grid	Years	High	Low	Pattern	Density	Sex	Notes	(Fig. 1)	References
OF	1971–74	45	5	Annual	Low		Mainland, B.C.	1	Sullivan and Krebs (1981)
		45	5	Annual	Low		OF, old field		
		70	?	Cycle?	30				
L	1971–74	90	15	Cycle?			Mainland, B.C.	1	Sullivan and Krebs (1981)
		40	15	Annual	Low		L, Ladner Grassland		
		40	15	Annual	Low		with *M. townsendii*		
		35	15	Annual	Low		and *Peromyscus maniculatus*		
G	1972–74	35	5	Annual	Low		Mainland, B.C.	1	Sullivan and Krebs (1981)
		20	5	Annual	Low		G, grassland with *M. townsendii* and *P. maniculatus*		
S	1975–80	15	0	Annual	Low		Mainland, B.C.	1	Sullivan and Krebs (1981)
		10	0	Annual	Low		S, shrub		
		35	0	Annual	Low		*P. maniculatus*		
		20	?	Annual?					

TABLE 6

POPULATION DENSITIES FROM LIVE-TRAPPING FOR *M. breweri*, *M. longicaudus*, *M. mexicanus*, AND *M. oeconomus*. SEE FOOTNOTES OF TABLE 1

Species	Grid	Years	Density/ha		Pattern	Spring dynamics		Notes	Map location (Fig. 1)	References
			High	Low		Density	Sex			
M. breweri	A	1972–75	125	96	Annual	Low	Both	Muskeget Island, Massachusetts; *Peromyscus leucopus*	7	Tamarin (1977)
			230	125						
			150	60						
	B	1972–75	115	40	Annual	Low	Both	Muskeget Island, Massachusetts; *P. leucopus*	7	Tamarin (1977)
			215	65	Annual	Low	Both			
			185	20	Annual					
M. longicaudus	1	1977–79	30	20	Annual	Low				
			30	5	Annual	Low				
	2	1977–79	50	20	Annual	Low		Mainland, Alaska; *P. maniculatus*, weasels; summer only	13	Van Horne (1982)
			50	30	Annual	Low				
	3	1977–79	45	5	Annual	Low				
			35	0	Annual	Low				
	4	1977–79	10	5	Annual	Low				
			15	0	Annual	Low				
M. longicaudus	C	1969–70	120	30	Cycle?	?	?	New Mexico; *M. mexicanus*	14	Conley (1976)
			30	20	Annual?	Low	Both			
M. mexicanus	C	1969–70	50	10	Annual	Low	Both	New Mexico; *M. longicaudus*		Conley (1976)
			50	15	Annual?	Low	Both			
M. oeconomus	A	1968–71	70	0	Cycle?	35		Mainland, Alaska; *Clethrionomys rutilus*	15	Whitney (1976)
	B	1968–71	80	0	Cycle?	—				
M. xanthognathus		1976	90	50	Annual	Low	Both	Mainland, Alaska	15	Wolff and Lidicker (1980)
		1977	110	60	Annual	Low	Both			

southwestern Yukon we found only one high-density population of *M. longicaudus* in 5 years of snap-trapping (Krebs, unpublished).

M. mexicanus

A single study of this interesting species by Conley (1976) suggested annual density fluctuations between a low of 15/ha and a high of 50/ha (Table 6).

M. oeconomus

This species fluctuates cyclically in Finland, and Whitney (1976) suggested one cyclic decline in central Alaska with a peak density around 70–80 voles/ha (Table 6).

M. xanthognathus

One 3-year study of this enigmatic vole by Wolff and Lidicker (1980) in central Alaska showed only annual density fluctuations and no evidence of cyclic changes.

General Conclusion

We present a synopsis of density changes in the species of *Microtus* for which the data indicate a clear population pattern in Table 7. Two major conclusions emerge from this analysis. First, annual fluctuations are common in most *Microtus* species. Of a grand total of 106 years of data on all species, 59% of the years had annual fluctuations and 41% were part of cycles. Second, both the amplitude and maximum density are higher in cyclic populations of a species than in annual fluctuations of the same species. The amplitude is always less than five-fold for annual fluctuations and usually well above 10-fold for cyclic fluctuations. The summary statistics given in Table 7 cannot be assumed to be more than general indications of the types of dynamics observed in each species. The available data show that *M. townsendii* sustains the highest average densities of any North American *Microtus,* closely followed by *M. californicus.* These trends do not apply to all populations of these species, as Krohne (1982) pointed out for *M. californicus.* We conclude that we must explain both patterns of fluctuation, especially because data for the two longest-term *Microtus* studies (Figs.

TABLE 7
SUMMARY OF POPULATION PATTERNS

Species	Pattern	Average density/ha Maximum	Average density/ha Minimum	Amplitude (max./min.)	No. years data	Proportion of years cyclic
M. townsendii	Annual	239	94	2.5	12	0.29
	Cycle	697	48	14.5	5	
M. pennsylvanicus	Annual	172	57	3.0	17	0.48
	Cycle	156	23	6.8	16	
M. ochrogaster	Annual	59	12	5.0	7	0.65
	Cycle	129	2	51.6	13	
M. californicus	Annual	167	38	4.4	7	0.50
	Cycle	427	12	35.6	7	
M. oregoni	Annual	32	7	4.6	10	<0.2?
M. breweri	Annual	170	68	2.5	3	0
M. longicaudus	Annual	33	11	3.0	2	0
M. mexicanus	Annual	50	15	3.3	2	0
M. oeconomus	Cycle	75	0	?	3	1.0
M. xanthognathus	Annual	100	55	1.8	2+	0

2, 3) show that individual populations can exhibit both patterns over time.

In the fifth column of Tables 1–6, we summarize the spring dynamics of each *Microtus* population study. The spring dynamics of *M. townsendii* show two patterns associated with the two forms of population fluctuation (Fig. 2). An annual fluctuation is preceded by a substantial spring decline. By contrast, in cyclic peak years (1975, 1977; Table 1) the spring decline is slight (Fig. 2). Taitt (in press) suggested that the form of the spring decline may indicate the type of population pattern shown by this species. A similar suggestion was made by Hansson (1971) for *M. agrestis* in south Sweden. The data for *M. townsendii* also indicate that the sexes have two patterns of spring decline: both male and female numbers decline in the spring of an annual fluctuation, but females do not decline in a cyclic peak spring (Fig. 2).

Spring densities of *M. pennsylvanicus* in Manitoba, Indiana, Massachusetts, Minnesota, and Illinois tend to be lower in years of annual fluctuation than in years of cycles (Table 2). This pattern also is seen in *M. ochrogaster* (Table 3), *M. californicus* (Table 4), and *M. breweri* (Table 6). Few of the studies in Tables 2–6 provided data on density change according to sex. But in six cases male *M. pennsylvanicus* declined more than females in the spring of cyclic years. Data for other species listed in Tables 5 and 6 are inadequate to establish whether this pattern is a general one. However, we know of no exceptions to the pattern of a strong spring decline being associated with annual fluctuations and weak spring declines being associated with cyclic peak populations.

Hypotheses to Explain Population Patterns

Since the review of Krebs and Myers (1974), there has been considerable development of hypotheses that account particularly for cyclic fluctuations in voles. We first state the hypotheses and then review the evidence in favor of each one.

Food Hypotheses

There are at least three food hypotheses now in the literature:

1) food quantity,
2) food quality,
3) secondary compounds.

The food-quantity hypothesis states that fluctuations in population size are produced by changes in the amount of available food. It was discussed by Elton (1942) and put forward by Lack (1954) as an explanation of cycles. In nutritional terms, it states that calories limit populations, and that malnutrition causes changes in birth and death rates.

The food-quality hypothesis arose in opposition to the simple world-is-green argument, and states that even though food supplies are abundant, they may be deficient in one or more nutrients that will stop reproduction and growth or accelerate mortality (Pitelka and Schultz, 1964). For example, Kalela (1962) postulated that fluctuations in boreal small rodents may be triggered by plant rhythms in production and growth. The food-quality hypothesis is now a family of hypotheses that explain population fluctuations by one or more macro- or micro-nutrients such as nitrogen, potassium, phosphorus, or sodium. For example, White (1978) argued that herbivores are limited by a relative shortage of nitrogenous food for young animals.

Plant secondary compounds can affect herbivores in three general ways. They can alter digestibility of forage and thus cause symptoms of food-quality deficiencies, they can be toxic directly and cause death, or they can inhibit (Berger et al., 1977) or stimulate (Berger et al., 1981) reproduction. Freeland (1974) was the first to suggest the toxic-compound hypothesis. General hypotheses about the role of plant secondary compounds were presented by Freeland and Janzen (1974). Haukioja and Hakala (1975) and Haukioja (1980) suggested that production of some compounds may be induced by herbivore grazing.

Predation Hypotheses

Predation on small mammals is postulated to determine the amplitude and timing of cycles (Pearson, 1971). Predation is not thought to act on increasing populations to stop their increase but rather to accelerate declines and hold numbers low. Mammalian predators are thought to be more effective than avian predators at hunting low-density populations (see Pearson, this volume).

Avian predation is one component of the effect of vegetative cover on vole populations. Birney et al. (1976) presented a two-threshold model called the "cover level hypothesis." Below the lower threshold of cover no population can exist. Non-cyclic populations with annual fluctuations are found at medium levels of cover. Cover can influence predation, available food supply, and behavioral interactions (Taitt and Krebs, 1983); it is reconsidered when we discuss multi-factor hypotheses.

Spacing-Behavior Hypotheses

The possibility that animals might limit their density by territorial behavior has been argued by ornithologists for 60 years. Wynne-Edwards (1962) elevated this idea to the general hypothesis that animals adjust their population density to available resources through social behavior. Watson and Moss (1970) provided an operational set of criteria that could be applied to field populations to determine whether breeding density is regulated by spacing behavior (Table 8).

The spacing-behavior hypothesis has been closely associated with

TABLE 8
THE CRITERIA SUGGESTED BY WATSON AND MOSS (1970) TO DETERMINE WHETHER SPACING BEHAVIOR LIMITS BREEDING DENSITY OF A POPULATION

A.	A substantial part of the population does not breed; they die, are unsuccessful at breeding, are inhibited from breeding, or they breed later.
B.	Such non-breeders are capable of breeding.
C.	Breeding animals are not resource limited.
D.	Spacing behavior is compensatory.
E.	If A to D are true, and densities change according to shifts in food availability, then both spacing behavior and food limit the number of breeders.

the role of dispersal in microtine population regulation. Spacing behavior in field populations produces dispersal. Lidicker (1975) recognized pre-saturation, saturation, and frustrated dispersal (Lidicker, this volume). Abramsky and Tracy (1979) suggested that immigration was necessary to produce population cycles. Populations with emigration but no immigration showed annual density fluctuations. Gaines and McClenaghan (1980) recently reviewed dispersal in small mammals. Anderson (1980) also reviewed dispersal in microtines but did not discuss how dispersal affects population fluctuations or cycles. The exact mechanism by which spacing behavior produces population declines has not been specified.

There are two other groups of social-behavior hypotheses which we call phenotypic-behavior and genotypic-behavior hypotheses. We tentatively separate these hypotheses from spacing behavior in this review because they suggest specific mechanisms for the cyclic decline. Watson and Moss (1970) discussed the important role of "surplus" animals in their criteria (Table 8), but neither Christian (1978) nor Chitty (1967) discussed them. We suggest that the criteria of Watson and Moss (1970) will be essential to testing both of these groups of hypotheses.

Phenotypic-Behavior Hypotheses

These hypotheses state that social behavior limits breeding density and that the relevant behaviors are under phenotypic (nonheritable), physiological control. The best known is the stress hypothesis or neurobehavioral-endocrine mechanism of regulation of population growth, which was discussed in detail by Christian

(1978, 1980). This hypothesis was the first proposed to explain population fluctuations by an intrinsic mechanism (Christian, 1950). At high density a high rate of interaction results in a stress response, which leads to increased mortality and decreased reproduction and hence to population declines.

Social behavior often is mistakenly identified with aggressive behavior, but it includes any type of dominance or spacing behavior that affects an individual's chances of surviving and breeding. Thus, social structure, as discussed by Getz (1978), can affect rates of sexual maturation through pheromones or can affect familiarity among individuals and dispersal (Bekoff, 1981). The problem is that social behavior can have such varied effects on animals that we cannot determine without field experiments whether the effects of social behavior are relevant to understanding population fluctuations. For example, in peak populations of *M. pennsylvanicus,* age at sexual maturity is increased. Is this increase due to malnutrition, to maturation-retarding pheromones, or to adrenal-pituitary stress? We must do field experiments to answer specific questions of this type.

Since the early work of Frank (1957), there have been suggestions that social organization changes during population cycles. Populations exist in socially-stable configurations (individual territories) or in unstable configurations (group territories or dominance hierarchies), which produce cyclic peaks and overpopulation. Getz (1978) suggested that *M. ochrogaster* changes from a monogamous, territorial system, to a polygamous mating system in the increase phase of a cycle. One difficulty of this model is that other *Microtus* species, such as *M. pennsylvanicus,* are polygamous at all times and yet also cycle (Getz et al., 1979). Nevertheless, the general hypothesis that a variable social system underlies the differences between annual and cyclic populations is an important one that needs testing.

Hamilton (1964) discussed how kin selection could affect the evolution of social behavior. Charnov and Finerty (1980) applied these ideas to vole cycles and argued that aggression should be low among close relatives and should become high when individuals interact with many non-relatives, as they would in a population with high dispersal rates. Note that this kin-selection hypothesis is not a genotypic-behavior hypothesis but a phenotypic one, because individual voles are not genetically programmed to act any differently in increasing or declining populations. Individuals simply apply a general rule at all times: be aggressive to non-relatives and docile to relatives.

Genotypic-Behavior Hypotheses

Genotypic-behavior hypotheses are similar to phenotypic ones in assuming that changes in population size are caused by changes in social behavior, but they differ in ascribing the changes to shifts in allelic frequencies of genes that affect behavior. Genotypic hypotheses do not deny the physiological machinery behind the behavioral changes but assume that there is an array of genotypes in natural populations with differing social behaviors and that these genotypes are alternately favored or disfavored by natural selection.

The Chitty hypothesis is the best known of the genotypic-behavior hypotheses (Chitty, 1967); the hypothesis was reviewed recently by Krebs (1978*a*). A second hypothesis involving heterozygosity was suggested by Smith et al. (1975). Increasing heterozygosity in natural populations is associated with outbreeding, population growth, and increasing aggressive behavior. Smith et al. (1978) discussed predictions that follow from their model.

If the genotypic-behavior hypothesis is correct, it allows us to predict which populations will show annual fluctuations and which will show cycles. Krebs (1979) suggested that there was a positive correlation between the amount of fluctuation in population density and the heritability of spacing behavior. Populations with strong cycles should show a high additive genetic variance in spacing behavior, and this genetic variance should provide the time lag necessary to generate a cycle.

Multi-factor Hypotheses

"In the case of every species, many different checks, acting at different periods of life, and during different seasons or years, probably come into play" (Darwin, 1859). The multi-factor hypothesis is an old idea which has become popular in vole research (Batzli, in press; Christian, 1978; Getz, 1978; Lidicker, 1973, 1978; Taitt, in press; Tamarin, 1978*a*). We recognize two variants of the multi-factor hypothesis. The Lidicker model is diagrammed in Lidicker (1978:135) and is a generalized version of the multi-factor hypothesis first suggested by Darwin. We do not accept this model as being useful for further research and agree with Tamarin's (1978*b*) criticism of Lidicker's model. We are not questioning the truth of the model but rather its utility.

Another variant of the multi-factor model was presented by Taitt (in press) and is shown in Fig. 4. The value of this model is two-fold. First, it integrates intrinsic and extrinsic variables through spacing behavior, and thus begins to specify a hierarchical type of systems model appropriate for explaining population changes. Second, it is experimentally oriented and suggests entry points for manipulation of populations. Thus, it avoids the major pitfall of most multi-factor models: they are a posteriori and untestable.

A general problem with many hypotheses in vole research is that they are often stated in vague terms. For example, Lidicker (1978: 135) stated that the multi-factor hypothesis can "explain densities" and population "regulation." We know of no hypothesis that can do this. Instead, we can only explain *changes* in density over time, or *differences* in density over space (Chitty, 1960).

Multi-factor approaches have been useful for recognizing the possible role of spatial heterogeneity in vole population fluctuations. Soviet ecologists have emphasized the role of spatial variation in habitat quality (for example, Naumov, 1972). A variety of terms has been used to describe habitat variations: central and marginal, optimal and suboptimal, primary and secondary, donor and receptor, survival and colonization (Anderson, 1980; Hansson, 1977; Smith et al., 1978; Wolff, 1981). The major distinction is whether the habitat is permanently occupied or not. There is no agreement about the role of chance in spatial heterogeneity, and this has led to circularity. Do we distinguish optimal habitats by their vegetation characteristics or by the fact that they always contain voles? Is it possible in a cyclic population to have empty primary habitats and occupied secondary habitats simultaneously? As Hansson (1977) recognized, only a spatially extensive mark-recapture program can answer these questions about the role of spatial variation.

Tests of Hypotheses

In the last decade, numerous experimental studies have been conducted on *Microtus* populations in an attempt to test explicitly some of the hypotheses outlined above.

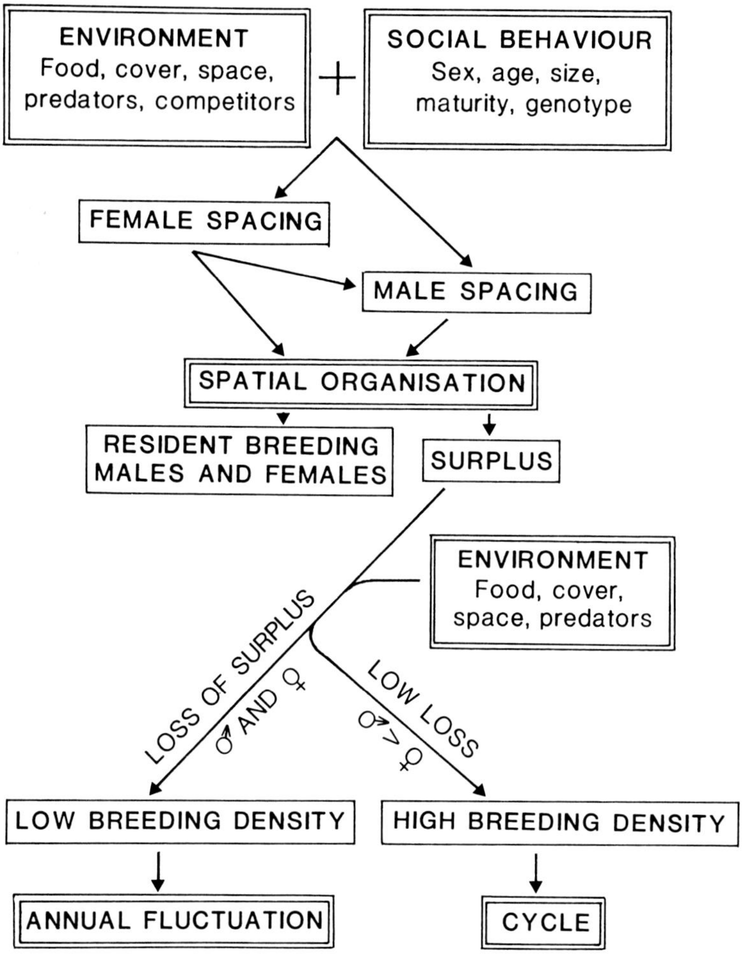

FIG. 4. General model of population dynamics for *Microtus townsendii* indicating how sex-specific spacing behavior may "decide" the potential surplus and how environmental conditions may "determine the fate" of the surplus and hence the population pattern (modified from Taitt, 1978, in press).

Food Experiments

Three food-addition experiments were conducted recently on *Microtus* populations. In spring 1973, we added two levels of food to populations of *M. townsendii* (Taitt and Krebs, 1981). The control population was fluctuating at low density, but experimental populations reached and maintained densities two (low food addition) and five times (high food addition) that of the control. An intermediate level of food the following year resulted in a doubling of density over the control, even though the control was then increasing to a cyclic peak density. Voles with extra food increased in weight and more were reproductive, and they had reduced home ranges in proportion to the level of food added. It is fairly certain (see density-controlled food experiment by Mares et al., 1982) that the reduction of resident home ranges in response to food enabled immigrants to settle on food grids and colonize new habitat in proportion to the extra food available.

A single level of extra food was supplied to *M. ochrogaster* (Cole and Batzli, 1978) and *M. pennsylvanicus* (Desy and Thompson, 1983) with similar results. But in both studies the control population cycled and, although grids with extra food reached higher densities, they declined at the same time as the controls. Cole and Batzli (1978) noted that erratic declines on their high-density food grid were associated with periodic concentrations of predators; however, they did not mention this as a cause of the severe cyclic decline. If feeding experiments are done on other cyclic species, attempts should be made to have a replicate food grid from which all predators are removed.

We conclude that these *Microtus* species do respond to an increase in food. They reach higher densities than controls because of increased growth, reproduction, and immigration. But so far extra food has not prevented cyclic declines in density.

Six 1-ha plots of shortgrass prairie were manipulated for 6 years in eastern Colorado as part of the IBP Grassland Biome study (Abramsky and Tracy, 1979; Birney et al., 1976). *M. ochrogaster* density on the control remained low (average maximum of 3.5/ha) throughout. No *Microtus* were trapped on plots receiving 50 kg/ha of ammonium nitrate. Grids treated with water had 14 *M. ochrogaster*/ha by the fourth year of treatment. Plots with both nitrogen and water added maintained the highest density (average maximum of 80/ha) of *M. ochrogaster* and had three times as much cover as the control. However, voles simply may have responded to cover and not to food quality (Birney et al., 1976).

In Fennoscandia, long-term monitoring studies indicate that peaks of plant flowering coincide with cyclic increases of rodent numbers

(Laine and Hettonen, 1983). It is not known if this correlation is a causal one or not.

The role of plant secondary compounds in vole population dynamics is difficult to assess. Although voles show food preferences (Batzli, in press), it is difficult to decide what is toxic to voles (Batzli and Pitelka, 1975; Freeland, 1974). Schlesinger (1976) challenged Freeland's (1974) first tenet, that voles must prefer non-toxic plants. But he agreed that *M. pennsylvanicus* (Thompson, 1965) and *M. californicus* (Batzli and Pitelka, 1971), both cited by Freeland, avoid toxic plants. The only other *Microtus* data considered by Schlesinger (1976) was for *M. ochrogaster,* which did not avoid toxic plants. However, Zimmerman (1965) found that *M. pennsylvanicus* avoided three toxic plant species. Problems of sample size, and the fact that seeds (which made up 66–86% of stomach contents) were not identified to species (Batzli and Pitelka, 1975) have made tests of Freeland's (1974) hypothesis inconclusive. Bergeron (1980) reported that *M. pennsylvanicus* increases its consumption of toxic plants at peak densities, as Freeland (1974) predicted, but whether these toxic food items are responsible for cyclic declines in numbers is not clear.

Details of the factors controlling reproduction and growth are discussed in other chapters (see Keller, this volume; Batzli, this volume). Since the duration of the breeding season is an important variable that can affect population changes, we need to know what factors start and stop breeding in *Microtus.* Negus and Berger (1977) reported that *M. montanus* populations given access to sprouted wheatgrass in mid-winter became reproductive in two weeks while controls remained non-reproductive. They isolated the causal chemical as 6-methoxybenzoxalinone (6-MBOA). Rose et al. (in press) fed oats impregnated with 6-MBOA to a *M. pennsylvanicus* population in January and reported 42% of females pregnant compared with 10% in a control population 5 weeks later. No field tests have been conducted on the phenolic compounds that inhibit reproduction in *M. montanus* (Berger et al., 1977).

Induction of secondary chemicals in plants eaten by *Microtus* has not been demonstrated. However, Haukioja (1980) suggested that induction of such chemicals could be ruled out if a vole population was able to increase immediately after being transferred to an area that previously had been heavily grazed. Myers and Krebs (1974) introduced *M. ochrogaster* into a fenced enclosure in which a population of this species had previously reached 5-times natural density (caused by a fence effect). The new *M. ochrogaster* population increased in 1 year to more than 10 times the density of the unenclosed control. Krebs (1966) showed that, if new voles were introduced, a population increase of *M. californicus* could be induced in an area that had just suffered a decline in density.

In summary, three *Microtus* species responded to experimental addition of food. Increases in other rodent populations were correlated with improved plant quality. Reproduction of *M. montanus* and *M. pennsylvanicus* was stimulated by the presence of 6-MBOA. Grazing-induced secondary compounds appear not to be important in two *Microtus* species. No data indicate that food is more than a necessary condition for *Microtus* population increase. Future research needs to determine whether changes in food quantity or quality are sufficient to cause cycles.

Evidence for Predation

Recent work on predation has taken into account the importance of cover as protection against predation. Reduced cover caused by cattle grazing results in low-density *Microtus* populations (Birney et al., 1976). Baker and Brooks (1981) observed high raptor densities in habitats with high numbers of *M. pennsylvanicus,* but the amount and distribution of cover affected prey availability. We experimentally increased cover by adding straw (Taitt et al., 1981), with the result that *M. townsendii* populations increased. We also reduced cover by mowing (Taitt and Krebs, 1983), and populations declined.

Avian predation is easier to quantify than mammalian predation because bird pellets tend to be localized at roosts. The most useful data on predation combine field studies of vole demography (where voles are identified by metal ear tags) and collection of as many pellets as possible in the immediate area of the vole grids. Two studies on *M. townsendii* (Beacham, 1979*b*; Boonstra, 1977*a*) indicate that avian predators take more males than females and select small voles. Still, such studies are limited because one can never find all predator pellets or scats, so the estimates of predation will always underestimate the impact of predation on tagged animals. However, Beacham (1979*b*) recorded an impressive 25% loss of *M. townsendii* to avian predation in a 1-week period of his study. Beacham found a density-dependent correlation ($r = 0.99$; $P < 0.02$) between avian predation and densities of *M. townsendii.*

Pearson (1971, this volume) argued that carnivore predation on *M. californicus* operated in an inverse density-dependent manner, so that the major effects were on low-density populations. Erlinge et al. (1983) measured both avian and mammalian predation of *M. agrestis* populations in south Sweden. They calculated that total annual predation was of the same magnitude as annual rodent production. Their result confirms Hansson's (1971) suggestion that small rodents in south Sweden are prevented from cycling by predation. Future predation studies must include both avian and mammalian species. Attempts should be made to experimentally manipulate predation, particularly at important periods during vole demographic changes (for example, at the onset of breeding; Taitt and Krebs, 1983); only then will we be able to judge the true impact of predation on vole population dynamics.

Spacing-Behavior Experiments

Krebs et al. (1976) were the first to apply the Watson and Moss (1970) criteria to determine whether spacing behavior limits the breeding density of a microtine population. They demonstrated that surplus *M. townsendii* existed that were capable of breeding (Condition A and B, Table 8) but did not do so. We now discuss briefly other recent *Microtus* studies that support the criteria of Watson and Moss (1970) in Table 8. A more detailed review recently was published by Tamarin (1983).

Condition A.—Voles occupy home ranges. If residents are removed, new voles colonize the vacant area (Baird and Birney, 1982; Krebs et al., 1976; Myers and Krebs, 1971). It is not certain whether colonizers are surplus from resident populations, but Krebs et al. (1978) found that new colonizers showed more subordinate behavior than control residents.

Condition B.—If new colonizers are allowed to remain in an area, they establish a breeding population (*M. ochrogaster* [Gaines et al. 1979]; *M. townsendii* [Krebs et al., 1978]).

Condition C.—No direct evidence has been collected for this condition in *Microtus* species. But when a vole population is fenced in, the enclosed habitat supports a much higher population than unenclosed controls (*M. pennsylvanicus* [Krebs et al., 1969]; *M. townsendii* [Boonstra and Krebs, 1977]). This suggests that food, space, and nest sites are not limiting voles directly in open control populations.

Condition D.—It is difficult to demonstrate behaviorly induced mortality in voles. If a vole ceases becoming trapped, it may have emigrated or died, or it simply may be avoiding traps. However, in a recent experiment on *M. townsendii* (Taitt and Krebs, 1983), we counted all such voles as "disappeared," and found that the number of voles that "disappeared" from five populations over the month of onset of breeding in females was correlated ($r = 0.93$; $P < 0.05$) with density of voles. Reproduction is compensatory (presumably behaviorally induced) in several species (*M. californicus* [Batzli et al., 1977]; *M. montanus, M. ochrogaster, M. pennsylvanicus* [Schaffer and Tamarin 1973]). We believe that these observations indicate that voles may show compensatory spacing behavior.

Condition E.—In one species (*M. townsendii*), we have some evidence for conditions A to D. Watson and Moss (1970) suggested that, if these populations respond to changes in food, they are regulated by both spacing behavior and food. Populations of *M. townsendii* increased to different densities in response to the amount of food added, and also colonized new habitat in response to food levels (Taitt and Krebs, 1981).

If we use the criteria in Table 8, populations of *M. townsendii* appear to be regulated by both spacing behavior and food. This, and the fact that females were more responsive to food availability, led to the formulation of the model in Fig. 4. The habitat patchiness (induced by winter rainfall) may be unique, but we feel that some of the mechanisms invoked (for example, cessation of reproduction through increased interaction as a result of winter flooding [Taitt and Krebs, 1981], and perhaps simultaneous settlement of breeding females in spring of cyclic years [Taitt and Krebs, 1983]), may be of general importance in other annual-cyclic species.

A study in Finland by Pokki (1981) on *M. agrestis* is particularly interesting because it is suggests the possible influence of dispersal on the fate of surplus animals and population fluctuations. Pokki (1981) observed that island colonization was by inter-island dispersal from small islands (isolated patches of grassland) over as much as 1 km of open water. However, dispersal on large islands was within islands between grassland and marginal habitat (woodland). Also, more inter-island dispersers colonized large islands than small ones. Pokki (1981) did not observe cycles on small islands, but *M. agrestis* appeared to be cyclic on the largest islands. This study gives a dramatic illustration of the dispersal ability of *M. agrestis,* and may provide evidence for an hypothesis about cycles (Fig. 4). If dispersers are surplus animals, can the observed population patterns be partly the result of elimination of surplus voles (on small islands), which leads to an absence of cycles, whereas survival of surplus voles (on large islands) results in cycles? Tamarin (1978*a*) suggested that the presence of a vole surplus explained the absence of cycling in *M. breweri* populations on Muskeget Island, but the two situations may not be comparable. Muskeget is isolated, and has been for 2,000–3,000 years. Experimental work is needed on island populations to test these interpretations.

Phenotypic-Behavior Experiments

A premise for both the phenotypic- and genotypic-behavior hypotheses is that the rate of interaction of individuals increases with population density. Pearson (1960) reported that *M. californicus* built more runways as numbers increased. Carroll and Getz (1976) also found that the number of active runways was correlated with population density of *M. ochrogaster.* However, it is not known if voles confine all their activities to runways. In fact, Crawford (1971) observed *M. ochrogaster* climbing low branches of trees and engaging in fighting outside burrows during a cyclic peak. In addition, interactions need not always be through direct contact, because voles probably use indirect methods such as marking (Richmond and Stehn, 1976) and vocalizations that enable them to react to increases in density.

Adrenocortical function has been evaluated indirectly in *Microtus* populations by measuring adrenal weight. But adrenal weight varies with sex, season, maturity, diet, and body weight. To and Tamarin (1977) found that adrenal weights of sexually mature *M. breweri* from non-cyclic, island populations were significantly influenced by population density. But mainland, cyclic *M. pennsylvanicus* showed no clear adrenal response to population density in their study. However, Geller and Christian (1982) found that "mean relative adrenal weight" of mature female *M. pennsylvanicus* was correlated with mean population density in spring (April to June). It is difficult to compare densities in these studies, but it appears that To and Tamarin's (1977) *M. pennsylvanicus* densities were lowest, their *M. breweri* densities were higher, and Geller and Christian's (1982) *M. pennsylvanicus* densities were highest. An interesting common trend in these studies is that, in populations where there is a relationship between adrenal weight and density, mature females showed a stronger relationship than males. Geller and Christian (1982) speculated that pregnant females, in populations at different densities, may affect fetal immune development.

Field studies on *Antechinus stuartii* in Australia indicate that males are extremely aggressive toward one another during mating (Braithwaite, 1974). This behavior is correlated with a marked increase in blood androgen (Moore, 1974). Bradley et al. (1980) showed that high free glucocorticoid concentrations in plasma result from increased total glucocorticoid and reduced plasma corticosteroid binding which, in turn, suppress the immune and inflammatory system. The consequence is that all males die after mating from gastro-intestinal hemorrhage and infection from parasites and microorganisms. No field studies on *Microtus* have demonstrated death on this scale from these causes. But such physiological responses to stress have been reported for *M. montanus* in the laboratory (Forslund, 1973). The period of spring decline is probably stressful in *M. townsendii* (coincides with a peak in male wounding and pregnancy of the first females). McDonald and Taitt (1982) found that a small sample of voles from such a population had high levels of free corticosteroids, but the highest levels were found in mature females.

Hormonal manipulation of behavior in the field has been attempted in *M. townsendii* (Gipps et al., 1981; Krebs et al., 1977; Taitt and Krebs, 1982). Pellets or silastic implants of testosterone in males had no significant effect on demography. But silastic implants of scopolamine HBr, which have been shown to reduce male aggressive behavior in *M. townsendii* (Gipps, 1982), reduced the rate of spring decline in males. Males also survived better in a population in which females were fed a synthetic steroid (mestranol), which rendered them anestrous. Female wounding is uncommon in *M. townsendii,* but females with implants of testosterone had more wounds than males, and, like males, had low survival in spring. These results suggest that male *M. townsendii* are responsive to the level of overt aggression (male or female). Normally, females may rely less on overt aggression (Caplis, 1977) and more on site-specific defensive behavior. If true, it might explain, for example, why females respond more quickly to increased food. Also, if increased vole density means more challenges to site-specific individuals, then females may be stressed more by increased population density than males.

Behavioral interactions may affect density through reproductive effects as well as through survival. The Bruce effect (pregnancy blockage) is perhaps the best known. Keller (this volume) reviewed these mechanisms and concluded that they may be important in field populations but that the evidence does not suggest a major role in generating population fluctuations. Taitt and Krebs (1981) suggested that *M. townsendii* may be driven to an annual fluctuation in most years because of winter cessation of reproduction. They hypothesized that rain causes the water table to rise to the point that voles cannot maintain deep burrows; they are forced into less space, which results in increased interaction, weight loss, and cessation of reproduction.

Social suppression of growth and reproduction may vary in different species of *Microtus* (Facemire and Batzli, 1983). Species like *M. californicus* and *M. ochrogaster,* which have a monogamous social system, show social suppression of growth when siblings are caged together. Species like *M. oeconomus* and *M. pennsylvanicus,* which are promiscuous and show no male parental care, do not exhibit social suppression of growth and reproduction. The possibility that social suppression changes over the period of a population cycle needs investigation in these species.

Future research on phenotypic behavior should concentrate more on female behavior (see section on Multi-factor Tests). Manipulations of behavior should be attempted in the field to increase or decrease stress. The consequences of such experiments may shed more light on the possibility of phenotypic maternal transfer of stressed conditions.

Genotypic-Behavior Experiments

Tests of the polymorphic behavior hypothesis typically have proceeded in two steps. First, measurable behavioral differences are demonstrated between populations changing over time. Standardized laboratory tests of agonistic or exploratory behavior are done. Second, these behaviors are shown to be heritable so that natural selection can operate on them.

Both agonistic and exploratory behavior changed with population density in *M. ochrogaster* and *M. pennsylvanicus* in Indiana (Krebs, 1970). Myers and Krebs (1971) found behavioral differences between resident and dispersing individuals of these same species. Hofmann et al. (1982) tried to repeat these observations on both species in Illinois but were unable to verify changes in behavior over a cycle. Rose and Gaines (1976) failed to find a relationship between wounding and density during a population cycle of *M. ochrogaster* in Kansas. Rasmuson et al. (1977) measured locomotory behavior in *M. agrestis* from cyclic and non-cyclic populations in Sweden and found strong differences between populations. They also demonstrated that locomotor activity was highly heritable. Anderson (1975) estimated heritability of agonistic behavior in *M. townsendii* as zero. There are no other estimates of the heritability of any component of spacing behavior in any *Microtus* species. Consequently, it is not yet possible to test the suggestions of Krebs (1979) that annual fluctuations are associated with low heritabilities of agonistic behavior and that cyclic fluctuations are associated with high heritabilities.

Several attempts have been made to test Chitty's (1967) hypothesis with electrophoretic markers in blood proteins. But because we do not understand the physiological effects associated with most electrophoretic markers or their linkage groups, changes in electrophoretic allele frequencies may no longer be necessary or sufficient to verify the hypothesis. At best, electrophoretic markers indicate the intensity of selection in field populations. LeDuc and Krebs (1975) manipulated the frequency of a leucine-aminopeptidase marker in field populations of *M. townsendii* and found no measurable effects of altered allelic frequencies on population density. We now think that experiments of this type are unlikely to be fruitful because of the difficulty of assessing linkage groups in natural vole populations.

Several attempts have been made to determine if dispersers differ in allelic frequencies from resident voles. Gaines and McClenaghan (1980) recently reviewed these studies, and concluded that electrophoretic markers are not likely to be useful in determining whether dispersal behavior is heritable. Three attempts to estimate the heritability of dispersal tendencies in *Microtus* populations produced suggestions of high heritability (Anderson, 1975; Beacham, 1979*c*; Hilborn, 1975), but the results may have been caused by maternal effects. If dispersal tendency is highly heritable and dispersal is critical for population fluctuations, we will have strong support for the polymorphic behavior hypothesis.

Chitty (in press) suggested that adult body size in *M. townsendii* is controlled by a single major gene; large voles are homozygotes (*AA*) and so are small voles (*aa*). If this simple major gene effect can be shown to underlie cyclic changes of body size in *Microtus,* it will be critical to study spacing behavior of these genotypes. Chitty (in press) suggested that the large-bodied homozygotes are in fact the hypothesized docile genotypes that dominate populations undergoing density increases. These ideas have not been confirmed for any *Microtus* species.

Attempts to test the genotypic-behavior hypothesis must rest on an estimation of the heritability of traits of dominance and spacing behavior for which few data exist at present. The most critical experimental approach would be to conduct an artificial selection experiment in a natural population, selecting for or against some form of spacing behavior and observing the demographic consequences.

Multi-factor Tests

In practice, those who invoke multi-factor hypotheses fall into two general groups. To the first group a multi-factor model comprises food and predators almost exclusively, with perhaps some climatic effects included (for example, Keith, 1974; Oksanen and Oksanen, 1981; Stenseth, 1978). In principle, there is no difficulty in testing such two-factor hypotheses experimentally, but no one seems to have done so.

To the second goup a multi-factor model involves food, predators, and social behavior. Lidicker's (1973) discussion on *M. californicus* dynamics is a good example of this approach. Social behavior can be looked at in two ways when it is part of a multi-factor hypothesis. Some authors view social behavior as a way of partitioning resources, so that it is the resources (usually food) that are critical (Lack, 1954). Others view social behavior as part of the life-history strategy in which individuals are trying to maximize their fitness.

In these situations individuals may compete for "social status," which is related only tenuously to resources (Wynne-Edwards, 1962). The central issue has become whether social behavior can regulate density below the carrying capacity dictated by food and predators (Łomnicki, 1978; Verner, 1977). Since social behaviors can be influenced by many variables (both phenotypic and genotypic), some population changes may occur in ways unrelated to resource levels.

It is difficult to test multi-factor models that include social behavior. Getz (1978) and his research group tested social-behavior hypotheses on laboratory populations of *M. ochrogaster* and are now applying them to field populations. Taitt and Krebs (1981, 1982, 1983) tried to test a complex multi-factor model on *M. townsendii* directly in field populations (Fig. 4). We do not know what factors determine the number of surplus voles in field populations or what factors determine the fate of surplus animals. We can gain insight by measuring social behavior while manipulating food and predators, and vice versa. Because dispersal is a critical element in these population systems, open populations must be the experimental units.

In what follows we consider two features associated with vole population dynamics for which multi-factor considerations may be most appropriate. The first, body weight, has a long association with the literature on small mammal cycles; the second, the role of females, has begun to receive attention over the last decade.

Body weight.—Chitty (1952) observed that peak-density populations of *M. agrestis* contained individuals of high body weight that were absent in low-density populations. All but one of the studies on *Microtus* listed as reporting cycles in abundance (Tables 1–6) found larger animals in peak populations. The exception was Gaines and Rose (1976), who reported no shift to heavier *M. ochrogaster* in a peak population. We do not know what the adaptive advantage of large size is for voles (Boonstra and Krebs, 1979); two contradictory hypotheses involving r-selection (Chitty, 1967) and α-selection (Stenseth, 1978) have been suggested.

Recent studies indicate that growth in voles is influenced by extrinsic factors. Iverson and Turner (1974) showed that mature *M. pennsylvanicus* lost weight in winter. Petterborg (1978) reported that *M. montanus* grew at a slower rate under a short photoperiod than under a long photoperiod. Beacham (1980) found that *M. townsendii* born in spring had higher growth rates than voles born in any other season. *M. townsendii* in open populations grew 20% faster than voles in enclosures (Beacham, 1979*b*); the density in the enclosures was higher than in the open populations (Beacham, 1979*a*). Finally, Batzli et al. (1977) found that growth was suppressed by social conditions in *M. californicus* and *M. ochrogaster*. These results indicate that weight cannot be correlated simply with age. However, Mallory et al. (1981) used lens weight to age *Dicrostonyx* and found that lemmings in the peak year were significantly older and heavier than lemmings in low years, suggesting that high body weights in the peak year could be the result of age.

Anderson (1975) did not find a strong genetic influence on growth rate or maximum body size in *M. townsendii*. Instead, she found that environmental effects made siblings resemble one another in growth rate, and that maximum size of offspring correlated with size of mothers. Further, female body weight is correlated positively with litter size in this species (Anderson and Boonstra, 1979).

Iverson and Turner (1974) suggested that loss of weight in old and lack of weight gain in young *M. pennsylvanicus* in winter were adaptive responses possibly cued by day length. They suggested that these were general phenomena among north temperate small rodents. But both deermice (*Peromyscus maniculatus*; Taitt, 1981) and Townsend's voles (*M. townsendii*; Taitt and Krebs, 1981) responded immediately to extra food in winter by gaining weight, suggesting that winter weight loss simply could be a proximate response to food availability. Beacham (1980) reported that "heavy" male *M. townsendii* (using ≥70 g as peak weights) in his cyclic population were animals that had gained weight throughout the preceeding ("increase") winter. Yet *M. townsendii*, given extra oats in late winter, gained weight so that mean weights of males and females were significantly higher than those on the control after only 2 weeks. In this short period, 63% of the males became "heavy" (≥70 g) compared with 23% on the control (Taitt and Krebs, 1983).

These results indicate that growth rates are highly labile. Work on *M. townsendii* indicates that animals with sufficient food can maintain positive growth rates in winter and become "heavy" animals. Because the spring decline in numbers in the peak year is slight, many of these animals may survive so that some voles in the peak population are older and heavier, whereas animals born at the peak have reduced growth rates because of high population density.

Such an explanation does not rule out a genetic basis for the morphs in peak populations (Chitty, in press). It could be that genotypes yielding potentially large body weight are not expressed phenotypically until food conditions are adequate, particularly in the winter preceeding a peak. Body weight in laboratory mice is highly heritable, but Roberts (1981) suggested that there may be a range of variation in weight over which there is little natural selection in wild populations. Also, Fulker (1970) suggested that maternal effects (behavioral and endocrine) could act as a buffering mechanism on the expression of offspring genotypes in rodents.

The phenomenon of body-weight changes in cyclic populations of *Microtus* will be understood only when both environmental and genetic influences on growth and weight are measured.

Role of females.—"Little work has been done on female aggressive behaviour . . . ." (Krebs and Myers, 1974). This situation has begun to change in the last decade, although the challenge to do so had been made much earlier. Frank (1957) made the following observations on *M. arvalis* in Germany: 1) breeding females occupied a range around their burrows from which they drove out all other voles; 2) females tolerated a strange male in their home ranges only when they were in heat; 3) males inhabited irregular large areas in which they wandered from female to female in order to mate; 4) in spring, young males without exception disappeared from their mothers' territory, but young females settled in the immediate vicinity; and 5) "great families" arose every autumn when the last two to three litters remained in the maternal home range to overwinter. In addition, Frank (1957) suggested that the social behavior of females—their tendency to remain together even if they move—might explain how peak populations arise.

One way to determine the role of females in natural populations is to alter sex ratios by removal experiments. Redfield et al. (1978) began sex-specific removal experiments on field populations of *M. townsendii* in 1972. They found that female recruitment was reduced in a population containing a majority of females and that there was an inverse relationship between the number of young voles recruited and the density of mature females (but not males). Further experiments on *M. townsendii* showed that juvenile survival was dependent on female (not male) densities (Boonstra, 1978), and that females responded before males to the addition of food (Taitt and Krebs, 1981, 1983). Also, males exhibited better survival in a population of "passive" females (Taitt and Krebs, 1982) and "passive" males (Gipps et al., 1981).

Research on other *Microtus* species also indicates that Frank's (1957) observations may apply to species other than *M. arvalis*. Radiotelemetry work by Madison (1980) showed that mature female *M. pennsylvanicus* occupy exclusive home ranges. Males, on the other hand, had large, overlapping, and more variable home ranges. Males also moved temporarily into areas occupied by estrous females. These observations were confirmed by Webster and Brooks (1981) for *M. pennsylvanicus* in Ontario. Field observations on other small mammals indicate that mature females exert control on population growth by excluding subordinates (Leuze, 1976; Viitala, 1977), or tolerating those that delay maturity (Bujalska, 1973; Jannett, 1978; Saitoh, 1981). In the laboratory, Batzli et al. (1977) found that females had more influence than males on the suppression of growth in *M. californicus* and *M. ochrogaster*. Finally, recent results on stress responses at high density also indicate that females are more responsive to stress and may subsequently affect their offspring accordingly (Geller and Christian, 1982).

Perhaps mature females in the breeding season can be considered the equivalent of territorial male birds. They secure an area for raising young (Boonstra, 1977*b*; Jannett, 1978), including ample food for lactation and space free from intraspecific intrusion. Pheromones may be the advertising currency equivalent to bird song. Male *Microtus* are forced to forage in the interstices of these female territories (Madison, 1980) and compete among themselves for estrous females (Boonstra, 1978; Krebs, 1978*b*; Madison, 1980; Webster and Brooks, 1981). Although these features suggest a polygamous mating system, the degree of polygyny could be dependent on population density (Getz, 1978).

Greenwood (1980) suggested that philopatry favors the evolution of cooperative traits between members of the sedentary sex. One such trait may be the phenomenon described by Frank (1957) in *M. arvalis* in which sisters from "great families," and sometimes their mother, remain together and breed on a common territory when conditions are optimal. Frank (1957) postulated that this "condensation potential" enabled *M. arvalis* populations to reach outbreak densities. Taitt and Krebs (1983) suggested another female behavior that might contribute to outbreaks. They argued that if conditions were favorable, all females may become reproductive simultaneously and that this might precipitate simultaneous settlement at higher than normal density, as observed in the spring of cyclic years in *M. townsendii* (Fig. 2). Large simultaneous pulses of young could be produced; the offspring, in turn, might simultaneously colonize any available habitat and so result in a spreading outbreak. Simultaneous settlement has been observed in territorial male birds by Knapton and Krebs (1974) and Tompa (1971).

Female behavior, like growth rates, appears to be influenced by extrinsic and intrinsic variables. Do Frank's (1957) observations apply to all species of *Microtus*? If so, what changes in territorial social organization precipitate a cycle in abundance? How do females respond to stress at peak density, and how does this affect survival of offspring? We suggest that answers to these questions will probably be needed before we can understand cyclic fluctuations.

Mathematical Models

In spite of the recent increase in mathematical modeling of biological populations, little work has been done on models of rodent populations. May (1981) summarized models for single-species populations. Beginning with a simple logistic model, one can add a time-lag and produce population curves that vary from stable to cyclic. The critical parameter is the time delay in the feedback mechanism that regulates population size. If the time delay is 9–12 months, the resulting populations trace cycles with a period of 3–4 years. The simple message is that for voles, which have a similar range of values for innate capacity for increase (r), we are looking for a delayed density-dependent factor that lags 9–12 months behind population density in order to establish a cyclic population. For shorter time lags an annual cycle would be produced. The problem with this simple approach is that we cannot evaluate easily any of the suggested biological mechanisms producing time delays in real vole populations.

Models of the food hypothesis were suggested by Rosenzweig and Abramsky (1980) based on a predator-prey interaction between voles and their food plants. Batzli (in press) used loop analysis to analyze the brown-lemming cycle in northern Alaska and suggested that, if vegetation quality is important in generating population cycles, it is likely to be a function of plant secondary compounds rather than delays in nutrient recycling. Stenseth et al. (1977) produced the most comprehensive and realistic model for a *Microtus* population. This model was based on the nutritional balance of individuals and how nutrition affects birth, death and dispersal. It includes some effects of predation and habitat heterogeneity, and thus begins to approach a multi-factor model. However, the model is intractable because it "is impossible to analyze in a manner providing intelligible results or predictions" (Stenseth, pers. comm.).

Models of the Chitty (1967) hypothesis have been analyzed recently by Stenseth (1981) to see if population cycles could be generated by a genetic polymorphism. Stenseth (1981) argued that intrinsic factors alone cannot generate a cycle, and that the only tenable hypothesis is that population cycles are caused by the interaction of intrinsic and extrinsic factors. Stenseth (1978) shows how this type of model can lead to cycles or annual fluctuations. The relevant extrinsic factors are not identified in his model; presumably weather, food, predators, or parasites could be involved.

The general tendency in population modeling has been to make the models more complex and include many factors. The result has not been very useful for guiding field work on *Microtus*. The most comprehensive recent effort by Finerty (1980) on population cycles includes the use of loop analysis. But almost none of these modelling studies has suggested a critical experiment, and they remain largely a posteriori analyses.

Discussion

In their review, Krebs and Myers (1974) challenged the existence of non-cycling populations of microtines. However, the pattern of fluctuations revealed in the present review indicate that field populations of *Microtus* in North America (Tables 1–6) show annual fluctuations, multi-annual cycles, and sometimes both in combination (Figs. 2, 3). We must, therefore, search for hypotheses which will allow a range of possible outcomes for density changes.

We are now more knowledgeable of the affect of temporal heterogeneity in population dynamics, but we are less well versed in understanding spatial heterogeneity. This is partly because most studies have been carried out in favorable habitats, and because it is difficult to trap in areas large enough to encompass several habitats. Habitat variation is interwoven with dispersal in population dynamics (Hansson, 1977), so it is not surprising that both these elements are poorly understood in vole populations.

The history of *Microtus* population studies is checkered by a series of arguments about the role of single factors in causing population fluctuations. We think that perhaps these arguments should be left to the past and that a new synthesis should be attempted. Perhaps this synthesis could be based on the premise that both extrinsic and intrinsic factors are involved in *Microtus* population fluctuations. A second premise could be that dominance and spacing behavior play a central role by potentially apportioning resources differentially among members of the population.

The investigation of *Microtus* population dynamics, and rodents in general, is still an expanding field of ecological research. Useful advances in the future will come largely from field experiments designed with a strong hypothesis-testing structure. Many of these tests will be difficult to formulate because they must be done on a complex system and we do not, in general, know the degree of complexity.

The present review of *Microtus* population dynamics reveals that: 1) annual fluctuations reach maximum densities typically one-third of cyclic densities; 2) the amplitude of an annual fluctuation tends to be less than five-fold, whereas that of a cycle can be more than ten-fold; and 3) substantial spring declines (of both sexes) may be characteristic of annual fluctuations, whereas reduced spring declines (sometimes confined to males) accompany cycles.

A number of specific questions has arisen from this review. Do dominance and spacing behaviors limit the breeding density of all *Microtus* populations? What restricts a population to a five-fold increase in density one year and yet allows it to reach a ten-fold increase to cyclic density in another year? If surplus voles are produced by spacing behavior, is it simply their fate at the onset of breeding that produces the two patterns of spring decline? What is the role of environmental factors on the fate of surplus animals and what bearing does this have on the population dynamics exhibited by a population? Why is body-weight distribution different in the two population patterns? Are "heavy" voles genetically different or do favorable conditions prior to peak density contribute to weight gain and longer lifespan? Are females more sensitive than males to environmental conditions such as food and cover? If so, is the spacing behavior of mature females the proximate mechanism of *Microtus* population regulation? Can maternal responses to stress be transferred to offspring? If so, what are the consequences at cyclic peak densities, and what is the time-lag of such responses?

Answers to these questions may be incomplete if they ignore the possible genetic basis of the relevant ecological variables—growth, reproduction, response to stress, dominance and dispersal behavior. Future research should emphasize the heritability of these variables in individuals from populations exhibiting both annual fluctuations and cycles in abundance (for example, see Rasmuson et al., 1977).

The paradigm suggested by this review is that future studies of *Microtus* population dynamics must address the two patterns of fluctuation. Field manipulations should be designed to test the interactions suggested, particularly between spacing behavior, food, and predation. The results should be related to the dispersal abilities of voles that enable them to exploit temporally favorable habitat, and to their potential to reach outbreak densities.

Literature Cited

ABRAMSKY, Z., AND C. R. TRACY. 1979. Population biology of a non-cycling population of prairie voles and a hypothesis on the role of migration in regulating microtine cycles. Ecology, 60:349–361.

ANDERSON, J. L. 1975. Phenotypic correlates among relatives, and variability in reproductive performance in populations of the vole, *Microtus townsendii*. Unpubl. Ph.D. dissert., Univ. British Columbia, Vancouver, 207 pp.

ANDERSON, J. L. AND R. BOONSTRA. 1979. Some aspects of reproduction in the vole *Microtus townsendii*. Canadian J. Zool., 57:18–24.

ANDERSON, P. 1980. Evolutionary implications of microtine behavioural systems on the ecological stage. The Biologist, 62:70–88.

BAIRD, D. D., AND E. C. BIRNEY. 1982. Pattern of colonization in *Microtus pennsylvanicus*. J. Mamm., 63:290–293.

BAKER, J. J., AND R. J. BROOKS. 1981. Distribution patterns of raptors in relation to density of meadow voles. Condor, 83:42–47.

BATZLI, G. O. In press. The role of nutrition in population cycles of microtine rodents. Acta Zool. Fennica.

BATZLI, G. O., AND F. A. PITELKA. 1971. Condition and diet of cycling populations of the California vole *Microtus californicus*. J. Mamm., 52:141–163.

———. 1975. Vole cycles—test of another hypothesis. Amer. Nat., 109:482–487.

BATZLI, G. O., L. L. GETZ, AND S. S. HURLEY. 1977. Suppression of growth and reproduction of microtine rodents by social factors. J. Mamm., 58:583–591.

BEACHAM, T. D. 1979*a*. Dispersal, survival, and population regulation in the vole *Microtus townsendii*. Unpubl. Ph.D. dissert., Univ. British Columbia, Vancouver, 226 pp.

———. 1979*b*. Selectivity of avian predation in declining populations of the vole, *Microtus townsendii*. Canadian J. Zool., 57:1767–1772.

———. 1979*c*. Dispersal tendency and duration of life of littermates during population fluctuations of the vole, *Microtus townsendii*. Oecologia, 42:11–21.

———. 1980. Growth rates of the vole *Microtus townsendii* during a population cycle. Oikos, 35:99–106.

BEACHAM, T. D., AND C. J. KREBS. 1980. Pitfall versus live-trap enumeration of fluctuating populations of *Microtus townsendii*. J. Mamm., 61:486–499.

BEKOFF, M. 1981. Vole population cycles: kin-selection or familiarity? Oecologia, 48:131.

BERGER, P. J., E. H. SANDERS, AND P. D. GARDNER. 1981. Chemical triggering of reproduction in *Microtus montanus*. Science, 214:69–70.

BERGER, P. J., E. H. SANDERS, P. D. GARDNER, AND N. C. NEGUS. 1977. Phenolic plant compounds functioning as reproductive inhibitors in *Microtus montanus*. Science, 195:575–577.

BERGERON, J. 1980. Importance des plantes toxiques dans le régime alimentaire de *Microtus pennsylvanicus* à deux étapes opposées de leur cycle. Canadian J. Zool., 58:2230–2238.

BIRNEY, E. C., W. E. GRANT, AND D. D. BAIRD. 1976. Importance of vegetative cover to cycles of *Microtus* populations. Ecology, 57:1043–1051.

BLAUSTEIN, A. R. 1980. Behavioral aspects of competition in a three species rodent guild of coastal southern California. Behav. Ecol. Sociobiol., 6:247–255.

———. 1981. Population fluctuations and extinctions of small rodents in coastal southern California. Oecologia, 48:71–78.

BOONSTRA, R. 1977*a*. Predation on *Microtus townsendii* populations: impact and vulnerability. Canadian J. Zool., 55:1631–43.

———. 1977*b*. Effect of conspecifics on survival during population declines in *Microtus townsendii*. J. Anim. Ecol., 46:835–851.

———. 1978. Effect of adult townsend voles (*Microtus townsendii*) on survival of young. Ecology, 59:242–248.

BOONSTRA, R., AND C. J. KREBS. 1976. The effect of odour on trap response in *Microtus townsendii*. J. Zool., 180:467–476.

———. 1977. A fencing experiment on a high-density population of *Microtus townsendii*. Canadian J. Zool., 55:1166–1175.

———. 1978. Pitfall trapping of *Microtus townsendii*. J. Mamm., 59:136–148.

———. 1979. Viability of large- and small-sized adults in fluctuating vole populations. Ecology, 60:567–573.

BOONSTRA, R., AND F. H. RODD. 1983. Regulation of breeding density in *Microtus pennsylvanicus*. J. Anim. Ecol., 52:757–780.

BOONSTRA, R., F. H. RODD, AND D. J. CARLETON. 1982. Effect of *Blarina brevicauda* on trap response of *Microtus pennsylvanicus*. Canadian J. Zool., 60: 438–442.

BRADLEY, A. J., E. R. MCDONALD, AND A. K. LEE. 1980. Stress and mortality in a small marsupial (*Antechinus stuartii,* Macleay). Gen. Comp. Endocrinol., 40:188–200.

BRAITHWAITE, R. W. 1974. Behavioural changes associated with the population cycle of *Antechinus stuartii*. Australian J. Zool., 22:45–62.

BUJALSKA, G. 1973. The role of spacing behaviour among females in the regulation of reproduction in the bank vole. J. Reprod. Fert., Suppl., 19:465–474.

CAPLIS, P. 1977. Neighbour recognition by the meadow vole (*Microtus pennsylvanicus*) and the role of olfactory cues. Unpubl. M.S. thesis, McGill Univ., Montreal, 60 pp.

CAROTHERS, A. D. 1973. The effects of unequal catchability on Jolly-Seber estimates. Biometrics, 29:79–100.

———. 1979. Quantifying unequal catchability and its effect on survival estimates in an actual population. J. Anim. Ecol., 48:863–869.

CARROLL, D., AND L. L. GETZ. 1976. Runway use and population density in *Microtus ochrogaster*. J. Mamm., 57:772–776.

CHARNOV, E. L., AND J. FINERTY. 1980. Vole population cycles: a case for kin-selection. Oecologia, 45:1–2.

CHITTY, D. 1952. Mortality among voles (*Microtus agrestis*) at Lake Vyrnwy, Montgomeryshire, in 1936–39. Phil. Trans. Roy. Soc. London, Ser. B, 236:505–552.

———. 1960. Population processes in the vole and their relevance to general theory. Canadian J. Zool., 38:99–113.

———. 1967. The natural selection of self-regulatory behaviour in animal populations. Proc. Ecol. Soc. Australia, 2:51–78.

———. In press. Fluctuations in numbers and body weight of the vole *Microtus townsendii*. Acta Zool. Fennica.

CHITTY, D., AND D. A. KEMPSON. 1949. Prebaiting small mammals and a new design of live trap. Ecology, 30:536–542.

CHITTY, D., AND E. PHIPPS. 1966. Seasonal changes in survival in mixed populations of two species of vole. J. Anim. Ecol., 35:313–331.

CHRISTIAN, J. J. 1950. The adreno-pituitary system and population cycles in mammals. J. Mamm., 31:247–259.

———. 1978. Neuro-behavioural-endocrine regulation of small mammal populations. Pp. 143–158, *in* Populations of small mammals under natural conditions (D. P. Snyder, ed.). Pymatuning Lab. Ecol. Spec. Publ. 5:1–237.

———. 1980. Endocrine factors in population regulation. Pp. 367–380, *in* Biosocial mechanisms of population regulation (M. N. Cohen, R. S. Malpass, and H. G. Klein, eds.). Yale Univ. Press, New Haven, Connecticut, 406 pp.

COLE, F. R., AND G. O. BATZLI. 1978. Influence of supplemental feeding on a vole population. J. Mamm., 59:809–819.

CONLEY, W. 1976. Competition between *Microtus*: a behavioral hypothesis. Ecology, 57:224–237.

CRAWFORD, R. D. 1971. High population density of *Microtus ochrogaster*. J. Mamm., 52:478.

DARWIN, C. 1859. On the origin of species by means of natural selection, or the preservation of favoured races in the struggle for life. John Murray, London, 502 pp.

DELONG, K. T. 1966. Population ecology of feral house mice: interference by *Microtus*. Ecology, 47:481–484.

DESY, E. A., AND C. F. THOMPSON. 1983. Effects of supplemental food on a *Microtus pennsylvanicus* population in central Illinois. J. Anim. Ecol., 52:127–140.

DUESER, R. D., M. L. WILSON, AND R. K. ROSE. 1981. Attributes of dispersing meadow voles in open-grid populations. Acta Theriol., 26:139–162.

ELTON, C. 1942. Voles, mice and lemmings. Clarendon Press, Oxford, 496 pp.

ERLINGE, S., ET AL. 1983. Predation as a regulating factor on small rodent populations in southern Sweden. Oikos, 40:36–52.

FACEMIRE, C. F., AND G. O. BATZLI. 1983. Suppression of growth and reproduction by social factors in microtine rodents: tests of two hypotheses. J. Mamm., 64:152–156.

FINERTY, J. P. 1980. The population ecology of cycles in small mammals. Yale Univ. Press, New Haven, Connecticut, 234 pp.

FORSLUND, L. G. 1973. Adrenocortical and reproductive adjustments in laboratory and natural populations of *Microtus montanus*. Abstr. of papers, Amer. Soc. Mamm., 53rd Ann. Meeting, Asilomar, California.

FRANK, F. 1957. The causality of microtine cycles in Germany. J. Wildl. Mgmt., 21:113–121.

FREELAND, W. J. 1974. Vole cycles: another hypothesis. Amer. Nat., 108:238–245.

FREELAND, W. J., AND D. H. JANZEN. 1974. Strategies in herbivory by mammals: the role of plant secondary compounds. Amer. Nat., 108:269–289.

FULKER, D. W. 1970. Maternal buffering of rodent genotypic responses to stress: a complex genotype-environment interaction. Behav. Genet., 1:119–124.

GAINES, M. S., AND L. R. MCCLENAGHAN, JR. 1980. Dispersal in small mammals. Ann. Rev. Ecol. Syst., 11:163–196.

GAINES, M. S., AND R. K. ROSE. 1976. Population dynamics of *Microtus ochrogaster* in eastern Kansas. Ecology, 57:1145–1161.

GAINES, M. S., A. M. VIVAS, AND C. L. BAKER. 1979. An experimental analysis of dispersal in fluctuating vole populations: demographic parameters. Ecology, 60:814–828.

GARSD, A., AND W. E. HOWARD. 1982. Microtine population fluctuations: an ecosystem approach based on time-series analysis. J. Anim. Ecol., 51:208–225.

GASHWILER, J. S. 1972. Life history notes on the Oregon vole, *Microtus oregoni*. J. Mamm., 53:558–569.

GELLER, M. D., AND J. J. CHRISTIAN. 1982. Population dynamics, adreno-cortical function, and pathology in *Microtus pennsylvanicus*. J. Mamm., 63:85–95.

GETZ, L. 1978. Speculation on social structure and population cycles of microtine rodents. The Biologist, 60:134–147.

GETZ, L. L., F. R. COLE, L. VERNER, J. E. HOFMANN, AND D. AVALOS. 1979. Comparisons of population demography of *Microtus ochrogaster* and *M. pennsylvanicus*. Acta Theriol., 24:319–349.

GIPPS, J. H. W. 1982. The effects of testosterone and scopolamine HBr on the aggressive behaviour of male voles, *Microtus townsendii*. Canadian J. Zool., 60:946–950.

GIPPS, J. H. W., M. J. TAITT, C. J. KREBS, AND Z. DUNDJERSKI. 1981. Male aggression and the population dynamics of the vole, *Microtus townsendii*. Canadian J. Zool., 59:147–157.

GREENWOOD, P. J. 1980. Mating systems, philopatry and dispersal in birds and mammals. Anim. Behav., 28:1140–1162.

HAMILTON, W. D. 1964. The genetical evolution of social behaviour. J. Theor. Biol., 7:1–16.

HANSSON, L. 1971. Habitat, food and population dynamics of the field vole *Microtus agrestis* (L.) in south Sweden. Viltrevy, 8:267–378.

———. 1977. Spatial dynamics of field voles *Microtus agrestis* in heterogeneous landscapes. Oikos, 29:539–544.

HAUKIOJA, E. 1980. On the role of plant defences in the fluctuation of herbivore populations. Oikos, 35:202–213.

HAUKIOJA, E., AND T. HAKALA. 1975. Herbivore cycles and periodic outbreaks. Formulation of a general hypothesis. Rep. Kevo Subarctic Res. Sta., 12: 1–9.

HAWES, D. B. 1975. Experimental studies of competition among four species of voles. Unpubl. Ph.D. dissert., Univ. British Columbia, Vancouver, 107 pp.

HILBORN, R. 1975. Similarities in dispersal tendency among siblings in four species of voles (*Microtus*). Ecology, 56:1221–1225.

HILBORN, R., J. A. REDFIELD, AND C. J. KREBS. 1976. On reliability of enumeration for mark and recapture census of voles. Canadian J. Zool., 54:1019–1024.

HOFMANN, J. E., L. L. GETZ, AND B. J. KLATT. 1982. Levels of male aggressiveness in fluctuating populations of *Microtus ochrogaster* and *M. pennsylvanicus*. Canadian J. Zool., 60:898–912.

IVERSON, S. L., AND B. N. TURNER. 1974. Winter weight dynamics in *Microtus pennsylvanicus*. Ecology, 55:1030–1041.

JANNETT, F. J. 1978. Density-dependent formation of extended maternal families of the montane vole *Microtus montanus nanus*. Behav. Ecol. Sociobiol., 3:245–263.

JOLLY, G. M. 1965. Explicit estimates from capture-recapture data with both death and immigration—stochastic model. Biometrika, 52:225–247.

JOLLY, G. M., AND J. M. DICKSON. 1983. The problem of unequal catchability in mark-recapture estimation of small mammal populations. Canadian J. Zool., 61:922–927.

KALELA, O. 1962. On the fluctuations in the numbers of arctic and boreal small rodents as a problem of production biology. Ann. Acad. Sci. Fennica, Series A, IV, 66:1–38.

KEITH, L. B. 1974. Some features of population dynamics in mammals. Proc. Internatl. Congr. Game Biol., 11:17–58.

KNAPTON, R. W., AND J. R. KREBS. 1974. Settlement patterns, territory size, and breeding density in the song sparrow (*Melospiza melodia*). Canadian J. Zool., 52:1413–1420.

KOTT, E. 1965. Factors affecting estimates of meadow mouse populations. Unpubl. Ph.D. dissert., Univ. Toronto, Toronto, Ontario, 136 pp.

KREBS, C. J. 1966. Demographic changes in fluctuating populations of *Microtus californicus*. Ecol. Monogr., 36:239–273.

———. 1970. *Microtus* population biology: behavioral changes associated with the population cycle in *Microtus ochrogaster* and *M. pennsylvanicus*. Ecology, 51:34–52.

———. 1977. Competition between *Microtus pennsylvanicus* and *Microtus ochrogaster*. Amer. Midland Nat., 97:42–49.

———. 1978*a*. A review of the Chitty hypothesis of population regulation. Canadian J. Zool., 56:2463–2480.

———. 1978*b*. Aggression, dispersal, and cyclic changes in populations of small rodents. Pp. 49–60, *in* Aggression, dominance, and individual spacing (L. Krames, P. Pliner, and T. Alloway, eds.). Plenum Publ. Corp., New York, 173 pp.

———. 1979. Dispersal, spacing behaviour, and genetics in relation to population fluctuations in the vole *Microtus townsendii*. Fortschr. Zool., 25:61–77.

KREBS, C. J., AND J. H. MYERS. 1974. Population cycles in small mammals. Adv. Ecol. Res., 8:267–399.

KREBS, C. J., Z. T. HALPIN, AND J. N. M. SMITH. 1977. Aggression, testosterone, and the spring decline in populations of the vole, *Microtus townsendii*. Canadian J. Zool., 55:430–437.

KREBS, C. J., B. L. KELLER, AND R. H. TAMARIN. 1969. *Microtus* population biology: demographic changes in fluctuating populations of *Microtus ochrogaster* and *M. pennsylvanicus* in southern Indiana. Ecology, 50:587–607.

KREBS, C. J., J. A. REDFIELD, AND M. J. TAITT. 1978. A pulsed-removal experiment on the vole, *Microtus townsendii*. Canadian J. Zool., 56:2253–2262.

KREBS, C. J., ET AL. 1976. *Microtus* population biology: dispersal in fluctuating populations of *M. townsendii*. Canadian J. Zool., 54:79–95.

KROHNE, D. T. 1982. The demography of low-litter-size populations of *Microtus californicus*. Canadian J. Zool., 60:368–374.

LACK, D. 1954. The natural regulation of animal numbers. Oxford Univ. Press, Oxford, 343 pp.

LAINE, K., AND H. HETTONEN. 1983. The role of plant production in microtine cycles in northern Fennoscandia. Oikos, 40:407–418.

LEDUC, J., AND C. J. KREBS. 1975. Demographic consequences of artificial selection of the LAP locus in voles (*Microtus townsendii*). Canadian J. Zool., 53:1825–1840.

LESLIE, P. H., D. CHITTY, AND H. CHITTY. 1953. The estimation of population parameters from data obtained by means of the capture-recapture method. III. An example of the practical applications of the method. Biometrika, 40:137–169.

LEUZE, C. C. K. 1976. Social behaviour and dispersion in the water vole, *Arvicola terrestris*, Lacepede. Unpubl. Ph.D. dissert., Univ. Aberdeen, Aberdeen, 243 pp.

LIDICKER, W. Z. 1966. Ecological observations on a feral house mouse population declining to extinction. Ecol. Monogr., 36:27–50.

———. 1973. Regulation of numbers in an island population of the California vole: a problem in community dynamics. Ecol. Monogr., 43:271–302.

———. 1975. The role of dispersal in the demography of small mammals. Pp. 103–128, *in* Small mammals: their productivity and population dynamics (F. B. Golley, K. Petrusewicz and L. Ryszkowski, eds.). Cambridge Univ. Press, London, 451 pp.

———. 1978. Regulation of numbers in small mammal populations—historical reflections and a synthesis. Pp. 122–141, *in* Populations of small mammals under natural conditions (D. P. Snyder, ed.). Pymatuning Lab. Ecol. Spec. Publ., 5:1–237.

ŁOMNICKI, A. 1978. Individual differences between animals and the natural regulation of their numbers. J. Anim. Ecol., 47:461–475.

MADISON, D. M. 1980. Space use and social structure in meadow voles, *Microtus pennsylvanicus*. Behav. Ecol. Sociobiol., 7:65–71.

MALLORY, F. F., J. R. ELLIOT, AND R. J. BROOKS. 1981. Changes in body size in fluctuating populations on the collared lemming: age and photoperiod influences. Canadian J. Zool., 59:174–182.

MARES, M. A., ET AL. 1982. An experimental analysis of social spacing in *Tamias striatus*. Ecology, 63:267–273.

MARTIN, E. P. 1956. A population study of the prairie vole (*Microtus ochrogaster*) in N.E. Kansas. Univ. Kansas Publ., Mus. Nat. Hist., 8:361–416.

MAY, R. M. 1981. Models for single populations. Pp. 5–29, *in* Theoretical ecology: principles and applications. Second ed. (R. M. May, ed.). Sinauer Assoc., Sunderland, Massachusetts, 489 pp.

MCDONALD, I. R., AND M. J. TAITT. 1982. Steroid hormones in the blood plasma of Townsend's vole (*Microtus townsendii*). Canadian J. Zool., 60:2264–2269.

MIHOK, S. In press. Life history profiles of boreal meadow voles (*Microtus pennsylvanicus*). Bull. Carnegie Mus. Nat. Hist.

MOORE, G. H. 1974. Aetiology of the die-off of male *Antechinus stuartii*. Unpubl. Ph.D. dissert., Australian Natl. Univ., Canberra.

MORRIS, R. D. 1968. A comparison of capture success between Sherman and Longworth live traps. Canadian Field-Nat., 82:84–88.

MYERS, J., AND C. KREBS. 1971. Genetic, behavioural, and reproductive attributes of dispersing field voles *Microtus pennsylvanicus* and *Microtus ochrogaster*. Ecol. Monogr., 41:53–78.

MYERS, J. H., AND C. J. KREBS. 1974. Population cycles in rodents. Sci. Amer., 230:38–46.

NAUMOV, N. P. 1972. The ecology of animals. Univ. Illinois Press, Urbana, 650 pp.

NEGUS, N. C., AND P. J. BERGER. 1977. Experimental triggering of reproduction in a natural population of *Microtus montanus*. Science, 196:1230–1231.

OKSANEN, L., AND T. OKSANEN. 1981. Lemmings (*Lemmus lemmus*) and grey-sided voles (*Clethrionomys rufocanus*) in interaction with their resources and predators on Finnmarksuidda, northern Norway. Rept. Kevo Subarctic Res. Sta., 17:7–31.

PEARSON, O. P. 1960. Habits of *Microtus californicus* revealed by automatic photographic recorders. Ecol. Monogr., 30:231–249.

———. 1971. Additional measurements of the impact of carnivores on California voles (*Microtus californicus*). J. Mamm., 52:41–49.

PETTERBORG, L. J. 1978. Effect of photoperiod on body weight in the vole *Microtus montanus*. Canadian J. Zool., 56:431–435.

PETTICREW, B. G., AND R. M. F. S. SADLEIR. 1974. The ecology of the deermouse *Peromyscus mainculatus* in a coastal coniferous forest. I. Population dynamics. Canadian J. Zool., 52:107–118.

PITELKA, F. A., AND A. M. SCHULTZ. 1964. The nutrient-recovery hypothesis for arctic microtine cycles. Pp. 55–68, *in* Grazing in terrestrial and marine environments (D. J. Crisp, ed.). Blackwell Sci. Publ., Oxford, 322 pp.

POKKI, J. 1981. Distribution, demography and dispersal of the field vole, *Microtus agrestis,* in the Tvärminne archipelago, Finland. Acta Zool. Fennica, 164: 1–48.

RASMUSON, B., M. RASMUSON, AND J. NYGREN. 1977. Genetically controlled differences in behaviour between cycling and noncycling populations of field vole (*Microtus agrestis*). Hereditas, 87:33–42.

REDFIELD, J. A., M. J. TAITT, AND C. J. KREBS. 1978. Experimental alteration of sex ratios in populations of *Microtus townsendii,* a field vole. Canadian J. Zool., 56:17–27.

RICHMOND, M., AND R. STEHN. 1976. Olfaction and reproductive behavior in microtine rodents. Pp. 197–217, *in* Mammalian olfaction, reproductive processes, and behavior (R. Doty, ed.). Academic Press, New York, 344 pp.

ROBERTS, R. C. 1981. Genetical influences on growth and fertility. Pp. 231–254, *in* Biology of the house mouse (R. J. Berry, ed.). Symp. Zool. Soc. London, 47:1–715.

ROSE, R. K., AND M. S. GAINES. 1976. Levels of aggression in fluctuating populations of the prairie vole, *Microtus ochrogaster,* in eastern Kansas. J. Mamm., 57:43–57.

ROSE, R. K., R. K. EVERTON, AND G. G. GLASS. In press. Experimentally induced winter breeding in populations of small mammals. Acta Zool. Fennica.

ROSENZWEIG, M. L., AND Z. ABRAMSKY. 1980. Microtine cycles: the role of habitat heterogeneity. Oikos, 34:141–146.

SAITOH, T. 1981. Control of female maturation in high density populations of the red-backed vole, *Clethrionomys rufocanus bedfordiae.* J. Anim. Ecol., 50: 79–87.

SCHAFFER, W. M., AND R. H. TAMARIN. 1973. Changing reproductive rates and population cycles in lemmings and voles. Evolution, 27:111–124.

SCHLESINGER, W. H. 1976. Toxic foods and vole cycles: additional data. Amer. Nat., 110:315–317.

SEBER, G. A. F. 1982. The estimation of animal abundance and related parameters. Second ed. Charles Griffin, London, 654 pp.

SMITH, M. H., C. T. GARTEN, AND P. R. RAMSEY. 1975. Genic heterozygosity and population dynamics in small mammals. Pp. 85–102, *in* Isozymes, IV. Genetics and evolution (C. L. Markert, ed.). Academic Press, New York, 965 pp.

SMITH, M. H., M. N. MANLOVE, AND J. JOULE. 1978. Spatial and temporal dynamics of the genetic organization of small mammal populations. Pp. 99–113, *in* Populations of small mammals under natural conditions (D. P. Snyder, ed.). Pymatuning Lab. Ecol. Special Publ., 5:1–237.

STENSETH, N. C. 1978. Demographic strategies in fluctuating populations of small rodents. Oecologia, 33:149–172.

———. 1981. On Chitty's theory for fluctuating populations: the importance of genetic polymorphism in the generation of regular density cycles. J. Theor. Biol., 90:9–36.

STENSETH, N. C., L. HANSSON, A. MYLLYMÄKI, M. ANDERSSON, AND J. KATILA. 1977. General models for the population dynamics of the field vole, *Microtus agrestis*, in central Scandinavia. Oikos, 29:616–642.

STODDART, D. M. 1982. Does trap odour influence estimation of population size of the short-tailed vole *Microtus agrestis*? J. Anim. Ecol., 51:375–386.

SULLIVAN, T. P., AND C. J. KREBS. 1981. *Microtus* population biology: demography of *M. oregoni* in southwestern British Columbia. Canadian J. Zool., 59: 2092–2102.

TAITT, M. J. 1978. Population dynamics of *Peromyscus maniculatus austerus* and *Microtus townsendii* with supplementary food. Unpubl. Ph.D. dissert., Univ. British Columbia, Vancouver, 180 pp.

———. 1981. The effect of extra food on small rodent populations: I. Deermice (*Peromyscus maniculatus*). J. Anim. Ecol., 50:111–124.

———. In press. Cycles and annual fluctuations: *Microtus townsendii* and *Peromyscus maniculatus*. Acta Zool. Fennica.

TAITT, M. J., AND C. J. KREBS. 1981. The effect of extra food on small rodent populations: II. Voles (*Microtus townsendii*). J. Anim. Ecol., 50:125–137.

———. 1982. Manipulation of female behaviour in field populations of *Microtus townsendii*. J. Anim. Ecol., 51:681–690.

———. 1983. Predation, cover, and food manipulations during a spring decline of *Microtus townsendii*. J. Anim. Ecol., 52:837–848.

TAITT, M. J., J. H. W. GIPPS, C. J. KREBS, AND Z. DUNDJERSKI. 1981. The effect of extra food and cover on declining populations of *Microtus townsendii*. Canadian J. Zool., 59:1593–1599.

TAMARIN, R. H. 1977. Demography of the beach vole (*Microtus breweri*) and the meadow vole (*M. pennsylvanicus*) in southeastern Massachusetts. Ecology, 58:1310–1321.

———. 1978*a*. Dispersal, population regulation, and K-selection in field mice. Amer. Nat., 112:545–555.

———. 1978*b*. A defense of single-factor models of population regulation. Pp. 159–162, *in* Populations of small mammals under natural conditions (D. P. Snyder, ed.). Pymatuning Lab. Ecol. Spec. Publ., 5:1–237.

———. 1983. Animal population regulation through behavioral interactions. Pp. 698–720, *in* Advances in the study of mammalian behavior, (J. F. Eisenberg, and D. G. Kleiman, eds.). Spec. Publ., Amer. Soc. Mamm., 7:1–753.

THOMPSON, D. Q. 1965. Food preferences of the meadow vole (*Microtus pennsylvanicus*) in relation to habitat affinities. Amer. Midland Nat., 74:75–86.

TO, L. P., AND R. H. TAMARIN. 1977. The relation of population density and adrenal weight in cycling and non-cycling voles (*Microtus*). Ecology, 58: 928–934.

TOMPA, F. 1971. Catastrophic mortality and its population consequences. Auk, 88: 753–759.

VAN HORNE, B. 1982. Demography of the longtailed *Microtus longicaudus* in seral stages of coastal coniferous forest, southeast Alaska. Canadian J. Zool., 60:1690–1709.

VERNER, J. 1977. On the adaptive significance of territoriality. Amer. Nat., 111: 769–775.

VIITALA, J. 1977. Social organization in cyclic subarctic populations of the voles *Clethrionomys rufocanus* (Sund.) and *Microtus agrestis* (L.). Ann. Zool. Fennica, 14:53–93.

WATSON, A., AND R. MOSS. 1970. Dominance, spacing behaviour and aggression in relation to population limitation in vertebrates. Pp. 167–218, *in* Animal populations in relation to their food resources (A. Watson, ed.). Blackwell Sci. Publ., Oxford, 477 pp.

WEBSTER, A. B., AND R. J. BROOKS. 1981. Social behavior of *Microtus pennsylvanicus* in relation to seasonal changes in demography. J. Mamm., 62:738–751.

WHITE, T. C. R. 1978. The importance of a relative shortage of food in animal ecology. Oecologia, 33:71–86.

WHITNEY, P. 1976. Population ecology of two sympatric species of subarctic microtine rodents. Ecol. Monogr., 46:85–104.

WOLFF, J. O. 1981. Refugia, dispersal, predation, and geographic variation in snowshoe hare cycles. Pp. 441–449, *in* Proceedings of the world lagomorph conference, Guelph (K. Myers and C. D. MacInnes, eds.). Univ. Guelph, Ontario, 983 pp.

WOLFF, J. O., AND W. Z. LIDICKER, JR. 1980. Population ecology of the taiga vole, *Microtus xanthognathus,* in interior Alaska. Canadian J. Zool., 58: 1800–1812.

WYNNE-EDWARDS, V. C. 1962. Animal dispersion in relation to social behaviour. Oliver and Boyd, Edinburgh, 653 pp.

ZIMMERMAN, E.G. 1965. A comparison of habitat and food of two species of *Microtus.* J. Mamm., 46:605–612.

MANAGEMENT AND CONTROL

ROSS E. BYERS

Abstract

CURRENT *Microtus* control technology is reviewed with specific information on rapid population monitoring methods; chemical, cultural, and biological control methods; economic threshold levels, rodenticide residues and environmental hazards. The merits of control methods based on barriers, habitat manipulation, repellents, predators, grazing of hoofed animals, trapping, baits, and ground-cover sprays are discussed.

Introduction

The national economic impact of vole damage to trees, shrubs, and agronomic crops has been a significant factor in crop production. Most of the information presented in this chapter pertains to the technology developed for controlling the pine vole (*Microtus pinetorum*) in apple orchards.

From a control point of view there are two classes of voles infesting orchards: 1) subterranean voles which burrow deep in the soil and which damage the plant below the soil level such as the pine vole (*Microtus pinetorum*) in the eastern U.S., and 2) surface running voles that damage at or above the soil level, such as the meadow vole (*Microtus pennsylvanicus*), montane vole (*Microtus montanus*), and the California vole (*Microtus californicus*). The prairie vole (*Microtus ochrogaster*) of the midwestern states develops runs on the surface similar to the meadow vole but also has a deep tunnel system similar to the pine vole. Vole feeding habits, however, vary considerably depending on availability of cover, loose soil for tunnelling, and the location and type of desirable food supplies (Bailey, 1924; Byers, 1979*a*; Dimmick, 1978; Hamilton, 1938; White, 1965). For example, *M. californicus* in plowed potato, sugarbeet, or artichoke fields is found largely underground or in the plants, whereas in orchards where tilling is minimal, in alfalfa, or in herbaceous cover, *M. pennsylvanicus* feeds largely along runways on the surface. Control and management of any vole species often requires an integrated knowledge of the crop being protected, the habits of the animals in the cultural system, the control methods available, and the potential hazard to man or non-target animals.

Numerous reports indicate that voles may cause serious economic losses to apple, peach, pear, citrus, blueberry, nursery, ornamental, and strawberry crops by girdling the roots and stems, causing plant death. By direct feeding, voles may also cause serious damage to flower bulbs, tubers, vegetables, sugar beets, grain, sagebrush, alfalfa, pasture land, and hay crops (Bailey, 1924; Batzli and Pitelka, 1970; Cummings and Marsh, 1978; Dana and Shaw, 1958; Littlefield et al., 1946; Morrison, 1953; Mueggler, 1967; Piper, 1908, 1928; Sartz, 1970; Spencer, 1959; Spencer et al., 1958).

Ferguson (1980) estimated from a 1978 national survey that apple growers lost 123,000 trees to vole injury, of which 37% of the trees were of bearing age. In perennial crops the loss of an economic unit (such as an apple tree) influences the profitability of the planting for its productive life (Byers 1979*a*). Even sporadic annual losses of less than 1% in tree fruit crops can result in a 20–30% tree loss in the most profitable years for the crop which is at 25–30 years of age. In orchards, serious vole damage usually occurs in a single year when growers are unaware of rising vole populations. In these situations it is likely that 30% of the trees may be completely girdled in a single season while another 20% or more may be seriously injured. In plantings sustaining this level of damage, all trees (good ones as well) often must be removed (bulldozed) due to the uneconomical operation of the block. Thus, in many cases twice as many trees may be removed as are actually damaged. Assessment of long-term production losses from single season surveys are difficult because growers usually remove vole-damaged trees quickly. Good tree stands must be maintained throughout the life of an orchard, forest, or ornamental planting in order to remain an economic unit. In addition, replacement trees planted in older vole-infested orchards are very difficult to protect from vole injury. Replanted trees usually do not survive because inadequate attention is taken to prepare individual soil planting sites as is recommended for establishing new trees on old orchard sites.

Anthony and Fisher (1977) estimated that Pennsylvania apple growers spent approximately $270,000 in 1974 for control of pine and meadow voles. No estimate was made of the economic losses caused by vole damage to fruit trees for that year.

Byers (1974*a*) estimated that the national apple market value losses caused by pine-vole damage in the eastern and midwestern apple-producing areas were approximately $40 million in the geographic range of this species, while an additional $3.3 million was spent on control measures for that year.

The use of toxicants, habitat manipulations, and barriers have been the traditional methods of arresting damage over the last 50 years for most agricultural crops (Hamilton, 1935). The use of predators, repellents, and trapping have had limited use as commercially acceptable agricultural practices; however, trapping can be quite useful to home owners and small orchardists with fewer than three acres.

For most agricultural crops the presence of voles may or may not pose an immediate threat. In many fruit-tree and ornamental plantings, vole damage is restricted to the dormant period from November through April except during a drought or extremely high population levels. In the late spring, summer, or early fall, more desirable food sources than tree roots and bark are plentiful. More important, however, may be more desirable temperatures which allow voles to forage over a greater range, accessing more desirable plant material, thus making the crop plant less vulnerable to damage. With monocultured crops such as vegetable or hay crops, damage is usually dependent on vole population levels and the developmental stage of the crop. In orchards, if control measures are not taken, vole damage is likely to occur annually. For this reason, the development of control methodology for eastern voles has been more intensive for apple orchards than for any other crop.

History of Vole Control in Orchards

Prior to 1935 voles were controlled largely through clean cultivation of the entire orchard floor, tree guards, and hand-placed poison baits made of strychnine or arsenic (Hamilton, 1935). Bait-carriers composed of fresh vegetable matter were thought to be more desirable than grain or oat carriers for toxicants. Although repellents, natural enemies, trapping, and gassing were suggested methods for the period, rarely were these methods relied upon as the sole commercially acceptable vole control measure.

Monitoring

Regular assessment of vole populations in crops susceptible to vole damage requires rapid assessment of large acreages in short intervals of time. In high-valued crops, a preventive vole control program should be followed because the economic threshold for damage is at low population levels. The loss of a single 15-year-old apple tree in a 50-ha block may reduce the gross value of the crop by $2,500 over the subsequent 20 years of the planting. If season-long control can be achieved by a single rodenticide treatment costing $25/ha, 100 ha of this age tree could be treated to prevent the loss of a single tree. As the age of the planting gets older, the value of trees decreases, and thus the economic threshold. Since a single animal residing at or near a tree may cause significant damage or tree loss, the economic threshold population is at a very low level. Thus, a highly effective and reliable preventative program is essential for avoiding damage to perennial tree crops (Byers, in press). Regular monthly inspections just prior to the damaging period and after treatments can provide the grower with an accurate view of future potential hazard (Barden et al., 1982).

Examination of the ground cover for vole runways and holes can quickly give an indication of the recent presence of voles. Observations based on vole signs (fresh digging, trails, feeding on plant material, defecation) are not adequate, because immediately after treatment runways and holes still may appear to be active but voles, in fact, may be eliminated. If voles are present in the runway systems, it must be assumed that a potential for vole damage exists in high-valued crops. Vole population levels and damage potential can change rapidly because of increased animal survival rates, increased reproduction levels, or changes in other environmental stress factors (snow, drought, soil freezing, ground-cover dormancy), and a simple, rapid, and accurate method for determining animal presence is desirable for researchers and growers as well.

The apple indexing method has been used in orchards for many years to determine the percentage of trees infested with voles (Barden et al., 1982). An apple with a 2.5-cm diameter slice removed from the cheek may be placed in a run or a hole for meadow voles or 5–15 cm below the soil surface in a tunnel for pine voles. Apples

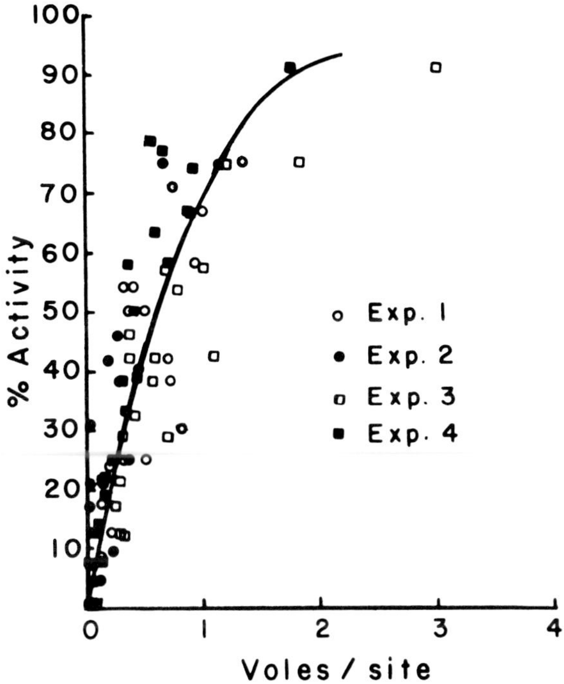

FIG. 1. Regression of percent activity on pine voles/site based on percent of apples having vole tooth-marks when placed 2/tree in runways 24 h previous. Plots (87 plots in four experiments in 1975 and 1976) were snap-trapped for a 5-day period following apple-activity reading. The apple-monitoring method was highly correlated with pine-vole population densities ($R^2 = 0.77$, $y = 7.5 + 78.0x - 17.7x^2$; from Byers, 1981).

can be observed for vole tooth-marks 24 h after placement and the percentage of trees infested can be calculated easily. This calculation can give a direct estimate of the percentage of trees that could be damaged, given the proper environmental conditions. In addition, vole population densities correlate strongly with the percentage of active sites (Fig. 1). This method has been used to evaluate experimental plots and general orchard populations pre- and post-treatment (Byers, 1975*a,* 1978, 1981). When assessing chemical control treatments, a reading of pre-treatment activity taken prior to and again approximately 3 weeks after treatment can be used to determine if a reduction in the percentage of infested trees has occurred.

In order to increase the quantitative measure of the number of animals at each feeding station, the apples are weighed prior to placement and after 24 h. Weighing the apple gives the grams of apples consumed on an individual tree basis. We determined that the amount of apple consumed for pine and meadow voles/24 h is approximately 0.5 g of apple per gram of body weight. The average pine vole should consume approximately 13 g/animal and the average meadow vole about 20 g/animal.

Barriers

Currently, tree guards are used to control damage from prairie and meadow voles but not pine voles, since the latter species can easily tunnel under barriers (Caslick and Decker, 1978; Hamilton, 1935; Hunter and Tukey, 1977). Crushed stone is used when installing tree guards so that nesting and trailing near the tree trunk is discouraged (Bode et al., 1981). In conjunction with tree guards, clean herbicide culture of 1.2 to 2-m wide strips in young plantings inhibits meadow voles from ranging near the tree trunk. As the tree enlarges, removal of the tree guard becomes necessary in order to prevent the guard from girdling the tree. The tree then becomes vulnerable to vole attack, particularly under snow cover.

Habitat Manipulation

In orchards the major food sources for voles are normally not apple trees, but include roots, stems, petioles, and leaves of a diversity of plants living on or below the soil surface (Cengel et al., 1978). Laboratory studies showed that, given sufficient water, pine voles cannot survive for more than about 4 days on 1-year-old stem or root tissue from apple trees (Byers, 1974*b*). Logically, if voles under field conditions cannot survive without a supplementary food source to apple trees, "clean culture" should reduce vole populations.

Fifty years ago the term "clean culture" referred to total destruction of the orchard-floor plant material through cultivation techniques. However, today, herbicide or cultivated strips from 5 to 12 ft wide within the tree rows and close mowing between rows is classified as clean culture (Byers and Young, 1978; Davis, 1976*a*, 1976*b*).

Field experiments have shown that clean culture can greatly assist in reducing existing pine vole population levels (Byers and Young, 1974, 1978; Byers et al., 1976). Techniques used to achieve

TABLE 1
EFFECT OF AN ANNUALLY-APPLIED HERBICIDE STRIP ON AVERAGE PINE-VOLE ACTIVITY PER TREE AFTER THE TENTH YEAR IN A COMMERCIAL APPLE ORCHARD (AFTER BYERS AND YOUNG, 1974)*

	No. sites		No. active sites		No. voles caught	
Tree no.	Control	Herbi-cide	Control	Herbi-cide	Control	Herbi-cide
1	2.00	0.75	1.00	0.25	1.50	0.50
2	2.00	0.00	1.75	0.00	1.50	0.00
3	2.00	0.00	1.50	0.00	1.50	0.00
4	1.75	0.75	1.75	0.25	2.00	0.25
Average	1.96	0.40	1.50	0.13	1.64	0.20

* Treatments and controls were initiated in the first year of planting and monitored for vole activity after the tenth annual application of herbicide culture. Eight blocks of four tree spaces each were alternated in a single row; thus tree 1 and 4 were adjacent to the other treatment. There were 15 trees in the herbicide treatment group and 14 controls (no herbicide). A site refers to a vole run or hole below the soil level which appeared to be active. A limit of two sites/tree was counted. Active sites were those having characteristic vole tooth-marks on an apple placed in a run or hole approximately 24 h previous.

clean culture vary considerably between orchardists and years. Some of the variables are related to type of equipment used, frequency of the practice, soil characteristics (particularly rockiness, depth of friable soil, terrain), tree age, planting distances, width of herbicide (or cultivated) band, ground-cover flora, and weather conditions (Byers and Young, 1978).

The use of clean culture may provide some degree of *preventive* protection from voles when 1) started in the first year of orchard planting, 2) the planting site has never been previously infested, 3) a wide strip of herbicide or cultivation is maintained in the tree row, and 4) regular close mowing of middles is practiced.

The use of wide-band cultivation can be advantageous for the control of pine voles (Byers and Young, 1978; Byers et al., 1976). However, the tilling of soil usually provides conditions for meadow voles to tunnel in the loose soil; thus the animals obtain a below-soil accessibility to roots and trunk (Byers, 1979*c*).

Three experiments at different locations showed that clean culture achieved with wide-band residual herbicides (Table 1), wide-band cultivations (Fig. 2), or combinations of the two (Fig. 3), in conjunction with regular mowing between rows, can greatly reduce

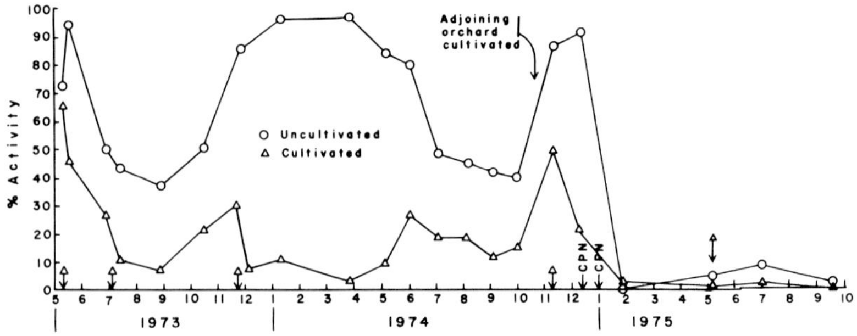

FIG. 2. Effect of wide-band cultivation and chlorophacinone (CPN) hand-placed bait on pine-vole activity. Symbols with arrows refer to time of application. Percent activity refers to percent of apples having vole tooth-marks when placed in runways 24 h previous (from Byers et al., 1976).

existing vole populations and subsequent hazard to trees. However, some locations are apparently more amenable to control of voles through cultural means than others (Byers and Young, 1974, 1978; Figs. 2, 3). If regular mowing is not practiced, voles may become abundant in row middles and may easily move under snow cover to damage tree trunks.

Costs of maintaining clean culture are almost prohibitive and were determined to be as much as three times as costly as a hand-placed toxicant or broadcast-bait program (Byers, 1977*a*, in press; Sullivan, 1979).

Hoofed Animals

Cattle, sheep, and swine have been used to a limited extent for control of pine and meadow voles in eastern U.S. orchards (Horsfall, 1953; Woodside et al., 1942). The disadvantages usually greatly outweigh advantages. Spray materials used in orchards may contaminate the ground cover so that meat or milk cannot be used for human consumption. Action by hoofed animals is usually incomplete, slow, and swine or cattle may severely damage trees.

Repellents

Repellents have been extensively used for rabbit, deer, and woodchuck damage control, but seldom used for vole control. Repellents were shown to be superior to rodenticides in tank studies where rodents were confined to repellent-treated trees, including roots

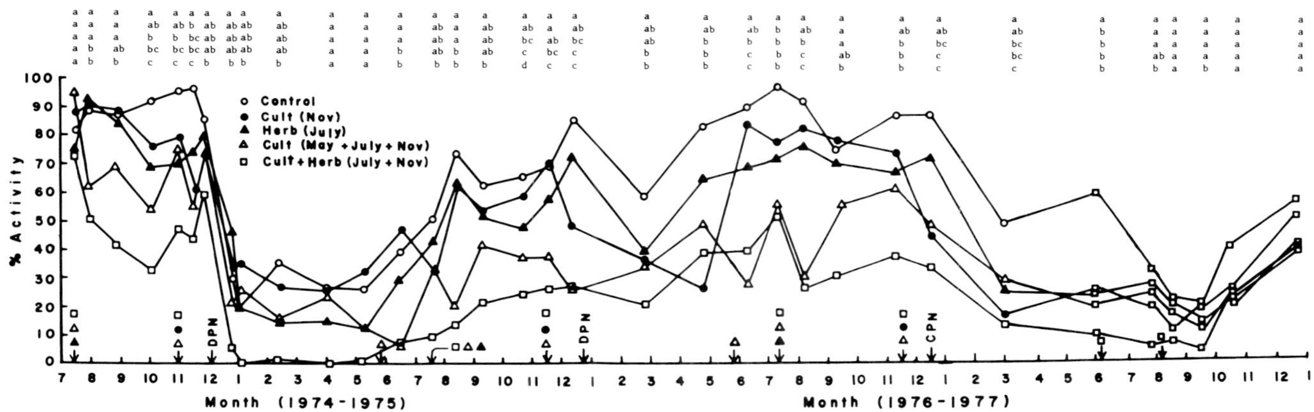

FIG. 3. Effect of orchard culture, and diphacinone (DPN) and chlorophacinone (CPN) hand-placed baits, on percent activity (percent of apples having vole tooth-marks when placed in runways 24 h previous). Symbols with arrows refer to time of application. Note the cultivation-plus-herbicide treatment gave better control of pine voles than either cultivation or herbicide treatments alone. Also note poor control with the herbicide-only treatment. Points within columns having the same letter are not statistically different by Duncan's multiple range test ($P > 0.05$) (from Byers and Young, 1978).

(Luke and Snetsinger, 1975). In practical use, however, tunnelling voles gnaw on roots and stems below soil level where repellents cannot be applied. In addition, repellents may wash off during the course of the winter or may not be reapplied if snow is present.

Horticulturists recognize that fruit tree species are different in their susceptibility to vole damage. Hunter and Tukey (1977) rated apple, pear, peach, cherry, apricot, and plum in descending order of preference, but no definitive data are available in the literature. Laboratory studies showed that a great deal of difference existed between susceptibility of various clones to vole damage. Crosses of R5 or PI 286613 with *Malus pumila* Mill were found to be less susceptible to damage when compared to Golden Delicious apple stems (Byers and Cummins, 1977; Cummins et al., 1983; Geyer and Cummins, 1980; Wysolmerski et al., 1980).

Predators

Because the economic threshold for vole damage occurs at very low population levels (Byers, in press) and because predator populations (snakes, owls, hawks, skunks, etc.; see Pearson, this volume) usually lag behind the prey, natural predatory control never has been considered commercially important. Vole populations are usually lowest in late winter and early spring when predators are reproducing and defining territories. Thus when voles are increasing during late summer and fall, predators may no longer be reproducing (Hamilton, 1935; Howard et al., 1982).

Mowing, spraying, picking, and post-harvest removal of dropped apples interefere with predator population increases. These activities disturb all types of wildlife, including voles. Rotary mowers are particularly devastating to snake populations and larger mammals within an orchard.

Trapping

Snap-traps have been used extensively for estimating vole populations (Chapman and Overton, 1966) in experimental plots because almost complete removal of all animals can be achieved in a 3–5 day period (Byers, 1975*a*, 1978, 1981) if done at critical periods when voles are susceptible to trapping. Many vole species, however, may not be as susceptible to trapping in summer when temperatures are high, during dry conditions, or when underground burrow systems have been developed. In fall when temperatures are ideal for vole movements, and in late winter while the soil is thawing, even pine voles can be trapped easily. Trapping success can be enhanced by pre-baiting with apples, using covers over traps, and by placing traps in active runs at intervals (for example, at every tree, 100/ha). Split tires can be used satisfactorily as trapping stations because they are convex and may be easily located in the fall when leaves may cover other types of flat stations. Because tires are black they retain heat, thus providing a warm, protected location for voles in adverse weather. Tires may be obtained without cost at many auto service centers or from commercial dumps where tires are split before covering. Commercial tire-splitting equipment is also available for purchase.

Chemical Controls

During the post-1935 period, zinc-phosphide grain and vegetable baits developed by the U.S. Fish and Wildlife Service were important for the control of meadow voles in many agronomic and tree-fruit crops. Zinc-phosphide grain formulations, however, have not given adequate control of pine voles under most circumstances (Byers et al., 1976, 1982; Merson and Byers, 1981). Broadcast baiting with zinc-phosphide (Zn_3P_2) grain baits was found to kill only 50–60% of pine voles in a population (Byers et al., 1982). The failure of Zn_3P_2 to adequately control pine voles was previously thought to be related to the differences between the two species, their acceptance of grain carriers, or the inadequate exposure of pine voles to surface applied bait.

Recent laboratory and field evaluations of zinc-phosphide pelleted bait show that wide differences exist between formulations. At least 27 formulations of Zn_3P_2 are now listed with the Environmental Protection Agency, but very few have been compared for their lethality to any species in the laboratory or field. Greater differences in mortality have been shown to exist between formulations than between species for a number of Zn_3P_2 formulations (Merson and Byers, 1981). The zinc-phosphide Rodent Bait AG formulation made by Bell Laboratories, Inc., recently has become extremely important to the fruit industry as a hand-placed and broadcast bait against both meadow and pine voles. Further improvement of zinc-phosphide formulations through encapsulation of the Zn_3P_2 or changes in inert ingredients may continue to improve the lethality of this old toxicant and provide a different mode of action from the anticoagulants.

In 1955 endrin became available to the apple industry as a ground-cover spray at the rate of 2.4 lbs/acre. Horsfall (1956*a,* 1956*b*) was instrumental in determining rates, application techniques, and the significance of the ground-cover plant communities in the successful application of ground-cover sprays (Horsfall et al., 1974). After 10 years of annual endrin use, growers complained about inadequate vole control and subsequent tree losses. Investigations in Virginia showed that some vole strains were 10 times more resistant to endrin than voles taken from untreated orchards (Hartgove and Webb, 1973; Webb and Horsfall, 1967; Webb et al., 1972, 1973). However, in other eastern U.S. states (North Carolina, Pennsylvania, New York) where endrin was less frequently used, resistance was not reported to be a major problem in most orchards by the early 1980s (Byers 1979b, 1980).

By the late 1960s the vole problem became a major threat to the Virginia apple industry because of the development of endrin resistant pine voles. Since no alternative measure existed for the control of the pine vole, Horsfall et al. (1974) investigated a number of toxicants and found the anticoagulant, chlorophacinone, was effective at 0.2 lbs/acre and above as a ground-cover spray. Since anticoagulants were rather expensive, the lowest rate of chlorophacinone (CPN) that gave control was given use clearances by several states in 1974. Inconsistent results were obtained with CPN ground sprays in the years following its initial introduction (Byers, 1975*a,* 1975*b*; Byers et al., 1976). By the early 1970s the Environmental Protection Agency was not favorable toward the clearance of new ground-sprayed rodenticides for replacement of endrin. In addition, changes in orchard spray equipment for insect and disease control from high-pressure machines to low pressure and low-water volumes caused an increase in the costs of rodenticide applications and lower cost methods were developed.

During the 1970s new bait formulations, cultural control methods, and animal habits and biology were under intensive investigation with emphasis on finding new solutions to the tree damaging problem (Byers, 1977*b*). Rodenticide-bait formulations developed by chemical companies for the commensal rodent trade were adapted for use in agriculture. This resulted in state approval for many anticoagulant baits and caused a return to hand-placed and broadcast baiting followed by an understanding of the failure of previous zinc-phosphide bait programs. Excellent control with broadcast anticoagulent bait programs showed that the failure of Zn_3P_2 broadcast baiting programs was related to poor acceptance of the formulation and not access of animals to bait (Byers, 1981; Byers et al., 1982; Merson and Byers, 1981).

Great differences between toxicants, formulations, and consumption time required for lethal doses resulted in some formulations outperforming others in vole field tests (particularly anticoagulants; Byers, 1978, 1981; Table 2; Fig. 4). Due to lack of laboratory methods for testing formulations, the evaluations of toxic baits were conducted primarily in the field where population levels, weather, and animal access to highly preferred alternate food sources (apples and lush ground cover) were a part of the testing program (Byers, 1978, 1981; Byers and Young, 1975). However, concurrent laboratory studies could have provided much useful information relative to quantities and exposure times required to achieve lethal doses from various bait formulations.

Since the hoarding of toxic-pelleted baits by pine voles was quite strong in the field, this behavioral characteristic was incorporated into control methodology (Byers et al., 1976). Using radiotelemetry techniques, transmitters were implanted in pelletized Chlorophacinone baits and placed in pine-vole runway systems. Pelleted bait placed with the transmitter was removed from the placement sites to more centralized caches near the pine-vole nests and located 25 cm or more below the soil surface (Byers et al., 1976). Wax-block formulations (2.5 × 5 × 5 cm) used in rat-control programs were found less effective presumably because the bait was fed upon only at the placement site (Byers et al., 1976). Pelletized baits became accepted by the fruit industry very quickly because of their relatively low cost, ease of handling, and the need for more effective control measures.

It was not until the 1980s that field experiments were conducted to determine if the caching behavior differed between pine and meadow voles. Laboratory-tank tests and caged trials showed both species exhibited a strong caching behavior (Merson and Byers, in press). However, in one field experiment three different pellet sizes were placed at 20 sites each. Using live-trap, toe-clip, and release methods, sixty pine voles were trapped over a 5-day period in one

TABLE 2

FIELD EVALUATION OF BROADCAST AND HAND-PLACED RODENTICIDES FOR PINE VOLE CONTROL IN ORCHARDS TREATED NOVEMBER 14–15, 1979

Treatment	Rate (kg/ha)	Rate (lbs/ac)	% Activity[4] Nov. 9	% Activity[4] Nov. 30	Voles/plot (December 3–7)	Voles/site (December 3–7)	% Control
1. Control	—	—	89 a[3]	87 a[3]	31.7 a[3]	1.25 a[3]	0
2. Volak[1]—0.005% BFC	21	19	88 a	15 def	0.7 d	0.03 d	98
3. Volak[1]—0.0025% BFC	20	18	85 a	6 ef	0.3 d	0.01 d	99
4. Volak[1]—0.001% BFC	19	17	88 a	5 ef	0.7 d	0.02 d	98
5. Volak[1]—0.0005% BFC	29	26	85 a	5 ef	0.3 d	0.02 d	98
6. Volak[2]—packet 0.005% BFC	8	7[2]	87 a	4 ef	1.0 d	0.03 d	98
7. Rozol[1]—0.005% CPN (French)	25	22	88 a	0 f	0.3 d	0.01 d	99
8. Rozol[1]—0.005% CPN (USA)	24	21	88 a	33 bcd	2.7 d	0.11 d	91
9. Maki[1]—0.005% BDL	22	20	87 a	44 bcd	4.7 cd	0.19 cd	85
10. Ramik[1]—0.005% DPN	24	21	84 a	51 bc	6.0 cd	0.24 bcd	81
11. Ramik—0.005% DPN	11	10[2]	85 a	40 bcd	10.7 bc	0.41 bc	67
12. ZnP[1]—2% Corn + Oats	21	19	85 a	67 ab	14.0 b	0.49 b	61
13. ZnP—2% Corn + Oats	6	5[2]	85 a	59 abc	11.0 bc	0.42 bc	66
14. ZnP[1]—2% Pellet (Bell Labs)	28	25	89 a	29 cde	2.7 d	0.10 d	92
15. ZnP—2% Pellet (Bell Labs)	6	5[2]	89 a	19 def	1.7 d	0.07 d	94

Treatment abbreviations: BFC, bromodialone; CPN, chorophacinone; DPN, diphacinone; ZnP, zinc phosphide.

[1] Treatment was broadcast in a band under tree limbs.

[2] Treatment was hand-placed at two locations under shingles at each tree.

[3] Numbers within columns followed by the same letter are not statistically different by Duncan's multiple range test ($P > 0.05$); three replicate plots per treatment.

[4] Apples placed in two holes or runs 5–15 cm below the soil surface on opposite sides of a tree trunk were examined 24 h after placement. Percent activity refers to all sites at which there were vole tooth-marks on the apple.

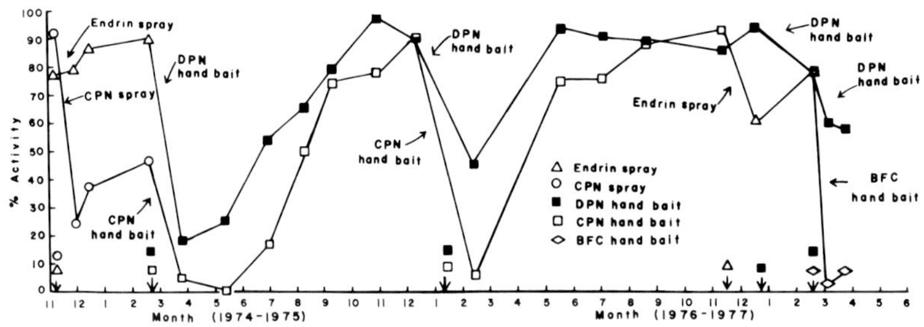

FIG. 4. Endrin applied at 2.7 kg/ha (2.4 lb/acre) did not control pine voles (probably because of endrin resistance). Symbols with arrows refer to time of treatment. Percent activity is percent of apples having vole tooth-marks when placed in runways 24 h previous. Chlorophacinone (CPN) ground spray applied at 0.2 kg/ha (0.2 lb/acre) gave some control. Both chlorophacinone and diphacinone (DPN) hand-baits at 11.2 kg/ha (10 lbs/acre) were effective when applied in Feburary 1975. Endrin applied in November 1976 did not give adequate control. Two applications of DPN bait did not give adequate control in 1977 but bromodialone (BFC) gave excellent control (from Byers, 1978).

orchard and in another orchard 50 meadow voles were trapped. (Using the Schnabel estimator 91 [60 to 136] pine voles and 47 [36 to 62] meadow voles existed in the plots, respectively). In the pine-vole orchard approximately 60% of the sites had animals which cached half or more of the 50 g placed at the sites within a 24-h period. Less than 1% of the sites in the meadow-vole orchard had cached bait. This study took place in December 1980 near the end of the normal fall control period when caching by both species should have been strong (Merson and Byers, in press). Obviously, if the majority of meadow voles are sporadic feeders (not feeding from cached bait), they probably would not obtain a lethal dose of weak multi-dose anticoagulants if bait were placed at only one or two sites within the vole range. Anticoagulants such as chlorophacinone or diphacinone may be expected to give better control of pine voles since they could be fed upon from bait cached near nests. Much work on the caching response under field conditions is needed to understand better the success and failure of different toxicants and pelleted formulations for each species.

Recent data have shown that both acute and chronic baits control voles equally well when used against pine voles, whether applied as a broadcast or a hand-placed bait (Table 2). When baits are broadcast, the quantity of bait required on the orchard floor may depend on the lethality of the bait as well as pellet density. The notion that pine voles do not sufficiently surface and thus do not retrieve sufficient surface-applied bait has been disproven in recent years in Virginia orchards (Byers et al., 1982; Table 2). The generalization that broadcast applications are effective in all orchard or agricultural situations for microtines can be seen from these experiments to be an over-simplification. For example, voles cannot be controlled by surface-broadcast baits in bluegrass sods that promote trailing below a thatch cover.

Pelletized-bait formulations absorb moisture readily and are more susceptible to water deterioration in rainy weather than whole or cracked grains. Laboratory data have shown that 3 days of continuous feeding and consumption of approximately 10 g of chlorophacinone bait/pine vole are required for 90% of animals to receive a lethal dose (Byers, 1976*b*, 1978). Field results have shown reduced control where chlorophacinone (CPN) bait has been broadcast 1 day prior to a rain, and 3 days without rain are thought to be required for adequate pine vole exposure and caching of bait. Residue analysis of voles from an orchard treated with the single-dose anticoagulant, brodifacoum (BFC) bait, showed that 95% of the meadow voles contained a detectable level of toxicant 1 day following treatment (Merson et al., 1984). Toxicants such as warfarin, which require numerous days of continuous feeding, probably would have limited usage when applied as hand-placed or broadcast baits because spoilage probably would occur before voles received a lethal dose.

In order to develop low-cost and effective bait formulations for field use, these factors must be considered: 1) the time required for the population to contact the bait, 2) the consumption required to deliver a lethal dose, 3) weatherability of the bait in the field, and 4) pellet sizes and density for optimum caching and feeding. Acute baits like 2% zinc phosphide, which have a quick action and taste aversion, have the advantage of low consumption for lethality (0.25 g/vole) but the disadvantage of poor acceptance. Theoretically, the "acute" baits should require rates that are sufficient only to expose the vole to a single pellet within its home range (5 kg/ha or less), whereas bait that requires relatively large consumptions over a period of days may be more dependent on the quantities presented within the home range of the vole.

Spoilage of bait in the field within 2 weeks after application has both advantages and disadvantages. Hazard to non-target species is increased with highly weather-resistant formulations, which might last months or years, but reduced effectiveness may occur if weatherability is not adequate. Packaging of bait in plastic packages has been shown to repel moisture while still being available to the voles. Placement of packaged bait under substantial bait-station covers (e.g., split tires, rubber mats, shingles) is desirable to prevent a non-target primary hazard. Testing of two packet types against pine voles in field trials showed that voles did not open packets at approximately 5% of the placement sites even though animals were known to be present (Byers, 1981; Byers et al., 1982). Sufficient numbers of animals appeared to be present to repopulate the orchard because packets were continuously being opened in the post treatment period (Fig. 5). The use of automobile tires split longitudinally and small open-top plastic cups to prevent soil contact with bait promotes good baiting conditions for at least 6 months (Merson and Byers, unpubl. observ.). Shingles or rubber mats that lay flat on the soil are easily covered by leaves, making baiting difficult. Since tire stations may be 6–10 cm above the soil level they may be easily located by personnel, but may cause difficulty for close mowing or cultivation operations. The use of smaller, compact automobile tires allows closer and less inhibited mowing operations. The black automobile tire retains heat and provides an ideal location for placement of bait in winter.

Some orchardists place tires in the tree row while using band-herbicide applications wider than the tire. The disadvantage of this system is the poor exposure of voles to tires, because voles are seldom active in the herbicide band. If the herbicide band is narrower than the tire, some of the tire extends into the vegetation strip where the voles range. If a wide band herbicide strip is used, movement of the tire into adjacent cover is necessary when baiting.

Invasion of voles from nearby fields can be reduced by perimeter baiting of orchards with tire stations. This system also provides some year-round protection even under heavy snow cover. If acute, rapid-kill baits are used, as little as 1 lb of formulated material/acre (Byers et al., 1982) is required. However, the potential for bait shyness with toxicants like zinc phosphide requires rotation to toxicants that do not promote this characteristic.

Several chemicals have potential use as rodenticides for vole control. Their eventual commercial use depends upon several factors: 1) clearance from federal and state agencies, 2) non-target hazards, 3) effectiveness, 4) profit potential as a world wide vertebrate con-

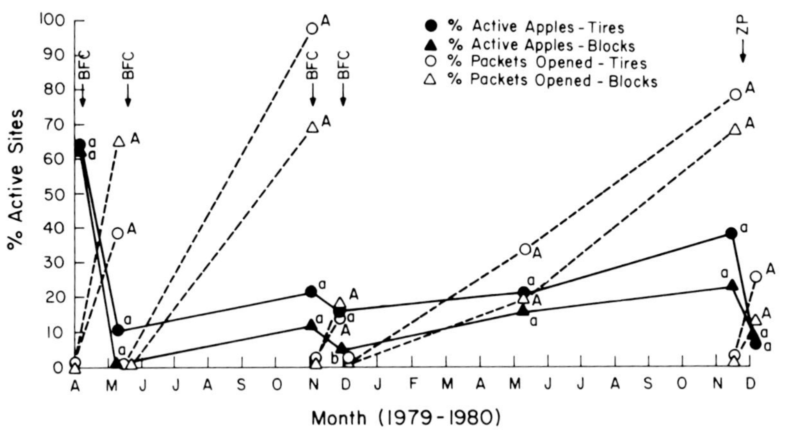

FIG. 5. Effect of bromodialone (BFC) and Zn_3P_2zp packets on percent activity, which refers to percent apples with vole tooth-marks (——) or percent packets opened (- - -) by voles when either was placed under cinder blocks or split-tires 24 h previous. Note that pine-vole populations were maintained uniformly low, but were not eliminated. In addition, a large percentage of packets was opened during summer, which indicates presence of voles under most trees and the annual need for placement of packets. Points followed by the same letter for percent activity (small letters) or percent packets opened (capital letters) are not statistically different for each sample date by Duncan's multiple range test ($P > 0.05$) (from Byers et al., 1982).

trol agent, and 5) consistent supply. In recent years, antimetabolites of vitamins B, C, and K, anticoagulants, chlorinated hydrocarbons, chemosterilants, inorganic toxicants, fumigants, organic phosphates, narcotics and inhibitors of feeding and functions of heart, muscle, and immune systems, intestinal microflora inhibitors, and mechanical action materials that cause a blockage in the digestive system have been studied for their rodenticide potential (Benjamini, 1982; Gutteridge, 1972; Marsh and Howard, 1976; Meehan, 1980*a*, 1980*b*; Merson and Byers, unpubl. observ.; Stehn et al., 1908; Tietjen, 1969). Many of these chemicals have great potential as safe and reliable rodenticides, but many have been discarded because of taste aversion and bait shyness.

Mechanical Spreaders

The degree of control achieved by broadcasting bait with a ground or aerial spreader may be quite variable since the types of distribution equipment vary greatly in 1) placement accuracy under tree limbs where vole runways exist, 2) rate of distribution when weight of bait in the hopper changes, 3) degree of pulverization of pelletized bait before distribution, 4) precision of control over hopper opening of the distribution box, 5) clogging of hopper opening by irregular pellet sizes, and 6) throwing distance and pattern of distribution by the spreader.

Burrow-builder equipment has been used successfully in some forest and agronomic crops for distribution of grain bait (Anonymous, 1957, 1968); however, they have not been very useful in orchards because of the wide variation in soil type, sod density, and rock content.

Combination of Control Methods

The use of toxicants, cultivation, herbicide strips, barriers, close mowing, and predators may have additive or counterproductive effects on reducing populations. The application of broadcast bait or ground-cover sprays to cultivated or herbicided strips may greatly reduce the exposure of the population to the chemical. Integration of the rodenticide program with regard to the cultural system is extremely important for good results. Even though the use of cultural programs may reduce the vole hazard, the costs associated with the cultural program are questionable if chemical control is required (Byers, in press).

Environmental Hazards and Chemical Residues

The hazards of using rodenticides in low-acreage, high-valued crops is often confused with large acreage usage such as in forest or other areas where wildlife may have a high priority in the scheme of things (Anthony and Fisher, 1977; Bailey et al., 1970). Simply plowing a field, cultivating an orchard, or picking fruit in an orchard interrupts and disturbs more existing wildlife than the application of a rodenticide. Only recently has man become aware or concerned about the encroachment of houses, buildings, and concrete on agricultural crop and forest lands. Orchard acreage has not changed in the U.S. in the last 30 years even though production has increased. I suggest that the problems associated with wildlife are much more affected by housing, industrial zoning, highway construction, and increasing human population levels than the use of rodenticides for a specific low-acreage high-valued crop. Toxicants used to kill mammalian pests may have some degree of risk, depending on how they are used, to other wildlife present. We must recognize that cultural practices may affect wild animal populations to a much greater extent than chemicals; overreaction to some wildlife kill may not be justified. Proper labelling and use-patterns of rodenticides may require the acceptance of some reasonable risks when costs or production benefits are significant.

The current use of most rodenticides in orchards during the dormant season has been classified as non-food usage because they are not applied directly to the edible plant part during the growing season and are not translocated through plants. Some crops such as artichokes, vegetables, grains, and hay require food-usage labels or specific application directions to avoid contact with the food product.

Of the toxicants used as a ground-cover spray in orchards, Endrin has been the most toxic and persistent. Much controversy surrounded the use of this material after its clearance in 1956 (Driggers, 1972; Eadie, 1961). Regardless, Endrin was used widely throughout the world for about 15–20 years. Many European countries and some states of the United States since banned its use for vole control. Poor handling of empty containers and Endrin spills into farm ponds or streams leading to larger bodies of water resulted in some fish kills and a "bad name" for this material. However, when Endrin was used according to labeled directions, few if any problems were documented.

The acute toxicant Zn_3P_2 has been considered one of the more safe secondary hazard toxicants. Bell and Dimmick (1975) showed little hazard to red and gray foxes and great horned owls that fed on prairie voles poisoned with Zn_3P_2. This compound was limited in its use for vole control to a single treatment because of its taste-aversion properties, which produce bait shyness in the surviving population. In addition, only recently have formulations of Zn_3P_2 been available (ZP Rodent Bait from Bell Labs) that are sufficiently effective to be considered good field rodenticides.

The potential for primary or secondary hazards of the anticoagulants to non-target animals was demonstrated in the laboratory (Evans and Ward, 1967; Mendenhall and Pank, 1980), but evidence for significant primary or secondary hazards to pets and wildlife under proper label use patterns in the field has not been demonstrated nor compared to existing toxicants such as zinc phosphide (Kaukeinen, 1982). Certainly any toxicant poses a risk or hazard under some circumstances or with improper usage. The degree of hazard and its value to society must be kept in proper perspective with existing technology.

Because of the increased cost of obtaining federal approval for minor-use rodenticides and the low potential profit for chemical companies, the continued development of safer and more effective rodenticides has been greatly curtailed in the last 10–15 years. Obviously, when new rodenticide development is inhibited, older and inferior technology must be relied upon.

Increasing EPA requirements for chemical-fate and non-target hazard evaluation of agricultural rodenticides has caused chemical companies to apply for state permits. Because of the sporadic use pattern of most agricultural rodenticides on high-valued, low-acreage crops, state labels have been important to the introduction of new toxicants, which allows companies to sell the product while continuing to collect data on various aspects of its use pattern.

Concluding Remarks

Effective rodent-control methodology for use in agriculture has not developed as rapidly as insect, disease, and weed-control methodology for several reasons. First, rodents affect crops more sporadically and inflict less damage in major agricultural crops. Second, because rodents are on a high evolutionary scale, chemical-control agents are more likely to be hazardous to other mammals or man. Third, the profitability of a new agricultural rodenticide may not warrant chemical-company research and development costs considering the limited and diverse markets for such products. Fourth, the organization of animal control agencies with the U.S. government is within the Department of Interior, whose primary responsibility is conservation of wildlife. The U.S. Department of Agriculture has the primary responsibility to develop methods for crop protection from pests but does not have the responsibility in cases in which wildlife is involved. In the past, most rodent-control efforts have been crash programs designed to find an immediate and economical solution to an agricultural pest problem. Even though overlapping responsibility should exist between the U.S. Department of Agriculture (USDA) and the U.S. Department of Interior (USDI), the USDA does not have a pest-mammal control section. Instead, commodity-oriented specialists within the Land Grant state universities have been pressured in the past by agricultural groups to find methods of control. Even though animal biologists and ecologists may be equipped better to develop new and innovative technology, in the past they did not address the problem with vigor. The organization of wildlife damage-control responsibilities within the universities also does not encourage the development of control technology since most wildlife departments are more conservation minded. In addition, since no direct relationship exists between professional wildlife specialists and growers, the luxury of not having to solve an immediate pest problem exists. If effective animal control methods are to be developed, we must recognize that long periods of time, financial commitment, and priority reorganization will be required before cost effective, easily applied methods are available.

Literature Cited

Anonymous. 1957. Orchard mouse control. U.S. Dept. Interior, U.S. Fish Wildl. Serv., Boston, Massachusetts, 13 pp.

———. 1968. Orchard mice . . . the underground suboteurs. Amer. Fruit Grower, 88:17–19, 26.

Anthony, R. G., and A. R. Fisher. 1977. Wildlife damage in orchards—a need for better management. Wildl. Soc. Bull., 5:107–112.

Bailey, S., P. J. Bunyan, C. M. Jennings, and A. Taylor. 1970. Hazards to wildlife from the use of DDT in orchards. Pesticide Sci., 1:66–69.

Bailey, V. 1924. Breeding, feeding, and other life habits of meadow voles (*Microtus*). J. Agric. Res., 27:523–541.

Barden, J. A., et al. 1982. Virginia spray bulletin for commercial tree fruit growers. Virginia Polytech. Inst. and State Univ. Coop. Ext. Serv. Bull., 219: 15–16.

Batzli, G. O., and F. A. Pitelka. 1970. Influence of meadow mouse populations on California grassland. Ecology, 51:1027–1039.

Bell, H. B., and R. W. Dimmick. 1975. Hazard to predators feeding on prairie voles killed with zinc phosphide. J. Wildl. Mgmt., 39:816–819.

Benjamini, L. 1982. Biocontrol of rodents: the use of immunosuppressants as a control agent. Pp. 22, *in* Abstracts of papers, Third Internatl. Theriol. Congr. (A. Myllymäki and E. Pulliainen, eds.). Helsinki, Finland, 313 pp.

Bode, W. M., et al. 1981. Tree fruit production guide. Pennsylvania State Univ. Coop. Ext. Bull., 88 pp.

Byers, R. E. 1974*a*. Pine mouse control in apple orchards. Mountaineer Grower, 335:3–13.

———. 1974*b*. Susceptibility of apple and peach stems to attack by pine voles. Hortscience, 9:190–191.

———. 1975*a*. A rapid method for assessing pine vole control in orchards. Hortscience, 10:391–392.

———. 1975*b*. Effect of hand baits and ground sprays on pine vole activity. Hortscience, 10:122–123.

———. (ed.). 1977*a*. Proceedings of the first eastern pine and meadow vole symposium (R. Byers, ed.). Winchester, Virginia, 113 pp.

———. 1977*b*. Pine vole control research in Virginia. Pp. 88–100 *in* Proceedings of the first eastern pine and meadow vole symposium (R. Byers, ed.). Winchester, Virginia, 113 pp.

———. 1978. Performance of rodenticides for the control of pine voles in orchards. J. Amer. Soc. Hort. Sci., 103:65–69.

———. 1979*a*. Highlights of pine vole research in Virginia. Mountaineer Grower, 394:12–15.

———. 1979*b*. Highlights of the third eastern pine and meadow vole symposium. P. i, *in* Proceedings of the third eastern pine and meadow vole symposium (R. Byers, ed.). New Paltz, New York, 86 pp.

———. 1979*c*. Controls to stop voles. Amer. Fruit Grower, 99:14–15, 22–23.

———. 1980. Highlights of the fourth eastern pine and meadow vole symposium. P. i, *in* Proceedings of the fourth eastern pine and meadow vole symposium (R. Byers, ed.). Hendersonville, North Carolina, 91 pp.

———. 1981. Pine vole control with anticoagulant baits in orchards. J. Amer. Soc. Hort. Sci., 106:101–105.

———. In press. Economics of *Microtus* control in eastern U.S. orchards. *In* The organization and practice of vertebrate pest control (Tropical Pest Management, ed.). Center Overseas Pest Res., London, England.

Byers, R. E., and J. N. Cummins. 1977. Variations in susceptibility of apple stems to attack by pine voles. J. Amer. Soc. Hort. Sci., 102:201–203.

Byers, R. E., and R. S. Young. 1974. Cultural management of pine voles in apple orchards. Hortscience, 9:445–446.

———. 1975. Pine vole control with anticoagulant baits. J. Amer. Soc. Hort. Sci., 100:691–694.

———. 1978. Effect of orchard culture on pine vole activity. J. Amer. Soc. Hort. Sci., 103:625–626.

Byers, R. E., M. H. Merson, and S. D. Palmateer. 1982. Control of orchard voles with broadcast baits. J. Amer. Soc. Hort. Sci., 107:631–637.

Byers, R. E., R. S. Young, and R. D. Neely. 1976. Review of cultural and other control methods for reducing pine vole populations in apple orchards. Pp. 242–253, *in* Proceedings of the seventh vertebrate pest conference (C. Siebe, ed.). Monterey, California, 323 pp.

Caslick, J. W., and D. J. Decker. 1978. Control of wildlife damage in orchards and vineyards. Cornell Univ. Coop. Ext. Inf. Bull., 146:1–18.

Cengel, D. J., J. Estep, and R. L. Kirkpatrick. 1978. Pine vole reproduction in relation to food habits and body fat. J. Wildl. Mgmt., 42:822–833.

Chapman, D. G., and W. S. Overton. 1966. Estimating and testing differences between population levels by the Schnabel estimation method. J. Wildl. Mgmt., 30:173–180.

Cummings, M. W., and R. E. Marsh. 1978. Vertebrate pests of citrus. *In* The citrus industry (W. Reuther, L. D. Batchelor, and H. J. Webber, eds.). Univ. California Press, Berkeley, 4:237–273.

Cummins, J. N., H. S. Aldwinckle, and R. E. Byers. 1983. 'Novole,' an apple stock resistant to environmental hazards. Hortscience, 18:772–774.

DANA, R. H., AND D. H. SHAW. 1958. Meadow mouse control in holly. Bull. California Dept. Agric., 48:224-226.

DAVIS, D. E. 1976*a*. Management of pine voles. Pp. 270-275, *in* Proceedings of the seventh vertebrate pest conference (C. Siebe, ed.). Monterey, California, 323 pp.

———. 1976*b*. Management of pine voles. North Carolina Agric. Ext. Serv., Zool. Series, 9:1-2.

DIMMICK, R. W. 1978. Microtine rodents in Virginia pine plantations: their ecology and measures for population control. *In* Proceedings of the symposium on management of pine of the interior south, Knoxville, Tenn. USDA Forest Serv. Tech. Publ., SATP2:130-134.

DRIGGERS, B. F. 1972. Ground spraying with endrin to control orchard mice may result in severe tree damage by the meadow mouse, *Microtus*. Hort. News, 52:18-20.

EADIE, W. R. 1961. Control of wildlife damage to orchards. Cornell Univ. Ext. Bull., 1055:1-16.

EVANS, J., AND A. L. WARD. 1967. Secondary poisoning associated with anticoagulant-killed *Nutria*. J. Amer. Vet. Med. Assoc., 151:856-861.

FERGUSON, W. L. 1980. Rodenticide use in apple orchards. Pp. 1-8, *in* Proceedings of the fourth eastern pine and meadow vole symposium (R. Byers, ed.). Hendersonville, North Carolina, 91 pp.

GEYER, L. A., AND J. N. CUMMINS. 1980. Textural and taste influences on gnawing by pine voles. Pp. 43-49, *in* Proceedings of the fourth eastern pine and meadow vole symposium (R. Byers, ed.). Hendersonville, North Carolina, 91 pp.

GUTTERIDGE, N. J. A. 1972. Chemicals in rodent control. Chem. Soc. Rev., 1:381-409.

HAMILTON, W. J., JR. 1935. Field mouse and rabbit control in New York orchards. New York (Cornell) Ext. Bull., 338:1-24.

———. 1938. Life history notes on the northern pine mouse. J. Mamm., 19:163-170.

HARTGROVE, R. W., AND R. E. WEBB. 1973. The development of benzyprene hydrolase activity in endrin susceptible and resistant pine mice. Pesticide Biochem. Physiol., 3:61-65.

HORSFALL, F., JR. 1953. Mouse control in Virginia orchards. Virginia Polytech. Inst. Agric. Exp. Sta. Bull., 465:1-26.

———. 1956*a*. Pine mouse control with ground-sprayed endrin. Proc. Amer. Soc. Hort. Sci., 67:68-74.

———. 1956*b*. Rodenticidal effect on pine mice of endrin used as a ground spray. Science, 123:61.

HORSFALL, F., JR., R. E. WEBB, AND R. E. BYERS. 1974. Dual role of forbes and rodenticides in the ground spray control of pine mice. Pp. 112-125, *in* Proceedings of the sixth vertebrate pest conference (R. Marsh, ed.). Anaheim, California, 299 pp.

HOWARD, W. E., R. E. MARSH, AND C. W. CORBETT. 1982. Raptor perches: their influence on crop protection. P. 107, *in* Abstracts of papers, Third Internatl. Theriol. Congr. (A. Myllymäki and E. Pulliainen, eds.). Helsinki, Finland, 313 pp.

HUNTER, R. E., AND R. B. TUKEY. 1977. Mouse control in Washington orchards. Washington State Univ. Coop. Ext. Serv., EM 2650:1-9.

KAUKEINEN, D. 1982. A review of the secondary poisoning hazard potential to wildlife from the use of anticoagulant rodenticides. Pp. 151-158, *in* Proceedings of the tenth vertebrate pest conference (R. Marsh, ed.). Monterey, California, 245 pp.

LITTLEFIELD, E. W., W. J. SCHOOMAKER, AND D. B. COOK. 1946. Field mouse damage to coniferous plantations. J. Forestry, 44:745–749.

LUKE, J. E., AND R. J. SNETSINGER. 1975. Apple trees protected from voles with thiram. Science in agriculture, Pennsylvania State Univ. Agric. Exp. Sta., 23:7–8.

MARSH, R. E., AND W. E. HOWARD. 1976. New perspectives in rodent and mammal control. Pp. 317–329, *in* Proceedings of the third international biodegradation symposium (J. M. Sharpley and A. M. Kaplan, eds.). Applied Sci. Publ. Ltd., London, 1138 pp.

MEEHAN, A. P. 1980*a*. The rodenticidal activity of reserpine and related compounds. Pesticide Sci., 11:555–561.

———. 1980*b*. Effect of temperature, body size, bait age and long-term feeding response of mice to reserpine. Pesticide Sci., 11:562–567.

MENDENHALL, V. M., AND L. F. PANK. 1980. Secondary poisoning of owls by anticoagulant rodenticides. Wildl. Soc. Bull., 8:311–315.

MERSON, M. H., AND R. E. BYERS. 1981. Laboratory efficacy of some commercial zinc phosphide baits used for control of meadow and pine voles in orchards. Hortscience, 16:49–51.

———. In press. Pellet size and the effectiveness of rodenticides against orchard *Microtus*. *In* The organization and practice of vertebrate pest control (Tropical Pest Management, eds.). Center Overseas Pest Res., London, England.

MERSON, M. H., R. E. BYERS, AND D. KAUKEINEN. 1984. Residues of the rodenticide brodifacoum in voles and raptors after orchard treatment. J. Wildl. Mgmt., 48:212–216.

MORRISON, H. E. 1953. The meadow mouse (*Microtus californicus*) problem in Sacramento County. California Dept. Agric. Bull., 42:59–62.

MUEGGLER, W. F. 1967. Voles damage big sagebrush in southwestern Montana. J. Range Mgmt., 20:88–91.

PIPER, S. E. 1908. Mouse plagues and their control and prevention. Yearb. U.S. Dept. Agric., Government Printing Office, Washington, D.C., pp. 301–310.

———. 1928. The mouse infestation of Buena Vista Lake basin. Monthly Bull., California Dept. Agric., Sacramento, California, 17:538–560.

SARTZ, R. S. 1970. Mouse damage to young plantations in southwestern Wisconsin. J. Forestry, 68:88–89.

SPENCER, D. A. 1958. Preliminary investigation of the Northwestern *Microtus* irruption. Special Rept., Denver Wildl. Res. Lab., 13 pp. mimeo.

———. 1959. Biological and control aspects, the Oregon meadow vole irruption 1957–1958. Oregon State Coll., Corvallis, Oregon, 9 pp. mimeo.

STEHN, R. A., E. A. JOHNSON, AND M. E. RICHMOND. 1980. An antibiotic rodenticide for pine voles in orchards. J. Wildl. Mgmt., 44:275–280.

SULLIVAN, W. T. 1979. Cost of controlling pine voles by different methods. Pp. 66–68, *in* Proceedings of the third eastern pine and meadow vole symposium (R. Byers, ed.). New Paltz, New York, 86 pp.

TIETJEN, H. P. 1969. Orchard mouse control—a progress report. Ann. Rept., Massachusetts Fruit Growers Assoc., North Amherst, Massachusetts, 7:60–66.

WEBB, R. E., AND F. HORSFALL, JR. 1967. Endrin resistance in the pine vole. Science, 156:1762.

WEBB, R. E., W. C. RANDOLPH, AND F. HORSFALL, JR. 1972. Hepatic benzpyrene hydroxylase activity in endrin susceptible and resistant pine mice. Life Sci., 11:477–483.

WEBB, R. E., R. W. HARTGROVE, W. C. RANDOLPH, V. J. PETRELLA, AND F. HORSFALL, JR. 1973. Toxicity studies in endrin-susceptible and resistant strains of pine mice. Toxicol. Appl. Pharmacol., 25:42–47.

WHITE, L. 1965. Biological and ecological considerations in meadow mouse population management. Bull. California Dept. Agric., 54:161–171.

WOODSIDE, A. M., R. N. JEFFERSON, R. C. MOORE, AND E. H. GLASS. 1942. Control of field mice in apple orchards. Virginia Polytech. Inst., Virginia Agric. Exp. Sta. Bull., 344:1–16.

WYSOLMERSKI, J. C., R. E. BYERS, AND J. N. CUMMINS. 1980. Laboratory evaluation of some *Malus* clones for susceptibility to girdling by pine voles. J. Amer. Soc. Hort. Sci., 105:675–677.

LABORATORY MANAGEMENT AND PATHOLOGY

FRANK F. MALLORY AND

ROBERT A. DIETERICH

Abstract

THIS chapter discusses and describes laboratory management procedures and possible pathogens associated with the genus *Microtus*.

The successful maintenance of active breeding colonies is outlined with respect to housing, cleaning, feeding, breeding and photoperiod, temperature, and humidity. Surgical procedures are discussed also.

A literature survey indicates that this genus may be host to a wide variety of pathogens, including 15 viral diseases, 13 bacterial diseases, three protozoal diseases, and one fungal disease. In addition, 28 varieties of neoplasms and approximately 22 constitutional disorders have been described.

Although the number of pathogens associated with these microtines should concern us all, ten years of laboratory experience supports the conclusion that pathogenic problems in colonies and personnel are minimal, and that voles have many characteristics which make them ideal laboratory mammals.

Introduction

Although small mammal populations have been studied since the turn of the century under natural conditions (Elton, 1942), the last decade has witnessed a major shift in research emphasis. Increasingly, wild species have been introduced to the laboratory and raised under artificial conditions. Among the more popular are a group of rodents of the subfamily *Microtinae,* genus *Microtus,* which are readily available by live-trapping. As indicated in Table 1, almost

TABLE 1
LABORATORY MANAGEMENT OF *Microtus* SPECIES

Species	Caging (cm)	Bedding	Nesting material	Frequency of cleaning	Photoperiod	Temperature (C°)	Food	References
M. abbreviatus	20.3 × 20.3 × 7.6 fiberglass	Sawdust	Facial tissue	Weekly	16L:8D	20	Barley, sprouts, carrots, sunflower seeds	Morrison et al. (1977*a*)
M. californicus	23 × 38 × 23 metal	Sawdust	Cotton	ND	12L:12D	21–27	Rabbit pellets	Batzli et al. (1977)
	Metal tubs	Soil and peat	Cotton	3–6 weeks	17L:7D	4.4–27	Mouse breeder chow, barley, carrots, lettuce, sunflower seeds, apples	Colvin and Colvin (1970)
M. longicaudus	Gallon cans, metal terraria	Soil	Cotton	ND	16L:8D	−12–17	Rabbit chow, apples	Jannett (1974)
	Metal tubs	Soil and peat	Cotton	3–6 weeks	17L:7D	4.4–27	Mouse breeder chow, barley, carrots, lettuce, sunflower seeds, apples	Colvin and Colvin (1970)
M. miurus	20.3 × 20.3 × 7.6 fiberglass	Sawdust	Facial tissue	Weekly	16L:8D	20	Barley sprouts	Morrison et al. (1977*a*)
M. montanus	29 × 19 × 13	ND	ND	ND	16L:8D	ND	Rabbit pellets	Kenney et al. (1977)

TABLE 1
CONTINUED

Species	Caging (cm)	Bedding	Nesting material	Frequency of cleaning	Photoperiod	Temperature (C°)	Food	References
	29 × 19 × 13	San-i-cel	Nestlet	ND	16L:8D (Day-night reversal)	Constant	Rabbit pellets, lettuce	Gray et al. (1976)
	Metal tubs	Soil and peat	Cotton	3–6 wks	17L:7D	4.4–27	Mouse breeder chow, barley, carrots, lettuce, sunflower seeds, apples	Colvin and Colvin (1970)
	ND	ND	ND	ND	Constant	Constant	Wheat sprouts, rat chow	Hinkley (1966)
M. ochrogaster	33 × 20.3 × 27.9 metal	Sawdust	Grass, hay	As necessary	12L:12D	22.2	Rabbit chow, lettuce, grass, clover	Richmond and Conaway (1969)
	20 × 35 × 15 metal	Sawdust	Cotton	ND	12L:12D	21–27	Rabbit pellets	Batzli et al. (1977)
	56 × 18 × 12 plastic	Sawdust	Cotton, straw	ND	16L:8D	ND	Rat chow, rabbit pellets	Stehn and Jannett (1980)
	ND	ND	ND	2 weeks	16L:8D	ND	Mouse chow, lettuce, oats	Kenney et al. (1977)

TABLE 1
CONTINUED

Species	Caging (cm)	Bedding	Nesting material	Frequency of cleaning	Photo-period	Tempera-ture (C°)	Food	References
	40 × 25 × 15	Sawdust	Straw	ND	ND	ND	Rabbit chow	Martin et al. (1976)
	20 × 20 × 40 wire	Sawdust	Cotton	ND	16L:8D	ND	Rabbit chow	McGuire and Getz (1981)
M. oeconomus	85 × 16 × 15 fiberglass	Sawdust	Facial tissue	Weekly	16L:8D	20	Mouse breeder chow, wheat germ, oats, carrots, barley sprouts	Dieterich and Preston (1977*b*)
M. oregoni	Metal tubs	Soil peat	Cotton	3–6 weeks	17L:7D	4.4–27	Mouse breeder chow, barley, carrots, lettuce, sunflower seeds, apples	Colvin and Colvin (1970)
M. pennsylvanicus	85 × 16 × 15 fiberglass	Sawdust	Facial tissue	Weekly	16L:8D	20	Mouse breeder chow, oats, wheat germ, barley sprouts, carrots	Dieterich and Preston (1977*a*)
	ND	ND	ND	ND	14L:10D	22	Rat, mouse and hamster chow	Imel and Amann (1979)

TABLE 1
CONTINUED

Species	Caging (cm)	Bedding	Nesting material	Frequency of cleaning	Photoperiod	Temperature (C°)	Food	References
	28.5 × 17.5 × 12.5 plastic	Sawdust	Cotton	Biweekly	18L:6D	25	Rat chow, oats, carrots	Clulow and Mallory (1970, 1974)
	29 × 19 × 13 plastic	Corn grit	Cotton	Biweekly	14L:10D	22	Alfalfa pellets, salt cubes	Lee et al. (1970)
	ND	ND	ND	2 weeks	16L:8D	ND	Mouse chow, lettuce, oats	Kenney et al. (1977)
	Gallon cans, metal terraria	Soil	Cotton	ND	16L:8D	−12–17	Rabbit chow, apples	Jannett (1974)
	ND	ND	ND	ND	14L:10D	24	Mouse chow, sunflower seeds	Pasley and McKinney (1973)
	29 × 18 × 12.5 plastic	Corn grit	None	ND	16L:8D	20	Guinea pig chow	Webster et al. (1981)
M. pinetorum	56 × 18 × 12 plastic	Sawdust	Cotton, straw	ND	16L:8D	ND	Rat chow, rabbit pellets	Stehn and Jannett (1980)
	30 × 62 × 41 glass	Sawdust	None	ND	12L:12D	16–18	Rat chow, guinea pig pellets, sunflower seeds	Schadler (1980)

Abbreviation: ND, no data.

half of all the Nearctic species, as defined by Hall (1981), have been reared successfully in the laboratory during the past ten years. In view of the current interest in rodent population fluctuations, detailed information on demographic parameters is needed. Although certain aspects of changes in abundance can be studied in the field, information on genetic, physiologic, reproductive, and behavioral indices can often be understood best from breeding and experimentation in captivity (Richmond and Conaway, 1969). Thus, the first objective of this chapter is to review the current practices of laboratory management for the genus *Microtus* and to make recommendations that can be used as a general guide for future researchers. The second objective is to examine our knowledge of pathogens and pathogenic conditions associated with *Microtus,* which, in addition to being a requirement for sound laboratory management, is especially important as more and more people may be exposed to these pathogens under confined conditions.

Laboratory Management

The easiest means of transport from the field is to carry the animal in the live-trap in which it was caught; however, if long distances are involved, special transport cages may be necessary. On reaching the laboratory, animals should be housed individually in cages containing bedding and cover. Additional cover appears to reduce the incidence of stress-related mortality, which can affect up to 50% of the animals within the first 2 weeks after capture. Animals housed together often fight, aggravating stress-related problems (Mallory, pers. observ.). A variety of both dry and fresh foods should be introduced to the cage, including the commercial chow on which the colony is maintained. Over a 2-week period, selection of foods should be reduced to that of the commercial chow. Water should be provided in a bottle with a lick tube and in a small dish in the cage, as it takes a little time for some individuals to learn to use standard water bottles. After a few days the dish can be removed. Recently captured animals should be quarantined from the colony for a 2-week period, during which time the cages should be cleaned twice a week. This procedure removes most ectoparasites, which are discarded in bedding, and allows one to assess the health of individual animals. Handling should be kept to a minimum, and photoperiod and temperature should be intermediate between that of the colony and the field situation.

Records

Although recorded information will vary with the desires and needs of each researcher, a general description of standard procedure may be of value. Records should be kept in both a daily log book and on cards attached to each cage. This duplication, though tedious, is often invaluable when important data are lost in one or the other system (most frequently the card is lost). Generally, each individual is identified by species, number, and sex, and where known, date of birth, date of weaning, and number of mother. In females, dates of pairing with males, dates of parturition, and litter sizes at parturition and weaning are important, and in males, pairing dates and offspring produced are often of value. Records should be used by the researcher to minimize inbreeding and genetic drift within the colony, unless otherwise desired. Wild caught animals should be introduced to the colony at regular intervals to keep it as representative of the natural population as possible.

Housing, Cleaning, and Food

As evident from Table 1, microtines have been maintained successfully in a wide array of containers, ranging from gallon cans (Jannett, 1974) to glass aquaria (Schadler, 1980). However, the majority of researchers have found standard plastic mouse cages with wire tops and a floor area ranging between 500 to 1,000 cm^2 most convenient.

In addition, breeding pairs and nursing females with litters should be placed in larger cages; solid bottom cages are preferred over those with wire (Richmond and Conaway, 1969). Sawdust or wood shavings approximately 2 cm deep is the most common bedding, although other absorbent materials such as San-i-cel, corn grit, hay, peat, and soil may be used. Because these animals are semi-fossorial and spend a considerable amount of time digging, the finer bedding materials have the disadvantage of creating a dust problem (Mallory, pers. observ.).

The most commonly used material for nesting and cover is cotton batting, although facial tissue (Dieterich and Preston, 1977*a*) and straw (Stehn and Jannett, 1980) have been employed. A number of recent researchers have refrained from using nesting material (Schadler, 1980; Webster et al., 1981), which has been our preference for the past five years, because cotton can become wrapped around the limbs of neonates resulting in amputation or maiming (Mallory, pers. observ.).

The frequency of cage cleaning (Table 1) may be from twice a week (Clulow and Mallory, 1970) to whenever necessary (Richmond and Conaway, 1969). Problems associated with changing cages are generally ones of disturbance and the negative effect it has on the pregnancy rate in the colony and the survival of neonates. Richmond and Conaway (1969) noted that female *M. ochrogaster* with neonates often killed their offspring after having their cage cleaned. In their laboratory, the incidence of this phenomenon was lowered by leaving a small amount of soiled bedding in the new cage. Mallory and Brooks (1980) demonstrated that handling gravid females of the lemming, *Dicrostonyx groenlandicus* (as one would do during cage changes), significantly reduced the number of pregnancies reaching parturition. Although the frequency of cage cleaning may vary with researcher and experimental design, current data suggest that colony productivity will be increased if gravid and lactating females are disturbed as little as possible. Cages should be washed according to standard mouse-colony procedure with a disinfecting detergent and rinsing (Les, 1966).

In all colonies studied, food and water were provided ad lib., and the majority of researchers provided their animals with both dry and fresh food (Table 1). Commercial dry food is more convenient than other combinations, and a number of different types have proved successful, including standard mouse chow, mouse breeder chow, rat and hamster chow, and rabbit and guinea-pig pellets. Batzli (pers. comm.) has suggested that rabbit and guinea-pig pellets, composed largely of alfalfa and having high fiber and low fat content, are preferable to rat or mouse chows (Batzli, this volume). Fresh food may include barley, oats, barley and wheat sprouts, sunflower seeds, carrots, lettuce, and apples. Supplements of fresh food are recommended, because reproduction is enhanced in *M. montanus* fed fresh plant greens or their extracts (Berger et al., 1981; Hinkley, 1966; Negus and Pinter, 1965, 1966; Pinter and Negus, 1965; Sanders et al., 1981). In one colony of *M. pennsylvanicus,* salt cubes were made available (Lee et al., 1970).

Photoperiod, Temperature, and Humidity

Control of photoperiod is essential if high rates of reproduction and sexual maturity are to be sustained throughout the year. The majority of successful colonies have been maintained on a long-day photoperiod ranging between 14 and 18 h of light/24-h period (Table 1). No colonies were given less than 12 h of light/day. Imel and Amann (1979) demonstrated that reproductive function and body weight in *M. pennsylvanicus* were significantly greater at a 16L:8D photoperiod, and were more favorable than 14L:10D and 18L:6D, at 22°C. Because evidence supports the conclusion that members of the genus *Microtus* are long-day breeders (Clarke and Kennedy, 1967; Iverson and Turner, 1974; Petterborg, 1978; Vaughan et al., 1973), the 16L:8D photoperiod may be best for most mid-latitude species. Light intensities inside cages of 40–75 lux and 100 lux were reported by Lee et al. (1970) and Imel and Amann (1979), respectively. Virtually no work has been done on the effect of different spectral emissions. Temperature of colonies generally varied between 20 and 25°C (range −12 to 27°C); Richmond and Conaway (1969) maintained a constant humidity of 65 ± 5%.

Breeding and Weaning Procedures

A survey of the literature indicates that most laboratories house their breeders as single pairs rather than in mixed groups. Stud males have been left successfully with gravid females throughout gestation and lactation (Morrison et al., 1977*a*, 1977*b*), often in the presence of previous litters. Other researchers removed the males on day 7 post coitum (Imel and Amann, 1979) or after the birth of the litter (Batzli et al., 1977). Maintaining a pair together is advantageous in that females most often mate at post-partum estrus, which occurs on the first day after parturition (Hasler, 1975). Two other factors that can reduce reproductive output in microtine colonies are pregnancy failure, which occurs when pregnant females are exposed to strange males (Clulow and Langford, 1971; Mallory and Clulow, 1977; Schadler, 1981; Stehn and Richmond, 1975), and infanticide, which can occur when strange males or females are introduced into cages holding females and their neonates (Mallory and Brooks, 1978, 1980; Webster et al., 1981). Laboratory personnel should be aware of these potential problems, which may become important during cage changes, when establishing new pairings, or when introducing new animals to the colony.

Weaning young from the maternal cage usually is accomplished at approximately 3 weeks post partum (range 17 to 35 days); however, in some instances up to three successive litters were left with the parents (Richmond and Conaway, 1969). The size and composition of post-weaning groups of immature animals has been shown to significantly influence rate of maturation and propensity to mate. Immature *M. californicus, M. ochrogaster* (Batzli et al., 1977), and *M. pinetorum* (Schadler, 1980) exhibited suppressed sexual development and growth when housed in groups. In addition, female *M. ochrogaster* developed the least when paired with littermate weanling males as compared to non-littermate adult males (Hasler and Nalbandov, 1974), and incest avoidance may occur in this species when siblings are housed together (McGuire and Getz, 1981). Thus, to maximize colony productivity, immature males should be housed individually and immature females should be paired with non-related adult males or non-littermate immature males (Baddaloo and Clulow, 1981; Batzli et al., 1977).

Other Procedures

Surgical procedures such as adrenalectomy, splenectomy, vasectomy, and castration have been successfully performed on microtines with minimum equipment (Richmond and Conaway, 1969). Both ether and sodium pentabarbital have been used successfully as anesthetics. Sodium pentabarbital at a dosage of 0.06 mg/g body weight administered intraperitoneally is sufficient to keep an animal immobilized for 3 h. Lower dosages have little effect and higher dosages increase mortality. Post-operative care requirements are minimal; however, a heat lamp over recovering animals increases survival.

Although ectoparasites are generally eliminated by the cleaning procedures described above, the follicle-inhabiting mite, *Psorergates simplex,* has been a problem on occasion (Lee and Horvath, 1969). Infestations can be suppressed successfully by treating animals and cages with a 2% aqueous solution of a wetable powder containing 15% Aramite [2-(p-tertbutylphenoxy)isopropyl 2-chloroethyl sulfite] or low-toxicity flea powder (Dieterich, pers. observ.).

Finally, all personnel regularly exposed to microtine breeding colonies should be required to wear lab coats and gloves for handling animals and washing cages. Standard tetanus-polio combination and rabies inoculations should be given to reduce risk of infection.

Pathology

Although *Microtus* is the most widely studied genus of microtines in North America, there is a surprising paucity of information concerning pathogens associated with these rodents. Indeed, in Europe and the USSR, a much greater effort has been made to understand the etiology and epizootics of infectious diseases and the role microtines play as vectors or reservoirs. Because most small mammals are studied by mammalogists lacking training in medical procedures, and because veterinarians and medical personnel tend to apply their energy and resources to more economically important species, the majority of specimens collected are discarded before a pathological examination is made, resulting in the loss of information in a potentially important area.

Viral Infections

Rabies.—Rabies is an acute and usually fatal infectious disease of the central nervous system caused by a virus which travels from the site of infection via the peripheral nervous system to the central nervous system; it appears to persist as a salivary gland infection in nature. All warm-blooded animals are susceptible (Sikes, 1970). The virus is usually transmitted by biting; however, infection through aerosol, nasal, and oral exposure also has been confirmed in both carnivores and rodents (Casals, 1940; Fischman and Ward, 1968; Ramsden and Johnston, 1975; Soave, 1966).

The symptoms of the disease may take one of two forms. Animals exhibiting the furious form of rabies initially become anorexic, apprehensive, and nervous prior to an excitatory phase during which they become restless and vicious. They bite most objects in the immediate vicinity, although they have difficulty chewing and swallowing. During this time the saliva contains the greatest amount of virus, although it is usually present throughout the entire course of the disease. Subsequently, the strong furious actions slowly subside and incoordination and muscle tremors are often apparent. The final stage usually includes convulsions, followed by paralysis and death. Animals with the dumb form of rabies usually exhibit the later symptoms of the disease, incoordination, paralysis, and death.

Post-mortum examination of the central nervous system usually identifies histopathologic lesions concentrated in the pons, medulla, brain stem, and thalamus (Sikes, 1970). Negri bodies, which are cytoplasmic inclusions in the neurons, are considered positive proof of rabies infection. Without these inclusions, a definite diagnosis cannot be made as lesions produced by other viral encephalitides are similar.

Considerable attention has been given to epizootological studies of rabies in both domestic and large wild mammals, and current evidence suggests that the disease is largely transmitted by direct contact with, and wounds from, infected individuals, during high population densities (Sikes, 1970). However, very little research has been conducted on species that may be permanent asymptomatic hosts of the virus. Although our literature survey found no information associating rabies with *Microtus* in North America, significant research has been done in Europe. Rabies virus has been isolated in small mammals in Czechoslovakia, from a region where fox epizootics occurred frequently, and from another area where rabies was not reported for a considerable time (Sodja et al., 1971). In this study, 103 of 556 *M. arvalis* and 14 of 29 *M. agrestis* were found to be rabies carriers, although symptoms were not apparent. In the enzootic and control areas, respectively, 22.5% and 12.8% of *M. arvalis* were diagnosed as positive; the incidence appeared to be higher in animals caught during the winter months. In a subsequent 4-year study, Sodja et al. (1973) isolated 28 rabies virus strains from the brain, salivary glands, and brown fat of 2,162 small rodents (88% *Microtus arvalis*). The identity of the isolates with rabies virus was demonstrated by a positive direct immunofluorescence reaction, inhibition by specific serum, and a serum neutralization test. The various strains were both cerebrally and extraneurally pathogenic for the usual laboratory animals and for dogs and foxes. Ramsden and Johnston (1975) demonstrated that red foxes (*Vulpes vulpes*) and striped skunks (*Mephitis mephitis*), which feed largely on small mammals, died or developed serum neutralizing antibody when fed mice infected with rabies virus. In addition, tooth-marks from small mammals have been observed on dead fox carcasses later diagnosed as rabid (D. H. Johnston, pers. comm.). From these results it is reasonable to hypothesize that *Microtus* and other microtines may be an asymptomatic reservoir for rabies, which can be transmitted to predators by ingestion, causing major outbreaks and epizootics to occur in these populations.

Rabies has public-health as well as agricultural-economic significance. In 1966–1967, 1,336 rabies-caused human deaths were reported; 1,980,238 people received post-exposure antirabies prophylaxis, and 175 paralytic accidents were attributed to vaccine treatment (World Health Organization, 1967). In addition, hundreds of millions of dollars are lost annually owing to loss of livestock. For these reasons, researchers working with microtines should take appropriate precautions and a major effort should be made to assess the role of microtines in the epidemiology of this disease.

Lymphocytic choriomeningitis (LCM).—This disease appears to be worldwide in distribution and occurs naturally in mice and other wild rodents (Hotchin and Benson, 1970; Morris and Alexander, 1951). It is occasionally transmitted to man, causing a nonfatal meningitis. Susceptible animals infected with LCM virus often die from meningeal or visceral causes, although the carrier condition is often common and the virus may become disseminated throughout a breeding colony, with most infections being subclinical (Maurer, 1964).

Symptoms appear in susceptible *Mus* after 5–6 days of inoculation. The animal becomes hunched in posture, eyes half-closed, and often has convulsions. The rear limbs often become paralyzed and rigid prior to death. Naturally infected animals may show little or no illness or a temporary wasting syndrome as has been demonstrated in *M. agrestis* and *Clethrionomys glareolus* (Dalldorf, 1943; Findlay and Stern, 1936). The virus is distributed widely in the infected host and has been recovered from most tissues including brain, blood, spleen, lungs, blood marrow, adrenal glands, lymph nodes, kidney, liver, and testes. Wild rodents appear to be the primary vertebrate host with ticks, mites, fleas, mosquitos, and other bloodsucking arthropods acting as vectors. LCM virus also has been transmitted to mice by direct contact with the conjunctiva, respiratory and digestive tracts, and intact skin (Maurer, 1964), and in man, handling of, or bites from, infected animals often produces infection. LCM is best controlled by sanitary measures in the colony and care taken in washing after handling animals.

Eastern (equine) encephalitis (EEV).—This virus is known to infect a wide range of mammals, birds, and reptiles; several species of mosquitos are believed to be the main arthropod vectors. Karstad (1970) found neutralizing antibody to EEV in six species of wild rodents; experimental inoculation of eight species of rodents from Wisconsin demonstrated that infections were readily induced when small doses of virus were administered by routes simulating natural exposure (Karstad et al., 1961). Sign of illness was absent and viremia was rare but detectable. Karstad (1970) concluded that eastern equine-encephalitis virus should be considered a possible cause of encephalitis in wild rodents, which may act as reservoirs for the disease.

Mice inoculated with equine encephalitis virus become paralytic and die between 2 and 6 days later. This disease is of significant socioeconomic importance because it can cause severe and often fatal encephalitis in man and horses, and epizootics in pheasants have been reported. Infants and children are most susceptible; symptoms include high fever, vomiting, drowsiness or coma, and severe convulsions (Feemster, 1938; Gittner and Shakan, 1933). In the most severe cases, death occurs within 3–5 days from onset; it also may occur later from complications. Survivors under 5 years of age often have mental retardation, periodic convulsions, and paralysis; survivors over 40 generally recover completely (James and Harwood, 1969).

Western (equine) encephalitis (WEV).—WEV is similar to EEV in its epidemiology and transmission (Karstad, 1970); however, it generally is not fatal in man. High mortality occurs in equines. Initially thought to be limited to the western United States, it now has been shown to be present from eastern Canada to Brazil. Symptoms of the disease are difficult to distinguish from other arbovirus-caused encephalitides. However, fever and drowsiness often accompanied by convulsions are common (James and Harwood, 1969).

St. Louis encephalitis (SLE).—Similar to the two previous forms of encephalitis, SLE has an active bird-mosquito cycle; wild rodents are implicated as secondary hosts (Henderson et al., 1962). The largest epidemic occurred in St. Louis in 1933, with 1,100 cases and more than 200 deaths; however, other outbreaks have occurred in most regions of the United States. The symptoms are similar to other encephalitides and in the east, older age groups appear more susceptible (James and Harwood, 1969).

Powassan virus.—This virus was first isolated in Ontario, Canada, from a fatal encephalitis case in 1958. Though widely distributed foci are recognized in nature, no subsequent clinical cases have been verified. The virus has been isolated from ticks of the genera *Dermacentor* and *Ixodes,* which are common throughout North America (Timm, this volume). Isolates and serological sampling reinforce the conclusion that wild rodents and lagomorphs are a major reservoir of this pathogen (James and Harwood, 1969).

Colorado tick fever virus (CTF).—CTF virus occurs in the Rocky Mountain states, the Black Hills of South Dakota, and in western Canada. It is transmitted by ticks of the genus *Dermacentor,* which are a common ectoparasite of mammals, including small rodents (James and Harwood, 1969; Timm, this volume). Clark et al. (1970) successfully isolated CTF virus from ticks collected on *Clethrionomys gapperi* and *Microtus longicaudus* in southwestern Montana, supporting the conclusion that small mammals may be reservoirs for the disease. Although no information was found describing the symptoms of this virus in microtines, humans experience fever, headache, and severe muscle pains 3–6 days after exposure to ticks. In children complications in the form of encephalitis and severe bleeding may occur. No lasting complications are reported (James and Harwood, 1969).

Enterovirus.—Main et al. (1976) reported the isolation of six viruses from *Clethrionomys gapperi* trapped in Massachusetts in 1969, two of which were similar to those identified from the same species by Whitney et al. (1970) from New York state. These isolates were related to an enterovirus isolated from *Microtus montanus* (Johnston, pers. comm.) trapped in Klamath County, Oregon, but were distinct from a strain found in *M. pennsylvanicus* in New York (Whitney et al., 1970). The pathology of these virions has not been described, however; generally, enteroviruses infect the gastro-intestinal tract and may cause diarrhea.

Herpesvirus.—A herpesvirus has been isolated and characterized from the kidney of *M. pennsylvanicus* (Melendez et al., 1973) and may be associated with interstitial nephritis in this species (Dieterich and Preston, 1977*b*).

Ectromelia virus (mouse pox).—Kaplan et al. (1980) reported the presence of this virus, which is highly contagious and often fatal in laboratory mice, in *Microtus agrestis* from Britain, where over half of the wild animals sampled had neutralizing antibodies. During the course of the disease in *Mus,* the virus multiplies in the cells of most organs. In the acute form, visceral lesions and hepatic necroses occur, with the animal dying within days, showing few external signs of illness. In susceptible colonies, 50–95% of the animals die.

Sendai virus (parainfluenza type I).—Antibodies were present in a large proportion of animals examined from Britain, including *M. agrestis* (Kaplan et al., 1980). Sendai virus infections of the respiratory tract destroyed the ciliated epithelium and caused congestion (Fenner et al., 1974); in the gastro-intestinal system it may produce diarrhea.

Theiler's mouse encephalomyelitis virus (GDIII).—Antibodies reacting to GDIII were detected in *M. agrestis* (Kaplan et al., 1980). In laboratory mice, infection usually causes unapparent intestinal infection.

Pneumonia virus of mice (PVM).—PVM antibodies have been identified in *M. agrestis* in Britain (Kaplan et al., 1980) and may be responsible for producing this disease in voles.

Reovirus III.—Antibodies which neutralize reovirus III have been identified in *M. agrestis* (Kaplan et al., 1980).

Bacterial Infections

Tularemia.—Tularemia is an acute, moderately severe infectious septicemia caused by the bacterium *Francisella tularensis.* It appears to be almost worldwide in distribution, affecting many species of mammals including man (Reilly, 1970). In the genus *Microtus,* it has been identified in *M. pennsylvanicus, M. californicus, M. montanus, M. oeconomus,* and *M. arvalis* (Murray, 1965; Rausch et al., 1969; Reilly, 1970). Clinical manifestations of tularemia are seldom evident and opportunities to observe the signs in nature are very limited, because infected animals are usually moribund or dead (Murray, 1965). In general, the gross and histopathological lesions from tularemia are tubercle-like nodules scattered in the liver, spleen, and lymph nodes, varying from pin-point size to large irregular foci, several mm in diameter. The liver may be dark bluish-red, enlarged; small white plaques may be evident in the lungs. Thromboses of small blood vessels are frequent.

Transmission of tularemia usually occurs as a result of blood sucking ectoparasites, especially mites and ticks (James and Harwood, 1969); however, flies, midges, fleas, mosquitoes, and lice also have been implicated (Reilly, 1970). Infection also has occurred owing to contact with infected vertebrates, inhalation of feces-contaminated dust, and ingestion of infected carcasses and contaminated water (Burroughs et al., 1945; Gorham, 1950; Maisky, 1945). In humans, the disease may take the form of a sudden fever, with severe pain affecting the lymph nodes. In susceptible individuals, septicemia may result in death from 4 to 14 days after exposure and pneumonic complications also may occur. Streptomycin is the usual antibiotic agent used to combat the disease (James and Harwood, 1969).

Sylvatic plague.—Plague is an acute infectious disease caused by the bacterium *Pasteurella pestis*; it primarily afflicts wild rodents. Few descriptions of the pathologic changes that occur in wild rodents have been published; however, it has been noted that a variety of manifestations of the disease result from the interaction of different hosts, vectors, and environmental conditions. McCoy (1911) defined three categories in the California ground squirrel (*Spermophilus beecheyi*): 1) acute plague—the animal dies in 3–5 days with hemorrhagic buboes and an enlarged spleen, but no macroscopic lesions develop on internal organs; 2) subacute plague—the animal dies at 6 or more days with caseous buboes, in the absence of hemorrhaging but in the presence of pinpoint nodular, necrotic foci in the spleen, liver, and lungs; and 3) residual plague—individuals survive and have enlarged lymph glands containing yellow purulent foci. Since McCoy's (1911) work, a latent form of plague has been described, which is characterized by an absence of gross lesions (Pollitzer, 1954); such asymptomatic infections are believed to be common especially among resistant genera like *Microtus*.

Microtus californicus and *M. montanus* are both susceptible to invasions of the organism but usually do not succumb either to natural or experimental inoculation of large numbers of plague bacilli (Olsen, 1970). Bacilli persist in *Microtus* and may produce unapparent infections. They often are taken up by the lymph nodes and transported to the viscera where they multiply prior to appearing in the blood and blood-filtering organs. Voles likely act as permanent reservoirs for this pathogen from which fleas become infected (Quan and Kartman, 1962). Studies of *M. californicus* have demonstrated that the proportion of individuals with positive sera can approach 100% in plague-prevalent regions (Hudson et al., 1972).

Sylvatic plague was first discovered in California; it now has been isolated from 57 rodent species in 15 western states as far east as Kansas, Oklahoma, and Texas, as well as Alberta, Saskatchewan, and northern Mexico (Olsen, 1970). Although plague is a disease of rodents and is transmitted by fleas, it has had a great influence on the course of history in the form of bubonic plague, characterized by epidemics that have decimated human populations of entire continents (James and Harwood, 1969). For this reason, all microtines should be handled with this in mind. Both sulfonamides and streptomycin are effective for treating the disease once contracted.

Pasteurellosis.—Pasteurellosis is an infectious disease of wild and domestic animals caused by the bacterium *Pasteurella multocida.* Its clinical manifestations vary, ranging from hemorrhagic septicemia to pneumonia, meningitis, mastitis, and arthritis (Rosen, 1970). Although it usually is associated with larger mammals, it was isolated from voles in the USSR (Ponomareva and Rodkevich, 1964), and epizootics were reported in *M. montanus* in Oregon (Murray, 1965). Clinical symptoms in wild animals are rarely observed and most infected animals are found dead, with nasal and oral mucous discharges. It most often affects the respiratory system, producing pneumonia and hemorrhages in the lungs, trachea, and nasal mucosa. If the bacterium enters the circulatory system, septicemia occurs and, on occasion, meningitis. The mode of transmission is not understood; however, it may be transmitted by carriers, or be present generally and only become pathogenic when individuals become stressed. Human infections develop when individuals are bitten (Rosen, 1970). Pasteurellosis is worldwide in distribution and of great importance to poultry, livestock, and mink industries. Antibiotics are used to treat individuals contracting this disease.

Pseudotuberculosis.—Pseudotuberculosis is an infectious disease caused by the bacterium *Pasteurella pseudotuberculosis,* which affects many visceral organs, especially the spleen, liver, lungs, and small intestine. Although Holarctic in distribution and found in most species of *Microtus,* including *M. mexicanus* (Wetzler, 1970), very little is known about its symptoms. Few wild animals become ill, or they die without notice, and as a result most information comes from zoological gardens or research institutions. Outbreaks in chinchillas were characterized by marked depression of activity, inappetence, anorexia, diarrhea, and death within several days. Histopathogenic observations indicate that hypertrophy of the mesenteric lymphatics occurs, and visceral nodules develop in the spleen, liver, ileocecal junction, and occasionally the lungs. Serofibrinous peritoneal fluid often is present. Diagnosis from clinical signs is virtually impossible; however, treatment is successful with a broad-spectrum antibiotic. Transmission appears to be via oral-fecal routes.

Tuberculosis.—Tuberculosis is a chronic infection due to the bacillus *Mycobacterium tuberculosis* and related species. The organism has a broad host range, including man, domestic animals, poultry, and many wild species (Winkler and Gale, 1970). Geographic distribution is essentially worldwide, although it is most predominant in temperate regions. Three varieties of *Mycobacterium tuberculosis* are recognized: *M. t. hominis, M. t. bovis,* and *M. t. avium.* There also is a vole bacillus, *Mycobacterium mycroti,* isolated from *Microtus agrestis* by Wells and Oxon (1937). The first description of tuberculous lesions in a wild vole (*M. arvalis*) was by Koch (1884). Tuberculosis starting with pulmonary infection results in multiple lesions in lung parenchyma and is accompanied by respiratory distress. Tuberculous bronchitis may progress to broncho-pneumonia and fatal respiratory collapse. Lymph glands often enlarge in the viscera and emaciation may be observed. Bacilli can be disseminated by infected animals via exhaled air, sputum, feces, urine, or milk. Jespersen (1975, 1976) has demonstrated that both *Microtus arvalis* and *M. agrestis* developed the disease when inoculated with *M. t. hominis* and *M. t. bovis,* although susceptibility was higher for *M. t. bovis.* Autopsy showed that infections of *M. t. bovis* caused lymph glands to be affected, and tubercles were frequently observed in the lungs but seldom the liver, spleen, or kidneys. Large numbers of bacilli were found in several organs, especially the lymph glands. *M. t. hominis* had little effect on lymph glands and the number of bacteria was few. Comparative experimental infection of voles with vole bacilli and the bovine tuberculosis organism produced similar generalized symptoms, except that bovine infections were of shorter duration and characterized by caseous lesions. Vole bacilli ran a longer course and produced non-caseated subcutaneous lesions (Winkler and Gale, 1970).

Tuberculosis is of significant socioeconomic importance. For this reason proper administration of laboratory procedures should be followed. Authorities generally agree that elimination rather than treatment of tuberculin-positive animals is the proper procedure. Standard tuberculin tests can be used to identify tuberculin-positive animals.

Erysipelas.—Erysipelas is a disease caused by the bacterium *Erysipelothrix rhusiopathiae.* This organism infects a large number of animals, domestic and wild, causing septicemia. The disease is of socioeconomic importance because it affects domestic sheep, pigs, turkeys, ducks, and pheasants, and should be a concern of those responsible for maintaining captive animals (Shuman, 1970). There are no specific symptoms associated with the disease except signs of acute illness (prostration, a thick exudate around the eyes, and a history of sudden death). Cutaneous lesions sometimes occur in domestic and wild animals and diagnosis requires post-mortem examination of infected tissue.

An epizootic of erysipelas was reported in *M. californicus* (Wayson, 1927); it has since been found in other North American rodents (Connell, 1954). Old World reports indicate that it has been identified in *M. oeconomus* (Khomyakov et al., 1970) and *M. arvalis,* in which it often reaches epizootic proportions (Shuman, 1970). It is not known specifically how the disease is transmitted; however, evidence suggests that direct ingestion may occur because it can persist free in nature. Ticks of the genera *Dermacentor* and *Ixodes,* mites, lice, house flies, and other insect vectors are implicated. Erysipelas appears to be worldwide in distribution and human infection can occur. Penicillin has been used successfully in treating domestic animals and would probably be suitable for wild species (Shuman, 1970).

Listeriosis.—As a zoonotic disease, listeriosis is becoming recognized as an important bacterial disease of man and domestic and wild animals. It is caused by the bacterium *Listeria monocytogenes,* which can produce a variety of pathologies, and is worldwide in distribution. The bacterium may cause encephalitis in domestic ruminants, septicemia in monogastric animals and birds, meningitis in man, abortion in many mammalian species, and other lesser disorders. It is found in 42 different mammals, 22 species of birds, in addition to fish, crustaceans, ticks, house flies, sewage sludge, and soil (Eveland, 1970). Isolates have been identified in the voles *M. montanus* (Bacon and Miller, 1958), *M. agrestis* (Levy, 1948), *M. arvalis* (Kratokhvil, 1953), and the lemmings *Lemmus trimu-*

cronatus and *Dicrostonyx groenlandicus* (Barrales, 1953; Magus, 1955; Nordland, 1959; Plummer and Byrne, 1950).

The characteristic lesions of the infection are well-defined, whitish-gray foci on the liver and spleen, lungs, and heart (Eveland, 1970). However, these are not essentially different from those of tularemia or pseudotuberculosis. Evidence suggests that listeriosis may be carried by many organisms and may become pathogenic only under stressful conditions (Barker et al., 1978; Nordland, 1959). Thus, the disease may be asymptomatic in most wild populations, which act as carriers, and only appear when occasional epizootics are triggered by demographic or environmental factors. Treatment is best accomplished by using broad-spectrum antibiotics.

Bordetella.—Bordetella bronchiseptica is a common infectious agent in domestic and laboratory animals, sometimes as the primary disease agent and other times as a secondary invader. The small bacillus can cause broncho-pneumonia and other respiratory infections and often is reported to complicate other diseases such as chronic pneumonia, canine distemper, and atrophic rhinitis in swine. In man, it occasionally causes a syndrome similar to whooping cough. In 1973, it was isolated from *M. montanus* found dead or dying in northern Utah (Jensen and Duncan, 1980). At necropsy, gross pathologic changes were confined to the lungs, which were congested and edematous. Histopathologic examination disclosed a considerable degree of atelectasis, and alveoli contained fluid, fibrin, inflammatory cells, and in some cases erythrocytes. Bacteria isolated from the voles killed seven of eight laboratory mice when one drop of broth culture was given by intranasal instillation. Although the data support the conclusion that *B. bronchiseptica* was the primary etiological agent, the outbreak of pulmonary disease may have been associated with other pathogens. The distribution of this pathogen is unknown (Jensen and Duncan, 1980).

Leptospirosis.—Leptospirosis is a group of infectious diseases of man and animals caused by small, coiled, actively motile spirochetes of the genus *Leptospira.* The disease can be unapparent or fatal, depending on the host and infecting serotypes. Wildlife may serve as sources of infection for domestic animals and man.

Leptospira bullum has been isolated from *M. pennsylvanicus* but was infrequent in the population (Clark et al., 1961). *L. icterohaemorrhagiae* was found in *M. montebelli* from Japan (Kitaoka and

Fujikura, 1975), and other serotypes were identified in *M. agrestis* and *Clethrionomys glareolus* in Britain (Twigg et al., 1968). The Japanese and European researchers considered the reservoir of leptospirosis in wildlife of considerable importance to the health and performance of domestic animals and man.

Very little is known about the symptoms of this disease in wild mammals; but they include anorexia, anemia, hemoglobinuria, fever, and death (Roth, 1970). The organism usually gains entrance through mucous membranes or broken skin and generally can be isolated from the blood from 4 to 9 days after infection. This condition precedes the febrile state by several days and by the time the fever subsides, the spirochetes no longer can be isolated from the blood. Antibodies normally appear about 10 days after infection and may persist for several months. Diagnosis usually requires serologic and bacteriologic methods (Roth, 1970). Treatment in humans normally requires antibiotics.

Relapsing fever.—Relapsing fever is a bacterial infection caused by spirochetes of the genus *Borrelia*; it is worldwide in distribution with the exception of Australia. It is transmitted mainly by ticks and lice and is an important infection of domestic animals and man. Experimental infection of *B. hermsii* in *M. pennsylvanicus* has been demonstrated (Burgdorfer and Mavros, 1970). Voles were shown to develop spirochetemias of various intensities and lengths. However, they experienced no signs of illness. All animals exhibited three periods of spirochetemia which lasted from 1 to 7 days, with the longest periods occurring early in the infection. Human cases of relapsing fever from Spokane, Washington, revealed that the tick *Ornithodoros hermsi* was the vector, and that it commonly was associated with a number of rodents, including *M. pennsylvanicus* (Burgdorfer and Mavros, 1970). In humans, an acute onset of fever occurs 3–10 days after infection and large numbers of spirochetes are present in the blood; they then disappear. Febrile attacks may recur three to 10 times and mortality rates of 50% have been reported. Penicillin and other antibiotics are an effective treatment (James and Harwood, 1969).

Rocky mountain spotted fever.—This disease is caused by infection of *Rickettsia rickettsi*, which is one member of a group of rickettsial zoonoses. The common name is misleading as the disease is found in most states, with 25% of cases reported in Virginia (Bell, 1970).

Indeed, members of this genus appear to be ubiquitous in temperate regions of the world (Asanuma et al., 1972; Burgdorfer et al., 1979; Tarasevich et al., 1976).

Transmission regularly occurs because of bites from ticks of the genera *Dermacentor, Amblyoma, Rhipicephalus,* and *Ixodes* (Bell, 1970). Ectoparasites other than ticks are not known to be vectors. The organism has been identified in a large number of rodents, including *M. pennsylvanicus* (Burgdorfer et al., 1975; Jellison, 1934), *M. agrestis* (Peter et al., 1981), *M. arvalis,* and *C. glareolus* (Rehacek et al., 1977), which may act as reservoirs of the disease.

Symptoms in wild animals are virtually unknown. Experimental infections of *M. pennsylvanicus* have shown that the response to the infection varies between individuals. Burgdorfer et al. (1966) observed that voles were not severely affected but the pathogens produced a microscopically detectable infection in the tunica vaginalis of the testes. Jellison (1934) found fever, swelling, and discoloration of the scrotum with adhesion formation, enlarged spleens, and moribund conditions developing in some individuals. Proper diagnosis requires laboratory analysis. Human symptoms include rashes on the wrists and ankles, headaches, backaches, and marked malaise with fever. In fatal infections death usually occurs between days 9 and 15. Broad-spectrum antibiotics are usually employed as treatment (James and Harwood, 1969). Other forms of rickettsieae, including coxiellosis, rickettsial pox, and eperythrozoonis, also may infect voles (Bell, 1970).

Other bacterial diseases.—Salmonella and *Streptococcus* infections have been reported in many small mammals (James and Harwood, 1969), transmitted by lice or other insect vectors. Murray (1965) reported the presence of these potential pathogens in *M. montanus* in Oregon and California during a population outbreak in 1957 and 1958. *Salmonella enteridis* was found in live and dead voles and their associated fleas. One juvenile *M. montanus* was diagnosed as having "big foot," a beta-hemolytic (*Streptococcus*) Group-A infection and another individual, which exhibited paralysis, difficult breathing, and had an open wound, was found positive for non-typable, Group-A *Streptococcus.* Both these pathogens have been reported in small-mammal breeding colonies causing morbidity and death (Haleermann and Williams, 1958). Broad-spectrum antibiotics have been used with some success.

Protozoan Infections

Babesiosis.—This is an infectious disease caused by protozoa of the genus *Babesia,* which are intraerythrocytic except during peaks in parasitemia, when they are liberated from ruptured red blood cells (Van Peenen and Healy, 1970). The life cycle and identity of these blood parasites still are not settled (James and Harwood, 1969), and their distribution appears to be wide ranging. Piroplasms of *Babesia microti* were found and observed in *M. californicus, M. ochrogaster, M. pennsylvanicus, M. oeconomus, M. arvalis, M. agrestis,* and *Lemmus lemmus* (Fay and Rausch, 1969; Krampitz, 1979; Mahnert, 1972; Van Peenen and Healy, 1970; Wiger, 1978*a*). The course of infection is extremely variable, with peak parasitemias occurring 7–20 days after inoculation in *M. ochrogaster.* Parasites usually could not be detected in the blood after 3–4 weeks, but sub-patent infections were evident for up to 3 months. No deaths occurred among intact *Microtus,* but splenectomized, infected animals often died as did intact *Lemmus lemmus* (Wiger, 1978*b*). All infected animals developed anemia, hemoglobinuria, splenomegaly, and deposition of hematin in the reticuloendothelial system. In Germany, Krampitz (1979) found *B. microti* most frequently associated with *M. agrestis,* with prevalence being greatest in early summer when 71% of the voles were infected. Ticks of the genera *Dermacentor* and *Ixodes* appear to be the main vectors for this disease, and in eastern United States *M. pennsylvanicus* appears to be the primary reservoir (McEnroe, 1977). Recent human cases of babesiosis infection from Nantucket Island, off the southeastern Massachusetts coast (Healy et al., 1976), support the conclusion that babesiosis could become an important public health problem. Symptoms are malaria-like and are characterized by chills, fever, headache, lethargy, and myalgia. Diagnosis depends on recognition of trophozoites of *Babesia* in the blood. No information on treatment is available. Other piroplasms with similar effects associated with microtines include *Hepatozoon* and *Grahamella* (Wiger, 1979).

Trypanosomes.—The term trypanosomiasis applies to all infections with flagellate protozoal parasites of the genus *Trypanosoma.* These parasites invade the blood, lymph, cerebrospinal fluid, and various organs in the body (liver and spleen) in many vertebrates from fish to man, in which they may produce sleeping sickness (James and Harwood, 1969).

The first record of a trypanosome from a species of the genus

Microtus was made by Laveran and Pettit (1909) when they described *Trypanosoma microti* from *M. arvalis*. Since that time, trypanosomes have been found to be almost worldwide in distribution, isolated from a large number of microtines including *M. pennsylvanicus, M. ochrogaster, M. oeconomus, M. californicus, M. agrestis, M. nivalis, Lemmus lemmus,* and *Dicrostonyx torquatus* (Fay and Rausch, 1969; Jolivet, 1970; McGeachin et al., 1970; Mahnert, 1972; Molyneux, 1969; Quay, 1955; Wiger, 1978*b*; Woo et al., 1980). Although symptoms may vary with species and individuals, and often are not apparent, trypanosome infections frequently cause anemia, hypoglycemia, and adrenal and splenic hypertrophy (Fay and Rausch, 1969; Wiger, 1978*b*). Experimental infections with *T. lewisi* in rats produced anemia, fetal resorption, abortion, and occasionally maternal death (Shaw and Dusanec, 1973), and Wiger (1977) suggested that these characteristics may apply to microtines. Transmission appears to occur from ticks and other blood-sucking insects (Liebisch, 1980); infestations tend to be highest at the end of the summer (Wiger, 1979).

Chagas disease caused by the trypanosome, *T. cruzi,* is common in the southern United States, Mexico, and South America. Symptoms include fever, facial edema, adenitis, anemia, and often death, and many species of mammals in this region have been implicated as reservoirs (James and Harwood, 1969).

Lyme disease.—Lyme disease is an epidemic inflammatory condition which starts with skin lesions and may be followed by neurologic and cardiac abnormalities and arthritis. Originally reported in Wisconsin, it is now known from throughout the northern states. A treponema-like spirochete that recently was isolated from the tick *Ixodes dammini,* a common associate of *Microtus,* strongly suggests that microtines may be a reservoir for this pathogen (Burgdorfer et al., 1982).

Fungal Diseases

The single fungal-caused disease in *Microtus,* adiasperomyiosis, is caused by members of the genus *Emmonsia,* and is usually a benign, self-limiting, mycotic infection in the lungs of wild animals. Experimental infections can be established in any tissue and animals given large enough doses succumb after weeks or months (Jellison, 1970).

The fungus has been isolated from the lungs of rodents through-

TABLE 2
SPONTANEOUS NEOPLASMS IN COLONY-REARED MICROTINES

Tumor	Species	References
Gastric squamous papillomas	*Dicrostonyx groenlandicus*	Barker et al. (1982); Dieterich (pers. observ.)
	M. pinetorum	Cosgrove and O'Farrell (1965)
	Microtus spp.	Lindsay (1976)
	Lemmus trimucronatus	Leininger et al. (1979); Raush and Rausch (1975)
Mammary adenocarcinomas	*D. groenlandicus*	Barker et al. (1982); Lindsay (1976)
	Clethrionomys rutilus	Dieterich (pers. observ.); Lindsay (1976)
	M. miurus	Dieterich (pers. observ.)
	Lemmus sp.	Lindsay (1976)
Pancreatic islet cell tumor	*D. groenlandicus*	Barker et al. (1982)
Pancreatic adenocarcinoma	*D. groenlandicus*	Barker et al. (1982)
	M. abbreviatus	Dieterich (pers. observ.)
Adrenal cortical adenoma	*D. groenlandicus*	Barker et al. (1982); Dieterich (pers. observ.)
Hardian gland adenocarcinoma	*D. groenlandicus*	Barker et al. (1982); Lindsay (1976)
	Microtus spp.	Lindsay (1976)
	C. rutilus	Lindsay (1976)
Inguinal adnexal carcinoma	*C. rutilus*	Dieterich (pers. observ.)
Subcutaneous sarcoma	*C. rutilus*	Dieterich (pers. observ.)
Sarcoma	Not reported	Lindsay (1976)
Alveolar rhabdomyo sarcoma	*C. rutilus*	Dieterich (pers. observ.)
Retrobulbar squamous cell carcinoma	*D. groenlandicus*	Dieterich (pers. observ.)
Retrobulbar adenocarcinoma	*D. groenlandicus*	Dieterich (pers. observ.)
Uterus choriocarcinoma	*D. groenlandicus*	Dieterich (pers. observ.)
Sweat gland adenocarcinoma	*D. groenlandicus*	Dieterich (pers. observ.)
Mesothelioma	*L. lemmus*	Dieterich (pers. observ.)
Vaginal adnexal carcinoma	*L. lemmus*	Dieterich (pers. observ.)
Leiomyosarcoma	*L. lemmus*	Dieterich (pers. observ.)
Sebaceous adenoma	*M. miurus* × *M. abbreviatus*	Dieterich (pers. observ.)
Labial squamous cell carcinoma	*M. oeconomus*	Dieterich (pers. observ.)
Perianal gland adenocarcinoma	*M. pennsylvanicus*	Dieterich (pers. observ.)
Pancreatic and bile duct adenocarcinoma	*M. abbreviatus*	Dieterich (pers. observ.)

TABLE 2
CONTINUED

Tumor	Species	References
Hepatic tumor	*Dicrostonyx* sp. *C. rutilus* *M. miurus* *M. abbreviatus* *L. sibiricus* *L. lemmus*	Lindsay (1976)
Preputial gland carcinoma	*Microtus* sp. *C. rutilus* *Dicrostonyx* sp.	Lindsay (1976)
Salivary gland carcinoma	Microtines	Lindsay (1976)
Melanoma	Microtines	
Chlolangiocarcinoma	Microtines	
Seminoma	Microtines	
Gastric squamous cell carcinoma	*M. abbreviatus*	Rausch and Rausch (1968)

out North America and appears to be Holarctic in distribution. It is especially common in microtine rodents, including *Microtus*. Inhalation is the only natural route of infection and histopathogenic examination should show the presence of numerous spherules in the lungs. McDiarmid and Austwick (1954) found evidence of pneumonia associated with this disease in dead and dying moles.

Neoplasms

Tumors are abnormal masses of tissue, whose growth exceeds, and is uncoordinated with, that of the normal parental stock, persisting after cessation of the stimuli that initiated their development. In most tumors, the neoplastic tissue consists of cells of a single type, which usually are classified histogenetically according to the tissues from which they arose. In addition, oncologists attempt to predict the behavior of tumors from their morphology, and classification can range from benign to malignant (Willis, 1960). Tumors are classified further according to their stage of development.

Viral, bacterial, nutritional, and other factors may act as etiologic agents, and genetic predisposition strongly influences the incidence and response to different carcinogens (Heston, 1963).

Although published information on microtine neoplasms is

sparse, they do occur, especially under laboratory conditions and should be a concern of those individuals managing breeding colonies (Table 2).

The etiology of neoplasms in laboratory microtines is unknown; however, gastric parasites have been associated with hyperkeratosis in the stomach of *M. ochrogaster* (Dunaway et al., 1968) and with papillomas in muskrats (Cosgrove et al., 1968). Gastric squamous hyperplasia and dysplasia were found in *Lemmus trimucronatus* infected with the parasite *Candida* (Leininger et al., 1979), and Rausch and Rausch (1968) reported gastric papillomas and carcinomas associated with these organisms. Lindsay (1976) found hamster type-H viruses and adenovirus associated with tumors in northern microtines, and Dieterich (pers. observ.) identified a type-R virus from mammary tumors. Although a number of possible etiologic agents have been identified, no direct cause-effect relationship has been established in laboratory animals.

Field data indicate that neoplasms occur rarely in natural populations, and are not an important factor in microtine demography. Rausch (1967), in a study of 9,376 wild arvicoline rodents from Alaska, found a single mammary tumor in *M. oeconomus*. This work was undertaken from 1949 to 1966, and included *M. oeconomus, M. miurus, M. longicaudus, M. xanthognathus, Clethrionomys rutilus, Dicrostonyx* spp., *Lemmus sibiricus,* and *Synaptomys borealis.*

Although neoplasms are relatively rare in wild populations, possibly because of the short lifespan of most small mammals (Mallory et al., 1981), they are present in significant numbers in longer-lived laboratory populations and etiologic agents may be a threat to laboratory personnel (Barker et al., 1982).

Constitutional and Other Diseases

Constitutional diseases are generally defined as malfunctions or pathological lesions whose etiology depends to a significant degree upon the action of genetic factors. The problem of delineating these conditions is that most diseases are a result of environmental and genetic interactions, and it is very difficult to separate the two. In this section we attempt to describe those conditions that do not fall into the previous categories.

Although information is not abundant, a number of pathologies have been mentioned in the literature (Table 3). Richmond and Conaway (1969) reported the occurrence of malocculusion of the incisors in *M. ochrogaster* which ultimately resulted in death. The

TABLE 3
PATHOLOGICAL FINDS OF A CONSTITUTIONAL NATURE FOUND IN MICROTINES FROM LABORATORY COLONIES

Species	Condition	References
M. oeconomus	Hepatic fatty infiltration, atherosclerosis, pulmonary congestion, pneumonia, pulmonary edema, renal lipidosis, hepatitis, nephrotic syndrome, lipidosis, myocarditis.	Dieterich and Preston (1979)
	Pulmonary hemorrhage, myocarditis, endocarditis, anemia, hepatic necrosis, enteritis, impacted stomach, impacted intestine, metritus, nephritis, otitis media, malnutrition.	Dieterich and Preston (1977*a*)
M. pennsylvanicus	Hepatic fatty infiltration, subacute interstitial pneumonia.	Dieterich et al. (1973)
	Musculoskeletal inflammation, bronchopneumonia, lobar pneumonia, pulmonary congestion and edema, enteritis, hypoplasia, endometritis, interstitial nephritis, glomerulonephritis, renal tubular degeneration, malnutrition.	Dieterich and Preston (1977*b*)
	Labyrinthitis.	Mallory (pers. observ.)
Clethrionomys rutilus	Pulmonary congestion, hepatic fatty infiltration, atherosclerosis, nephritis, renal lepidosis, nephrotic syndrome, interstitial pneumonia.	Dieterich and Preston (1979)
Dicrostonyx stevensoni	Atherosclerosis, hepatic fatty infiltration, pulmonary congestion, esophagitis, esophageal lipidosis, lipidosis of feet, pulmonary edema, nephrotic syndrome, cystitis, interstitial pneumonia, otitis media.	Dieterich and Preston (1979)
D. rubricatus	Atherosclerosis, hepatic fatty infiltration, esophageal lipidosis, pulmonary congestion, interstitial pneumonia, fat infiltration, cystitis, lipid pneumonitis, pneumonia, pulmonary edema.	

prevalence of this condition was greater when they started their colony and were bringing voles in from the wild. Similar conditions were observed in *M. pennsylvanicus* and *Dicrostonyx groenlandicus* under laboratory conditions, and may be associated with problems of diet (pers. observ.). Gill and Bolles (1982), however, described elongate and distorted root development in the molars of *M. californicus,* which they believed was heritable.

In a study of the effects of high cholesterol diets on microtines, Dieterich and Preston (1979) reported that the voles *Clethrionomys rutilus* and *Microtus oeconomus,* and the lemmings *Dicrostonyx stevensoni* and *D. rubricatus,* had marked increases in serum cholesterol causing lesions of atherosclerosis and hepatic fatty infiltration. *D. rubricatus* had the greatest increase in serum cholestrol (llx), significantly more lesions, and all animals that died spontaneously had pathologic lesions associated with hepatic fatty infiltration. Similar results were observed in *M. pennsylvanicus* and *D. groenlandicus* fed the same diet (Dieterich et al., 1973).

Summary

Although microtines of the genus *Microtus* are associated with a large number of diseases, personal experience and discussion with colleagues support the conclusion that pathogenic problems in laboratory colonies are relatively rare. Indeed, no instances of infection of laboratory personnel nor epidemics among animals have come to our attention.

The many breeding colonies of microtines that have been maintained successfully during the past 10 years (Table 1) have demonstrated that voles have many characteristics desirable of laboratory mammals. Members of the genus *Microtus* are maintained easily and inexpensively, are relatively easy to handle, have high reproductive rates that can be sustained year-round, have good pre- and post-operative survival, are generally non-aggressive toward familiar conspecifics, appear to be relatively free from disease, and in most instances are obtained easily. In addition, compared to *Mus,* they are virtually odorless. These characteristics and others make *Microtus* ideal animals for the study of parameters influencing demography and other mammalian phenomena under controlled laboratory conditions.

Acknowledgments

We thank Drs. E. Kott and R. M. Simm for reviewing the manuscript and L. Spoltore for technical assistance. This work was supported by a National Sciences and Engineering Research Council of Canada grant (No. A7241) to F. F. Mallory.

Literature Cited

ASANUMA, K., M. KITAOKA, AND K. OKUBO. 1972. Enzootic occurrence and possible vector of *Rickettsia orientalis* in Noppore, Hokkaido, the northern limit of geographic distribution of the agent in Japan. J. Med. Entomol., 9:593.

BACON, M., AND N. G. MILLER. 1958. Two strains of *Listeria monocytogenes* (Pirie) isolated from feral sources in Washington. Northwest Sci., 32:132–139.

BADDALOO, E. G. Y., AND F. V. CLULOW. 1981. Effects of the male on growth, sexual maturation and ovulation of young female meadow voles *Microtus pennsylvanicus*. Canadian J. Zool., 59:415–421.

BARKER, I. K., F. F. MALLORY, AND R. J. BROOKS. 1982. Spontaneous gastric squamous cell carcinomas and other neoplasms in Greenland collared lemmings (*Dicrostonyx groenlandicus*). Canadian J. Comp. Med., 46:307–313.

BARKER, I. K., I. BEVERIDGE, A. J. BRADLEY, AND A. K. LEE. 1978. Observations on spontaneous stress-related mortality among males of the dasyurid marsupial *Antechinus stuarti* Macleay. Australian J. Zool., 26:435–447.

BARRALES, D. 1953. Listeriosis in lemmings. Canadian J. Public Health, 44:180–184.

BATZLI, G. O., L. L. GETZ, AND S. S. HURLEY. 1977. Suppression of growth and reproduction of microtine rodents by social factors. J. Mamm., 58:583–591.

BELL, J. F. 1970. Rocky Mountain spotted fever. Pp. 324–331, *in* Infectious diseases of wild mammals (J. W. Davis, L. H. Karstad, and D. O. Trainer, eds.). Iowa State Univ. Press, Ames, 421 pp.

BERGER, P. J., N. C. NEGUS, E. H. SANDERS, AND P. D. GARDNER. 1981. Chemical triggering of reproduction in *Microtus montanus*. Science, 214:69–70.

BURGDORFER, W., AND A. J. MAVROS. 1970. Susceptibility of various species of rodents to the relapsing fever spirochete, *Borrelia hermii*. Infect. Immunity, 2:256–259.

BURGDORFER, W., K. T. FRIEDHOFF, AND J. L. LANCASTER. 1966. Natural history of tick-borne spotted fever in the U.S.A. II. Susceptibility of small mammals to virulent *Rickettsia rickettsi*. Bull. World Health Organ., 35:149–153.

BURGDORFER, W., A. AESCHLIMANN, O. PETER, S. F. HAYES, AND R. N. PHILIP. 1979. *Ixodes ricinus*: vector of a hitherto undescribed spotted fever group agent in Switzerland. Acta Trop., 36:357–367.

BURGDORFER, W., ET AL. 1975. *Rhipicephalus sanguineus*: Vector of a new spotted fever group *Rickettsia* in the United States. Infect. Immunity, 5:205–210.

BURGDORFER, W., ET AL. 1982. Lyme disease—A tick-borne spirochetosis? Science, 216:1317–1319.

BURROUGHS, A. L., R. HOLDENREID, D. S. LONGANECKER, AND K. F. MEYER. 1945. A field study of latent tularemia in rodents with a list of all known naturally infected vertebrates. J. Infect. Dis., 76:115–119.

CASALS, J. 1940. Influence of age factors on susceptibility of mice to rabies virus. J. Exp. Med., 72:445–451.

CLARK, G. M., C. M. CLIFFORD, L. V. FADNESS, AND E. K. JONES. 1970. Contributions to the ecology of Colorado tick fever virus. J. Med. Entomol., 7:189–197.

Clark, L. G., J. I. Kresse, R. R. Marshak, and C. J. Hollister. 1961. Natural occurrence of leptospirosis in the meadow vole, *Microtus pennsylvanicus*. Amer. J. Vet. Res., 22:949.

Clarke, J. R., and J. P. Kennedy. 1967. Effect of light and temperature upon gonad activity in the vole (*Microtus agrestis*). Gen. Comp. Endocrinol., 8: 474–488.

Clulow, F. V., and P. E. Langford. 1971. Pregnancy-block in the meadow vole, *Microtus pennsylvanicus*. J. Reprod. Fert., 24:275–277.

Clulow, F. V., and F. F. Mallory. 1970. Oestrus and induced ovulation in the meadow vole, *Microtus pennsylvanicus*. J. Reprod. Fert., 23:341–343.

———. 1974. Ovaries of meadow vole *Microtus pennsylvanicus* after copulation with a series of males. Canadian J. Zool., 52:265–267.

Colvin, M. A., and D. V. Colvin. 1970. Breeding and fecundity of six species of voles (*Microtus*). J. Mamm., 51:417–419.

Connell, R. 1954. *Erysipelothrix rhusiopathiae* infection in a northern chipmunk *Eutamias minimus borealis*. Canadian J. Comp. Med., 18:22–23.

Cosgrove, G. E., and T. P. O'Farrell. 1965. Papillomas and other lesions in the stomach of pine mice. J. Mamm., 46:510–513.

Cosgrove, G. E., W. B. Lushbaugh, G. Humason, and M. G. Anderson. 1968. *Synhimantus* (Nematoda) associated with gastric squamous tumors in muskrats. Bull. Wildl. Res., 4:54–57.

Dalldorf, G. 1943. Lymphocytic choriomeningitis of dogs. Cornell Vet., 33:347–350.

Dieterich, R. A., and D. J. Preston. 1977*a*. The tundra vole (*Microtus oeconomus*) as a laboratory animal. Lab. Anim. Sci., 27:500–506.

———. 1977*b*. The meadow vole (*Microtus pennsylvanicus*) as a laboratory animal. Lab. Anim. Sci., 27:494–499.

———. 1979. Atherosclerosis in lemmings and voles fed a high fat, high cholesterol diet. Atherosclerosis, 33:181–189.

Dieterich, R. A., R. W. Van Pelt, and W. A. Galster. 1973. Diet-induced cholesteremia and atherosclerosis in wild rodents. Atherosclerosis, 17:345–352.

Dunaway, P. B., G. E. Cosgrove, and J. D. Story. 1968. Capillaria and trypanosoma infestations in *Microtus ochrogaster*. Bull. Wildl. Dis., 4: 18–20.

Elton, C. 1942. Voles, mice and lemmings. Oxford Univ. Press, Oxford, 496 pp.

Eveland, W. C. 1970. Listeriosis. Pp. 273–282, *in* Infectious diseases of wild mammals (J. W. Davis, L. H. Karstad, and D. O. Trainer, eds.). Iowa State Univ. Press, Ames, 421 pp.

Fay, F. H., and R. L. Rausch. 1969. Parasitic organisms in the blood of arvicoline rodents in Alaska. J. Parasitol., 55:1258–1265.

Feemster, R. F. 1938. Outbreak of encephalitis in man due to the eastern virus of equine encephalomyelitis. Amer. J. Public Health, 28:1403–1410.

Fenner, F., B. R. McAuslan, C. A. Mims, J. Sambrook, and D. O. White. 1974. The biology of animal viruses. Second ed. Academic Press, New York, 546 pp.

Findlay, G. M., and R. O. Stern. 1936. Pathological changes due to infection with virus of LCM. J. Pathol. Bacteriol., 43:327–338.

Fischman, H. R., and F. E. Ward, III. 1968. Oral transmission of rabies virus in experimental animals. Amer. J. Epidemiol., 88:132–138.

Gill, A. E., and K. Bolles. 1982. A heritable tooth trait varying in two subspecies of *Microtus californicus* (Rodentia:Cricetidae). J. Mamm., 63:96–103.

GITTNER, L. T., AND SHAKAN, M. S. 1933. The 1933 outbreak of infectious equine encephalomyelitis in the eastern states. N. Amer. Vet., 14:25–27.

GORHAM, J. R. 1950. Tularemia kills mink too! Amer. Fur. Breeder, 23:15.

GRAY, G. D., H. N. DAVIS, A. MCM. KENNEY, AND D. A. DEWSBURY. 1976. Effect of mating on plasma levels of LH and progesterone in montane voles (*Microtus montanus*). J. Reprod. Fert., 47:89–91.

HALEERMANN, R. T., AND F. P. WILLIAMS JR. 1958. Salmonellosis in laboratory animals. J. Natl. Cancer Inst., 20:933–947.

HALL, E. R. 1981. The mammals of North America. Second ed. John Wiley and Sons Inc., New York, 2:601–1181 + *90*.

HASLER, J. F. 1975. A review of reproduction and sexual maturation in the microtine rodents. The Biologist, 57:52–86.

HASLER, M. J., AND A. V. NALBANDOV. 1974. The effect of weanling and adult males on sexual maturation in female voles (*Microtus ochrogaster*). Gen. Comp. Endocrinol., 23:237–238.

HEALY, G. R., A. SPIELMAN, AND N. GLEASON. 1976. Human babesiosis: reservoir of infection on Nantucket Island. Science, 192:479–480.

HENDERSON, J. R., N. KARABATSOS, A. T. C. BOURKE, R. C. WALLIS, AND R. M. TAYLER. 1962. A survey for arthropod-borne viruses in south-central Florida. Amer. J. Trop. Med., 11:800–810.

HESTON, W. E. 1963. Genetics of neoplasia. Pp. 247–268, *in* Methodology in mammalian genetics (W. J. Burdette, ed.). Holden-Day, San Francisco, 568 pp.

HINKLEY, R., JR. 1966. Effects of plant extracts in the diet of male *Microtus montanus* on cell types of the anterior pituitary. J. Mamm., 47:396–400.

HOTCHIN, J. E., AND L. M. BENSON. 1970. Lymphocytic choriomeningitis. Pp. 153–172, *in* Infectious diseases of wild mammals (J. W. Davis, L. H. Karstad, and D. O. Trainer, eds.). Iowa State Univ. Press, Ames, 421 pp.

HUDSON, B. W., M. I. GOLDENBERG, AND T. J. QUAN. 1972. Serologic and bacteriologic studies on the distribution of plague infection in a wild rodent plague pocket in the San Francisco Bay area of California. J. Wildl. Dis., 8:278–287.

IMEL, K. J., AND R. P. AMANN. 1979. Effects of duration of daily illumination on reproductive organs and fertility of the meadow vole (*Microtus pennsylvanicus*). Lab. Anim. Sci., 9:182–185.

IVERSON, S. L., AND B. N. TURNER. 1974. Winter weight dynamics in *Microtus pennsylvanicus*. Ecology, 55:1030–1041.

JAMES, M. T., AND R. F. HARWOOD. 1969. Medical Entomology. Sixth ed. MacMillan, Collier-MacMillan Ltd., London, 484 pp.

JANNETT, F. J. JR. 1974. "Hip glands" of *Microtus pennsylvanicus* and *M. longicaudus* (Rodentia: Muridae), voles "without" hip glands. Syst. Zool., 24: 171–175.

JELLISON, W. L. 1934. Rocky Mountain spotted fever. The susceptibility of mice. Public Health Rept., 49:363–367.

———. 1970. Adiasperomyiosis. Pp. 321–323, *in* Infectious diseases of wild mammals (J. W. Davis, L. H. Karstad, and D. O. Trainer, eds.). Iowa State Univ. Press, Ames, 421 pp.

JENSEN, W. I., AND R. M. DUNCAN. 1980. *Bordetella bronchiseptica* associated with pulmonary disease in mountain voles (*Microtus montanus*). J. Wildl. Dis., 16:11–14.

JESPERSEN, A. 1975. Infection of *Microtus arvalis* (common vole) with *Mycobacte-*

rium tuberculosis and *Mycobacterium bovis*. Acta Path. Microbiol. Scand., Sect. B, 83:201–210.

———. 1976. Multiplication of *Mycobacterium tuberculosis* and *Mycobacterium bovis* in *Microtus agrestis* (field vole). Acta Path. Microbiol. Scand., Sect. B, 84:57–60.

JOLIVET, A. 1970. *Trypanosoma petymydis* n.sp., protozoaire flagelle parasite de *Pitymys multiplex* (Fatio 1905) =*P. incertus* (De Selep-Longchamps) (Rongeur microtide). Protistologica, 6:53–55.

KAPLAN, C., T. D. HEALING, N. EVANS, L. HEALING, AND A. PRIOR. 1980. Evidence of infection by viruses in small British field rodents. J. Hyg. (Camb.), 84:285–294.

KARSTAD, L. H. 1970. Arboviruses. Pp. 60–67, *in* Infectious diseases of wild mammals (J. W. Davis, L. H. Karstad, and D. O. Trainer, eds.). Iowa State Univ. Press, Ames, 421 pp.

KARSTAD, L. H., J. SPALATIN, AND R. P. HANSON. 1961. Natural and experimental infections with the virus of eastern encephalitis in wild rodents from Wisconsin, Minnesota, Michigan and Georgia. Zoonoses Res., 1:87–96.

KENNEY, A. MCM., R. L. EVANS, AND D. A. DEWSBURY. 1977. Post implantation pregnancy distribution in *Microtus ochrogaster, M. pennsylvanicus* and *Peromyscus maniculatus*. J. Reprod. Fert., 49:365–367.

KHOMYAKOV, A. I., R. N. SADOVNIKOVA, N. A. FETISOVA, AND O. A. FETISOVA. 1970. Natural nidality of erysipeloid at the south-east of the Ryazan district. J. Microbiol. Epidemiol. Immunobiol. (U.S.S.R.), 47:131–134.

KITAOKA, M., AND T. FUJIKURA. 1975. Isolation of icterohaemorrhagiae from *Microtus montebelli* trapped at the Nagaoka area, Niigata prefecture in Japan. Internatl. J. Zoonoses, 2:100–104.

KOCH, R. 1884. The etiology of tuberculosis. New Sydenham Soc. Publ., 115:67–201.

KRAMPITZ, H. E. 1979. *Babesia microti*: morphology, distribution and host relationship in Germany. Zbl. Bakt. Hyg., I. Abt. Orig. A, 244:411–415.

KRATOKHVIL, N. I. 1953. Excretion of *Listeria* by field voles and ticks *Ixodes ricinus*. Zh. Microbiol. Epidemiol. Immunobiol., 24:60–61.

LAVERAN, A., AND A. PETTIT. 1909. Sur un trypanosome d'un campagnol *Microtus arvalis* Pallas. C.R. Seanc. Soc. Biol., 67:798.

LEE, C., AND D. J. HORVATH. 1969. Management of the meadow vole (*Microtus pennsylvanicus*). Lab. Anim. Sci., 19:88–91.

LEE, C., D. J. HORVATH, R. W. METCALFE, AND E. K. INSKEEP. 1970. Ovulation in *Microtus pennsylvanicus* in a laboratory environment. Lab. Anim. Sci., 20:1098–1102.

LEININGER, J. R., G. E. FOLK, AND P. S. COOPER. 1979. Gastric candiasis in laboratory-reared brown lemmings. J. Amer. Vet. Med. Assoc., 175:990–991.

LES, E. P. 1966. Husbandry. Pp. 29–37, *in* Biology of the laboratory mouse. Second ed. (E. L. Green, ed.). McGraw-Hill, New York, 204 pp.

LEVY, M. I. 1948. *Listeria monocytogenes* in voles. Vet. J., 104:310–312.

LIEBISCH, G. W. 1980. Untersuchungen zur Okologie einiger Blutprotozoen bei wildlebenden Kleinsäugern in Norddeutschland. Acta Trop., 37:31–40.

LINDSAY, J. W. 1976. Spontaneous occurrence of tumors in laboratory-reared arvicoline rodents. Cancer Res., 36:4092–4098.

MAGUS, M. 1955. Listeriosis in lemmings. Canadian J. Public Health, 45:27.

MAHNERT, V. 1972. Grahamella und Sporozoa als Blutparasiten alpiner Kleinsauger. Acta Trop., 29:88–100.

MAIN, A. J., R. E. SHOPE, AND R. C. WALLIS. 1976. Characterization of Whitney's *Clethrionomys gapperi* virus isolates from Massachusetts. J. Wildl. Dis., 12:154–164.

MAISKY, I. M. 1945. Tularemia outbreaks of murine origin. Zh. Mikrobiol. Epidemiol. Immunobiol., 8:32–38.

MALLORY, F. F., AND R. J. BROOKS. 1978. Infanticide and other reproductive strategies in the collared lemming, *Dicrostonyx groenlandicus*. Nature, 273: 144–146.

———. 1980. Infanticide and pregnancy failure: reproductive strategies in the female collared lemming (*Dicrostonyx groenlandicus*). Biol. Reprod., 22: 192–196.

MALLORY, F. F., AND F. V. CLULOW. 1977. Evidence of pregnancy failure in the wild meadow vole, *Microtus pennsylvanicus*. Canadian J. Zool., 55:1–17.

MALLORY, F. F., J. R. ELLIOTT, AND R. J. BROOKS. 1981. Changes in body size in fluctuating populations of the collared lemming: age and photoperiod influences. Canadian J. Zool., 59:174–182.

MARTIN, K. H., R. A. STEHN, AND M. E. RICHMOND. 1976. Reliability of placental scar counts in the prairie vole. J. Wildl. Mgmt., 40:264–271.

MAURER, F. B. 1964. Lymphocytic choriomeningitis. Lab. Anim. Care, 14:415–419.

MCCOY, G. W. 1911. Studies upon plague in ground squirrels. Public Health Bull., 43.

MCDIARMID, A., AND P. K. C. AUSTWICK. 1954. Occurrence of *Haplosporangium parvum* in the lungs of the mold (*Talpa europaea*). Nature, 174:843.

MCENROE, W. D. 1977. Human babesiosis. Science 195:506.

MCGEACHIN, W. T., F. H. WHITTAKER, AND F. W. QUICK, JR. 1970. Record of occurrence of a trypanosome infection in the prairie vole, *Microtus ochrogaster*, in Jefferson County, Kentucky. Kentucky Acad. Sci., 31:64–65.

MCGUIRE, M. R., AND L. L. GETZ. 1981. Incest taboo between sibling *Microtus ochrogaster*. J. Mamm., 62:213–215.

MELENDEZ, L. V., M. D. DANIEL, AND N. W. KING. 1973. Isolation and *in vitro* characterization of a herpesvirus from field mouse (*Microtus pennsylvanicus*). Lab. Anim. Sci., 23:385–390.

MOLYNEUX, D. H. 1969. The morphology and life-history of *Trypanosoma (Herpetosoma) microti* of the field-vole, *Microtus agrestis*. Ann. Trop. Med. Parasitol., 63:229–244.

MORRIS, A. J., AND A. D. ALEXANDER. 1951. LCM virus from gray mice trapped in a rural area. Cornell Vet., 41:122–123.

MORRISON, P., R. DIETERICH, AND D. PRESTON. 1977*a*. Body growth in sixteen rodent species and subspecies maintained in laboratory colonies. Physiol. Zool., 50:294–310.

———. 1977*b*. Longevity and mortality in 15 rodent species and subspecies maintained in laboratory colonies. Acta Theriol., 22:317–335.

MURRAY, K. F. 1965. Population changes during the 1957–1958 vole (*Microtus*) outbreak in California. Ecology, 46:163–171.

NEGUS, N. C., AND A. J. PINTER. 1965. Litter size in *Microtus montanus* in the laboratory. J. Mamm., 46:434–437.

———. 1966. Reproductive responses of *Microtus montanus* to plants and plant extracts in the diet. J. Mamm., 47:596–601.

NORDLAND, O. S. 1959. Host-parasite relations in initiation of infection. I. Occurrence of listeriosis in arctic mammals, with a note on its possible pathogenesis. Canadian J. Comp. Med., 23:393–400.

OLSEN, P. F. 1970. Sylvatic (wild rodent) plague. Pp. 200–213, *in* Infectious diseases of wild mammals (J. W. Davis, L. H. Karstad, and D. O. Trainer, eds.). Iowa State Univ. Press, Ames, 421 pp.

PASLEY, J. N., AND T. D. MCKINNEY. 1973. Grouping and ovulation in *Microtus pennsylvanicus*. J. Reprod. Fert., 34:527–530.

PETER, O., W. BURGDORFER, AND A. AESCHLIMANN. 1981. Enquête épidémiologique dans un foyer naturel de Rickettsies à *Ixodes ricinus* du plateau Suisse. Ann. Parasitol., 56:1–8.

PETTERBORG, L. J. 1978. Effects of photoperiod on body weight in the vole, *Microtus montanus*. Canadian J. Zool., 56:431–435.

PINTER, A. J., AND N. C. NEGUS. 1965. Effects of nutrition and photoperiod on reproductive physiology of *Microtus montanus*. Amer. J. Physiol., 208:633–638.

PLUMMER, P. J. G., AND J. L. BYRNE. 1950. *Listeria monocytogenes* in the lemming. Canadian J. Comp. Med. Vet. Sci., 14:214–217.

POLLITZER, R. 1954. Plague. World Health Organ. Monogr., Ser. 22, Geneva, Switzerland, 83 pp.

PONOMAREVA, T. N., AND L. V. RODKEVICH. 1964. *Pasteurella multocida* infection among rodents in a large city. J. Microbiol. Epidemiol. Immunobiol. (USSR), 41:144–145.

QUAN, S. F., AND L. KARTMAN. 1962. Ecological studies of wild rodent plague in the San Francisco Bay area of California. VIII. Susceptibility of wild rodents to experimental plague infection. Zoonoses Res., 1:121–144.

QUAY, W. B. 1955. Trypanosomiasis in the collared lemming, *Dicrostonyx torquatus* (Rodentia). J. Parasitol., 41:562–565.

RAMSDEN, R. O., AND D. H. JOHNSTON. 1975. Studies on the oral infectivity of rabies virus in Carnivora. J. Wildl. Dis., 11:318–324.

RAUSCH, R. L. 1967. On the ecology and distribution of *Echinococcus* spp. (Cestoda: Taeniidae), and characteristics of their development in the intermediate host. Ann. Parasitol. Human Comp., 42:19–63.

RAUSCH, R. L., AND V. R. RAUSCH. 1968. On the biology and systematic position of *Microtus abbreviatus* Millar, a vole endemic to the St. Matthew Islands, Bering Sea. Z. Saugetierk., 33:65–99.

———. 1975. Taxonomy and zoogeography of *Lemmus* spp (Rodentia: Arviodinae) with notes on laboratory-reared lemmings. Z. Saugetierk., 40:8–34.

RAUSCH, R. L., B. E. HUNTLEY, AND J. G. BRIDGENS. 1969. Notes on *Pasteurella tularensis* isolated from a vole, *Microtus oeconomus* Pallas, in Alaska. Canadian J. Microbiol., 15:47–55.

REHACEK, J., J. URBOLGYI, AND E. KOVACOVA. 1977. Massive occurrence of Rickettsiae of the spotted fever group in fowl tampan, *Argas persicus*, in the Armenian S.S.R. Acta Virol., 21:431–438.

REILLY, J. R. 1970. Tularemia. Pp. 175–199, *in* Infectious diseases of wild mammals (J. W. Davis, L. H. Karstad, and D. O. Trainer, eds.). Iowa State Univ. Press, Ames, 421 pp.

RICHMOND, M., AND C. H. CONAWAY. 1969. Management, breeding and reproductive performance of the vole, *Microtus ochrogaster* in a laboratory colony. Lab. Anim. Sci., 19:80–87.

ROSEN, M. N. 1970. Pasteurellosis. Pp. 214–223, *in* Infectious diseases of wild mammals (J. W. Davis, L. H. Karstad, and D. O. Trainer, eds.). Iowa State Univ. Press, Ames, 421 pp.

ROTH, E. E. 1970. Leptospirosis. Pp. 293–303, *in* Infectious diseases of wild mammals (J. W. Davis, L. H. Karstad, and D. O. Trainer, eds.). The Iowa State Univ. Press, Ames, 421 pp.

SANDERS, E. H., P. D. GARDNER, P. J. BERGER, AND N. C. NEGUS. 1981. Methoxybenzoxazolinone: a plant derivative that stimulates reproduction in *Microtus montanus*. Science, 214:67–69.

SCHADLER, M. H. 1980. The effect of crowding on the maturation of gonads in pine voles, *Microtus pinetorum*. J. Mamm., 61:769–774.

———. 1981. Post implantation abortion in pine voles (*Microtus pinetorum*) induced by strange males and pheromones of strange males. Biol. Reprod., 25:295–297.

SHAW, G. L., AND D. G. DUSANEC. 1973. *Trypanosoma lewsi*: termination of pregnancy in the infected rat. Exp. Parasitol., 33:46–55.

SHUMAN, R. D. 1970. Erysipelas. Pp. 267–272, *in* Infectious diseases of wild mammals (J. W. Davis, L. H. Karstad, and D. O. Trainer, eds.). Iowa State Univ. Press, Ames, Iowa, 421 pp.

SIKES, R. K., SR. 1970. Rabies. Pp. 3–19, *in* Infectious diseases of wild mammals (J. W. Davis, L. H. Karstad, and D. O. Trainer, eds.). Iowa State Univ. Press, Ames, 421 pp.

SOAVE, O. A. 1966. Transmission of rabies to mice by ingestion of infected tissue. Amer. J. Vet. Res., 27:44–46.

SODJA, I., D. LIM, AND O. MATOUCH. 1971. Isolation of rabies virus from small wild rodents. J. Hyg. Epidemiol. Microbiol. Immunol., 15:271–277.

———. 1973. Isolation of rabies strains from small wild rodents and their biological properties. Folia Microbiol., 18:182.

STEHN, R. A., AND F. J. JANNETT, JR. 1980. Male-induced abortion in various microtine rodents. J. Mamm., 62:369–372.

STEHN, R. A., AND M. E. RICHMOND. 1975. Male-induced pregnancy termination in the prairie vole, *Microtus ochrogaster*. Science, 187:1211–1213.

TARASEVICH, I. V., V. A. MAKAROVA, AND L. F. PLOTNIKOVA. 1976. Studies of the antigenic properties of the newly isolated strains of Rickettsiae and their relation to Spotted Fever Group. Folia Microbiol., 4:503.

TWIGG, G. I., C. M. CUERDEN, AND D. M. HUGHES. 1968. Leptospirosis in British wild mammals. Symp. Zool. Soc. London, 24:75–98.

VAN PEENEN, P. F. D., AND G. R. HEALY. 1970. Infection of *Microtus ochrogaster* with piroplasms isolated from man. J. Parasitol., 56:1029–1031.

VAUGHAN, M. K., G. M. VAUGHAN, AND R. J. REITTER. 1973. Effect of ovariectomy and constant dark on the weight of reproductive and certain other organs in the female vole, *Microtus montanus*. J. Reprod. Fertil., 32:9–14.

WAYSON, N. E. 1927. An epizootic among meadow mice in California, caused by the bacillus of mouse septicema or of swine erysipelas. Public Health Rept., 42:1489–1493.

WEBSTER, A. B., R. G. GARTSHORE, AND R. J. BROOKS. 1981. Infanticide in the meadow vole, *Microtus pennsylvanicus*: significance in relation to social system and population cycling. Behav. Neur. Biol., 31:342–347.

WELLS, A., AND D. OXON. 1937. Tuberculosis in wild voles. Lancet, 1:1221.

WETZLER, T. F. 1970. Pseudotuberculosis. Pp. 224–235, *in* Infectious diseases of wild mammals (J. W. Davis, L. H. Karstad, and D. O. Trainer, eds.). Iowa State Univ. Press, Ames, 421 pp.

WHITNEY, E., A. P. ROZ, AND G. A. RAYNER. 1970. Two viruses isolated from rodents (*Clethrionomys gapperi* and *Microtus pennsylvanicus*) trapped in St. Lawrence County, New York. J. Wildl. Dis., 6:48–55.

WIGER, R. 1977. Some pathological effects of endoparasites on rodents with special reference to the population ecology of microtines. Oikos, 29:598–606.

———. 1978*a*. Fatal experimental *Babesia microti* infections in the Norwegian lemming, *Lemmus lemmus* (L.). Folia Parasitol., 25:103–108.

———. 1978*b*. Hematological, splenic and adrenal changes associated with natural and experimental infections of *Trypanosoma lemmi* in the Norwegian lemming, *Lemmus lemmus* (L.). Folia Parasitol., 25:295–301.

———. 1979. Seasonal and annual variations in the prevalence of blood parasites in cyclic species of small rodents in Norway with special reference to *Clethrionomys glareolus*. Holarctic Ecol., 2:169–175.

WILLIS, R. A. 1960. Pathology of tumors. Third ed. Butterworth, Washington, D.C., 189 pp.

WINKLER, W. G., AND N. B. GALE. 1970. Tuberculosis. Pp. 236–248, *in* The infectious diseases of wild mammals (J. W. Davis, L. H. Karstad, and D. O. Trainer, eds.). Iowa State Univ. Press, Ames, 421 pp.

WOO, P. T. K., D. R. GRANT, AND L. MCLEAN. 1980. Trypanosomes of small mammals in southern Ontario. Canadian J. Zool., 58:567–571.

WORLD HEALTH ORGANIZATION. 1967. World Survey of Rabies 9. Veterinary Public Health Unit, Geneva, Switzerland, 127 pp.

ENDOCRINOLOGY

ROBERT W. SEABLOOM

Abstract

THE endocrinology of North American *Microtus* is not well known. Most studies have involved certain aspects of the female reproductive system and the adrenopituitary system; limited data are available on the male reproductive system and on thyroid function. Comparative data are sparse; endocrine studies have been conducted on only six species.

Annual reproduction in *Microtus* results from the interaction of an endogenous annual rhythm with several known exogenous factors, including photoperiod, light intensity, temperature, nutrition, and social cues. Of special interest is the recent identification of plant substances that can stimulate or inhibit reproduction.

Microtus exhibits a pheromonally induced estrus and coitus-induced ovulation. Successful ovulation can also be facilitated by pheromonal and other contact factors. A post-partum estrus occurs in all species. Extended copulatory stimulation or contact with the stud male enhances establishment of corpora lutea and the pre-implantation stages of pregnancy. The presence of a strange male can result in blockage of any stage of pregnancy (Bruce effect), or even impair litter survival. This phenomenon has been suggested as a side effect of induced estrus and ovulation.

Estrogen and glucocorticoid-binding macromolecules have been demonstrated in the lactating mammary gland of *Microtus*. There is some indication of hypothalamic inhibition of prolactin secretion subsequent to exposure to a strange male, thus extending the Bruce effect to post-partum events.

Adrenal weights of *Microtus* fall within the range of variation for other small mammals, but secretory activity is relatively high. A high level of 11β-dehydrogenase activity occurs in the adrenal cortex of *M. pennsylvanicus*. This activity appears to vary seasonally, being highest in fall and winter. The level of corticosterone secretion exhibits a marked daily periodicity, normally reaching a peak during late afternoon, prior to the peak of motor activity. Secretory activity also varies seasonally, and is highest during the spring breeding season.

Adrenal-gonadal interactions have been demonstrated in New World *Microtus.* At puberty, high testosterone levels in males inhibit adrenal enlargement and corticosterone secretion, whereas estrogens have the opposite effect on females. High progesterone levels during pregnancy appear to inhibit adrenal response. ACTH administration inhibits ovarian and uterine development, but the specific pathway of action is not known.

Introduction

Much of the research dealing with endocrine mechanisms in New World *Microtus* has emanated from widespread interest in the remarkable population phenomena exhibited by microtine rodents. Consequently, the status of our knowledge of *Microtus* endocrinology has been tempered by an ecological-behavioral perspective. Certain aspects of adrenocortical function and female reproductive physiology have received significant attention in some species, while other endocrine systems have been relatively unstudied. Nevertheless, work to date on the genus has made highly significant contributions to comparative endocrinology and indicates important directions for future research.

Timing of Reproductive Function

Sexual Maturation

In an extensive review of reproduction in microtines, Hasler (1975) noted that most species, including North American *Microtus,* mature earlier than other rodents, with females frequently attaining puberty at about 30 days of age. However, along with adult reproductive development, the specific age of puberty appears to be related to both endogenous and exogenous factors, including nutrition, social factors, and light.

Seasonality

With the exception of species living in warmer climates, North American *Microtus* exhibit variable breeding seasons that generally run from early spring until late summer or fall (Asdell, 1964). In some species, however, reproductive activity has been recorded during all months (Keller, this volume), with a variety of exogenous factors having the capability of maintaining an endocrinological balance favoring reproduction. Seasonal reproduction tends to occur in northern latitudes, whereas more southern species frequently breed throughout the year.

Bailey (1924), along with numerous subsequent workers, observed *M. pennsylvanicus* females carrying embryos at all seasons. However, winter breeding in northern populations of this species is unusual, except under conditions of heavy snow (Beer and MacLeod, 1961) or during periods of cyclic population increase (Krebs et al., 1973). Sexual activity occurs throughout the year in *M. ochrogaster* (Fitch, 1957), but there is a seasonal incidence of enhanced reproduction in response to heavy precipitation and abundant new grass. *M. californicus* also breeds throughout the year (Greenwald, 1957). Early litters have the capability of mating in their first year, but late spring animals will not attain puberty until the following year.

Adams et al. (1980) reported that initiation of spermatogenesis in *Microtus breweri* coincides with spring increases in daily photoperiod and temperature. Plasma androgen levels were highest from April to June and lowest in October. Like other *Microtus,* early litters of *M. breweri* may become sexually mature during the season of their birth, but late litters delay puberty through the winter and become mature prior to the subsequent spring breeding season.

The existence of an endogenous circannual rhythm of reproductive development must be considered for the North American *Microtus.* These voles may undergo a refractory period after the breeding season in which the gonads regress while under the same light regimen providing the original stimulus (van Tienhoven, 1968). Grocock (1980) reported that the British vole, *Microtus agrestis,* undergoes spontaneous gonadal recrudescence after a 6-month period of inhibition following short daylengths. *M. pennsylvanicus* captured during the late summer or fall generally does not come into breeding condition in the laboratory until the following spring, in spite of maintenance of favorable photoperiods (Seabloom, pers. observ.).

Photic Cues

In *Microtus,* as with many other rodents, light exerts a major influence over sexual maturation and gonadal recrudescence. Specific components may include length of daily photoperiod, light intensity, and wavelength. Reproductive development of both New World and Old World microtines is positively correlated with increased photoperiods. Pinter and Negus (1965) reported that litter size in *M. montanus* is greater under 18-h versus 6-h photoperiods. However, optimal daylengths may exist, above or below which there are adverse effects on gonadal development and production of young. In *M. pennsylvanicus,* reproductive function is optimal under a 16:8 light-dark cycle (Imel and Amann, 1979). Shorter (12:12) or longer (18:6) photoperiods have an adverse effect on female fertility.

Despite behavioral preferences for low light intensities, there appears to be a positive correlation between intensity of lighting and reproductive development in microtines. Geyer and Rogers (1979) compared litter production in *M. pinetorum* raised under high (75–200 lumens) and low (0–75 lumens) light intensities. Litter production and litter size were approximately doubled under the high intensities. Vaughan et al. (1973) reported that female *M. montanus* held in constant dark exhibited suppressed body size along with low ovarian, uterine, adrenal, and Harderian gland weights. They further suggested that the influence of constant dark may be mediated through the pineal gland. Darkness has been demonstrated to stimulate the pineal gland to produce the antigonadotrophin, melatonin, in laboratory rats. Both ovariectomy and constant dark inhibited thymic involution in *M. montanus,* suggesting that constant dark stimulates pineal production of melatonin which, in turn, inhibits the action of follicle-stimulating hormone (FSH) on ovarian secretion of thymolytic steroids. Earlier Vaughan et al. (1972) demonstrated the action of melatonin in blocking the effect of FSH on compensatory ovarian hypertrophy of unilaterally ovariectomized laboratory mice and *M. montanus.*

There have been no studies of the effects of wavelength on reproductive development of New World *Microtus,* and reports involving other microtines are inconclusive. There is some indication that exposure to only the longer (red) wavelengths may result in delayed puberty, at least in females (Hasler, 1975).

Nutritional Cues

While the status of the food resource has long been recognized as having a major influence on reproductive performance, only in recent years have nutritional cues and their regulation of specific endocrine pathways been studied intensively. Much of the relevant work on wild species has dealt with North American *Microtus* (see Batzli, this volume).

Initiation of breeding seasons has long been associated with fresh production of green plants, and many species experience reduced fertility during periods of drought. Some authors postulated that in certain rodents the timing of breeding seasons may be in response to the appearance of new vegetation rather than to photoperiodic cues, because the nutritional stimulus may be more appropriate in harsh environments (Labov, 1977). Greenwald (1957) observed a close association between breeding activity by *M. californicus* and the occurrence of new vegetative growth. Pinter and Negus (1965) discussed the interaction of diet and photoperiod in regulation of reproduction in *M. montanus*. They suspected the existence of a specific dietary cue rather than direct effects of changes in nutritional levels.

A series of studies on *M. montanus* demonstrated that small dietary supplements of plants and plant extracts have marked effects on rate of growth, endocrine development, and reproductive performance (Negus and Berger, 1977; Negus et al., 1977). Sprouted wheat supplied in the diet increased growth rates and reduced the time to onset of puberty (Pinter, 1968). Weight decreases of the pineal gland, and increases of uterus and adrenal gland followed dietary supplements of fresh lettuce, sprouted wheat, or spinach extract (Berger and Negus, 1974; Negus and Berger, 1971; Negus and Pinter, 1966). Supplements of spinach extracts resulted in increased numbers of ovarian follicles (Negus and Pinter, 1966). However, overall enhanced reproductive performance following such supplements appeared to be via increased frequency of post-partum matings and decreased rates of litter loss rather than through increased litter size (Negus and Pinter, 1966; Pinter and Negus, 1965).

Recently, 6-methoxybenzoxazolinone (6-MBOA) was identified

as a stimulant of reproductive activity in *M. montanus* (Sanders et al., 1981). This naturally occurring plant-derived cyclic carbamate is a non-estrogenic compound, which, when added to a laboratory diet, resulted in significantly increased uterine and ovarian weights. Enlarged ovaries were due primarily to increased numbers of antral follicles. Although Sanders et al. (1981) noted that it is yet to be demonstrated whether this plant-derived cue is widespread among herbivorous mammals, equivalent response of laboratory mice (*Mus musculus*) indicates that at least it is not restricted to microtines.

To test the capability of 6-MBOA in triggering reproduction of *M. montanus,* Berger et al. (1981) provided treated and untreated supplements of rolled oats to reproductively inactive populations during winter. After three weeks of treatment, males from the experimental plots exhibited testicular hypertrophy and females a 70% incidence of pregnancy. No pregnancies occurred on control plots. Consequently, they concluded that 6-MBOA provides an ultimate cue for reproduction in this species, and suggested that it may play a more widespread role in other microtines.

Berger et al. (1981) suggested that 6-MBOA operates at the neural or pituitary rather than gonadal level, and available evidence tends to support this hypothesis. Hinkley (1966) observed an increase in delta basophil cells in the pituitaries of *Microtus montanus* that received dietary supplements of extracts from wheat sprouts. Delta cells are known to secrete gonadotropins. Negus and Berger (1971) reported a significant decrease in pineal weight of *M. montanus* following dietary supplements of fresh lettuce, and later Berger and Negus (1974) added experimental evidence that the compound operates at the pineal-hypothalamic-pituitary level. It would appear, therefore, that the microtine pineal gland may utilize dietary as well as photoperiodic cues in its regulation of pituitary secretion of gonadotropins.

In addition to the utilization of dietary cues in initiation of its breeding season, *Microtus montanus* apparently relies on other naturally occurring compounds to signal termination of reproduction. Negus et al. (1977) provided data correlating initiation and cessation of reproduction with seasonally varying chemical composition of vegetation. Furthermore, Berger et al. (1977) identified cinnamic acids and related vinylphenols as reproductive inhibitors in *M. montanus.* Dietary supplements of these compounds resulted in decreased uterine weight, inhibition of follicular development, and diminished reproductive activity. These compounds are most abundant in vegetation subsequent to flowering, senescence, and browning. The physiological site of activity of these inhibitors has yet to be identified.

Social Cues

Population density.—High population densities apparently inhibit sexual maturation and adult female reproduction in both North American and Old World microtines. Crowding was proposed by Christian (1961, 1963, 1971, 1975) to result in social pressures affecting natality as well as mortality. Pasley and McKinney (1973) reported that female *M. pennsylvanicus* that were housed in groups of eight from weaning until pairing exhibited lighter ovaries and uteri and fewer corpora lutea than those that were housed singly. They noted prior work by Christian et al. (1965) and Christian and Davis (1966), in which increased secretory activity of the pituitary-adrenal axis was implicated as providing density-dependent negative feedback inhibiting reproduction.

The pine vole (*M. pinetorum*), in contrast to *M. pennsylvanicus,* exhibits a relatively low reproductive rate and stable populations in nature. Schadler (1980) examined the histology of testes and ovaries of pine voles raised under varying conditions of crowding. Testes of crowded males weighed 41% less than uncrowded and exhibited low spermatogenic indices. None of the crowded females ovulated, in contrast to a 21% frequency of corpora lutea observed in uncrowded voles. Crowded voles exhibited premature formation of antra, a small proportion of mature preovulatory follicles, and increased atresia of undeveloped follicles.

Pheromones and neuroendocrine response.—The total social environment, as well as density per se, functions as an external variable in regulation of rate of sexual maturation and development of breeding condition. There has been considerable work on the influence of conspecifics and pheromonal factors influencing reproduction in murids, but relatively little on microtines.

Pheromonal inhibition of sexual maturation by littermates occurs in some species of *Microtus.* In *M. ochrogaster,* vaginal opening is earliest in weanling females paired with non-littermate adult males, intermediate with non-littermate weanling males, and slowest with littermate weanlings (Hasler and Nalbandov, 1974). Hasler and Nalbandov noted that age and degree of "strangeness" had two distinct effects. Vaginal opening was influenced by both factors, but litter production was only affected by strangeness. Batzli et al. (1977) found that both sexual maturation and growth were suppressed by littermates in *M. californicus* and *M. ochrogaster,* but not in *M. pennsylvanicus.* A pheromone was implicated because suppression also occurred in voles isolated except for air supply. Normal development resumed when voles were housed with strangers of the opposite sex. McGuire and Getz (1981) obtained similar results with *M. ochrogaster,* but their data suggest that the activation pheromone must be transmitted by naso-genital grooming rather than through the air.

Age-related olfactory cues may change with the onset of testosterone production and attainment of puberty in the male. Richmond and Stehn (1976) questioned, however, if early maturation merely involved early induction of estrus or might be "further regulated by prepuberal exposure to males or other conspecifics." They noted that the stimulus provided by male exposure might have been preconditioned by a brief prepuberal exposure to another male. If so, then seasonal occurrence of delayed maturation characteristic of many microtines may be related to the seasonal absence of stimuli provided by sexually active males.

Baddaloo and Clulow (1981) exposed laboratory-raised female meadow voles (*M. pennsylvanicus*) to mature males (with and without physical contact), virgin and multi-parous females, male urine, and empty cages. Exposure to males or male urine accelerated maturation, whereas female exposure had no effect. Consequently, Baddaloo and Clulow (1981) concluded that male mediation was pheromonal and that the active compound was in the urine.

Recent studies have further documented the existence of a pheromone in male urine having the capability of activating female reproduction. Carter et al. (1980) reported that virgin female *M. ochrogaster* over 20 days of age exhibited uterine growth and other indications of reproductive activity following exposure to male-related stimuli. Exposure to an unfamiliar adult male for less than 1 h induced uterine weight increases within 48 h and lasted at least 10 days. Exposure to male urine induced similar reproductive development. In contrast to Baddaloo and Clulow's (1981) study, Carter et al. (1980) reported that physical contact with an intact male or male urine was essential for reproductive activation, thus eliminating visual and airborne cues. Although sibling pairs normally did not reproduce, estrus could be induced by direct application of a sibling male's urine to the female's upper lip, thus indicating a behavioral barrier to reproduction.

In a related study elucidating the physiological pathways for reproduction in *M. ochrogaster,* Dluzen et al. (1981) exposed females to a single drop of male urine on the upper lip. This produced a significant increase in serum luteinizing hormone (LH) in less than 1 min. The exposure also resulted in changes in luteinizing hormone-releasing hormone (LHRH) and norepinephrine (NE) in the tissue of the posterior olfactory bulb. They noted that most studies of LHRH release implicated the preoptic-hypothalamic areas, but that nerve terminals containing LHRH are found in the olfactory bulb. The catecholamines norepinephrine and dopamine are also reproductive regulators found in the olfactory bulb. Norepinephrine may be implicated in synthesis or release of LHRH, while dopamine is an inhibitor of reproductive processes. Dluzen et al. (1981) suggested that the observed increase in LHRH and its concentration in the posterior olfactory bulb of the prairie vole implicated a neuroendocrine link between the external environment and reproductive activation.

Estrus and Ovulation

The social cues discussed above appear to be instrumental in regulation of estrous cycles and ovulation in most microtines. Hasler (1975) discussed the problems associated with some of the early studies based upon females permanently paired with males or histological studies of wild-caught animals. Neither approach allowed examination of a recurrent cycle. Consequently, many reports in the literature yielded contradictory results.

Older reports suggest that estrous cyles in New and Old World microtines are similar to those of laboratory mice and rats. Asdell (1964) cited unpublished data for *M. pennsylvanicus* indicating spontaneous changes in the vaginal smear typical of *Rattus* and *Mus*. Similar cycles were reported for *M. oeconomus* (Hoyte, 1955) and *M. pinetorum* (Kirkpatrick and Valentine, 1970).

A preponderance of recent studies, however, indicate that experimentally isolated microtine females are capable of remaining in diestrus for extended periods. In contrast to the earlier report on

M. pinetorum (Kirkpatrick and Valentine, 1970), Schadler and Butterstein (1979) found no pattern of vaginal cyclicity. Female pine voles housed adjacent to males exhibited 1–22 days of continuous estrus followed by 1–9 days of diestrus. Similar patterns also have been described for *M. pennsylvanicus, M. montanus,* and *M. ochrogaster.* Clulow and Mallory (1970) could not demonstrate any regular cyles of vaginal smear patterns from wild-caught *M. pennsylvanicus.* In addition, isolated females exhibited constant diestrus, whereas those housed with castrate males exhibited constant estrus. Similarly, isolated *M. townsendii* were found to delay maturation and extend diestrus prior to their first estrus (MacFarlane and Taylor, 1981). Both diestrus and estrus may be extended up to 18 days, but isolated females do not ovulate or form corpora (MacFarlane and Taylor, 1982*a*).

Regular estrous cycles do not occur in *M. montanus* that have been isolated or housed adjacent to males (Gray et al., 1974*a*). Isolated *M. ochrogaster* held under a 12-h photoperiod remain in continuous diestrus, but altering housing conditions can have varying effects on reproductive activity and receptivity (Richmond and Conaway, 1969*a*). Richmond and Conaway found that 71–83% of the females attained estrus within a week if moved adjacent to males or allowed direct contact with males.

Hasler and Conaway (1973) further studied the effect of males in inducing estrus in *M. ochrogaster.* In tests of the effect of the presence or absence of the male on the female reproductive state they found a 72-h exposure to be maximally effective in inducing estrus. Injections of low levels of estradiol cyclopentylpropionate in castrated females resulted in vaginal mucification, whereas higher levels resulted in cornification. Their data supported the hypothesis that among species exhibiting induced estrus and ovulation, it would be advantageous for development of the uterine epithelium or vaginal opening to occur only in the presence of a strong estrus inducer. Vaginal epithelial hyperplasia, vaginal opening, and uterine epithelial hyperplasia would represent successive stages with increasing levels or more prolonged exposure to estrogen stimulation.

In addition to pheromonally induced estrus, ovulation induced by coitus further maximizes reproductive efficiency. This phenomenon is widespread among mammalian orders, and microtine rodents are not exceptions. Indeed, Jöchle (1973) noted that "The

TABLE 1
TYPE OF OVULATION IN NORTH AMERICAN *Microtus* (IN PART, AFTER HASLER, 1975)

Species	Type of ovulation	Time of ovulation	References
M. californicus	Induced	15 h post-coitus	Greenwald (1956)
M. montanus	Induced	8 h post-coitus	Cross (1972)
	Induced	8 h post-HCG	Gray et al. (1974*a*)
M. ochrogaster	Induced	9–10 h post-coitus	Richmond and Conaway (1969*b*)
	Induced	—	Gray et al. (1974*b*)
M. oeconomus	Spontaneous	—	Hoyte (1955)
	Spontaneous	—	Asdell (1964)
M. pennsylvanicus	Induced	12–18 h post-coitus	Lee et al. (1970)
	Induced	—	Clulow and Mallory (1970)
M. pinetorum	Induced	—	Kirkpatrick and Valentine (1970)

system is so effective in coordinating all necessary steps for the assurance of fertility, in so many species of different orders, families, and genera, that it makes one wonder why its principles, in toto or at least partially, have not found an even wider distribution in mammalian evolution."

Induced ovulation appears to be the rule in *Microtus,* and although there are reports to the contrary, Breed (1967) suggested that there is only circumstantial evidence for spontaneous ovulation in the genus. To date, induced ovulation has been demonstrated for six species of North American *Microtus* (Table 1).

Post-copulatory ovarian changes have been reported for several species of *Microtus,* but the associated requisite neurohormonal pathways involved must be inferred from studies of other species. Jöchle (1973) summarized the known neurohormonal connections between the genital tract, hypothalamus, pituitary, and ovaries for a variety of spontaneous and induced ovulators. In rats and mice the pelvic nerves are involved, with the coital stimulus eventually reaching the preoptic region of the hypothalamus. The stimulus may activate the cyclic ovulatory center or descend to the median

TABLE 2
MEAN (±*SE*) PLASMA LEVELS OF LH AND PROGESTERONE IN MONTANE VOLES, *Microtus montanus* (FROM GRAY ET AL., 1976)

Reproductive state	LH (nanograms/ml)	Progesterone (nanograms/ml)
Females		
Diestrus	20.6 ± 5.9	9.0 ± 0.9
Estrus, unmated	23.1 ± 2.5	14.0 ± 1.1
Estrus, mated	896.1 ± 136.7	22.0 ± 1.5
Males		
Unmated	28.8 ± 3.6	
Mated	123.0 ± 40.5	

eminence, eventually resulting in triggering an ovulatory LH discharge from the adenohypophysis.

Few data are available on precise hormonal changes in *Microtus* following copulation. Gray et al. (1976) reported plasma levels of LH and progesterone for different reproductive states of *M. montanus* (Table 2). In females, mating resulted in a nearly 40-fold increase in LH, and a 57% increase in progesterone within 1 h. This response was similar to that observed for Old World *M. agrestis.* In addition to the post-coital increase in progesterone, there is an accompanying decrease in serum estradiol. Estrous *M. ochrogaster* have serum E_2 levels around 78 picograms/ml, which decline to 57 picograms/ml by 48 h post-coitum (Prentice and Shepherd, 1978).

Post-copulatory ovarian changes have been reported for several species of *Microtus.* Following copulation there is usually significant follicular enlargement. Follicular diameter of *M. californicus* enlarges from 500–600 μm to 900 μm, a 70–80% increase (Greenwald, 1956). Post-copulatory follicles of *M. ochrogaster* average about 1,000 μm (Richmond, 1967). Cross (1972) observed follicular enlargement in *M. montanus* of 623–722 μm. However, Gray et al. (1974*a*) did not observe any pre-ovulatory swelling in that species.

In *M. californicus,* subsequent to pre-ovulatory swelling, there is a breakdown of the granulosa cells surrounding the ovum until it is free in the antrum, surrounded only by the corona radiata

(Greenwald, 1956). Ova of all reported *Microtus* are of similar size, averaging about 60 μm (Cross, 1971; Greenwald, 1956; Richmond, 1967). By contrast, mature ova of *Mus* average 95 μm (Rugh, 1968).

Varying frequencies of copulatory activity can affect the probability of ovulation and implantation. In *M. ochrogaster,* only one ejaculatory series is sufficient to induce ovulation and implantation, but the probability of ovulation increases with the number of intromissions and intravaginal thrusts (Gray et al., 1974*b*). Similar results have been reported for *M. montanus* (Davis et al., 1974). Kenney et al. (1977*b*) found that *M. ochrogaster,* like *M. agrestis,* ovulated in response to artificial vaginal-cervical stimulation, but only subsequent to one intromission from a male. However, unlike *M. agrestis,* less copulatory stimulation was required and there was no apparent dissociation between ovulation and subsequent formulation of a functional corpus luteum resulting from minimal mechanical stimulation. They also suggested that pheromonal or contact factors are a prerequisite to ovulation. This was supported recently by Dluzen et al. (1981), who found that exposure of females to a single drop of male urine on the upper lip results in a rapid increase in LHRH in the olfactory bulb and LH in the serum.

Formation and Duration of Corpus Luteum

In *Microtus,* new corpora lutea are formed 15–18 h post-coitum, and are completely solid between 48 and 72 h (Greenwald, 1956; Lee et al., 1970). The corpus luteum forms from both thecal and granulosa cells but at the time it differentiates into luteal cells the distribution of the two components cannot be determined.

The life of the corpus luteum in those New World *Microtus* in which it has been studied is similar to that described for *Mus* (Rugh, 1968). Lee et al. (1970) mated mature female *M. pennsylvanicus* with vasectomized males, and observed persistent corpora lutea up to 9 days post-coitum. These corpora lutea had well-defined, functional luteal cells with small fat particles. Regression began on days 10–11, as evidenced by the presence of vacuolization, connective tissue cells, and large fat particles.

Corpora lutea are functional throughout pregnancy, reaching maximum size near the end of gestation (Greenwald, 1956; Lee et al., 1970; Richmond, 1967). Some females possess large numbers of corpora (up to 29), most of which are regarded as accessory corpora (Greenwald, 1956).

Limited copulatory stimuli, while sufficient to induce ovulation (Gray et al., 1974*b*), may result in short-lived corpora lutea. Kenney and Dewsbury (1977) subjected *M. montanus* females to only one ejaculatory series prior to examination for CL on days 3 and 8 after mating. Seven of 10 females had well developed CL on day 3, while only one of 10 had CL and implanted embryos by day 8. This rapid degeneration of CL following limited mating is similar to reports for the Old World *M. agrestis* (Milligan, 1974, 1975), and may represent an additional type of reproductive cycle for the non-pregnant female mammal.

Gestation

Most small microtines have gestation periods averaging 20–25 days (Hasler, 1975). However, various endocrine mechanisms can influence gestation, up to and including its termination.

Although lactational delay of gestation has been reported for a variety of microtines (Hasler, 1975), it has not been found in New World *Microtus.* Reports for *M. montanus* (Pinter and Negus, 1965) and *M. ochrogaster* (Richmond and Conaway, 1969*a*) specifically indicated no lactational delay of gestation. Data on litter intervals for *M. pennsylvanicus, M. oeconomus, M. miurus,* and *M. abbreviatus* also tend to support this conclusion (Morrison et al., 1976).

Subsequent to fertilization, continued tactile and olfactory stimulation by the stud male can be important in reinforcing the neuroendocrine pathways requisite to the pre-implantation stages of pregnancy. Richmond and Stehn (1976) reported that in *M. ochrogaster,* between 1 and 4 days of cohabitation were required to achieve a maximum (over 90%) incidence of successful pregnancies. In *M. montanus,* removal of the stud male within 24 h of mating caused a significant incidence of pregnancy terminations (Berger and Negus, 1982). However, continued mating activity for up to 48 h enhanced the maintenance of pregnancy. Similar results were reported for Old World *M. agrestis* by Milligan (1975) who indicated that, although limited mating can induce ovulation, the resulting corpora lutea degenerate rapidly and cannot maintain a decidual reaction.

The termination of pregnancy by pheromonal influence of a strange male (Bruce effect) has been demonstrated for both Old World and New World *Microtus*. Male-induced abortion has been reported for *M. pennsylvanicus, M. ochrogaster, M. montanus,* and *M. pinetorum*. Clulow and Langford (1971) demonstrated a depressed pregnancy rate of 20% in female *M. pennsylvanicus* exposed to strange males 3 days or less after coitus with an original stud. Clulow and Mallory (1974) further demonstrated that the pregnancies of *M. pennsylvanicus* can be terminated repeatedly when exposed to a series of strange males, each subsequently inducing ovulation and initiating a further pregnancy. Mallory and Clulow (1977) studied normal and blocked pregnancy in *M. pennsylvanicus* in the laboratory, and compared blockage with the incidence of pregnancy failure in the wild. Females were susceptible to blockage on days 2 and 5 post-coitum. Occurrence of a second set of corpora lutea apparently did not accelerate involution of the first set. Lactating females were not susceptible to male-induced blockage. The latter observation was consistent with Bruce's (1966) conclusion that blockage is dependent on hypothalamic inhibition of prolactin secretion. Apparently, the neural stimulus provided by nursing young overrides the pheromonally-induced blocking action provided by the strange male.

Pre-implantation pregnancy blockage can apparently be induced by heterospecific as well as conspecific strange males. In *M. montanus,* blockage was induced by male *Lagurus curtatus* (Jannett, 1979).

Male-induced pregnancy blockage has now been demonstrated for post-implantation as well as pre-implantation stages of pregnancy. Blockage was induced in *M. ochrogaster* during most stages of pregnancy with no reduction in incidence until after day 15 (Stehn and Richmond, 1975). Kenney et al. (1977*a*) reported pregnancy blockage by day 14 in *M. ochrogaster* and *M. pennsylvanicus,* as well as in the cricetid, *Peromyscus maniculatus*. The incidence of blockage was lower than that reported for *M. ochrogaster* by Stehn and Richmond, but may have been due to higher levels of prolactin in recently lactating females of the latter study. Stehn and Jannett (1981) further reported on the incidence of pregnancy blockage in *M. ochrogaster, M. montanus, M. pinetorum,* and *Lagurus curtatus.*

Abortions occurred in all species tested except *L. curtatus*. Concurrent lactation did not reduce abortion in *M. ochrogaster* or *M. montanus* in contrast to that reported for *M. pennsylvanicus* (Mallory and Clulow, 1977) and to the earlier suggestion that the low incidence of blockage in *M. ochrogaster* was associated with recent lactation (Kenney et al., 1977*a*).

Schadler (1981) reported an incidence of 87–88% blocked pregnancies in *M. pinetorum* when females were exposed to a strange male on day 10 or 15. A high incidence of post-implantation abortion also occurred when females were only exposed to cage litter soiled by strange males. Consequently, these data support the conclusion that odor alone is sufficient to induce blockage at any stage of pregnancy in *Microtus*.

Male-induced pregnancy blockage in microtines may be a side effect of induced estrus and ovulation (Stehn and Richmond, 1975). Stehn and Jannett (1981) further suggested that strong selection for acceleration of puberty and estrus may exist in microtines, and that the occasional loss of a litter through male-induced estrus may be a relatively unimportant consequence. However, Kenney et al. (1977*a*) detected no significant differences in the incidence of pregnancy blockage between spontaneous and induced ovulators. They concluded that the data did not suggest an association between increased male-induced pregnancy blockage and induced ovulation. Nevertheless, there appears to be a definite association of the incidence of pregnancy blockage with a variety of species in which the induction of estrus and ovulation plays an overriding role.

Post-partum Events

Post-partum Estrus

All microtines apparently experience a post-partum estrus, becoming receptive shortly after giving birth (Hasler, 1975). North American *Microtus* for which post-partum estrus has been described or implied include *M. abbreviatus* (Morrison et al., 1976), *M. californicus* (Greenwald, 1956), *M. miurus* (Morrison et al., 1976), *M. montanus* (Gray et al., 1974*a*; Pinter and Negus, 1965), *M. ochrogaster* (Richmond and Conaway, 1969*a*, 1969*b*), *M. pennsylvanicus* (Lee et al., 1970; Morrison et al., 1976), *M. pinetorum* (Kirkpatrick and Valentine, 1970; Schadler and Butterstein, 1979), and *M. townsendii* (MacFarlane and Taylor, 1982*b*).

In *M. pennsylvanicus,* estrus occurs on the day of parturition, with copulation inducing ovulation on the same day (Lee et al., 1970). Richmond and Conaway (1969*a*) observed *M. ochrogaster* females copulating before completion of all births of a litter. *M. ochrogaster* females may remain in continuous estrus throughout lactation, or if separated from a male, for about 4 days following parturition.

Lactation

There has been very little research on lactation per se in microtine rodents. What little has been done indicates that mammary physiology may be comparable to that described for laboratory rats and mice. However, some neuroendocrine pathways controlling lactation may be somewhat distinct.

Hormone receptor proteins have been identified and partially characterized in the lactating mammary gland of *M. montanus*. Specific estrogen receptor proteins were demonstrated by Beers and Wittliff (1973) in mammary and uterine cytosol. Hydrocortisone had no effect on the binding of ^{3}H-estradiol-17β to mammary or uterine receptors, but later work (Turnell et al., 1974) reported the presence of distinct glucocorticoid-binding macromolecules in the lactating mammary gland. These protein receptors have similar characteristics to those identified in the lactating mammary gland of *Rattus* and *Mus*. Estrogens and progesterone function in proliferation of mammary cells, whereas glucocorticoids, along with insulin and prolactin, are required for cell differentiation (Bentley, 1976).

There is some indication that the neuroendocrine influences associated with male-induced pregnancy blockage now may be extended into the period of lactation. Schadler (1982) recently reported that removal of a stud *M. pinetorum* which was paired to a nursing female, and replacement with a strange male, resulted in high litter mortality and poor weight gain in surviving young. This implies an extension of the Bruce effect into post-partum events via hypothalamic inhibition of prolactin secretion resulting in failure or impairment of lactation. Under this scheme, the olfactory stimulus provided by a strange male would result in hypothalamic production of FSH-RH and subsequently high estrogen levels associated with estrus. In addition, the same olfactory stimulus would provide for hypothalamic production of prolactin release-inhibiting hormone (P-R-IH), with resulting diminished mammary cell differentiation and secretion.

Testicular Activity

In contrast to the bulk of research on reproductive physiology of female *Microtus,* relatively little has been done on the male. The morphology of the male reproductive tract of *M. ochrogaster* was described by Janes (1963). The testis is comparable to that of other mammals, and is very similar to Old World *M. arvalis.* Secretory interstitial cells are of variable shape and occur in groups of 1–10 in angular spaces between the seminiferous tubules. Other morphological features of the testes (seminiferous tubules, rete testis, efferent ducts) are all characteristic of other small rodents. Relative testicular size in microtines appears to be high compared to other rodents. In *M. pennsylvanicus,* relative weight of the testis is about double that of the laboratory mouse (Dieterich and Preston, 1977).

Although testicular morphology is similar to other species, testicular activity in *Microtus* is relatively high. *Microtus ochrogaster* exhibited the shortest known spermatogenic cycle (7.2 days) of seminiferous epithelium (Schuler and Gier, 1976). The entire process of spermatogenesis in *M. ochrogaster,* including meiotic stages, encompassed 28.7 days. The durations of spermatogenic cycles for other microtines have not been reported to date.

Data on circulating androgens are limited to two species of North American *Microtus,* the beach vole (*M. breweri*) and Townsend's vole (*M. townsendii*). Plasma androgens of *M. breweri* were highest (>2 nanograms/ml) during April–June, the period of greatest testicular weight (1,300–1,600 mg) and spermatogenic activity (Adams et al., 1980). Androgen levels were minimal (<1 nanogram/ml) during October when testes were smallest (43 mg) and spermatogenic activity was nil. Intraperitoneal administration of 10 μg of either ovine or murine LH resulted in a two- to three-fold increase in plasma androgens.

Total androgens of male *M. townsendii* during a spring population decline were reported by McDonald and Taitt (1982). Androgen levels of larger (>80 gm) voles averaged about 2.6 nanograms/ml. Smaller males had levels averaging 1.25 nanograms/ml. Androgen levels reported for other rodents were highly variable (Gustafson and Shemesh, 1976), but those indicated for *M. breweri* and *M. townsendii* appear to be in the low range. However, those values should not necessarily be regarded as representative of microtines until data are available involving seasonal and diurnal variation in other more widely distributed species.

Thyroid

Thyroid activity has not been extensively studied in *Microtus*. Those studies which have been conducted indicate similar responses to various stressors, photoperiod, and temperature to those observed for laboratory rodents.

In *M. californicus*, thyroid activity can be inhibited by various stressors, including high population density, food depletion, and harassment (Houlihan, 1963). In a penned experiment, voles in the control group (low density) accumulated 20.7% of administered ^{131}I after 24 h. Thyroidal ^{131}I uptake by voles in the experimental (high density) pen was 14.4%. The observed diminished thyroidal activity is consistent with results of experiments by other workers using a variety of stresses on laboratory rats.

Circulating levels of thyroxine have been reported for *M. montanus* and *M. ochrogaster*. In *M. montanus* maintained under a 16-h photoperiod, T_4 levels averaged from 4.4 to 4.6 μg/dl (Petterborg, 1978). These levels were suppressed under short (8-h) photoperiods, concomitant with loss of body weight. Similar photoperiodic effects on growth and thyroid activity in *M. pennsylvanicus* were reported by Pistole and Cranford (1982). Subadult voles gained weight more rapidly under 18-h than 6-h photoperiods, and adults lost weight under the shorter photoperiods. Relative thyroid weights were similar under the two light regimes, but thyroid activity was significantly higher in voles held under the 18-h photoperiods. Thyroid uptake of ^{125}I and circulating thyroxine were both significantly higher than in voles held under 6 h of light. These data, along with those of Petterborg (1978) have been interpreted as indicative of a metabolic adjustment resulting in reduced body size and lowered energy demands in preparation for winter.

Serum T_4 in *M. ochrogaster* averaged 4.8 μg/dl (Hudson, 1980), a level comparable to that in *M. montanus*. Thyroid secretion was inhibited by Tapazole but there was no effect on standard metabolism. Tapazole blockage of thyroxine resulted in a 3°C increase in the highest air temperature tolerated without stress. In subsequent experiments, there were no significant differences in Serum T_4 in voles exposed to a variety of air temperatures from 5 to 35°C. However, there was a high correlation between ^{125}I clearance and air temperature. The half-life of ^{125}I labeled T_4 was 20.2 days at 35°C, but this decreased to 4.3 days at 5°C. The conflicting data between thyroxine levels and rate of radioiodine release caused Hudson (1980) to question the reliability of using circulating thyroxine as an indicator of thyroid secretory activity.

Adrenal Cortex

Adrenal Morphology

Adrenal weight has long been utilized as a convenient indicator of the functional state of cortical activity. In the absence of other differential influences, there is a positive logarithmic relationship between adrenal weight and body size which holds for a variety of mammals, including *Microtus* (Christian, 1953). Adrenal weight relationships have been published for a variety of species of New World *Microtus,* including *M. breweri* (To and Tamarin, 1977), *M. californicus* (Mullen, 1960), *M. montanus* (McKeever, 1959; Pinter, 1968), *M. oeconomus* (Dieterich et al., 1973), *M. pennsylvanicus* (Christian, 1953; Christian and Davis, 1966; Dieterich et al., 1973; Quiring, 1951; Seabloom et al., 1978; To and Tamarin, 1977), and *M. pinetorum* (Christian, 1953). Dieterich et al. (1973) compared adrenal and other organ weights of *M. pennsylvanicus, M. oeconomus,* and seven other species of myomorph rodents including laboratory mice (*Mus musculus*). Adrenal weights averaged from 0.05 to 0.09% of body weight and were greater than values for *Mus* or most of the other species examined. Although the values were within the published range of averages for various species of *Microtus,* they do not reflect the known range of variation due to age, sex, reproductive condition, and response to external stimuli.

Significant changes in adrenal size occur with sexual maturation. In *M. montanus* and *M. pennsylvanicus,* adrenal size is not significantly different in juvenile males and females (McKeever, 1959; Seabloom et al., 1978). With sexual maturity, however, there is a decrease in relative adrenal size in males, but in females relative

TABLE 3
ANNUAL VARIATION IN ADRENAL WEIGHT [MG/100 G BODY WEIGHT ± *SE* (*N*)] OF *Microtus pennsylvanicus* FROM PINAWA, MANITOBA (FROM SEABLOOM ET AL., 1978)

Season	Males		Females	
	Age class	Adrenal weight	Age class	Adrenal weight
Late summer 1971	J	65.0 ± 5.1 (4)	J	70.6 ± 31.8 (2)
	A	28.3 ± 2.1 (7)	A	107.4 ± 9.7 (5)
			P	71.4 ± 0.0 (2)
Fall 1971	J	47.3 ± 4.8 (11)	J	43.6 ± 4.8 (6)
	A	29.3 (1)	A	88.2 ± 13.7 (2)
Winter 1971–72	I	33.8 ± 3.4 (5)	I	46.4 ± 5.7 (2)
Spring 1972	A	35.1 ± 2.5 (17)	A	76.0 ± 6.0 (5)
			P	98.5 ± 7.6 (11)
Early summer 1972	SA	41.3 ± 5.4 (6)		
	A	35.3 ± 4.7 (20)	A	107.4 ± 6.7 (4)
			P	115.2 ± 8.5 (15)

Abbreviations of age classes are: J, juvenile; SA, subadult; A, adult; P, pregnant; I, inactive.

weight may be doubled (Table 3). Christian (1975) reviewed reported causal factors for the observed shifts in relative size, and noted that immature male *Microtus* along with many other species have an X-zone which is involuted by increased testosterone levels at puberty. Delost (1952) reported that the X-zone of Old World *M. arvalis* regenerates during periods of sexual inactivity. However, Seabloom et al. (1978) did not observe any adrenal enlargement of *M. pennsylvanicus* during winter, the only period when sexually inactive adult voles occurred.

Females of many species of small mammals have heavier adrenals than males (Chester Jones, 1957), but in *Microtus* the differences are especially pronounced (Christian and Davis, 1964, 1966). In the laboratory rat (*Rattus norvegicus*) the female adrenal may average 20–50 percent larger than that of the male (Chester Jones, 1957); sexually mature female *M. pennsylvanicus* may have adrenals two to four times as heavy as those of mature males (Table 3). This sexual dimorphism was attributed by Christian (1975) to: 1) different configurations of social stimuli between sexes; 2) estrogenic stimulation resulting in higher levels of corticosteroid binding proteins in mature females; and 3) greater rates of hepatic metabolism and clearance of corticosteroids in females. Christian suggested that the lowering of free corticosteroids resulted in decreased inhibition of pituitary secretion of ACTH causing adrenal enlargement and increased secretion rate.

There has been some disagreement as to the nature of the X-zone in female *Microtus* and its contribution to adrenal size. In contrast to the situation in the male, the X-zone of female *Microtus* apparently persists until involution during the first pregnancy (Christian, 1956; Christian and Davis, 1964; Delost and Chirvan-Nia, 1956). However, Chitty and Clarke (1963) reported a persistent X-zone in females of the British vole, *M. agrestis,* which enlarges during pregnancy, thus accounting for the marked sexual dimorphism in adrenal size. This contention was refuted by Christian and Davis (1964), who cited evidence indicating that the inner juxtamedullary zone of the adrenal cortex of female *M. pennsylvanicus* is an "inner-fasciculata-reticularis" rather than an X-zone. Christian (1975) further suggested that X-zone involution in the female may be brought about by ovarian secretion of testosterone during pregnancy.

Secretory Products

The fluorometric characteristics of adrenocortical secretory products from *Microtus* have indicated corticosterone to be the major hormone produced (Olsen and Seabloom, 1973; Seabloom, 1965). Chromatographic evidence subsequently verified corticosterone as the major endogenous steroid produced from in vitro incubation of adrenals from *M. pennsylvanicus* and the British vole, *M. agrestis* (Ogunsua et al., 1971; Ungar et al., 1973, 1978). In addition to corticosterone, six other steroids have been identified in small amounts from in vitro metabolism of progesterone-4^{14}C or pregnenolone-4-^{14}C by *Microtus* adrenals (Table 4).

Ungar et al. (1973) initially identified 11-dehydrocorticosterone (Compound A) and other 11-keto rather than 11β-hydroxysteroids as the major products of incubation of adrenals from *M. pennsylvanicus.* This finding was not reported for other species and conflicted with fluorometric and other data implicating corticosterone (Compound B) as the major steroid produced. The presence of the 11-keto forms is indicative of a high level of 11β-hydroxysteroid dehydrogenase activity in the *Microtus* adrenal. Under the condi-

TABLE 4
STEROID PRODUCTS FROM METABOLISM OF RADIOACTIVE PRECURSORS BY *Microtus* ADRENALS (FROM OGUNSUA ET AL., 1971; UNGAR ET AL., 1973, 1978)

Product	*Microtus agrestis*	*Microtus pennsylvanicus*
Corticosterone	X	X
11-Dehydrocorticosterone	X	X
11-Deoxycorticosterone	X	
18-Hydroxycorticosterone	X	
18-Hydroxy-11-dehydrocorticosterone		X
Tetrahydro-11-dehydrocorticosterone		X
Aldosterone	X	

tions of in vitro incubation in a closed system, Ungar et al. (1973) concluded that Compound B and other 11β-hydroxysteroids were formed and oxidized to the 11-keto form. They also noted that, whereas low levels of Compound A were detected in many species, significant levels were only found in incubations of rabbit adrenal.

In a subsequent study, Ungar et al. (1978) established Compound B as the major conversion product from steroid precursors incubated with homogenates of *Microtus* adrenals, and that Compound A formed a secondary conversion product via action of 11β-OHD (11β-hydroxysteroid dehydrogenase). They further noted a significant seasonal variation in 11β-OHD activity in *M. pennsylvanicus* and *M. ochrogaster*. Peak activity occurred during fall and winter and dropped markedly during spring and summer. They suggested that, in light of prior association of other components of adrenal function with reproductive activity, there may be a significant negative correlation between 11β-OHD activity and seasonal reproductive development.

Level of Secretion

Serum corticosterone levels averaged 50.4 (34.0 to 69.7) μg/100 ml in lab-raised male *M. pennsylvanicus* and 71.4 (58.5 to 83.9) μg/100 ml in females (Seabloom, 1965). Plasma levels reported for *M. townsendii* averaged 27 μg/100 ml in males and 234 μg/100 ml in females (McDonald and Taitt, 1982). Corticosterone concentrations in *Microtus* were three to six times greater than those reported for laboratory mice and rats. However, studies of steroid levels in *Rattus* and *Mus* have been confined essentially to inbred domestic strains. The wild Norway rat (*Rattus norvegicus*) has adrenal glands several times larger than those of its domestic counterpart. While severity of daily living can be a factor in determination of adrenal size and secretion rate, Seabloom and Seabloom (1974) suggested that "if smaller size is related to reduced adrenal function, it is possible that in the process of selection for 'tameness' and in the absence of natural selective pressures certain genetic shifts, including those affecting adrenocortical function, may occur." Superfused adrenals of wild and domestic house mice exhibited significantly different levels of response to ACTH stimulation. Adrenals of wild house mice (*Mus musculus*) reared from birth by domestic mothers responded in the same manner as their wild-caught counterparts, indicating genetic differences between wild and domestic stocks rather than response to the stimuli of capture and handling.

Corticosterone levels in wild-caught *M. pennsylvanicus* were markedly higher than in laboratory-reared voles (Seabloom, 1965). Certainly, the captive environment does not provide the configurations of stimuli for adrenal response comparable to that occurring in the wild. However, the data also indicate that in the process of selection for domestication the responsiveness of the adrenal cortex in a wild species may be greatly diminished.

The initial exposure to the captive environment provides a significant stimulus for prolonged, elevated secretion of corticosterone in *M. pennsylvanicus* (Olsen and Seabloom, 1973). Both adrenal and serum corticosterone were highest on day 1 of captivity, declined rapidly until day 30, and then went into a more gradual decline until they appeared to stabilize around day 70 (Table 5). Regression coefficients of logs of adrenal and serum corticosterone levels on time were significantly different from zero in both males and females. Furthermore, the slopes of the regressions were significantly steeper in males than females. Consequently, wild *Microtus* must make profound physiologic adjustments during the first few weeks of captivity. The alteration in level of adrenocortical secretion subsequent to capture appears to provide an indicator of acclimation, and is also indicative of the difficulty in obtaining valid estimates of secretion in wild voles. Estimates of levels of secretion in captive colonies are subject to question because of selection for

TABLE 5

CORTICOSTERONE LEVELS [($\bar{X} \pm SE$ (N))] IN *Microtus pennsylvanicus* AFTER VARYING PERIODS OF CAPTIVITY (AFTER OLSEN AND SEABLOOM, 1973)

Day	Adrenal (nanograms/100 g body wt)		Serum (nanograms/ml)	
	Males	Females	Males	Females
1	9,051 ± 1,469 (6)	8,360 ± 1,083 (6)	1,397 ± 131 (6)	1,562 ± 470 (6)
10	3,733 ± 979 (5)	4,291 ± 737 (5)	915 ± 152 (5)	907 ± 247 (5)
20	2,855 ± 1,228 (5)	4,150 ± 463 (7)	773 ± 211 (5)	883 ± 155 (7)
30	1,567 ± 264 (10)	4,214 ± 521 (10)	494 ± 94 (9)	776 ± 119 (10)
40	1,044 ± 130 (11)	3,607 ± 721 (9)	496 ± 57 (10)	972 ± 156 (7)
50	2,054 ± 329 (10)	3,525 ± 653 (10)	418 ± 47 (10)	660 ± 87 (9)
60	1,056 ± 209 (10)	4,633 ± 1,193 (10)	304 ± 52 (10)	992 ± 251 (10)
70	675 ± 126 (9)	1,784 ± 424 (10)	300 ± 49 (10)	590 ± 150 (10)

tameness, while determination of normal secretion rates in wild-caught stocks appear to require extensive periods of acclimation.

Periodicity

The adrenal-cortical function of *M. pennsylvanicus* exhibits a marked daily periodicity, and can fluctuate as much as 157% around the 24-h mean (Fig. 1). Peaks of both serum and adrenal corticosterone occur in mid-afternoon and lows during hours of darkness. The daily rhythm is similar to that demonstrated for laboratory mice (*Mus musculus*), where the adrenal peak precedes the motor-activity peak by about 4 h. However, unlike *Mus, M. pennsylvanicus* does not exhibit a well-defined rhythm of daily motor activity (Seabloom, 1965). Under controlled conditions, there are successive short bursts of motor activity throughout the 24-h period. However, these bursts are more numerous and of longer duration during hours of darkness. Consequently, as with more distinctive nocturnal species, the *Microtus* adrenal cortex appears to be activated in anticipation of the onset of increased motor activity. Meier (1975) reviewed work on the functions of corticoid rhythms in a variety of vertebrates and concluded that the daily light-dark cycle is the principal entrainer of the daily adrenal cycle. The daily adrenal cycle in turn functions in entraining many metabolic and behavioral rhythms, including that of motor activity.

The superfused adrenal of *M. pennsylvanicus* exhibits an annual periodicity in response to ACTH stimulation which can be correlated with the animal's behavioral and reproductive state (Seabloom et al., 1978). Although there are no significant changes in adult male adrenal weight throughout the year, there is a gradual increase in magnitude of response to ACTH which peaks in spring, followed by a sharp drop during early summer (Table 6). A high level of secretory responsiveness occurs in pre-pubescent subadults during early summer. This peak, along with that exhibited by spring adults occurs in animals that have recently entered or are reaching breeding condition. Spring adults are in the process of establishing territories during a period of high aggression, whereas summer subadults represent inexperienced young interacting with a population of established intolerant adults. Consequently, the adrenal response in these cohorts of the population may be attributed to their behavioral state.

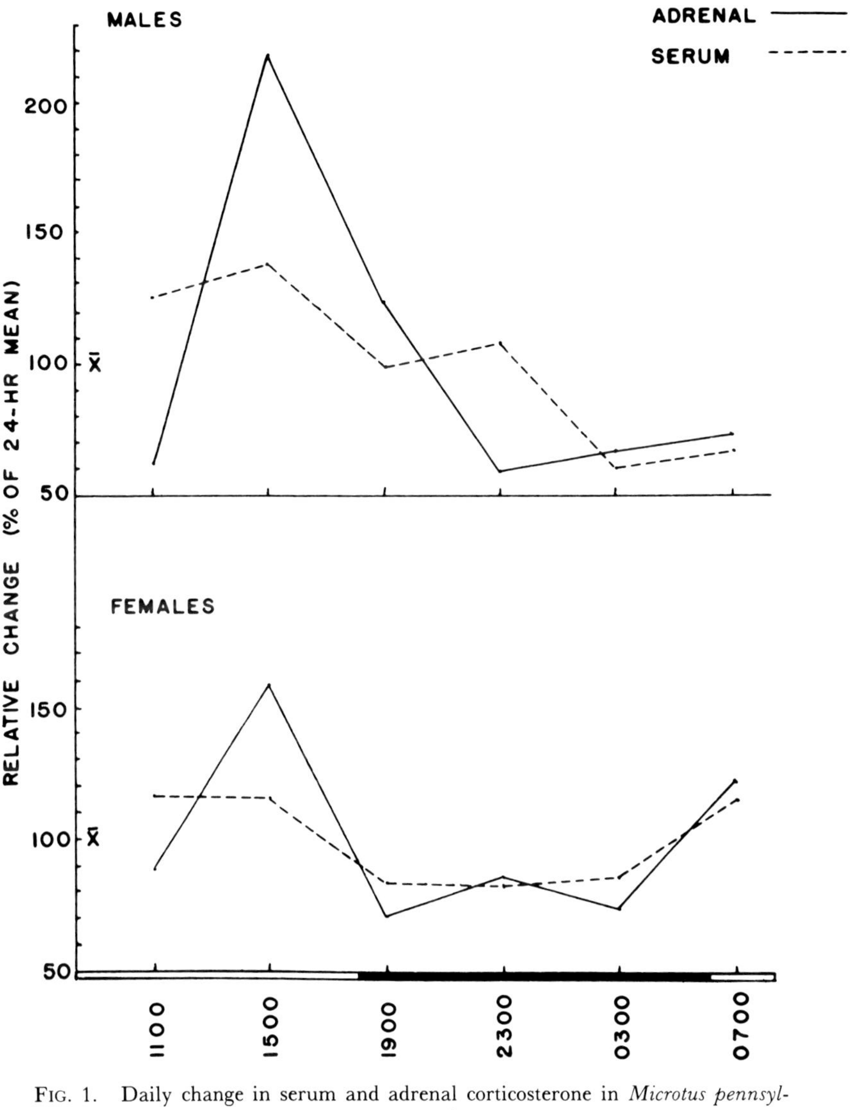

FIG. 1. Daily change in serum and adrenal corticosterone in *Microtus pennsylvanicus* (from Seabloom, 1965, with permission).

TABLE 6

CORTICOSTERONE LEVELS (NANOGRAMS/5 ML SUPERFUSATE/100 G BODY WEIGHT) FOLLOWING SUPERFUSION OF ACTH-STIMULATED ADRENALS OF *Microtus pennsylvanicus* (AFTER SEABLOOM ET AL., 1978)

Season	Age class	Adrenal response	Late summer 1971		Fall 1971		Winter 1971–1972	Spring 1972	Early summer 1972	
			J	A	J	A	I	A	SA	A
Males										
Late summer 1971	J	326								
	A	413								
Fall 1971	J	373								
	A	331								
Winter 1971–1972	I	450								
Spring 1972	A	500	X*		X					
Early summer 1972	SA	486								
	A	374								

Season	Age class	Adrenal response	Late summer 1971			Fall 1971		Winter 1971–1972	Spring 1972		Early summer 1972	
			J	A	P	J	A	I	A	P	A	P
Females												
Late summer 1971	J	468										
	A	492										
	P	401										
Fall 1971	J	317		X								
	A	955	X	X	X	X						
Winter 1971–72	I	396					X					
Spring 1972	A	778	X	X	X	X		X				
Early summer 1972	A	439					X		X	X		
	P	386					X		X	X		

Abbreviations of age classes are: J, juvenile; SA, subadult; A, adult; P, pregnant; I, inactive.
* Denotes significant differences between responses ($P < 0.05$).

In adult and pregnant females, there is a marked peak adrenal response to ACTH which occurs in spring, but the increase in weight of the gland appears to lag, reaching maximum size during summer and fall (Tables 3 and 6). Estradiol enhances ACTH secretion (Coyne and Kitay, 1969), and estrogen dependent increases in corticoid binding during the breeding season result in compensatory adrenal growth and secretion (Christian, 1975). In *Microtus,* the time-lag between the peaks of adrenal responsiveness and glandular size increase appears to be significant, however, and complete dependence on adrenal weight as an index of seasonal changes in secretion may result in considerable timing error.

Response to Stimuli

Secretions of the adrenal cortex are involved in metabolic regulation and play a significant role in acclimation to environmental change. There is a plethora of reports involving adrenocortical response of laboratory species, especially mice and rats, to a variety of stimuli. However, in-depth studies involving wild species, including *Microtus,* are uncommon.

The duration of daily illumination appears to have an indirect effect on development and secretion of the adrenal cortex. In *M. montanus,* typical sexual dimorphism in adrenal size (see Adrenal Morphology) was masked in animals kept under short photoperiods (Pinter, 1968). Normal development of the adrenal, however, is probably more a direct function of reproductive status than photoperiod, whereas the daily light-dark cycle functions in entraining the 24-h corticoid rhythm (Meier, 1975).

The stimulus of captivity results in significant increases in serum and adrenal corticosterone in *M. pennsylvanicus* (see Level of Secretion). The relative response of males to captivity appears to be greater than that of females, but the total period of acclimation is about the same. After at least 70 days of confinement, corticosterone levels were considered to represent "complete" acclimation to the captive environment. However, it is not known if these levels were representative of those exhibited by free-living meadow voles in the wild.

There is a considerable body of evidence correlating adrenocortical activity with social or behavioral stimuli. The spring peak adrenal response to ACTH in adult male *M. pennsylvanicus* reported by Seabloom et al. (1978) (see Periodicity) is associated with the season of elevated levels of male aggression (Turner and Iverson, 1973). Interactions between different behavioral components and the functioning of the adrenal-pituitary axis have been reviewed by Brain (1972), Bronson and Desjardins (1971), and Davidson and Levine (1972). Brain (1972) noted the difficulty in separating behavioral and physiological (gonadal) influences on adrenal function, but it generally is agreed that routine activity, fighting, sexual activity, and fear-motivated responses all cause elevated secretion of corticosteroids. These behaviors are at their peak during spring and are associated with territorial establishment and other events of the early breeding season. In like manner, the elevated adrenal response of subadult males during early summer may result from the stresses involved in recruitment of inexperienced pubescent animals into an established territorial population.

Population density may, in conjunction with other social factors, elicit increased rates of corticosteroid secretion. However, documentation of the effect of such factors on adrenocortical function has been extremely difficult because of the rapid and stereotyped response of the cortex to many different stimuli, and the consequent problem of distinguishing the response to the density-dependent stimulus from that to trapping and handling. Even though much has been written on correlation of adrenal function with fluctuations in population density in *Microtus,* there have been very few in-depth studies dealing with confined or wild populations of this or any other genus of small mammal.

Studies of confined and free-living New World *Microtus* to date have correlated high population density with decreased eosinophil counts, an indicator of increased cortical activity (Louch, 1956, 1958), and increased adrenal weight (Christian, 1959; Christian and Davis, 1966). Subsequently, Christian (1975) presented data indicating significant positive correlations between adrenal weight and population size for female *M. pennsylvanicus,* but not for males. However, adrenal size in males was significantly correlated with degree of scarring (presumably from fighting). Using data from a variety of sources, Christian (1975) proposed that endocrine behavioral feedback mechanisms can operate in mammalian populations through aggressive encounters, resulting in increased pituitary-adrenal activity and diminished pituitary-gonadal activity "by peripheral feedbacks in the form of adrenal androgens and possibly progesterone, or by a short loop feedback in the form of ACTH inhibition of gonadotrophin secretion."

Adrenocortical-Gonadal Interaction

Adrenals of adult female *Microtus* may be two to four times larger than those of adult males, while levels of circulating corticosterone and adrenal response to ACTH can average 150–200% of observed values for adult males (see Adrenal Morphology, Levels of Secretion, Periodicity). Furthermore, response to ACTH by adrenals of pregnant female meadow voles is suppressed when compared to nonpregnant adults (Table 6; Seabloom et al., 1978).

Although the female-male and pregnant-nonpregnant cohorts are certainly exposed to differing configurations of social stimuli, there is overwhelming evidence based largely on work with other species for significant negative feedback between the pituitary-adrenal and pituitary-gonadal axes. Testosterone inhibits ACTH secretion, whereas estradiol is a known stimulus (Coyne and Kitay, 1969, 1971). Furthermore, progesterone inhibits corticosterone secretion (Rodier and Kitay, 1974). Consequently, adrenal enlargement and secretion in the male are inhibited with sexual maturation; secretory activity in the female is modulated by the relative levels of the principal gonadal hormones present at various stages of estrus and pregnancy. Hunter and Hunter (1972) noted that adrenal function may shift with stage of pregnancy, again a correlation with estrogen-progesterone balance. Therefore, the differing levels of ACTH responsiveness in non-pregnant and pregnant meadow voles can be interpreted in terms of estrogen and progesterone domination.

Conversely, a high level of adrenocortical activity can affect reproductive function. Christian (1975) noted that increased secretion of adrenal corticoids, androgens, progesterone, and other steroids is associated with inhibition of reproductive activity. Increased levels of adrenal androgens and progesterone may inhibit secretion of gonadotrophins. Christian also suggested that ACTH per se can act as a short-loop feedback inhibiting gonadotrophin releasers at the hypothalamic level. Pasley and Christian (1971) found that exogenous ACTH administration inhibited ovarian development, uterine development, and spermatogenesis in *M. pennsylvanicus*, effects similar to those observed in *Mus* and *Peromyscus*. In a subsequent study, Pasley (1974) stimulated endogenous production of ACTH in *M. pennsylvanicus* through administration of metyrapone, an 11β-hydroxylase inhibitor. Following daily metyrapone injections, compensatory increase in ACTH production occurred, resulting in depressed body, uterine, and ovarian weights of females, and decreased seminal-vesicle weights of males. Pasley further noted that, in the absence of 11β-hydroxylation, ACTH stimulation enhances secretion of adrenal androgens, thus providing additional inhibition of gonadotrophin secretion.

Summary and Conclusions

Detailed knowledge to date of the endocrinology of the North American *Microtus* is limited to certain aspects of the reproductive and adrenopituitary systems, involving six species. Comparative data are sparse; indeed, the literature indicates that values and mechanisms described for one species have been extrapolated readily to the entire genus and beyond.

North American representatives of the genus generally exhibit an annual periodicity of reproductive activity that results from a balance between an endogenus circannual rhythm and several known exogenous factors, including daily photoperiod, light intensity, temperature, nutritional cues, and social factors. The recent identification of naturally occurring plant compounds that can stimulate or inhibit reproduction in *M. montanus* has major significance in comparative physiology and ecology. If their effects can be demonstrated in other species, a new chapter will have been written in our understanding of the regulation of breeding cycles.

Olfactory cues involving pheromones contained in male urine have important regulatory effects on female maturation and induction of estrus. Recent studies have implicated the posterior olfactory bulb as providing a neuroendocrine link between the external environment and secretion of the reproductive regulators LHRH and norepinephrine.

Coitus-induced ovulation appears to be well established in both New World and Old World *Microtus* as an important phenomenon maximizing reproductive efficiency. Vaginal-cervical stimulation alone may be sufficient to induce ovulation, but there is also indication that pheromonal or other contact factors may play a role. Limited copulatory stimulation may result in formation of abnormally short-lived corpora lutea.

Male-induced pregnancy blockage in *Microtus* has been documented for pre-implantation and post-implantation stages, and there has been recent evidence for the "strange male" or Bruce effect resulting in poor litter survival following parturition. Odor alone is sufficient to effect blockage, and there is evidence that the phenomenon may be a side effect of induced estrus and ovulation.

All microtines studied go through a post-partum estrus, which occurs between one and four days following parturition. In some cases, estrus and ovulation may occur on the day of parturition.

Little work has been done on the control of lactation in *Microtus,* but estrogen and glucocorticoid-binding macromolecules have been demonstrated in the lactating mammary gland. There is some indication that the "strange male" or Bruce effect can apply to post-partum events, such as lactation, via hypothalamic inhibition of prolactin secretion.

In contrast to female *Microtus,* there has been little attention paid to male reproductive physiology. The morphology of the male reproductive tract has been described. The spermatogenic cycle has been described for *M. ochrogaster,* and circulating androgen levels are reported for *M. breweri* and *M. townsendii.*

Thyroid activity has been studied in four species of North American *Microtus.* Generally, activity is suppressed by high population density, food depletion, harassment, and shortened photoperiods. Serum thyroxine and rates of radioiodine release have been studied in *M. montanus, M. ochrogaster,* and *M. pennsylvanicus.* Blockage of thyroid secretion results in a 3°C increase in the highest air temperature tolerated without stress in *M. ochrogaster.* Serum thyroxine does not change with alteration of air temperature, but rate of radioiodine uptake is reciprocally related to air temperature.

Adrenal-weight relations have been recorded for six species of North American *Microtus,* and generally fall within the range of variation for other small mammals. With maturation, there is a significant sexual dimorphism in adrenal size. Relative adrenal weight in females is doubled; a decrease occurs in males that is associated with involution of the X-zone. In females, adrenal enlargement is associated with increase in inner cortical mass in response to greater rates of binding in plasma and hepatic clearance of corticosteroids.

Corticosterone is the major steroid secreted by the *Microtus* adrenal, but small amounts of other steroids also have been recorded. The occurrence of Compound A (11-dehydrocorticosterone) in *Mi-*

crotus adrenal-incubates indicates a very high level of 11β-hydroxysteroid dehydrogenase activity. There is indication that the level of dehydrogenase activity varies seasonally, being highest during fall and winter.

Levels of corticosterone secretion are significantly higher than those recorded for laboratory rats and mice, in spite of comparable relative adrenal size. These secretion rates may be attributed to the stimulus of capture and confinement, and to genetic adaptation of a wild species to its natural environment.

The adrenal cortex exhibits both daily and seasonal periodicity in secretion rate. The daily rhythm can fluctuate as much as 157% around the 24-h mean, with a peak in the afternoon and a low during hours of darkness. Seasonal adrenal response to ACTH stimulation is highest during spring (the early breeding season).

As with other species, *Microtus* adrenal function is influenced by many exogenous stimuli, including light, captivity, aggression, and population density. However, specific documentation of each response has been very difficult because of the sterotyped, high-magnitude response of the gland to all stimuli.

Adrenal-gonadal interactions have been demonstrated in New World *Microtus*. Adrenal enlargement and secretion in males is inhibited by high testosterone levels at puberty. Secretory activity in females is modulated by increased levels of gonadal hormones during estrus and pregnancy. At puberty and estrus, there is adrenal enlargement and a high secretion rate in the estrogen-dominated female, whereas high progesterone levels during pregnancy appear to inhibit adrenal response.

Conversely, ACTH administration has been shown to inhibit spermatogenesis and ovarian and uterine development in *M. pennsylvanicus*. The effect can be direct or via ACTH stimulation of adrenal androgen secretion, which in turn inhibits secretion of gonadotrophins.

Literature Cited

Adams, M. R., R. H. Tamarin, and I. P. Callard. 1980. Seasonal changes in plasma androgen levels and the gonads of the beach vole, *Microtus breweri*. Gen. Comp. Endocrinol., 41:31–40.

Asdell, S. A. 1964. Patterns of mammalian reproduction. Third ed. Cornell Univ. Press, Ithaca, New York, 670 pp.

BADDALOO, E. G. Y., AND F. V. CLULOW. 1981. Effects of the male on growth, sexual maturation, and ovulation of young female meadow voles, *Microtus pennsylvanicus*. Canadian J. Zool., 59:415–421.

BAILEY, V. 1924. Breeding, feeding, and other life habits of meadow mice (*Microtus*). J. Agric. Res., 27:523–537.

BATZLI, G. O., L. L. GETZ, AND S. S. HURLEY. 1977. Suppression of growth and reproduction of microtine rodents by social factors. J. Mamm., 58:583–591.

BEER, J. R., AND C. F. MACLEOD. 1961. Seasonal reproduction in the meadow vole. J. Mamm., 42:483–489.

BEERS, P. C., AND J. L. WITTLIFF. 1973. Identification and partial characterization of specific estrogen receptors in the vole (*Microtus montanus*). Comp. Biochem. Physiol., 46B:647–652.

BENTLEY, P. J. 1976. Comparative vertebrate endocrinology. Cambridge Univ. Press, London, 415 pp.

BERGER, P. J., AND N. C. NEGUS. 1974. Influence of dietary supplements of fresh lettuce on ovariectomized *Microtus montanus*. J. Mamm., 55:747–750.

———. 1982. Stud male maintenance of pregnancy in *Microtus montanus*. J. Mamm., 63:148–151.

BERGER, P. J., N. C. NEGUS, E. H. SANDERS, AND P. D. GARDNER. 1981. Chemical triggering of reproduction in *Microtus montanus*. Science, 214:69–70.

BERGER, P. J., E. H. SANDERS, P. D. GARDNER, AND N. C. NEGUS. 1977. Phenolic plant compounds functioning as reproductive inhibitors in *Microtus montanus*. Science, 195:575–577.

BRAIN, P. F. 1972. Mammalian behavior and the adrenal cortex—a review. Behav. Biol., 7:453–477.

BREED, W. G. 1967. Ovulation in the genus *Microtus*. Nature, 214:826.

BRONSON, F. H., AND C. DESJARDINS. 1971. Steroid hormones and aggressive behavior in mammals. Pp. 43–63, *in* The physiology of aggression and defeat (B. E. Eleftheriou and J. P. Scott, eds.). Plenum Publ. Corp., New York, 312 pp.

BRUCE, H. M. 1966. Smell as an exteroceptive factor. J. Anim. Sci., 25:83–87.

CARTER, C. S., L. L. GETZ, L. GAVISH, J. L. MCDERMOTT, AND P. ARNOLD. 1980. Male-related pheromones and the activation of female reproduction in the prairie vole (*Microtus ochrogaster*). Biol. Reprod., 23:1038–1045.

CHESTER JONES, I. 1957. The adrenal cortex. Cambridge Univ. Press, London, 316 pp.

CHITTY, H., AND J. R. CLARKE. 1963. The growth of the adrenal gland of laboratory and field voles, and changes in it during pregnancy. Canadian J. Zool., 41:1025–1034.

CHRISTIAN, J. J. 1953. The relation of adrenal weight to body weight in mammals. Science, 117:78–80.

———. 1956. Adrenal and reproductive responses to population size in mice from freely growing populations. Ecology, 37:258–273.

———. 1959. The roles of endocrine and behavioral factors in the growth of mammalian populations. Pp. 71–97, *in* Comparative endocrinology (A. Gorman, ed.). John Wiley and Sons, New York, 746 pp.

———. 1961. Phenomena associated with population density. Proc. Natl. Acad. Sci., 47:428–448.

———. 1963. Endocrine adaptive mechanisms and the physiologic regulation of population growth. Pp. 189–353, *in* Physiological mammalogy (W. V. Mayer and R. G. Van Gelder, eds.). Academic Press, New York, 1:1–381.

———. 1971. Population density and reproductive efficiency. Biol. Reprod., 4:248–294.

———. 1975. Hormonal control of population growth. Pp. 205–274, *in* Hormonal correlates of behavior (B. E. Eleftheriou and R. L. Sprott, eds.). Plenum Publ. Corp., New York, 806 pp.

CHRISTIAN, J. J., AND D. E. DAVIS. 1964. Endocrines, behavior, and population. Science, 146:1550–1560.

———. 1966. Adrenal glands in female voles (*Microtus pennsylvanicus*) as related to reproduction and population size. J. Mamm., 47:1–18.

CHRISTIAN, J. J., J. A. LLOYD, AND D. E. DAVIS. 1965. The roles of endocrines in the self-regulation of mammalian populations. Recent Prog. Horm. Res., 21:501–578.

CLULOW, F. V., AND P. E. LANGFORD. 1971. Pregnancy block in the meadow vole, (*Microtus pennsylvanicus*). J. Reprod. Fert., 24:275–277.

CLULOW, F. V., AND F. F. MALLORY. 1970. Oestrus and induced ovulation in the meadow vole, *Microtus pennsylvanicus*. J. Reprod. Fert., 23:341–343.

———. 1974. Ovaries of meadow voles, *Microtus pennsylvanicus,* after copulation with a series of males. Canadian J. Zool., 52:265–268.

COYNE, M. D., AND J. I. KITAY. 1969. Effect of ovariectomy on pituitary secretion of ACTH. Endocrinology, 85:1097–1102.

———. 1971. Effect of orchiectomy on pituitary secretion of ACTH. Endocrinology, 89:1024–1028.

CROSS, P. C. 1971. The dictyate oocyte of *Microtus montanus*. J. Reprod. Fert., 25:291–293.

———. 1972. Observations on the induction of ovulation in *Microtus montanus*. J. Mamm., 53:210–212.

DAVIDSON, J. M., AND S. LEVINE. 1972. Endocrine regulation of behavior. Ann. Rev. Physiol., 34:375–407.

DAVIS, H. N., G. D. GRAY, M. ZERYLNICK, AND D. A. DEWSBURY. 1974. Ovulation and implantation in montane voles (*Microtus montanus*) as a function of varying amounts of copulatory stimulation. Horm. Behav., 5:383–388.

DELOST, P. 1952. Le cortex surrenal du campagnol des champs (*Microtus arvalis*) et ses modification apres castration. Compt. Rend. Soc. Biol., 146:27–31.

DELOST, P., AND P. CHIRVAN-NIA. 1956. Donnes experimentales compares sur la zone X surrenalienne. Action de la cortisone et de la testosterone. Compt. Rend. Soc. Biol., 150:1330–1332.

DIETERICH, R. A., AND D. J. PRESTON. 1977. The meadow vole (*Microtus pennsylvanicus*) as a laboratory animal. Lab. Anim. Sci., 27:494–499.

DIETERICH, R. A., P. R. MORRISON, AND D. J. PRESTON. 1973. Comparative organ weights for eight standardized wild rodent species. Lab. Anim. Sci., 23:575–581.

DLUZEN, D. E., V. D. RAMIREZ, C. S. CARTER, AND L. L. GETZ. 1981. Male vole urine changes luteinizing hormone-releasing hormone and norepinephrine in female olfactory bulb. Science, 212:573–575.

FITCH, H. S. 1957. Aspects of reproduction and development in the prairie vole (*Microtus ochrogaster*). Misc. Publ. Mus. Nat. Hist., Univ. Kansas, 10: 129–161.

GEYER, L. A., AND J. G. ROGERS, JR. 1979. The influence of light intensity on reproduction in pine voles, *Microtus pinetorum*. J. Mamm., 60:839–841.

GRAY, G. D., H. N. DAVIS, A. M. KENNEY, AND D. A. DEWSBURY. 1976. Effect of mating on plasma levels of LH and progesterone in montane voles (*Microtus montanus*). J. Reprod. Fert., 47:89–91.

GRAY, G. D., H. N. DAVIS, M. ZERYLNICK, AND D. A. DEWSBURY. 1974*a*. Oestrus and induced ovulation in montane voles. J. Reprod. Fert., 38:193–196.

GRAY, G. D., M. ZERYLNICK, H. N. DAVIS, AND D. A. DEWSBURY. 1974*b*. Effects of variations in male copulatory behavior on ovulation and implantation in prairie voles, *Microtus ochrogaster*. Horm. Behav., 5:389–396.

GREENWALD, G. S. 1956. The reproductive cycle of the field mouse, *Microtus californicus*. J. Mamm., 37:213–222.

———. 1957. Reproduction in a coastal California population of the field mouse, *Microtus californicus*. Univ. California Publ. Zool., 54:421–446.

GROCOCK, C. A. 1980. Effects of age on photo-induced testicular regression, recrudescence, and refractoriness in the short-tailed field vole *Microtus agrestis*. Biol. Reprod., 23:15–20.

GUSTAFSON, A. W., AND M. SHEMESH. 1976. Changes in plasma testosterone levels during the annual reproductive cycle of the hibernating bat, *Myotis lucifugus lucifugus,* with a survey of plasma testosterone levels in adult male vertebrates. Biol. Reprod., 15:9–24.

HASLER, J. F. 1975. A review of reproduction and sexual maturation in the microtine rodents. The Biologist, 57:52–86.

HASLER, M. J., AND C. H. CONAWAY. 1973. The effect of males on the reproductive state of female *Microtus ochrogaster*. Biol. Reprod., 9:425–436.

HASLER, M. J., AND A. B. NALBANDOV. 1974. The effect of weanling and adult males on sexual maturation in female voles (*Microtus ochrogaster*). Gen. Comp. Endocrinol., 23:237–238.

HINKLEY, R., JR. 1966. Effects of plant extracts in the diet of male *Microtus montanus* on cell types of the anterior pituitary. J. Mamm., 47:396–400.

HOULIHAN, R. T. 1963. The relationship of population density to endocrine and metabolic changes in the California vole *Microtus californicus*. Univ. California Publ. Zool., 65:327–362.

HOYTE, H. M. D. 1955. Observations on reproduction in some small mammals of arctic Norway. J. Anim. Ecol., 24:412–425.

HUDSON, J. W. 1980. The thyroid gland and temperature regulation in the prairie vole, *Microtus ochrogaster,* and the chipmunk, *Tamias striatus*. Comp. Biochem. Physiol., 65A:173–179.

HUNTER, J. S., AND F. HUNTER. 1972. Ovarian-adrenal-liver interactions during pregnancy and lactation in the rat. Endokrinologie, 59:1–47.

IMEL, K. J., AND R. P. AMANN. 1979. Effects of duration of daily illumination on reproductive organs and fertility of the meadow vole (*Microtus pennsylvanicus*). Lab. Anim. Sci., 29:182–185.

JANES, D. W. 1963. The reproductive system of the prairie vole, *Microtus ochrogaster*. Unpubl. Ph.D. dissert., Kansas State Univ., Manhattan, 110 pp.

JANNETT, F. J., JR. 1979. Experimental laboratory studies on the interactions of sympatric voles (Microtinae). Amer. Zool., 19:966.

JÖCHLE, W. 1973. Coitus-induced ovulation. Contraception, 7:523–564.

KENNEY, A. M., AND D. A. DEWSBURY. 1977. Effect of limited mating on the corpora lutea in montane voles, *Microtus montanus*. J. Reprod. Fert., 49: 363–364.

KENNEY, A. M., R. L. EVANS, AND D. A. DEWSBURY. 1977*a*. Postimplantation pregnancy disruption in *Microtus ochrogaster, M. pennsylvanicus,* and *Peromyscus maniculatus*. J. Reprod. Fert., 49:365–367.

KENNEY, A. M., D. L. LANIER, AND D. A. DEWSBURY. 1977*b*. Effects of vaginal-cervical stimulation in seven species in muroid rodents. J. Reprod. Fert., 49:305–309.

KIRKPATRICK, R. L., AND G. L. VALENTINE. 1970. Reproduction in captive pine voles, *Microtus pinetorum*. J. Mamm., 51:779–785.

KREBS, C. J., M. S. GAINES, B. L. KELLER, J. H. MEYERS, AND R. H. TAMARIN. 1973. Population cycles in small rodents. Science, 179:35–41.

LABOV, J. B. 1977. Phytoestrogens and mammalian reproduction. Comp. Biochem. Physiol., 57A:3–9.

LEE, C., D. J. HORVATH, R. W. METCALF, AND E. K. INSKEEP. 1970. Ovulation in *Microtus pennsylvanicus* in a laboratory environment. Lab. Anim. Care, 20:1098–1102.

LOUCH, C. D. 1956. Adrenocortical activity in relation to the density and dynamics of three confined populations of *Microtus pennsylvanicus*. Ecology, 37:701–713.

———. 1958. Adrenocortical activity in two meadow vole populations. J. Mamm., 39:109–116.

MACFARLANE, J. D., AND J. M. TAYLOR. 1981. Sexual maturation in female Townsend's voles. Acta Theriol., 26:113–117.

———. 1982*a*. Nature of estrus and ovulation in *Microtus townsendii* (Bachman). J. Mamm., 63:104–109.

———. 1982*b*. Pregnancy and reproductive performance in the Townsend's vole, *Microtus townsendii* (Bachman). J. Mamm., 63:165–168.

MALLORY, F. F., AND F. V. CLULOW. 1977. Evidence of pregnancy failure in the wild meadow vole, *Microtus pennsylvanicus*. Canadian J. Zool., 55:1–17.

MCDONALD, I. R., AND M. J. TAITT. 1982. Steroid hormones in the blood plasma of Townsend's vole (*Microtus townsendii*). Canadian J. Zool., 60:2264–2269.

MCGUIRE, M. R., AND L. L. GETZ. 1981. Incest taboo between sibling *Microtus ochrogaster*. J. Mamm., 62:213–215.

MCKEEVER, S. 1959. Effects of reproductive activity on the weight of adrenal glands in *Microtus montanus*. Anat. Rec., 135:1–5.

MEIER, A. H. 1975. Chronoendocrinology of vertebrates. Pp. 469–549, *in* Hormonal correlates of behavior (B. E. Eleftheriou and R. L. Sprott, eds.). Plenum Publ. Corp., New York, 806 pp.

MILLIGAN, S. R. 1974. Social environment and ovulation in the vole, *Microtus agrestis*. J. Reprod. Fert., 41:35–47.

———. 1975. Mating, ovulation and corpus luteum function in the vole, *Microtus agrestis*. J. Reprod. Fert., 42:35–44.

MORRISON, P. R., R. A. DIETERICH, AND D. J. PRESTON. 1976. Breeding and reproduction of fifteen wild rodents maintained as laboratory colonies. Lab. Anim. Sci., 26:232–243.

MULLEN, D. A. 1960. Adrenal weight changes in *Microtus*. J. Mamm., 41:129–130.

NEGUS, N. C., AND P. J. BERGER. 1971. Pineal weight response to a dietary variable in *Microtus montanus*. Experientia, 27:215–216.

———. 1977. Experimental triggering of reproduction in a natural population of *Microtus montanus*. Science, 196:1230–1231.

NEGUS, N. C., AND A. J. PINTER. 1966. Reproductive responses of *Microtus montanus* to plants and plant extracts in the diet. J. Mamm., 47:596–601.

NEGUS, N. C., P. J. BERGER, AND L. G. FORSLUND. 1977. Reproductive strategy of *Microtus montanus*. J. Mamm., 58:347–353.

OGUNSUA, A. O., A. F. DENICOLA, H. TRAIKOV, M. K. BIRMINGHAM, AND S. LEVINE. 1971. Adrenal steroid biosynthesis by different species of mouselike rodents. Gen. Comp. Endocrinol., 16:192–199.

OLSEN, D. E., AND R. W. SEABLOOM. 1973. Adrenocortical response to captivity in *Microtus pennsylvanicus*. J. Mamm., 54:779–781.

PASLEY, J. N. 1974. Effects of metyrapone on reproductive organs of the meadow vole, *Microtus pennsylvanicus*. J. Reprod. Fert., 40:451–453.

PASLEY, J. N., AND J. J. CHRISTIAN. 1971. Effects of ACTH on voles (*Microtus pennsylvanicus*) related to reproductive function and renal disease. Proc. Soc. Exp. Biol. Med., 137:268–272.

PASLEY, J. N., AND T. D. MCKINNEY. 1973. Grouping and ovulation in *Microtus pennsylvanicus*. J. Reprod. Fert., 34:527–530.

PETTERBORG, L. J. 1978. Effect of photoperiod on body weight in the vole, *Microtus montanus*. Canadian J. Zool., 56:431–435.

PINTER, A. J. 1968. Effects of diet and light on growth, maturation, and adrenal size of *Microtus montanus*. Amer. J. Physiol., 215:461–466.

PINTER, A. J., AND N. C. NEGUS. 1965. Effects of nutrition and photoperiod on reproductive physiology of *Microtus montanus*. Amer. J. Physiol., 208:633–638.

PISTOLE, D. H., AND J. A. CRANFORD. 1982. Photoperiodic effects on growth in *Microtus pennsylvanicus*. J. Mamm., 63:547–553.

PRENTICE, R. C., AND B. A. SHEPHERD. 1978. The relationship between the ovarian vesicular follicle population and serum estradiol-17β concentration in *Microtus ochrogaster ochrogaster*. Trans. Illinois State Acad. Sci., 71:286–290.

QUIRING, D. P. 1951. A comparison between *Microtus drummondi* (Aud. & Bach.) and *Microtus pennsylvanicus pennsylvanicus*. Growth, 15:101–120.

RICHMOND, M. E. 1967. Reproduction of the vole, *Microtus ochrogaster*. Unpubl. Ph.D. dissert., Univ. Missouri, Columbia, 108 pp.

RICHMOND, M. E., AND C. H. CONAWAY. 1969*a*. Management, breeding, and reproductive performance of the vole, *Microtus ochrogaster*, in a laboratory colony. Lab. Anim. Care, 19:80–87.

———. 1969*b*. Induced ovulation and oestrous in *Microtus ochrogaster*. J. Reprod. Fert. Suppl., 6:357–376.

RICHMOND, M. E., AND R. A. STEHN. 1976. Olfaction and reproductive behavior in microtine rodents. Pp. 198–217, *in* Mammalian olfaction, reproductive processes and behavior (R. L. Doty, ed.). Academic Press, New York, 344 pp.

RODIER, W. I., AND J. I. KITAY. 1974. The influence of progesterone on adrenocortical function in the rat. Proc. Soc. Exp. Biol. Med., 146:376–380.

RUGH, R. 1968. The mouse: its reproduction and development. Burgess, Minneapolis, 430 pp.

SANDERS, E. H., P. D. GARDNER, P. J. BERGER, AND N. C. NEGUS. 1981. 6-methoxybenzoxazolinone: a plant derivative that stimulates reproduction in *Microtus montanus*. Science, 214:67–69.

SCHADLER, M. H. 1980. The effect of crowding on the maturation of gonads in pine voles, *Microtus pinetorum*. J. Mamm., 61:769–744.

———. 1981. Postimplantation abortion in pine voles (*Microtus pinetorum*) induced by strange males and pheromones of strange males. Biol. Reprod., 25:295–297.

———. 1982. Strange males block pregnancy in lactating pine voles, *Microtus pinetorum*, and effect survival and growth of nursing young. Proceedings of the eastern pine and meadow vole symposium, 6:132–138.

SCHADLER, M. H., AND G. M. BUTTERSTEIN. 1979. Reproduction in the pine vole, *Microtus pinetorum*. J. Mamm., 60:841–844.

SCHULER, H. M., AND H. T. GIER. 1976. Duration of the cycle of the seminiferous epithelium in the prairie vole (*Microtus ochrogaster*). J. Exp. Zool., 197: 1–12.

SEABLOOM, R. W. 1965. Daily motor activity and corticosterone secretion in the meadow vole. J. Mamm., 46:286–295.

SEABLOOM, R. W., AND N. R. SEABLOOM. 1974. Response to ACTH by superfused adrenals of wild and domestic house mice (*Mus musculus*). Life Sci., 15: 73–82.

SEABLOOM, R. W., S. L. IVERSON, AND B. N. TURNER. 1978. Adrenal response in a wild *Microtus* population: seasonal aspects. Canadian J. Zool., 56:1433–1440.

STEHN, R. A., AND F. J. JANNETT, JR. 1981. Male-induced abortion in various microtine rodents. J. Mamm., 62:369–372.

STEHN, R. A., AND M. E. RICHMOND. 1975. Male-induced pregnancy termination in the prairie vole, *Microtus ochrogaster*. Science, 187:1211–1213.

TO, L. P., AND R. H. TAMARIN. 1977. The relation of population density and adrenal gland weight in cycling and non-cycling voles (*Microtus*). Ecology, 58:928–934.

TURNELL, R. W., P. C. BEERS, AND J. L. WITTLIFF. 1974. Glucocorticoid-binding macromolecules in the lactating mammary gland of the vole. Endocrinology, 95:1770–1773.

TURNER, B. N., AND S. L. IVERSON. 1973. The annual cycle of aggression in male *Microtus pennsylvanicus,* and its relation to population parameters. Ecology, 54:967–981.

UNGAR, F., R. GUNVILLE, AND R. W. SEABLOOM. 1973. 11-dehydrocorticosterone (Compd. A) formation by the *Microtus* adrenal. Steroids, 22:503–514.

———. 1978. Seasonal variation in adrenal 11β-hydroxysteroid dehydrogenase activity in the meadow vole (*Microtus pennsylvanicus*). Gen. Comp. Endocrinol., 36:111–118.

VAN TIENHOVEN, A. 1968. Reproductive physiology of vertebrates. Saunders, Philadelphia, 498 pp.

VAUGHAN, M. K., G. M. VAUGHAN, AND R. J. REITER. 1973. Effect of ovariectomy and constant dark on the weight of reproductive and certain other organs in the female vole, *Microtus montanus*. J. Reprod. Fert., 32:9–14.

VAUGHAN, M. K., R. J. REITER, G. M. VAUGHAN, L. BIGELOW, AND M. D. ALTSCHULE. 1972. Inhibition of compensatory ovarian hypertrophy in the mouse and vole: a comparison of Altschule's pineal extract, pineal indoles, vasopressin, and oxytocin. Gen. Comp. Endocrinol., 18:372–377.

REPRODUCTIVE PATTERNS

Barry L. Keller

Abstract

Variation in breeding duration, breeding intensity, and litter size of New World voles is reviewed. Most species appear to follow a facultative strategy with regard to environmental cues that mediate onset and duration of breeding. Eight species (*Microtus californicus, M. oregoni, M. townsendii, M. montanus, M. ochrogaster, M. oeconomus, M. pennsylvanicus,* and *M. pinetorum*) show considerable variation in their breeding periods, whereas six (*M. breweri, M. chrotorrhinus, M. longicaudus, M. mexicanus, M. richardsoni,* and *M. xanthognathus*) appear to have restricted breeding seasons. Early termination or late initiation of breeding are found in species displaying either annual or multi-annual cycles, and it is still not clear why such breeding variations occur. Pregnancy rate does not appear to vary in predictable patterns among species or years, but seasonal variations are apparent. It is unclear whether success of copulation and capacity of a strange male to block pregnancy are important in natural populations, as contrasted to effects documented for laboratory populations. Age at maturation may directly affect breeding intensity, whereas minor variations in sex ratio appear unimportant. Significant changes in breeding intensity can be affected by major disruption of the sex ratio such that the social structure of populations is affected. Age at sexual maturation and length of breeding season may change with such perturbations, but it is not clear whether such effects occur in all species. Small differences in litter size appear to be a phenotypic rather than a genotypic response to environmental variation. *M. pinetorum* has the smallest litter size, *M. xanthognathus* the largest; but it is not clear why litter sizes differ between species. Contrasts within and among species are encumbered because of differences in seasons of collection of specimens, sampling intensity, and inappropriate use of statistical techniques. Age and parity of the female and a variety of other factors may affect litter size. Pre- and post-implantation losses do not appear to significantly affect the reproductive output for the few species studied, but temporal or geographic differences in litter size may contribute to the capacity of a population to cycle.

A plea is made for development of corroborative experiments that critically test the importance of reproductive patterns detailed in descriptive studies. Some experiments are suggested that would increase our understanding of the importance of seasonal and annual differences in reproductive patterns among species.

Introduction

Reproductive attributes of microtine rodents have been investigated widely, but the genus *Microtus* has been studied most extensively (Hasler, 1975). Laboratory or field studies have been reported for 18 species, although reproductive data are available for *M. abbreviatus, M. canicaudus,* and *M. miurus,* largely as a result of studies associated with laboratory colonies. No field studies are published for *M. coronarius, M. guatemalensis, M. nesophilus, M. oaxecensis, M. umbrosus, M. quasiater,* and *M. abbreviatus. Microtus californicus, M. longicaudus, M. montanus, M. ochrogaster, M. pennsylvanicus,* and *M. pinetorum* have been studied at widely separated geographical locations, whereas geographical variation in reproductive patterns of *Microtus agrestis* have received the most attention in Europe. I include, for contrast, some information on winter breeding for the field vole (*M. agrestis*), because Ellerman and Morrison-Scott (1951:702) suggested and Klimkiewicz (1970) presented morphometric evidence that *Microtus agrestis* is conspecific with *M. pennsylvanicus.* By contrast, Matthey (1952) noted chromosomal differences and Johnson (1968) showed that serological differences exist between *M. agrestis* and *M. pennsylvanicus.* Thus, I treat *M. pennsylvanicus* as a distinct species. Additionally, I include winter-breeding information from the Old World literature for *M. oeconomus* (European root vole), although the North American tundra vole (*M. ratticeps*?) may not be conspecific with the root vole (Hall, 1981).

This chapter is limited to a consideration of factors known or suspected, on the basis of field and laboratory evidence, to affect reproductive performance of voles in natural populations. I avoid review of evolutionary implications and anatomical and endocrinological aspects of reproduction, as they are considered elsewhere (see Carleton, this volume; Phillips, this volume; Seabloom, this volume). I have considered environmental factors known to influence the breeding effort.

Laboratory studies of endogenous factors known to affect reproductive performance of voles suggest many predictions that could be field-tested. Unfortunately, definitive evidence is lacking as to whether these processes, particularly pheromonally mediated events, are important controls of reproductive tactics for natural populations. I have assumed reproductive, aggressive, and recognition behavior of individual voles is mediated at least partially by pheromones distributed from specialized glands (Quay, 1962, 1965, 1968). Certain olfactory cues can moderate behavior (Beard, 1978; Jannett, 1981*a*; Lyons, 1979) and these substances may be found to be important for integration of breeding.

Only recently have we begun to recognize that the social fabric of vole populations may be important in the integration of reproductive processes (Anderson, 1980; Getz, 1978; Jannett, 1980; Lidicker, 1980; Madison, 1980; Wolff, 1980). This adds confusion to the literature because many field studies have described reproductive patterns without regard for reproductive mechanisms disrupted through data collection procedures or experimental manipulation. For example, we do not know if post-partum breeding in a pair-bonding species such as *M. ochrogaster* (Getz et al., 1981) is permanently disrupted by removing females to determine litter size in conjunction with experiments (see Cole and Batzli, 1978). Can reproductive estimates be compared in populations subjected to disruption of incest taboos (McGuire and Getz, 1981) or maturation controls (Hasler and Nalbandov, 1974)? Clearly, removal of a sample of individuals to assess reproductive parameters by autopsy (Keller and Krebs, 1970; Rose and Gaines, 1978) may significantly affect the remaining social structure and reproductive pattern owing to action through the Whitten effect (Whitten, 1956) or the Bruce effect (Bruce, 1959) on breeding performance. Rose and Gaines (1978) certainly altered the breeding intensity of their selectively trapped populations by removing only animals weighing >20 g, and their subsequent samples, taken at approximately 2-month intervals, probably reflected enhanced reproductive effort, lowered ages at sexual maturity, and altered reproductive fitness of individuals.

Infrequent disruptions of social or age structure of voles may be unimportant. However, we presently lack carefully graded and replicated experiments that would separate effects disruptive to reproductive processes, as observed in the laboratory, from processes that occur naturally under field conditions. The extent to which variation in reproductive patterns of voles is due to investigator-induced changes in field populations and to artifacts caused by modifications of social structure in the laboratory must be clarified.

This chapter is subsectioned in accord with the early studies of Hamilton (1937, 1941), who suggested that changes in density for *M. pennsylvanicus* were fostered by: 1) increased duration of the reproductive season such that females produced more litters; 2) an acceleration of the rate of breeding; and 3) an increase in the number of young produced by pregnant females. These initial premises have been used as focal points in many field studies of voles. Only now are variations in reproductive performance among individual voles and heritability of litter size, age at sexual maturity, and ability to breed during winter beginning to be investigated under field conditions. More research needs to be concentrated on this aspect of microtine reproductive biology.

Length of Breeding Season

Seasonal rhythms in reproduction in New World voles may result from a variety of factors, including temperature, dehydration, photoperiod, nutrition (see Batzli, this volume), and chemical cues. Additionally, both phenotypic (Christian, 1971) and genotypic (Clarke, 1977; Keller and Krebs, 1970) differences among individuals may affect reproductive capabilities of voles. Further, spacing behavior, which may be mediated partially by pheromones, may alter reproductive performance. It remains to be discovered, however, which pheromones are released in response to exogenous or endogenous factors in natural populations. In the laboratory, their release has been related to endogenous hormone production (Milligan, 1976), but endocrine responses leading to initiation of breeding appear to be intimately related to environmental cues (Seabloom, this volume). Thus, environmental cues may control the onset and perhaps the duration of the breeding effort, but a network of intrinsic cues may integrate breeding processes. This network may very well be tied to behavioral systems.

Environmental Cues

Baker and Ranson (1932) suggested that photoperiod was a synchronizing agent in voles. During their studies on *M. oregoni,* Cowan and Arsenault (1954) suggested that both temperature and photoperiod operated in combination to initiate breeding. Greenwald (1957) and Hoffmann (1958) noted a correspondence between green vegetation and reproduction in *Microtus californicus,* a relationship also suggested by Batzli and Pitelka (1971) on the basis of extensive analysis of the diet of this species. Subsequently, Lidicker (1976) studied *M. californicus* in artificially watered enclosures during the California dry season and concluded that water and vegetation determined the length of the breeding season. Pinter and Negus (1965), studying the effect of photoperiod and a supplement of sprouted wheat, concluded that reproduction in *M. montanus* was enhanced by a combined action of diet, photoperiod, and other environmental variables. Negus and Pinter (1966) subsequently suggested that "phytoestrogens" constituted an important environmental stimulus for reproduction in montane voles, but Berger and Negus (1974) demonstrated that the stimulatory plant substances were not estrogenic. Rather, they appear to act through the pineal-hypothalamic-pituitary axis, increasing the production of substances that elicit steroid production by the ovaries and testes (Seabloom, this volume). The induction of reproductive activity by a "start cue" has been demonstrated in field populations of *M. montanus* during two winters (Negus and Berger, 1977). Conversely, Sanders (1976) extracted cinnamic acids and their related vinylphenols, which are naturally occurring plant compounds, and concluded that they inhibited reproduction in montane voles but that the physiological response times were longer for males than for females. Berger et al. (1977) suggested that these compounds serve as stop cues, indicating the termination of a food supply conducive to breeding activity. Most recently, Sanders et al. (1981) identified a compound (6-MBOA) that can trigger reproduction in *Microtus montanus*; Berger et al. (1981) suggested that this compound may be generally important in cueing reproduction in other species.

It seems doubtful that all New World species have adopted a strategy of using vegetation as an ultimate Zeitgeber, because a varied diet is known to exist for different species (Batzli, this volume). Negus et al. (1977) proposed that voles in highly predictable environments may be selected for stereotyped breeding seasons. In such environments, the central cue might consist of a fixed parameter such as photoperiod. By contrast, species requiring a facultative reproductive strategy may be selected to cue, although not necessarily completely, on substances available during periods favorable for breeding.

It seems to me, because environments tend to vary in plant composition on a temporal basis, that mid-continental populations of vole species with broad distributions might possess differing cue sensitivities based upon the predictability of the environment in which they live. Studies are needed to quantify variations in response to a variety of environmental cues among individuals of single species collected along geographical and altitudinal gradients. Perhaps the quantities of plant cues or the nutritional value of vegetation mediate the integrity of the breeding process by altering sensitivities to other cues, but we lack quantitative information on response to cues for any geographic area.

Breeding Duration

New World voles possess considerable variation in their periods of reproduction. This variation may result in differences in amplitude displayed by populations that undergo either annual or multiannual cycles, although other influences could be important as well. Birney et al. (1976) suggested that cover, especially because it affects a variety of factors that impinge upon voles, may affect amplitude, and Krebs et al. (1969) noted that frustration of dispersal also affected amplitude.

Two patterns of variation in the duration of the reproductive period are commonly reported for New World voles. First, peak density populations often appear to terminate breeding early in the summer of peak numbers and initiate breeding late the following spring. Secondly, at least nine species are known to occasionally extend reproduction into the dry or winter season. Keller and Krebs (1970) suggested that the progeny of winter breeders might be at a selective advantage. However, only a limited amount of information has been developed on the extent, success, and causes of extended reproduction. Early investigators often attributed winter breeding to the quantity (Bailey, 1924; Fitch, 1957; Hamilton, 1937) or quality (Fuller, 1967) of the food supply. Unfortunately, only Anderson (1975) has attempted to determine whether individual aseasonal breeders (winter breeders in her study) are genetically distinct. Her results for *Microtus townsendii* indicate a lack of heritability for this trait. Similarly, Clarke (1977) speculated that sexual development in winter-breeding *M. agrestis* may be due to the prevalence of genetically distinct individuals that have a greater tendency to breed under short photoperiods.

Our knowledge of the importance of winter breeding is fragmentary for a number of reasons. The preponderance of studies completed in areas of snowfall have been conducted during summers. Further, repeatability has rarely been measured where winter breeding has been documented, and the causes for breeding often have been evaluated post hoc (but see Getz et al., 1979). Some of the difficulty in obtaining such information results from a lack of employment of sampling systems now available or recently developed (Fay, 1960; Iverson and Turner, 1969; Keller et al., 1982; Larsson and Hansson, 1977; Merritt and Merritt, 1978; Pruitt, 1959), but the winter ecology of small mammals is now receiving increased attention.

Species with Restricted Breeding Periods

Recognizing that further study may demonstrate substantial shifts in the breeding seasons of all species, I would presently list five species (*M. breweri, M. longicaudus, M. mexicanus, M. richardsoni,* and *M. xanthognathus*) as seasonally restricted breeders. The breeding season of *M. breweri* generally extends from April through October. Tamarin (1977*a*) suggested that the duration of the breeding effort for this species was consistent during his 3-year study and that a delay of breeding during one spring was followed by an extension of breeding the following fall. Goldberg et al. (1980) noted significant dietary shifts in the beach vole (*M. breweri*) that appeared to correspond with the non-breeding period, but a cause–effect relationship has not been demonstrated.

Some data are available on the breeding habits of *M. longicaudus* and *M. mexicanus.* As a result of his 61-week study in New Mexico, Conley (1976) suggested that the breeding season for the long-tailed vole ceased in October and was resumed during spring. *M. mexicanus* trapped in the same area were breeding from May through November. Based upon lack of recruitment the following year, Conley (1976) suggested that the Mexican vole did not breed during winter, but he did not sample his area from mid-November to May. He suggested *M. longicaudus* populations were completing a peak-decline phase and *M. mexicanus* a low phase during his study, but his data from *M. mexicanus* actually suggest that the Mexican vole is an annual cyclic species. Baker (1956), by contrast, found pregnant Mexican voles during January in Coahuila, Mexico. Thus, without further data, the characterization of this species as a seasonally restricted breeder should be considered tentative. Farris (1971) found *Microtus longicaudus* breeding from March through October in Washington and cited 17 years of snap-trapping samples collected between October 12 and November 9 in which only two of 93 adult females were pregnant. It is of interest to note that he suggested long-tailed voles on his study area were seed (*Rosa*) and bark (*Symphoricarpos albus*) feeders during fall and winter (Farris 1971:74). Van Horn (1982) observed breeding from mid-May through mid-September in long-tailed voles found in coniferous forest in southeast Alaska. *Microtus longicaudus* did not appear to exhibit a multi-annual cycle during the combined 3-year study of Farris (1971) and Wright (1971), or during Van Horn's (1982) 3-year study.

Subdivision of populations of the water vole, *M. richardsoni,* into small isolated groups (Anderson et al., 1976) and the sociobiology of the yellow-cheeked vole, *Microtus xanthognathus* (Douglass, 1977; Wolff and Lidicker, 1980), would appear to preclude extension of their respective breeding seasons. In Alberta, the water vole bred from June through August, but only the first litters matured in their season of birth. No winter breeding was evident in summer samples of overwintered individuals during a 1-year study by Anderson et al. (1976). The yellow-cheeked vole bred from early May to July and young did not breed during their season of birth (Wolff and Lidicker, 1980; Youngman, 1975). Males initiated breeding approximately 1 month before females (Wolff and Lidicker, 1980), a condition also observed by Douglass (1977) during a 3-year live-trapping study. Douglass (1977), however, found females breeding in August, but none in September. Wolff and Lidicker (1980) also noted that males achieved maximum seminal-vesicle length 2 weeks to 1 month after the testis size declined in this species, a condition that may be important to social integration of non-breeding individuals that form midden groups (Wolff and Lidicker, 1981) during winter. We do not know how the duration of breeding would be affected during periods of irruption in either the yellow-cheeked or water vole; however, Youngman (1975) suggested such irruptions occur about every 20 years in *M. xanthognathus*. The intervals between irruptions are unknown in *M. richardsoni* (Anderson et al., 1976).

In summary, significant variations in length of breeding season appear to be largely absent in five species of New World voles studied over periods of one to several years. I would tentatively add that, although annual or multi-annual live-trapping studies are not available for rock voles (*M. chrotorrhinus*), museum and field-collection data suggest that this species has a restricted breeding season extending from March to mid-October (Kirkland, 1977; Martin, 1971; Timm et al., 1977). It remains to be established if rock voles undergo cycles in optimal habitat (species review: Kirkland and Jannett, 1982).

Species with Variable Breeding Periods

Considerable variation occurs in length of the breeding season of voles found in both snow-free areas and areas covered by moderate or limited snow. Extension of the breeding season has been found under both conditions and at least one species that does not usually demonstrate multi-annual cycles, *M. townsendii,* occasionally undergoes extension of the breeding season into winter (Krebs, 1979; Taitt and Krebs, this volume).

In snow-free areas, *M. californicus* displays both annual (Krohne, 1982; Lidicker, 1973) and multi-annual cycles (Krebs, 1966). Lidicker (1973) suggested that this species usually shows a monotonous pattern of breeding that begins several months after autumn rains (September to December) and terminates with the desiccation of vegetation (usually June). Batzli and Pitelka (1971), Bowen (1982), Greenwald (1957), Hoffmann (1958), Lidicker and Anderson (1962), Pearson (1963), and others have also proposed that breeding closely corresponds to wet seasons for the California vole. However, Lidicker (1973) noted one multi-annual cycle that was associated with a continued breeding effort during the dry season, which he attributed to high-quality habitat and an unusual early rainfall in September. Krohne (1982), who studied a northern coastal population for several years, found that breeding extended well into summer in a population that did not cycle, and Batzli and Pitelka (1971), Greenwald (1957), Krebs (1966), and Krebs and DeLong (1965) found that breeding can be extended during dry seasons in populations displaying multi-annual fluctuations. Krebs (1966) also failed to find breeding females for over 2 months following an October rain that produced green vegetation. Lidicker (1976) subsequently analyzed breeding variation by artificially watering enclosures containing voles during dry periods. He suggested that adequate food was required for reproduction; available moisture, including dew, was the most important factor controlling length of the breeding season, and individuals subjected to dehydration delayed reproduction in spite of adequate food.

Microtus oregoni appears to vary its breeding habits with the quality of the habitat it occupies. Gashwiler (1972) suggested that creeping voles breed from mid-February to mid-September in clearcut and virgin Douglas fir forests in western Oregon. By contrast, Sullivan (1980) suggested that these voles breed from April to August on both burned and unburned cutover areas in British Columbia. Redfield et al. (1978*a*) showed that experimental disruption of the sex ratio affects the duration of breeding (see below). In a study of five populations of *M. oregoni,* Sullivan and Krebs (1981) failed to find a consistent pattern of breeding in four different types of habitat. It is noteworthy that the highest vole densities achieved during their study (Sullivan and Krebs, 1981:Fig. 5) occurred on an area suggested to be optimal habitat, and that a short burst of breeding following a mild winter occurred on this area. Breeding rapidly terminated, but resumed earlier than that observed on a similar old-field grid where *M. townsendii* was present and may have been a competitor.

Microtus townsendii populations in coastal British Columbia have been studied very thoroughly by experimentation. Perhaps with one or two exceptions, they did not display multi-annual cycles (Krebs, 1979; Taitt and Krebs, this volume). Breeding duration, although not reported by a long-term autopsy study, usually began early in spring and terminated in fall, but a number of exceptions were documented. Winter breeding (December to February), as assessed by the presence of lactating females, was documented for three populations (two control, one experimental) at a reduced level (18–22%), whereas seven populations displayed limited breeding (1–10%), and three others none at all (Krebs, 1979). No commonality was found among populations breeding during winter, but two of the three populations displaying limited winter breeding achieved higher peak densities the following year. The third population (experimental) was subjected to a pulse-removal experiment that may have affected the speed of growth; enumeration was not carried out beyond May (Krebs, 1979:Fig. 5). Thus, we do not know the ultimate density that this population might have achieved. Anderson (1975) showed that the tendency of breeding in winter is not inherited to any extent in Townsend's voles.

Besides extensions of the breeding season, early cessation and late initiation of breeding periods also have been noted (Anderson and Boonstra, 1979; Beacham, 1980; LeDuc and Krebs, 1975). Beacham (1980) suggested that dispersal and death of fast-growing, early-maturing Townsend's voles may result in a shortened breeding season during summers of peak density. Other variations also have been documented. Boonstra and Krebs (1977) noted reduction to near zero in mid-summer breeding in an enclosed population at peak density, and Taitt and Krebs (1981) were able to shorten non-breeding periods with extra food. Taitt et al. (1981) achieved the same effect with extra cover. Neither female nor male enrichment of the sex ratio (see below) significantly altered length of the breeding season (Redfield et al. 1978*b*).

In areas that usually receive snowfall, inconsistent patterns of winter breeding occur. In their review of winter breeding in *Microtus*, Keller and Krebs (1970) suggested that individuals of high body weight continue to breed during the winter months of population increase and that this breeding appeared to lead to population peaks. Subsequent studies suggest that winter breeding is not always associated with periods of population expansion in at least six species.

Microtus montanus was found to undergo multi-annual fluctuations in three cycles monitored over a 10-year period by Negus in Wyoming (*in* Jannett, 1977) and one cycle monitored by Hoffmann (1958) in California. Pattie (1967) and Hoffmann (1974) both suggested that alpine populations do not cycle, however. Hoffmann (1958) concluded after a 3-year summer study in mountain meadows that montane voles showed a reasonably consistent pattern of breeding from June to August. Reproduction, as assessed by back-dating pregnancies, was initiated earlier during the year of peak numbers and terminated earlier in the summer preceding a decline.

Farris (1971) found pregnant females in every month except December, but suggested the main breeding season occurred from mid-February through November. The limited winter breeding he observed appears to have occurred during a Type-H decline. Working in the same area in Washington, Wright (1971) found individuals breeding from early February through December during his 18-month study, but his data cannot be separated for individual years and his samples for January and February were limited to a total of two adults. I documented (pers. observ.) winter breeding in enclosed, expanding populations of *M. montanus* near Pocatello, Idaho, during experiments conducted over several years, and Groves and Keller (1983) found that montane voles continued breeding during a period of winter population expansion at the Idaho National Engineering Laboratory. Negus et al. (1977) noted natural late-winter breeding in saltgrass marshes bordering the Great Salt Lake during February for 1 of 6 years; they attributed this breeding to the presence of fresh green vegetation. As noted above, Negus and Berger (1977) were able to trigger reproduction in sexually quiescent montane voles by use of sprouted wheatgrass and 6-MBOA (Berger et al., 1981).

Prairie voles (*M. ochrogaster*) breed throughout the year in some areas, although the intensity of the effort varies seasonally and may be reduced during winters or summers. Fitch (1957), Gaines and Rose (1976), Jameson (1947), Martin (1956), and Rose and Gaines (1978) have documented varied patterns in populations near Lawrence, Kansas, but these studies largely suggest that winter breeding, if it occurs, is most pronounced prior to peak years and is highly unpredictable. By contrast, Rolan and Gier (1967) did not obtain pregnant females during December, January, or February in their sample of 198 female prairie voles trapped on native Kansas prairies over an 11-year period. Abdellatif et al. (1982) were able to cause more intensive mid-summer breeding in females residing in an artificially watered, enclosed population, but despite this breeding increase, the population continued to decline.

In Indiana, Corthum (1967) and Keller and Krebs (1970) found that winter breeding in prairie voles occurred prior to peak densities, but Quick (1970) found winter breeding following a period of population decline in Kentucky. Fisher (1945) suggested that winter breeding can occur during mild but prolonged winters, and Richmond (1967) also noted winter breeding during studies in Missouri; however, neither author documented the breeding durations of populations that were sampled. DeCoursey (1957) noted a very reduced level of winter breeding during what appears to have been a period of population expansion in Ohio. Meserve (1971) noted perforate females in Nebraska during winter. Cole and Batzli (1978) were able to extend the breeding period for an Illinois population of prairie voles all months of one winter by supplemental feedings with rabbit pellets. They suggested that food availability affected both the length of breeding and its intensity (see below) which, in turn, affected the amplitude of cycles.

Abramsky and Tracy (1979) studied the effects of various combinations of water and soil-mineral nitrogen treatments on Colorado prairie-vole populations and suggested that unusually high reproductive activity during winter, prior to peak densities, was not necessary to produce high numbers. During an extensive analysis of live-trapped prairie vole populations in Illinois, Getz et al. (1979), concluded that a gradient for habitat qualities was responsible for significant variations in the length of breeding periods they encountered. Reproduction continued during two winters of decline in two independent cycles but failed to occur during a winter of heavy snow prior to a spring where breeding was delayed. *M. ochrogaster* populations expanded following this delay, but failed to achieve peak amplitudes equivalent to those reached during a previous cycle.

Microtus oeconomus (=*M. ratticeps*?) breeds from approximately April to September during a period of cyclic peak, but in one study showed a delay in the initiation of breeding until early May and ceased breeding in mid-August during a period of low numbers (Whitney 1976). Whitney (1976) suggested that the tundra vole displayed a multi-annual cycle during his studies. The weight distributions (Whitney 1976:Fig. 10) provided for this species suggest that these voles were breeding during the winter of increase when snow depth prevented Whitney from sampling. Tast and Kaikusalo (1976) suggested that the European root vole normally breeds from May to late September, but recorded winter reproduction following an exceptionally warm summer in Finland that induced fall rather than spring shoot development of some plants.

Winter breeding in *Microtus pennsylvanicus* occurs in a variety of distinctly different habitats and widely separated geographical areas. Hamilton (1937), Beer and MacLeod (1961), Krebs et al. (1969), and Keller and Krebs (1970) found winter breeding to be associated with periods of population expansion in *M. pennsylvanicus* in New York, Minnesota, and Indiana. Subjective evaluation of Linduska's (1942, 1950) statements about densities of meadow voles also suggests that this pattern occurs in Michigan. Christian (1971) suggested that winter breeding occurred in Pennsylvania whenever mature individuals were available to breed. From 4 years of necropsy data for meadow voles collected in Manitoba, Iverson and Turner (1976) found a 4-month spread in the occurrence of positive epididymal sperm smears during winter for males initiating breeding. The last pregnancy recorded over a 6-year period occurred in August or September, but during one winter, males with *abdominal* testes had positive sperm smears and pregnancy was noted in females from November through February. This unusual period of winter reproduction occurred in animals of lower weight than that observed for individuals during summers, as contrasted to the results of Keller and Krebs (1970). From live-trapping studies, Iverson and Turner (1974) suggested that lower weights were a result of winter weight loss experienced by individuals until snow cover was established. Peak densities were achieved following the period of winter breeding, but breeding occurred when this population was at low density (Mihok, pers. comm.). More recently, Tamarin (1977*a*) found a limited amount of winter breeding in *M. pennsylvanicus* in Massachusetts among populations interpreted to have reached peak densities, and Getz et al. (1979) found few meadow voles breeding during a winter of population expansion in Illinois.

Microtus agrestis also breeds during winter months (for example, see Raynaud, 1951; Thibault et al., 1966). Tast and Kaikusalo (1976) and Larsson and Hansson (1977) called special attention to this condition in Finland and Sweden, but Chitty (*in* Krebs and Myers, 1974) reported complete cycles in England in which winter breeding was absent.

Hamilton (1938) initially proposed that *Microtus pinetorum* was a cyclic species, but Horsfall (1963) suggested that pine voles maintained relatively stable densities. No subsequent studies indicate that pine voles display multi-annual fluctuations. During a 3-year study of pine voles in New York orchards, Benton (1955) found that reproduction occurred from late December or January through October. During a 3-year live-trapping study in Connecticut, Miller and Getz (1969) found breeding individuals from May through September, but their trapping was not conducted during all months each year. Paul (1966:73) found pregnant females during all months on one study area in North Carolina. During an 18-month study in Oklahoma, Goertz (1971) detected no pregnant female pine voles during May to August in the first summer of his study, but caught pregnant females the following summer in June and July. He suggested reproduction was curtailed during summer.

Pine voles appear to breed year-round in Virginia (Horsfall, 1963), although Cengel et al. (1978) failed to obtain pregnant females in samples taken in November and January for a maintained and abandoned orchard, respectively. Valentine and Kirkpatrick (1970) concluded that reproduction occurred from March through October. However, the results from the latter 1-year study may have been confounded by a change in sampling sites (Valentine and Kirkpatrick, 1970).

In summary, for the 15 species examined above, neither snow cover nor periods of prolonged breeding effort are necessary and sufficient to produce rapid population expansion. Amplitudes achieved by individual species, however, may be affected by duration of breeding, but not invariably so (Abramsky and Tracy, 1979). Food quality or cues in food may be sufficient to explain periods of extended breeding, but prolonged periods of high food quality have not been established as causative agents under natural conditions. Alternately, breeding can be re-initiated or extended, at least in *Microtus montanus,* by experimentally supplying a population with 6-MBOA, or in *M. ochrogaster* with food; but we do not know whether the quantity consumed produces effects similar to those achieved through consumption of natural vegetation.

Early terminations or late initiations of breeding may be associated with earlier dispersal of individuals capable of breeding, genotypic or phenotypic differences among individuals in ability to respond to environmental cues, phenotypic effects that regulate social structure, or physiological mechanisms. It is not clear which of these factors, either singly or in consort, are necessary and sufficient to stop breeding efforts in natural populations of any species, but we cannot eliminate the possibility that cessations and late initiations of breeding efforts are regulated by one mechanism, especially since both patterns are common in different species.

Breeding Intensity

Since Hamilton (1937, 1941) first suggested that population expansion in meadow voles (*M. pennsylvanicus*) was caused partially by an increased rate of breeding, numerous investigators have sought to document pregnancy rates and their seasonal, temporal, and geographic variation. Three observations can be drawn from these data for New World voles: 1) pregnancy rates vary seasonally but are generally greatest at the midpoint of the breeding season and are generally lower if extensions (winter breeding) occur; 2) pregnancy rates vary geographically among conspecific populations; and 3) pregnancy rates lack a consistent pattern of change during the generalized breeding periods among years. In short, pregnancy rates are as likely to be high in a summer of low density as they are in a summer of high density, and population declines are not necessarily associated with low pregnancy rates (but see Getz et al., 1979). Unfortunately, these observations are probably confounded by shifts in age at sexual maturity, which affects calculation of the rate of breeding.

Operationally, four parameters interact and can potentially affect the observed variation: 1) the frequency of consecutive pregnancies; 2) the ratio of pregnant to non-pregnant females; 3) the age at sexual maturity; and 4) the sex ratio. Each of these factors is important, but data on consecutive interbirth intervals have not been separated from the ratio of pregnant to non-pregnant females such that we can deduce the importance of any single parameter on the variation observed in field populations (Keller and Krebs, 1970). Thus, in this section I look at the implications of the variability in the first two parameters combined.

Pregnancy

Changes in the interval between consecutive pregnancies (interbirth interval) are a function of variation in post-partum receptivity of females and the probability that coitus will produce a conception that ends in parturition. Greenwald (1956) concluded that *Microtus californicus* underwent induced ovulation and Breed (1967, 1969, 1972) subsequently suggested that *M. agrestis* was an induced ovulator. The pattern has now been confirmed for *M. canicaudus* (Tyser, 1975), *M. ochrogaster* (Richmond and Conaway, 1969), *M. penn-*

sylvanicus (Clulow and Mallory, 1970; Lee et al., 1970), *M. pinetorum* (Kirkpatrick and Valentine, 1970), *M. montanus* (Cross, 1972), *M. richardsoni* (Jannett, 1979), and *M. townsendii* (MacFarlane and Taylor, 1982*a*). Breed (1967) suggested that induced ovulation is probably prevalent in all species for the genus *Microtus*. Because estrus appears to be induced within several days by contact with males or their urine (for example, see Carter et al., 1980; Clulow and Mallory, 1970; Gray et al., 1974; and others), it is also reasonable to assume that male-induced estrus (Whitten effect), given that it is the pattern for the genus, should prevent prolonged periods of anestrus if infertile matings occur. Further, all members of the genus appear to undergo a post-partum estrus (Hasler, 1975). Thus, extended intervals between consecutive pregnancies in natural populations should constitute an unusual condition and pregnancy rates of females should approach maximal limits. If true, these conditions differ markedly from laboratory litter intervals during which some permanently paired females fail to conceive after parturition and enter temporary periods of anestrus or pseudopregnancy. I know of no field evidence that suggests this occurs for long intervals during normal breeding periods, except in *M. richardsoni* (Anderson et al., 1976).

Pregnancy can be determined at approximately 6 days post-coitum in necropsy samples (Hoffmann, 1958) or at about 9 days by abdominal palpation of living voles (Innes, 1978*a*), although some authors suggest longer periods (for example, see Cole and Batzli, 1978; Stehn and Jannett, 1981). Thus, pregnancy rates (fraction of females pregnant) should approach 0.71 (15/21) in necropsy and 0.57 (12/21) in field samples of voles that have gestation periods of approximately 21 days. Only *Microtus oregoni* (23.5 to 25 days; Cowan and Arsenault, 1954), *M. pinetorum* (24 to 25 days; Schadler and Butterstein, 1979), and *M. townsendii* (21 to 24 days; MacFarlane and Taylor, 1982*b*) have slightly longer gestation periods, which raises overall values to a maximum of 0.76 (19/25, laboratory) and 0.64 (16/25, field). Sufficient data exist from both necropsy and palpation to suggest that often not all adult females are pregnant even if they are reproductively mature and environmental conditions are conducive for reproduction. Additionally, pregnancy rates occasionally exceed these upper limits, perhaps owing to sampling error or as a result of synchronous breeding. Consequently, we need to ask why this variation exists.

Success of copulation.—Successful initiation of pregnancy in voles, based upon laboratory evidence, may be related to whether copulation occurs during male-induced estrus or post-partum estrus and the duration of the normal mating sequence (to satiety). Pregnancy in *Microtus ochrogaster* and *M. montanus* occurring during post-partum estrus is significantly less successful when numbers of copulations are restricted than when they are unrestricted (Dewsbury et al., 1979). Additionally, the presence of two male prairie voles (*M. ochrogaster*) caused a decrease in the number of mounts, intromissions, and thrusts prior to the first ejaculation (Evans and Dewsbury, 1978). In species where pair-bonding occurs, such as in *M. ochrogaster* (Getz et al., 1981), successful post-partum breeding seemingly should be maintained and pregnancy assured. Perhaps this explains why more complex mating sequences are required to maximize pregnancy in *M. montanus,* which is polygamous. Further, Gavish et al. (1981) noted that forced non-sib monogamous pairings of *M. ochrogaster* resulted in production of more pups than forced polygamous pairings. However, these laboratory data may be of limited value for ascertaining conditions in natural situations where more complex social interactions may occur. If disruptions to the mating sequence are an important factor, then pregnancy rate might be expected to be lowest during initiation and cessation of the breeding season when territorial boundaries are not fully established. Additionally, early reduction or termination of breeding during periods of peak density may be related partially to reduced mating success in multiparous females. Sterile breeding cycles may be rare in *M. townsendii* (MacFarlane and Taylor, 1981), but Westlin (1982) and Westlin and Nyholm (1982) suggested sterile matings may be a general feature in overwintered females caught at the beginning of the breeding season. Additionally, they might be more common in autumn populations containing largely subadult individuals. *M. californicus* (Greenwald, 1956), *M. oeconomus* (Hoyte, 1955), and *M. pinetorum* (Kirkpatrick and Valentine, 1970) are known to have sterile matings. It would be of interest to learn if the success of copulatory acts varies in relation to seasonal changes in density or social groupings and to the degree of successful insemination based upon the estrous condition of the female in field situations. Few data are available on these aspects and more laboratory information is needed for many species.

Pregnancy failure.—Pregnancy rate in natural populations could also be affected by inhibition of implantation or premature terminations of gestation. For voles, in which the lifespan is typically short, both types of failure only slightly affect field assessments of pregnancy rates in populations, but they potentially lower the reproductive fitness of females through reduction in the potential number of young that could be delivered and weaned. However, terminations occurring in late stages of pregnancy, as described for *M. ochrogaster* (Stehn and Richmond, 1975), would be especially significant if they occurred toward the end of conditions favorable to breeding.

The capacity of a conspecific strange male to block pregnancy of a female mated with a stud of proven fertility (Bruce effect) has been reported from laboratory experiments with *M. agrestis* (Clulow and Clarke, 1968), *M. montanus* (Berger and Negus, 1982; Jannett, 1980), *M. ochrogaster* (Stehn, 1978; Stehn and Richmond, 1975), *M. pennsylvanicus* (Clulow and Langford, 1971; Mallory and Clulow, 1977), and *M. pinetorum* (Schadler, 1981; Stehn, 1978). The Bruce effect is known to be mediated via olfaction of urine, although other environmental factors, such as disturbance, can produce blockage (Stehn and Jannett, 1981). Additionally, both parity and the continued presence of the male appear to be important (Milligan, 1976). Lastly, blockage may be related to the social status of an individual. Labov (1981) presents data that refute this possibility in *Mus,* but comparative and contrasting studies that consider the status of the female have not been undertaken on voles.

Mallory and Clulow (1977) suspected that pregnancy blockage occurred in eight females from field populations of *M. pennsylvanicus* and suggested that incidence of blockage was related to density. Subsequently, Mallory (in litt.) concluded from studies of Milligan (1975) that three of those females developed corpora lutea as a result of an insufficient number of copulations with males. Reevaluation of the importance of Mallory and Clulow's (1977) remaining five animals is necessary because it may be impossible to distinguish sets of luteinized corpora lutea produced during the Bruce effect from those developed from a penultimate sterile mating (Westlin and Nyholm, 1982). Thus, further studies are needed to establish if the Bruce effect occurs in wild populations of *Microtus.* Milligan (1976) suggested that, in general, short-lived corpora lutea represent limited matings rather than pregnancy blockage. Further, pregnancy failures of *M. californicus,* described by Greenwald (1956) and thought to be due to blockage by Mallory and Clulow (1977), may have resulted from males completing an insufficient number of mounts and copulations.

Based upon laboratory studies of the Bruce effect, several postulates can be suggested for assessment in field studies where pregnancy rates appear variable.

1) The duration of contact with strange males in the absence of the original stud appears to be related to the probability that disruption will occur. Therefore, populations that are subjected to frustrated dispersal or increasing immigration should be more prone to display the Bruce effect. Additionally, populations seeded with conspecific strange males should display proportionally more blocked individuals.
2) Lactation, parity, or age appears to somewhat reduce the probability of a Bruce effect for some species (Kenney et al., 1977). Therefore, nulliparous mature females will be more prone to disruption of their first pregnancy when the social fabric of the population is changing or becoming established during the autumn of peak density and the spring of decline, respectively. Thus, the Bruce effect may account, at least in part, for ineffective breeding following a population peak. (Other hypotheses exist; for example, see Beacham, 1980; Christian, 1971; Lidicker, 1976).
3) The presence of a group of females with a female exposed to a strange male inhibits blockage. Therefore, communally grouping species, especially those in which previous pair-bonding has been present, will be less prone to undergo the Bruce effect. Thus, blockage may be more common in species in which family groups do not form.

Other hypotheses are also possible for field populations. But until further evidence is accumulated on the occurrence of the Bruce effect for field populations in species known to display it under laboratory conditions, and pending further elaboration of the social structure for natural populations, field studies may prove of limited value. Non-histological methods to assess disrupted pregnancies need to be developed and used for field studies.

Aside from the fact that pregnancy disruption may play a role in affecting changes in the interbirth interval, it may be important as a mechanism to effect genetic changes in populations. Unfortunately, few studies have attempted to consider the reproductive contribution of individual pairs (Krebs, 1979); techniques developed to trace parentage (Tamarin et al., 1983) may be of value. Contributions of individual parents may prove difficult to document if multiple paternity, such as observed for laboratory *M. ochrogaster* (Dewsbury and Baumgardner, 1981), occur in field situations. Further research on this aspect is clearly warranted. Finally, the evolution of the Bruce effect, especially as it relates to reproductive strategies for voles, is of considerable interest. Schwagmeyer (1979) and Labov (1981) reviewed the purported advantages to species that exhibit the Bruce effect. Dawkins' (1976) hypothesis that there is a mutual advantage to both sexes appears most probable for members of the genus *Microtus*. Boonstra (1980) presented compelling evidence that nestling mortality is not related to density in four species of voles, and he suggested disruption of pregnancies was unimportant on the basis of limited evidence from studies of reproduction by necropsy. Based upon laboratory evidence, the Bruce effect clearly is important in the reproductive tactics of at least five species of *Microtus*, but it remains to be established why this is so and whether or not this factor significantly affects pregnancy rates in field populations.

Sexual Maturity

Undoubtedly, much of the variation in pregnancy rates is a result of difficulties in measuring attainment of puberty (Leslie et al., 1952) in young females, except by autopsy. In live-trapping studies, investigators commonly have employed fixed-weight criteria or have used external reproductive characteristics that may or may not identify breeding individuals. In females, mid-winter nipple size suggests active reproduction by a limited number of females, whereas autopsy samples indicate reproductive quiescence (compare Tamarin, 1977*a* and Tamarin, 1977*b*). Further development of criteria to assess which portion of a necropsy sample is mature can involve circular reasoning (Keller and Krebs, 1970), and juvenile mice that are capable of induced ovulation may be excluded because of lack of appropriate signs of maturity (Hasler, 1975). Further, if females undergo sterile breeding cycles at the termination of the breeding season, necropsy may suggest they were mature. Thus, it is not clear how much of the variation in pregnancy rates can be attributed to pregnancy failure in females as contrasted to inappropriate assessment of the number of mature breeding females.

In general, it appears that field criteria used in identifying maturity in female voles may be more accurate than criteria used for males, because several measures such as weight change, known pregnancy, suspected lactation, condition of the pubic symphysis (open), perforation of the vaginal orifice, and the presence of a litter in a trap can be combined for assessment. Although a series of combined criteria can be used to establish fecundity in female voles, external reproductive characteristics of males may be poor indicators of fecundity (for example, see Batzli and Pitelka, 1971; Iverson and Turner, 1976). Thus, determination of temporal changes in the age at maturity and identification of individual males remaining reproductively active during "quiescent" periods may require estimation of plasma androgen levels. Although these data are available for *M. breweri* (Adams et al., 1980), continuous assessments on individuals remaining alive in natural populations have not been sought because adequate techniques have not been available.

Assessment of temporal changes in age of sexual maturity are important factors affecting the rate of population growth (Cole, 1954; Schaffer and Tamarin, 1973; Stearns, 1976). Many factors are known to affect sexual maturation in voles, (see reviews by Hasler, 1975; Nadeau, this volume) as ascertained from laboratory studies. In natural populations, the social structure and condition of the food supply are known to affect age at puberty; both factors are subject to change as a result of changes in population density. Laboratory studies suggest that estrous suppression of grouped females (Lee and Boot, 1955) and male-induced estrus (Whitten effect), which may simply be expression of the Bruce effect, leads to seasonal changes in age (weight) at which sexual maturity is achieved in field populations of voles. Batzli et al. (1977) examined attainment of sexual maturity in *M. californicus, M. ochrogaster,* and *M. pennsylvanicus,* and concluded that suppression, which they observed for sib-held *M. californicus* and *M. ochrogaster* but not for *M. pennsylvanicus* or *M. oeconomus* (Facemire and Batzli, 1983), was probably related to behavioral strategies initially proposed by Christian (1970). But, it remains to be established whether or not suppression operates as a result of urine-behavioral interactions for field populations. *M. xanthognathus* (Wolff and Lidicker, 1980), *M. ochrogaster* (Getz, 1978; Getz et al., 1981), *M. montanus* (Jannett, 1978), and *M. miurus* (Murie, 1961; Quay, 1951) have family groups where suppression might occur.

Seasonal and temporal shifts in the age at sexual maturity have been assessed for several species of voles, both on live-trapped samples and by necropsy. Since the age of individuals is difficult to determine, body weight or length has been substituted as an index for age, but both of these measures must be viewed with caution because of variations in growth rates known to occur among individuals born at different times (Krebs and Myers, 1974). Comparisons have been sought by computing a median weight at sexual maturity (Leslie et al., 1945) for four species.

From necropsy samples of *M. ochrogaster,* Keller and Krebs (1970) found that both males and females matured at approximately equal weights, but that maturity was achieved at higher weights during years of peak density than during years of increasing or low density. Further, weights at sexual maturity were found to vary seasonally. By contrast, Rose and Gaines (1978) found a trend toward reduction in weight during peak density and greater weights in females present in declining populations of Kansas prairie voles. Additionally, Rose and Gaines (1978) found lower weights at sexual maturity for Kansas prairie voles than those documented in Indiana by Keller and Krebs (1970). In *M. pennsylvanicus,* Keller and Krebs (1970) found seasonal increases in weight at sexual maturity and slightly higher median weights at sexual maturity during periods of peak density. Tamarin (1977*a*) computed median weights at sexual maturity for *M. breweri.* Maturity in Brewer's vole was achieved at much greater weights than in *M. ochrogaster* and *M. pennsylvanicus,* seasonal trends were apparent, and females matured at lighter weights than males during the early portion of the breeding season. *M. breweri* populations did not cycle during Tamarin's (1977*a*) 4-year study; thus, seasonal trends could not be contrasted to different densities during different years of a cycle.

Although assessment of temporal changes in age at sexual maturity may be encumbered by assumptions about the reproductive competency of individuals during quiescent reproductive periods, estimates have been developed for shifts in weight at sexual maturity in *M. townsendii* during the usual breeding seasons. Beacham (1980) and Krebs et al. (1976) found a spring-to-fall increase in weight at sexual maturity in *M. townsendii,* which Boonstra (1980) suggested was density dependent. Boonstra and Krebs (1977) documented a significant autumn decrease in weight at sexual maturity for each sex in both an enclosed and control peak population exposed to a large flush of green vegetation. Based on studies of families of *M. townsendii* in small pens, Anderson (1975) suggested that some component common to the environment of individual pups prior to weaning influenced sexual maturation such that size at maturation was more similar among sibs than among unrelated individuals. However, Anderson's (1975) studies were not completed in the normal complex social situation in which individuals freely mix. Under these circumstances, alterations of sex ratios (see below) of voles appear to affect social structure, and maturity occurs earlier. Both the immediate family environment and the social structure of populations appear to affect maturation in this species.

In summary, variations in pregnancy rate appear to be common. Although Krebs and Myers (1974) treated pregnancy rate as an unimportant factor in cyclic fluctuations in voles, changes in social structure that in turn influence age at sexual maturation affect our ability to determine how much variation in this parameter is necessary to significantly alter reproductive output. Thus, until we understand the social structure of New World voles, attempts to generalize about the importance of pregnancy to production levels may be counterproductive.

Sex Ratio

Variations in sex ratio may have important demographic and genetic consequences if the operational adult sex ratio does not approach unity. Such a condition may result from disparate sex ratios at birth that are subsequently maintained in breeding adults, or may develop through differential survival, movement, trappability, or growth. As an initial premise, a population with an adult sex ratio favoring females will have a potentially higher reproductive output; populations having more breeding females should reach peak densities more frequently (Stenseth, 1977).

Myers and Krebs (1971) have modeled the demographic consequences of variations in sex ratio of populations of *M. ochrogaster* and *M. pennsylvanicus* live-trapped in Indiana. They found that a significant excess of males was recruited into populations, but attributed this excess to increased trappability of males because of their more rapid growth. By contrast, the live-trapping data, at any instant in time, usually showed a slight deficiency in males except during a period of decline (Myers and Krebs, 1971:Figs. 1, 2).

From their simulations, increased male recruitment was found to lower population growth, and they concluded that populations maintained approximately equal numbers of males and females.

Some New World voles have sex ratios that deviate significantly from unity, but the reproductive consequences of these deviations are poorly understood. Further, it is difficult to ascertain whether these variations are a result of sampling error owing to different factors affecting susceptibility of males and females to being captured, or to differences related to production or survival. Two studies suggest that unusually large disparities can exist in adult vole sex ratios without significant demographic consequences. Anderson et al. (1976) found that the first litter of *M. richardsoni* was composed only of females, but this observation needs further evaluation because they did not provide information on whether or not males were actually produced. Redfield et al. (1978*a*) studied a non-manipulated population of *M. oregoni* where the sex ratio was 21% males, a significant deviation from the sex ratio reported elsewhere (for example, see Gashwiler, 1972).

Alternatively, Jannett (1981*b*) argued that sampled sex ratios and operational sex ratios may differ. He found that, in *M. montanus,* the ratio of older males to older females in high-density populations significantly favored females as a result of territoriality by breeding males. Further, territorial males remained in breeding condition. Therefore, the total number of males, which includes non-territorial males, becomes irrelevant to the breeding pattern for this species.

Deliberate manipulation of the sex ratio has important consequences to the breeding structure of voles. Redfield et al. (1978*b*) artificially manipulated the sex ratio of *M. townsendii* on unenclosed grids to determine if the demographic performance of these populations was altered by a greatly disparate sex ratio. Their results suggested that an enrichment of the proportion of males produced no significant differences in the percentage of adult or subadult males with scrotal testes. Further, no significant difference was detected in lactation between the female-enriched and control grids. However, weight at sexual maturity for the rarer sex on both enriched grids was *lower* than the value for the same sex on the control.

Microtus oregoni also was subjected to manipulation (Redfield et al., 1978*a*) during the above studies on *M. townsendii,* and a sum-

TABLE 1

SUMMARY OF CHANGES IN THE BREEDING PATTERN OF *Microtus oregoni* ON 0.64-HA UNENCLOSED STUDY AREAS WHERE THE SEX RATIO OF THE EXPERIMENTAL POPULATION WAS MANIPULATED (REDFIELD ET AL., 1978*a*)

		Experimental populations	
	Control population	Male-enriched	Female-enriched
Main breeding season	Adult ♂♂ enter breeding condition 6 weeks before ♀♀, 1973; not clear for 1972	More scrotal ♂♂ than control	♀♀ breed more intensively and longer than control
Winter breeding season	Adult ♂♂ enter breeding condition 6 weeks before ♀♀ (February vs March) but no winter breeding in adults	Higher percent ♂♂ breeding; breed longer, and in winter	Higher percent ♀♀ lactating; breed longer (October), but not in winter
Sexual maturity	Subadult ♂♂ mature before subadult ♀♀ but are not mature in winter	Subadult ♂♂ mature during winter	Subadult ♀♀ do not mature during winter
Recruitment of sexes		More ♂♂ and ♀♀ recruited than control	More ♂♂ and ♀♀ recruited than control

mary of the changes that occurred in the creeping vole is presented in Table 1. Although the initial populations were found to be distorted (21% males), further distortion of the sex ratio produced a profound change in the demographic pattern of the enriched populations. With regard to reproduction, no winter breeding occurred in the control population. However, breeding continued in the male-enriched population (at a reduced level by both adults and subadults). Females also continued to breed for a longer period during the first winter. Although Redfield et al. (1978*a*) did not comment on age at sexual maturation, their data suggests that males on the male-enriched grid initiated breeding at lighter body weights. Additionally, other components in the reproductive process were subjected to alteration (fine-tuning changes), but the potential effects of these changes in relation to subsequent changes in density are not clear.

In summary, sex ratios for many species of New World voles have been documented over extended periods, but only two studies have dealt with the potential effects on reproductive processes if these ratios are significantly altered experimentally. From these studies, it appears that changes in the breeding potential can be induced, but it is neither clear what range of disruption is required to significantly alter this potential nor how disruption affects the social structure of populations. Krebs (1964) proposed that the sex ratio only affected the number of breeding animals in polyestrous mammals, but a significant disruption of this ratio also appears to alter the social structure of populations such that age at sexual maturity and length of the breeding season may be affected.

Litter Size

A comparison of interspecific and intraspecific variation in litter size for New World voles is difficult for several reasons. Presently it is not possible to assess the amount of variation that is genetically determined in each species. Where phenotypic differences have been noted, either geographically or temporally, the statistical treatments are often inadequate, largely as a result of small samples. Additionally, because parity, season of collection, weight, age, and physiological condition of females are all subject to variation, assessment of geographical variation among conspecific populations may be of limited value. Presently, we lack adequate estimates for the proportion of variation in litter size produced by each of these factors.

Table 2 gives the mean litter size and pertinent data on sampling durations and locations for 18 species of New World *Microtus*. Except as noted, I excluded studies in which counts of placental scars were included with counts of embryos because placental scar counts are not always reliable (Corthum, 1967; Martin et al., 1976; Rolan and Gier, 1967). In some cases, I computed grand mean values by pooling data for individual periods. Additionally, I excluded data for individual species in which sample size was <10 unless the data base was found limited or the locality distinct. Thus, more data are available, especially for *M. californicus, M. ochrogaster, M. pennsylvanicus*, and *M. pinetorum*, but they are largely anecdotal or are presented in regional works in which samples were pooled from broad geographical areas.

TABLE 2

LITTER SIZE DATA, AS DETERMINED FROM EMBRYO COUNTS OR YOUNG DELIVERED, FOR NEW WORLD *Microtus*

Species	Mean litter size*	Ex-tremes*	N	Duration years	Months sampled†	Geographical location(s)	Source
Subgenus *Microtus*							
M. breweri	3.4	1–6[1]	102	3	32C	Muskeget Island, Massa-chussetts	Tamarin (1977*a*)
M. californicus	4.20	1–9	154	2	21C	Marin Co., California	Greenwald (1957)
	4.94	1–10	73	3	9VAY	Contra Costa Co., California	Hoffmann (1958)
	5.05	1–10	280	13	VAY	Brooks Island, California	Lidicker (1973)
	4.4[2]	1–10	33	2	25C	Contra Costa Co., California	Krohne (1980)
	3.36[3]	1–8	44	2	25C	Sonoma Co., California	Krohne (1980)
	4.7	1–9	42			Laboratory colony	Colvin and Colvin (1970)
	4.25[2]	1–10	65			Laboratory colony	Krohne (1980)
	5.23[2]	1–10	42			Experimental enclosures	Krohne (1980)
	4.17[3]	1–10	220			Laboratory colony	Krohne (1980)
	3.45[3]	1–7	20			Experimental enclosures	Krohne (1980)
M. canicaudus	3.23[4]	2–10[5]	44			Laboratory colony	Tyser (1975)
M. chrotorrhinus	3.56	2–5	9	Several		Temagami, Ontario	Coventry (1937)
	3.71	1–7	52			Largely museum study	Martin (1971)
	2.88	2–5	8	2	2S	Pocahontas, Randolph, and Tucker Cos., West Virginia	Kirkland (1977)
	3.5		4	1	1S	Cook Co., Minnesota	Timm et al. (1977)

TABLE 2
CONTINUED

Species	Mean litter size*	Ex-tremes*	N	Duration years	Months sampled†	Geographical location(s)	Source
M. longicaudus	4.9	4–6	10	2	1S	Graham Co., Arizona	Hoffmeister (1956)
	3.85[6]	2–7	25	1†	7NC	Whitman Co., Washington	Wright (1971)
	3.8[7]		23	2	8C	Whitman Co., Washington	Farris (1971); Wright (1971)
	4.7	4–6	15		15VAY	Pennington Co., South Dakota	Turner (1974)
	3.7	2–5	9		3S	Yukon Territory	Youngman (1975)
	5.0		26		2S	Prince of Wales Island, Alaska	Van Horne (1982)
	4.0	1–7	37			Laboratory colony	Colvin and Colvin (1970)
M. mexicanus	2.7	1–4	15		1S	Coahuila, Mexico	Baker (1956)
	2.23	1–4	22		2S	Coconino Co., Arizona	Brown (1968)
	2.25	1–3	8		1S	Otero Co., New Mexico	Brown (1968)
M. montanus	5.60	3–8	41		1S	Mono Co., California	Howell (1924)
	6.47	2–10	109	4	3S	Nevada Co., California	Hoffmann (1958)
	5.72[6]		18		4S	Modoc Co., California	Murray (1965)
	5.8	2–10	46	3	3S	Grand Co., Colorado	Vaughan (1969)
	4.08[6]		38	2	18C	Whitman Co., Washington	Wright (1971)
	6.32[6]		65	3	2S	Teton Co., Wyoming	Negus et al. (1977)
	4.5	3–6				Laboratory colony	Seidel and Booth (1960)

TABLE 2
CONTINUED

Species	Mean litter size*	Ex-tremes*	N	Duration years	Months sampled†	Geographical location(s)	Source
	4.05	1–10	253			Laboratory colony	Negus and Pinter (1965)
	6.0	3–9	42			Laboratory colony	Colvin and Colvin (1970)
M. ochrogaster	3.4	1–7	58	1	9C	Mostly Douglas Co., Kansas	Jameson (1947)
	3.18	1–6	65	3	30C	Douglas Co., Kansas	Martin (1956)
	3.37	2–5	82	7	12P & Y	Douglas Co., Kansas	Fitch (1957)
	3.89	2–7	134	1	13C	Vigo Co., Indiana	Corthum (1967)
	4.19		198	11	2W & 2SP	Variable, Kansas	Rolan and Gier (1967)
	3.27	1–6[1]	160	2+	32C	Monroe and Brown Cos., Indiana	Keller and Krebs (1970)
	3.35	1–6	31	2	8C	Jefferson Co., Kentucky	Quick (1970)
	3.43[6]		181	2	24C	Douglas Co., Kansas	Rose and Gaines (1978)
	5.11[8]$\theta\theta$		19	1	SP & S	Champaign Co., Illinois	Cole and Batzli (1978)
	4.25$\theta\theta$		28	1	SP & S	Champaign Co., Illinois	Cole and Batzli (1978)
	3.77	1–8	280			Laboratory colony	Richmond (1967)
	3.9	1–7	28			Laboratory colony	Colvin and Colvin (1970)

TABLE 2
CONTINUED

Species	Mean litter size*	Ex-tremes*	N	Duration years	Months sampled†	Geographical location(s)	Source
M. oeconomus	6.9		91		3S	Arctic slope, Alaska	Bee and Hall (1956)
	5.58[6]		40		2S	Yukon Territory	Youngman (1975)
	6.9		7	4	VAY	Fairbanks, Alaska	Whitney (1977)
	3.9		98			Laboratory colony	Dieterich and Preston (1977*a*)
M. oregoni	3.11	1–8	18	16	VAY	Clackamas, Lane, and Linn Cos., Oregon	Gashwiler (1972)
	3.11	1–5	26	1	12	British Columbia?	Cowan and Arsenault (1954)
	2.79	1–5	28			Laboratory colony	Cowan and Arsenault (1954)
	3.8	1–16	15			Laboratory colony	Colvin and Colvin (1970)
M. pennsylvanicus	5.07	2–9	41	3	VAY	Onondaga Co., New York	Townsend (1935)
	5.83	3–9	18	1	4VS	Toronto, Ontario	Coventry (1937)
	4.35	3–7	23	1	4VS	Temagami and Algonquin Park, Ontario	Coventry (1937)
	5.07	1–11		4	55C	Tompkins Co., New York	Hamilton (1937)
	6.05	1–8	24	1+	6VS	Crawford Co., Pennsylvania	Goin (1943)
	3.65		16	3	4VS + W	Dorchester Co., Maryland	Harris (1953)
	5.03	1–9	246	23	10P	Aweme District, Manitoba	Criddle (1956)

TABLE 2
CONTINUED

Species	Mean litter size*	Extremes*	N	Duration years	Months sampled†	Geographical location(s)	Source
M. pennsylvanicus	6.9	4–12	17	4	5S	Churchill, Manitoba	Smith and Foster (1957)
	5.31	2–10	13	2	6P	Otsego and Schoharie Cos., New York	Connor (1960)
	5.72	1–11	251	6	12C	Dakota, Lake Co., Minnesota	Beer and MacLeod (1961)
	4.9[9]	3–8	37	5	4S	Toronto, Ontario	Kott and Robinson (1963)
	5.5	1–8	124	5	5S	Toronto, Ontario	Kott and Robinson (1963)
	4.68[6]		76	4	12NC	Franklin Co., Pennsylvania	Christian and Davis (1966)
	4.46	1–9	153	1	11C	Vigo Co., Indiana	Corthum (1967)
	4.54	1–7[1]	154	3	31C	Monroe and Brown Cos., Indiana	Keller and Krebs (1970)
	5.3	2–10	76		4S	Yukon Territory	Youngman (1975)
	3.82	1–11	312	6	VAY	Pinawa, Manitoba	Iverson and Turner (1976)
	4.5	2–8[1]	57	3	27C	Middleborough and Barnstable Cos., Massachusetts	Tamarin (1977*a*)
	5.5	2–8	31			Laboratory colony	Colvin and Colvin (1970)

TABLE 2
CONTINUED

Species	Mean litter size*	Ex-tremes*	N	Duration years	Months sampled†	Geographical location(s)	Source
	4.1		66			Laboratory colony	Dieterich and Preston (1977*b*)
M. townsendii	5.10		278	2	19C	Westham Island and Haney, British Columbia	Anderson and Boonstra (1979)
	6.0	5–7	20			Ladner, British Columbia	MacFarlane and Taylor (1982*b*)
M. xanthognathus	8.0	7–10	11	1	1S	Yukon Territory	Youngman (1975)
	8.8	6–13	71	3	3S + 1W	150 km NW Fairbanks and Lake Minchumina, Alaska	Wolff and Lidicker (1980)
Subgenus *Pitymys*							
M. pinetorum	2.0	1–4	149	1	12C	Botetourt and Roanoke Cos., Virginia	Horsfall (1963)
	2.24	1–5	138	2	30P	8 counties, North Carolina	Paul (1966)
	1.90	1–3	51	1	12C	Pittsylvania Co., Virginia	Valentine and Kirkpatrick (1970)
	2.54	2–5	16	2	6VAY	Payne Co., Oklahoma	Goertz (1971)
	2.0[10]		35	1	11C	Rappahannock Co., Virginia	Cengel et al. (1978)

TABLE 2
CONTINUED

Species	Mean litter size*	Ex-tremes*	N	Duration years	Months sampled†	Geographical location(s)	Source
	1.6[11]		11	1	11C	Rappahannock Co., Virginia	Cengel et al. (1978)
	3.11	1–6	150			Laboratory colony	Shadler and Butterstein (1979)
M. quasiater	2.2	1–4	11			Jalapa, Veracruz	Hall and Kelson (1959)
Subgenus *Stenocranius*							
M. abbreviatus	3.0					Laboratory colony	Morrison et al. (1976)
M. miurus	8.2	4–12	46			Alaska	Bee and Hall (1956)
	3.9		43			Laboratory colony	Morrison et al. (1976)
Subgenus *Arvicola*							
M. richardsoni	6.0	5–9	10		2S	Fremont Co., Wyoming	Negus and Findley (1959)
	5.45		16			Carbon Co., Montana, and Park Co., Wyoming	Pattie (1967)
	7.85	6–10	26		2S	Northwestern Montana	Brown (1977)

TABLE 2
CONTINUED

* Coding, litter size:

[1] Unpublished, courtesy of original author(s)
[2] Annual grassland
[3] Perennial grassland
[4] Repeated samples of some females
[5] From Maser and Storm, 1970
[6] Data pooled from several years
[7] Data from two studies pooled
[8] Food added to population
[9] Born in traps
[10] Maintained orchard
[11] Abandoned orchard
θθ Mean number of placental scars or embryos

† Abbreviations, months sampled:

C, consecutive months sampled
NC, non-consecutive months sampled
P, pooled values
S, summer samples
SP, spring samples
VAY, months sampled variable among years
VS, months sampled variable in year
W, winter months
Y, yearly values

The smallest mean litter sizes shown are for *M. pinetorum* (Cengel et al., 1978), *M. quasiater* (Hall and Kelson, 1959), and *M. mexicanus* (Brown, 1968), whereas the largest is reported for *M. xanthognathus* (Wolff and Lidicker, 1980). Values provided in the table for laboratory colonies are lower than the highest values observed under field conditions, excepting those in *M. oregoni* and *M. pinetorum*.

Genotypic and Phenotypic Variation

Innes (1978*b*) reviewed the relation between embryo counts and latitude and elevation for 42 independent literature samples of *Microtus* species. Although he found a significant correlation ($r = 0.77$, $P < 0.01$) between litter size and these variables when values for several species were pooled, no correlation could be demonstrated for each of four species with sufficient sample sizes for contrasts. Thus, Innes (1978*b*) concluded that the relationship of latitude and altitude, or both, were of questionable importance for explaining litter size in voles. Kenney et al. (1979) suggested litter size in voles is related to persistence of copulatory behavior. However, subsequent consideration of several untested species failed to support this hypothesis (Dewsbury and Hartung, 1982). Lord (1960) suggested large litter size compensated for presumed higher winter mortality in northern areas. Spencer and Steinhoff (1968) suggested that larger litters were favored as a result of short breeding seasons. But the two latter studies failed to differentiate litter size at birth and recruitment. Thus, voles with larger litters would only be at reproductive advantage if their young have larger litters and are recruited in at least proportionate numbers of if they breed for longer durations. The relative contribution of young by individual females remains largely unknown for any species of *Microtus,* but Anderson (1975) documented high repeatability for litter size in female *M. townsendii* studied in breeding enclosures. Unfortunately, the degree of similarity of litter sizes between breeding adults and recruited young could not be measured in her experimental enclosures. Anderson and Boonstra (1979) also were unable to demonstrate a relationship between maternal body size or parity and litter size at recruitment. Thus, it is not clear how selection for litter size operates on voles under natural conditions, and its role within and between different species of voles remains an enigma.

Statistical Considerations

In voles, phenotypic rather than genotypic responses to environmental variation probably produce the intraspecific differences in litter size observed geographically, altitudinally, and temporally (Krohne, 1980). Unfortunately, appropriate statistical treatments are difficult to make for a number of reasons. Pelikán (1979) noted that many of the comparisons made for litter size in small mammals are derived from sample sizes that do not provide reliable mean estimates and that increasing litter size is correlated with increasing standard deviations. Thus, in species with large embryo counts, greater sample sizes are required to distinguish between alternative hypotheses. For example, in *M. pinetorum,* which has a litter size approximately equivalent to *Pitymys subterranus,* between 30 and 40 pregnant females were required to obtain a reliable mean for contrast (Pelikán, 1979). For species with mean litter sizes of 4.91 to 6.20, 90 to 120 pregnant females were needed to estimate a mean with the same reliability (Pelikán, 1979).

The above observations are important in assessing differences among species, such as the contrast provided by Innes (1978*b*), because assumptions of ANOVA procedures are violated when cross-species comparisons are sought with samples that are heteroscedastic. Additionally, Pelikán's (1979) analyses clearly indicate that conspecific contrasts require complete monthly seasonal data sets for comparisons, because mid-season means differ statistically from whole-season means owing to greater variability in embryo counts at the beginning and end of breeding periods. Because relatively few studies have separated peak seasonal data into blocks for comparisons among years of treatments, and because data blocks are often developed with limited samples, most of the litter-size values that now exist are not commensurable. In order to improve future commensurability, data should be displayed by week for individual months.

Pelikán (1979) did not address the question of the effect of parity and weight on mean values of litter size, but this variation also affects comparability. A number of studies for voles indicate that litter size varies with the age (weight) of females and their parity.

Age (Weight) and Parity

Leslie and Ranson (1940) first noted an association between increased litter size and age in *Microtus agrestis*; Hasler (1975) reviewed the literature on the effect of parity. A relationship between parity and litter size has not been found for *M. chrotorrhinus* (Martin, 1971), *M. canicaudus* (Tyser, 1975), *M. townsendii* (Anderson and Boonstra, 1979), or *M. xanthognathus* (Wolff and Lidicker, 1980). Exceptions have been noted in *M. longicaudus* (Wright, 1971), *M. ochrogaster* (Rose and Gaines, 1978), and *M. breweri* (Tamarin, 1977*a*).

When the weight of females, which may or may not relate to parity, affects litter size, and breeding is not synchronized like that observed in *M. xanthognathus,* significant differences in litter size among years or between areas being sampled may be distinguished only on the basis of covariance analyses (Keller and Krebs, 1970). Thus, the different contributions of weight (age) and parity, because they are rarely detailed, renders many estimates of embryo counts difficult to compare on a geographical basis.

Some investigators have made contrasts of embryo counts after adjusting for parity and weight differences among samples. Keller and Krebs (1970) and Tamarin (1977*a*) were unable to demonstrate significant differences in embryo counts for primiparae and multiparae female *M. pennsylvanicus* in Indiana and Massachusetts. No significant depression in embryo counts among years for cycling meadow voles was found by these authors.

Keller and Krebs (1970) found that multiparous and primiparous female *M. ochrogaster* differed in their embryo counts; the former contained embryo counts depressed by 25% during periods of peak density. By contrast, Rose and Gaines (1978) were unable to demonstrate significant weight-embryo regressions for prairie voles in Kansas, but the absence of light females may have influenced their results as females <20 g were not collected. Marked seasonal effects on living embryo counts were observed, but a reduction in litter size was not found at the peak density (Rose and Gaines, 1978).

No significant differences in embryo counts among years have been found for non-cyclic species. Tamarin (1977*a*) was unable to demonstrate a significant relationship between parity or weight and embryo count in *Microtus breweri,* but Anderson and Boonstra (1979) found that litter size for *M. townsendii* is influenced by weight and not parity and that embryo counts were significantly larger in spring than summer or fall.

Other Factors

Many authors attribute differences in litter size to nutritional deficiencies (Batzli, this volume), endocrine responses related to density (Seabloom, this volume), or physiological responses related to the presence of chemical substances that stimulate reproduction (Negus et al., 1977). Given that substances such as 6-MBOA (Berger et al., 1981; Sanders et al., 1981) stimulate rapid reproductive development of reproductively quiescent voles other than *M. montanus,* we would expect populations exposed to greater quantities of stimulatory chemicals to display larger litters at the height of the breeding season. Although this supposition awaits a critical evaluation, studies exist which demonstrate that litter size differs significantly in qualitatively different habitats for other species. Cengel et al. (1978) suggested that food quality affected litter size in *M. pinetorum.* Krohne (1981) was able to eliminate effects of parity and age on embryo counts in *M. californicus* populations trapped in annual and perennial grasslands. In a series of replicated studies in enclosures, he was able to establish that embryo-count differences in voles occupying the two habitats were the result of responses to vegetation (Krohne, 1980). Since these populations were established with a pair of sibs, a genetic basis for these differences seems unlikely, although Krohne (1981) noted that genetically based dissimilarities in embryo production occurred among conspecifics raised under laboratory conditions. Additionally, replicated experiments all demonstrated similar patterns. Krohne (1982) suggested that reduced litter size in California voles in perennial grasslands was partially responsible for the lack of a multi-annual cycle in his population.

Cole and Batzli (1978) observed greater production of young *M. ochrogaster* fed rabbit pellets under field conditions. Although sample sizes used for comparison were small and the parity-weight relationships of these samples were not reported, the results are suggestive; concurrent studies in dissimilar habitats suggested dissimilar embryo counts (Cole and Batzli, 1979).

Prenatal Mortality

The potential litter size in voles, as contrasted to the number of embryos that develop, can only be determined by autopsy. Rela-

TABLE 3

Summary of Mean Pre- and Post-Implantation Mortality in Four Species of Voles. Values are Grand Estimates for Studies in Which Prenatal Loss was Assessed over One to Several Years, as Noted in the Text

Species	Percent ova lost	N	Percent resorbing embryos	N	Mean egg loss before implantation	Mean litter loss after implantation	Total realized prenatal mortality	Source
M. breweri	14.2	102	8.1	102	0.52	0.27	0.79	Tamarin (1977*a*)
M. montanus	5.9	110	3.7	110	0.42	0.23	0.65	Hoffmann (1958)
M. ochrogaster	6.56	148	6.9	151	0.23	0.25	0.48	Keller and Krebs (1970)
	10.0	182	1.6	187	0.38	0.05	0.43	Rose and Gaines (1978)
M. pennsylvanicus	6.3	251	1.9	251	0.38	0.11	0.49	Beer et al. (1957)
	9.5	152	6.2	159	0.51	0.28	0.79	Keller and Krebs (1970)
	6.4	57	2.8	57	0.32	0.12	0.44	Tamarin (1977*a*)

tively few studies have been undertaken on New World voles to assess the degree of prenatal mortality associated with changes in density, although some seasonal assessments are available. Table 3 shows the pooled values of pre- and post-implantation loss for four species of voles. I included the results of Beer et al. (1957) for contrast, although the data were produced from a variety of locations and from unknown population densities. The data from Tamarin (1977*a*) are restricted to peak periods of density for *M. pennsylvanicus*. Data for *M. californicus* were excluded, because accessory corpora lutea develop in this species (Greenwald, 1956; Hoffmann, 1958; Lidicker, 1973), a condition that prevents assessment of total loss because pre-implantation mortality cannot be determined. Post-implantation mortalities (percent resorbing embryos) for *M. californicus* in the three studies were 7.2, 3.9, and 4.7, respectively. Post-implantation resorptions in laboratory *M. ochrogaster* exceeded field resorptions (32/278 = 11.5%; Stehn, 1978). On the basis of these studies, levels of prenatal mortality do not appear related to changes in density. Total losses appear highest in *M. breweri* (Table 3), but comparative data are lacking for most species.

In voles, pre-implantation losses can be determined by computing the difference between implantations (living and resorbing) and the number of corpora lutea (except in *M. californicus*). Cases of presumed polyovuly or polyembryony (twinning) range from approximately 2% to 13% and the values appear to be relatively consistent within two species where independent determinations have been made. The lowest values, 1.2% (2/170) and 1.6% (3/185), were reported for *Microtus ochrogaster* by Keller and Krebs (1970) and Rose and Gaines (1978). Beer et al. (1957) reported 6.8% (17/251), Keller and Krebs (1970) 4.3% (7/162), and Tamarin (in litt.; 1977*a*) 5.3% (3/57) for *M. pennsylvanicus*. The value for *M. breweri* (Tamarin, 1977*a*) was 3.9% (4/102) (Tamarin, in litt.). Hoffmann (1958) found the largest value (13.0%; 14/108) in *Microtus montanus*. Tamarin (in litt.) did not find twinning in either *M. breweri* or *M. pennsylvanicus*, but Beer et al. (1957) noted that approximately 30% (5/17) of their results could be attributed to twinning.

In cases in which the number of implants exceeds the number of corpora lutea, and twinning is excluded, corpora lutea may be counted incorrectly. Snyder (1969) sectioned ovaries of *M. pennsylvanicus* and found that one corpus luteum in a sample of 24 ovaries was overlooked. Values for polyovuly or polyembryony should be viewed as conservative estimates because they are underestimated if corpora lutea and implant counts are identical and early resorption of one or more embryos is missed. Additionally, total pre-implantation losses (already noted in conjunction with potential changes in the interbirth interval) are missed frequently because corpora lutea rapidly undergo involution following blockage by strange males (Bruce effect).

Post-implantation losses result from failure of one or more embryos, but we are unable to separate genetic failure of individual implants from failures due to exogenous or endogenous factors that affect the physiology of female voles. Total losses are rarely encountered in necropsy samples. The loss may be total where stress (Seabloom, this volume) or the Bruce effect occur, but the opportunity to observe male-induced abortion, because of its rapid completion, is unlikely in kill-trap samples. Stehn and Richmond (1975) documented the sequence of events for male-induced abortion in *M. ochrogaster.* They noted that termination was accompanied by a mucilaginous bloody discharge that contained amorphic pieces of debris. Although we cannot determine whether live-trapped populations display these symptoms because of handling or the Bruce effect, I have observed female discharges composed of debris similar in composition to the placental sign described by Venable (1939), in *M. montanus, M. ochrogaster,* and *M. pennsylvanicus.*

In summary, it is not presently possible to separate the factors that have led to variation in litter size for New World voles. Phenotypic plasticity appears to account for much of the variation observed for conspecific populations living in qualitatively dissimilar habitats. The number of living embryos shows seasonal peaks that may be related to the size, age, weight, or parity of females. Many statistical treatments can be faulted where these relationships are not considered. No compelling evidence suggests embryo production is lower during periods of population decline, but the number of embryos is generally lower in females pregnant early or late in the breeding season.

Discussion

Since Hasler's (1975) excellent review of the literature on reproduction in the subfamily Microtinae was published, most field studies have continued to assess variation in breeding patterns without corroborative experiments. More emphasis needs to be placed on reproductive analyses in which suspected variables are manipulated experimentally. Describing relationships between breeding intensity and environmental parameters in contrast to testing necessary and sufficient agents responsible for breeding patterns seems to me to be a self-defeating task; further description may add little to our knowledge of how reproductive parameters affect population changes. Years ago, Chitty (1952) tried to convince us that social factors affect reproductive status and fertility of individuals. It appears that in our haste to describe why populations decline, cycle, and disperse, we often ignored the reproductive success of individuals and remained content to consider only the average of the masses. If we find that some species adjust their breeding seasons as a result of chemicals in vegetation, then we must immediately ask about individual variation in responsiveness to limited cues. Pheromones and social learning seem to play a synergistic role in behavior of voles. Do all individuals respond to these cues in a similar manner? I stress the importance of individual variation in reproductive adaptations in voles, but it is evident that we also are unable to directly relate reproductive variation, as measured in field populations, to subsequent population patterns. Much remains to be learned. In summary, the following list illustrates some experimental manipulations that should increase our understanding of intraspecific reproductive processes for populations of New World voles: 1) chemical identification and field experimental studies of pheromones that may serve to integrate environmental cues with the social organization required for breeding in voles; 2) field experiments with voles unable to smell their conspecifics (see Horton and Shepherd, 1979; Richmond and Stehn, 1976); 3) application of graded doses of 6-MBOA in a variety of species over an entire winter non-breeding period; 4) 6-MBOA enhancement of breeding in early-stop peak and late-start declining populations; 5) quantification of seasonal and altitudinal variation in 6-MBOA content of vegetation; 6) sex-ratio enrichment experiments for species other than *M. townsendii* and *M. oregoni*, especially in single-species populations; 7) extensive heritability analyses for age at sexual maturity, growth potentials, and winter breeding in species known to cycle; 8) analyses of reproductive success in marginal habitats for colonizing individuals; 9) assessment of the degree of reliability between necropsy and field assessment of fecundity, especially for "winter" breeders; 10) deliberate introduction of unknown conspecifics into known populations in large enclosures where breeding can be carefully assessed prior to introduction and can be followed subsequently for Bruce-Whitten effects; 11) initiation of large, enclosed field populations with females having small litters versus females having large litters previously housed in laboratory situations. Age, weight, and pairs must be equalized.

Acknowledgments

This chapter was made possible through a grant to the Idaho State University Foundation provided through the offices of Kirkland Ellis, Chicago, Illinois. I especially want to thank Mrs. Joan Downing, Assistant Librarian, Idaho State University, and the staff of the libraries of Idaho State University and the University of Utah who went to great lengths to be helpful and provide space during development of this chapter. I thank Bonnie Bowen for offering comment on the final manuscript and the reviewers who offered comment on the initial draft.

Literature Cited

Abdellatif, E. A., K. B. Armitage, M. S. Gaines, and M. L. Johnson. 1982. The effect of watering on a prairie vole population. Acta Theriol., 18:243–255.

Abramsky, Z., and C. R. Tracy. 1979. Population biology of a "noncycling" population of prairie voles and a hypothesis on the role of migration in regulating microtine cycles. Ecology, 60:349–361.

Adams, M. R., R. H. Tamarin, and I. P. Callard. 1980. Seasonal changes in plasma androgen levels and the gonads of the beach vole, *Microtus breweri*. Gen. Comp. Endocrinol., 41:31–40.

Anderson, J. L. 1975. Phenotypic correlations among relatives and variability in reproductive performance in populations of the vole *Microtus townsendii*. Unpubl. Ph.D. dissert., Univ. British Columbia, Vancouver, 207 pp.

Anderson, J. L., and R. Boonstra. 1979. Some aspects of reproduction in the vole *Microtus townsendii*. Canadian J. Zool., 57:18–24.

Anderson, P. K. 1980. Evolutionary implications of microtine behavioral systems on the ecological stage. The Biologist, 62:70–88.

Anderson, P. K., P. H. Whitney, and J-P Huang. 1976. *Arvicola richardsoni*: ecology and biochemical polymorphism in the front ranges of southern Alberta. Acta Theriol., 21:425–468.

Bailey, V. 1924. Breeding, feeding, and other life habits of meadow mice (*Microtus*). J. Agric. Res., 27:523–535.

BAKER, J. R., AND R. M. RANSON. 1932. Factors affecting the breeding of the field mouse (*Microtus agrestis*). Part I. Light. Proc. Roy. Soc. London, Ser. B, 110:313–322.

BAKER, R. H. 1956. Mammals of Coahuila, Mexico. Univ. Kansas Publ., Mus. Nat. Hist., 9:125–335.

BATZLI, G. O., AND F. A. PITELKA. 1971. Condition and diet of cycling populations of the California vole, *Microtus californicus*. J. Mamm., 52:141–163.

BATZLI, G. O., L. L. GETZ, AND S. S. HURLEY. 1977. Suppression of growth and reproduction of microtine rodents by social factors. J. Mamm., 58:583–591.

BEACHAM, T. D. 1980. Breeding characteristics of Townsend's vole (*Microtus townsendii*) during population fluctuations. Canadian J. Zool., 58:623–625.

BEARD, H. B. 1978. Hormonal influence on the social behavior of the vole, *Microtus ochrogaster*: effect of photoperiod, temperature, gonadectomy, preputialectomy and oral angle gland removal. Unpubl. Ph.D. dissert., Iowa State Univ., Ames, 232 pp.

BEE, J. W., AND E. R. HALL. 1956. Mammals of northern Alaska. Misc. Publ., Mus. Nat. Hist., Univ. Kansas, 8:1–309.

BEER, J. R., AND C. F. MACLEOD. 1961. Seasonal reproduction in the meadow vole. J. Mamm., 42:483–489.

BEER, J. R., C. F. MACLEOD, AND L. D. FRENZEL. 1957. Prenatal survival and loss in some cricetid rodents. J. Mamm., 38:392–402.

BENTON, A. H. 1955. Observations on the life history of the northern pine mouse. J. Mamm., 36:52–62.

BERGER, P. J., AND N. C. NEGUS. 1974. Influence of dietary supplements of fresh lettuce on ovariectomized *Microtus montanus*. J. Mamm., 55:747–750.

———. 1982. Stud male maintenance of pregnancy in *Microtus montanus*. J. Mamm., 63:148–151.

BERGER, P. J., N. C. NEGUS, E. H. SANDERS, AND P. D. GARDNER. 1981. Chemical triggering of reproduction in *Microtus montanus*. Science, 214:69–70.

BERGER, P. J., E. H. SANDERS, P. D. GARDNER, AND N. C. NEGUS. 1977. Phenolic plant compounds functioning as reproductive inhibitors in *Microtus montanus*. Science, 195:575–577.

BIRNEY, E. C., W. E. GRANT, AND D. D. BAIRD. 1976. Importance of vegetative cover to cycles of *Microtus* populations. Ecology, 57:1043–1051.

BOONSTRA, R. 1980. Infanticide in microtines: importance in natural populations. Oecologia, 46:262–265.

BOONSTRA R., AND C. J. KREBS. 1977. A fencing experiment on a high-density population of *Microtus townsendii*. Canadian J. Zool., 55:1166–1175.

BOWEN, B. S. 1982. Temporal dynamics of microgeographic structure of genetic variation in *Microtus californicus*. J. Mamm., 63:625–638.

BREED, W. G. 1967. Ovulation in the genus *Microtus*. Nature, 214:826.

———. 1969. Oestrus and ovarian histology in the lactating vole (*Microtus agrestis*). J. Reprod. Fert., 18:33–42.

———. 1972. The question of induced ovulation in wild voles. J. Mamm., 53: 185–187.

BROWN, L. N. 1968. Smallness of mean litter size in the Mexican vole. J. Mamm., 49:159.

———. 1977. Litter size and notes on reproduction in the giant water vole *Arvicola richardsoni*. Southwestern Nat., 22:281–282.

BRUCE, H. M. 1959. An exteroceptive block to pregnancy in the mouse. Nature, 184:105.

CARTER, C. S., L. L. GETZ, L. GAVISH, J. L. MCDERMOTT, AND P. ARNOLD. 1980. Male related pheromones and the activation of female reproduction in the prairie vole (*Microtus ochrogaster*). Biol. Reprod., 23:1038–1045.

CENGEL, D. J., J. E. ESTEP, AND R. L. KIRKPATRICK. 1978. Pine vole reproduction in relation to food habits and body fat. J. Wildl. Mgmt., 42:822–833.

CHITTY, D. 1952. Mortality among voles (*Microtus agrestis*) at Lake Vyrnwy, Montgomeryshire in 1936–39. Phil. Trans. Roy. Soc. London, Ser. B, 236:505–552.

CHRISTIAN, J. J. 1970. Social subordination, population density and mammalian evolution. Science, 168:84–90.

———. 1971. Population density and reproductive efficiency. Biol. Reprod., 4: 248–294.

CHRISTIAN, J. J., AND D. E. DAVIS. 1966. Adrenal glands in female voles (*Microtus pennsylvanicus*) as related to reproduction and population size. J. Mamm., 47:1–18.

CLARKE, J. R. 1977. Long and short term changes in gonadal activity of field voles and bank voles. Oikos, 29:457–467.

CLULOW, F. V., AND J. R. CLARKE. 1968. Pregnancy-block in *Microtus agrestis* an induced ovulator. Nature, 219:511.

CLULOW, F. V., AND P. E. LANGFORD. 1971. Pregnancy-block in the meadow vole, *Microtus pennsylvanicus*. J. Reprod. Fert., 24:275–277.

CLULOW, F. V., AND F. F. MALLORY. 1970. Oestrus and induced ovulation in the meadow vole, *Microtus pennsylvanicus*. J. Reprod. Fert., 23:341–343.

COLE, F. R., AND G. O. BATZLI. 1978. Influence of supplemental feeding on a vole population. J. Mamm., 59:809–819.

———. 1979. Nutrition and population dynamics of the prairie vole, *Microtus ochrogaster*, in central Illinois. J. Anim. Ecol., 48:455–470.

COLE, L. C. 1954. The population consequences of life history phenomena. Quart. Rev. Biol., 29:103–137.

COLVIN, M. A., AND D. V. COLVIN. 1970. Breeding and fecundity of six species of voles (*Microtus*). J. Mamm., 51:417–419.

CONLEY, W. 1976. Competition between *Microtus*: a behavioral hypothesis. Ecology, 57:224–237.

CONNOR, P. F. 1960. The small mammals of Otsego and Schoharie counties, New York. New York State Mus. Sci., Serv. Bull., 382:1–84.

CORTHUM, D. W., JR. 1967. Reproduction and duration of placental scars in the prairie vole and the eastern vole. J. Mamm., 48:287–292.

COVENTRY, A. F. 1937. Notes on the breeding of some cricetidae in Ontario. J. Mamm., 18:489–496.

COWAN, I. MCT., AND M. G. ARSENAULT. 1954. Reproduction and growth in the creeping vole, *Microtus oregoni serpens* Merriam. Canadian J. Zool., 32: 198–208.

CRIDDLE, S. 1956. Drummond's vole in Manitoba. Canadian Field-Nat., 70: 78–84.

CROSS, P. C. 1972. Observations on the induction of ovulation in *Microtus montanus*. J. Mamm., 53:210–212.

DAWKINS, R. 1976. The selfish gene. Oxford Univ. Press, New York, 224 pp.

DECOURSEY, G. E., JR. 1957. Identification, ecology and reproduction of *Microtus* in Ohio. J. Mamm., 38:44–52.

DEWSBURY, D. A., AND D. J. BAUMGARDNER. 1981. Studies of sperm competition in two species of muroid rodents. Behav. Ecol. Sociobiol., 9:121–133.

DEWSBURY, D. A., AND T. G. HARTUNG. 1982. Copulatory behavior of three species of *Microtus*. J. Mamm., 63:306–309.

DEWSBURY, D. A., R. L. EVANS, AND D. G. WEBSTER. 1979. Pregnancy initiation in postpartum estrus in three species of muroid rodents. Horm. Behav., 13:1–8.

DIETERICH, R. A., AND D. J. PRESTON. 1977*a*. The tundra vole (*Microtus oeconomus*) as a laboratory animal. Lab. Anim. Sci., 27:500–506.

———. 1977*b*. The meadow vole (*Microtus pennsylvanicus*) as a laboratory animal. Lab. Anim. Sci., 27:494–499.

DOUGLASS, R. J. 1977. Population dynamics, home ranges, and habitat associations of the yellow-cheeked vole, *Microtus xanthognathus,* in the Northwest Territories. Canadian Field-Nat., 91:237–247.

ELLERMAN, J. R., AND T. C. S. MORRISON-SCOTT. 1951. Checklist of Palaearctic and Indian mammals, 1758 to 1946. British Mus. Nat. Hist., London, 810 pp.

EVANS, R. L., AND D. A. DEWSBURY. 1978. Copulatory behavior of prairie voles (*Microtus ochrogaster*) in a two-male situation. Behav. Biol., 24:498–508.

FACEMIRE, C. F. AND G. O. BATZLI. 1983. Suppression of growth and reproduction by social factors in microtine rodents: tests of two hypotheses. J. Mamm., 64:152–156.

FARRIS, A. L.. 1971. Population dynamics and habitat distribution of *Microtus longicaudus, Microtus montanus,* and *Peromyscus maniculatus* in southeastern Washington. Unpubl. Ph.D. dissert., Washington State Univ., Pullman, 94 pp.

FAY, F. H. 1960. Technique for trapping small tundra mammals in winter. J. Mamm., 41:141–142.

FISHER, H. J. 1945. Notes on voles in central Missouri. J. Mamm., 26:435–437.

FITCH, H. S. 1957. Aspects of reproduction and development in the prairie vole (*Microtus ochrogaster*). Univ. Kansas Publ., Mus. Nat. Hist., 10:129–161.

FULLER, W. A. 1967. Ecologie hivernale des lemmings et fluctuations de leurs populations. Terre et Vie, 2:97–115.

GAINES, M. S., AND R. K. ROSE. 1976. Population dynamics of *Microtus ochrogaster* in eastern Kansas. Ecology, 57:1145–1161.

GASHWILER, J. S. 1972. Life history notes on the Oregon vole *Microtus oregoni.* J. Mamm., 53:558–569.

GAVISH, L., C. S. CARTER, AND L. L. GETZ. 1981. Further evidences for monogamy in the prairie vole. Anim. Behav., 29:955–957.

GETZ, L. L. 1978. Speculation on social structure and population cycles of microtine rodents. The Biologist, 60:134–147.

GETZ, L. L., C. S. CARTER, AND L. GAVISH. 1981. The mating system of the prairie vole, *Microtus ochrogaster*: field and laboratory evidence for pair-bonding. Behav. Ecol. Sociobiol., 8:189–194.

GETZ, L. L., L. VERNER, F. R. COLE, J. E. HOFMANN, AND D. E. AVALOS. 1979. Comparisons of population demography of *Microtus ochrogaster* and *Microtus pennsylvanicus.* Acta Theriol., 24:319–349.

GOERTZ, J. W. 1971. An ecological study of *Microtus pinetorum* in Oklahoma. Amer. Midland Nat., 86:1–12.

GOIN, O. B. 1943. A study of individual variation in *Microtus pennsylvanicus pennsylvanicus.* J. Mamm., 24:212–223.

GOLDBERG, M., N. R. TABROFF, AND R. H. TAMARIN. 1980. Nutrient variation in beach grass in relation to beach vole feeding. Ecology, 61:1029–1033.

GRAY, G. D., H. N. DAVIS, M. ZERYLNICK, AND D. A. DEWSBURY. 1974. Oestrus and induced ovulation in montane voles. J. Reprod. Fert., 38:193–196.

GREENWALD, G. S. 1956. The reproductive cycle of the field mouse, *Microtus californicus.* J. Mamm., 37:213–222.

———. 1957. Reproduction in a coastal California population of the field mouse *Microtus californicus*. Univ. California Publ. Zool., 54:421–446.

Groves, C. R., and B. L. Keller. 1983. Ecological characteristics of small mammals on a radioactive waste disposal area in southeastern Idaho. Amer. Midland Nat., 109:253–265.

Hall, E. R. 1981. The mammals of North America. John Wiley and Sons, New York, 2:601–1181 + *90*.

Hall, E. R., and K. R. Kelson. 1959. The mammals of North America. Ronald Press Co., New York, 2:547–1083 + *79*.

Hamilton, W. J., Jr. 1937. The biology of microtine cycles. J. Agric. Res., 54: 779–790.

———. 1938. Life history notes on the northern pine mouse. J. Mamm., 19:163–170.

———. 1941. Reproduction of the field mouse *Microtus pennsylvanicus* (Ord.). Cornell Univ. Agric. Exp. Sta. Mem. 237:1–23.

Harris, V. T. 1953. Ecological relationships of meadow voles and rice rats in tidal marshes. J. Mamm., 34:479–487.

Hasler, J. F. 1975. A review of reproduction and sexual maturation in the microtine rodents. The Biologist, 57:52–86.

Hasler, M. J., and A. V. Nalbandov. 1974. The effect of weanling and adult males on sexual maturation in female voles (*Microtus ochrogaster*). Gen. Comp. Endocrinol., 23:237–238.

Hoffmann, R. S. 1958. The role of reproduction and mortality in population fluctuations of voles (*Microtus*). Ecol. Monogr., 28:79–109.

———. 1974. Terrestrial vertebrates. Pp. 475–568, *in* Arctic and alpine environments (J. D. Ives and R. G. Berry, eds.). Methuen, London, 999 pp.

Hoffmeister, D. F. 1956. Mammals of the Graham (Pinaleno) Mountains, Arizona. Amer. Midland Nat., 55:257–288.

Horsfall, F., Jr. 1963. Observations on fluctuating pregnancy rate of pine mice and mouse feed potential in Virginia orchards. Amer. Soc. Hort. Sci., 83: 276–279.

Horton, L. W., and B. A. Shepherd. 1979. Effects of olfactory bulb ablation on estrus-induction and frequency of pregnancy. Physiol. Behav., 22:847–850.

Howell, A. B. 1924. Individual and age variation in Microtus montanus Yosemite. J. Agric. Res., 28:977–1015.

Hoyte, H. M. D. 1955. Observations on reproduction in some small mammals of arctic Norway. J. Anim. Ecol., 24:412–425.

Innes, D. G. L. 1978*a*. The reproductive tactics of two sympatric microtines. Unpubl. M.S. thesis, Univ. Western Ontario, London, 84 pp.

———. 1978*b*. A reexamination of litter size in some North American microtines. Canadian J. Zool., 56:1488–1496.

Iverson, S. L., and B. N. Turner. 1969. Under-snow shelter for small mammal trapping. J. Wildl. Mgmt., 33:722–723.

———. 1974. Winter weight dynamics in *Microtus pennsylvanicus*. Ecology, 55: 1030–1041.

———. 1976. Small mammal radioecology: natural reproductive patterns of seven species. Atomic Energy of Canada Limited Report. Whiteshell Nuclear Research Establishment, Pinawa, Manitoba, AECL-5393, 53 pp.

Jameson, E. W., Jr. 1947. Natural history of the prairie vole (Mammalian Genus *Microtus*). Univ. Kansas Publ., Mus. Nat. Hist., 1:125–151.

Jannett, F. J., Jr. 1977. On the sociobiology of the montane vole, *Microtus montanus nanus* (Rodentia: Muridae). Unpubl. Ph.D. dissert., Cornell Univ., Ithaca, New York, 167 pp.

———. 1978. The density-dependent formation of extended maternal families of the montane vole, *Microtus montanus nanus*. Behav. Ecol. Sociobiol., 3:245-263.

———. 1979. Notes on reproduction in captive *Arvicola richardsoni*. J. Mamm., 60:837-838.

———. 1980. Social dynamics of the montane vole, *Microtus montanus,* as a paradigm. The Biologist, 62:3-19.

———. 1981*a*. Scent mediation of intraspecific, interspecific, and intergeneric agonistic behavior among sympatric species of voles (Microtinae). Behav. Ecol. Sociobiol., 8:293-296.

———. 1981*b*. Sex ratios in high-density populations of the montane vole, *Microtus montanus,* and the behavior of territorial males. Behav. Ecol., Sociobiol., 8:297-307.

JOHNSON, M. L. 1968. Application of blood protein electrophoretic studies to problems in mammalian taxonomy. Syst. Zool., 17:23-30.

KELLER, B. L., AND C. J. KREBS. 1970. *Microtus* population biology III. Reproductive changes in fluctuating populations of *M. ochrogaster* and *M. pennsylvanicus* in southern Indiana, 1965-67. Ecol. Monogr., 40:263-294.

KELLER, B. L., C. R. GROVES, E. J. PITCHER, AND M. J. SMOLEN. 1982. A method to trap rodents in snow, sleet, or rain. Canadian J. Zool., 60:1104-1106.

KENNEY, A. MCM., R. L. EVANS, AND D. A. DEWSBURY. 1977. Postimplantation pregnancy disruption in *Microtus ochrogaster, Microtus pennsylvanicus* and *Peromyscus maniculatus*. J. Reprod. Fert., 49:365-367.

KENNEY, A. MCM., T. G. HARTUNG, AND D. A. DEWSBURY. 1979. Copulatory behavior and the initiation of pregnancy in California voles (*Microtus californicus*). Brain Behav. Evol., 16:176-191.

KIRKLAND, G. L., JR. 1977. The rock vole, *Microtus chrotorrhinus,* (Miller) (Mammalia:Rodentia) in West Virginia. Ann. Carnegie Mus., 46:45-53.

KIRKLAND, G. L., JR., AND F. J. JANNETT. 1982. Microtus chrotorrhinus. Mamm. Species, 180:1-5.

KIRKPATRICK, R. L., AND G. L. VALENTINE. 1970. Reproduction in captive pine voles, *Microtus pinetorum*. J. Mamm., 51:779-785.

KLIMKIEWICZ, M. K. 1970. The taxonomic status of the nominal species *Microtus pennsylvanicus* and *Microtus agrestis* (Rodentia: Cricetidae). Mammalia, 34:640-665.

KOTT, E., AND W. L. ROBINSON. 1963. Seasonal variation in litter size in the meadow vole in southern Ontario. J. Mamm., 44:467-470.

KREBS, C. J. 1964. The lemming cycle at Baker Lake, Northwest Territories, during 1959-62. Arctic Inst. N. Amer. Tech. Paper, 15:1-104.

———. 1966. Demographic changes in fluctuating populations of *Microtus californicus*. Ecol. Monogr., 36:239-273.

———. 1979. Dispersal, spacing behaviour, and genetics in relation to population fluctuations in the vole *Microtus townsendii*. Fortschr. Zool., 25:61-77.

KREBS, C. J., AND K. T. DELONG. 1965. A *Microtus* population with supplemental food. J. Mamm., 46:566-573.

KREBS, C. J., AND J. H. MYERS. 1974. Population cycles in small mammals. Adv. Ecol. Res., 8:267-399.

KREBS, C. J., B. L. KELLER, AND R. H. TAMARIN. 1969. *Microtus* population biology: demographic changes in fluctuating populations of *M. ochrogaster* and *M. pennsylvanicus* in southern Indiana. Ecology, 50:587-607.

KREBS, C. J., ET AL. 1976. *Microtus* population biology: dispersal in fluctuating populations of *M. townsendii*. Canadian J. Zool., 54:79-95.

KROHNE, D. T. 1980. Intraspecific litter size variation in *Microtus californicus* II. Variation between populations. Evolution, 34:1174–1182.

———. 1981. Intraspecific litter size variation in *Microtus californicus*: variation within populations. J. Mamm., 62:29–40.

———. 1982. The demography of low-litter size populations of *Microtus californicus*. Canadian J. Zool., 60:368–374.

LABOV, J. B. 1981. Pregnancy blocking in rodents: adaptive advantages for females. Amer. Nat., 118:361–371.

LARSSON, T. B., AND L. HANSSON. 1977. Sampling and dynamics of small rodents under snow cover in northern Sweden. Z. Saugetierk., 42:290–294.

LEDUC, J., AND C. J. KREBS. 1975. Demographic consequences of artificial selection at the LAP locus in voles (*Microtus townsendii*). Canadian J. Zool., 53:1825–1840.

LEE, D. C., J. HORVATH, R. W. METCALFE, AND E. K. INSKEEP. 1970. Ovulation in *Microtus pennsylvanicus* in a laboratory environment. Lab. Anim. Care, 20:1098–1102.

LEE, S. VANDER, AND L. M. BOOT. 1955. Spontaneous pseudo-pregnancy in mice. Acta Physiol. Pharmacol. Neerl., 4:442–443.

LESLIE, P. H., AND R. M. RANSON. 1940. The mortality, fertility and rate of natural increase of the vole (*Microtus agrestis*) as observed in the laboratory. J. Anim. Ecol., 9:27–52.

LESLIE, P. H., J. S. PERRY, AND J. S. WATSON. 1945. The determination of the median body-weight at which female rats reach maturity. Proc. Zool. Soc. London, 115:473–488.

LESLIE, P. H., U. M. VENABLES, AND L. S. V. VENABLES. 1952. The fertility and population structure of the brown rat (*Rattus norvegicus*) in corn-ricks and some other habitats. Proc. Zool. Soc. London, 122:187–238.

LIDICKER, W. Z., JR. 1973. Regulation of numbers in an island population of the California vole, a problem in community dynamics. Ecol. Monogr., 43: 271–302.

———. 1976. Experimental manipulation of the timing of reproduction in the California vole. Res. Population Ecol., 18:14–27.

———. 1980. The social biology of the California vole. The Biologist, 62:46–55.

LIDICKER, W. Z., JR., AND P. K. ANDERSON. 1962. Colonization of an island by *Microtus californicus*, analyzed on the basis of runway transects. J. Anim. Ecol., 31:503–517.

LINDUSKA, J. P. 1942. Winter rodent populations in field-shocked corn. J. Wildl. Mgmt., 6:353–363.

———. 1950. Ecology and land-use relationships of small mammals on a Michigan farm. Game Div., Dept. Conserv., Lansing, Michigan, 144 pp.

LORD, R. D., JR. 1960. Litter size and latitude in North American mammals. Amer. Midland Nat., 63:488–499.

LYONS, T. J. 1979. Hip gland occurrence and function in *Microtus montanus*. Unpubl. M.S. thesis, Idaho State Univ., Pocatello, 50 pp.

MACFARLANE, J. D., AND J. M. TAYLOR. 1981. Sexual maturation in female Townsend's voles. Acta Theriol., 26:113–117.

———. 1982*a*. Nature of estrus and ovulation in *Microtus townsendii* (Bachman). J. Mamm., 63:104–109.

———. 1982*b*. Pregnancy and reproductive performance in the Townsend's vole, *Microtus townsendii* (Bachman). J. Mamm., 63:165–168.

MADISON, D. M. 1980. An integrated view of the social biology of *Microtus pennsylvanicus*. The Biologist, 62:20–33.

MALLORY, F. F., AND F. V. CLULOW. 1977. Evidence of pregnancy failure in the wild meadow vole, *Microtus pennsylvanicus*. Canadian J. Zool., 55:1-17.

MARTIN, E. P. 1956. A population study of the prairie vole (*Microtus ochrogaster*) in northeastern Kansas. Univ. Kansas Publ., Mus. Nat. Hist., 8:361-416.

MARTIN, K. H., R. A. STEHN, AND M. E. RICHMOND. 1976. Reliability of placental scar counts in the prairie vole. J. Wildl. Mgmt., 40:264-271.

MARTIN, R. L. 1971. The natural history and taxonomy of the rock vole, *Microtus chrotorrhinus*. Unpubl. Ph.D. dissert., Univ. Connecticut, Storrs, 123 pp.

MASER, C., AND R. M. STORM. 1970. A key to Microtinae of the Pacific Northwest (Oregon, Washington, Idaho). Oregon State Univ. Bookstores, Corvallis, 162 pp.

MATTHEY, R. 1952. Chromosomes de muridae (Microtinae et Cricetinae). Chromosoma, 5:113-138.

MCGUIRE, M. R., AND L. L. GETZ. 1981. Incest taboo between sibling *Microtus ochrogaster*. J. Mamm., 62:213-214.

MERRITT, J. F., AND J. M. MERRITT. 1978. Population ecology and energy relationships of *Clethrionomys gapperi* in a Colorado subalpine forest. J. Mamm., 59:576-598.

MESERVE, P. L. 1971. Population ecology of the prairie vole, *Microtus ochrogaster*, in the western mixed prairie of Nebraska. Amer. Midland Nat., 86:417-433.

MILLER, D. H., AND L. L. GETZ. 1969. Life-history notes on *Microtus pinetorum* in central Connecticut. J. Mamm., 50:777-784.

MILLIGAN, S. R. 1975. Mating, ovulation and corpus luteum function in the vole, *Microtus agrestis*. J. Reprod. Fert., 42:35-44.

———. 1976. Pregnancy blocking in the vole, *Microtus agrestis*. I. Effect of the social environment. J. Reprod. Fert., 46:91-95.

MORRISON, P., R. DIETERICH, AND D. PRESTON. 1976. Breeding and reproduction of fifteen wild rodents maintained as laboratory colonies. Lab. Anim. Sci., 26:237-243.

MURIE, A. 1961. A naturalist in Alaska. Devin-Adair, New York, 302 pp.

MURRAY, K. F. 1965. Population changes during the 1957-1958 vole (*Microtus*) outbreak in California. Ecology, 46:163-171.

MYERS, J. H., AND C. J. KREBS. 1971. Sex ratios in open and enclosed vole populations: demographic implications. Amer. Nat., 105:325-344.

NEGUS, N. C., AND P. J. BERGER. 1977. Experimental triggering of reproduction in a natural population of *Microtus montanus*. Science, 196:1230-1231.

NEGUS, N. C., AND J. S. FINDLEY. 1959. Mammals of Jackson Hole, Wyoming. J. Mamm., 40:371-381.

NEGUS, N. C., AND A. J. PINTER. 1965. Litter sizes of *Microtus montanus* in the laboratory. J. Mamm., 46:434-437.

———. 1966. Reproductive responses of *Microtus montanus* to plants and plant extracts in the diet. J. Mamm., 46:596-601.

NEGUS, N. C., P. J. BERGER, AND L. G. FORSLUND. 1977. Reproductive strategy of *Microtus montanus*. J. Mamm., 58:347-353.

PATTIE, D. L. 1967. Dynamics of alpine small mammal populations. Unpubl. Ph.D. dissert., Univ. Montana, Missoula, 103 pp.

PAUL, J. R. 1966. Observations on the ecology, populations and reproductive biology of the pine vole, *Pitymys p. pinetorum* in North Carolina. Unpubl. Ph.D. dissert., North Carolina State Univ., Raleigh, 98 pp.

PEARSON, O. P. 1963. History of two local outbreaks of feral house mice. Ecology, 44:540-549.

PELIKÁN, J. 1979. Sufficient sample size for evaluating the litter size in rodents. Folia Zool., 28:289–297.

PINTER, A. J., AND N. C. NEGUS. 1965. Effects of nutrition and photoperiod on reproductive physiology of *Microtus montanus*. Amer. J. Physiol., 208:633–638.

PRUITT, W. O., JR. 1959. A method of live-trapping small taiga mammals in winter. J. Mamm., 40:139–143.

QUAY, W. B. 1951. Observations on mammals of the Seward Peninsula, Alaska. J. Mamm., 32:88–99.

———. 1962. Apocrine sweat glands in the angulus oris of microtine rodents. J. Mamm., 43:303–310.

———. 1965. Comparative survey of the sebaceous and sudoriferous glands of the oral lips and angle in rodents. J. Mamm., 46:23–37.

———. 1968. The specialized posterolateral sebaceous glandular regions in microtine rodents. J. Mamm., 49:427–445.

QUICK, F. W., II. 1970. Small mammal populations in an old field community. Unpubl. Ph.D. dissert., Univ. Louisville, Louisville, Kentucky, 152 pp.

RAYNAUD, A. 1951. Reproduction, en hiver, des campagnols agrestis (*Microtus agrestis* L.) dans le département du Tarn. Bull. Soc. Zool., France, 76: 188–200.

REDFIELD, J. A., M. J. TAITT, AND C. J. KREBS. 1978*a*. Experimental alterations of sex-ratios in populations of *Microtus oregoni*, the creeping vole. J. Anim. Ecol., 47:55–69.

———. 1978*b*. Experimental alteration of sex ratios in populations of *Microtus townsendii*, a field vole. Canadian J. Zool., 56:17–27.

RICHMOND, M. E. 1967. Reproduction of the vole, *Microtus ochrogaster*. Unpubl. Ph.D. dissert., Univ. Missouri, Columbia, 100 pp.

RICHMOND, M. [E.], AND C. H. CONAWAY. 1969. Induced ovulation and oestrus in *Microtus ochrogaster*. J. Reprod. Fert., Suppl., 6:357–376.

RICHMOND, M. E., AND R. STEHN. 1976. Olfaction and reproductive behavior in microtine rodents. Pp. 197–216, *in* Mammalian olfaction, reproductive processes and behavior (R. L. Doty, ed.). Academic Press, New York, 344 pp.

ROLAN, R. G., AND H. T. GIER. 1967. Correlation of embryo and placental scar counts of *Peromyscus maniculatus* and *Microtus ochrogaster*. J. Mamm., 48: 317–319.

ROSE, R. K., AND M. S. GAINES. 1978. The reproductive cycle of *Microtus ochrogaster* in eastern Kansas. Ecol. Monogr., 48:21–42.

SANDERS, E. H. 1976. Reproductive responses of *Microtus montanus* to phenolic compounds in the diet. Unpubl. Ph.D. dissert., Univ. Utah, Salt Lake City, 81 pp.

SANDERS, E. H., P. D. GARDNER, P. J. BERGER, AND N. C. NEGUS. 1981. 6-Methoxybenzoxazolinone: a plant derivative that stimulates reproduction in *Microtus montanus*. Science, 214:67–69.

SCHADLER, M. H. 1981. Postimplantation abortion in pine voles (*Microtus pinetorum*) induced by strange males and pheromones of strange males. Biol. Reprod., 25:295–297.

SCHADLER, M. H., AND G. M. BUTTERSTEIN. 1979. Reproduction in the pine vole, *Microtus pinetorum*. J. Mamm., 60:841–844.

SCHAFFER, W. M., AND R. H. TAMARIN. 1973. Changing reproductive rates and population cycles in lemmings and voles. Evolution, 27:111–124.

SCHWAGMEYER, P. L. 1979. The Bruce effect: an evaluation of male/female advantages. Amer. Nat., 114:932–938.

SEIDEL, D. R., AND E. S. BOOTH. 1960. Biology and breeding habits of the meadow mouse, *Microtus montanus,* in eastern Washington. Walla Walla College Publ., Dept. Biol. Sci., Biol. Sta., 29:1-14.

SMITH, D. A., AND J. B. FOSTER. 1957. Notes on the small mammals of Churchill, Manitoba. J. Mamm., 38:98-115.

SNYDER, D. B. 1969. Corpora bodies in the ovaries of meadow voles (*Microtus pennsylvanicus*) by serial sectioning versus gross examination. Amer. Midland Nat., 81:594-595.

SPENCER, A. W., AND H. W. STEINHOFF. 1968. An explanation of geographical variation in litter size. J. Mamm., 49:281-286.

STEARNS, S. C. 1976. Life-history tactics: a review of the ideas. Quart. Rev. Biol., 51:3-47.

STEHN, R. A. 1978. Characterization of the male-induced abortion response in the prairie vole, *Microtus ochrogaster.* Unpubl. Ph.D. dissert., Cornell Univ., Ithaca, New York, 125 pp.

STEHN, R. A., AND F. J. JANNETT, JR. 1981. Male-induced abortion in various microtine rodents. J. Mamm., 62:369-372.

STEHN, R. A., AND M. E. RICHMOND. 1975. Male-induced pregnancy termination in the prairie vole, *Microtus ochrogaster.* Science, 187:1211-1213.

STENSETH, N. C. 1977. Evolutionary aspects of demographic cycles: the relevance of some models of cycles for microtine fluctuations. Oikos, 29:525-538.

SULLIVAN, T. P. 1980. Comparative demography of *Peromyscus maniculatus* and *Microtus oregoni* populations after logging and burning of coastal forest habitats. Canadian J. Zool., 58:2252-2259.

SULLIVAN, T. P., AND C. J. KREBS. 1981. *Microtus* population biology: demography of *M. oregoni* in southwestern British Columbia. Canadian J. Zool., 59: 2092-2102.

TAITT, M. J., AND C. J. KREBS. 1981. The effect of extra food on small rodent populations: II. Voles (*Microtus townsendii*). J. Anim. Ecol., 50:125-137.

TAITT, M. J., J. H. W. GIPPS, C. J. KREBS, AND Z. DUNDJERSKI. 1981. The effect of extra food and cover on declining populations of *Microtus townsendii.* Canadian J. Zool., 59:1593-1599.

TAMARIN, R. H. 1977*a*. Reproduction in the island beach vole, *Microtus breweri,* and the mainland meadow vole, *Microtus pennsylvanicus* in southeastern Massachusetts. J. Mamm., 58:536-548.

———. 1977*b*. Demography of the beach vole (*Microtus breweri*) and the meadow vole (*Microtus pennsylvanicus*) in southeastern Massachusetts. Ecology, 58: 1310-1321.

TAMARIN, R. H., M. SHERIDAN, AND C. K. LEVY. 1983. Determining matrilineal kinship in natural populations of rodents using radionuclides. Canadian J. Zool., 61:271-274.

TAST, J., AND A. KAIKUSALO. 1976. Winter breeding of the root vole, *Microtus oeconomus,* in 1972/1973 at Kilpisjarvi, Finnish Lapland. Ann. Zool. Fennica, 13:174-178.

THIBAULT, C., ET AL. 1966. Regulation of breeding season and estrous cycles by light and external stimuli in some mammals. J. Anim. Sci., Suppl., 25: 119-142.

TIMM, R. M., L. R. HEANEY, AND D. D. BAIRD. 1977. Natural history of rock voles *Microtus chrotorrhinus* in Minnesota. Canadian Field-Nat., 91:177-181.

TOWNSEND, M. T. 1935. Studies on some of the small mammals of central New York. Roosevelt Wildl. Ann., 4:1-20.

TURNER, R. W. 1974. Mammals of the Black Hills of South Dakota and Wyoming. Misc. Publ., Mus. Nat. Hist., Univ. Kansas, 60:1–178.

TYSER, R. W. 1975. Taxonomy and reproduction of *Microtus canicaudus*. Unpubl. M.S. thesis, Oregon State Univ., Corvallis, 67 pp.

VALENTINE, G. L., AND R. L. KIRKPATRICK. 1970. Seasonal changes in reproductive and related organs in the pine vole, *Microtus pinetorum,* in southwestern Virginia. J. Mamm., 51:553–560.

VAN HORNE, B. 1982. Demography of the longtail vole *Microtus longicaudus* in seral stages of coastal coniferous forest, southeast Alaska. Canadian J. Zool., 60:1690–1709.

VAUGHAN, T. A. 1969. Reproduction and population densities in a montane small mammal fauna. Misc. Publ. Mus. Nat. Hist., Univ. Kansas, 51:51–74.

VENABLE, J. H. 1939. Intra-uterine bleeding in the pregnant albino rat. Anat. Rec., 74:273–295.

WESTLIN, L. M. 1982. Sterile matings at the beginning of the breeding season in *Clethrionomys rufocanus* and *Microtus agrestis.* Canadian J. Zool., 60:2568–2571.

WESTLIN, L. M., AND E. NYHOLM. 1982. Sterile matings initiate the breeding season in the bank vole, *Clethrionomys glareolus.* A field and laboratory study. Canadian J. Zool., 60:387–391.

WHITNEY, P. 1976. Population ecology of two sympatric species of subarctic microtine rodents. Ecol. Monogr., 46:85–104.

———. 1977. Seasonal maintenance and net production of two sympatric species of subarctic microtine rodents. Ecology, 58:314–325.

WHITTEN, W. K. 1956. Modification of the oestrous cycle of the mouse by external stimuli associated with the male. J. Endocrinol., 13:399–404.

WOLFF, J. O. 1980. Social organization of the taiga vole (*Microtus xanthognathus*). The Biologist, 62:34–45.

WOLFF, J. O., AND W. Z. LIDICKER, JR. 1980. Population ecology of the taiga vole, *Microtus xanthognathus,* in interior Alaska. Canadian J. Zool., 58: 1800–1812.

———. 1981. Communal winter nesting and food sharing in taiga voles. Behav. Ecol. Sociobiol., 9:237–240.

WRIGHT, V. L. 1971. Population dynamics of cricetids in southeastern Washington. Unpubl. Ph.D. dissert., Washington State Univ., Pullman, 110 pp.

YOUNGMAN, P. M. 1975. Mammals of the Yukon Territory. Natl. Mus. Nat. Sci. (Ottawa), Publ. Zool., 10:1–189.

NUTRITION

GEORGE O. BATZLI

Abstract

SEVERAL characteristics of the gastro-intestinal tracts of microtine rodents appear to be adaptations for use of high-fiber, low-protein, and low-mineral diets, which are consistent with the observation that most microtine species eat primarily the vegetative parts of plants. The exact compositions of diets are a function of the availability of food items and the nutritional adaptations of individual species; the same species in different habitats and different species in the same habitat eat different food items. Food-item preference seems to depend upon a combination of the positive (water and nutrient content) and negative (fiber content and plant secondary compounds) characteristics of the item, and different microtine species have different tolerances for specific secondary compounds. Performances of microtines on particular food items, as measured by food intake and body growth, parallel their food preferences.

Although little is known about nutrient requirements of microtine rodents, they seem to require lower concentrations of digestible energy and protein in their diets than do laboratory rodents. Mineral requirements are similar to those of laboratory rodents, but concentrations in natural diets may often be low. Increased intake can compensate for low-quality food (low digestibility or low-nutrient content) so that requirements for energy and nutrients are met. But this compensation is not always sufficient, and mounting evidence indicates that the quality of available forage can help to explain differences in the densities of microtine populations among habitats, among seasons, and among years.

Introduction

Because all the life processes of organisms depend upon the acquisition of energy and nutrients, the topic of nutrition can be expanded to include much of biology. However, the scope of this chapter is restricted to the more traditional topics of nutrition—food habits, food quality, nutritional physiology, and nutritional ecology. My approach is functional and comparative; my goals are to understand the mechanisms behind and the implications of the patterns that we see. The chapter treats microtine rodents as a group because our understanding of *Microtus* can be greatly enhanced by considering additional information from closely related genera.

Microtine rodents have evolved morphological characteristics that can be interpreted as adaptations to high-fiber, low-nutrient diets. In general, they possess high-crowned molars with enamel loops that provide prismatic grinding surfaces (Guthrie, 1965; Hinton, 1926). This allows reduction of vegetative material to fine particles without wearing teeth down to the gums. As a further adaptation, genera that take large amounts of fibrous and siliceous material (*Lemmus* and *Microtus*) have rootless molars that continue to grow through life.

The morphology of microtine stomachs is extremely variable and overlaps broadly with other muroid rodents. Vorontsov (1962, 1967) argued that the tendency to a chambered stomach and a reduced glandular zone is analogous to stomach development in ruminants, but Carleton (1973, 1981) pointed out the varied nature of microtine stomachs and diets and challenged this view.

The cecum and large intestine of microtines are among the largest and most elaborate of all muroid rodents (Vorontsov, 1962, 1967). Cecal size and the post-cecal spiral are particularly well developed in the most herbivorous species (Lange and Staaland, 1970). The enlarged cecum seems to function as a chamber for digestion of fiber and for production of protein and B-vitamins (McBee, 1970, 1971), and the post-cecal spiral may be a mechanism for mineral retention, particularly sodium (Staaland, 1975). Because the cecum occurs at the juncture of the small and large intestines, feces must be reingested if the microbial protein and vitamins are to be absorbed. At least one microtine (*Microtus pennsylvanicus*) is known to practice coprophagy in a manner similar to rats and rabbits (Ouellette and Heisinger, 1980). Thus, although the functional significance of morphological peculiarities of the gastro-intestinal tract of microtines cannot be specified with certainty, most evidence points to adaptation for handling high-fiber (and silica), low-protein, and low-mineral diets.

In the discussion that follows, it becomes clear that the diet and nutritional adaptations of microtines vary considerably among species, although most species are primarily herbivorous. Because the nutrition of microtines per se is poorly understood, many of the principles developed from studies of domesticated animals (Maynard et al., 1979) and wildlife (Robbins, 1983) must be applied to them. But this should be done with caution, for we must expect nutritional systems of ruminants (cattle, sheep, and deer) or omnivorous rodents (laboratory rats and mice) to be somewhat different from those of herbivorous rodents such as microtines. Lagomorphs (rabbits and hares) seem to be the group whose nutritional characteristics are most similar to those of microtine rodents; both groups are small, monogastric herbivores with enlarged cecae.

The Diets of Microtines

Food Habits

Although it is common knowledge among mammalogists that microtine rodents are herbivores, there have been relatively few reliable, quantitative studies of food habits. The most accurate estimates of diet composition for microtine rodents seem to be volumetric estimates based upon microscopic examination of stomach contents (Batzli and Pitelka, 1971; Hansson, 1970; Neal et al., 1973; Williams, 1962). Estimates based on frequency overestimate the importance of items taken regularly in small amounts. Differential digestibility of epidermal cells, which bear the distinctive characteristics that allow identification, causes errors in estimates based upon fecal samples. Items with relatively thin cell walls (dicotyledons) tend to be underestimated, and items with thick cell walls (monocotyledons and mosses) tend to be overestimated. Correction factors can be calculated for a particular population by comparing the abundance of items in stomachs with the abundance of the same items in fecal pellets from the colon of the same animals (Batzli and Pitelka, 1971, 1983), but this is seldom done. Another source of error may be the underestimation of seeds and arthropods in the diet because much of the material in these items lacks distinctive characteristics (Fish, 1974); only the seed coat and chitinous exoskeletons are easily detected. Finally, there is substantial variability in the relative abundance of items in individual stomachs,

TABLE 1
COMPARISON OF DIETS (PERCENT COMPOSITION) OF SOME NORTH AMERICAN MICROTINE RODENTS. DATA ARE BASED ON STOMACH OR CORRECTED FECAL CONTENTS WITH TEN OR MORE SAMPLES FOR EACH SEASON AND SITE

Species, location, season	Food items					Source
	Monocotyledon leaves, stems, roots	Dicotyledon leaves, stems, roots	Seeds or fruit	Arthropods	Other	
M. californicus						
California, annual grassland						Batzli and Pitelka (1971)
Summer	6	20	73	0	1	
Winter	88	10	1	0	1	
M. ochrogaster						
Indiana, old fields						Zimmerman (1965)
All year	27	40	4	5	24[a]	
Central Illinois						Cole and Batzli (1979)
Prairie						
Summer	20	38	35	7	0	
Winter	22	38	30	5	5	
Old bluegrass pasture						
Summer	11	48	23	8	10	
Winter	55	12	23	1	9	
Old alfalfa field						
Summer	11	65	12	3	9	
Winter	50	32	12	0	6	

TABLE 1
CONTINUED

Species, location, season	Food items: Monocotyledon leaves, stems, roots	Dicotyledon leaves, stems, roots	Seeds or fruit	Arthropods	Other	Source
M. oeconomus						
Alaska, arctic tundra						Batzli and Jung (1980)
Summer	56	36	3	+	5[c]	
Northern Finland, bogs and meadows						Tast (1974)
Summer	47	28	0	+	25[d]	
Winter	96	2	0	0	2[c]	
Microtus pennsylvanicus						
Indiana, old fields						Zimmerman (1965)
All year	73	14	0	4	9[a]	
Northern Illinois, prairie						Meserve (in litt.)
Summer	47	46	2	2	3[b]	
Autumn	6	70	18	+	6[b]	
Central Illinois Prairie						Lindroth and Batzli (1984*b*)
Spring	25	55	7	1	12[b]	
Summer	28	65	1	5	2[b]	
Autumn	17	40	16	4	23[b]	
Winter	19	44	36	2	0	

TABLE 1
CONTINUED

Species, location, season	Food items: Monocotyledon leaves, stems, roots	Dicotyledon leaves, stems, roots	Seeds or fruit	Arthropods	Other	Source
Old bluegrass pasture						
Spring	50	41	1	3	6[b]	
Summer	27	60	9	0	4[b]	
Autumn	20	66	2	2	10[b]	
Winter	63	21	13	2	1[b]	
M. xanthognathus						
Alaska, taiga						Wolff and Lidicker (1980)
Summer	38	7	12	0	43[d]	
Winter	13	12	1	0	74[d]	
Clethrionomys rutilis						
Alaska, taiga						West (1982)
Spring	0	8	73	+	19[b]	
Summer	0	4	62	4	30[c]	
Autumn	0	+	92	6	2[b]	
Dicrostonyx torquatus						
Alaska, arctic tundra						Batzli and Jung (1980)
Varied habitats						
Summer	11	83	1	+	5[c]	
Winter	10	70	+	0	20[c]	

TABLE 1
CONTINUED

Species, location, season	Food items: Monocotyledon leaves, stems, roots	Dicotyledon leaves, stems, roots	Seeds or fruit	Arthropods	Other	Source
Ridges						Batzli and Pitelka (1983)
Summer	12	83	+	+	5[c]	
Lemmus sibiricus						
Alaska, arctic tundra						Batzli and Jung (1980)
Varied habitats						
Summer	82	3	5	+	10[c]	
Low polygons						Batzli (1975)
Summer	60	13	1	0	26[c]	
Winter	55	5	+	0	40[c]	
High polygons						Batzli and Pitelka (1983)
Summer	69	5	+	0	26[c]	
Winter	54	4	0	0	42[c]	
Ridges						
Summer	63	4	+	0	33[c]	

+ Trace amounts (<1%).
[a] Unidentified vegetation.
[b] Lichens and fungi.
[c] Mosses.
[d] Horsetails (*Equisetum* spp.).

so population estimates for a particular time and place should be based upon at least 10, and preferably 20, samples (Batzli and Pitelka, 1983).

To reduce potential error the dietary information reviewed here is restricted to studies based upon adequate numbers of stomachs (or corrected fecal samples) for which volumetric estimates were made of all types of food items. In general, these data support the notion that microtine rodents are primarily herbivorous; all species take <10% animal material (Table 1). However, if we distinguish true herbivores (those that consume vegetative parts of plants) from granivores (seed eaters) and frugivores (fruit eaters), then clear differences between species and populations can be seen. *Microtus ochrogaster* takes variable amounts of seeds (up to 35% of its diet) depending upon location, and *M. californicus* switches to a predominantly seed diet (73%) during summer (Table 1). *Clethrionomys rutilis* in Alaskan taiga takes mostly fruit throughout the year, supplemented by substantial amounts of fungi or moss at different seasons.

Although the two lemmings (*Lemmus* and *Dicrostonyx*) and all *Microtus* species consume mostly vegetative plant parts, the types of plants taken vary within and between species. Thus *M. pennsylvanicus* takes mostly monocotyledons or mostly dicotyledons depending on location and season; fungi and seeds make up about 20 to 40% of their diet in prairie habitats during autumn and winter. In non-prairie habitats both *M. pennsylvanicus* and *M. ochrogaster* shift from favoring dicotyledons in summer to monocotyledons in winter. Both *M. xanthognathus* and *M. oeconomus* (when not in tundra) eat substantial amounts of horsetails (*Equisetum* spp.), and both favor rhizomes in winter. In arctic tundra, *Lemmus* strongly and consistently favors monocotyledons, *Dicrostonyx* strongly and consistently favors dicotyledons (particularly willow), and *M. oeconomus* takes large amounts of both, although it takes more monocotyledons. All three microtines also eat mosses; both *Lemmus* and *Dicrostonyx* increase their consumption of mosses in winter, but *Lemmus* eats more moss year-round.

Given that all these species are plant eaters, why this bewildering variety of dietary patterns? Three main factors are probably involved: 1) the relative abundance of some items in the diet of microtines simply reflects the availability of those items in the local habitat; 2) the nutritional adaptations of microtine species differ owing to their different evolutionary histories; 3) microtines show strong preferences for different items depending on the quality of that item in relation to the nutritional adaptations of the species. The last point is particularly important; the quality of plant material as food is not only a function of the plant's physical and chemical characteristics but also a function of the herbivore's requirements, abilities, and tolerances. The most certain assay of the quality of a food item is the performance of the herbivore in question when fed that food item, and even then some results may be artifacts of experimental conditions that affect feeding behavior.

Food Selection

Clear differences in food habits occur between pairs of species living in the same habitat, such as *Lemmus* and *Dicrostonyx* in arctic tundra, *Clethrionomys* and *Microtus* in taiga, and *M. ochrogaster* and *M. pennsylvanicus* in central Illinois prairie and old bluegrass pasture (Table 1). These differences between species confronted with the same array of vegetation indicate that the species have specialized preferences, even though all still take a wide variety of food items and all show strong shifts in their diet with location and season. Narrow specialization on very few species of plants has been reported only for two microtine populations: *M. breweri* on Muskeget Island, Massachusetts, eat almost only beach grass (*Ammophila breviligulata*) and bayberry (*Myrica pennsylvanica*) (Rothstein and Tamarin, 1977), and *M. montanus* at Tempe Springs, Utah eat primarily (>90% of diet) *Distichlis stricta* (Berger et al., 1977). Both species live in habitats with very low vegetational diversity, and both show seasonal shifts in the parts of plant taken.

If an animal shows a consistent response to a particular food item, then diet composition will be related to availability of that item. Although there are several ways to make this comparison (Lechowicz, 1983) a simple preference index (PI = proportion of diet/proportion of forage) allows one to assess a variety of patterns (Batzli, 1983). If the herbivore responds to availability of the food item, there will be a positive correlation between percent of diet and percent of forage accounted for by that item; PI > 1 if consistently preferred, PI < 1 if consistently avoided, or PI = 1 if taken in the same amount as available. Alternatively, an item may be taken erratically or in relatively constant amounts no matter what its availability (no consistent preference or PI decreases with increased availability, respectively). This type of analysis requires multiple samples from a variety of sites with different availability of food items, and given the paucity of quantitative analyses of diets, it is not surprising that there have been few such studies. Analyses that have been done show three general types of responses of herbivorous microtines to food items: consistent preference, consistent avoidance, or relatively constant intake (Batzli and Jung, 1980; Batzli and Pitelka, 1983).

Preferences shown by analyses of diets in the field generally, but not always, agree with palatability measured by intake in the laboratory. Thus Batzli and Jung (1980) reported that *Lemmus* and *Microtus* strongly preferred cotton grasses (*Eriophorum* spp., PI ~ 5) in their diet near Atkasook, Alaska, and these were among the most palatable foods in the laboratory. *Dicrostonyx* and *Microtus* strongly preferred willows (*Salix* spp., PI ~ 5) and forbs (PI ~ 10) and found them palatable in the laboratory; *Lemmus* avoided willows (PI ~ $\frac{1}{5}$) and forbs (PI ~ $\frac{1}{2}$) in the field, and both had low palatability ratings for *Lemmus*. Certain evergreen shrubs (*Ledum, Cassiope,* and *Empetrum*) were avoided by all microtines in the field (PI < $\frac{1}{10}$) and were generally unpalatable in the lab. On the other hand, no microtines showed any consistent preference for the most common plants, sedges in the genus *Carex*. Whatever the availability of *Carex, Lemmus* consistently took large amounts (30 to 60% of diet), *Microtus* took substantial amounts (about 20% of diet), and *Dicrostonyx* took small amounts (<10% of diet). Although palatability was highest for *Lemmus,* it was also high for the other microtines. Apparently, *Carex* was a staple food item for *Lemmus* no matter what its availability (it was relatively common in all habitats), and other palatable foods (*Eriophorum,* some grasses, and some mosses) filled in the diet in relation to their availability. *Dicrostonyx* had a strong preference for other foods that were usually available (*Eriophorum, Salix,* and forbs), and *Carex* simply acted as a filler. The pattern for *Microtus* fell between the other two species. Clearly, these microtine species responded very differently to the same food items, presumably because these items affected them differently; that is, the quality of each food item varied with the species consuming it.

What aspects of forage do rodents respond to when selecting their diet? Probably they respond to the same factors that humans do:

aroma, texture, and flavor. But these are merely cues that indicate to the vole that the food is good or of poor quality. The value of cues lies in their correlation with underlying determinants of quality, such as digestibility, nutrient content, and plant secondary compounds.

Three studies looked at forage palatability to voles in relation to nutrient concentrations. Hansson (1971) compared the rank order of palatability for seven species of monocotyledons at three seasons to results from a proximate chemical analysis (organic matter, crude protein, ether extract [total lipid], crude fiber, N-free extract, ash, and kcal/g). He found positive correlations between ranks for palatability and those for protein and ether extract and a negative correlation between palatability and fiber, but none was significant. Nevertheless, it was probably no coincidence that the most utilized species under natural conditions, *Agrostis tennuis,* had high-protein and low-fiber content. Meade (1975) compared intake of 27 plant species by *M. pennsylvanicus* under laboratory conditions with their water, nitrogen, phosphorus, and potassium contents. Using only species that were acceptable forage, he found significant positive correlations between intake and all of the nutrients, but the strongest relationship by far was for water ($R^2 = 0.75$). Multiple regression techniques revealed that only the relationships with water and nitrogen content remained significant when effects of other nutrients were removed. Finally, Goldberg et al. (1980) reported on variation in nutrients (proximate chemical analysis and calcium, magnesium, and phosphorus) in relation to seasonal shifts in preference for parts of beach grass (*A. breviligulata*). In spring and summer voles chose leaf blades, which had the highest concentrations of all nutrients and the lowest fiber concentrations; in late summer and early autumn voles chose roots, which had the lowest fiber at that time; in winter voles chose stems, which then had the lowest fiber content and the highest phosphorus content. Water content was generally similar in all plant parts in all seasons except winter when water in leaf blades was half that (34%) of the other parts.

Thus, it seems that voles use fiber content (poorly digestible and tough), water, and nutrient content (particularly protein and phosphorus) when selecting among palatable plant parts or species, but some other factor(s) is involved in determining palatability as well. As suggested by numerous authors, one such factor is likely to be plant secondary compounds (see Harborne, 1982 for review). In the last 10 years a variety of secondary plant compounds has been implicated as factors affecting food intake by microtine rodents (Table 2). Apparently intake is depressed as a result of strong odor (terpenes; Batzli and Jung, 1980), bitter taste (alkaloids; Kendall and Sherwood, 1975), or astringency (quebracho; Lindroth and Batzli, 1984*b*). Effects of these compounds on performance are considered below.

In general then, both availability and quality of individual food items affect the diet composition of herbivores. For example, Lindroth and Batzli (1984*b*) show that important food items of *M. pennsylvanicus* may be either poor in quality but highly available (taken in large amounts even though they are selected against) or high in quality but poorly available (taken in large amounts because they are strongly selected).

Intake, Forage Quality, and Individual Performance

General Considerations

Forage quality can affect three basic aspects of microtine performance: growth, reproduction, and survival. These effects may occur because of low concentrations of digestible nutrients in the forage, because of physical or chemical characteristics of the forage that reduce intake or digestibility, because of toxins in the forage, or because of a combination of these factors.

Whatever its diet, an organism must consume enough to meet its long-term metabolic requirements, including both energy and nutrients. Energetic considerations have usually been emphasized by biologists, perhaps because energy is relatively easy to measure and bears a clear relationship to performance for all organisms. Nutrient requirements vary widely among species and general patterns are more difficult to discern. Nevertheless, nutrient requirements for any herbivore are closely linked to energy requirements and digestibility of the forage. This is because nutrient turnover is directly related to metabolic rate and the amount of material passing through the gut (Barkley et al., 1980). In the discussion that follows I sometimes adjusted body mass in relation to metabolic rates to facilitate comparisons among animals of different sizes; however, I

TABLE 2
SECONDARY PLANT COMPOUNDS LIKELY TO BE DELETERIOUS TO MICROTINE RODENTS

Species of microtine	Compound and plant species	Effect	References
Microtus pennsylvanicus	β-nitroproprionic acid in crown vetch (*Coronilla varia*)	Depressed intake, growth, and survival	Barnes et al. (1974); Gustine et al. (1974); Kendall et al. (1979); Shenk (1976); Shenk et al. (1970, 1974)
	Saponins in alfalfa (*Medicago sativa*)	Depressed intake and growth	Kendall and Leath (1976); Marcarian (1972)
	Alkaloids in reed canary grass (*Phalaris arundinacea*)	Depressed intake, increased reticulocytes, and kidney lesions	Goelz et al. (1980); Kendall and Sherwood (1975); Kendall et al. (1979)
M. montanus	Cinnamic acids and related vinyl phenols in wheat and salt grass (*Distichlis stricta*)	Depressed reproduction	Berger et al. (1977)
M. ochrogaster	Flavonoid (quercetin) and tannins (tannic acid and quebracho) in artificial diet	Depressed growth by quercetin and tannic acid, depressed intake by quebracho	Lindroth and Batzli (1984*a*)
M. oeconomus	Ethanol extracts of Laborador tea (*Ledum palustre*)	Terpenes depress intake and unidentified compounds depress growth and survival	Batzli and Jung (1980); Jung and Batzli (1981)
Lemmus sibiricus	Ethanol extracts of willow (*Salix pulchra*) and Labrador tea	Terpenes depress intake and unidentified compounds depress growth and survival	Batzli and Jung (1980); Jung and Batzli (1981)

TABLE 2
CONTINUED

Species of microtine	Compound and plant species	Effect	References
Dicrostonyx torquatus	Ethanol extracts of sedge (*Carex aquatilus*) and Labrador tea	Terpenes depress intake and unidentified compounds depress growth	Batzli and Jung (1980); Jung and Batzli (1981)

do not review the bioenergetics of microtine rodents because that is done elsewhere in this book (Wunder, this volume).

Digestibility and Intake

Intake of food and output of feces and urine can be measured by placing animals in metabolic cages. Intake and apparent digestibility of forage can then be compared to weight change of the animal. Animals do not always respond well to confined conditions, and there are often great individual differences in their performance. Nevertheless, some reassuring patterns emerge. First, as expected, change in body mass is directly related to intake of digestible dry matter (or energy) on a given diet (Fig. 1; Shenk, 1976). The better performance of *M. ochrogaster* in Fig. 1 occurred because the artificial diet was of higher quality for them (greater growth on the same intake as the other species). The generally low intake by *Lemmus* compared to *Microtus* indicates lower palatability of the diet to them. Second, intake of palatable food decreases as digestibility of the food increases (Fig. 2). This trend results from compensation for low digestible energy and nutrient content by increased intake so that nutritional requirements are met, a phenomenon that will be discussed in more detail below. Third, the digestibility of food items is related to the general type of food over a wide variety of plant and microtine species. A review by Batzli and Cole (1979) showed that, on average, microtines digested 89% of the energy in seeds and garden vegetables, 74% of dicotyledon stems (non-woody) and leaves, and 54% of monocotyledon stems and leaves. Digestible dry matter (DDM) followed a similar trend, but fewer data were available.

Digestibility of forage for herbivores is generally negatively cor-

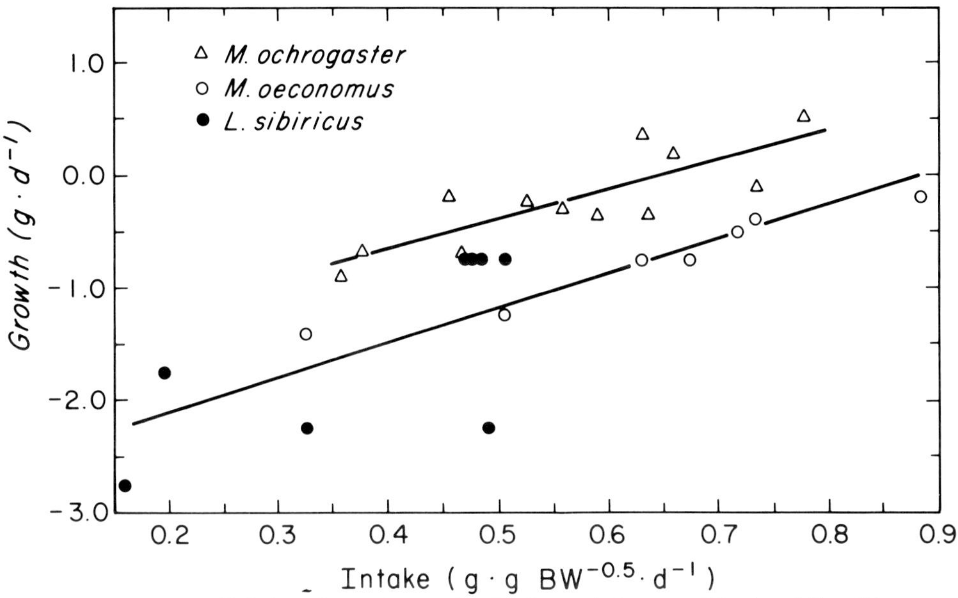

FIG. 1. Relation of growth rate of animals to relative rate of intake of digestible dry matter on an artificial diet. Data for *Microtus oeconomus* and *Lemmus sibiricus* are combined because regressions were not significantly different. Regression equations with 95% C.L.: Y = 2.61 ± 1.21 X − 1.70 ± 0.70 ($R^2 = 0.70$) for *M. ochrogaster,* and Y = 3.05 ± 1.21 X − 2.70 ± 0.67 ($R^2 = 0.68$) for *M. oeconomus* and *L. sibiricus.* See Lindroth et al. (1984) for methods.

related with fiber content (hemicellulose, cellulose, and lignin), and weight gain of voles on grass diets may also be negatively correlated with fiber content (Russo et al., 1981). Nevertheless, intake and weight gain improved when weanling meadow voles ate cereal diets with 18% cellulose (alphacel) compared to the same diets without cellulose. Chemically isolated cellulose (alphacel) is essentially undigested by voles (Shenk et al., 1970) and the improved performance with alphacel in the diet may simply reflect a need for bulk. Apparently 10 to 30% of natural fiber can be digested by voles (Keys and Van Soest, 1970). Most of this digestion is probably done by microbes in the cecum, but cellulolytic bacteria and fermentation products have also been found in the stomach (Kudo et al., 1979; McBee, 1970). Toughness and texture of the diet also are related to the amount and arrangement of fiber, and too much fiber may inhibit intake of forage (Ulyatt, 1973).

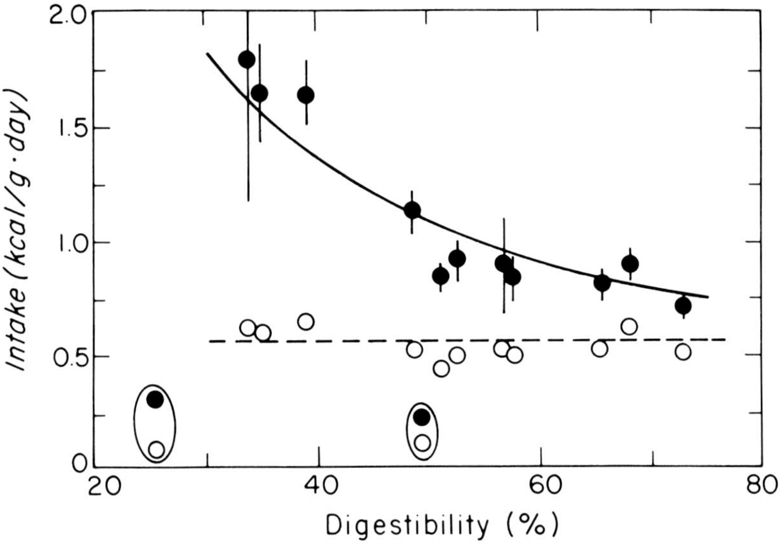

FIG. 2. Comparison of total intake of energy (solid points and solid line) to intake of digestible energy (open points and dashed line) in relation to digestibility of forage by *Microtus ochrogaster, M. californicus,* and *Lemmus sibiricus.* Circled points represent unpalatable food; vertical lines give 95% confidence intervals (after Batzli and Cole, 1979).

The compensatory increase of intake for less digestible food is well known for ruminants (Ulyatt, 1973), laboratory rats (Adolf, 1947), and laboratory mice (Dalton, 1963). Of course, lower digestibility of forage must be compensated by greater intake if the animal is to survive. Although the size of a single meal for voles may be limited by gastro-intestinal fill (Kendall et al., 1978), total daily intake appears to be adjusted depending upon digestible energy or nutrients. For many foods intake may compensate completely so that the consumption of digestible energy and dry matter remains relatively constant (Fig. 2). But some foods, usually those of low quality, simply are not palatable enough to be taken in large amounts. Thus, although mosses may form up to 40% of the diet of *L. sibiricus,* they are poorly digested compared to monocotyledons (23% DDM and 33–37% DDM, respectively), and voluntary intake of mosses alone is not sufficient to maintain the animals. Similarly, *M. ochrogaster* does not consume enough bluegrass to

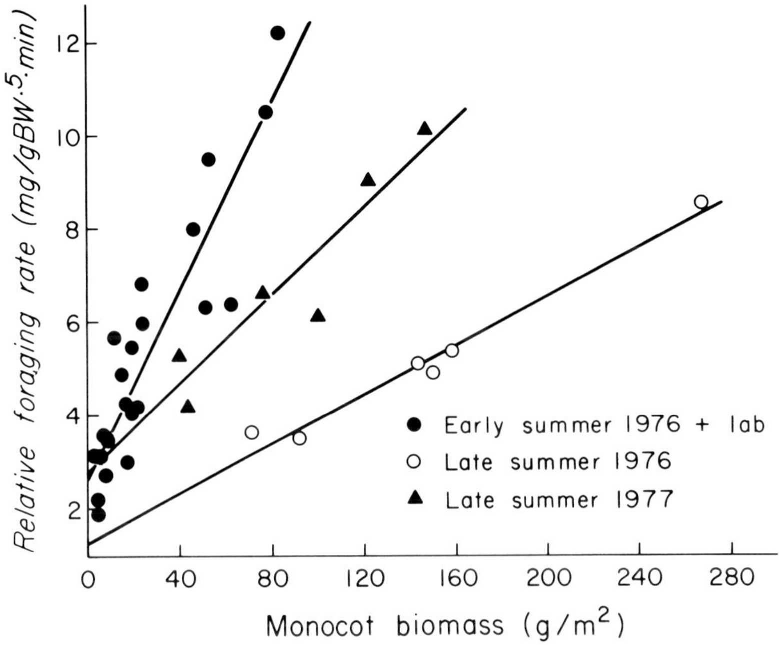

FIG. 3. Relative foraging rates for brown lemmings (*Lemmus sibiricus*) in relation to forage availability (from Batzli et al., 1981).

maintain its body weight, and bluegrass is relatively poorly digested (51% DDM) compared to more palatable dicotyledons (61 to 69% DDM).

It is difficult to assess how herbivores would perform on food they will not eat, but it is clear that different species of microtines show different physiological responses to the same food. Whereas *Lemmus* only digested 33–37% of the dry matter in tundra monocotyledons, *M. ochrogaster* digested 52% of the same plants (Batzli and Cole, 1979). Similar differences can be seen on laboratory diets. Two microtines that prefer monocotyledons (*L. sibiricus* and *M. californicus*) digested only 53–54% of the dry matter in commercial rabbit chow (largely alfalfa meal), whereas a dicotyledon eater (*M. ochrogaster*) digested 68% (Batzli and Cole, 1979). On an artificial diet made with chemically defined materials, *Lemmus* and *M. oeconomus* digested 54%, whereas *M. ochrogaster* digested 61% of the dry matter (Lindroth et al., 1984).

In nature, of course, it takes time to select and harvest food, and it is not surprising that foraging rate (rate of intake) varies with availability of palatable food (Fig. 3). Stage of growth and year-to-year variability in growth form also affect foraging rates; older, larger plants are consumed more slowly (Batzli et al., 1981). Thus, as quality and availability of food items change, herbivores must change their diet in order to maintain high rates of intake. If they cannot switch diets, they must spend more time foraging, and this means greater exposure to the physical environment and to predation. Hence, seasonal changes in food selection can be viewed as the expected response to seasonal changes in availability and quality of food items. In order to track this changing quality a herbivore must continually sample available forage, which accounts for the wide variety of food items taken in small amounts by most generalist herbivores (Westoby, 1978).

Flexible turnover times of gut contents exist in most species so that less digestible forage is processed more rapidly (Batzli and Cole, 1979), but whatever the demand for nutrients, intake of food can be no faster than the gut can process it. Traditional wisdom says that smaller ruminants must eat a more highly digestible diet to survive—the Jarman-Bell principle (Geist, 1974; Janis, 1975; Jarman, 1974; Parra, 1978). The argument goes as follows: 1) smaller animals have similar relative gut size but larger relative metabolic rates and more rapid turnover of gut contents than do larger animals; 2) for a given diet, a decrease in turnover time is also associated with a decrease in digestibility; 3) mathematical relationships are such that for a given diet smaller animals get less energy relative to their metabolic requirements than do larger animals; and 4) therefore smaller animals must eat more digestible food.

When fed similar forage, the gut turnover time for a wide variety of herbivores decreases in a regular way with body size (Fig. 4). Monogastric animals have a shorter turnover time than ruminants, but the rate of decline with body size (slope of the line) is the same. Given the same general relationship (even with different parameter values) for monogastric herbivores as for ruminants, the same arguments should apply to ruminant and monogastric herbivores. However, it is clear that many small herbivores, including some microtine rodents, eat large amounts of poorly digestible food (Batzli and Cole, 1979). Furthermore, some microtines can digest hay almost as well as horses, even though they are several orders of

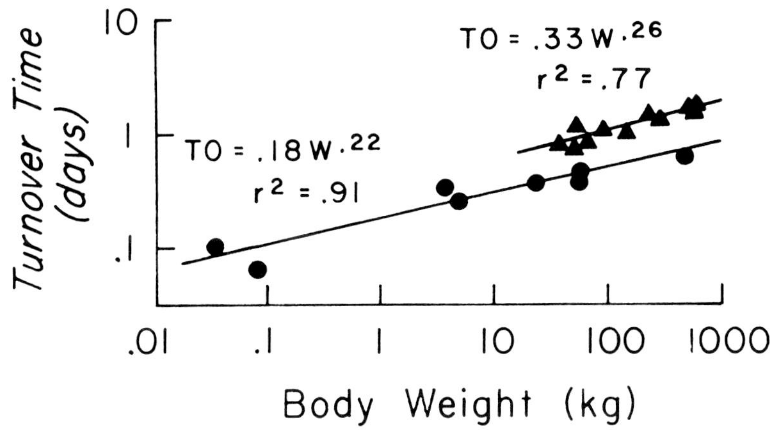

FIG. 4. Turnover time of gut contents in relation to body size for ruminant (triangles) and non-ruminant (circles) animals (from Batzli, unpubl. observ.).

magnitude smaller (Batzli, pers. observ.). How can this be? The traditional analysis assumes that digestion proceeds as a simple exponential function of time in the gut, a model proposed by Blaxter et al. (1956). In fact, it is more likely that small molecules in cell contents are absorbed very quickly by the gut, non-fibrous polymers (proteins, glucans, and pectin) require moderate processing, and fibrous polymers (cellulose and lignin) require much longer processing (Hungate, 1966). Thus, digestibility is a mixed function of time; small animals that chew forage very finely, thereby rupturing the cells and releasing cell contents, can reduce turnover time without suffering the full consequences expected based upon a simple continuous function (Batzli, pers. observ.).

Nutrients and Performance

The exact nutrient requirements of organisms are difficult to specify because of the large number of required nutrients, interactions among nutrients, and substantial individual differences within a species. As a result only the nutritional requirements of domesticated rodents are very well known. Because of the increasing use of voles for bioassays in agricultural research, they have now been included in the group of laboratory animals covered by the National Research Council's publication on nutrient requirements of domes-

TABLE 3
RECOMMENDED NUTRIENT CONTENT OF DIETS FOR GROWTH AND REPRODUCTION OF RODENTS AND RABBITS

	Rabbit[a]	Rat[a]	Mouse[a]	Guinea pig[a]	Hamster[a]	Vole
Digestible energy (kcal/kg)	2,500	3,800	3,700	3,000	4,200	3,750[a] 2,000–3,000[b]
Protein (%)	16.0–17.0	15.1	18.0	18.0	15.0	13.0[a] 8.0[b]
Calcium (%)	0.4–0.7	0.5	0.4	0.8–1.0	0.6	0.3–0.5[b]
Phosphorus (%)	0.2–0.5	0.4	0.4	0.4–0.7	0.3	0.2–0.4[b]
Sodium (%)	0.20	0.05	0.08	?	0.15	>0.02[b]

[a] Based upon National Research Council publication on nutrient requirements for domestic animals and references cited therein (National Research Council, 1977, 1978).

[b] Based upon data for voles and lemmings (Batzli, unpubl. observ.; Batzli and Cole, 1979; Lindroth et al., 1984).

tic animals (National Research Council, 1978). As can be seen in Table 3, requirements of microtines appear to be similar to laboratory rodents and rabbits, but many nutrient requirements have not been studied. Recent work indicates that digestible energy requirements of voles are more similar to rabbits than to laboratory rodents (Table 3) and that *Lemmus sibiricus* may only require 70% as much digestible energy in its diet as does *M. ochrogaster* (Batzli and Cole, 1979). Data for an artificial diet (Lindroth et al., 1984) suggest that the protein requirement for maximal growth of young *M. ochrogaster* is only 8% or less of dry matter (Lindroth and Batzli, 1984*a*), rather than the 13% suggested by data for *M. pennsylvanicus* (Shenk et al., 1970). Other requirements of different species of microtines also may differ. Species with the same intake of digestible dry matter on the same diet may show significantly different growth rates (Fig. 1).

The nutrients that appear to be most critical for microtine rodents in their natural food are digestible energy, protein (organic N), calcium (Ca), phosphorus (P), and sodium (Na), but this may be an artifact of the paucity of studies involving other nutrients. Requirements for nutrients are greatest for lactating females; in microtine rodents the mass of the litter at weaning is often greater than that of the female (Batzli and Jung, 1980; Batzli et al., 1974). Thus, it is not surprising that the breeding season for most herbivorous microtines coincides with the growing season, the period when the quality of available food is usually highest (Fleming, 1973; Goldberg et al., 1980). For most temperate species this means spring, summer, and fall (*M. montanus, M. ochrogaster, M. pennsylvanicus*), although in a Mediterranean climate the growing season is reversed and breeding stops during the dry summer (*M. californicus*). As plants age, their quality as forage for microtines declines (Hansson, 1970; Martinet and Daketse, 1976; Martinet and Meunier, 1969; Myllymäki, 1977). Thus, during the breeding season the diets of these herbivores are mostly fresh stems and leaves, whereas they gradually shift to seeds, stem bases, and roots as the above-ground parts of the plants age and die back. After a breeding pause, when quality of available food is low (Batzli, in press), reproduction recommences with the first appearance of high-quality green shoots (Batzli and Pitelka, 1971; Negus et al., 1977). Apparently the animals respond to a chemical cue (6-MBOA) in the developing plants (Berger et al., 1981; Sanders et al., 1981). Provision of high-quality food can maintain breeding during the cold winter (Cole and Batzli, 1978) or dry summer (Ford, 1978).

Length of reproductive season, litter size, body growth, and survival rates all correlate with nutrient content of natural forage (Cole and Batzli, 1979; Hoffmann, 1958), and laboratory feeding trials indicate that growth and reproduction are direct responses to nutrient content of the diet. Cole and Batzli (1979) reported that *M. ochrogaster* grew more rapidly on natural diets with higher nutrient concentration, and Batzli (in press) found that summer diets for *M. californicus* (grass seeds) are deficient in Ca and Na, both of which affect reproductive success.

The role of sodium in microtine nutrition has been of particular interest. Aumann and Emlen (1965) found that reproductive output (number of young) of *M. pennsylvanicus* in small pens increased when a sodium supplement was added to their water, and that animals increased their sodium intake as conditions became more crowded. Normal sodium levels in urine of voles (*M. arvalis*) and lemmings (*L. lemmus*), and sodium levels in the feces of lemmings

(*L. lemmus*), are extremely low (DeKock and Robinson, 1968; Lange and Staaland, 1970). Apparently these patterns of sodium conservation occur because of the low sodium content in the diet of these herbivores and the evolution of efficient mechanisms for absorption of sodium in the colon of microtines, but social stress upsets endocrine balance and can result in unusually high loss of sodium in urine.

The nutrients that are most important for microtines probably vary with season and location. A simulation model of N, Ca, and P nutrition for *L. sibiricus* indicated that for lactating females N was in short supply in winter, P was limiting in early summer, and a high Ca/P ratio caused difficulties in late summer (Barkley et al., 1980). But nutrient content of the major food type, monocotyledon stems and leaves, varied by a factor of 2 from year to year, and nutritional difficulties only occurred in low-nutrient years. As already mentioned, Ca and Na availability seem to limit summer breeding by *M. californicus,* and no doubt other nutrients are important in other places.

Secondary Plant Compounds and Performance

For microtines, negative nutritional factors other than high fiber appear to consist largely of secondary plant compounds. The same compounds that reduce intake of particular plant species also reduce growth, survival, and reproduction if given in amounts equivalent to expected dietary levels (Table 2). Thus, saponins, alkaloids, and phenolic compounds have all been shown to be detrimental to voles when ingested, and no doubt other classes of compounds, such as terpenes, also will prove to be detrimental. Terpenes do disrupt digestive processes in ruminants (Oh et al., 1970).

Not all secondary compounds affect microtines in the same way, nor does the same compound affect different species of microtines in the same way. Evaporation of ethanol extracts of plant tissue on laboratory diets produced a variety of effects on growth, body composition, and organ weight of arctic microtines (Jung and Batzli, 1981). Performance on diets containing extracts of three foods—a sedge (*Carex aquatilis*) that was highly palatable to *L. sibiricus* and *M. oeconomus,* a willow (*Salix pulchra*) that was highly palatable to *D. torquatus* and *M. oeconomus,* and Labrador tea (*Ledum palustre*) that was palatable to none of the microtines—were entirely consistent with results of palatability trials. Willow extract contained compounds that reduced growth and body fat of *Lemmus* but not *Microtus* or *Dicrostonyx*; sedge extract reduced growth and body fat of *Dicrostonyx,* but only body fat of *Lemmus* and *Microtus*; and *Ledum* extract reduced growth and body fat of all three microtines (and caused the death of *Lemmus* even though food intake was normal).

Some secondary compounds act as toxins (β-nitroproprionic acid, alkaloids) when absorbed, but others may act by reducing the digestibility of important dietary components, for instance complexing of protein by some phenolics (Rhoades and Cates, 1976). Thus, voles (*M. ochrogaster*) fed artificial diets containing two kinds of phenolics had poorer growth on low-protein diets than on high-protein diets (Lindroth and Batzli, 1984*a*). Protein digestibility was also lower for voles on low-protein diets with high levels of tannic acid, but these voles also had higher intake so that they digested equivalent total amounts of protein on low- and high-phenolic diets. The level of detoxication products (glucuronides) in urine also suggested that the depression of growth by phenolics was the result of a toxic effect and not because of lowered protein digestibility. High levels of protein may have protected the voles from the toxic effect by binding with the tannic acid. This interaction between protein levels and phenolic levels is probably not unique, and it seems likely that the quality of forage is a product of multiple interactions between positive and negative chemical factors.

Optimal Foraging

Given a complex array of forage that varies in availability and quality through time and space, herbivores must somehow decide what to eat. If we assume that animals eat so as to maximize their performance under a given set of conditions, and if we understand how these conditions influence performance, then we should be able to predict how an animal will forage and what it will eat. This is the basis for optimal foraging theory, most of which has been developed for predators (Krebs, 1978). Much of this theory requires that food items be ranked according to their net value, which usually is couched in terms of net energy yield and does not seem directly applicable to herbivores.

One optimization model that has been applied to microtine herbivores is the graphical model developed by Stenseth and Hansson (1979), which predicts the net fitness gain from food in relation to its value (digestible energy content). Net gain for each food type is a function of the direct cost of foraging activities (which increases with decreasing availability of an item), maintenance cost (which increases with the time spent foraging), and the distribution of values for the food type (not all items of the same type have the same value). Thus, the net gain from a food type increases as the values and densities for items in a type increase. If the distributions of net gains (items with different values within a type have different net gains) for different food types overlap substantially, the animal maximizes its net gain by taking a mixed diet. Unlike most of the optimization models developed for predators, this model predicts that relative densities of food items (not just absolute densities) influence diet choice and that partial preferences (not all or none responses) for food items will occur. However, like other models, Stenseth and Hansson's (1979) model requires a currency. The currency they favor is energy, although they acknowledge that others might be used.

Stenseth et al. (1977) used the graphical model outlined above to predict diets of *M. agrestris* in Sweden and Finland. They included four food types (grass, forbs, seeds, and bark) and assigned the value of items by digestible energy content. They successfully predicted nearly equal use of grass and forbs in spring in northern Sweden, but predictions for other seasons and for two communities in Finland depended upon somewhat arbitrary evaluations. In addition, they needed to invoke "search images" and polymorphic behavior, for which they presented no evidence, to reconcile predictions and observed diets.

A different approach to optimal foraging, the use of linear programming, was suggested by Westoby (1974) and Pulliam (1975). In this technique constraints (such as minimal nutrient intake) are established; the combination of food items that satisfies those constraints and maximizes or minimizes some other factor (for instance energy or foraging time) is sought. The most successful use of this technique to date has been that of Belovsky (1978) with moose. He used constraints of 1) minimal energy and sodium requirements for maintenance and reproduction, 2) maximal times allowed to spend foraging in water (because of heat loss) and on land (owing to time needed for rumination), and 3) maximal amount of bulk in the diet (rumen capacity is more quickly filled by aquatic plants with high water content). Then he predicted the amount of aquatic plants, forbs, and leaves of shrubs in the diet if energy intake were maximized or foraging time were minimized. Actual diets almost exactly matched those predicted by the strategy of energy maximization. Of course, not all plant species within these general food categories were taken, and predicting which species would be taken was more difficult (Belovsky, 1981). Selection of aquatic plants seemed clearly related to their sodium content, but use of terrestrial plants did not depend simply on their nutrient content or availability.

It seems likely that positive and negative nutritional factors (such as secondary compounds) need to be balanced by herbivores when selecting their diet (Lindroth, 1979). Certainly, the information available to date for microtine rodents suggests that this is so (see above). Thus, a model that predicts the diet of microtine rodents probably will need to include multiple constraints within which there is very little room to maximize nutrient or energy intake. Indeed this may explain why the performance of animals and populations varies so with habitat type and, therefore, quality of available food.

Forage Quality and Population Characteristics

Habitat Differences

That population densities and demography differ in different habitats is well known, but the causes of these differences generally are not. Most microtines require a minimal amount of cover, presumably as protection against predation, and Birney et al. (1976) have suggested that response to cover explains many of the differences in density among habitats. Addition of water and fertilizer to shortgrass prairie markedly increased the density of *M. ochrogaster*, but it is not clear how much of the response was due to increased cover and how much was due to improved nutrition (Grant et al., 1977).

Two studies have shown that the quality of diet differs in different habitats, and because of the effects of diet quality on growth, reproduction, and survival, the population dynamics in the habitats varied. Cole and Batzli (1979) found low, moderate, and high densities of *M. ochrogaster* in tallgrass prairie, abandoned bluegrass pasture, and abandoned alfalfa fields. Growth of young, litter size, length of breeding season, and survival were all clearly related to the quality of different diets in three study areas, and these differences accounted for the different densities reached in the populations. Krohne (1980, 1982) found that litter sizes of *M. californicus* were greater and that penned populations had greater reproductive output and rates of growth when fed annual grasses compared to perennial grasses. These results corresponded to different population dynamics found in the field: seasonal fluctuations at low densities in perennial grassland and multi-annual fluctuations reaching high densities in annual grasslands. In neither of these studies could the differences between habitats be explained by availability of cover.

It is not clear how often differences in populations between habitats can be related to available food because most studies do not examine nutrition adequately. Collared lemmings and brown lemmings in arctic Alaska have strong habitat preferences that are associated with concentration of preferred foods (Batzli and Jung, 1980; Batzli et al., 1983), and Batzli (1983) suggested that the wide variability in the population densities of lemmings in different geographical regions of tundra is a function of the quality of available food. Because cover and food often are contributed by the same plants, the two are not always separable, but it seems clear that given a minimal amount of cover (and therefore food), the quality of available food accounts for many of the observed differences in microtine rodent populations in different habitats.

Population Dynamics

Because the reproductive season of microtines is often linked to available food, it follows that seasonal changes in density (increases during the reproductive season and declines during the non-breeding season) are also a function of nutrition. Thus, every summer when vegetation dries, the voles shift to grass seeds that are deficient in Ca and Na, reproduction ceases and population densities of *M. californicus* decline (Batzli, in press; Batzli and Pitelka, 1970, 1971). Most temperate species show a similar pattern of shifting food habits and a reproductive pause during winter, although the population of trappable animals does not always decline immediately (Gaines and Rose, 1976; Getz et al., 1979; Krebs et al., 1969; Negus et al., 1977; Tamarin, 1977; Whitney, 1976; Wolff and Lidicker,

1980). Winter breeding may occur in some species if high-quality forage is accessible under the snow (Batzli et al., 1980), and winter breeding can be maintained if supplemental food is given (Cole and Batzli, 1978).

In addition to seasonal changes, many microtine species go through extreme multi-annual fluctuations in density (cycles). Because these fluctuations are analyzed in another chapter of this book (Taitt and Krebs, this volume), and because I recently reviewed the role of nutrition in these cycles (Batzli, in press), I only make a few comments here.

First, the data on habitat effects summarized above indicate that only when high-quality forage is available can microtine rodents reach the high densities associated with cyclic peak populations. Second, theoretical analyses and empirical data (Batzli, in press; Batzli et al., 1980) indicate that neither the food-shortage hypothesis of Lack (1954) nor the nutrient-recovery hypothesis of Pitelka (1964) and Schultz (1964) are likely to account for cycles. The plant-production hypothesis of Kalela (1962) recently was both supported (Laine and Henttonen, 1983) and rejected (Andersson and Jonasson, in litt.) for two areas in northern Fennoscandia. Third, manipulations of natural populations by providing fertilizer or supplementary food all indicate improved reproduction, growth, and survival during the population increase (Cole and Batzli, 1978; Desy and Thompson, 1983; Krebs and DeLong, 1965; Schultz, 1969; Taitt and Krebs, 1981), but none prevented the population decline. However, these experiments were flawed because they did not monitor or prevent an influx of predators to the small experimental sites when all other nearby populations declined. One experiment on penned populations that included predator control did prevent a population crash by provision of food and water (Ford, 1978). Fourth, a theoretical analysis of the implications of positive nutrient feedback versus negative nutrient feedback (secondary plant compounds) suggested that, whereas strong positive nutrient feedback leads to instability or stability of a soil-plant-herbivore-predator trophic system, inducible secondary compounds acting as proposed by Haukioja (1980) may lead to oscillatory instability (Batzli, in press). Thus, if changes in nutrition are sufficient to produce population cycles, it is most likely because food plants respond to damage with lowered quality, probably because of production of secondary plant compounds.

On the whole I doubt that any single factor, including nutrition, will be sufficient to explain population cycling. Environmental factors, such as nutrition and weather, and responses of organisms, such as aggressive behavior and dispersal, interact in complex ways, and it is those interactions that need to be examined.

Conclusions

It seems clear that nutrition plays a large role in the well-being, habitat preference, and successful reproduction by microtine rodents. Thus, much of the morphology, physiology, and behavior of these animals should be interpretable in relation to the availability, quality, and processing of forage. A thorough analysis of such patterns awaits the development of much better information on diet, gut morphology, and nutritional physiology for a wider variety of species. Only then will the relationships among these variables, and the evolutionary response of microtine species to the variable nutritional conditions found in their habitats, become clear.

Literature Cited

ADOLF, E. F. 1947. Urges to eat and drink in rats. Amer. J. Physiol., 151:110–125.

AUMANN, G. D., AND J. T. EMLEN. 1965. Relation of population density to sodium availability and sodium selection in microtine rodents. Nature, 208:198–199.

BARKLEY, S., G. O. BATZLI, AND B. COLLIER. 1980. Nutritional ecology of microtine rodents: a simulation model of mineral nutrition for brown lemmings. Oikos, 34:103–114.

BARNES, R. F., G. W. FISSEL, AND J. S. SHENK. 1974. Comparison of ethanol-extracted and unextracted forage fed to weanling meadow voles. Agron. J., 66:72–75.

BATZLI, G. O. 1975. The role of small mammals in arctic ecosystems. Pp. 243–268, *in* Small mammals: their productivity and population dynamics (F. Golley, K. Petrusewicz, and L. Ryszkowski, eds.). Cambridge Univ. Press, London, 451 pp.

———. 1983. Responses of arctic rodent populations to nutritional factors. Oikos, 40:396–406.

———. In press. The role of nutrition in population cycles of microtine rodents. Acta Zool. Fennica.

———. In press. The effects of food quality on reproduction of California voles. Ecology.

BATZLI, G. O., AND F. R. COLE. 1979. Nutritional ecology of microtine rodents: digestibility of forage. J. Mamm., 60:740–750.

BATZLI, G. O., AND H. G. JUNG. 1980. Nutritional ecology of microtine rodents: resource utilization near Atkasook, Alaska. Arctic Alpine Res., 12:483–499.

Batzli, G. O., and F. A. Pitelka. 1970. Influence of meadow mouse populations in California grassland. Ecology, 51:1027–1039.

———. 1971. Condition and diet of cycling populations of the California vole, *Microtus californicus*. J. Mamm., 52:141–163.

———. 1983. Nutritional ecology of microtine rodents: food habits of lemmings near Barrow, Alaska. J. Mamm., 64:648–655.

Batzli, G. O., H. G. Jung, and G. Guntenspergen. 1981. Nutritional ecology of microtine rodents: linear foraging rate curves for brown lemmings. Oikos, 37:112–116.

Batzli, G. O., F. A. Pitelka, and G. W. Cameron. 1983. Habitat use by lemmings near Barrow, Alaska. Holarctic Ecol., 6:255–262.

Batzli, G. O., N. C. Stenseth, and B. M. Fitzgerald. 1974. Growth and survival of suckling brown lemmings, *Lemmus trimucronatus*. J. Mamm., 55:828–831.

Batzli, G. O., R. G. White, S. F. MacLean, Jr., F. A. Pitelka, and B. Collier. 1980. The herbivore-based trophic system. Pp. 335–410, *in* An arctic ecosystem: the coastal plain of northern Alaska (J. Brown et al., eds.). Dowden, Hutchinson and Ross, Stroudsburg, Pennsylvania, 571 pp.

Belovsky, G. E. 1978. Diet optimization in a generalist herbivore: the moose. Theor. Population Biol., 14:105–134.

———. 1981. Food plant selection by a generalist herbivore: the moose. Ecology, 62:1020–1030.

Berger, P. J., N. C. Negus, E. H. Sanders, and P. D. Gardner. 1981. Chemical triggering of reproduction in *Microtus montanus*. Science, 214:69–70.

Berger, P. J., E. H. Sanders, P. D. Gardner, and N. C. Negus. 1977. Phenolic plant compounds functioning as reproductive inhibitors in *Microtus montanus*. Science, 195:575–577.

Birney, E. C., W. E. Grant, and D. D. Baird. 1976. Importance of vegetative cover to cycles of *Microtus* populations. Ecology, 57:1043–1051.

Blaxter, K. L., N. M. Graham, and F. W. Wainman. 1956. Some observations on the digestibility of food by sheep and on related problems. Nutrition, 10:69–91.

Carleton, M. D. 1973. A survey of the gross stomach morphology in New World Cricetinae (Rodentia: Muroidea), with comments on functional interpretation. Misc. Publ. Mus. Zool., Univ. Michigan, 146:1–43.

———. 1981. A survey of gross stomach morphology in Microtinae (Rodentia: Muroidea). Z. Saugetierk., 46:93–108.

Cole, F. R., and G. O. Batzli. 1978. The influence of supplemental feeding on a population of the prairie vole *Microtus ochrogaster*. J. Mamm., 59:809–819.

———. 1979. Nutrition and population dynamics of the prairie vole, *Microtus ochrogaster*, in central Illinois. J. Anim. Ecol., 48:455–470.

Dalton, D. C. 1963. Effect of dilution of the diet with an indigestible filler on feed intake in the mouse. Nature, 197:909–910.

DeKock, L. L., and A. E. Robinson. 1968. Individual sodium and potassium excretion patterns in rodents during certain life situations. Z. Tierpsychol., 25:811–824.

Desy, E. A., and C. F. Thompson. 1983. Effects of supplemental food on a *Microtus pennsylvanicus* population in central Illinois. J. Anim. Ecol., 52: 127–140.

Fish, P. G. 1974. Notes on the feeding habits of *Microtus ochrogaster* and *Microtus pennsylvanicus*. Amer. Midland Nat., 96:460–461.

Fleming, G. A. 1973. Mineral composition of herbage. Pp. 529–566, *in* Chemistry and biochemistry of herbage, Vol. I (G. W. Butler and R. W. Bailey, eds.). Academic Press, New York, 639 pp.

FORD, R. G. 1978. Computer enhancement of mark-recapture data and its application to the role of food supply in declining populations of *Microtus*. Unpubl. Ph.D. dissert., Univ. California, Berkeley, 177 pp.

GAINES, M. S., AND R. K. ROSE. 1976. Population dynamics of *Microtus ochrogaster* in eastern Kansas. Ecology, 51:1145–1161.

GEIST, V. 1974. On the relationship of social evolution and ecology in ungulates. Amer. Zool., 4:205–220.

GETZ, L. L., L. VERNER, F. R. COLE, J. E. HOFMANN, AND D. E. AVALOS. 1979. Comparisons of population demography of *Microtus ochrogaster* and *M. pennsylvanicus*. Acta Theriol., 24:319–349.

GOELZ, M. F. B., H. ROTHENBACHER, J. P. WIGGINS, W. A. KENDALL, AND T. V. HERSHBERGER. 1980. Some hematological and histopathological effects of the alkaloids gramine and hordenine on meadow voles (*Microtus pennsylvanicus*). Toxicology, 18:125–131.

GOLDBERG, N., N. R. TABROFF, AND R. H. TAMARIN. 1980. Nutrient variation in beach grass in relation to beach vole feeding. Ecology, 61:1029–1033.

GRANT, W. E., N. R. FRENCH, AND D. M. SWIFT. 1977. Response of a small mammal community to water and nitrogen treatments in a shortgrass prairie ecosystem. J. Mamm., 58:637–652.

GUSTINE, D. L., J. S. SHENK, B. G. MOYER, AND R. F. BARNES. 1974. Isolation of β-nitroproprionic acid from crownvetch. Agron. J., 66:636–639.

GUTHRIE, R. D. 1965. Variability in characters undergoing rapid evolution, an analysis of *Microtus* molars. Evolution, 19:214–233.

HANSSON, L. 1970. Methods of morphological diet micro-analysis in rodents. Oikos, 21:255–266.

———. 1971. Habitat, food and population dynamics of the field vole *Microtus agrestis* (L.) in south Sweden. Viltrevy, 8:268–378.

HARBORNE, J. B. 1982. Introduction to ecological biochemistry. Second ed. Academic Press, New York, 278 pp.

HAUKIOJA, E. 1980. On the role of plant defences in the fluctuation of herbivore populations. Oikos, 35:202–213.

HINTON, M. A. C. 1926. Monograph of the voles and lemmings (Microtinae) living and extinct. Vol. I. British Mus. Nat. Hist., London, 488 pp.

HOFFMANN, R. S. 1958. The role of reproduction and mortality in population fluctuations of voles (*Microtus*). Ecol. Monogr., 28:79–109.

HUNGATE, R. E. 1966. The rumen and its microbes. Academic Press, New York, 533 pp.

JANIS, C. 1975. The evolutionary strategy of the Equidae and the origins of rumen and cecal digestion. Evolution, 30:757–774.

JARMAN, P. J. 1974. The social organization of antelope in relation to their ecology. Behaviour, 48:215–268.

JUNG, H. G., AND G. O. BATZLI. 1981. Nutritional ecology of microtine rodents: effects of plant extracts on the growth of arctic microtines. J. Mamm., 62: 286–292.

KALELA, O. 1962. On the fluctuations in the numbers of arctic and boreal small rodents as a problem of production biology. Ann. Acad. Sci. Fennica A, IV Biol., 66:1–38.

KENDALL, W. A., AND K. T. LEATH. 1976. Effects of saponins on palatability of alfalfa to meadow voles. Agron. J., 68:473–476.

KENDALL, W. A., AND R. T. SHERWOOD. 1975. Palatability of leaves of tall fescue and reed canarygrass and some of their alkaloids to meadow voles. Agron. J., 67:667–671.

KENDALL, W. A., R. R. HILL, JR., AND J. S. SHENK. 1978. Regulation of intake and utilization of carbohydrates by meadow voles. J. Anim. Sci., 46:1641–1647.

———. 1979. Inhibition by some allelochemicals of intake of individual meals by meadow voles. Agron. J., 71:613–616.

Keys, J. E., Jr., and P. J. Van Soest. 1970. Digestibility of forages by the meadow vole (*Microtus pennsylvanicus*). J. Dairy Sci., 53:1502–1508.

Krebs, C. J., and K. T. DeLong. 1965. A *Microtus* population with supplemental food. J. Mamm., 46:566–573.

Krebs, C. J., B. L. Keller, and R. H. Tamarin. 1969. *Microtus* population biology: demographic changes in fluctuating populations of *M. ochrogaster* in southern Indiana. Ecology, 50:587–607.

Krebs, J. R. 1978. Optimal foraging: decision rules for predators. Pp. 23–63, *in* Behavioural ecology—an evolutionary approach (J. R. Krebs and N. B. Davies, eds.). Sinauer Assoc., Sunderland, Massachusetts, 494 pp.

Krohne, D. T. 1980. Intraspecific litter size variation in *Microtus californicus*. II. Variation between populations. Evolution, 34:1174–1182.

———. 1982. The demography of low-litter-size populations of *Microtus californicus*. Canadian J. Zool., 60:368–374.

Kudo, H., Y. Oki, and H. Minato. 1979. *Microtus* species as laboratory animals. I. Bacterial flora of the esophageal sac of *Microtus montebelli* fed different rations and its relationship to the cellulolytic bacteria. Bull. Nippon Veterin. Zootech. Coll., 28:13–19.

Lack, D. 1954. The natural regulation of animal numbers. Oxford Univ. Press, London, 343 pp.

Laine, K., and H. Henttonen. 1983. Plant production and population cycles of microtine rodents in Finnish Lapland. Oikos, 40:407–418.

Lange, R., and H. Staaland. 1970. Adaptations of the caecum-colon structure of rodents. Comp. Biochem. Physiol., 35:905–919.

Lechowicz, M. 1983. The sampling characteristics of electivity indices. Oecologia, 52:22–30.

Lindroth, R. L. 1979. Diet optimization by generalist mammalian herbivores. The Biologist, 61:41–58.

Lindroth, R. L., and G. O. Batzli. 1984*a*. Plant phenolics as chemical defenses: the effects of natural phenolics on survival and growth of prairie voles. J. Chem. Ecol., 10:229–244.

———. 1984*b*. Food habits of the meadow vole (*Microtus pennsylvanicus*) in bluegrass and prairie habitats. J. Mamm., 65:600–606.

Lindroth, R. L., G. O. Batzli, and G. R. Guntenspergen. 1984. An artificial diet for use in nutritional studies with microtine rodents. J. Mamm., 65: 139–143.

Marcarian, V. 1972. Characterization of certain active components limiting nutritional efficiency from alfalfa. Unpubl. Ph.D. dissert., Michigan State Univ., East Lansing, 88 pp.

Martinet, L., and M.-J. Daketse. 1976. Effect of temperature on survival during the first month of life in the field vole, *Microtus arvalis,* raised under different conditions of daylight ratio and feeding. Ann. Biol. Anim. Biochem. Biophys., 16:773–782.

Martinet, L., and M. Meunier. 1969. Influence des variations saisonnières de la luzerne sur la croissance, la mortalité et l'établissement de la maturité sexuelle chez le campagnol des champs (*Microtus arvalis*). Ann. Biol. Anim. Biochem. Biophys., 9:451–462.

Maynard, L. A., J. K. Loosli, H. F. Hintz, and R. G. Warner. 1979. Animal nutrition. Seventh ed. McGraw-Hill, New York, 602 pp.

McBee, R. H. 1970. Metabolic contributions of the caecal flora. Amer. J. Clin. Nutr., 23:1514–1518.

———. 1971. Significance of intestinal microflora in herbivory. Ann. Rev. Ecol. Syst., 2:165–176.

Meade, J. B. 1975. Food selection and turnover of nitrogen, phosphorus, and potassium by *Microtus pennsylvanicus.* Unpubl. Ph.D. dissert., Cornell Univ., Ithaca, New York, 142 pp.

Myllymäki, A. 1977. Demographic mechanisms in the fluctuating populations of the field vole *Microtus agrestis.* Oikos, 29:468–493.

National Research Council. 1977. Nutrient requirements of rabbits. Second ed. Nutrient requirements of domestic animals. Natl. Acad. Sci., Washington, D.C., 30 pp.

———. 1978. Nutrient requirements of laboratory animals. Third ed. Nutrient requirements of domestic animals, No. 10. Natl. Acad. Sci., Washington, D.C., 96 pp.

Neal, B. R., D. A. Pulkinen, and B. D. Owen. 1973. A comparison of faecal and stomach content analysis in the meadow vole. Canadian J. Zool., 51: 715–721.

Negus, N. C., P. J. Berger, and L. G. Forslund. 1977. Reproductive strategy of *Microtus montanus.* J. Mamm., 58:347–353.

Oh, H. K., M. B. Jones, W. M. Longhurst, and G. E. Connelly. 1970. Deer browsing and rumen microbial fermentation of Douglas fir as affected by fertilization and growth stage. Forest Sci., 16:21–27.

Oullette, D. E., and J. F. Heisinger. 1980. Reingestion of feces by *Microtus pennsylvanicus.* J. Mamm., 61:366–368.

Parra, R. 1978. Comparison of foregut and hindgut fermentation in herbivores. Pp. 205–229, *in* The ecology of arboreal folivores (G. G. Montgomery, ed.). Smithsonian Inst. Press, Washington, D. C., 573 pp.

Pitelka, F. A. 1964. The nutrient-recovery hypothesis for arctic microtine cycles. I. Introduction. Pp. 55–56, *in* Grazing in terrestrial and marine environments (D. Crisp, ed.). Blackwell Sci. Publ., Oxford, 573 pp.

Pulliam, H. R. 1975. Diet optimization with nutrient constraints. Amer. Nat., 109:765–768.

Rhoades, D. F., and R. G. Cates. 1976. Towards a general theory of plant antiherbivore chemistry. Recent Adv. Phytochem., 10:168–213.

Robbins, C. T. 1983. Wildlife feeding and nutrition. Academic Press, New York, 343 pp.

Rothstein, B. E., and R. H. Tamarin. 1977. Feeding behavior of the insular beach vole, *Microtus breweri.* J. Mamm., 58:84–85.

Russo, S. L., J. S. Shenk, R. F. Barnes, and J. E. Moore. 1981. The weanling vole as a bioassay of forage quality of temperate and tropical grasses. J. Anim. Sci., 52:1205–1210.

Sanders, E. H., P. D. Gardner, P. J. Berger, and N. C. Negus. 1981. 6-methoxybenzoxazolinone: a plant derivative that stimulates reproduction in *Microtus montanus.* Science, 214:67–69.

Schultz, A. M. 1964. The nutrient recovery hypothesis for arctic microtine cycles. II. Ecosystem variables in relation to arctic microtine cycles. Pp. 57–68, *in* Grazing in terrestrial and marine environments (D. Crisp, ed.). Blackwell Sci. Publ., Oxford, 573 pp.

———. 1969. A study of an ecosystem; the arctic tundra. Pp. 77–93, *in* The ecosystem concept in natural resource management (G. Van Dyne, ed.). Academic Press, New York, 372 pp.

Shenk, J. S. 1976. The meadow vole as an experimental animal. Lab Anim. Sci., 26:664–669.

Shenk, J. S., F. C. Elliot, and J. W. Thomas. 1970. Meadow vole nutrition studies with semisynthetic diets. J. Nutr., 100:1437–1446.
Shenk, J. S., M. L. Risius, and R. F. Barnes. 1974. Weanling vole responses to crownvetch forage. Agron. J., 66:13–15.
Staaland, H. 1975. Absorption of sodium, potassium and water in the colon of the Norway lemming *Lemmus lemmus* (L.). Comp. Biochem. Physiol., 52A:77–80.
Stenseth, N. C., and L. Hansson. 1979. Optimal food selection: a graphic model. Amer. Nat., 113:373–389.
Stenseth, N. C., L. Hansson, and A. Myllymäki. 1977. Food selection of the field vole *Microtus agrestis*. Oikos, 29:511–524.
Taitt, M. J., and C. J. Krebs. 1981. The effect of extra food on small rodent populations: II. Voles (*Microtus townsendii*). J. Anim. Ecol., 50:125–137.
Tamarin, R. H. 1977. Demography of the beach vole (*Microtus breweri*) and the meadow vole (*Microtus pennsylvanicus*) in southeastern Massachusetts. Ecology, 58:1310–1321.
Tast, J. 1974. The food and feeding habits of the root vole, *Microtus oeconomus,* in Finnish Lapland. Aquilo Ser. Zool., 15:25–32.
Ulyatt, M. J. 1973. The feeding value of herbage. Pp. 131–178, *in* Chemistry and biochemistry of herbage, Vol. III (G. W. Butler and R. W. Bailey, eds.). Academic Press, New York, 295 pp.
Vorontsov, N. 1962. The ways of food specialization and evolution of the alimentary system in Muroidea. Pp. 360–377, *in* Symposium theriologicum. Publ. House Czech. Acad. Sci., Praha.
———. 1967. Evolution of the alimentary system of myomorph rodents (transl.). Indian Nat. Sci. Doc. Centre, New Dehli, 346 pp.
West, S. D. 1982. Dynamics of colonization and abundance in central Alaskan populations of the northern red-backed vole, *Clethrionomys rutilus.* J. Mamm., 63:128–143.
Westoby, M. 1974. An analysis of diet selection by large generalist herbivores. Amer. Nat., 108:290–304.
———. 1978. What are the biological bases of varied diets? Amer. Nat., 112:627–631.
Whitney, P. 1976. Population ecology of subarctic microtine rodents. Ecol. Monogr., 46:85–104.
Williams, O. 1962. A technique for studying microtine food habits. J. Mamm., 43:365–368.
Wolff, J. O., and W. Z. Lidicker, Jr. 1980. Population ecology of the taiga vole, *Microtus xanthognathus,* in interior Alaska. Canadian J. Zool., 58:1800–1812.
Zimmerman, E. G. 1965. A comparison of habitat and food of two species of *Microtus.* J. Mamm., 46:605–612.

ENERGETICS AND THERMOREGULATION

BRUCE A. WUNDER

Abstract

In general, *Microtus* species live in cool environments, are thought to have a boreal origin, and are small. They feed primarily upon vegetative plant parts which have relatively high fiber and low digestibility. Thus, voles should have high energy needs while feeding on an energetically dilute, but abundant, food; yet none shows any form of torpor. This review covers the manner in which voles accumulate and allocate energy and the environmental and social factors which affect those processes.

Digestibility of food by voles varies between species and is affected by season and plant or plant part, but it does not seem to be affected by increased energy flow drains from cold stress or reproduction. *Microtus* species regulate body temperature (T_B) well but generally have not been tested at extremely low ambient temperatures. The data available make it difficult to conclude whether they regulate at high T_B or not. *Microtus* species can vary insulation relative to habitat and season but do not show high insulation as a group. Basal metabolism (BMR) of *Microtus* species is about 20–40% greater than expected from allometry (but not the 70–80% greater that is now given in the literature). The effects of food, photoperiod, and temperature on BMR and non-shivering thermogenesis are discussed.

When expressed as exponential growth constants, but not when summed as growth during lactation, growth rates of *Microtus* species are high. However, many environmental factors affect these rates and the energy required for them. Gestation and lactation necessitate about 35% and 100–120% increases in energy flow, respectively, although values for *M. pinetorum* are low. Population energy considerations are briefly discussed.

Introduction

To exist as homeotherms and continue as populations or as species, mammals must acquire and expend energy. There are several reviews of the general concepts of how and what avenues are used by animals in general, and mammals in particular, to do this (Calow, 1977; Slobodkin, 1962; Townsend and Calow, 1981). There are also several reviews of energetics in small mammals in particular (Ferns, 1980; Gessaman, 1973; Grodziński and Wunder, 1975).

To exist and to maintain body mass and body temperature a vole must balance energy gain with energy expenditures. We can envision such balance and the avenues for exchange in Fig. 1. I discussed these balance factors before as representing a cascade of priorities for energy use (Wunder, 1978*a*). First, a vole initially must allocate enough energy for thermoregulation to maintain body temperature; otherwise it will become hypothermic and can do nothing else. Second, because foraging is the only feedback for energy acquisition, that need must be met, and will vary depending upon the animal's total energy needs. Once these two functions are met, excess energy can be stored (fat) or used for other activities. One important aspect of this view, and implied in the model, is that energy allocated to one function generally cannot be used for another. In order to reproduce, a vole must accumulate enough energy to thermoregulate, feed, and then meet all the physiological and behavioral requirements for reproduction. Another assumption made in considering the importance of energetics for organisms is that energy may be limiting at certain times for certain activities during an animal's life (for example, during winter there may not be enough energy for both thermoregulation and reproduction).

There are several ways of looking at energy limitations. I previously discussed some of these such as total needs and turnover needs (Wunder, 1978*a*). In addition, energy availability in the environment (food density) may limit an animal's capacity to acquire and use energy. Another limiting factor that is seldom considered by ecologists is the limitation imposed by the morphology and physiology of the gut. An animal's acquisition of energy is limited by the volume of food it can process per unit time and the efficiency of energy extraction from that volume. Thus, even though energy may be available in the environment, it can only become chemically

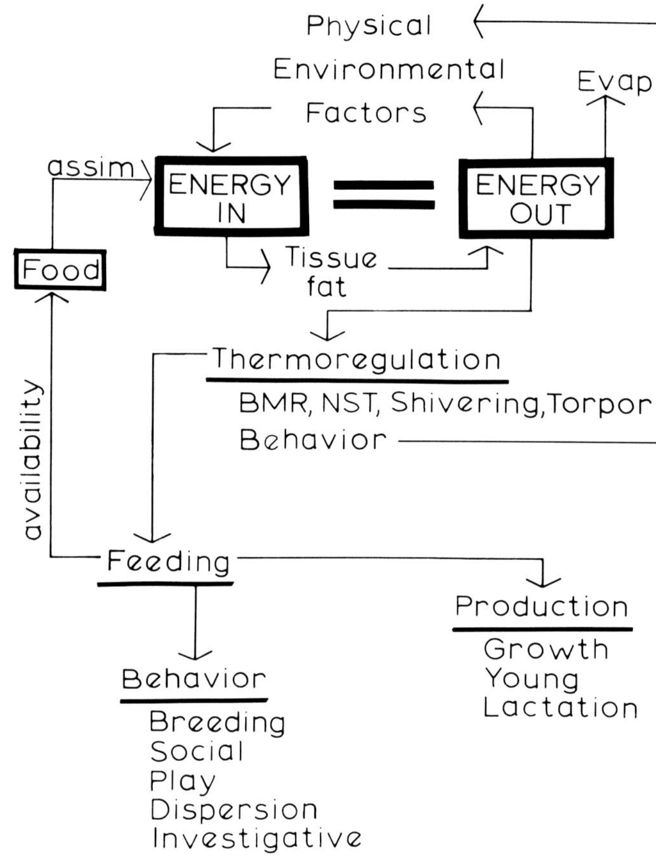

FIG. 1. A conceptual model of energy balance for a small mammal, indicating a priority cascade for energy allocation. Lines represent both total energy flow and rate functions (from Wunder (1978*a*), with permission). Abbreviations are: BMR, basal metabolism; NST, non-shivering thermogenesis; Evap, evaporation; assim, assimilation.

available for an organism within certain limits. White (1978) discussed this as a relative shortage of food.

Energy limitation is significant in the life histories of *Microtus*. In general, *Microtus* species live in cool environments, are thought to have a boreal origin (Hooper, 1949; Zakrzewski, this volume; Hoffmann and Koeppl, this volume), and they are small. They feed primarily on vegetative plant parts, which have high fiber and low digestibility (Grodziński and Wunder, 1975). They are the only small mammals that do not regularly feed on a calorically dense food (flesh, seeds, or fruits) and that do not show any form of torpor. Most cricetines or other small mammals, by contrast, hibernate (for example, *Zapus*) or at least show daily torpor (for example, *Peromyscus*). Thus, voles have high energy needs yet feed on an energetically inferior but abundant food type. Most of this review considers energy balance at the individual level and how *Microtus* species solve these problems. In this discussion I emphasize New World *Microtus*; however, reference to Old World forms is necessary because much work has been done with them.

From studies of ecosystem function ecologists have developed an interest in the concept of ecosystem energy flow (from Lindemann, 1942, to recent IBP studies). Thus, there is an interest in how small mammals like *Microtus* may be involved. Because there have not been many detailed studies of this type (but see Ferns, 1980; French et al., 1976; Golley, 1960; Whitney, 1977), I only cover this subject lightly.

Methods

A variety of techniques has been used to investigate the bioenergetics of small mammals (Grodziński and Wunder, 1975; Grodziński et al., 1975; Petrusewicz and MacFadyen, 1970). Basically they consist of respirometry trials, which give information about maintenance costs or food consumption trials that include both maintenance and production costs. Respiration trials cannot give information about energy tied up in production because they only measure consumption or production of gases associated with respiration (oxygen, carbon dioxide) as an index to heat production.

There is a certain terminology used in bioenergetics and since I use it throughout the chapter, I discuss it here. Food energy that is ingested is called *ingestion* (I) or *consumption*. Energy that is not absorbed through the gut is lost in the feces and called *egested energy* (F). Food absorbed into the blood may be stored or utilized. When utilized, most carbon is ultimately lost as CO_2. When protein is catabolized, nitrogen is released and forms urea. This is voided in urine and the energy lost in these chemical bonds is *excretory energy* (U). Since it is now used throughout the ecological literature, I use

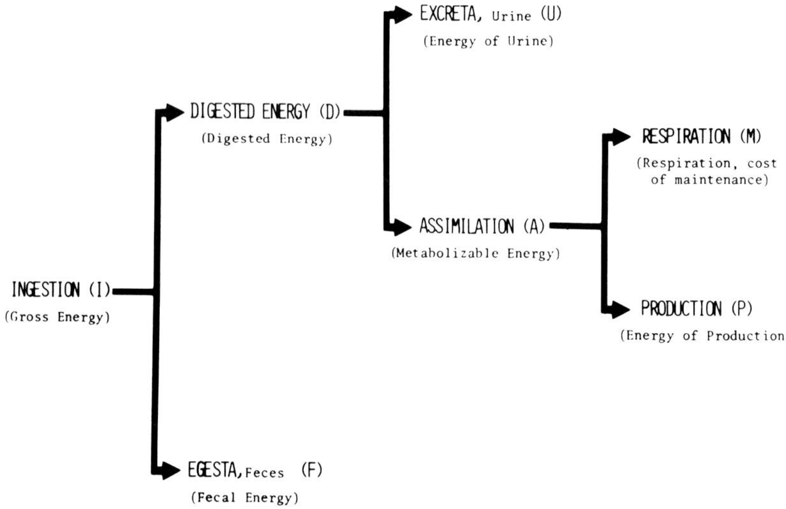

FIG. 2. Conceptual relation of energy compartmentalization in mammals. Terminology is from Petrusewicz (1967).

the terminology of Petrusewicz (1967). In his terminology the portion of consumption remaining after deducting egestion and excretion is called *assimilation* (A). This definition differs from that normally used by physiologists and animal nutritionists who define assimilation as consumption minus egestion (Brody, 1945). This latter quantity is called *digestion* (D) by Petrusewicz. Fig. 2 outlines the relation between these parameters.

Energy balance of an individual can be represented by the following equation:

$$A = I - (F + U) = M + P \tag{1}$$

where A equals energy assimilated into the body for use by an animal, I is total energy ingested, and F and U are energy lost in feces and urine, respectively. M is energy used for maintenance functions and P is energy expended and stored due to production (this may include growth of an individual and development of embryos and young). Digestibility refers to the amount of energy (or any nutrient under consideration) digested relative to that ingested and is usually referred to as a percent, which can be represented by the equation:

$$\text{Percent digestibility} = \frac{D}{I} \times 100 \qquad (2)$$

where D = (I − F). This is a useful concept because it gives an index to how much of the energy in a volume of food can be extracted. For *Microtus,* such an index can be important because many voles eat vegetative plant parts which are not as highly digestible as fruit or seeds (Grodziński and Wunder, 1975). When reading the literature one must be careful to note whether digestibility includes or excludes urinary energy loss. Not all authors use the term the same way; however, urinary energy loss is usually no more than 2–4% of total ingestion (Grodziński and Wunder, 1975).

For estimating maintenance costs several approaches are used. In some energetics models standard metabolic rate (SMR—resting metabolic rate in thermoneutrality; see Bartholomew, 1977) multiplied by some constant (usually 2 or 3) is used as an index to total energy costs (see Gessaman, 1973). Another approach devised by Grodziński (see Grodziński and Wunder, 1975) is to use the Average Daily Metabolic Rate (ADMR). This is determined by measuring metabolic rate (usually oxygen consumption) for 24 h from an animal in a cage with food, water, nesting material, and occasionally an exercise wheel. The idea is that this better approximates field conditions because the animal can be active and feeding (Grodziński and Wunder, 1975) and different temperatures can be used to simulate different seasons. The use of radioisotopes or other tracers has been used to estimate metabolism of mammals in the field (Mullen, 1973), but they have not been used with *Microtus.* A last approach is to combine field-time budget data with a metabolic model, which allows estimates of instantaneous rates of metabolism (Wunder, 1975). The first two methods give an integrated single value for metabolism over some time period (usually 24 h). Thus, there is no easy way to test the effects of environmental change or animal activity. By using a mechanistic model (Wunder, 1975), sensitivity analyses can be made to test for effects of changes in activity level or period and changes in nest or air temperature for various periods over a 24-h day.

Energy Acquisition

Mammals may use solar energy as a means of increasing their surface temperature and hence effectively increase insulation, thus sparing energy needed for thermoregulation (Campbell, 1977); but they cannot gain useful energy (for biochemical processes) from the sun or other sources of radiant energy (houses, barns, etc.). Given that they inhabit environments with grasses or other types of closed microcanopies, *Microtus* species probably use the sun little, if at all, for behavioral thermoregulation. Thus, accumulating food energy is the primary mode of energy acquisition for *Microtus*. This involves two general processes. Voles must find, handle, and chew food, and they need to digest and assimilate this food.

Gathering Food

Gathering food involves a variety of activities and the associated costs are not simply energetics, but include risks (ecological costs such as predation and social interaction). There are numerous reviews on foraging strategies (Charnov, 1976; Pyke et al., 1977; Schoener, 1971); most theories consider the time and energy costs involved in finding and handling food. For *Microtus,* these may not be significant because most voles feed on grasses or dicot leaves; hence, finding food may not be a major energetic challenge for them (but see Batzli, this volume; Madison, this volume; Wolff, this volume).

Furthermore, there are few references to species of *Microtus* storing food as is frequently the case with cricetines and other small granivores (Barry, 1976). However, Wunder (1978*a*) suggested that clipped vegetation left by *Microtus* may be used as a nutrient (especially protein) source in winter. Wolff and Lidicker (1980) reported that yellow-cheeked voles (*M. xanthognathus*) store rhizomes for winter.

Digestibility and Processing

Although *Microtus* feed primarily upon vegetative plant parts, which are relatively easy to find, this does not necessarily mean that acquiring energy is not a problem for them because there is another step involved in "gaining" energy: digestion and processing. *Microtus* species may be food limited in how well and how fast they can digest and assimilate energy from a food source (White, 1978; Wunder, 1978*a*). In this regard, energy acquisition entails three functions: 1) how well food can be processed (what is the digestibility), 2) how fast a unit volume can be processed, and 3) how much volume can be processed per unit time. For *Microtus,* there is in-

TABLE 1
DIGESTIBILITY OF DIFFERENT FOODS BY *Microtus*

Species	Season and food	Digestibility (%)	Reference
M. californicus	Rabbit chow	52.8	Batzli and Cole (1979)
	Bromegrass	48.8	
	Ryegrass	73.0	
	Lab chow	77.4	Bradley (1976)
M. mexicanus	Lab chow	76.5	Bradley (1976)
M. ochrogaster	Summer; rat chow	72.7	Cherry and Verner (1975)
	Winter; rat chow	65.3	
	Rabbit chow	68.2	Batzli and Cole (1979)
	Alfalfa	65.5	
	Rabbit chow and alfalfa	57.9	
	Bluegrass	49.6	
	Tundra monocots	51.3	
	Rat chow	74.4	Bradley (1976)
M. oeconomus (European populations)	Spring; mixed grasses and herbs	69.7	Gebczyńska (1970)
	Summer; mixed grasses and herbs	68.7	
	Autumn; mixed grasses and herbs	73.7	
	Autumn; as above plus beets and roots of parsnip and carrots	91.4	
M. pennsylvanicus	Oatmeal, lettuce, carrots	82.2	Golley (1960)
	Alfalfa	89.8	
	Bluegrass, white clover	61.5	Cowan et al. (1968)
	Rat chow	81.1	Johnson and Groepper (1970)
	Bluegrass	46.0	Johanningsmeier and Goodnight (1969)
	Red top (*Agrostis stolonifera*)	40.0	
	Rat chow	77.7	Bradley (1976)
M. pinetorum	Lab chow	79.9	Bradley (1976)
	Lab chow	81.0	Lochmiller et al. (1982)
M. richardsoni	Lab chow	80.5	Bradley (1976)

formation available on digestibility, but relatively little information is available on the latter two components. They are areas in need of much more study.

The ability of small mammals to extract energy from food varies as a function of food type (animal matter, fruits, and seeds are more digestible than vegetative plant parts such as leaves and stems); it has been discussed by Grodziński and Wunder (1975). Since most *Microtus* species are grazing herbivores (but see Batzli, this volume), in contrast to other small mammals, they should have lower digestibility, and must process more food to gain similar amounts of energy. Therefore one might predict that in times of energy stress microtines should change digestive efficiency, food type (to one more digestible), food volume processed per unit time, or some combination.

Unfortunately, most studies on digestibility have been performed with artificial diets (for example, lab chows), which don't really tell us much about how much energy wild *Microtus* species may be getting from natural diets. What information there is in the literature suggests that digestibilities for grazing herbivores range from 60 to 70% (Grodziński and Wunder, 1975); however, recently Batzli and Cole (1979) cautioned that these values actually range from 30 to 90% depending upon species of herbivore and the plant material consumed. Table 1 compares some of the data from the literature for digestibility in New World *Microtus* (Old World forms show similar values; Batzli and Cole, 1979; Grodziński and Wunder, 1975). As an example of this variability, Cole and Batzli (1979) found that the digestibilities of alfalfa and bluegrass, which have similar energy densities, were quite different (67% and 50%, respectively) in *M. ochrogaster*. Thus, we really need more careful studies of digestibility for natural diets of species of *Microtus*.

Seasonal changes in plant composition can affect digestibility. Keys and Van Soest (1970) showed that digestibility decreased as the amount of cell-wall (fiber) content in the diet increased for *M. pennsylvanicus*. Thus, it is interesting to note that, although beach voles (*M. breweri*) eat primarily beach grass, they eat different parts at different seasons (Goldberg et al., 1980). In their study, Goldberg et al. (1980) noted that voles did not always choose those portions of the plant with the highest energy content. However, they did note that voles usually chose those plant parts which had the lowest cell-wall content (determined by neutral detergent fiber analysis) and speculated that beach voles ". . . probably realize the advantage of increased assimilation of energy and nutrients . . . ." by selecting such foods. Energy content was not studied in that investigation but it poses the interesting possibility that energy levels (through digestibility) may have varied. More studies of a similar sort are needed to see whether *Microtus* species can select more digestible food at energetically stressful times of year.

Certain chemicals in food affect digestibility. Kendall et al. (1979) found that certain allelochemicals in forage plants can inhibit forage intake by meadow voles (*M. pennsylvanicus*). Negus (pers. comm.) also found that the compound 6-MBOA in green vegetation increases growth in *M. montanus* (Sanders et al., 1981) without necessitating significant increases in food intake over controls, implying that some digestive or processing changes are occurring. And energy density in food itself may influence intake. Although Batzli and Cole (1979) suggested that microtines do not regulate food intake on the basis of energetic considerations alone, Kendall et al. (1978) and Shenk et al. (1970) showed that individual meal size in *M. pennsylvanicus* is regulated by energy content when energy concentration in the food is high and by gastrointestinal fill when it is low. This suggests that energy density in food can be an important factor limiting energy accumulation and should be investigated more critically in *Microtus,* especially because there may be species differences in food digestibility.

The only data relating to seasonal changes in digestibility independent of food type are those of Cherry and Verner (1975) for *M. ochrogaster* eating lab chow. Digestibility was 73% in summer and 65% in winter. For Old World *M. agrestis,* Hansson (1971) also found digestibility of a mixed grass diet to be slightly lower in winter than in summer.

Energy Allocation

Maintenance

Temperature regulation.—Since there are no reports of any species of *Microtus* (or any microtine) showing torpor either on a seasonal basis (hibernating) or for a shorter term (daily), they must always expend energy for thermoregulation. In contrast, many cricetines and other small mammals in similar habitats are capable of daily torpor, if not hibernation, when thermal stress is high (cold) or energy difficult to find (Wunder, 1978*a*). Thus, thermoregulation is a major maintenance cost for species of *Microtus,* but one which allows them to be active throughout the year.

Microtus species studied to date are able to regulate body temperature (T_B) well. Their patterns of regulation relative to ambient temperature (T_A) exposures are similar to other small placental mammals. In most studies, voles were not exposed to T_A much below 0°C and all species studied were able to maintain T_B at that exposure (Beck and Anthony, 1971; Bradley, 1976; Hart, 1971; Packard, 1968; Wunder et al., 1977). In a study of microtine rodents, Bradley (1976) found that six species of *Microtus* (*pennsylvanicus, ochrogaster, mexicanus, californicus, pinetorum, richardsoni* [=*Arvicola richardsonii*]) were able to maintain T_B constant between T_A exposures of 2–34°C. Above 34°C some species showed loss of T_B regulatory ability. Beck and Anthony (1971) noted that at high T_A (34 to 36°C) *M. longicaudus* showed obvious heat stress, but unlike some other small mammals (for example, *Peromyscus*), it did not show saliva-spreading to increase heat dissipation. They suggested that *Microtus* may not handle heat stress as well as other forms. However, this needs to be investigated more closely because results of Bradley (1976) and Wunder et al. (1977) suggest that many species of *Microtus,* as well as other small mammals, regulate at these high T_As.

There are no data suggesting that the level at which T_B is regulated changes seasonally; Wunder et al. (1977) showed that it definitely does not change in *M. ochrogaster.*

Bradley (1976) concluded that *Microtus* species regulate T_B at a high level. Using a review table from Hudson and Brower (1971), he calculated the mean T_B for 36 species of non-microtine rodents to be 37.3°C, whereas the mean T_B for six species of *Microtus* that he studied was 38.4°C. However, Wunder et al. (1977) did not find that *M. ochrogaster* regulated at such high levels. Prairie voles brought in from the field regulated at 37.8°C both in summer and winter. Perhaps this difference was due to technique. Our animals were fresh from the field and Bradley's *M. ochrogaster* were from a lab colony at Cornell University. Interestingly, our animals, which were held for warm (30°C) or cold (5°C) acclimation in the lab for 2 weeks, maintained higher T_B (38.3°C) following acclimation (similar to Bradley's voles in the lab). However, following lab acclimation and exposure to various T_As, *M. montanus* showed a T_B of 37.8°C (Packard, 1968), and *M. longicaudus* showed a T_B of 37.7°C (Beck and Anthony, 1971). Obviously, more studies need to investigate the level of T_B regulation more rigorously.

Thus, species of *Microtus* regulate T_B well, and none appear to resort to torpor. Considering that many species live in relatively cool regions or areas with cold winters, they have three methods to assist in maintaining T_B. They can 1) select warmer microclimates to reduce cold stress (for example, they can confine most activities to subnivean areas; Wolff, this volume); 2) increase insulation to reduce heat loss; and 3) increase thermogenic capacity.

Insulation is the inverse of thermal conductance (TC); hence, the values of TC can be used as an index to insulation (Bartholomew, 1977). Thermal conductances in New World *Microtus* are slightly less than those predicted by the allometric equation of Herreid and Kessel (1967; Table 2). However, they are generally not different from values for other similar sized cricetid rodents (Bradley, 1976). New world *Microtus* appear to show insulation values that are generally as expected for their body sizes, or slightly lower. In any case, they are not insulated extraordinarily for their size.

There have not been many studies which investigated factors affecting insulation in species of *Microtus*. However, Bradley (1976) found that habitat influences insulative values. *M. richardsoni* had the lowest thermal conductance; it occurs in a cold, aquatic environment. *M. pinetorum* had the value closest to that predicted by allometry; it has somewhat semi-fossorial habits in a potentially more stable microhabitat. Wunder et al. (1977) found that thermal conductance varied seasonally in *M. ochrogaster* (Table 2)—it was higher in winter than in summer—and it was not affected by heat or cold acclimation in either season. Much of the change was due to body-size changes. Interestingly, Cherry and Verner (1975), using different techniques, did not find significant seasonal changes in thermal conductance of *M. ochrogaster* in Illinois.

In summary, there appears to be some capacity for modification of thermal conductance in relation to habitat and season, but, in general, New World *Microtus* do not show any strong adaptive trends in insulation as might be expected for a small, boreal, non-hibernating mammal.

Insulation can also effectively be modified by nest behavior. *M. xanthognathus* (Wolff and Lidicker, 1980) and *M. pinetorum* are

TABLE 2

THERMAL CONDUCTANCE IN NEW WORLD *MICROTUS*. SPECIES ARE LISTED APPROXIMATELY IN ASCENDING ORDER OF BODY MASS

Species	Body mass (g)	Thermal conductance[1] Measured	Predicted[2]	Deviation from prediction (%)	Reference
M. longicaudus	25	0.87	0.97	−10	Beck and Anthony (1971)
M. pinetorum	26	0.92	0.95	−3	Bradley (1976)
M. mexicanus	27	0.81	0.93	−13	Bradley (1976)
M. montanus	31	0.82	0.87	−6	Packard (1968)
M. ochrogaster (summer)	37	0.75	0.79	−5	Cherry and Verner (1975)
M. ochrogaster (winter)	39	0.73	0.77	−5	Cherry and Verner (1975)
M. ochrogaster (summer)	48	0.56	0.70	−20	Wunder et al. (1977)
M. ochrogaster (winter)	38	0.71	0.78	−9	Wunder et al. (1977)
M. ochrogaster	50	0.61	0.68	−10	Bradley (1976)
M. pennsylvanicus	37	0.72	0.79	−9	Bradley (1976)
M. pennsylvanicus	51	0.67	0.67	0	Morrison and Ryser (1951)
M. californicus	43	0.66	0.73	−10	Bradley (1976)
M. richardsoni	51	0.56	0.67	−16	Bradley (1976)

[1] Units of thermal conductance are cal g^{-1} h^{-1} $°C^{-1}$.

[2] Predicted values were calculated using the allometric relation of Herreid and Kessel (1967): thermal conductance = $4.91(g)^{-.505}$.

social species which nest in groups during winter; thus, they may reduce their maintenance costs.

Thermogenesis.—The other principal means *Microtus* species have to combat winter cold is to increase metabolism. There are two metabolic components. One is minimal energy turnover, basal metabolism. In small mammals minimal energy needs are more appropriately described by standard metabolism (SMR; see Bartholomew, 1977) because the conditions necessary for defining basal metabolism are seldom met; yet the values reported are usually called basal as often as standard (see Grodziński and Wunder, 1975). The second component is the increase in metabolism above standard in response to low T_A (thermoregulatory response), which involves shivering and non-shivering thermogenesis (Janský, 1973; Wunder, 1979, 1984).

The pioneering studies of Kleiber (1932) and Brody (1945) established that metabolism in mammals is related to body size. In their classic paper, Scholander et al. (1950) suggested that basal metabolism (BMR) is not adaptive and the major means of adaptation to harsh environments is through thermal conductance (or insulation). More recently, however, several studies have shown that basal metabolism may be more adaptive than Scholander and his colleagues concluded. Many desert species show reduced BMRs (see Bartholomew, 1977; Hudson and Brower, 1971; Hudson et al., 1972) and some mammals have high BMRs (insectivores: Morrison et al. [1959], Neal and Lustick [1973]; *Lepus americanus*: Hart et al. [1965]; *Tamiasciurus hudsonicus*: Irving et al. [1955]; some pinnipeds and cetaceans: Hart and Irving [1959], Kanwisher and Sundes [1965]).

It is frequently stated that microtines have high BMRs (Grodziński and Wunder, 1975; Hart, 1971). This conclusion is based primarily upon the paper by Packard (1968) in which he reported a BMR (SMR) for *M. montanus* of 75% greater than that predicted by the allometric equation of Kleiber (1961). He also reviewed the literature available at that time and reported high BMR from other studies of microtines. Subsequently Beck and Anthony (1971), following Packard's methods, reported the SMR of *M. longicaudus* to be 75% greater than predicted. However, these values are all artificially high (Wunder et al., 1977). Most of the earlier reports dealt with animals that were not tested in thermoneutrality and hence had high responses because of added thermoregulatory costs (values can be found in Bradley, 1976, or Hart, 1971). Further, it is now well known that cold acclimation will cause an increase in SMR of many small mammals (Hart, 1971; Wunder, 1979). In attempting to maintain *M. montanus* and *M. longicaudus* on "natural" environmental conditions in the lab both species were actually cold acclimated, which probably accounts for the higher value (75%) than predicted. Wunder et al. (1977) found that the SMR of *M. ochrogaster* freshly captured from the field varied with season; the effects of cold or heat acclimation also varied with season (Table 3). Interestingly, when prairie voles (Wunder et al., 1977) were cold acclimated in winter (as in Packard's [1968] study), they too showed SMRs 80% greater than predicted. Nevertheless SMR val-

TABLE 3

METABOLISM OF PRAIRIE VOLES DURING SUMMER AND WINTER. DATA ARE FROM WUNDER ET AL. (1977), WITH METABOLISM MEASURED AT 27.5°C. VALUES GIVEN ARE MEANS ±1 *SD*. NUMBERS IN PARENTHESES ARE SAMPLE SIZES

Treatment[1]	Body mass (g)	Metabolism O_2 g^{-1} h^{-1} (ml)	Deviation from predicted[2] (%)
Winter, field	38.5 ± 4.5 (15)	2.16 ± 0.34 (15)	+41
Winter, 5°	41.0 ± 5.6 (8)	2.72 ± 0.40 (8)	+81
Winter, 30°	48.4 ± 8.9 (10)	2.19 ± 0.25 (10)	+52
Summer, field	47.4 ± 8.9 (9)	1.74 ± 0.20 (9)	+20
Summer, 5°	50.0 ± 4.7 (11)	1.76 ± 0.12 (11)	+23
Summer, 30°	48.5 ± 8.7 (10)	1.40 ± 0.15 (10)	0

[1] Treatments are voles fresh from the field or temperature acclimated at 5°C or 30°C during winter or summer.

[2] The following equation was used to estimate predicted metabolism: $O_2\ g^{-1}\ h^{-1} = 3.8\ W^{-0.25}$, in ml (modified from Morrison et al., 1959) for calculation of percent deviation.

ues for field animals were still higher than predicted by the Kleiber equation (20% in summer and 41% in winter). In addition, Bradley (1976) found that SMRs of the six *Microtus* species he studied (all under identical lab conditions) never deviated by more than 37% from the Kleiber prediction (Table 4), and *M. ochrogaster* was right on the predicted value. Thus, I conclude that SMRs of New World *Microtus* are higher than allometric predictions but only by 20–40%, not the 70–80% now given in the literature.

Packard (1968) argued that since the subfamily Microtinae apparently evolved in boreal regions, it is reasonable to postulate that high metabolic rates are adaptive to allow for increased thermogenesis during acute low-temperature stress. Janský (1966) and Lechner (1978) independently showed that maximal metabolism in mammals is generally not greater than 7–10 times the basal rate. If such is the case then increases in SMR may allow for a higher maximal thermogenesis and hence tolerance to lower T_A exposures.

The ambient temperature at which a mammal maintains T_B, given a particular metabolic rate, can be calculated by rearranging the following equation (Bartholomew, 1977):

$$MR = TC(T_B - T_A) \qquad (3)$$

TABLE 4

STANDARD METABOLIC RATES (SMRS) OF NEW WORLD *Microtus* STUDIED IN THE SAME LABORATORY (DATA FROM BRADLEY, 1976). SPECIES ARE LISTED IN DESCENDING ORDER OF SMR

Species	Body mass (g)	SMR $O_2\ g^{-1}\ h^{-1}$ (ml)	Predicted SMR	Deviation from predicted (%)
M. pinetorum	25	1.98	1.60	+24
M. pennsylvanicus	39	1.93	1.41	+37
M. richardsoni	51	1.74	1.31	+33
M. mexicanus	29	1.63	1.53	+6
M. californicus	44	1.55	1.37	+13
*M. ochrogaster**	54	1.18	1.29	−9

* See Table 3.

$$T_A = T_B - \frac{MR}{TC} \tag{4}$$

where T_A is ambient temperature, T_B is body temperature, TC is minimal thermal conductance, and MR is mass-specific metabolic rate. Using the allometric equations of Kleiber (1961) for SMR and Herreid and Kessel (1967) for TC, we can calculate the above values for any given body mass. If we assume maximal metabolism is seven times SMR (Lechner, 1978) and T_B is 38°C, then we can use equation (4) to calculate the minimal T_A which could be tolerated without a drop in T_B. For a 40-g mammal this would be −37.4°C. If SMR were increased by 30% and maximal metabolism is seven times that value, then the lower temperature at which the mammal could maintain T_B would be reduced to −60°C.

Thus, increasing SMR could be an effective means of lowering the lower lethal temperature. However, energetically it is rather expensive because there is the increased metabolic cost in thermoneutrality; that may be manifest all year although cold stress may only occur in winter. In fact, King and Farner (1961) argued that increased SMR for birds would not be adaptive because of the increased energy cost in thermoneutrality. Wunder et al. (1977) argued much the same for mammals (in that paper we incorrectly referred to seasonal changes in SMR as non-shivering thermogenesis; see below). It may well be that during their evolution, microtines moved from a calorically dense, hard-to-find food (seeds) to a calorically more dilute but easy-to-find food (vegetative plant parts). Thus, if the processing capacity of the gut existed (see below), readily available food could be used, allowing for high metabolism. But, of course, the argument does not provide an explanation for why high metabolic rates exist. There may be several reasons why *Microtus* species have slightly high rates of metabolism, and adaptation to cold may be only one. McNab (1980) recently argued that mammals with high metabolic turnover rates (see Kleiber [1975] for discussion of terminology) also show high potential for reproduction and hence population growth. Obviously this area needs more attention.

An important factor involved in acclimatization to winter cold is the increased capacity for thermoregulatory non-shivering thermogenesis (Janský, 1973; Wunder, 1979, 1984). As discussed in Janský (1973), a mammal metabolizes at the level of SMR in thermoneutrality, but when exposed to lower ambient temperatures, it must increase thermogenesis. In small forms (<5 to 10 kg) the first mechanism used is non-shivering thermogenesis (NST); they then turn to shivering when NST capacity is nearly exhausted. The advantage of NST over increases in SMR for increasing metabolic capacity is that it is only used at low T_A and hence does not increase energetic costs when not in use (for example, in thermoneutrality). The capacity for NST in small mammals can be enhanced following cold exposure or in response to photoperiod changes so that total metabolic capacity can be increased during colder times of year and as needed. I (Wunder, 1981, 1984) found that *M. ochrogaster* changed capacity for NST from essentially no capacity to 17.1 cal g^{-1} h^{-1} following cold (5°C) acclimation in the lab. When tested fresh from the field in July prairie voles had no significant NST. The capacity increased during fall and animals caught in December showed 10.5 cal g^{-1} h^{-1}. This represented an increase of 136% over SMR, a significantly greater addition to thermogenesis than increased SMR following cold exposure. These winter NST values varied from year to year and probably depend upon the T_A to which the voles were exposed before capture (Wunder, 1978*b*, 1984).

Since most *Microtus* species are seasonally exposed to cold it would seem adaptive to stimulate NST capacity prior to cold exposure. It is now well established (Heldmaier et al., 1982) that short photoperiods can stimulate NST capacity in dwarf hamsters (*Phodopus sungorus*) and *Peromyscus leucopus* (Lynch and Gendler,

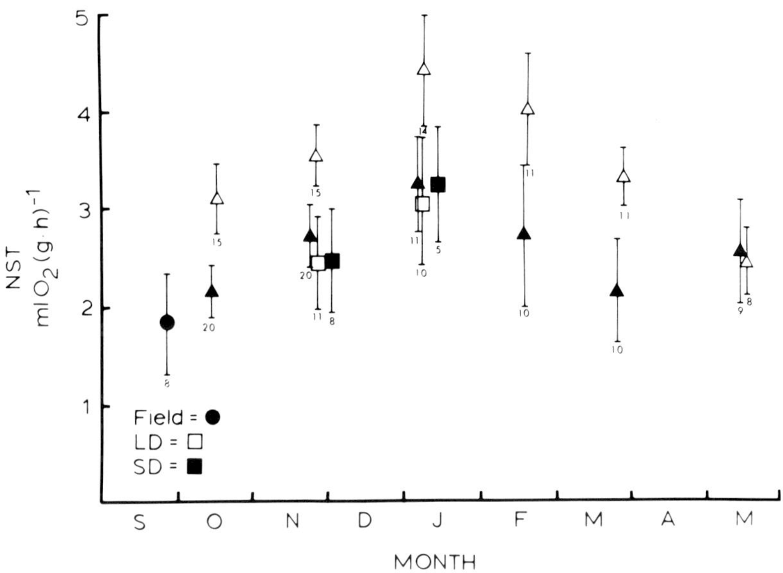

FIG. 3. Seasonal changes in non-shivering thermogenesis (NST) of *M. ochrogaster*. Symbols designate means; numbers are sample sizes; vertical lines represent ±2 *SE*. Unshaded triangles are voles held outside, and shaded triangles voles held at a constant lab temperature (23°C) but with a seasonally changing photoperiod. The shaded circle indicates animals fresh from the field in September; unshaded and shaded squares are animals held on long-day (15L:9D) or short-day (9L:15D) photoperiods, respectively, captured in September and tested in November and January.

1980; Lynch et al., 1978). Initial experiments suggested that *M. ochrogaster* also was sensitive to photoperiod (Wunder, 1984). However, voles were studied throughout the year only on natural photoperiods at a constant lab temperature of 23°C. Subsequent studies with voles exposed to long (15L:9D) and short (9L:15D) photoperiods throughout fall and winter suggested that they did not cue on photoperiod but had an endogenous rhythm for changes in NST (Wunder, pers. observ.; Fig. 3). Voles held on either photoperiod increased NST into winter just like the animals on natural photoperiods, with no statistically significant differences among the groups.

Thus, NST is a powerful means whereby *Microtus* species enhance their capacity for thermogenesis at low T_A exposures without increasing energetic costs in thermoneutrality. The capacity can be enhanced by low T_A exposure either chronically (Wunder, pers. observ.) or by short daily exposure to low T_A (Wunder, 1981, pers. observ.). Although *Phodopus sungorus* and *Peromyscus leucopus* change NST capacity in response to short-day photoperiods in fall, it is still unclear whether *M. ochrogaster* does so or whether it has an endogenous rhythm for seasonal changes in NST.

Activity.—The energetic costs of activity in species of *Microtus* are largely unknown. To estimate such costs we need to know the cost of locomotion per unit time or speed and the amount of time spent in such activity each day (or year, depending upon the time frame). There are many studies of activity patterns and time spent active by *Microtus* for laboratory, enclosures, and field circumstances (Wolff, this volume; Madison, this volume). The energetic costs of locomotion can be estimated from the allometric relations published by Taylor et al. (1982), but no *Microtus* species have been studied in this manner. Given that species of *Microtus* are active so often throughout a 24-h period, they should be good experimental subjects for studies of activity costs.

Production

Growth.—The energetic consequences and costs of growth in New World *Microtus* have received some attention. Growth ties up energy in tissue and includes the energetic cost of building such tissue. The cost for energy in tissue is relatively easy to measure and calculate; it is the product of the mass of tissue accumulated multiplied by its caloric density:

$$\begin{matrix}\text{Energy accumulated in}\\ \text{tissue during growth}\end{matrix} = \begin{matrix}\text{increase}\\ \text{in mass}\end{matrix} \times \text{caloric density.}$$

In mature animals this tissue is usually fat; in young animals it reflects a combination of body components. But these potential differences have not been well studied. The costs for growth were reviewed by Grodziński and Wunder (1975) and their conclusions remain unaltered. Energy content of tissue in *Microtus* species is 1.03 kcal/g (Górecki, 1965), so growth, at a minimum, costs that much per gram to produce.

The other cost of growth is the metabolic cost of building additional tissue. This topic has been addressed critically in the animal production literature but has not been pursued by ecologists, perhaps because it is not easy to measure. Theoretical considerations of the energy contained in, and biochemical processes associated with, fat disposition suggest that deposition of fat should cost little more than a 2% increase over normal metabolic costs (Baldwin and Smith, 1974). However, Jagosz et al. (1979) estimated empirically that tissue deposition costs are 8.57 kcal g^{-1} in *Microtus agrestis,* and that overall cost of depositing and subsequently using energy stored in tissue (versus catabolizing the original foodstuffs) is 35% greater. Rock and Williams (1979) proposed that fat levels may serve as an index to the "condition" of an animal. They stressed *M. montanus* with low-food rations, low temperature, or both, and showed that fat reserves seem to serve as an energy store used in response to environmental stress.

Rapid growth rates have been suggested as important features of animal life histories because they allow animals to reach maturity faster (see Case, 1978, for discussion). In addition, McNab (1980) argued that increased metabolic turnover rate (Kleiber, 1975) allows for faster individual growth which, in turn, allows for faster population growth. Thus, it seems important to ask whether species of *Microtus* have increased growth rates compared to other similar-sized small mammals, because they can attain high population densities rapidly. Table 5 summarizes growth data for different species of *Microtus* during lactation; this is usually the period of fastest growth. Using this index, most species are comparable to other similar-sized small mammals (Table 5; Morrison et al., 1977). However, using a logistic growth constant (Ricklefs, 1967), McNab (1980) argued that microtines have higher growth rates than similar-sized cricetines.

There are several factors which affect growth rates. They can be categorized as physical factors in the environment and social factors. There are numerous reports in the literature that many small mammals from boreal regions show lower body masses in winter than in summer (Brown, 1973, and references therein; Dehnel, 1949; Fuller et al., 1969; Schwarz et al., 1964). A number of species of *Microtus* are included in these studies. For a long while it was proposed that the reason lower average body mass was found in winter was because older, heavier individuals died, leaving only younger cohort animals. We now know that individual animals actually lose mass in winter or change growth rates. This was shown clearly in field studies with marked individuals of *M. pennsylvanicus* (Brown, 1973; Iverson and Turner, 1974). Season appears to affect growth in this species. Several factors could be im-

TABLE 5
GROWTH IN MALE AND FEMALE *Microtus*

Species	Adult body mass (g)	Growth rate[1] (g/d)	Growth rate[1] % Adult body mass	Lab or field study	Season of birth	Reference
M. abbreviatus	56	0.82	1.5	L	—	
M. californicus	53	0.83	1.6	L	—	Hatfield (1935)
	62	0.98	1.6	L	—	Selle (1928)
M. miurus	36	0.56	1.6	L	—	Morrison et al. (1977)
M. montanus	40	0.63	1.6		—	Seidal and Booth, *in* Innes and Millar (1979)
M. oregoni	22	0.61	2.8	L	—	Cowan and Arsenault (1954)
M. ochrogaster	—	0.61	—	L	—	Fitch (1957)
	—	0.81	—	L	—	Richmond and Conaway (1969)
	45	0.83	1.8	?	—	Cooksey, *in* Innes and Millar (1979)
	—	0.73	—	L	—	Kruckenberg et al. (1973)
M. oeconomus	45	0.79	1.8	L	—	Morrison et al. (1954)
	32	0.67	2.1	L	—	Morrison et al. (1977)
M. pennsylvanicus	35	0.40	1.1	F	June–Aug	Barbehenn (1955)
	35	0.20	0.6	F	July–Sept	
	48	0.80	1.7	L	—	Hamilton (1937)
	29	0.67	2.2	L	—	Innes and Millar (1979)
	40	0.65	1.6	L	—	Morrison et al. (1977)
M. pinetorum[2]	28	0.52	1.8	L	—	Hamilton (1938)
	29	0.35[3]	1.2	L	—	Lochmiller et al. (1982)

[1] Growth rates were usually calculated to 20 days of age.
[2] Value of growth calculated to weaning at age of 17 days.
[3] Growth rates were calculated as the average, for the average litter size (2.2), because growth varied with litter size.

portant in causing (ultimate factors) or cueing (proximate factors) such changes. Two obvious factors that affect growth (and hence the energy costs of it) during winter are decreased quality of food and an increased proportion of energy intake necessary for thermoregulation. These suppositions have not been tested directly; however, some component parts have. There have been no careful studies of the effects of temperature on growth in New World *Microtus*; however, Daketse and Martinet (1977) studied its effects on young *M. arvalis* and found (contrary to the suppositions above) that the young grow faster and larger when raised at lower temperatures (5°C) rather than at higher temperatures (22 or 33°C). We also know that lab animals (rats, pigs, etc.) grow larger when raised at low T_A with plenty of food available. Thus, this growth may be due to high food availability (and high-quality food) while at low T_A.

It is also known that food quality or some factor in food may affect growth rates of *Microtus* species. Daketse and Martinet (1977) found that voles fed alfalfa harvested in spring grew faster and heavier than those exposed to the same conditions except fed alfalfa harvested in summer. In field and enclosure studies, Cole and Batzli (1979) demonstrated that *M. ochrogaster* grew faster and attained higher body mass when fed alfalfa than when sustained on bluegrass or prairie habitats. It is not known whether such effects are due to some special nutrient, to a caloric deficiency, or to some digestive difference. However, Batzli and Cole (1979) showed that *M. ochrogaster* does not do as well on monocots as do other *Microtus* species, but does grow better on dicots. It also may be that these forage effects are due to chemicals in the food acting as cueing agents to affect the animals' physiology. Negus and his colleagues showed that specific chemicals in plants eaten by *M. montanus* can affect reproduction and growth (Berger et al. 1981; Negus, pers. comm.).

One other physical environmental factor that may affect growth is photoperiod. Although growth of certain *Microtus* species varies with season (see above), the factors affecting such growth are not known. Pinter (1968) showed that photoperiod affected growth of *M. montanus,* and Petterborg (1978) showed that photoperiod may be the most important factor that affects differential growth (and hence maturation) in different seasonal cohorts for this species. More recently, Pistole and Cranford (1982) found that photoperiod affects growth in *M. pennsylvanicus.* In both species, young animals on long-day photoperiods grew faster than those on short-day photoperiods, and adult animals on long days maintained a higher body mass than those on short days. Further, adults on short days lost body mass, whereas long days stimulated growth to, or maintenance of, high mass. When animals in any treatment were switched to the alternate photic conditions they reversed their mass dynamics to reflect their photic environment. The energetic consequences of such changes are that animals on short days have less body mass to maintain, or with lower growth rates they have a lower energetic commitment to growth.

Several studies suggest that social factors affect growth in species of *Microtus*. Batzli et al. (1977) found that when *M. ochrogaster* were raised in the laboratory in the same cage as littermates, they showed suppressed growth and maturation compared to controls raised alone in cages or when raised with strangers of the opposite sex. The pattern was not clear with *M. pennsylvanicus,* which the authors attributed to differences in habitat type and use. Baddaloo and Clulow (1981) subsequently showed that female *M. pennsylvanicus* grew faster (compared to controls) when exposed to males or male urine, even if separated by a wire barrier. They proposed that growth may be controlled by a pheromone in male urine.

Beacham (1980) also reported that growth may be influenced by population density in *M. townsendii* and that this effect may be influenced by differential growth rate of "behavioral types" in the population. In this field study he showed that voles born in spring had higher growth rates than those born in any other season and that growth rates decreased in summer and autumn (a photoperiod effect?). He also found that heavy males present in peak populations gained mass throughout the previous winter, whereas all other males lost body mass. Beacham and Krebs (1980) categorized voles as docile or aggressive and found that "docile" *M. townsendii* under 50 g had faster growth rates than similar-sized aggressive ones. The energetics of these changes in growth have not been investigated so we do not know whether the changes are simply the consequence of changes in food consumption, changes in relative efficiencies, or due to differential hormone levels. These studies clearly indicate that once voles are weaned and exposed to the physical and biological environment many factors may affect their growth rates.

Reproduction.—A convenient way to envision the costs of reproduction is to divide them into those occurring during gestation and those during lactation. Such a division allows one to separate better the adaptive responses shown in mammals. Costs incurred during each phase of reproduction are quite different, both in magnitude and mechanism.

TABLE 6
INCREASE IN ENERGY CONSUMPTION FOR REPRODUCTION IN SPECIES OF *Microtus*

Species	Body size (g)	Litter size	Increase over non-reproductives (%) Gestation	Lactation	Reference
Microtus arvalis	25.3[1]	4.25	32	133	Migula (1969)
Microtus pennsylvanicus	29.4[2]	5.05	36	122	Innes and Millar (1981)
Microtus pinetorum	28.9[3]	2.20	—	47.5	Lochmiller et al. (1982)

[1] Body mass of non-pregnant female.
[2] Post-partum body mass.
[3] Mean mass throughout lactation.

In both cases energy needs can be divided into two categories: 1) increased energy needed to gather more energy from the environment; and 2) increased energy to digest food and form the compounds used by the embryo or young for growth and maintenance. During gestation the embryo essentially uses the same foodstuffs as the mother because transfer is via the vascular system, and since the embryo is inside the female, she need not produce extra heat to keep it warm. Once the embryo is born there should be increased costs for maintenance because the young is outside the female and must be brooded for thermoregulation. Also, as the embryo becomes larger, its total energy needs for continued growth will be greater.

To my knowledge there have been only two studies of the direct energetic costs for reproduction in New World *Microtus* (Innes and Millar, 1981; Lochmiller et al., 1982) and three for one species of Old World *Microtus* (Kacmarski, 1966; Migula, 1969; Trojan and Wojciechowska, 1967). In all cases the actual costs can't be fractionated further than increased costs due to gestation and those due to lactation. In these studies food consumption of pregnant or lactating females was simply compared to similar-sized non-reproductive females in the laboratory. Thus, we really have no estimates of the increased cost for gathering food during reproduction and in no studies were the animals on natural diets.

Both gestation and lactation are energetically expensive. Although there are few data for *Microtus,* energy needs during gestation increase with larger litter sizes (Grodziński and Wunder, 1975), and the same is true for lactation in many species, including *Microtus pinetorum* (Lochmiller et al., 1982). Table 6 summarizes the increased energy requirements from reproduction in voles. Gestation increases costs 30% or more and lactation usually entails increases of more than 100–120% over non-lactation. This appears true not only for *M. arvalis* and *M. pennsylvanicus,* but also many other small mammals (Mattingly and McClure, 1982; Millar, 1979; Randolph et al., 1977). However, Lochmiller et al. (1982) reported a somewhat low value for *M. pinetorum,* which characteristically has small litter sizes; that may be the reason for the low increase in total energy needs. Lochmiller et al. (1982) suggested that this trait, along with efficiency of energy conversion to young, may allow pine voles to breed throughout winter in some years. However, voles and lemmings with larger litter sizes and masses also occasionally breed in winter (Taitt and Krebs, this volume).

Many incidental observations and studies suggest that species of *Microtus* may be near their limits for food gathering and processing during reproduction. Although not rigorously tested, modelling of energy flow for *M. arvalis* suggests this (Stenseth et al., 1980). Molt-pattern changes in reproductive and non-reproductive *M. breweri* also suggest that reproduction cannot be maintained at the same time as certain molts (Rowsemitt et al., 1975). And the observation that many species do not breed in winter when thermoregulatory costs are high suggests that added costs during reproduction cannot be met (Millar, 1978; Wunder, 1978*a*).

Given those constraints, it is interesting that, although small mammals in general, and *Microtus* species in particular, increase energy intake during reproduction, there are no indications that process time is decreased (energy cannot be gained more quickly from a unit of food). And there is good evidence that percent digestion and assimilation do not increase in *Microtus* during reproduction (Innes and Millar, 1979; Johnson and Groepper, 1970; Lochmiller et al., 1982; Migula, 1969). Thus, the only means species of *Microtus* appear to use to increase energy accumulation for reproduction is increased food intake.

Energy-Flow Models: Individuals and Populations

To describe energy flow through an individual mammal, one simply integrates the metabolic costs discussed in this chapter over some unit of time. This can be done using an Average Daily Metabolic Rate model or some combination of models to integrate metabolic costs (Wunder, 1975) with a time budget (see Methods). For mammals in general this approach is well described in Grodziński and Wunder (1975) and Ferns (1980).

To discuss the effects of small mammal populations on community function and the role of energetics in such functions, investigators occasionally have generated energy flow models for populations. These models give some insight into: 1) how much of the energy flowing through a community is channeled through small mammals (voles for our purposes), and hence how voles may influence production or community processes; 2) how seasonal bottlenecks in energy availability or need may influence population processes; and 3) how patterns of community function vary in different ecotypes. The models are essentially population integrations of the energy costs associated with individuals. Although these models are discussed in Grodziński and Wunder (1975), a more complete and lucid discussion is given by Ferns (1980) using *M. agrestis* as an example.

There have been very few studies of the population energetics of New World *Microtus*. Golley (1960) published the earliest study on population energetics in *M. pennsylvanicus*. Grodziński (1971) undertook studies on population energetics of *M. oeconomus* in Alaska. Studying the energetics of small mammals in grassland ecosystems, French et al. (1976) found highest energy turnover (172×10^3 kcal/ha) in tallgrass prairie systems dominated by *M. ochrogaster*. However, the efficiency of biomass supported was not as great as in northern shortgrass prairie systems that did not have any species of *Microtus*. Using *Clethrionomys rutilus* and *Microtus oeconomus,* Whitney (1977) tested the hypothesis that arctic and subarctic communities have low production, and found the hypothesis unsupported. He also found that maintenance energy costs for both species during winter were double summer costs (despite reproduction only in summer), in contrast to findings of Gebczyńska (1970). Using population energetics, Stenseth et al. (1980) suggested that energy considerations limit reproduction in *M. agrestis*. In analyzing a number of small mammal energy models including some for *M. oeconomus*, *M. pennsylvanicus*, and several Old World species, Ferns (1980) suggested that populations inhabiting open habitats (such as species of *Microtus*) have higher annual energy flow than those in more mature habitats. Production efficiency and ecological efficiency of his *M. agrestis* population were about 1%.

Englemann (1966) suggested that there is a linear relationship between annual production and respiration per unit area in animal populations. McNeill and Lawton (1970) and Humphreys (1980) re-examined that suggestion and found that it is apparently true. Based on these relations, Humphreys (1980) separated homeotherms into four groups, one of which is "small mammal communities." *Microtus* are not notably different from other small mammals in this relationship.

Future Studies

I have indicated throughout the text where knowledge is lacking; I only highlight certain questions here. *Microtus* species provide excellent models for studies of small mammal energetics because they are the smallest mammals that eat relatively high-fiber (energetically dilute) food and yet live in cool environments. So why, and by what mechanism, do they have BMRs 20–40% greater than expected? Is it related to thyroxine and high cellular metabolism, or do voles simply carry more gut (a metabolically active tissue) to digest their food than similar-sized mammals? McNab (1980) observed that populations of mammals with high BMRs have high rates of natural increase. Perhaps these mammals have more gut to process more food for allocation to production, and increased BMR relates to more gut tissue. Or is BMR simply related to thermoregulatory needs? We need detailed, long-term studies on the balance of energy gain and loss. Are voles limited, temporarily or seasonally, in their capacity to find and process enough food for several simultaneous energy-demanding functions (for example, molt and reproduction, cold-induced thermogenesis and reproduction)? More data are needed on reproductive costs of populations with high and low litter sizes. The phenomenon of seasonal body-mass change needs long-term study because changes do not always occur (Wunder, 1978*b*). Such studies would allow better documentation of yearly patterns; then questions about the mechanism and significance of such changes could be better formulated. These studies should consider not only climatic factors but also fiber content of food and 6-MBOA levels (Sanders et al., 1981). Lastly, more detailed studies of limits to energy gain are needed. How important are behavioral-physiological factors in allowing voles to select low-fiber food (as in Goldberg et al., 1980) relative to their physiological ability to digest these foods (Batzli and Cole, 1979)? We know nothing at all about food passage rates or gut-size variation in voles and their effects on energy gain, although we are pursuing the latter.

Literature Cited

BADDALOO, E. G. Y., AND F. V. CLULOW. 1981. Effects of the male on growth, sexual maturation, and ovulation of young female meadow voles *Microtus pennsylvanicus*. Canadian J. Zool., 59:415–421.

BALDWIN, JR., R. L., AND N. E. SMITH. 1974. Molecular control of energy metabolism. Pp. 17–34, *in* The control of metabolism (J. D. Sink, ed.). Pennsylvania State Univ. Press, University Park, 267 pp.

BARBEHENN, K. R. 1955. A field study of growth in *Microtus pennsylvanicus*. J. Mamm., 36:533–543.

BARRY, W. J. 1976. Environmental effects on food hoarding in deermice (*Peromyscus*). J. Mamm., 57:731–746.

BARTHOLOMEW, G. A. 1977. Energy metabolism. Pp. 57–110, *in* Animal physiology: principles and adaptations (M. S. Gordon, ed.). Macmillan Publ. Co., Inc., New York, 699 pp.

BATZLI, G. O., AND F. R. COLE. 1979. Nutritional ecology of microtine rodents: digestibility of forage. J. Mamm., 60:740–750.

BATZLI, G. O., L. L. GETZ, AND S. S. HURLEY. 1977. Suppression of growth and reproduction of microtine rodents by social factors. J. Mamm., 58:583–591.

BEACHAM, T. D. 1980. Growth rates of the vole *Microtus townsendii* during a population cycle. Oikos, 35:99–106.

BEACHAM, T. D., AND C. J. KREBS. 1980. Growth rates of aggressive and docile voles, *Microtus townsendii*. Amer. Midland Nat., 104:387–389.

BECK, L. R., AND R. G. ANTHONY. 1971. Metabolic and behavioral thermoregulation in the long-tailed vole, *Microtus longicaudus*. J. Mamm., 52:404–412.

BERGER, P. J., N. C. NEGUS, E. H. SANDERS, AND P. D. GARDNER. 1981. Chemical triggering of reproduction in *Microtus montanus*. Science, 214:69–70.

BRADLEY, S. R. 1976. Temperature regulation and bioenergetics of some microtine rodents. Unpubl. Ph.D. dissert., Cornell Univ., Ithaca, New York, 153 pp.

BRODY, S. 1945. Bioenergetics and growth, with special reference to the efficiency complex in domestic animals. Reinhold Publ. Corp., New York, 1023 pp.
BROWN, E. B., III. 1973. Changes in patterns of seasonal growth of *Microtus pennsylvanicus*. Ecology, 54:1103–1109.
CALOW, P. 1977. Ecology, evolution and energetics: a study in metabolic adaptation. Adv. Ecol. Res., 10:1–62.
CAMPBELL, G. S. 1977. An introduction to environmental biophysics. Springer-Verlag Inc., New York, 159 pp.
CASE, T. J. 1978. On the evolution and adaptive significance of postnatal growth rates in the terrestrial vertebrates. Quart. Rev. Biol., 53:243–282.
CHARNOV, E. L. 1976. Optimal foraging: the marginal value theorem. Theor. Population Biol., 9:129–136.
CHERRY, R. H., AND L. VERNER. 1975. Seasonal acclimatization to temperature in the prairie vole, *Microtus ochrogaster*. Amer. Midland Nat., 94:354–360.
COLE, F. R., AND G. O. BATZLI. 1979. Nutrition and population dynamics of the prairie vole, *Microtus ochrogaster*, in central Illinois. J. Anim. Ecol., 48: 455–470.
COWAN, I. MCT., AND M. G. ARSENAULT. 1954. Reproduction and growth in the creeping vole, *Microtus oregoni serpens* Merriam. Canadian J. Zool., 32: 198–208.
COWAN, R. L., T. A. LONG, AND M. JARRETT. 1968. Digestive capacity of the meadow vole (*Microtus pennsylvanicus*). J. Anim. Sci., 27:1517.
DAKETSE, M., AND L. MARTINET. 1977. Effect of temperature on the growth and fertility of the field-vole, *Microtus arvalis*, raised in different day length and feeding conditions. Ann. Biol. Anim. Biochem. Biophys., 17:713–721.
DEHNEL, A. 1949. Studies on the genus *Sorex*. Ann. Univ. Mariae Curie-Sklodowska, Ser. C, 4:17–97.
ENGLEMANN, M. D. 1966. Energetics, terrestrial field studies and animal productivity. Adv. Ecol. Res., 3:73–115.
FERNS, P. N. 1980. Energy flow through small mammal populations. Mamm. Rev., 10:165–188.
FITCH, H. S. 1957. Aspects of reproduction and development in the prairie vole (*Microtus ochrogaster*). Univ. Kansas Publ., Mus. Nat. Hist., 10:129–161.
FRENCH, N. R., W. E. GRANT, W. GRODZIŃSKI, AND D. SWIFT. 1976. Small mammal energetics in grassland ecosystems. Ecol. Monogr., 46:201–220.
FULLER, W., L. L. STEBBINS, AND G. R. DYKE. 1969. Overwintering of small mammals near Great Slave Lake, northern Canada. Arctic, 22:34–55.
GEBCZYŃSKA, Z. 1970. Bioenergetics of a root vole population. Acta Theriol., 15: 33–66.
GESSAMAN, J. A. (ED.). 1973. Ecological energetics of homeotherms: a view compatible with ecological modeling. Utah State University Press, Logan, 155 pp.
GOLDBERG, M., N. R. TABROFF, AND R. H. TAMARIN. 1980. Nutrient variation in beach grass in relation to beach vole feeding. Ecology, 61:1029–1033.
GOLLEY, F. B. 1960. Energy dynamics of a food chain of an old-field community. Ecol. Monogr., 30:187–206.
GÓRECKI, A. 1965. Energy values of body in small mammals. Acta Theriol., 10: 333–352.
GRODZIŃSKI, W. 1971. Energy flow through populations of small mammals in the Alaskan taiga forest. Acta Theriol., 16:231–275.
GRODZIŃSKI, W., AND B. A. WUNDER. 1975. Ecological energetics of small mammals. Pp. 173–204, *in* Small mammals: their productivity and population

dynamics (F. B. Golley, K. Petrusewicz, and L. Ryszkowski, eds.). Cambridge Univ. Press, London, 451 pp.

GRODZIŃSKI, W., R. Z. KLEKOWSKI, AND A. DUNCAN (EDS.). 1975. Methods for ecological bioenergetics. Blackwell Sci. Publ., Oxford, 367 pp.

HAMILTON, W. J., JR. 1937. Growth and life span of the field mouse. Amer. Nat., 71:500–507.

———. 1938. Life history notes on the northern pine mouse. J. Mamm., 19:163–170.

HANSSON, L. 1971. Habitat, food, and population dynamics of the field vole *Microtus agrestis* L. in south Sweden. Viltrevy, 8:267–378.

HART, J. S. 1971. Rodents. Pp. 1–149, *in* Comparative physiology of thermoregulation (G. C. Whittow, ed.). Academic Press, New York, 410 pp.

HART, J. S., AND L. IRVING. 1959. The energetics of harbor seals in air and in water with special consideration of seasonal changes. Canadian J. Zool., 37:447–452.

HART, J. S., H. POHL, AND J. S. TENER. 1965. Seasonal acclimation in the varying hare (*Lepus americanus*). Canadian J. Zool., 43:731–744.

HATFIELD, D. M. 1935. A natural history study of *Microtus californicus*. J. Mamm., 16:261–271.

HELDMAIER, G., S. STEINLECHNER, AND J. RAFAEL. 1982. Nonshivering thermogenesis and cold resistance during seasonal acclimatization in the Djungarian hamster. J. Comp. Physiol., 149:1–9.

HERREID, C. F., AND B. KESSEL. 1967. Thermal conductance in birds and mammals. Comp. Biochem. Physiol., 21:405–414.

HOOPER, E. T. 1949. Faunal relationships of Recent North American rodents. Misc. Publ. Mus. Zool., Univ. Michigan, 72:1–28.

HUDSON, J., AND J. E. BROWER. 1971. Oxygen consumption, Part I. Mammals. Pp. 460–467, *in* Respiration and circulation. Biological handbooks (P. Altman and D. Dittmer, eds.). Fed. Amer. Soc. Exp. Biol., Bethesda, Maryland, 930 pp.

HUDSON, J., D. R. DEAVERS, AND S. R. BRADLEY. 1972. A comparative study of temperature regulation in ground squirrels with special reference to desert species. Symp. Zool. Soc. Lond., 31:191–213.

HUMPHREYS, W. F. 1980. Production and respiration in animal populations. J. Anim. Ecol., 48:427–453.

INNES, D. G. L., AND J. S. MILLAR. 1979. Growth of *Clethrionomys gapperi* and *Microtus pennsylvanicus* in captivity. Growth, 43:208–217.

———. 1981. Body weight, litter size, and energetics of reproduction in *Clethrionomys gapperi* and *Microtus pennsylvanicus*. Canadian J. Zool., 59:785–789.

IRVING, L., H. KROG, AND M. MONSON. 1955. The metabolism of some Alaskan animals in winter and summer. Physiol. Zool., 28:173–185.

IVERSON, S. L., AND B. N. TURNER. 1974. Winter weight dynamics in *Microtus pennsylvanicus*. Ecology, 55:1030–1041.

JAGOSZ, J., A. GORECKI, AND M. POSSI-CABAJ. 1979. The bioenergetics of deposit and utilization of stored energy in the common vole. Acta Theriol., 24: 391–397.

JANSKÝ, L. 1966. Body organ thermogenesis of the rat during exposure to cold and at maximal metabolic rate. Fed. Proc., 25:1297–1302.

———. 1973. Nonshivering thermogenesis and its thermoregulatory significance. Biol. Rev., 48:85–132.

JOHANNINGSMEIER, A. G., AND C. J. GOODNIGHT. 1969. Digestibility of nitrogen, cellulose, lignin, dry matter and energy in *Microtus pennsylvanicus* on *Agrostis stolonifera* and *Poa pratensis*. Agron. Abstr., 61:59.

JOHNSON, D. R., AND K. L. GROEPPER. 1970. Bioenergetics of north plains rodents. Amer. Midland Nat., 84:537–548.

KACMARSKI, F. 1966. Bioenergetics of pregnancy and lactation in the bank vole. Acta Theriol., 11:409–417.

KANWISHER, J., AND G. SUNDES. 1965. Physiology of a small cetacean. Hvalrad. Skr. Nor. Videskaps-Akod. Oslo, 48:45–53.

KENDALL, W. A., R. R. HILL, JR., AND J. S. SHENK. 1978. Regulation of intake and utilization of carbohydrates by meadow voles. J. Anim. Sci., 46:1641–1647.

———. 1979. Inhibition by some allelochemicals of intake of individual meals by meadow voles. Agron. J., 71:613–616.

KEYS, JR., J. E., AND P. J. VAN SOEST. 1970. Digestibility of forages by the meadow vole, *Microtus pennsylvanicus*. J. Dairy Sci., 53:1502–1508.

KING, J. R., AND D. S. FARNER. 1961. Energy metabolism, thermoregulation and body temperature. Pp. 215–288, *in* Biology and comparative physiology of birds, Vol. II (A. J. Marshall, ed.). Academic Press, New York, 467 pp.

KLEIBER, M. 1932. Body size and metabolic rate. Physiol. Rev., 27:511–541.

———. 1961. The fire of life: an introduction to animal energetics. John Wiley and Sons, New York, 454 pp.

———. 1975. Metabolic turnover rate: a physiological meaning of the metabolic rate per unit body weight. J. Theor. Biol., 53:199–204.

KRUCKENBERG, S. M., H. T. GIER, AND S. M. DENNIS. 1973. Postnatal development of the prairie vole, *Microtus ochrogaster*. Lab. Anim. Sci., 23:53–55.

LECHNER, A. J. 1978. The scaling of maximal oxygen consumption and pulmonary dimensions in small mammals. Respiration Physiol., 34:29–44.

LINDEMANN, R. L. 1942. The trophic-dynamic aspect of ecology. Ecology, 23:399–418.

LOCHMILLER, R. L., J. B. WHELAN, AND R. L. KIRKPATRICK. 1982. Energetic cost of lactation in *Microtus pinetorum*. J. Mamm., 63:475–481.

LYNCH, G. R., AND S. L. GENDLER. 1980. Multiple responses to different photoperiods occur in the mouse, *Peromyscus leucopus*. Oecologia, 45:318–321.

LYNCH, G. R., S. E. WHITE, R. GRUNDEL, AND M. S. BERGER. 1978. Effects of photoperiod, melatonin administration and thyroid block on spontaneous daily torpor and temperature regulation in the white-footed mouse, *Peromyscus leucopus*. J. Comp. Physiol., 125:157–163.

MATTINGLY, D. K., AND P. A. MCCLURE. 1982. Energetics of reproduction in large-littered cotton rats (*Sigmodon hispidus*). Ecology, 63:183–195.

MCNAB, B. K. 1980. Food habits, energetics, and the population biology of mammals. Amer. Nat., 116:106–124.

MCNEILL, S., AND J. H. LAWTON. 1970. Annual production and respiration in animal populations. Nature, 225:472–474.

MIGULA, P. 1969. Bioenergetics of pregnancy and lactation in Europeon common vole. Acta Theriol., 14:167–179.

MILLAR, J. S. 1978. Energetics of reproduction in *Peromyscus leucopus*: the cost of lactation. Ecology, 59:1055–1061.

———. 1979. Energetics of lactation in *Peromyscus maniculatus*. Canadian J. Zool., 57:1015–1019.

MORRISON, P. R., AND F. A. RYSER. 1951. Temperature and metabolism in some Wisconsin mammals. Fed. Proc., 10:93–94.

MORRISON, P. R., R. DIETERICH, AND D. PRESTON. 1977. Body growth in sixteen rodent species and subspecies maintained in laboratory colonies. Physiol. Zool., 50:294–310.

MORRISON, P. R., F. A. RYSER, AND A. DAWE. 1959. Studies on the physiology of the masked shrew (*Sorex cinereus*). Physiol. Zool., 32:256–271.

MORRISON, P. R., F. A. RYSER, AND R. L. STRECKER. 1954. Growth and development of temperature regulation in the tundra redback vole. J. Mamm., 35:376–386.

MULLEN, R. K. 1973. The $D_2{}^{18}O$ method of measuring the energy metabolism of free-living animals. Pp. 32–43, *in* Ecological energetics of homeotherms (J. Gessaman, ed.). Utah State Univ. Press, Monogr. Ser., 20:1–155.

NEAL, C. M., AND S. I. LUSTICK. 1973. Energetics and evaporative water loss in the short-tailed shrew, *Blarina brevicauda*. Physiol. Zool., 46:180–185.

PACKARD, G. C. 1968. Oxygen consumption of *Microtus montanus* in relation to ambient temperature. J. Mamm., 49:215–220.

PETRUSEWICZ, K. 1967. Suggested list of more important concepts in productivity studies (definitions and symbols). Pp. 51–80, *in* Secondary productivity of terrestrial ecosystems (K. Petrusewicz, ed.). Polish Acad. Sci., Warsaw, 379 pp.

PETRUSEWICZ, K., AND A. MACFADYEN. 1970. Productivity of terrestrial animals: principles and methods. Blackwell Sci. Publ., Oxford, 190 pp.

PETTERBORG, L. J. 1978. Effect of photoperiod on body weight in the vole, *Microtus montanus*. Canadian J. Zool., 56:431–435.

PINTER, A. J. 1968. Effects of diet and light on growth, maturation and adrenal size of *Microtus montanus*. Amer. J. Physiol., 215:461–466.

PISTOLE, D. H., AND J. A. CRANFORD. 1982. Photoperiodic effects on growth in *Microtus pennsylvanicus*. J. Mamm., 63:547–553.

PYKE, G. H., H. R. PULLIAM, AND E. L. CHARNOV. 1977. Optimal foraging: a selective review of theory and tests. Quart. Rev. Biol., 52:137–157.

RANDOLPH, P. A., J. C. RANDOLPH, K. MATTINGLY, AND M. M. FOSTER. 1977. Energy costs of reproduction in the cotton rat, *Sigmodon hispidus*. Ecology, 58:31–45.

RICHMOND, M., AND C. H. CONAWAY. 1969. Management, breeding and reproductive performance of the vole, *Microtus ochrogaster*, in a laboratory colony. Lab. Anim. Care, 19:80–87.

RICKLEFS, R. E. 1967. A graphical method of fitting equations to growth curves. Ecology, 48:978–983.

ROCK, P., AND O. WILLIAMS. 1979. Changes in lipid content of the montane vole. Acta Theriol., 24:237–247.

ROWSEMITT, C., T. H. KUNZ, AND R. H. TAMARIN. 1975. The timing and patterns of molt in *Microtus breweri*. Occas. Papers Mus. Nat. Hist., Univ. Kansas, 34:1–11.

SANDERS, E. H., P. D. GARDNER, P. J. BERGER, AND N. C. NEGUS. 1981. 6-Methoxybenzoxazolinone: a plant derivative that stimulates reproduction in *Microtus montanus*. Science, 214:67–69.

SCHOENER, T. 1971. Theory of feeding strategies. Ann. Rev. Ecol. Syst., 2:369–404.

SCHOLANDER, P. F., R. HOCK, V. WALTERS, AND L. IRVING. 1950. Adaptation to cold in arctic and tropical mammals and birds in relation to body temperature, insulation and basal metabolic rate. Biol. Bull., 99:259–271.

SCHWARZ, S. S., ET AL. 1964. Biological peculiarities of seasonal generations of rodents, with special reference to the problem of senescence in mammals. Acta Theriol., 8:11–43.

SELLE, R. M. 1928. *Microtus californicus* in captivity. J. Mamm., 9:93–98.

SHENK, J. S., F. C. ELLIOTT, AND J. W. THOMAS. 1970. Meadow vole nutrition studies with semisynthetic diets. J. Nutr., 100:1437–1446.

SLOBODKIN, L. B. 1962. Energy in animal ecology. Adv. Ecol. Res., 1:69–101.

STENSETH, N. C., E. FRANSTAD, P. MIGULA, P. TROJAN, AND B. WOJCIECHOWSKA-TROJAN. 1980. Energy models for the common vole *Microtus arvalis*: energy as a limiting resource for reproductive output. Oikos, 34: 1–22.

TAYLOR, C. R., N. C. HEGLUND, AND G. M. O. MALOIY. 1982. Energetics and mechanics of terrestrial locomotion. J. Exp. Biol., 97:1–21.

TOWNSEND, C. R., AND P. CALOW (EDS.). 1981. Physiological ecology: an evolutionary approach to resource use. Sinauer Associates, Inc., Sunderland, Massachusetts, 393 pp.

TROJAN, P., AND B. WOJCIECHOWSKA. 1967. Resting metabolic rate during pregnancy and lactation in the European common vole, *Microtus arvalis*. Ekologia Polska, Ser. A, 15:811–817.

WHITE, T. C. R. 1978. The importance of relative food shortage in animal ecology. Oecologia, 33:71–86.

WHITNEY, P. 1977. Seasonal maintenance and net production of two sympatric species of subarctic microtine rodents. Ecology, 58:314–325.

WOLFF, J. O., AND W. Z. LIDICKER, JR. 1980. Population ecology of the taiga vole, *Microtus xanthognathus*, in interior Alaska. Canadian J. Zool., 58: 1800–1812.

WUNDER, B. A. 1975. A model for estimating metabolic rate of active or resting mammals. J. Theor. Biol., 49:345–354.

———. 1978*a*. Implications of a conceptual model for the allocation of energy resources by small mammals. Pp. 68–75, *in* Populations of small mammals under natural conditions (O. Snyder, ed.). Pymatuning Lab. Ecology, Univ. Pittsburgh, Spec. Publ. Ser., 5:1–237.

———. 1978*b*. Yearly differences in seasonal thermogenic shifts of prairie voles (*Microtus ochrogaster*). J. Thermal Biol., 3:98 (Abst.).

———. 1979. Hormonal mechanisms. Pp. 143–158, *in* Comparative mechanisms of cold adaptation (L. S. Underwood et al., eds.). Academic Press, New York, 379 pp.

———. 1981. Effects of short-term, daily, cold exposure on brown adipose tissue and nonshivering thermogenesis in the house mouse and prairie vole. Acta Univ. Carolinea, 1979:315–318.

———. 1984. Strategies for, and environmental cueing mechanisms of, seasonal changes in thermoregulatory parameters of small mammals. Pp. 165–172, *in* Winter ecology of small mammals (J. F. Merritt, ed.). Spec. Publ. Carnegie Mus. Nat. Hist., 10:1–392.

WUNDER, B. A., D. S. DOBKIN, AND R. D. GETTINGER 1977. Shifts of thermogenesis in the prairie vole (*Microtus ochrogaster*), strategies for survival in a seasonal environment. Oecologia, 29:11–26.

GENETICS

MICHAEL S. GAINES

Abstract

DIFFERENT kinds of genetic variation in New World *Microtus* are reviewed. This variation ranges from traits controlled by single genes such as coat color and allozymes to those that are polygenic such as body weight and agonistic behavior. Coat color polymorphisms reported in the literature are unsatisfactory from a genetic standpoint because the mechanism of inheritance of most polymorphisms is unknown. At the karyotypic level, there is little variation in diploid chromosomal number or fundamental number. Karyotypic analyses have been used primarily as tools in elucidating systematic relationships within the genus. The frequency distributions of genic diversity values based on allozymic variation for *Microtus* and other mammal species indicate similar levels of genetic variation. There is some evidence from physiological components of fitness and perturbation experiments that natural selection maintains polymorphisms at a few electrophoretic loci. However, nonselective forces also play a significant role in gene-frequency change over short time periods. I conclude that changes in gene frequency at electrophoretic loci are effects of demographic changes and are not causally related to population cycles. There is a dearth of studies on the inheritance of quantitative traits in the genus. Heritabilities for dispersal behavior, aggressive behavior, growth rates, and age at sexual maturity have been estimated from full-sib analysis in *M. townsendii* populations. Three areas are profitable for future research: 1) the effect of social dynamics on genetic structure of populations; 2) inheritance and evolution of quantitative traits; and 3) the application of new molecular techniques to assess genetic variation.

Introduction

In a review of this scope an obvious starting point is to extoll the virtues of *Microtus* as a suitable organism for genetic investigations.

Because there is detailed information on the ecology of microtine rodents, it affords investigators the opportunity of combining genetics and ecology in the study of natural populations. This synthetic approach taken by ecological geneticists will enhance our understanding of evolutionary processes in natural populations. The periodic fluctuations in population density exhibited to some degree by most microtine species enable the ecological geneticist to measure the direction and intensity of natural selection during different phases of a population cycle that consists of an increase, peak, and decline phase. The synchrony in microtine fluctuations reported over large geographic areas (see Taitt and Krebs, this volume) also allows for spatial replication.

The major theme of this chapter is the kinds of genetic variation found in *Microtus*. The variation discussed spans the spectrum from traits controlled by single genes, such as coat color and electromorphs, to those that are polygenic, such as body weight and agonistic behavior. Wherever possible, I examine the evolutionary significance of the variation. I conclude with a section on areas of genetic research that may prove to be fruitful in the future.

Pelage Coloration

The pelage of *Microtus* varies from pale yellow to dark brown or black. Variation in coat color is due to differences in the number of completely black hairs and the width of a subapical band of yellow pigment on black hairs. A summary of coat-color variants reported in six species of *Microtus* is given in Table 1. The list is unsatisfactory from a genetic standpoint for several reasons. First, there may be problems with the nomenclature because few attempts have been made to cross-check new color morphs with actual specimens of similar phenotypes reported in the literature. Thus, either the same morph may be renamed by different investigators or different morphs may be given the same name. A case in point is the grey-eared morph in *M. ochrogaster* (Semeonoff, 1973), which is similar in overall appearance to a smoky morph in the same species reported by Pinter and Negus (1971). However, after direct comparison, Semeonoff concluded that the two morphs had very different phenotypes. Second, in only a few cases have investigators performed the appropriate breeding studies to determine the genetic basis of the color polymorphism.

TABLE 1
SUMMARY OF PELAGE-COLOR POLYMORPHISMS IN NEW WORLD *Microtus* SPECIES

Species	Pelage coloration	Origin of polymorphism	Breeding data	References
Microtus californicus	Buffy	Natural population	Yes	Lidicker (1963)
	Yellow	Natural population	No	Orr (1941)
	White spotting	Natural population	Yes	Gill (1976)
	White with brown ears	Natural population	No	Fisher (1942)
Microtus montanus	Albino	Natural population	Yes	Jannett (1981); Warren (1929)
	Yellow	Natural population	No	Maser et al. (1969)
	Pink-eye dilution	Laboratory	Yes	Pinter and Negus (1971)
	Hairless	Laboratory	Yes	Pinter and McLean (1970)
	White spotting	Natural population	Yes	Pinter (1979)
	Melanism	Natural population	No	Jewett (1955)
Microtus ochrogaster	Albino	Natural population	No	Hays and Bingham (1964)
	Grey-eared	Laboratory	Yes	Semeonoff (1973)
	Black	Natural population	Yes	Semeonoff (1973)
	Smoky	Laboratory	Yes	Pinter and Negus (1971)
	White spotting	Laboratory	Yes	Hartke et al. (1974)
Microtus oeconomus	Melanism	Natural population	No	Murie (1934)
Microtus pennsylvanicus	Albino	Natural population	No	Barrett (1975); Hatt (1930); Owen and Shackelford (1942)
	Yellow	Natural population	No	Owen and Shackelford (1942)
	Cream with dark eyes	Natural population	Yes	Clark (1938)
	Light cinammon with dark eyes	Natural population	Yes	Kutz and Smith (1945); Snyder (1930)
	White with buff underfur	Natural population	No	Snyder (1930)

TABLE 1
CONTINUED

Species	Pelage coloration	Origin of polymorphism	Breeding data	References
	Dark buff	Natural population	No	Snyder (1930)
	White spotting	Natural population	No	Owen and Shackelford (1942); Snyder (1930)
	Melanism	Natural population	No	Blossom (1942)
Microtus pinetorum	Albino	Natural population	No	Paul (1964); Schantz (1960)
	Yellow	Natural population	No	Owen and Shackelford (1942)
	Light brown	Natural population	No	Owen and Shackelford (1942)

Finally, there is little information on the adaptive significance of coat color polymorphisms in natural populations of *Microtus*. A notable exception is the buffy coat color in *Microtus californicus*. Lidicker (1963) found that buffy coat color is due to a single-locus recessive mutation. The wild type agouti allele (+) is completely dominant over the buffy allele (*bf*) so that the +/+ homozygote and *bf*/+ heterozygote are phenotypically indistinguishable. Lidicker (as reported by Gill, 1977) monitored the frequency of buffy in a population of *M. californicus* over a 7-year period on Brooks Island off the coast of California. Gill (1977) reported that the frequency of buffy individuals in the population fluctuated seasonally and was highest after the breeding season. Changes in the frequency of buffy individuals lagged behind changes in population density. In laboratory crosses, heterozygous females (*bf*/+) had a higher mean number of offspring born per month and mean number of offspring weaned than both homozygotes, and heterozygous males were more fertile than other males. Gill (1976) proposed that the seasonal decrease in the frequency of buffy homozygotes resulted from differential predation and that the subsequent increase during the breeding season resulted from the high fertility of heterozygotes. If Gill's proposition is correct, this form of overdominance could maintain the coat color polymorphism in this island population. In support of her hypothesis she noted that on the mainland where predation is high, the buffy phenotype is almost absent. Clearly, more studies of this type are necessary before we can begin to understand the mechanisms for maintenance of coat color polymorphisms in natural populations of *Microtus*.

Cytogenetics

Karyotypic analyses of new world *Microtus* have been used primarily as tools in elucidating systematic relationships within the genus. Many species of *Microtus* differ in both diploid chromosome number and fundamental number (Table 2). The latter is determined from the total number of autosomal chromosome arms, counting one for each telocentric or acrocentric chromosome and two for each metacentric chromosome. There is little variation in diploid chromosomal number and fundamental number within species because discoveries of this sort usually lead to new species assignations. For example, there was some disagreement whether

TABLE 2

DIPLOID AND FUNDAMENTAL CHROMOSOME NUMBERS OF NEW WORLD SPECIES OF *Microtus*. SOURCES ARE HSU AND BENIRSCHKE (1967–1975) AND MATTHEY (1973) UNLESS OTHERWISE NOTED

Species	Diploid number	Fundamental number
Microtus breweri[1]	46	50
Microtus californicus[2]	52, 53, 54	60, 61, 62
Microtus canicaudus	24	48
Microtus longicaudus	56	84
Microtus mexicanus	44	54
Microtus montanus[3]	22, 24	40, 44
Microtus ochrogaster	54	64
Microtus oeconomus	30	52
Microtus oregoni	17 ♀; 18 ♂	32
Microtus pennsylvanicus	46	50
Microtus pinetorum[4]	62	62
Microtus townsendii	50	48
Microtus xanthognathus[5]	54	62

[1] Fivush et al. (1975); [2] Gill (1982); [3] Judd et al. (1980); [4] Beck and Mahan (1978); [5] Rausch and Rausch (1974).

the species *M. canicaudus* and *M. montanus* should be considered as conspecific (Johnson, 1968). The former has a limited range in Oregon and Washington, whereas the latter is widely distributed throughout much of the western United States. The diploid number of both species is 24 and all the autosomes are metacentric. However, the X-chromosomes differ; they are acrocentric in *M. montanus* but metacentric in *M. canicaudus*. In addition, there are subtle differences in the structure of the autosomes: three pairs of smaller autosomes are similar in size in *M. canicaudus* but dissimilar in *M. montanus*. On the basis of these differences in karyotype, Hsu and Johnson (1970) supported the view that *M. canicaudus* should be given full species status.

There are a few exceptions to the rule of constant chromosomal number within species of North American *Microtus*. Geographic variation in diploid chromosomal number has been reported for *M. longicaudus* (Judd and Cross, 1980). Specimens examined from Arizona, Colorado, and New Mexico all have a diploid number of 56 with 10 pairs of medium- to large-sized biarmed chromosomes, 12 pairs of small to large acrocentric, and five pairs of small metacentric chromosomes. Six other chromosomal forms (2n = 57, 58, 59,

62, 66, and 70) were observed from southern Oregon and northern California. The major differences in the California and Oregon races compared with the 2n = 56 race were six pairs of metacentrics, only 11 pairs of acrocentrics, and variations in number of supernumerary or minute chromosomes. The absence of a pair of acrocentrics and an extra pair of metacentrics suggests that this was a result of a pericentric inversion. Although supernumerary chromosomes have been found in other rodent species (for instance, *Reithrodontomys* [Shellhammer, 1969] and *Perognathus* [Patton, 1977]), this is the only case reported to date for a *Microtus* species.

Gill (1982) found a polymorphism in chromosomal number in *M. californicus* populations. Individuals have diploid numbers of 52, 53, or 54 chromosomes with fundamental numbers ranging from 60 to 62. Furthermore, based on breeding data, Gill (1980) suggested that *M. californicus* is undergoing speciation. Finally, Fredga and Bergström (1970) reported a chromosomal polymorphism in *M. oeconomus* caused by a centric fission of one chromosome pair. In an isolated population in northern Europe, animals with 2n = 31 and 2n = 32 were captured. Although this is not a New World microtine, it is nominally the same species as that which occurs in North America.

The differential staining of specific regions of chromosomes also has been useful in determining differences and similarities between populations. In a thorough analysis of chromosomal variation in *M. montanus,* Judd et al. (1980) compared populations from Arizona and New Mexico (2n = 24) to a population from Oregon (2n = 22). One conspicuous difference between the two karyotypes was the absence of the smallest pair of metacentrics (pair 8) in the 22-chromosome form. The following differences were observed between the two forms with respect to constitutive heterochromatin (C-bands): 1) the 22-chromosome form had smaller C-bands compared to the 24-chromosome form; 2) in the 22-chromosome form, pair 5 had much less centromeric heterochromatin; and 3) in both forms, pairs 9, 10, and 11 had little or no heterochromatin, the C-banded X-chromosomes were identical, and the Y-chromosome was totally heterochromatic. The G-banding patterns of the two forms were almost identical; the only difference was in the short arms of chromosome 2. The location of nucleolar organizing regions (NORs), identified by the silver staining method of Hubbell and Hsu (1977), were invariable in both karyotypes; chromosomal pair

10 had NORs on the long arm and pair 11 had them on the short arm. On the basis of their karyotypic analysis, Judd et al. (1980) suggested that the two forms of *M. montanus* might be specifically distinct. Nadler et al. (1976) also used G-banding techniques to investigate interpopulational variation of Holarctic microtine species; they found similar patterns in Alaskan and Siberian populations of *M. oeconomus* and *Clethrionomys rutilus*.

Recently, there has been a considerable amount of interest in the rates of karyotypic change and direction of evolution. Maruyama and Imai (1981) estimated the evolutionary rates of change of mammalian karyotypes by making pairwise comparisons of chromosomal number and arm number of species belonging to each genus. They calculated probabilities, which decrease exponentially with time, that two randomly chosen species from a given genus would have the same karyotype. Assuming that the average divergence time of a mammalian species from a common ancestor is 2.5×10^6 years, they estimated the rate at which a karyotype changes in unit time for different genera. The genus *Microtus* had the highest rate of karyotypic change (8.18×10^{-7} chromosomal or arm number changes per year) of the 18 rodent genera included in the study.

Three hypotheses have been proposed for the mode and direction of chromosomal evolution in mammals: fusion hypothesis (Ohno, 1969), fission hypothesis (Todd, 1967), and the modal hypothesis (Matthey, 1973). The fusion hypothesis assumes that the ancestral karyotype consisted of a large number of acrocentric chromosomes which were reduced in number through a series of pericentric inversions and centric fusions. Fedyk (1970) proposed that in the *gregalis*-group of *Microtus* the primary mechanism of karyotypic evolution in the subarctic species involved centric fusions, whereas in the Nearctic species of the group, pericentric inversions were predominant. Conversely, the fission hypothesis assumes that ancestral mammals had a low diploid number which generally increased under the influence of centric fissions. The modal hypothesis assumes that ancestral mammals had a diploid number near the present mode and that chromosome numbers moved upward or downward.

Matthey (1973) suggested that the modal hypothesis best explains chromosomal evolution in the subfamily Microtinae because 32 of the 78 species examined have 54 or 56 chromosomes. Matthey (1973) stated that this subset is "exclusively found in the genera regarded by taxonomists as the most primitive on the basis of their morphology." Considering that only five species of microtines have diploid numbers greater than 56, most of the Robertsonian rearrangements occurring over evolutionary time had to be centric fusions. Matthey's hypothesis for chromosomal evolution in *Microtus* is reasonable only if fusions are the predominant Robertsonian rearrangement over evolutionary time. However, in a recent study, Imai and Crozier (1980) presented evidence from a statistical analysis of mammalian karyotypes which strongly supports fission rather than fusion as the predominant Robertsonian rearrangement. Needless to say, the directionality of karyotypic evolution in New World *Microtus* is still open to interpretation.

Karyotypic analyses promise to be useful tools for elucidating systematic relationships within the genus *Microtus* and assessing the amount of chromosomal variation within species. In many studies to date karyotypic analysis was performed on only a few individuals. Moreover, as one progresses to finer levels of karyotypic analysis (for example, C- and G-banding), sample sizes decrease, and in fact, some banding studies are based on only one individual from each species. As both the number of species studied and the sample sizes increase, karyotypic analysis, especially using differential staining techniques, will undoubtedly increase our understanding of the organization of the genetic material.

Allozymic Variation

With the widespread application of protein electrophoresis, estimates of genic variation have now been determined for hundreds of organisms (Nevo, 1978; Selander, 1976). Surprisingly, *Microtus* has been relatively neglected in surveys of allozymic variation. I have summarized the available data in Table 3. The most thoroughly studied *Microtus* species to date is *M. californicus* (Bowen and Yang, 1978) in which 28 proteins were examined. Fewer proteins are represented in the remaining studies in Table 3, primarily because allozymes were used as genetic markers in live-trapping programs that prohibited sacrificing animals. Thus, investigators relied exclusively on plasma or hemolysate, obtained from blood samples, for electrophoresis. More protein polymorphisms were revealed when a wider range of tissues was included in the analysis.

TABLE 3

PROTEIN POLYMORPHISMS IN SEVEN NEW WORLD SPECIES OF *Microtus*. THE MOLECULAR STRUCTURE, SOURCE OF TISSUE FOR ELECTROPHORESIS, GENIC DIVERSITY (*H*), AND THE NUMBER OF ELECTROMORPHS (NE) FOR 30 PROTIEN POLYMORPHISMS ARE PRESENTED

Species	Locus[1]	Molecular structure	Tissue	*H* (NE)[2]	References
M. breweri	TF	Monomer	Plasma	.100 (2)	Kohn and Tamarin (1978); Maurer (1967)
M. californicus	GPD	—	Kidney	.118 (2)	Bowen and Yang (1978); Gill (1980)
	LDH-A	Tetramer	Kidney	.012 (2)	
	LDH-B	Tetramer	Kidney	.059 (2)	
	ME-2	—	Kidney	.180 (2)	
	IDH-1	Dimer	Kidney	.020 (2)	
	6PGD	Dimer	Kidney, hemolysate	.194 (2)	
	GOT-1	Dimer	Kidney, hemolysate	.165 (2)	
	PGM-2	Monomer	Kidney	.281 (2)	
	ES-1	—	Hemolysate	—	
	ES-2	Monomer	Kidney	.611 (5)	
	ES-3	—	Plasma	—	
	ES-4	--	Hemolysate	—	
	LAP	Monomer	Plasma	.440 (2)	
	GPI	Dimer	Kidney, plasma	.091 (2)	
	PT-1	—	Plasma	—	
M. miurus	6PGD	Dimer	Hemolysate	.144 (2)	Nadler et al. (1978)
M. oeconomus	TF	Monomer	Plasma	.070 (3)	Nadler et al. (1978)
	LAP	Monomer	Plasma	.488 (2)	
	6PGD	Dimer	Hemolysate	.505 (2)	

TABLE 3
CONTINUED

Species	Locus[1]	Molecular structure	Tissue	H (NE)[2]	References
M. ochrogaster	TF	Monomer	Plasma	.214 (4)	Gaines et al. (1978); Semeonoff (1972)
	LAP	Monomer	Plasma	.325 (2)	
	6PGD	Dimer	Hemolysate	.159 (3)	
	ES-1	Monomer	Hemolysate	.365 (2)	
	ES-2	Monomer	Plasma	— (2)	
	ES-4	Monomer	Plasma	.448 (2)	
M. pennsylvanicus	TF	Monomer	Plasma	.472 (4)	Kohn and Tamarin (1978)
	LAP	Monomer	Plasma	.449 (3)	
	6PGD	Dimer	Hemolysate	—	
M. townsendii	LAP	Monomer	Plasma	.453 (2)	LeDuc and Krebs (1975)

[1] Abbreviations are: ACP, acid phosphatase; ALB, albumin; ADH, alcohol dehydrogenase; ALD, aldolase; ES, esterase; G6PD, glucose-6-phosphate dehydrogenase; GOT, glutamate-oxaloacetate transaminase; GPD, glycerol-3-phosphate dehydrogenase; αGPD, α-glycerophosphate dehydrogenase; G3PD, glyceraldehyde-3-phosphate dehydrogenase; HB, hemoglobin; IDH, isocitrate dehydrogenase; LDH, lactate dehydrogenase; LAP, leucine aminopeptidase; MDH, malate dehydrogenase; ME, malic enzyme; MPI, mannose phosphate isomerase; PEP, peptidase leucylalanine; PGM, phosphoglucomutase; 6PGD, 6-phosphogluconate dehydrogenase; PT, general protein; SORDH, sorbital dehydrogenase; SDH, succinate dehydrogenase; SOD, superoxide dimutase; TF, transferrin.

[2] $H = 1 - \sum_{i=1}^{k} \bar{x}_i^2$ where $\bar{x}_i$ is the mean frequency of the ith of k alleles.

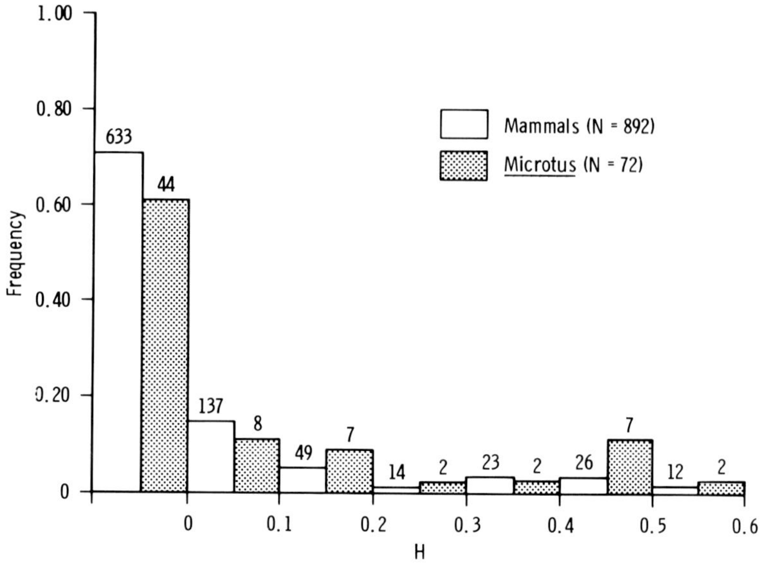

FIG. 1. The frequency distribution of genic diversity (*H*) for species of *Microtus* (see Table 3) compared to other mammals (from Smith et al., 1975). Abbreviation: N, number of loci.

For instance, Bowen and Yang (1978) found nine polymorphic proteins in kidney tissue alone (Table 3). However, the genus inherently may have low levels of variation because of periodic bottlenecks that occur during low phases of density cycles.

Frequency distributions of genic diversity values for *Microtus* and other mammal species (Smith et al., 1978) are presented in Fig. 1. The distributions are similar but there is a slight excess of loci with relatively high genic diversity (for example, 0.4–0.5) in *Microtus* species. Certain loci tend to appear in this range. In particular, leucine aminopeptidase has a genic diversity of about 0.45 in four of the seven species of *Microtus* included in Table 3. Several other loci have relatively high genic diversities, including the esterases, transferrin, and 6-phosphogluconate dehydrogenase. These genetically diverse polymorphisms have been studied more extensively to investigate the roles of different evolutionary forces in maintaining protein polymorphisms in *Microtus* populations.

Recently, some doubts have been raised about the reliability of certain electromorphs as genetic markers in *Microtus* populations. McGovern and Tracy (1981) exposed field caught *M. ochrogaster* in Colorado to different temperature regimes in the laboratory and found changes in the mobility of electromorphs at the TF and LAP locus. Although there is extensive mating data for both the LAP and TF systems (Gaines and Krebs, 1971), the results are inconclusive because animals were housed at a constant temperature. Mihok and Ewing (in press) found complete reliability in TF and LAP electromorphs in *M. pennsylvanicus*. Because McGovern and Tracy's results have serious implications on the interpretation at genic variation in the genus, their experiments need to be repeated further.

Several different approaches have been taken to measure the direction and intensity of selection on structural proteins in *Microtus* populations. Kohn and Tamarin (1978) plotted Δp_t ($=p_{t+1} - p_t$) against p_i from successive trapping periods at the TF and LAP loci in populations of *M. breweri* and *M. pennsylvanicus*. They argued that a significant negative regression around the point where $\Delta p_t = 0$ would be evidence for a stable polymorphism. They calculated regressions for *M. breweri* (for Tf^E) and for *M. pennsylvanicus* (for Tf^E and Lap^S) in four areas and by sex within each area. All 24 regression lines had negative slopes and ten were significantly different from 0. Thus, Kohn and Tamarin (1978) concluded that the polymorphisms were maintained by selection.

However, the method of regressing Δp on p has been shown to be inadequate for estimating selection pressures in populations. Kirby (1974) showed that the regression coefficient, calculated from data obtained from a sequential census of one population, does not provide an unbiased estimate of the amount of immigration or selection maintaining an equilibrium gene frequency. Furthermore, Whittam (1981) demonstrated that a negative regression coefficient is expected when sequential gene frequencies are simply random numbers from the interval [0, 1] of a uniform probability distribution. Using computer simulations, Whittam (1981) randomly sampled gene frequencies from a uniform probability distribution, plotted Δp versus p, and obtained a significant negative regression coefficient with the regression line explaining about 60% of the variance in Δp. A comparison of Kohn and Tamarin's (1978) results and the confidence limits for the regression coefficients indicated that about half of the slopes obtained from natural populations did not differ from the negative slopes obtained by the

TABLE 4

ESTIMATES OF THE DEVIATION OF PROPORTIONS OF HOMOZYGOTES FROM HARDY-WEINBERG PROPORTIONS ($\bar{H}$) DURING DENSITY FLUCTUATIONS OF *Microtus pennsylvanicus*. DATA ARE COMBINED FROM THREE LIVE-TRAPPING GRIDS. NUMBERS IN PARENTHESES ARE ESTIMATES OF THE STANDARD ERROR OF $\bar{H}$ (FROM BIRDSALL, 1974)

Phase of cycle	TF locus		LAP locus	
	Males	Females	Males	Females
Increase	.007 (.014)	−.009 (.015)	−.037* (.016)	−.021 (.018)
Peak	.005 (.013)	.004 (.014)	−.025 (.014)	−.002 (.016)
Decline	−.065* (0.24)	.050† (0.29)	.025 (.027)	.011 (.031)

* Significant deviation from Hardy-Weinberg proportions ($P < 0.05$).
† Significant difference in heterozygosity between males and females ($P < 0.05$).

simulation. A second analysis of genetic drift with a small amount of migration and different population sizes revealed many significant regression coefficients were negative and many were significant (357 out of 1,000 simulations) in the absence of selection. Thus, the interpretation of a negative slope as evidence for selection maintaining a polymorphism is questionable.

Birdsall (1974) used deviation of genotypic frequencies from Hardy-Weinberg equilibrium as evidence for selection acting on the TF and LAP loci in fluctuating populations of *M. pennsylvanicus*. He estimated the excess proportions of each homozygote, *H*, following the method of Smith (1970). Estimates of the deviation of the proportions of homozygotes from Hardy-Weinberg equilibrium during different phases of the density fluctuation for three trapping grids combined, treating sexes separately, are given in Table 4. Birdsall (1974) interpreted the deviations in the proportion of genotypes at the two loci as evidence for natural selection and not a consequence of non-selective forces because the two loci exhibited different patterns of deviation during the density cycle (Table 4). There was a significant excess of male TF heterozygotes in the decline phase, whereas there was a significant excess of male LAP heterozygotes in the increase phase. Furthermore, the significant difference between male and female heterozygosity at the TF locus during the decline phase is difficult to explain by non-selective forces because they should affect both sexes similarly.

TABLE 5

MINIMUM SURVIVAL RATES/14 DAYS OF TF AND LAP GENOTYPES IN *Microtus ochrogaster* POPULATIONS DURING PHASES OF INCREASING AND DECLINING DENSITY REPORTED IN TWO STUDIES IN SOUTHERN INDIANA AND ONE STUDY IN EASTERN KANSAS (FROM GAINES, 1981)

Locus and phase of cycle	Locality					
	Indiana (1965–1967)		Indiana (1967–1969)		Kansas (1970–1973)	
	Male	Female	Male	Female	Male	Female
Transferrin*						
Increase						
Fast homozygote	.84	.92	.78	.87	.82	.83
Heterozygote	.76	.76	.91	.85	.72	.85
Slow homozygote	—	—	—	—	.86	.87
Decline						
Fast homozygote	.59	.68	.70	.69	.65	.65
Heterozygote	.75	.33	.77	.74	.66	.69
Slow homozygote	—	—	—	—	.75	.82
Leucine aminopeptidase*						
Increase						
Fast homozygote	—	—	.60	.84	.80	.85
Heterozygote	—	—	.79	.91	.88	.87
Slow homozygote	—	—	.85	.86	.80	.86
Decline						
Fast homozygote	—	—	.70	.62	.51	.58
Heterozygote	—	—	.75	.58	.59	.58
Slow homozygote	—	—	.75	.77	.63	.63

* Genotypes for the TF locus were Tf^E/Tf^E, Tf^E/Tf^F, and Tf^F/Tf^F, and for the LAP locus were Lap^F/Lap^F, Lap^S/Lap^F, and Lap^S/Lap^S, respectively.

Another approach used in live-trapping studies is to measure physiological components of fitness (Gaines and Krebs, 1971; Gaines et al., 1978; Kohn and Tamarin, 1978; LeDuc and Krebs, 1975; Tamarin and Krebs, 1969). Because animals are marked in the field and their genotypes are known, one can estimate survival rates, growth rates, and breeding activity for each genotypic class. Minimum survival rates for TF and LAP genotypes during density fluctuations of *M. ochrogaster* are presented in Table 5. In spite of variation in survival rates over different studies, certain trends are apparent. At the TF locus, the Tf^F/Tf^F homozygote was extremely rare in Indiana populations. The Tf^E/Tf^F heterozygote generally had higher survival rates than Tf^E/Tf^E homozygotes during the decline phase in both Indiana studies, the only exception being females in the study of Tamarin and Krebs (1969). In declining Kansas populations, individuals with at least one Tf^F allele had higher survival rates than Tf^E/Tf^E homozygotes. Tf^F/Tf^F homozygotes had the highest survivorship of any genotype. In Indiana and Kansas, Lap^S/Lap^S homozygotes had the highest survival rates for males and females during population declines. In addition to survival rates, Gaines et al. (1978) found differences in the breeding activity and growth rates among TF and LAP genotypes in Kansas prairie-vole populations.

Perturbation experiments provide the strongest evidence for selection acting on electrophoretic loci. Gaines et al. (1971) introduced laboratory voles into a fenced enclosure so as to found the population with a Tf^E gene frequency of 0.50. Tf^E gene frequencies in natural populations in the area ranged from 0.80 to 0.90. Gene frequences of the enclosed and control populations were monitored every 14 days over a 16-week period. The experiment was replicated over three seasons. At the conclusion of each experiment all animals were removed from the enclosure and the new introduction was made. In all three replicates the Tf^E gene frequencies increased and approached values observed in open field populations.

Although natural selection may play a role in maintaining polymorphisms, not all observed gene-frequency changes necessarily result from the action of selection. Demographic changes also affect local population sizes and rates of migration, which in turn can lead to random fluctuations in allele frequencies. To assess the roles of selective and non-selective forces in gene-frequency change, Lewontin and Krakauer (1973) developed a statistical test that relies on a comparison of gene-frequency distributions for different loci. Their rationale is that alleles at all loci will be similarly affected by the breeding structure of the population and, thus, the effects of non-selective forces, such as genetic drift and migration, should be uniform over loci. However, natural selection, operating through differential fitness of genotypes, affects gene frequency only at specific loci. Therefore, a measure of genetic variation at each polymorphic locus over an ensemble of populations should be similar if only non-selective forces are operating but dissimilar when selection is acting upon alleles at specific subsets of loci. The measure chosen by Lewontin and Krakauer is a standardized variance of gene frequencies called the effective inbreeding coefficient, $\hat{F}_e$.

For a locus with two alleles, $\hat{F}_e$ is calculated as the ratio of the observed variance in allele frequency, s^2_p, to the maximum variance possible for the average allele frequency, $\bar{p}$, as follows:

$$\hat{F}_e = \frac{s^2_p}{\bar{p}(1 - \bar{p})} .$$

Note that $\hat{F}_e$ is the same as Wright's (1965) F_{st}. For neutral alleles, the $\hat{F}_e$ values calculated for each of many loci over an ensemble of populations will be statistically homogeneous, whereas if selection is occurring there will be heterogeneity in $\hat{F}_e$ values.

Heterogeneity in $\hat{F}_e$ values among loci can be tested from the ratio of the observed variance in $\hat{F}_e$'s over all loci to the theoretical variance. Lewontin and Krakauer (1973) found the theoretical variance of $\hat{F}_e$ over n subpopulations in the absence of selection to be a function of the average $\hat{F}_e$ as follows:

$$\sigma_F{}^2 = \frac{k\bar{F}_e{}^2}{(n - 1)} .$$

Through computer simulation, the limiting value of $k = 2$ was found for various underlying distributions of gene frequencies. The ratio of $s_F{}^2/\sigma_F{}^2$ is compared with an $F(n - 1, \infty)$ distribution. If the sampling variance is significantly greater than the theoretical variance, one can infer heterogeneity in $\hat{F}_e$'s among loci.

The Lewontin-Krakauer test (L-K test) has been criticized in its application to spatial distribution of gene frequencies. Ewens and Feldman (1976), Nei and Maruyama (1975), and Robertson (1975*a*, 1975*b*) contended that heterogeneity of $\hat{F}_e$ could result from factors other than selection (for example, different initial gene frequencies in each population). However, this problem is unlikely in tests of temporal distributions of gene frequencies within populations where the initial gene frequencies are known.

Gaines and Whittam (1980) used the L-K test to assess changes in gene frequencies at five polymorphic loci in fluctuating populations of *M. ochrogaster* in eastern Kansas. Although gene frequency data were available for 2-week samples (Gaines et al., 1978), they chose a 14-week interval to avoid confounding effects of the same individual being sampled more than once. Each of seven time pe-

TABLE 6

ESTIMATES (TOP) OF EFFECTIVE INBREEDING COEFFICIENTS ($\hat{F}_e$) CORRECTED FOR SAMPLING VARIANCE AT FIVE LOCI AMONG SUBPOPULATIONS DURING SEVEN TIME PERIODS ON EACH GRID, AND (BOTTOM) A SUMMARY OF HETEROGENEITY TESTS OF $\hat{F}_e$ VALUES. THE VARIANCE RATIO, $s_F{}^2/\sigma_F{}^2$, IS COMPARED WITH AN $F_{6,\infty}$ DISTRIBUTION (FROM GAINES AND WHITTAM, 1980). ALL RATIOS ARE NON-SIGNIFICANT

Locus/ statistic	Grid A	Grid B	Grid C	Grid D
TF	0.026	0.021	0.044	0.050
LAP	0.010	0.007	0.037	0.050
EST-1	0.034	0.072	0.036	0.104
EST-4	0.042	0.026	0.010	0.007
6-PGD	0.000	0.063	0.004	0.005
$\bar{F}_e$	0.023	0.038	0.027	0.042
$s_F{}^2$	0.0002	0.0006	0.0003	0.0006
$\sigma_F{}^2$	0.0002	0.0005	0.0002	0.0006
$s_F{}^2/\sigma_F{}^2$	1.000	1.200	1.500	1.000

Abbreviations are: $\bar{F}_e$, mean estimate of effective inbreeding coefficient; $s_F{}^2$, observed variance; $\sigma_F{}^2$, theoretical variance. For identities of proteins, see Table 3.

riods sampled was considered a subpopulation for calculations of the $\hat{F}_e$'s. They corrected for both sampling variance within time periods and correlations in alleles over sampling periods.

The $\hat{F}_e$ values, using the mean and variance in gene frequency over the seven time periods, for the five polymorphic loci on four live-trapped grids, are given in Table 6. The homogeneity of $\hat{F}_e$ values indicates that non-selective forces are primarily responsible for the changes in gene frequency through time.

The results of the L-K test conflicted with those of Gaines et al. (1978) who concluded from an analysis of the same data set that changes in gene frequency at the TF and LAP loci were probably due to selection. Their conclusion was based on differences in physiological components of fitness (see Table 5) among genotypes. Gaines and Whittam (1980) attributed these conflicting interpretations to a reductionist versus holistic approach. Physiological components of fitness were measured during each phase of the density fluctuation without considering the historical events that preceded them. On a micro-scale, Gaines et al. (1978) found statistically significant differences in fitness components among genotypes dur-

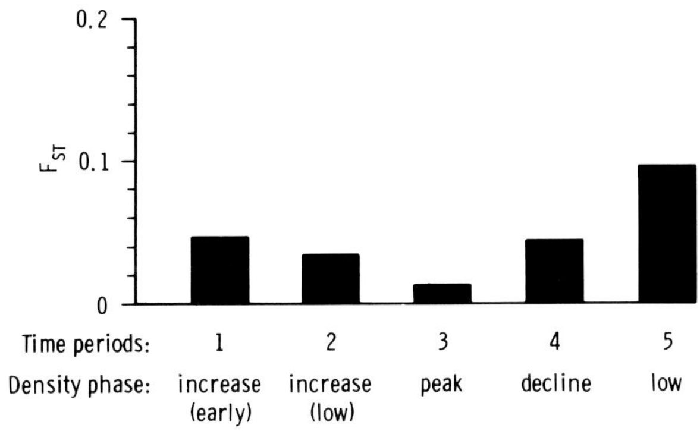

FIG. 2. F_{st} values for resident *M. californicus* from four subpopulations averaged over four loci (from Bowen, 1982).

ing phases of increasing density. However, assuming that the L-K test is valid for temporal variation in vole populations, the intensity of selection was not strong enough to counteract the effects of non-selective evolutionary forces, such as random genetic drift, which most likely predominate during the periodic bottlenecks of the low-density phase and lead to random changes in allelic frequencies observed over short time periods.

Bowen (1982) used F-statistics to measure genetic differentiation in a population of *M. californicus*. The population was subdivided into four 0.15-ha grids spaced 50 m apart. F_{st} values for four electrophoretic loci (PGD, GPI, GOT-1, and LAP) were calculated for five time periods during a 2-year density cycle. The average F_{st} values for the four loci over the cycle are presented in Fig. 2. The greatest genetic differentiation occurred during phases of the population cycle when density was low, whereas the population became relatively more homogeneous as density increased during the breeding season. Bowen interpreted the U-shaped distribution of F_{st} values in Fig. 2 as evidence for increased dispersal at the onset of the breeding season. Once migrants established themselves in existing patches of habitat, the genetic heterogeneity among patches would decrease as a result of gene flow. After the population density returns to a low phase, genetic heterogeneity would be reestablished as a result of genetic drift within isolated patches. Thus, Bowen (1982) related changes in the genetic structure of a population of *M. californicus* to changes in its population dynamics.

In summary, there is evidence that natural selection maintains polymorphisms at the TF and LAP locus in natural populations of *Microtus*. Significant differences were observed between genotypes in certain physiological components of fitness, and these observations were repeatable both in time and space. The most convincing evidence for selection comes from perturbation experiments in which enclosed field populations started with different initial frequencies converged to the frequencies found in natural populations. However, non-selective forces also play a significant role in gene-frequency change over short time periods as revealed by the L-K test on five polymorphic loci in *M. ochrogaster* populations, and by F_{st} values calculated for *M. californicus*.

Quantitative Genetics

There has been a dearth of studies on quantitative traits in *Microtus*. Guthrie (1965) related intrapopulational variation in dentition of the extinct *M. paroperarius* and the recent *M. pennsylvanicus* to the rapid evolution of microtine rodents in the late Pliocene and Pleistocene. Guthrie (1965) suggested that rapid evolution of the molars may have been a response to a major change in diet from fruit and seeds to grass and bark. Gill and Bolles (1982) found variation in the root length of teeth in two populations of *M. californicus*. Although the trait had some genetic component, its mode of inheritance was unclear. Hilborn (1974) studied the inheritance of three non-continuous skeletal variants (preorbital foramina, maxillary foramina, and sphenoid foramina) from a captive colony of *M. californicus*. Breeding data indicated some association between phenotype of parent and offspring for the preorbital foramina.

In all these studies it is difficult to assess the environmental and genetic components of each trait. Only a few attempts have been made to estimate the heritability of polygenic traits in *Microtus* populations. Heritability (h^2) in the narrow sense is defined as (Falconer, 1981):

$$h^2 = \frac{V_A}{V_P}$$

where V_A is the additive genetic variance, and V_P is the phenotypic variance. The V_P term is the sum of the environmental variance

(V_E) and the total genetic variance (V_G). The total genetic variance can be partitioned into the additive genetic variance (V_A), the variance due to dominance effects (V_D), and the variance resulting from epistatic interactions (V_I). The evolutionary response to natural selection depends primarily on the additive genetic variance.

Most methods used to estimate heritability rely upon phenotypic resemblances among relatives. If we know the expected phenotypic correlation between relatives based entirely on the additive effects of genes, then any deviation from the expected correlation is due to environmental effects. For example, since offspring share ½ their genes with their parents, the phenotypic covariance between offspring and one parent or offspring and the mean of both parents is ½. The slope of the regression line of offspring phenotypic values against phenotype values of a single parent is $\frac{1}{2}V_A/V_P$ or $\frac{1}{2}h^2$. In the case of midparent values the slope of the regression line would be $\frac{1}{2}V_A/\frac{1}{2}V_P$ or h^2. Estimation of heritability from sib analysis is more complicated (Falconer, 1981). The phenotypic covariance between half sibs is ¼, based on the additive effects of the genes they have in common. Full sibs share ½ their genes but are phenotypically similar due to effects of dominance and a common environment. Heritability of siblings can be estimated by the intrafamily correlation (t), which is defined as:

$$t = \frac{s^2(B)}{s^2(T)}$$

where $s^2(B)$ is the between-family component of variance and $s^2(T)$ is the total populational variance (the sum of between- and within-family components).

Dispersal Behavior

Howard (1965) codified dispersal behavior of rodents into two categories: innate dispersal and environmental dispersal. He suggested that the former is instinctive behavior governed by laws of heredity, whereas the latter is a behavioral response to overcrowding, food supply, mate selection, homing ability, and other environmental factors. The results from several electrophoretic studies of *Microtus* populations have indicated that dispersers are genetically different from residents at some loci, supporting Howard's innate dispersal hypothesis. Myers and Krebs (1971) found differences in genotypic frequencies between dispersers and residents in two species of *Microtus* in southern Indiana. In *M. pennsylvanicus,* Tf^E/Tf^E homozygotes were more common among dispersing males, compared to resident males, during the late population peak and decline phase of the density cycle. During periods of population increase, Tf^C/Tf^E heterozygotes were more common among dispersing females than in resident females. There was also increased dispersal of Lap^S/Lap^S males during the peak phase. In *M. ochrogaster* populations, the rare Tf^F/Tf^F homozygote was found only among dispersing males. Pickering et al. (1974) found differential dispersal of individuals with different esterase phenotypes in *M. ochrogaster* populations in Illinois. Dispersing *M. townsendii* individuals were not a genetically random subsample from a resident population at the LAP locus (Krebs et al., 1976). Keith and Tamarin (1981) found an excess of the Tf^C allele in dispersing individuals in *M. pennsylvanicus* and *M. breweri* populations. However, there was no evidence for differential dispersal of LAP and TF genotypes in *M. pennsylvanicus* and *M. ochrogaster* populations in Illinois (Verner, 1979), nor did the genetic composition of dispersers and residents differ at seven electrophoretic loci in *M. californicus* populations (Riggs, 1979). Although genetic differences at electrophoretic loci between dispersers and residents are consistent with an innate dispersal hypothesis, this result is not sufficient to conclude that dispersal behavior has a large genetic component because a causal relationship cannot be demonstrated.

There have been three attempts to estimate the heritability of dispersal tendency in *Microtus.* The most exciting work to date is from a Ph.D. thesis on *M. townsendii* by Judith Anderson (1975), which represents the first attempt to examine the inheritance of ecologically relevant traits. Anderson (1975) housed individual breeding pairs of *M. townsendii* in 16 small field enclosures (6 m × 6 m) surrounded by rodent-proof fences. After litters were weaned, siblings were tagged, removed from the small enclosure and released either in a larger 0.8-ha enclosure or in an unfenced grid. If dispersal tendency has a genetic component, there should be a higher within-family correlation for length of residence in the population on the unfenced grid where dispersal can occur than on the fenced grid where no dispersal is possible. Siblings resembled one another closely in duration of life on both unfenced (t = 0.62) and fenced grids (t = 0.37). Furthermore, the intrafamily correlation on the unfenced grid was significantly higher than on the fenced grid.

Hilborn (1975) analyzed differences in dispersal tendency within and between sibships in *M. californicus, M. ochrogaster, M. pennsylvanicus,* and *M. townsendii.* If dispersal tendency has a large genetic component, then members of a single sibship should be more similar in their dispersal behavior than individuals from different sibships. An analysis of variance indicated that within-litter variance for disappearance rates was significantly lower than between-litter variance. Because disappearance could be due to either dispersal or death in situ, the results were ambiguous. Beacham (1979) was able experimentally to separate disappearance into survivorship and dispersal components in enclosed populations of *M. townsendii,* and compare within- and between-litter variability for both parameters using an analysis of variance. Dispersers were identified as those individuals that crossed an 18.3-m mowed area and were captured in pitfall traps. An analysis of variance indicated that in increasing and peak populations, identifiable families tended to survive or disperse as a unit.

The results from these three studies suggest that sibs resemble one another in their tendency to disperse. However, estimates of heritability from full-sib analysis should be viewed as upper limits of the true heritability values because it includes both common environment and dominance effects. Another problem is the large standard errors associated with these heritability estimates. Finally, in the latter two studies, sibs were determined by their similarity in weight and proximity of their trapping locations. This indirect method may have led to incorrect assignations of some individuals to family units.

Aggressive Behavior

Anderson (1975) also estimated heritability of agonistic behavior in *M. townsendii.* Adult voles were brought into the laboratory from the field and each test animal was matched against an opponent of the same sex. All tests were performed in a neutral arena (61 cm × 30 cm). The two opponents were separated for five minutes by a partition. After this time period the barrier was lifted and for 10 min the number of different types of behavior was recorded. The following behavioral variables were scored in each bout: active threat, approach latency, initiate investigation, fight initiator, defensive posture, mutual upright, retaliation, submissive posture, and activity. Voles were returned to the field after testing. Heritability was measured from the regression of offspring scores on midparent scores for each behavioral variable separately. The slopes of all regression lines were not significantly different from 0. Correlation coefficients were then calculated between offspring and sire scores, and offspring and dam scores, for each behavioral variable. There was only one association that was statistically significant: offspring attacks versus dam's attacks ($r = 0.36$, $P < 0.05$). When stepwise multiple regression of offspring behavioral variables on all maternal variables was performed, four of the nine offspring variables could be predicted at a statistically significant level by varying combinations of the dam's variables. Conversely, the sire's behavior could not predict any of the offspring's behavioral variables. Thus, there is a large maternal effect contributing to offspring behavior.

Growth Rates

Anderson (1975) used changes in skull width to measure growth rates of juvenile *M. townsendii.* Growth rates of skull width were measured for juveniles captured at least twice within a 4-week period. After correcting for seasonal effects by regression analysis, adjusted growth rates were compared among sibs. The intrafamily correlation, t, among full sibs resulted in an estimate of $h^2 = 0.46$.

Estimating the heritability of maximum body size presents a special problem because voles in natural populations usually disappear before they reach an asymptote in size. Anderson (1975) arbitrarily used skull width at last capture as a measure of maximum size. Parents whose skull widths were still changing rapidly were excluded from the analysis. She was able to correct for age by regressing maximum size on age and obtaining an adjusted maximum size for different age classes. These standardized sizes were used in estimates of heritability. Neither slopes of the regressions of offspring's maximum size on midparent's maximal size, or on sire's maximum size, were significantly different from 0. However, there was a positive correlation between offspring's maximum size and the dam's size, suggesting a maternal influence.

TABLE 7
ESTIMATES OF HERITABILITY FROM INTRAFAMILY CORRELATIONS OF FULL SIBS FOR SIX QUANTITATIVE TRAITS IN *Microtus townsendii* (FROM ANDERSON, 1975)

Trait	Heritability	Standard error
Dispersal tendency (unfenced grid)	0.62	0.11
Duration of life (fenced grid)	0.37	0.08
Adult agonistic behavior	0.00	—
Juvenile growth rate	0.46	0.24
Maximum body weight	0.00	—
Age at sexual maturity	0.55	0.20

Age at Sexual Maturity

Because the time of birth of litters born in breeding enclosures was known, Anderson (1975) was able to estimate the age at puberty for most of them. After adjusting for seasonal effects, the estimate of the intrafamily correlation for age at puberty was 0.55. This estimate of heritability was based on data from 41 litters and 89 offspring.

General Evaluation

Anderson's (1975) attempt to elucidate the genetic control of quantitative traits in *M. townsendii* is a trailblazing effort in several respects. It represents the first attempt to measure heritability in natural populations of *Microtus*. By raising litters in small breeding enclosures and later releasing littermates in natural populations, she provided a realistic environment for estimating heritability. Furthermore, the traits she examined were all ecologically relevant in the context of population cycles. The heritabilities of these traits are summarized in Table 7. Because the estimates were based on full-sib analysis, phenotypic resemblance may have been due in part to a common environment and dominance effects. Separate analyses of sib's phenotype on dam's phenotype and on sire's phenotype indicated that most traits were influenced by a maternal effect. In spite of difficulties in interpretation of the results of studies of this kind, similar attempts need to be made in other microtine species. In the future, problems associated with maternal effects could be circumvented by the use of paternal half-siblings and cross-fostering experiments. At the very least, we should be able to obtain a range of estimates of heritabilities for traits in populations of the same species in different localities as well as across species.

Relationship between Genetics and Population Regulation

Chitty (1967) formulated a genetic-behavioral hypothesis to explain multiannual density cycles in microtine rodents. His hypothesis was originally based on an r- and α-selection argument (Stenseth, 1978) but was later modified by Krebs (1978) to include dispersal. The model assumes: 1) a trade off between reproductive capabilities and survivorship, and 2) that space becomes limiting at high population densities. When densities are low, mutual interference is minimal, and natural selection favors those genotypes with a high reproductive output. As density increases and resources and space become limited, genotypes that are aggressive and exhibit spacing behavior have a selective advantage. The agonistic interactions resulting from spacing behavior by aggressive individuals promote the dispersal of subordinates. Dominant individuals of both sexes may pay for their aggressiveness by sacrificing other components of fitness such as reproduction, which sets the stage for the population decline. The major tenet of Chitty's (1967) hypothesis is that demographic changes are mediated by natural selection operating on the genetic composition of the population.

Historically, the first step in testing Chitty's (1967) hypothesis was to determine whether genetic changes occurred in the population and if these changes were closely associated with density. In several studies changes in gene frequency at electrophoretic loci were correlated with changes in density. Changes in gene frequencies at the TF locus (Tamarin and Krebs, 1969) and the TF and LAP loci (Gaines and Krebs, 1971) were correlated with population density in *M. ochrogaster* and *M. pennsylvanicus* in southern Indiana. LeDuc and Krebs (1975), monitoring gene frequency at the LAP locus in a population of *M. townsendii,* found a positive association between changes in the Lap^F allele and changes in population density. Kohn and Tamarin (1978) reported that changes in gene frequency at the TF locus were correlated with changes in density in *M. pennsylvanicus* and *M. breweri* populations in Massachusetts.

TABLE 8

CORRELATION COEFFICIENTS FOR CHANGES IN GENE FREQUENCY AT TRANSFERRIN AND LEUCINE AMINOPEPTIDASE LOCI IN RELATION TO POPULATION DENSITY FOR *Microtus ochrogaster* IN KANSAS ON FOUR GRIDS DURING DIFFERENT PHASES OF THE POPULATION CYCLE, 1970–1973 (FROM GAINES, 1981)

Location and phase	Number of trapping periods	Tf^E allele		Lap^F allele	
		Male	Female	Male	Female
Grid A					
Increase	27	0.73**	0.56*	−0.37	0.17
Decline	9	−0.42	−0.56	0.89**	0.10
Grid B					
Increase	23	0.59**	0.67**	0.20	0.51*
Decline	14	−0.90**	−0.08	0.77**	0.71**
Grid C					
Increase	14	−0.14	0.06	−0.26	−0.88**
Decline	27	0.18	0.16	0.48*	0.16
Grid D					
Increase	13	0.61*	0.10	0.32	0.20
Decline	14	0.02	−0.04	0.72**	0.22

* $P < 0.05$.
** $P < 0.01$.

One shortcoming of the above studies is that only one or at most two loci were monitored. Gaines et al. (1978) expanded the scope of earlier studies by monitoring changes in gene frequency at five loci: TF, LAP, 6-PGD, EST-1, and EST-4. Four live-trapped grids of *M. ochrogaster* were monitored over a 3-year period in eastern Kansas. Densities and gene frequencies are presented in Gaines et al. (1978:Figs. 1–6). Three general patterns of changes in gene frequency emerged from the Kansas data. 1) One locus (6-PGD) had relatively stable gene frequencies over the population cycle. The common allele, $6\text{-}Pgd^B$, went to fixation during some trapping periods with the polymorphism being restored by immigration. 2) Two loci (EST-1 and EST-4) had changes in gene frequencies unrelated to density. The largest temporal changes in gene frequencies occurred at the two esterase loci and were quantified by calculating averages of absolute changes in gene frequency (Δp) over time (Gaines et al., 1978:Table 3). 3) Two loci (TF and LAP) had gene frequency changes correlated with density. Correlation coefficients for Tf^E and Lap^F gene frequencies versus density during different phases of the population cycle are given in Table 8.

I found a somewhat different pattern of temporal variation at the TF and LAP loci in southern Indiana populations. In Indiana, Tf^E frequencies in both sexes were positively correlated with density over the entire population cycle. In Kansas, except for grid C, changes in gene frequency in both sexes were positively correlated with density during the increase phase. Changes in Lap^F frequency in Indiana populations were negatively correlated with density of males over the entire cycle, whereas these two variables were positively correlated in males during the decline phase in Kansas populations. Thus, only changes in gene frequency at the TF locus are repeatable over time and space.

Correlations between changes in gene frequency and density are consistent with Chitty's (1967) hypothesis, but it is difficult to disentangle cause and effect. Genetic changes may cause demographic changes or may be an effect of density changes. Charlesworth and Giesel (1972) demonstrated with computer simulations that a correlation between gene frequency and density could be produced by a change in the rate of population growth. They define the Wrightian fitness w_{ij} of the genotype carrying alleles i and j in an equilibrium population as:

$$w_{ij} = \sum_{x=1}^{n} e^{-rx} l_{ij}(x) m_{ij}(x)$$

where r is the rate of population growth of an equilibrium population in its stable age distribution, $l_{ij}(x)$ is the probability of the ith genotype living to age x, and $m_{ij}(x)$ is the number of offspring produced by the ijth genotype per unit time at age x. It follows from the above equation that as r becomes increasingly positive, younger age classes make a proportionately greater contribution to fitness, and gene frequencies change in favor of the genotype that reproduces earliest. Conversely, as r becomes increasingly negative, older age classes will be weighted more heavily and gene frequencies will change in favor of late reproducing genotypes. Thus, fluctuations in population age structure can alter relative contributions of early and late reproducing genotypes to the gene pool. Charlesworth and Giesel (1972) assigned $m(x)$ functions to three genotypes, each having three age classes, such that one homozygote started reproducing earlier than the other. In each case the heterozygote started reproducing at the same age as the earlier homozygote. Fluctuations in population density were accomplished by changing the $m(x)$ schedules of all genotypes uniformly to produce the desired change in population growth-rate. This procedure is equivalent to an extrinsic factor that has an identical effect on fecundity of all genotypes and age classes. In simulations consisting of 400 time intervals, gene-frequency changes were closely associated with changes in density (Charlesworth and Giesel, 1972: Fig. 2). These results suggest that fluctuations in gene frequency could be a side effect of population cycles (also see Charlesworth, 1980).

There are several lines of evidence supporting Charlesworth and Giesel's (1972) contention that changes in gene frequency are effects of density changes. First, a number of protein polymorphisms have been shown to be correlated with population density in a variety of New World and Old World microtine species (Bowen, 1982; Gaines and Krebs; 1971; Gaines et al., 1978; Kohn and Tamarin, 1978; Mihok et al., 1983; Nygren, 1980; Semeonoff and Robertson, 1968; Tamarin and Krebs, 1969). It is exceedingly unlikely that all these loci chosen at random are causally related to population cycles. Second, a comparative study of changes in gene frequency at the TF locus revealed similar patterns of temporal variation in a noncycling island population of *M. breweri* and a cycling mainland population of *M. pennsylvanicus* (Kohn and Tamarin, 1978). Finally, the best evidence comes from two perturbation experiments. Gaines et al. (1971) introduced "pure stands" of three different TF genotypes of *M. ochrogaster* into three separate fenced enclosures. There was no significant effect of genotype on population growth rate, percentage of breeding females, recruitment index, or survival rate of voles. LeDuc and Krebs (1975) maintained divergent allelic frequencies at an LAP locus by selective removal and addition of genotypes in two field populations of *M. townsendii*. The altered allelic frequencies in the two populations did not have any consistent effects on demography.

Perturbation experiments suggest that genetic changes at a single locus are effects of demographic changes, but they were not designed to test whether changes in average heterozygosity over many loci were causing density changes. Smith et al. (1975) related average heterozygosity to fluctuations in rodent numbers. They suggested that at low density inbreeding decreases heterozygosity, whereas at high density there is increased dispersal and the population becomes relatively more outbred, leading to increased heterozygosity. Because Garten (1976) found an increase in aggressive behavior with increased heterozygosity in *Peromyscus polionotus* populations, it could be argued that an increase in heterozygosity owing to outbreeding, as the population increases, results in increased aggressive behavior, which in turn is followed by increased mortality, decreased reproduction, and a population decline. This scenario is consistent with Chitty's (1967) hypothesis. However, Gaines et al. (1978) found a greater deficiency of heterozygotes averaged over five electrophoretic loci, compared to the expected number based on Hardy-Weinberg equilibrium in prairie-vole populations, as density increased.

I suggested previously (Gaines, 1981) that if density and the genetic structure of a population are in a closed feedback loop as implied by Chitty's (1967) hypothesis, the cause and effect dilemma becomes a moot issue. In this self-regulatory model, genotypic fitness is a function of density and a change in density will change the fitness of genotypes, which in turn will act back on density. If the genetic structure of the population and its demography are intimately associated with one another, we would like to know whether there is a set of simultaneous equations that describes the interaction between these two variables. The challenging task is to determine the form and relevant parameters of these equations.

Stenseth (1981) modeled a self-regulatory system in accordance with assumptions implicit in Chitty's (1967) genetic-behavioral hypothesis. He used two behavioral morphs, a docile phenotype and an aggressive phenotype, which were under simple Mendelian control. The two morphs were assigned fitnesses such that the docile phenotype had a selective advantage at low population density because of its higher reproduction, whereas selection favored the aggressive phenotype as density increased because of its higher survivorship and its depressing effect on the reproduction of the docile form. Stenseth (1981) demonstrated formally, using several mating schemes, that one morph eliminated the other. The outcome of which form persisted was dependent upon the dominance relationship between the docile and aggressive allele. Stenseth (1981) concluded that stable limit cycles could be generated only by the intervention of extrinsic environmental factors. The major weakness of Stenseth's model is its over-simplification of the real world. A complex behavioral trait is assumed to be controlled by two alleles; time lags and age structure are ignored. Nevertheless, it does represent one of the first direct tests of Chitty's hypothesis from a purely theoretical standpoint.

We can increase the complexity of the genetic feedback model by incorporating extrinsic factors such as weather. For example, changes in climate may cause changes in density and concomitantly cause changes in the genetic structure of the population. The problem of distinguishing between cause and effect is now compounded even further; not only must we consider the interaction of genetics and density, but also how demographic and genetic changes covary with different combinations of extrinsic factors. Lidicker (1973) is the leading proponent of this multi-factorial approach to the study of population regulation (see Taitt and Krebs, this volume).

In summary, there is convincing evidence from a number of studies that genetic changes at electrophoretic loci are closely associated with density changes in *Microtus* populations. It is an error to interpret these associations as support for Chitty's (1967) hypothesis. Theoretical and field studies suggest that genetic changes at a single locus were effects of demographic changes rather than vice-versa. In the future, attempts to relate genetic structure to population regulation must focus on those traits deemed ecologically relevant. The first steps in this direction have been taken by Anderson (1975). Finally, Smith et al.'s (1975) hypothesis about the relationship between average genic heterozygosity over many loci and density needs to be explored in natural populations of *Microtus*. If there is a consistent association between the two variables, perturbation experiments should be done.

Conclusions

In this concluding section I identify areas for future research in the genetics of *Microtus*. Of course these selections reflect my personal bias. Three research areas that may prove to be profitable in the future are: 1) the effect of social dynamics on the genetic structure of populations; 2) inheritance and evolution of quantitative traits; and 3) the application of new molecular techniques to assess genetic variation in natural populations.

Mating systems can have profound effects on the genetic structure of populations. If a population is subdivided into small inbreeding units or demes, genotypic frequencies will deviate from the expected proportions based on Hardy-Weinberg equilibrium; there will be an excess of homozygotes and a deficiency of heterozygotes. Furthermore, a cohesive family unit will restrict gene flow between populations. Microtines present real difficulties in studying social behavior because individuals are nocturnal or crepuscular and occupy habitats which preclude direct observation (see Getz, this volume; Wolff, this volume). As a result of these difficulties most of the genetic studies referenced in this review have treated microtine populations as one large panmictic unit. However, Wolff's review (this volume) of social behavior in microtines indicates that mating systems can vary from monogamy to promiscuity. From a genetic interest, we need to know how social behavior changes as a function of different demographic parameters such as density and reproductive activity, and how the social dynamics relate to the temporal and spatial distribution of gene frequencies. Hopefully, we will be able to answer these questions as the technology for studying social behavior becomes better developed.

Future work in genetics should be directed towards the inheritance of quantitative traits. We now have estimates of heritability from full-sib analysis for several traits in *M. townsendii* (Anderson, 1975). Krebs (1979) has arranged microtine populations on a demographic continuum from strongly cyclic, exhibiting 3–4 year cycles at one end, to stable, exhibiting annual cycles at the other end. Krebs (1979) hypothesizes that this demographic continuum can be mapped directly on a genetic continuum of the heritability of spacing behavior, from high heritability in strongly cyclical populations to low heritability in stable populations. This hypothesis can be tested by estimating the heritability of behavioral traits in a variety of microtine species. The major obstacle is devising techniques to determine parentage in the field. Anderson (1975) housed breeding pairs in small field enclosures and subsequently released littermates in open field populations where traits were quantified. Because rates of disappearance of these young voles from open field populations were high, sample sizes were greatly reduced. Tamarin et al. (1983) developed a new technique for determining matrilineal kinship in natural populations of microtines that should be useful in estimating heritability. Pregnant females trapped in the field were injected with different gamma-emitting radionuclides and released. Young animals subsequently captured were subjected to whole-body gamma spectroscopy and identified by the spectral characteristics of the nuclides used to tag the mother. By combining this technique with electrophoresis of mothers, young, and potential fathers, the maternity and paternity of offspring may be determined in the field.

After obtaining estimates of heritability, it would be interesting to estimate genetic correlations between pairs of traits. For example, we could determine whether there is a genetic correlation between agonistic behavior and dispersal tendency. Genetic correlations can be calculated from the following formula:

$$r_A = \frac{COV_{XY}}{\sigma^2{}_X \sigma^2{}_Y}$$

where COV_{XY} is the among family component of covariance between the two traits and $\sigma^2{}_X$ and $\sigma^2{}_Y$ are the among-family components of variance for the two traits. Generally, data from paternal half-sib families are used in this formula but full-sib data can be used assuming no dominance effects. Genetic correlations between phenotypic variables could be due to pleiotropy or linkage. If selection is weak, pleiotropy will be the predominant cause of genetic covariance (Falconer, 1981).

As we accumulate more information on heritability and genetic correlation of phenotypic characters, it will eventually lead us to a point where we can make meaningful conclusions about multivariate phenotypic evolution. Lande (1979) provided a theoretical framework for the evolution of quantitative traits by examining the effects of natural selection on correlated characters within populations. Some progress is being made in this area by Atchley and his coworkers (Atchley and Rutledge, 1980; Atchley et al., 1981) on size and shape variation in the laboratory rat. In the future, quantitative genetic analysis of traits in microtine populations also may be a useful data base to test some of the predictions generated by Lande's (1979) theory.

After electrophoresis was first applied to natural populations of organisms by Lewontin and Hubby (1966), investigators relied exclusively on this technique to estimate levels of genetic variation in a multitude of species ranging from bacteria to humans. Recently, new techniques have become available from the field of molecular biology that are more sensitive in detecting genetic variation. One such method compares sequences of DNA segments obtained with the use of restriction endonucleases. These enzymes recognize specific nucleotide sequences and cleave the DNA at these sequences. Fragments can then be compared with electrophoresis. Avise et al. (1979) used six restriction endonucleases to measure mitochondrial (mtDNA) sequence relatedness in natural populations of *Peromyscus*. They found heterogeneity in mtDNA among individuals in the same population and among individuals from different populations. Individuals from the same population showed less than 0.5% sequence divergence, whereas those from different populations separated by 50–500 miles differ by 1.5%. Similar types of analyses could be done on microtine populations to get more reliable estimates of genetic variation. In addition, these new techniques will be extremely useful in determining phylogenetic relationships in the genus *Microtus* (see Anderson, this volume).

Acknowledgments

I am indebted to Thomas S. Whittam for the extraordinary amount of work that he did in improving the first draft of the manuscript. Also, I am grateful to Ayesha Gill who made many constructive comments and directed me to source material for this chapter. The following individuals read selected sections of the manuscript and made many helpful suggestions: W. Bloom, K. Hamrick, R. Lande, L. McClenaghan, Jr., and R. Tamarin. My own work on the genetics of *Microtus* has been supported by grants from the General Research Grant Fund of the University of Kansas and the National Science Foundation.

Literature Cited

ANDERSON, J. L. 1975. Phenotypic correlations among relatives and variability in reproductive performance in populations of the vole *Microtus townsendii*. Unpubl. Ph.D. dissert., Univ. British Columbia, Vancouver, 207 pp.

ATCHLEY, W. R., AND J. J. RUTLEDGE. 1980. Genetic components of size and shape. I. Dynamics of components of phenotypic variability and covariability during ontogeny in the laboratory rat. Evolution, 34:1161–1173.

ATCHLEY, W. R., J. J. RUTLEDGE, AND D. E. COWLEY 1981. Genetic components of size and shape. II. Multivariate covariance patterns in the rat and mouse skull. Evolution, 35:1037–1055.

AVISE, J. C., R. A. LANSMAN, AND R. O. SHADE. 1979. The use of restriction endonucleases to measure mitochondrial DNA sequence relatedness in natural populations. I. Population structure and evolution in the genus *Peromyscus.* Genetics, 92:279–295.

BARRETT, G. W. 1975. Occurrence of an albino *Microtus pennsylvanicus* in Ohio. Ohio J. Sci., 75:102.

BEACHAM, T. D. 1979. Dispersal tendency and duration of littermates during population fluctuations of the vole *Microtus townsendii.* Oecologia, 42: 11–22.

BECK, M. L., AND J. T. MAHAN. 1978. The chromosomes of *Microtus pinetorum.* J. Heredity, 69:343–344.

BIRDSALL, D. A. 1974. An analysis of selection at two loci in fluctuating populations of *Microtus.* Canadian J. Zool., 52:1457–1462.

BLOSSOM, P. M. 1942. Total melanism in *Microtus* from Michigan. J. Mamm., 23:214.

BOWEN, B. S. 1982. Temporal dynamics of microgeographic structure of genetic variation in *Microtus californicus.* J. Mamm., 63:625–638.

BOWEN, B. S., AND S. Y. YANG. 1978. Genetic control of enzyme polymorphisms in the California vole, *Microtus californicus.* Biochem. Genet., 16:455–467.

CHARLESWORTH, B. 1980. Evolution in age-structured populations. Cambridge Univ. Press, London, 300 pp.

CHARLESWORTH, B., AND J. T. GIESEL. 1972. Selection in populations with overlapping generations. II. Relations between gene frequency and demographic variables. Amer. Nat., 106:388–401.

CHITTY, D. 1967. The natural selection of self-regulatory behaviour in animal populations. Proc. Ecol. Soc. Australia, 2:51–78.

CLARK, F. H. 1938. Coat color in the meadow vole. J. Heredity, 29:265–266.

EWENS, W. J., AND M. FELDMAN. 1976. The theoretical assessment of selective neutrality. Pp. 303–338, *in* Population genetics and ecology (S. Karlin and E. Nevo, eds.). Academic Press, New York, 832 pp.

FALCONER, D. S. 1981. Introduction to quantitative genetics. Second ed. Ronald Press Co., New York, 340 pp.

FEDYK, S. 1970. Chromosomes of *Microtus (Stenocranius) gregalis major* (Ognev, 1923) and phylogenetic connections between sub-arctic representatives of the genus *Microtus* Schrank, 1798. Acta Theriol., 15:143–152.

FISHER, H. I. 1942. A white meadow mouse. J. Mamm., 23:336.

FIVUSH, B., R. PARKER, AND R. H. TAMARIN. 1975. Karyotype of the beach vole, *Microtus breweri,* an endemic island species. J. Mamm., 56:272–273.

FREDGA, K., AND U. BERGSTRÖM. 1970. Chromosome polymorphism in the root vole (*Microtus oeconomus*). Hereditas, 66:145–152.

GAINES, M. S. 1981. The importance of genetics to population dynamics. Pp. 1–27, *in* Mammalian population genetics (M. H. Smith and J. Joule, eds.). Univ. Georgia Press, Athens, 380 pp.

GAINES, M. S., AND C. J. KREBS. 1971. Genetic changes in fluctuating vole populations. Evolution, 25:702–723.

GAINES, M. S., AND T. S. WHITTAM. 1980. Genetic changes in fluctuating vole populations: selective vs nonselective forces. Genetics, 96:767–778.

GAINES, M. S., L. R. MCCLENAGHAN, JR., AND R. K. ROSE. 1978. Temporal patterns of allozymic variation in fluctuating populations of *Microtus ochrogaster.* Evolution, 32:723–729.

GAINES, M. S., J. H. MYERS, AND C. J. KREBS. 1971. Experimental analysis of relative fitness in transferrin genotypes of *Microtus ochrogaster.* Evolution, 25:443–450.

GARTEN, C. T., JR. 1976. Relationships between aggressive behavior and genetic

heterozygosity in the old field mouse, *Peromyscus polionotus.* Evolution, 30: 59–72.
GILL, A. E. 1976. White spotting in the California vole. Heredity, 51:113–128.
———. 1977. Maintenance of polymorphism in an island population of the California vole, *Microtus californicus.* Evolution, 31:512–525.
———. 1980. Partial reproductive isolation of subspecies of the California vole, *Microtus californicus.* Genetika, 52/53:105–117.
———. 1982. Variability in the karyotype of the California vole, *Microtus californicus. In* Abstracts of the Twentieth Annual Somatic Cell Genetics Conference, Lake Tahoe, Nevada.
GILL, A. E., AND K. BOLLES. 1982. A heritable tooth trait varying in two subspecies of *Microtus californicus* (Rodentia: Cricetidae). J. Mamm., 63:96–103.
GUTHRIE, R. D. 1965. Variability in characters undergoing rapid evolution, an analysis of *Microtus* molars. Evolution, 19:214–233.
HARTKE, G. T., H. W. LEIPOLD, K. HUSTON, J. E. COOK, AND G. SAPERSTEIN. 1974. Three mutations and the karyotype of the prairie vole. J. Heredity, 65:301–307.
HATT, R. T. 1930. Color varieties of Long Island mammals. J. Mamm., 11:322–323.
HAYS, H. A., AND D. BINGHAM. 1964. An albino prairie vole from Kansas. J. Mamm., 45:479.
HILBORN, R. 1974. Inheritance of skeletal polymorphism in *Microtus californicus.* Heredity, 33:87–89.
———. 1975. Similarities in dispersal tendency among siblings in four species of voles (*Microtus*). Ecology, 56:1221–1225.
HOWARD, W. E. 1965. Interaction of behavior, ecology, and genetics of introduced mammals. Pp. 461–484, *in* The genetics of colonizing species (H. G. Baker and G. L. Stebbins, eds.). Academic Press, New York, 588 pp.
HSU, T. C., AND K. BENIRSCHKE. 1967–1975. An atlas of mammalian chromosomes. Vols. 1–9. Springer-Verlag, New York.
HSU, T. C., AND M. L. JOHNSON. 1970. Cytological distinction between *Microtus montanus* and *Microtus canicaudus.* J. Mamm., 51:824–826.
HUBBELL, H. R., AND T. C. HSU. 1977. Identification of nucleolus organizer regions (NORs) in normal and neoplastic human cells by the silver-staining technique. Cytogenet. Cell Genet., 19:185–196.
IMAI, H. T., AND R. H. CROZIER. 1980. Quantitative analysis of directionality in mammalian karyotype evolution. Amer. Nat., 116:537–569.
JANNETT, F. J., JR. 1981. Albinism and its inheritance in populations of the montane vole. J. Heredity, 72:144–146.
JEWETT, S. G. 1955. Free-tailed bats and melanistic mice in Oregon. J. Mamm., 36:458–459.
JOHNSON, M. L. 1968. Application of blood protein electrophoretic studies to problems in mammalian taxonomy. Syst. Zool., 17:23–30.
JUDD, S. R., AND S. P. CROSS. 1980. Chromosomal variation in *Microtus longicaudus* (Merriam). Murrelet, 61:2–5.
JUDD, S. R., S. P. CROSS, AND S. PATHAK. 1980. Non-Robertsonian chromosomal variation in *Microtus montanus.* J. Mamm., 61:109–113.
KEITH, T. P., AND R. H. TAMARIN. 1981. Genetic and demographic difference between dispersers and residents in cycling and noncycling populations. J. Mamm., 60:713–725.
KIRBY, G. C. 1974. The bias in the regression of Δq on q. Heredity, 33:93–97.
KOHN, P. H., AND R. H. TAMARIN. 1978. Selection of electrophoretic loci for

reproductive parameters in island and mainland voles. Evolution, 32: 15–28.

KREBS, C. J. 1978. Aggression, dispersal and cyclic changes in populations of small mammals. Pp. 49–60, *in* Aggression, dominance and individual spacing (L. Krames, P. Pliner, and T. Alloway, eds.). Plenum, New York, 173 pp.

———. 1979. Dispersal, spacing behaviour, and genetics in relation to population fluctuations in the vole *Microtus townsendii*. Fortschr. Zool., 25:61–77.

KREBS, C. J., ET AL. 1976. *Microtus* population biology: dispersal in fluctuating populations of *M. townsendii*. Canadian J. Zool., 54:79–95.

KUTZ, H. L., AND R. H. SMITH. 1945. Breeding of abnormally colored meadow mice. J. Mamm., 26:307–308.

LANDE, R. 1979. Quantitative genetic analysis of multivariate evolution applied to brain:body size allometry. Evolution, 33:402–416.

LEDUC, J., AND C. J. KREBS. 1975. Demographic consequences of artificial selection at the LAP locus in voles (*Microtus townsendii*). Canadian J. Zool., 53:1825–1840.

LEWONTIN, R. C., AND J. L. HUBBY. 1966. A molecular approach to the study of genic heterozygosity in natural populations. II. Amount of variation and degree of heterozygosity in natural populations of *Drosophila pseudoobscura*. Genetics, 54:595–609.

LEWONTIN, R. C., AND J. KRAKAUER. 1973. Distribution of gene frequency as a test of the theory of the selective neutrality of polymorphisms. Genetics, 74:175–195.

LIDICKER, W. Z., JR. 1963. The genetics of a naturally occurring coat-color mutation in the California vole. Evolution, 17:340–346.

———. 1973. Regulation of numbers of an island population of the California vole, a problem in community dynamics. Ecol. Monogr., 43:271–302.

MARUYAMA, T., AND H. T. IMAI. 1981. Evolutionary rate of the mammalian karyotype. J. Theor. Biol., 90:111–121.

MASER, C. E., W. HAMMER, AND M. L. JOHNSON. 1969. Abnormal coloration in *Microtus montanus*. Murrelet, 50:39.

MATTHEY, R. 1973. The chromosome formulae of eutherian mammals. Pp. 39–81, *in* Cytotaxonomy and vertebrate evolution (A. B. Chiarelli and E. Capanna, eds.). Academic Press, London, 783 pp.

MAURER, F. W. 1967. Heritability of transferrin protein in three species of *Microtus*. Nature, 215:95–96.

MCGOVERN, M., AND C. R. TRACY. 1981. Phenotypic variation in electromorphs previously considered to be genetic markers in *Microtus ochrogaster*. Oecologia, 51:276–280.

MIHOK, S., AND D. EWING. 1983. Reliability of transferrin and leucine aminopeptidase phenotyping in wild meadow voles (*Microtus pennsylvanicus*). Biochem. Genet., 21:969–983.

MIHOK, S., W. A. FULLER, R. P. CANHAM, AND E. C. MCPHEE. 1983. Genetic changes at the transferrin locus in the red-backed vole (*Clethrionomys gapperi*). Evolution, 37:332–340.

MURIE, O. J. 1934. Melanism in an Alaskan vole. J. Mamm., 15:323.

MYERS, J. H., AND C. J. KREBS. 1971. Genetic, behavioral, and reproductive attributes of dispersing field voles *Microtus pennsylvanicus* and *Microtus ochrogaster*. Ecol. Monogr., 41:53–78.

NADLER, C. F., V. R. RAUSCH, E. A. LYAPUNOVA, R. S. HOFFMANN, AND N. N. VORONSTOV. 1976. Chromosomal banding patterns of the Holarctic rodents, *Clethrionomys rutilus* and *Microtus oeconomus*. Z. Saugetierk., 41: 137–146.

NADLER, C. F., ET AL. 1978. Biochemical relationships of the Holarctic vole genera (*Clethrionomys, Microtus,* and *Arvicola*) (Rodentia:Arvicolinae). Canadian J. Zool., 56:1564–1575.

NEI, M., AND T. MARUYAMA. 1975. Lewontin-Krakauer test for neutral genes. Genetics, 80:395.

NEVO, E. 1978. Genetic variation in natural populations: patterns and theory. Theor. Pop. Biol., 13:831–840.

NYGREN, J. 1980. Allozyme variation in natural populations of field vole (*Microtus agrestis* L.). III. Survey of a cyclically density-varying population. Hereditas, 93:125–136.

OHNO, S. 1969. The mammalian genome in evolution and conservation of the original X-linkage group. Pp. 18–29, *in* Comparative mammalian cytogenetics (K. Benirshke, ed.). Springer-Verlag, New York, 473 pp.

ORR, R. T. 1941. Yellow mutation in the California meadow mouse, *Microtus californicus*. Wasmann Collector, 4:129–130.

OWEN, R. D., AND R. M. SHACKELFORD. 1942. Color aberrations in *Microtus* and *Pitymys*. J. Mamm., 23:306–314.

PATTON, J. L. 1977. B-chromosome systems in the pocket mouse, *Perognathus baileyi*: meiosis and C-band studies. Chromosoma, 60:1–14.

PAUL, J. R. 1964. Second record of an albino pine vole. J. Mamm., 45:485.

PICKERING, J., L. L. GETZ, AND G. S. WHITT. 1974. An esterase phenotype correlated with dispersal in *Microtus*. Trans. Illinois State Acad. Sci., 67: 471–475.

PINTER, A. J. 1979. Dominant spotting in a natural population of the vole *Microtus montanus*. J. Heredity, 70:441–443.

PINTER, A. J., AND A. K. MCLEAN. 1970. Hereditary hairlessness in the montane vole. J. Heredity, 61:112–114.

PINTER, A. J., AND N. C. NEGUS. 1971. Coat color mutations in two species of voles (*Microtus montanus* and *Microtus ochrogaster*) in the laboratory. J. Mamm., 52:196–199.

RAUSCH, V. R., AND R. L. RAUSCH. 1974. The chromosomal complement of the yellow-cheeked vole, *Microtus xanthognathus* (Leach). Canadian J. Genet. Cytol., 16:267–272.

RIGGS, L. A. 1979. Experimental studies of dispersal in the California vole, *Microtus californicus*. Unpubl. Ph.D. dissert., Univ. California, Berkeley, 236 pp.

ROBERTSON, A. 1975*a*. Remarks on the Lewontin-Krakauer test. Genetics, 80:396.

———. 1975*b*. Gene frequency distribution as a test of selective neutrality. Genetics, 81:775–785.

SCHANTZ, V. S. 1960. Record of an albino pine vole. J. Mamm., 41:129.

SELANDER, R. K. 1976. Genic variation in natural populations. Pp. 21–45, *in* Molecular evolution (F. J. Ayala, ed.). Sinauer Assoc., Inc., Sunderland, Massachusetts, 277 pp.

SEMEONOFF, R. 1972. Esterase polymorphisms in *Microtus ochrogaster*. Biochem. Genet., 6:125–138.

———. 1973. Two coat color variants in the prairie vole. J. Heredity, 64:48–52.

SEMEONOFF, R., AND F. W. ROBERTSON. 1968. A biochemical and ecological study of plasma esterase polymorphism in natural populations of the field vole, *Microtus agrestis* L. Biochem. Genet., 1:205–227.

SHELLHAMMER, H. S. 1969. Supernumerary chromosomes of the harvest mouse, *Reithrodontomys megalotis*. Chromosoma, 27:102–108.

SMITH, C. A. B. 1970. A note on testing the Hardy-Weinberg law. Ann. Hum. Genet., 33:377–383.

SMITH, M. H., C. T. GARTEN, JR., AND P. R. RAMSEY. 1975. Genic heterozygosity and population dynamics in small mammals. Pp. 85–102, *in* Isozymes. IV. Genetics and evolution (C. L. Markert, ed.). Academic Press Inc., New York, 965 pp.

SMITH, M. H., M. N. MANLOVE, AND J. JOULE. 1978. Spatial and temporal dynamics of genetic organization of small mammal populations. Pp. 99–103, *in* Populations of small mammals under natural conditions (D. P. Snyder, ed.). Univ. Pittsburgh, Pittsburgh, 237 pp.

SNYDER, L. L. 1930. Color mutants in *Microtus*. J. Mamm., 11:83.

STENSETH, N. C. 1978. Demographic strategies in fluctuating populations of small rodents. Oecologia, 33:149–172.

———. 1981. On Chitty's theory for fluctuating populations: the importance of genetic polymorphism in the generation of regular density cycles. Theor. Biol., 90:9–36.

TAMARIN, R. H., AND C. J. KREBS. 1969. *Microtus* population biology. II. Genetic changes at the transferrin locus in fluctuating populations of two vole species. Evolution, 23:183–211.

TAMARIN, R. H., M. SHERIDAN, AND C. K. LEVY. 1983. Determining matrilineal kindship in natural populations of rodents using radionuclides. Canadian J. Zool., 61:271–274.

TODD, N. B. 1967. A theory of karyotypic fissioning, genetic potentiation and eutherian evolution. Mamm. Chromosomes Newsl., 8:268–279.

VERNER, L. 1979. The significance of dispersal in fluctuating populations of *Microtus ochrogaster* and *M. pennsylvanicus*. Unpubl. Ph.D. dissert., Univ. Illinois, Urbana, 86 pp.

WARREN, E. R. 1929. An albino field mouse. J. Mamm., 10:82.

WHITTAM, T. S. 1981. Is a negative regression of Δp on p evidence of a stable polymorphism? Evolution, 35:595–596.

WRIGHT, S. 1965. The interpretation of population structure by F-statistics with special regard to systems of mating. Evolution, 19:395–420.

INDEX*

Activity rhythms, 374–389, 412
  circadian, 381–382
  climate, 387–389
  competition, 386–387
  energetics, 384, 830
  genetics, 384
  infradian, 382–384
  parasitism, 386–387
  predation, 386
  sex, 385
  social factors, 385–386
  ultradian, 381
Adrenal gland
  endocrinology, 704–716
  ultrastructure, 241–243
Agonistic behavior, 360–364
  genetics, 867–869
Agricultural habitats, 304–305
Allophaiomys, 6, 8, 9, 11, 105
Allozymes (see Genetics, allozymic variation)
Amphibians, predation by, 558–559
Anatomy
  gross, 118–159
    circulatory system, 138–140
    digestive system, 140–155
    integument, 118–121
    musculature, 136–138
    reproductive system, 155–159
    skeleton, 121–136
    teeth, 140–150
  ultrastructure, 177–247
    adrenal gland, 241, 243
    brain, 179
    dentition, 196–202
    digestive tract, 216–240, 242, 244
    eyes, 180–193
    integumentary glands, 194–196
    pituitary gland, 179–180
    reproductive tracts, 243, 245–247
    salivary glands, 202–217
    tarsal (Meibomian) glands, 193–194
Arborimus, 91
Artichoke method in taxonomy, 75–76
Avian predation, 537–550

Baculum
  function, 159
  macroanatomy, 155–157
Baubellum, macroanatomy, 158
Beetles, as parasites, 481–482
Behavior, 340–366
  nonsocial, 341–344
  social, 344–366
    activity rhythms, 385–386
    agonistic, 360–364, 867–869
    communal nesting, 354–356
    copulatory, 353–354
    genotypic causes, 592, 602–604, 867–869
    mating systems, 344–353
    olfactory communication, 356–359
    phenotypic causes, 590–592, 600–602
    role in demography, 590–592, 600–604
    social structure, 344–353
    vocalization, 359–360
  spacing, 389–413
    climate, 409–411
    dispersal, 405, 432–434
    dispersion, 405–406
    energetics, 406–407

* This index is primarily a guide to subject areas covered in the text. Topics and species briefly mentioned in the text or in abstracts, summaries, figures, references, or appendices may not be indexed. Check CONTENTS for broad subject areas.

home range, 398–401
interspecific interactions, 409
movement types, 402–405
role in demography, 589–590, 598–600
sex, 407–408
social factors, 408–409
territoriality, 401–402
Biomes and biogeographical provinces, 85–105 (see also Zoogeography, ecological)
cloud forest, 101–102
grassland, 99, 101
shrubland and woodland, 97–99
taiga, 90–97
temperate deciduous forest, 101
tundra, 88–90
Body size
affect on competition, 327
demographic consequences, 605–607
Brain, ultrastructure, 179
Breeding season
length, 728–739
timing, 687–688
Bruce effect, 602, 699–700, 742–745
Burrowing, 332

Caecum
fermentation, 154, 780
macroanatomy, 153–155
osmoregulation, 238
ultrastructure, 238
Carnivore (mammalian) predation, 551–558
Cecum (see Caecum)
Chilotus, 91, 107
Chionomys, 108
Circadian rhythms, 381–382
Circulatory system, 138–140
Cladistics, 78
Cladograms, 61
Clethrionomys
distribution, 91
prenatal development, 257–262
systematics, 54, 56
taxonomic key, 62–66
Climate
effect on activity, 387–389
effect on spacing behavior, 409–411
effect on species diversity, 316–318
Cloud forest biome, 101–102
Communal food storing, 354–356
Communal nesting, 317, 354–356, 402
Communication
olfactory, 356–359
vocalization, 359–360
Community ecology, 310–334
biomass, 331–332
climate, 316–318
competition, 321–324
influence of *Microtus,* 325–329
predation, 324–325
role of *Microtus,* 329–332
species diversity, 310–316
substrate, 318–319
vegetation, 319–321
Competition, 297–300, 321–324
effect on activity, 386–387
effect on demography, 577
Control, 621–642
barriers, 626
chemicals, 631–639
environmental hazards, 639–641
habitat manipulation, 626–628
hoofed animals, 628
monitoring, 624–626
predators, 630
repellents, 628–630
trapping, 630
Coprophagy, 384, 780
Copulatory
behavior, 353–354
plugs, 159
success, 742
Corpus luteum, 697–698
Cranium, 121–135
foramina, 129–133
morphometrics, 121–129
Cycles (see Demography)
Cytogenetics, 849–853

Damage to agriculture, 621–623

Demography, 567–612
  causes, 588–609
    food, 588–589, 594–597, 804–806
    genotypic behavior,592, 602–604
    multifactorial, 592–594, 604–609
    phenotypic behavior, 590–592, 600–602
    predation, 589, 597–598
    quantitative inheritance, 870–875
    role of dispersal, 590
    spacing behavior, 589–590, 598–600
  effect on communities, 326–327
  fence effect, 440
  impact of predation, 556–563
  mathematical models, 609–610
  methods of study, 569–572
  patterns, 572–588
  relation to dispersal, 427, 430–432, 436–442
Dentition (see also Teeth)
  macroanatomy, 140–150
  ultrastructure, 196–202
Development, 255–280
  neonatal, 263–265
  post-implantation, 258–259
  postnatal, 270–277
  pre-implantation, 256–257
  stages, 262
Dicrostonyx
  systematics, 54, 56–57
  taxonomic key, 62–66
Diet, 329–332, 781–790 (see also Nutrition)
Digestive system
  macroanatomy, 140–155
  ultrastructure, 216–240, 242, 244
Diseases (see Pathology)
Dispersal, 420–448
  behavioral features, 432–434
  categories, 425–429
  demographic causes, 436–442
  demographic consequences, 436–442, 590
  demographic features, 427, 430–432
  evolutionary issues, 442–445
  fence effect, 440
  genetic features, 434–436, 865–867
  relation to spacing behavior, 405
  techniques of study, 422–425
Dispersion, 405–406

Ear, internal, macroanatomy, 133–135
Ectoparasites, 455–504 (see also Parasites)
Electrophoresis (see Genetics, allozymic variation)
Endocrinology, 685–718
  adrenal gland, 704–716
  Bruce effect, 699–700
  corpus luteum, 697–698
  estrus, 693–697
  gestation, 698–700
  lactation, 701–702
  ovulation, 693–697
  postpartum estrus, 700–701
  testicular activity, 702–703
  thyroid gland, 703–704
  timing of reproduction, 686–693
    nutritional cues, 689–691
    photic cues, 688–689
    seasonality, 687–688
    sexual maturation, 686
    social cues, 691–693
Endoparasites, 528–534 (see also Parasites)
Energetics, 812–839
  effect on activity, 384
  effect on spacing behavior, 406–407
  energy acquisition, 817–821
  energy allocation, 821–836
    activity, 830
    growth, 830–834
    reproduction, 834–836
    temperature regulation, 821–824
    thermogenesis, 824–830
  methods and terminology, 815–817

models, 814, 816, 837–838
role in community structure, 332
Esophagus, ultrastructure, 218–222
Estrus, 693–697, 700–701
Evolution (see also Fossil record, Systematics)
karyotypic, 852–853
of dispersal, 442–445
Eye, ultrastructure, 180–193

Fence effect, 440
Fish, predation by, 558–559
Fleas, 484–503
Flies, as parasites, 482–484
Food (see also Plant secondary compounds, Nutrition)
digestibility, 790–797, 818–821
gathering, 818
habits, 781–787
palatability, 789–790
reproductive cues, 689–691, 729–730
role in demography, 588–589, 594–597
role in litter size, 763
selection, 329–332, 787–790
Fossil faunas, 37–51
Fossil record
definition, 1–2
Microtus group, 15–29, 105–113
Pitymys group, 5–15
sites, 3
systematics, 5–29
time chart, 5

Gall bladder, macroanatomy, 153
Genetics, 845–878
allozymic variation, 853–864
natural selection, 857–864
polymorphisms, 853–857
cytogenetics, 849–853
pelage coloration, 846–849
quantitative genetics, 864–875
age at sexual maturity, 869
aggressive behavior, 867–869
dispersal, 865–867
growth rates, 868–869
heritability, 864–865
population regulation, 870–875
role in activity, 384
role in demography, 592, 602–604
role in dispersal, 434–436, 603–604
Gestation, 262–263, 698–700
Glans penis, macroanatomy, 156–157
Grassland biome, 99, 101
Growth
demographic consequences, 605–607
energetics, 830–834
genetics, 867–869
post-implantation, 256–258
postnatal, 270–275
pre-implantation, 256–257
Gut, macroanatomy, 152–155

Habitats, 287–305
agricultural, 304–305
cover, 298–299
graminoid, 291–292
human activities, 302–305
insular, 300–301
moisture regimes, 295–298
non-graminoid herbaceous, 293
nutritional differences, 803–804
patchiness, 301–302
rocky, 294–295
species diversity, 310–316
succession, 327–329
wooded, 293–294
Home range, 398–401
Hormones, affects on aggression, 601–602 (see also Endocrinology)

Infradian rhythms, 382–384
Insular forms, 85, 109
competition, 323–324
demography, 599–600
habitats, 300–301
Integument
macroanatomy, 118–121
Meibomian glands, 120

plantar foot pads, 120–121
skin glands, 118–120, 356–359
ultrastructure, 194–196
Interspecific interactions
effects on activity rhythms, 386–387
effects on spacing behavior, 409
Intestine
macroanatomy, 153–155
ultrastructure, 233–240, 242, 244

Karyotypes, 109–110 (see also Cytogenetics)
Kin selection, 591–592
Kite predation, 541–550

Laboratory management, 647–657
breeding, 655-656
housing, 653–657
records, 653
Lactation, 701–702
Lagurus
systematics, 54, 56
taxonomic key, 62–66
Lasiopodomys, 17
Lemmings, taxonomic key, 62–66
Lemmus
systematics, 54, 56–57
taxonomic key, 62–66
Lice, 478–481
Light cues, 688–689
Litter size, 266–268, 751–766
Liver, macroanatomy, 153

Macroanatomy, 116–169 (see also Anatomy)
Mammalian predation, 550–558
Mammary glands, macroanatomy, 157–158
Management (see Control)
Mating systems, 344–353, 591
Meibomian glands
macroanatomy, 120
ultrastructure, 193–194
Microanatomy, 177–247 (see also Anatomy)
Microtus
fossil record, 15–29
general characteristics, 59–60
skin glands, 118–120
taxonomic characters, 55–57, 166–167
taxonomic key, 62–66
zoogeography, 105–113
Microtus abbreviatus
distribution, 89
endoparasites, 529, 531
fleas, 491
mites, 461
Microtus agrestis
breeding season, 738
similarity to *Microtus pennsylvanicus,* 27, 55
Microtus breweri
adrenal glands, 243
breeding season, 731
caecum, 238
demography, 583, 585, 587
distribution, 90
endoparasites, 529
fleas, 491
lice, 480
ticks, 476
Microtus californicus
breeding season, 733–734
demography, 577, 580, 582–583, 587
distribution, 97, 100, 107
endoparasites, 529, 532
fleas, 491–493
fossil record, 20–21
lice, 480
mites, 461–462
pre-implantation development, 256
social organization, 346, 351–352
ticks, 476
Microtus canicaudus
distribution, 91, 94, 110
fleas, 493
prenatal mortality, 245
ticks, 476
Microtus chrotorrhinus
breeding season, 733
distribution, 95, 99, 108
endoparasites, 529, 532
fleas, 493–494
fossil record, 23–24

mites, 462–463
Old World affinities, 55
pelage, 118
ticks, 476
Microtus coronarius, distribution, 96
Microtus deceitensis, 16–17, 107–108
Microtus gregalis, distribution, 111
Microtus guatemalensis, distribution, 101, 106
Microtus llanensis, 8
Microtus longicaudus
breeding season, 731–732
demography, 583, 585, 587
distribution, 92, 95–96, 108
endoparasites, 529, 532
fleas, 494–495
fossil record, 22
lice, 480
mites, 463–464
Old World affinities, 55
skin glands, 119–120, 195–196
ticks, 476
Microtus mexicanus
breeding season, 731–732
demography, 585–587
distribution, 99, 102, 109–110
endoparasites, 529, 532
fleas, 495
fossil record, 20
karyotype, 109
lice, 480
mites, 464
Microtus miurus
communal nesting, 355–356
distribution, 89, 110–111
endoparasites, 529, 532, 533
fleas, 495–496
fossil record, 18, 20
lice, 480
Meibomian glands, 120
Old World affinities, 54
ticks, 476
Microtus montanus
breeding season, 735–736
distribution, 91–92, 94–95, 110
endoparasites, 529–530, 532, 534
fleas, 496–497
fossil record, 22–23
karyotype, 110
lice, 480
mites, 464–465
nutritional cues, 689–691, 729
pituitary gland, 179–180
skin glands, 118–120
social organization, 346–348
ticks, 476–477
Microtus nesophilus, distribution, 90
Microtus oaxacensis, distribution, 101, 106
Microtus ochrogaster (see also *Pitymys ochrogaster*)
breeding season, 736–737
communal nesting, 356
demography, 577, 581, 587
distribution, 99, 101, 103
endoparasites, 528, 530, 532
fleas, 497
lice, 480
mites, 465–466
retina, 185
social organization, 346, 348–349
ticks, 477
Microtus oeconomus
breeding season, 737
demography, 585–587
distribution, 88–90, 110–111
endoparasites, 530, 532, 534
fleas, 497–498
fossil record, 18
lice, 480–481
mites, 466
skin glands, 119–120, 195–196
ticks, 477
Microtus oregoni
breeding season, 734
demography, 583–584, 587
distribution, 91, 93, 107–108
fleas, 498
lice, 481
mites, 467
Microtus paroperarius, 17–18, 107
Microtus pennsylvanicus
activity rhythms, 381–384
adrenal glands, 241, 243
brain, 179
breeding season, 737–738

C-3 and C-4 grasses, 27
communal nesting, 354–355
demography, 575, 577–580, 587
digestive tract, 218–240, 242, 244
dispersion, 405–406
distribution, 89–91, 107, 109
endoparasites, 529, 530–531, 533, 534
eye, 180–193
fleas, 498–501
fossil record, 25, 27, 50–51
home range, 398–401
karyotype, 109
lice, 481
mites, 467–470
movement types, 402–405
salivary glands, 203–217
similarity to *Microtus agrestis,* 27, 55
skin glands, 119–120, 194–196
social organization, 345–347
teeth, 198–202
ticks, 477–478
wounding, 362

Microtus pinetorum (see also *Pitymys pinetorum*)
breeding season, 738–739
distribution, 101, 104
endoparasites, 529, 531, 533
fleas, 501–502
lice, 481
mites, 470–471
reproductive system, ultrastructure, 243, 245–246
social organization, 346, 350–351
ticks, 478

Microtus quasiater, distribution, 101–105 (see also *Pitymys quasiater*)

Microtus richardsoni
breeding season, 732–733
distribution, 95, 98, 108
endoparasites, 531, 533
fleas, 502
fossil record, 20
mites, 471
Old World affinities, 55
pelage, 118
social organization, 346, 351

Microtus sp.
fossil record, 28
mites, 472
ticks, 478

Microtus speothen, 18

Microtus townsendii
breeding season, 733–735
demography, 574–577
distribution, 91–92, 109
fleas, 502–503
karyotype, 109
lice, 481
mites, 471–472
ticks, 478

Microtus umbrosus, distribution, 101, 106

Microtus xanthognathus
breeding season, 732–733
communal nesting, 355
demography, 586–587
distribution, 95, 97, 108
endoparasites, 531
fossil record, 25–26
pelage, 118
social organization, 346, 349–350

Mimomys, 7, 64, 108
Mites, 457–472.
Molt, 273, 276
Mortality
postnatal, 273
prenatal, 259, 261–262
Movement types, 402–405
Multi-factorial demographic mechanism, 592–594, 604–609
Musculature, macroanatomy, 136–138

Neodon, 6, 55, 65, 106
Neofiber, systematics, 65, 71
Neonatal development, 263–265
Nesting, 343–344
Non-social behavior, 341–344
Nutrition, 779–806 (see also Diet, Food, Plant secondary compounds)
diet, 329–332, 781–790
digestibility, 790–797, 818–821
forage quality, 790–797

habitat differences, 803–804
nutrients, 797–800
optimal foraging, 801–803
role in population dynamics, 804–806

Ontogeny, 254–280
Olfactory communication, 356–359
Optimal foraging, 801–803
Oral cavity, macroanatomy, 150–151
Orientation, 181
Outbreaks, 304
Ovulation, 693–697

Parasites
ectoparasites, 455–504
beetles, 481–482
fleas, 484–503
flies, 482–484
lice, 478–481
mites, 457–472
ticks, 472–478
endoparasites, 528–534
acanthocephalans, 528–529
cestodes, 529–531
nematodes, 531–533
trematodes, 533–534
Parasitism, affects on activity rhythms, 386–387
Parental behavior, 270 (see also Social structure)
Parturition, 262–270
Pathology, 657–676
bacterial infections, 662–669
constitutional diseases, 674–676
fungal diseases, 671, 673
neoplasms, 672–674
protozoan infections, 670–671
viral infections, 657–662
Pedomys, 6, 9, 11, 13–14, 55, 66
Pelage coloration, 846–849
Phaiomys, 6, 9, 66, 106
Phallic morphology, 156–157
Phenacomys, taxonomic key, 62–66
Pheromones, 691–693
Pituitary gland, ultrastructure, 179–180
Pitymys
fossil record, 5–15
pelage, 118
Pleistocene distributions, 105–107
skin glands, 118–120
systematics, 54–57
taxonomic key, 62–66
teeth, 5–7
Pitymys aratai, 12
Pitymys cumberlandensis, 11
Pitymys dideltus, 12
Pitymys guildayi, 9–11
Pitymys hibbardi, 12
Pitymys involutus, 11–12
Pitymys llanensis, 12–13
Pitymys mcnowni, 13
Pitymys meadensis, 15
Pitymys ochrogaster, fossil record, 13–14, 49–50 (see also *Microtus ochrogaster*)
Pitymys pinetorum, fossil record, 14–15, 48–49 (see also *Microtus pinetorum*)
Pitymys quasiater, fossil record, 15 (see also *Microtus quasiater*)
Pitymys sp., fossil record, 7–9
Plant secondary compounds, 790–797, 800–801, 821 (see also Food)
role in demography, 588–589, 596–597
Plantar footpads, 120–121
Pleistocene distributions, 105–113
Population cycles (see Demography)
Population dynamics (see Demography)
Postcranial skeleton, 135–136
Postnatal development, 270–277
Postnatal mortality, 273
Postpartum estrus, 700–701
Predation, 535–563
by amphibians, 558–559
by birds, 537–550
by fish, 558–559
by mammals, 550–558
by reptiles, 558–559
during outbreaks, 304
effects on activity rhythms, 386
effects on demography, 589, 597–598

impact, 547–550
role in species diversity, 324–325
role of cover, 589, 597
Pregnancy, 740–745
Prenatal development, 255–262
Prenatal mortality, 259, 261–262, 763–766

r- and K-selection, 277–280, 332
Raptors, predation by, 538–550
Reproduction
energetics, 834–836
hormonal timing, 686–693 (see also Endocrinology, timing of reproduction)
Reproductive patterns, 725–768
breeding intensity, 740–751
pregnancy, 740–745
sex ratio, 748–751
sexual maturity, 745–748
breeding season, 728–739
duration, 730–731
environmental cues, 729–730
patterns, 731–739
litter size, 751–766
effect of age, 761–762
effect of parity, 761–762
mortality, 763–766
variation, 760
Reproductive system
female tract, 158–159
gross anatomy, 155–159
male accessory glands, 157, 159
Reptiles, predation by, 558–559
Retina, ultrastructure, 243, 245–247 (see also Eye, ultrastructure)
Runways, 343–344

Salivary glands, ultrastructure, 202–217
Scent marking, 357–359
Sebaceous glands (see Integument, Skin glands)
Secondary compounds (see Plant secondary compounds)
Sex
effects on activity rhythms, 385
effects on spacing behavior, 407–408
Sex ratio, 268–271
demographic consequences, 607–609
patterns, 748–751
Sexual maturation, 276–277, 745–748, 869
Shrew predation, 550–551
Shrubland and woodland biomes, 97, 99
Skeleton, 121–136
cranial, 121–135
postcranial, 135–136
Skin glands
in olfactory communication, 356–359
macroanatomy, 118–120
ultrastructure, 194–196
Social behavior (see Behavior, social)
Social organization (see Social structure)
Social structure, 344–353
Spacial heterogeneity, 593
Spacing behavior (see Behavior, spacing)
Species diversity, 310–321
role of climate, 316–318
role of competition, 321–324
role of predation, 324–325
role of substrate, 318–319
role of vegetation, 319–321
Stenocranius, 20, 54, 89
Stomach
macroanatomy, 152–153
ultrastructure, 221, 223–233
Stress hypothesis, 590–592, 600–602
adrenal gland, 704–716
Subspecies concept, 127–129
Substrate, role in species diversity, 318–319
Succession, role in species diversity, 327–329
Swimming, 296, 342–343
Synaptomys
systematics, 56
taxonomic key, 62–66
Systematics, 53–81
artichoke method, 75–76

cladograms, 61
fossil record, 5–29
historical viewpoints compared, 74–81, 159–169
history at the genus level, 55–68
history at the species level, 68–74
karyotypes, 853
synonyms, 57–59
using macroanatomy, 159–169

Taiga biome, 90–97
Tarsal glands (see Meibomian glands)
Taxonomic key, 62–66
Teeth
macroanatomy, 140–150
terminology, 4–5
ultrastructure, 196–202
Temperate deciduous biome, 101
Temperature regulation, 821–824
Territoriality, 401–402
Testicular activity, 702–703
Thermogenesis, 824–830
Thermoregulation, 812–839 (see also Energetics)
Thyroid gland, 703–704
Ticks, 472–478
Tongue, macroanatomy, 151
Tundra biome, 88–90
Tunnels, 343

Ultradian rhythms, 381
Ultrastructure (see Anatomy, Microanatomy)

Vegetation, role in species diversity, 319–321
Vocalization, 359–360

Weasel predation, 551–554
Wounding, 362–364

Zoogeography, 84–113
ecological, 85–105
historical, 105–113
species numbers, 84–85